CRITICAL PATHWAYS
in Therapeutic Intervention
EXTREMITIES AND SPINE

CRITICAL PATHWAYS
IN Therapeutic
Intervention

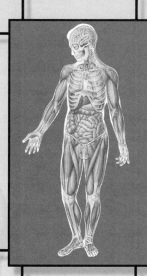

EXTREMITIES
AND
SPINE

DAVID C. SAIDOFF, BS, PT
Physical Therapist
Private Practice
West Hempstead, New York

ANDREW L. McDONOUGH, EdD, PT
Associate Professor
Department of Physical Therapy
New York University
New York, New York

Illustrated by **Laura Pardi Duprey**

with **834** *illustrations*

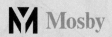 Mosby

St. Louis   London   Philadelphia   Sydney   Toronto

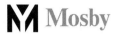

Publishing Director: John Schrefer
Acquisitions Editor: Kellie White
Developmental Editor: Christie M. Hart
Project Manager: Patricia Tannian
Production Editor: Larry State
Book Design Manager: Gail Morey Hudson
Cover Designer: Teresa Breckwoldt

Mosby, Inc.
11830 Westline Industrial Drive
St. Louis, Missouri 63146

Printed in United States of America

International Standard Book Number 0-323-00105-X

01   02   03   04   05   GW/RRD-W   9   8   7   6   5   4   3   2   1

I wish to dedicate this volume to

my best friend, my lovely wife Debby, and to my sons

Elisha, Jesse, and Robby

for their sacrifice and support over the many hours I spent away

from them while working on this project

DCS

To

Nancy and Amanda, the two women in my life.

You keep the fire burning in my soul and make life worth living . . .

I'm a lucky guy

DB

Foreword

The first *Critical Pathways* was a refreshing approach to textbooks in physical therapy because it presented teachers in the academic and especially in the clinical setting with a ready resource for identifying the principles of intervention. This new text expands the coverage to the spine and lower extremities, which provides the practitioner, student, and teacher with a fertile source of questions that are conducive to a Socratic approach to learning.

My teaching colleagues and I have found the choice of the clinical problems to be both applicable to and important in the clinical setting. The heavy emphasis on outcome assessment and patient satisfaction in the clinical setting of 21st-century physical therapy practice underscores the relevance of this text. The authors have provided readers with a wealth of information related to the questions raised. This can give read-

ers a systematic review of specific clinical problems and suggested interventions as a basis for the formulation of principles that can contribute to solving "real world" clinical problems.

The illustrations enhance the readers' ability to visualize the conceptual basis of the kinesiopathy and the intervention directed at its amelioration. Instructors have found these illustrations valuable in showing students the mechanism of injury, the assessment of kinesiologic or physiologic deviation, and the approach to take in rehabilitation. The authors are to be congratulated on formulating a most helpful and relevant case study approach that will increase awareness and therefore understanding of effective interventions in physical therapy.

Arthur J. Nelson, PhD, PT, FAPTA

Preface

Critical Pathways in Therapeutic Intervention was written to address the needs of health professionals who attempt to treat their patients with more conservative methods before resorting to referral for surgical intervention. To many professionals, the knowledge base so necessary for approaching given maladies becomes less familiar in direct proportion to the time away from schooling or from their last exposure to the disorder in question.

The scope of this book is generally restricted to those pathologic conditions that are amenable to conservative management. In addition, we have restricted our scope to the more common neuromusculoskeletal maladies and have intentionally left out some of the more unlikely or occult disorders. Moreover, the story line beginning many of the chapters is not always the most classic presentation, especially with regard to the age and gender distribution of given condition. These colorful anecdotes were intentionally structured to deviate somewhat from the standard clinical patient presentation. This is in keeping with our didactic philosophy that the student must learn to think, rather than try to memorize simple-fit solutions to a subject as complex as the pathologic process. Therapy is very much an art, despite its firm grounding in science.

I hope this text will serve as a bridge, bringing together ideas and concepts from fields as diverse as anatomy, kinesiology, orthopedics, rheumatology, neurology, sports medicine, physiatry, ergonomics, and geriatrics. While the information within these covers is not new, the organization and format of the material are novel in that they permit both student and clinician to home in on the information necessary for an understanding of each pathologic condition. Although students generally view textbooks as adversaries to conquer, information is presented here in a nonthreatening format. Each chapter is self-contained and does not require reading of the previous chapter. However, several chapters should be studied early on because they provide the keys to understanding the complex biomechanics of specific regions. These chapters include those on the cruciate ligament sprain at the knee and on ankle sprain for the foot and ankle, as well as three chapters on the spine, including degenerative disc disease, herniated disc, and spinal stenosis.

The story line of each chapter is followed by a paradigm of information and an occasional clue needed for the clinician's arrival at a conclusive diagnosis. We have adhered to this model except in chapters on such disorders as anterior shoulder dislocation, for which many of the early signs and symptoms have been omitted because management of the acute disorder is best performed by a physician.

Together, the chapters compose a volume that may be used as a guide, review, and reference for professionals and students alike. The actual ratiocination relevant to the encounter with each disorder is laid out for the benefit of the reader, with each question and answer in a sequence that encourages critical thinking. We have tried to make the chapters as eclectic as they are focused, so that they may stimulate and provoke thought, and perhaps even be entertaining.

In the words of 17th-century naturalist, John Ray, "He that useth many words for the explaining of any subject, doth like the cuttle-fish hide himself . . . in his own ink. Throughout this volume we have attempted to be terse and, in the tradition of the late E.B. White, not obfuscate the topics with excessive embellishment. We have tried to stay away from lofty "medicalese" when possible and to replace intimidating terms with simple, yet accurate explanations.

The idea of critical path thinking is used in the way Buckminster Fuller defined this term in his magnum opus *Synergetics 2* and in *Critical Path*. Much more than a simple list of linear thoughts required to arrive at a given objective or conclusion, "critical pathway" implies a complex of thoughts and concepts that come together to create something new that is much more than the mere sum of its parts.

The professional literature has long suffered a yawning gap because of the lack of a source book or compendium of the many rheumatologic, orthopedic, and neurologic maladies that are responsive to therapeutic intervention. Such intervention is not restricted to therapeutic exercise and other treatment modalities, but implies all the knowledge necessary in making an accurate assessment before rehabilitation. There is need for a text, comprehensive in scope, that contains a detailed description of the clinical presentation, pathokinesiology, and differential diagnosis. The latter is particularly important because therapists are increasingly assuming the role of primary care providers.

We have chosen some of the most common disorders encountered in outpatient clinics and private practice, recognizing that variations in pathologic conditions are all too common and that the responsible clinician must not pigeonhole his or her patients into preassumed disorders. Each patient is unique and must be looked upon during the initial evaluation in terms of his or her unique history and clinical presentation.

In the words of the late Isaac Asimov, "Originality consists in the organization and expression of facts, not the facts themselves" *(Opus 200)*. Although the format and spirit of this book are unique, the information contained therein has been compiled entirely from the many sources listed at the end of each chapter. I hope that this book helps to bridge the gap between theory and practice.

The immense effort dedicated toward creating a text of this scope was a joyful if not epiphanic experience. Preparation of these volumes is payback to the Creator on that precious altar of life. I thank God for a mind that understands, a heart that feels the pain of others, and hands that have learnt to heal their wounds.

David C. Saidoff

At the outset of this project I envisioned the book as a series of case reports that physical therapists, students, and others might find useful in recognizing and treating some common and not-so-common neuromuscular and musculoskeletal disorders. At the beginning of each chapter is a thorough review of pertinent anatomy, kinesiology, and biomechanics that I believe the reader will find to be a state-of-the-art reprise of structure and function. Each analysis is generously supported by current and past literature. The figures and illustrations facilitate the understanding of sometimes complicated structural and functional issues. I hope users of this book will appreciate it and use it as a high-level discussion of anatomy and kinesiology, suitable for advanced graduate study in clinical practice and research. I had not fully realized that this would be the outcome when we set out to write the book—I've been pleasantly surprised.

Andrew L. McDonough

ACKNOWLEDGMENTS

The primary motivation for writing this textbook originated in my wish that such a book were available to me when I began my studies in physical therapy. My temerity in undertaking the writing of such a book at a relatively early stage in my career stemmed from the intuition that I had to do this before I became too remote from the initial learning process and forgot the problems that had caused me difficulty. All this could not have been possible without the efforts of several colleagues whose encouragement and review contributed in the making of this volume. Foremost, I thank Andy McDonough, Ph.D., for his collaboration and editorial comments. His generous guidance evolved into a valued mentorship. I wish to take this opportunity to thank Sid Hershkowitz, P.T., for his many helpful suggestions, and David Nussbaum, P.T., for the many hours we discussed and clarified minutiae regarding many kinesiologic topics. Thanks to my good friend, Dr. Stuart Apfel for his generous time in discussing and clarifying of neurologic issues related to the low back and cervical spine. Thanks to my buddy, Dr. Charlie Barax for reviewing the many portions discussing radiology and other forms of imaging. Thanks also to Dr. Robert Koppel for his valuable input regarding pediatric matters and to Dr. Avi Schneider regarding his vast knowledge on cardiopulmonary topics; their overall support was much appreciated. Many thanks to my in-laws the late Mr. Ernest and Mrs. Edith Goldberger for their love and support.

Many thanks to the editorial staff at Mosby, especially Christie Hart and Kellie White for their guidance and extra effort in getting this project to completion. My deep thanks to Martha Sasser for believing in the premise of this book and in helping define its approach. Much thanks to Marcia Craig and her crew of Graphic World Publishing Services for their hard work in getting this work to print.

I thank Laura Pardi Duprey for her expert and beautiful illustrations. I consider myself fortunate to have worked together with so talented an artist. Thank you to Sherry Ickowicz, D.P.T., for helping with many of the endnotes.

I wish to acknowledge the many individuals who, over the years have contributed to my personal and professional growth. I hope this endeavor serves as a source of satisfaction and pride to my teachers and mentors. I offer thanks as a token of gratitude and appreciation for their efforts.

Above all, I am indebted to my wife Debby for bearing with me during the long and arduous effort involved in the conception, gestation, and birth of this book. The majority of the book was written at 2 or 3 AM several nights a week, over many years, after which I would go to work and have a normal day. Since at the same time I was building a career and being a full-time father to a growing family, I simply cannot imagine how everything got done. Debby was the glue that held it all together, and I thank her immeasurably.

David C. Saidoff
dsaidoff@netzero.net

Contents

xiii

PART I

HAND AND WRIST

1

Chilly Fingertips

An 18-year-old white woman is referred by your friend, a rheumatologist, with complaints of bilateral chilly index and middle fingers lasting for up to 10 minutes and precipitated by cold, vibration, or even emotional upset. The patient cannot remember when her symptoms started exactly but states that they have become more frequent over the past 4 months. At your request, the patient subjects herself to voluntary cold exposure by placing her hands flat up against the cold windowpane in your office. Over the next 10 minutes, you notice how the color of her hands dramatically changes from white to blue and finally to red. During this time the patient complains of numbness and cold. Upon communicating with the referring physician you learn that his associate, a vascular surgeon, has ruled out any vessel-obstructing disease. The presence of a cervical rib has also been ruled out. There is no history of injury or diabetes, though the patient reports that her mother occasionally suffers from the same malady. The patient smokes regularly, drinks three cups of coffee daily, and uses oral contraceptives.

OBSERVATIONS   There are no trophic changes observed.

PALPATION   The patient's hand (or hands) feels cold and then very warm over the course of 20 minutes.

RANGE OF MOTION   Within functional limits.

STRENGTH   Within normal limits.

FLEXIBILITY   Normal.

SENSATION   Normal to light touch, pressure, and proprioception as well as to two-point discrimination.

PULSES   Normal.

SPECIAL TESTS   Negative Allen test, negative Adson test and costoclavicular maneuver, negative compression or distraction of the cervical spine.

1. What is most likely causing this young woman's symptoms?
2. What is the body's reaction to cold exposure?
3. What stimuli may provoke an attack of symptoms?
4. What circulatory changes occur during an attack of Raynaud's syndrome?
5. What are the differences between primary and secondary Raynaud's syndrome?
6. What is the differential diagnosis?
7. What treatment strategy is indicated in Raynaud's syndrome?

---

1. What is most likely causing this young woman's symptoms?

Raynaud's syndrome (pronounced ray-NOZE) was first described in 1862 by the French physician Maurice Raynaud who postulated that exaggerated sensitivity to cold stemmed from an overly sensitive nervous system. Defining it as *cold-induced reflex digital vasoconstriction and ischemia,* Raynaud proposed a pathophysiology involving an exaggerated reflex sympathetic vasoconstriction.[3] This syndrome, mildly affecting 5% to 10% of the population, causes considerable discomfort and inconvenience and comes in two forms: (1) primary Raynaud's syndrome, or *Raynaud's disease,* and (2) secondary Raynaud's syndrome, or *Raynaud's phenomenon.*[2] An attack may occur after even the slightest provocation such as reaching into the refrigerator momentarily to remove an item or even grasping a cold metal doorknob. Arteriole spasm will follow, resulting in *pallor,* even *cyanosis,* and then *redness* of the digits, and this cycle may also occur in other acral parts such as the toes, nose, ears, or tongue when exposed to cold because these areas are located at the outer reaches of the circulatory system.

2. What is the body's reaction to cold exposure?

Physiologic thermoregulation is governed by the autonomic nervous system and responds to cold fingers by shunting blood to the core by means of a *countercurrent heat-exchange mechanism.*[1] This results in blood vessel constriction of distal, outlying areas of the body so as to divert blood away from the extremities, preventing heat loss by way of exposed hand and feet surfaces. Raynaud's syndrome more frequently involves the fingers than it does the toes.[3]

3. What stimuli may provoke an attack of symptoms?

In the majority of patients symptoms are precipitated by exposure to cold as insignificant as a cool breeze on a hot day, or just from sitting in a drafty room. Some patients' symptoms are triggered by emotional upset. Raynaud's is also common to individuals whose occupations subject hands to unusual wear and tear, such as typists, pianists, and meat cutters, and especially affects those persons using vibrating tools such as jackhammers, chain saws, pneumatic drills, riveting equipment, and mining, quarrying, and grinding machines. Exposure to certain chemicals such as vinyl chloride, commonly used in the rubber industry, may also increase susceptibility. Certain medications are potentially troublesome, and included in this category are oral contraceptives, ergot-containing drugs used to treat migraine headaches by way of vessel constriction, beta-adrenergic receptor blockers used in the treatment of high blood pressure, arrhythmias, or angina, as well as drugs used to treat cancer such as cisplatin, vinblastine, and bleomycinonicotine.[3]

4. What circulatory changes occur during an attack of Raynaud's syndrome?

Circulatory changes may be biphasic or triphasic. In the first stage an exaggerated shutdown in the form of sudden vasoconstriction, experienced as tingling, occurs as the body attempts to conserve heat and causes the fingers to turn pale or *white* (pallor). This is followed by *blueness* (cyanosis) resulting from sluggish flow of poorly oxygenated darker blood and is experienced as numbness. This is then followed by overwarming of the area at the end of the attack as the body overcompensates by way of exuberant blood flow rushing back into the fingers, manifesting as *redness* (rubor), throbbing, swelling, and a sensation of warmth (Fig. 1-1). When circulatory changes occur in a biphasic fashion, the fingers may seemingly bypass the middle cyanotic stage. This sequence may, in addition to cold exposure, be caused by stress, which triggers the release of hormones that initiate constriction. Regardless of the cause of this disorder, color changes do not occur above the metacarpophalangeal joints and rarely involve the thumb. This sharply demarcated pallor is reflective of spasm of the digital arteries. Usually, all digits are symmetrically affected. Although pain may occur, paresthesias are frequent during the attack, which typically lasts 20 to 30 minutes.

5. What are the differences between primary and secondary Raynaud's syndrome?

Primary Raynaud's syndrome (Raynaud's disease) is idiopathic and is five times more common in young women than in men,[3] with symptoms starting in females between 13 and 40 years of age. It occurs frequently in people who have migraine headaches or variant angina.[3] Most patients cannot precisely date the onset of symptoms. Mild symptoms may have been overlooked for years and recognized only in retrospect. Onset is gradual because the patient notices only an occasional mild and short-lasting attack during the winter season.[6] Over the subsequent years, the duration and severity of attacks may increase. Familial cases are not infrequent and this condition is not considered to be symmetric (such as involving the same fingers in both hands).

A diagnosis of primary Raynaud's is pronounced after a history of symptoms for at least 2 years without progression, no evidence of underlying cause, and absent or only minimal trophic changes. The physical examination is often entirely normal, as are the radial, ulnar, and pedal pulses. Between attacks, however, the fingers and toes may be cool and perspire excessively. Sclerodactyly is thickening and tightening of the digital subcutaneous tissue and develops in 10% of patients. Digital angiography for diagnostic purposes is not indicated as part of the medical work-up.[3]

The prognosis for Raynaud's disease is good. Some 50% of patients show improvement of this disorder, which may completely disappear after several years.

Secondary Raynaud's syndrome (Raynaud's phenomenon) may start in later years, usually after 50 years of age. It may also start more abruptly, occur on one side or one finger only, and be more severe. Here, signs and symptoms of the underlying disease occur within 2 years of the onset of symptoms, and painful ulcerations of the fingers and toes are more common and more troublesome because they may eventually become gangrenous and require amputation. Raynaud's disease in males is most often of this second variety. Secondary Raynaud's is associated with what were previously described as collagen vascular diseases (such as scleroderma, rheumatoid arthritis, and lupus). These diseases have in common vasculitis, a process that thickens the walls of blood vessels thus reducing blood flow. Raynaud's in such patients is attributable to both vessel disease and vessel spasm, a combination that may account for why the secondary form is more severe than the primary. Secondary Raynaud's may also be caused by diseases causing arterial blockage.

6. What is the differential diagnosis?

The differential diagnosis of Raynaud's syndrome includes thoracic outlet compression syndromes (see Chapter 18), primary pulmonary hypertension, acrocyanosis, a history of drug ingestion or exposure, and atherosclerosis. Although the former condition may be excluded by appropriate maneuvers, the latter is a frequent cause of Raynaud's disease in men over 50 years old. Thromboangiitis obliterans is an uncommon cause but should be considered in young men who smoke cigarettes. Approximately 15% of patient's exhibiting Raynaud's symptoms eventually develop a connective tissue disorder, particularly scleroderma. In fact, Raynaud's may be the only symptom for many years before the full-blown manifestation of systemic sclerosis. Prognosis of Raynaud's disease stemming from the latter condition is unsatisfactory, especially when the condition has progressed to ischemic digital ulceration. Gangrene and autoamputation may then follow.[3,6]

A diagnosis of primary Raynaud's is pronounced after a history of symptoms for at least 2 years without progression, no evidence of underlying cause, and absent or only minimal trophic changes.

7. What treatment strategy is appropriate in Raynaud's syndrome?

The following rehabilitative treatment strategy suffices for a patient with mild or infrequent attacks:

- Biofeedback teaches patients to "think" their fingers are warm by consciously wresting out of the uncon-

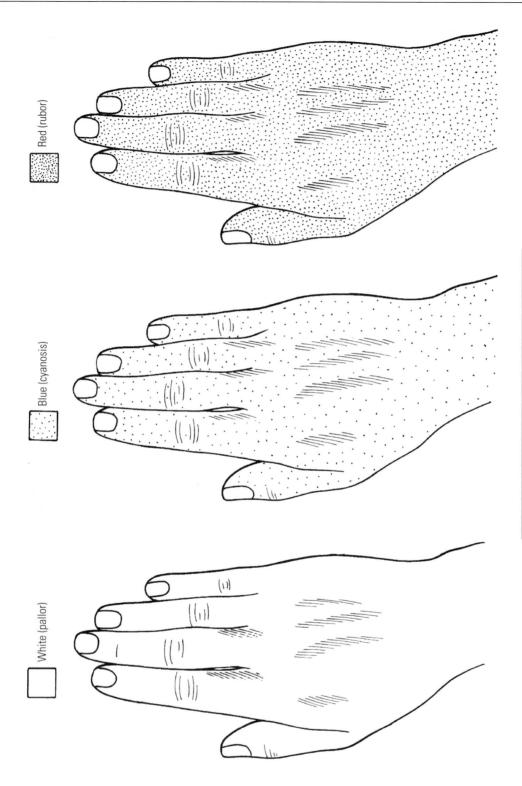

FIG. 1-1 Triphasic circulatory changes in Raynaud's phenomenon.

scious autonomic regulation of finger temperature so as to prevent and abort future attacks of Raynaud's syndrome. Training sessions typically last 30 to 60 minutes and are repeated twice a week for a total of 10 sessions. At each session the temperature of the patient's fingertips is recorded with the results visually displayed so that the patient can visually detect tiny increases in finger temperature.[5]

- Circulatory conditioning involves "teaching" the arteries to remain open despite the fact that the person is out in the cold. Treatment involves sitting outdoors in cool weather while placing one's hands in a pail of warm water. This is repeated several times a day, 10 minutes at a time, every other day over a period of 3 to 4 weeks.[3]
- One should eat a good breakfast. Skipping breakfast results in low blood glucose, which triggers epinephrine (adrenaline) release, which in turn causes small-vessel constriction.
- Keeping the chest warm is important because the body reacts to central warmth by shifting blood from the core to cooler peripheral areas.
- Mittens are better than lined gloves and are to be used when the patient is opening a refrigerator or freezer door, taking out the trash, or reaching for the outdoor mailbox.
- Use of earmuffs, muffler, and scarf.
- Use of electrically heated socks or mittens.
- Wearing layered clothing.
- Avoidance of nicotine and caffeine.
- Avoidance of smoking because smoking causes cutaneous vasoconstriction.
- Use of tepid water to wash vegetables or dishes, or while washing laundry by hand.
- Placement of rubber caps on keys and outside doorknobs.

- Letting the car warm up before driving.
- Fitting the steering wheel with an insulated cover, such as a fleece.
- Use of fabric seat covers.
- Use of cup warmers to hold cold drinks.
- Wearing of reflective inner soles in shoes.
- Learning stress-reducing relaxation techniques.

When Raynaud's syndrome is more frequent or severe, especially when trophic changes or ulcerations have occurred, conservative treatment is supplemented by drug therapy. Of the calcium-channel blockers, nifedipine is the drug of choice. Reserpine, a drug that interferes with sympathetic nerve activity, and topical nitroglycerin or prostaglandin ointment have also been found to be helpful in relieving ischemia during attacks. Preganglionic sympathectomy may be initially beneficial, but the long-term benefits have been disappointing.[6]

REFERENCES

1. Arms K, Camp PS: *Biology,* ed 2, Philadelphia, 1982, Saunders College Publishing.
2. Berkow R: *The Merck manual of diagnosis and therapy,* Rahway, NJ, 1987, Merck, Sharp and Dohme Research Laboratories.
3. Isselbacher KJ, editor: *Harrison's principles of internal medicine,* vol 1, ed 13, New York, 1994, Health Professions Div/McGraw-Hill.
4. Jobe JB et al: Home treatment for Raynaud's disease, *J Rheumatol* 12:953-956, 1985.
5. The New York Times: HEALTH, B2, Thursday, Dec 4, 1989.
6. Wyngaarden JB, Smith LH, Bennet JC: *Cecil textbook of medicine,* vol 1, Philadelphia, 1992, Saunders.

RECOMMENDED READING

Jobe JB et al: Home treatment for Raynaud's disease, *J Rheumatol* 12:953-956, 1985.

2

Volar Nodule and Flexion Contracture of Ring Finger

A 51-year-old jovial white man with a thick Scottish accent complains of no longer being able to clap his hands, put on his gloves, shake hands, or wash his face without sticking his right ring finger in his eye. His past medical history includes bouts of gout, non-insulin dependent diabetes, and a childhood history of epilepsy, and he mentions that his father was plagued by trigger finger and carpal tunnel syndrome. He also discloses that he had pulmonary tuberculosis approximately 18 years previously. He exhibits normal strength to all fingers including his involved ring finger, which is 70° flexed at the right metacarpophalangeal joint of the fourth finger without interphalangeal joint involvement. When asked, the patient reports that his finger remains flexed all day and all night. When questioned further, the patient admits to drinking three to four glasses of scotch vermouth per day since his wife was accidentally killed during a motor vehicle accident 7 years previously. He denies any other such manifestation elsewhere on his person.

OBSERVATION   Pitting, fissuring, puckering, and dimpling of skin over right distal palmar crease on the ulnar side of the hand, with the area corresponding to the ring finger drawn into pits and folds.

PALPATION   Prominent nodules are felt at the ring and little fingers of both hands, and the involved finger cannot be passively straightened.

MUSCLE STRENGTH   Normal.

? Questions

1. What is most likely this gentleman's diagnosis?
2. What is the evolution of this disease?
3. What is the pathogenesis of this disease?
4. What is the epidemiology of this disorder?
5. Is there a genetic component to this disorder?
6. Where else in the body does a similar disorder manifest?
7. Which fingers are most commonly involved?
8. How rapidly does this disease progress?
9. What conservative treatment is attempted for milder cases before surgical intervention?
10. What are two indications for surgery, and what is the therapist's responsibility for monitoring the progression of contracture?
11. What are the risks of surgery?
12. What type of operations are used in the surgical correction of this disease?
13. What postoperative therapy is indicated?
14. What other pathologic condition affecting the fingers involves nodular development?

1. What is most likely this gentleman's diagnosis?

In 1832 the Parisian surgeon Baron Dupuytren described a progressive nonpainful benign flexion deformity of the fingers caused by a contracture of the palmar and digital fasciae (that is, aponeurosis) as well as the adjacent digital flexor tendon sheaths. The *palmar aponeurosis* consists of four broad divergent bands that extend to the base of the fingers (Fig. 2-1). Early in the course of this disease there is painless proliferation of fibroblasts, histologically manifesting as a low-grade inflammatory fibrosis that results in the transformation of noncontractile tissue into contractile tissue. Diagnosis is made by visual inspection and palpation (Fig. 2-2).

2. What is the evolution of this disease?

The stages in the evolution of this disease are not distinct and begin as a tender[6] nodular thickening at the distal palmar crease of the ring finger that may spread to involve the middle finger. With the passage

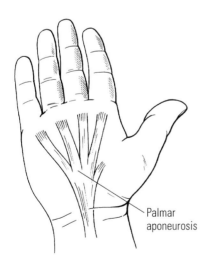

FIG. 2-1 The palmar aponeurosis is composed of four broad and divergent bands that extend to the base of the fingers.

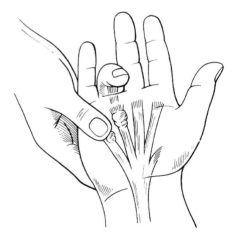

FIG. 2-2 In Dupuytren's contracture the fascia (comprising the palmar aponeurosis and natatory ligament) has palpable thickenings or nodules.

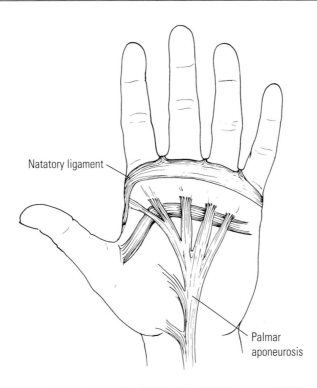

Natatory ligament

Palmar
aponeurosis

FIG. 2-3 The natatory ligament and palmar aponeurosis. Once the natatory ligament becomes fibrotic, fibrosis will soon spread to the adjacent fascia of the digital flexor tendon sheaths. Additionally, natatory ligament involvement precludes separation of the digits. (From McFarlane RM, Albion U: Dupuytren's disease. In Hunter JM, Schneider LH, Mackin EJ, Callahan AD, editors: *Rehabilitation of the hand: surgery and therapy*, ed 3, St Louis, 1990, Mosby.)

of time the nodules enlarge and spread longitudinally toward the proximal palmar crease as cordlike bands. As the tenderness subsides,[5] fibrosis expands to involve the surrounding adjacent digital flexor tendon sheaths; contracture develops in the form of subcutaneous cords that extend proximally to the base of the palm and, of greatest concern, distally to encompass the *natatory ligament*[4] (Fig. 2-3) at the base of the fingers.[6] Once the disease has migrated this far, it is only a matter of time before it involves the digital fascia. Subcutaneous cords are not to be confused with the more deeply located flexor tendons, since active finger flexion remains unaffected. The natatory ligament extends across the distal part of the palm, supporting each web space and ending in the first web at the base of the thumb. When this ligament is diseased, the digits cannot be separated.

As the flexion deformity continues, secondary contractures occur in the skin, nerves, blood vessels, and adjacent joint capsules,[6] with eventual articular cartilage destruction.[8] Extension of the involved fingers becomes impossible in advanced cases. The underlying fascia is normally attached to the skin so that gripping or pinching an object will occur without the skin or the grasped object sliding away. With Dupuytren's disease there is puckering and dimpling of the overlying skin in the area of the distal palmar crease on the *ulnar* side of the hand caused by adhesion of the skin to the underlying fascia.

3. What is the pathogenesis of this disease?

The cause of this disease remains unclear, though an association exists between Dupuytren's contracture and chronic alcoholism with liver cirrhosis or chronic use of anticonvulsant medication, suggestive of a hormonally affected enzyme abnormality permitting overactivity of myofibroblasts.[5] Gout and diabetes are also associated with this condition, as are tuberculosis, liver disease, chronic invalidism, epilepsy, and patients with pulmonary tuberculosis.[1] Repeated microtrauma may play a role. It is not understood why the ring or little fingers are most commonly involved or why thickening may be quiescent for years and then within a brief time cause symptomatic digital contracture.[5] This disorder may appear as a late sequel to shoulder-hand syndrome after myocardial infarction.

4. What is the epidemiology of this disorder?

Victims tend to be northern Europeans, particularly of Celtic descent.[5] This disorder is common to middle-aged white males to the extent that four out of every five patients are male[2] However, after menopause the sex ratio tends to equalize. In 5% of patients similar contractures occur in the feet.[6] One or both hands may be affected, whereas the right hand is more frequently affected when involvement is unilateral.

5. Is there a genetic component to this disorder?

The genetic profile of this condition implies mendelian dominance with incomplete penetrance. This means that family members may or may not be similarly affected.[5]

6. Where else in the body does a similar disorder manifest?

A similar pathologic process in the plantar fascia of the foot in which fascial thickening develops in the sole of the foot *(Lederhose disease)* as well as fibrous plaques within the fascia of the shaft of the penis *(Peyronie's disease)*.[4]

7. Which fingers are most commonly involved?

The disease affects the ulnar side of the hand with the ring finger most commonly affected; the fifth, third, second, and first fingers are then affected in decreasing order of frequency.[7] The latter two are more rarely involved.

8. How rapidly does this disease progress?

Some contractures develop quickly over a matter of weeks, whereas others may progress for years. Long remissions followed by exacerbation with increasing deformity may occur.[6] Thus, although it is a progressive disease, one cannot predict how rapidly the disease will progress from the appearance of the initial nodule to full-blown finger-joint contracture.

9. What conservative treatment is attempted for milder cases before surgical intervention?

Therapeutic intervention focuses on prevention of secondary joint contractures by means of:
- Orally administered vitamin E.[4]
- Iontophoresis over nodule with Iodex (iodine with methyl salicylate) using the negative pole.
- Ultrasound to follow iontophoresis so as to disperse Iodex within soft tissue, applied during passive stretch into extension.
- Posterior extension splints.[9]
- In the early stage of this disease teach the patient to stretch palm and fingers vigorously out into extension in an attempt to elongate the palmar fascia as fast as it contracts.[2]
- Moist heat before stretching, followed by cold application.[9]

10. What are two indications for surgery, and what is the therapist's responsibility for monitoring the progression of contracture?

The only way to alter the course of the disease process is to surgically remove diseased tissue.[4] However, surgical repair should not be performed before contractures develop.[6] Indications for surgery revolve around whether contracture has occurred at the metacarpophalangeal (MP) joint or the interphalangeal (IP) joint. MP joint contractures, regardless of severity, are usually correctable because the collateral ligaments and capsule of the MP joints are stretched taut when the joint is in flexion and therefore without restriction to full extension once the offending fascia is released.[4] Because of this, there is no urgency to operate when the MP joint alone is affected, and it is best to leave it alone until functional limitations have developed[5] for fear of leaving the patient with a worse hand than before.[5] It is best to wait to advise the patient to operate until the *MP joint contractures are at least 30°.*

Additionally, the collateral ligaments stabilizing the IP joints are such that any position of flexion will cause their quick foreshortening. *Fifteen degrees of proximal interphalangeal joint (PIP) contracture* is a definite indication for surgery,[4] whereas procrastination until contracture reaches 50° is too late because the joint will respond poorly to surgery.[5] Distal interphalangeal joint (DIP) flexion contracture is rare and, similar to the situation of contracture greater than 15° of the PIP, it is difficult to correct. In contrast, DIP hyperextension is more common, is most frequently seen in the little finger, and is compensatory to severe PIP flexion.[4]

11. What are the risks of surgery?

The shortcomings of surgery include:

- A triad of skin necrosis, skin infection, and hematoma.[4]
- Surgical injury that may itself generate scarring and joint stiffness.
- Risk of laceration of digital nerves because their course is frequently distorted by contracted fascia.
- Disease recurrence in operated areas or extension into previously undisturbed portions of the hand.[5]

12. What types of operations are used in surgical correction of this disease?

SURGICAL PROCEDURES

- ***Partial Palmar Fasciectomy.*** Removal of only the diseased fascia without excision of the uninvolved portion and effective in most instances. It should be made clear to the patient that the disease may indeed recur elsewhere in the palm. This procedure permits full correction of MP joint deformity.
- ***The More Radical Complete Fasciectomy.*** Removal of all palmar fascia in the palm and finger so as to preclude any source of recurrent contracture. Here maximum correction of the PIP joints is attempted, though with this procedure there is a greater risk for complications as well as prolonged if not permanent disability.[4]

By the time the finger is flexed down into the palm the joint has usually become frozen and uncorrectable. In some cases, the affected digit is amputated through the neck of the metacarpal.[3]

13. What postoperative therapy is indicated?

Prolonged postoperative care may be required for several months and is necessary to obtain optimal results. Recovery time is variable. With most patients, hand function will be incapacitated for 6 to 8 weeks.[4]

TREATMENT

- Initially record edema at same anatomic landmarks with circumferential measurements and progress to volumetric measurements once wounds have healed.
- Accurately measure the range of motion with a finger goniometer.

- Reassure patients that healing will progress over the coming weeks because patients are often startled by the horrible wound appearance.
- Active range of motion exercises begin the first postoperative day and include the following regimen performed for three or four sets of 10 repetitions per day:
    1. Thumb opposition to each fingertip, abduction, and extension
    2. Finger blocking (DIP joint flexion with the PIP joint and MP joint held in extension with the uninvolved hand, followed by PIP joint flexion with MP joint extension)
    3. Flexion of each finger to the thenar eminence
    4. Fist making
    5. Finger abduction and adduction
    6. Finger extension
    7. Full wrist motion and thumb range of motion
- Caution patient against overdoing his or her exercises, so as not to cause edema and pain.
- Tendon-gliding exercises may be begun by the second postoperative week.
- Instruct patients in gentle passive range of motion of all joints.
- Posterior extension splint fabricated at initial therapy session and necessary adjustments made with frequent visits. Splint removal is permitted only for wound care and exercise. Remember that the MP capsule and ligaments are taut in flexion, whereas the IP capsule and ligaments are taut in extension. In the event that a digit shows early signs of recurring contracture (most frequently seen in the little finger's PIP joint) a splint with a Velcro loop over the outrigger serves to provide extension force instead of a finger loop and rubber band. The Velcro provides a static pull and may be adjusted to provide increased tension as tolerated by the patient between treatments.
- If flexion is a problem, flexion splinting may be necessary and is worn by day; night splinting is reserved for extension.
- Scar management is by lanolin massage to both palm and digits with small, deep, circular strokes over the scar for 10 minutes before each exercise session. After massage, excess lanolin should be removed to prevent skin maceration.
- Desensitization is appropriate in the occasional patient experiencing hypersensitivity beginning with fur and progressing to vibration for 10 minutes each waking hour.
- Remove Velcro straps three or four times per day to flex fingers to distal phalanx crease actively or with

active assistance, as well as full extension, fist making, finger blocking, finger abduction and adduction, flexion of each finger to thenar eminence, as well as wrist and thumb circumduction for 10 repetitions per set.

- Whirlpool bath.
- Progress to more difficult exercises (such as crossing fingers, passing coin from finger to finger, using handgrips and putty, and functional exercises).
- Having regained full flexion and extension of the fingers, the patient is advised to continue to wear the night splint for 3 months. Despite this supervised splinting, scar contracture may cause 10% to 15% flexion contracture at the PIP joint.[4]

14. What other pathologic condition affecting the fingers involves nodular development?

Trigger finger is another disorder involving nodules as well as the digital flexor tendon sheaths and, unlike Dupuytren's disease, may also involve the synovial sheaths enveloping those tendons.[6] With Dupuytren's disease, active finger flexion remains complete but not so for trigger finger.[6]

The function of the digital flexor tendon retacular sheath (that is, the *annular ligament*) is to tightly restrain the tendon as it crosses the flexed MP joint, serving as a simple pulley to prevent bowstringing from origin to insertion during contraction.

Repetitive gliding of the tendon under the restraining sheath as from excessive repetitive handwork or unconscious fist clenching may exceed the lubricating capacity of synovial fluid. This may be worsened by the presence of a sesamoid bone, osteoarthritis,[7] or rheumatoid arthritis.[6] The resulting friction generates localized inflammation at the point where the tendon enters the sheath, causing swelling of the tendon[3] *(tendinitis)*, which over time irritates the opening of the sheath causing inflammation and thickening *(tenosynovitis)* (see page 16). This further restricts tendon gliding, and a vicious cycle is established in which swelling aggravates constriction, and the constriction aggravates the swelling.

Trigger finger progresses to the development of a fusiform swelling—a *nodule* in either the deep or the superficial flexor tendon or tendons at a *metacarpal head*[6] (Fig. 2-4). Palpation over the metacarpal head reveals a tender nodule that moves with the tendon. Early on, this thickened portion may pop in and out of the constricted sheath with a slightly painful click or grating when the finger is *flexed* or *extended,* akin to pulling a knotted rope through a narrow stretch of pipe[5] (Fig. 2-5). Although *the sensation is subjectively perceived at the proximal interphalangeal joint,*

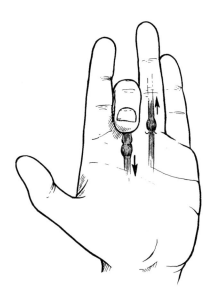

FIG. 2-4 Trigger finger. Locking may occur in either finger flexion or finger extension. (From Dandy DJ: *Essential orthopaedics and trauma,* Edinburgh, 1989, Churchill Livingstone.)

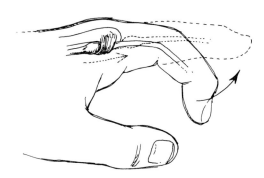

FIG. 2-5 The nodule within the tendon is restrained by the flexor retinaculum sheath on attempted extension. Persistent extension will result in a click sound as the nodular portion of the tendon is forced past the stricture. (From Meals RA: *One hundred orthopaedic conditions every doctor should understand,* St. Louis, 1992, Quality Medical Publishing.)

the nodule may be palpated just proximal to the metacarpophalangeal joint. The digit often locks in flexion when the patient arises from sleep.[7] As pathologic changes in the tendon and sheath progress, intermittent locking gives way to flexion of the IP joint on the MP joint arrested in midrange, since the flexors are stronger than the extensors. Extension becomes possible only when performed passively as when the nodule is forced through the stricture. The finger then extends with a click, imparting a crepitation to the examiner's hand.[6]

Early treatment consists in splinting the finger in extension at night along with nonsteroidal antiinflammatory medication. When more chronic, a steroid injection with a local anesthetic may be indicated. In recalcitrant cases surgical release of the tendon by longitudinal incision of the thickened sheath is indicated.

REFERENCES

1. Berkow R: *The Merck manual of diagnosis and therapy,* Rahway, NJ, 1987, Merck Sharp & Dohme Research Laboratories.
2. Cyriax J: *Textbook of orthopaedic medicine, vol 1: diagnosis of soft tissue lesions,* ed 8, London, 1988, Bailliere-Tindall.
3. Dandy DJ: *Essential orthopaedics and trauma,* Edinburgh, 1989, Churchill Livingstone.
4. McFarlane RM, Albion U: *Dupuytren's disease: rehabilitation of the hand: surgery and therapy,* ed 3, St Louis, 1990, Mosby.
5. Meals RA: *One hundred orthopaedic conditions every doctor should understand,* St Louis, 1992, Quality Medical Publishing.
6. Netter FH: *The CIBA collection of medical illustrations, vol 8: Musculoskeletal system, part 2,* Summit, NJ, 1990, CIBA-Geigy.
7. Rodnan GP, Schumacher HR: *Primer on the rheumatic diseases,* ed 8, Atlanta, 1983, The Arthritis Foundation.
8. Salter RB: *Textbook of disorders and injuries of the musculoskeletal system,* ed 2, Baltimore, 1990, Williams & Wilkins.
9. Saunders HD: *Evaluation, treatment, and prevention of musculoskeletal disorders,* Bloomington, Minn, 1985, Educational Opportunities.

RECOMMENDED READING

Hill N: Current concepts review: Dupuytren's contracture, *J Bone Joint Surg* 67A:1439-1443, 1985.
Hueston JT, Tubicra R: *Dupuytren's disease,* Edinburgh, 1985, Churchill Livingstone.
McFarlane RM, Albion U: Dupuytren's disease. In Hunter JM, Schneider LH, Mackin EJ, et al, editors: *Rehabilitation of the hand: surgery and therapy,* ed 3, St Louis, 1990, Mosby. See also McFarlane RM, MacDermid JC: Dupuytren's disease. In Hunter JM, Mackin EJ, Callahan AD, editors: *Rehabilitation of the hand: surgery and therapy,* ed 4, St Louis, 1995, Mosby.

3

Painful Thumb after Intense Bout of Hammering

An aspiring carpenter spent his first day of apprenticeship atop the roof of a refurbished two-family house, laying down precut planks in slanted fashion across the roof and hammering them down every 4 inches around their periphery using 5-inch nails. He would spend the next 5 months doing this work on six adjacent homes whose roofs were gutted by a fire that had spread from one to the other because of the proximity of homes in that neighborhood. Eager to impress his employer, he worked with gusto for 6 hours at a time without rest except for a quick 15-minute lunch break toward the end of each day. At the end of 1 week's work he was awakened at night by a searing hot pain at the base of his right thumb that came on gradually and partially abated when he wrung his hand. During the following week the same pain would occur after hammering for 2 hours and intensified as he attempted to ignore it.

MEDICAL HISTORY   Unremarkable, as was family history. No medications aside from aspirin. When asked, patient could not remember falling and landing on an outstretched hand in recent or past history.

SUBJECTIVE   Patient reports decrease in pain upon resting from work and upon taking one or two aspirins per day as needed. When asked, patient reported no numbness, excess sweating, hand color changes, tingling, or paresthesia. The patient was right handed.

OBSERVATION   No swelling, color changes, or atrophy.

PALPATION   Point tenderness at base of thumb. The skin was not excessively moist. Fine crepitus was noted over the length of tendons in the anatomical snuffbox.

RANGE OF MOTION   Grossly the range of motion was within functional limits though touching the tips of the thumb and small finger was slow and painful. Passive thumb extension and abduction beyond midrange was painful. All other fingers were within functional limits.

STRENGTH TESTING   All thumb movements were painful, and designation of muscle grade was deferred. All other fingers tested normal.

SENSORY   Intact to light touch, pinprick, and temperature to entire hand.

VOLUMETRIC MEASUREMENTS   No edema.

PULSES   Normal.

UPPER QUARTER SCREENING   No evidence of double-crush phenomenon, or of different site as cause of symptoms.

SPECIAL TESTS   Positive Finkelstein's test.

? Questions

1. **Based on the history and examination what is most likely wrong with this patient?**
2. **What is the difference between tendinitis, tenosynovitis, and tenovaginitis, and why are the latter two appropriate in describing this patient's condition?**
3. **What are three separate yet related sources of friction causing inflammation in this patient?**
4. **Which segments of the population are more prone to this condition?**
5. **Which predisposing movements identify the mechanism causing this overuse syndrome?**
6. **What signs and symptoms are common to this malady, and what provocative tests or movements elicit the latter?**
7. **How is concomitant inflammation of the tendon of the third dorsal compartment evaluated?**
8. **What other conditions must be ruled out upon eliciting pain and tenderness at the snuffbox?**
9. **Which metabolic abnormalities, though not causative, are associated with this condition?**
10. **What medical management is typical for this patient, and what, if any, are deleterious effects of this management?**
11. **What surgical management is appropriate for this patient, and what complications are associated with surgery?**
12. **What therapeutic intervention will best rehabilitate this patient?**

1. Based on the history and examination what is most likely wrong with this patient?

De Quervain's disease is tenosynovitis and tenovaginitis[5,19] at the base of the thumb involving the tendons of the first dorsal compartment (the abductor pollicis longus and the extensor pollicis brevis)[17] and forming the radial border of the anatomic snuffbox. The tendon of the extensor pollicis longus passing through the third dorsal compartment and defining the ulnar border of the snuffbox is less commonly involved (Fig. 3-1).

2. What is the difference between tendinitis, tenosynovitis, and tenovaginitis, and why are the latter two appropriate in describing this patient's condition?

Tendinitis occurs in sheath-lacking structures such as the Achilles tendon, supraspinatus tendon, or the bicipital aponeurosis on the ulna. Tendinitis is an inflammation of the tendon with subsequent scarring either (1) within the substance of the tendon or (2) at the insertion of tendon into bone (i.e., tenoperiosteal junction, TPJ).[5]

Tenosynovitis is an inflammation of synovial membrane with subsequent scarring (1) anywhere along the tendinosynovial complex or (2) at the insertion of tendon into bone, the tenoperiosteal junction; this may occur in the peroneal tendons, posterior tibialis tendon, or the distal biceps attachment on the radial tuberosity. Synovial sheaths are like bursae except that they are (1) tubular structures and (2) are found around superficial tendons and provide decreased friction in potentially high-friction areas; thus they are found mostly in hands and feet because these distal areas contain an excess of long superficial tendons.[8]

In addition, certain synovial sheath-tendon complexes are bound down and anchored by fibrous sheaths, or tunnels, and prevent bowstringing when the wrist is flexed.[8] These sheaths act as simple pulleys to divert the line of pull from the long axis of the arm to the plane of the long axis of the hand. This ensheath-

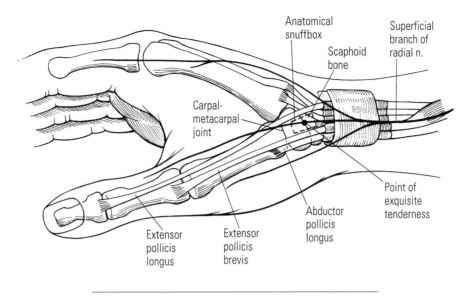

FIG. 3-1 Pertinent anatomy of de Quervain's disease.

ment may be a source of additional inflammation and thickening *(tenovaginitis).*

3. What are three separate yet related sources of friction causing inflammation in this patient?

In de Quervain's disease there is an additional factor contributing to friction: a fibro-osseous canal. The tendons of the abductor pollicis longus (APL) and of the extensor pollicis brevis (EPB) pass through a shallow groove on the lateral aspect of the radial styloid.[1] If movement through this tunnel as well as against other structures is constant and repetitive, a vicious cycle of inflammation leading to synovitis is encouraged by friction (1) between the tendons, (2) between the tendons and their common tendon sheath, and (3) between the sheath and the bony groove of the radius.[1] A loss of blood flow may affect the nutritional status of the area[18] and contribute to a self-perpetuating cycle of inflammation. Since these structures are additionally roofed by the fibrous extensor retinaculum of the first dorsal compartment, inflammation may spread causing thickening[17] and eventual stenosis[8] of that tunnel.

4. Which segments of the population are more prone to this condition?

During wrist motion the tendons of the first dorsal compartment undergo approximately 105° of angulation as they course over several joints to their distal attachment. These angulations are greatest in females and

may be viewed as an anatomic predisposing factor.[3] In addition, as much as 20% of the general population have an additional tendon passing through the first dorsal tunnel and attaching to a carpal bone.

5. Which predisposing movements identify the mechanism causing this overuse syndrome?

The most frequently documented occurrences of de Quervain's disease are in manual laborers who combine wrist motion and forearm rotation.[1,11] The classic case involves the carpenter who continuously hammers many nails, an action that involves repetitive and forceful ulnar deviation and flexion after radial deviation and extension of the wrist. Human tendons will not tolerate more than 1500 to 2000 manipulations per hour.[4] Bilaterally de Quervain's disease may occur in jackhammer operators[14] and is caused by bilateral symmetric trauma to both hands. A high incidence of de Quervain's disease occurs in women between 30 and 50 years of age,[17] three to 10 times more frequently than in men.[9,14,21]

6. What signs and symptoms are common to this malady, and what provocative tests or movements elicit the latter?

Symptoms include hot searing pain over the radial aspect of the wrist that may radiate up the forearm or distally to the fingers.[13] By mimicking the motion that caused the pain in the first place, *Finkelstein's test* (Fig. 3-2) elicits pain by passively stretching

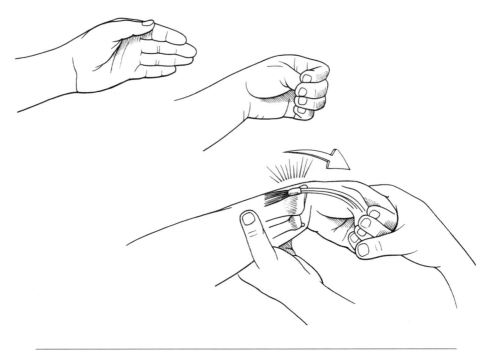

FIG. 3-2 Finkelstein's test. The wrist is sharply deviated ulnarly, provoking severe, sudden pain.

the inflamed tendons. All thumb motion, in particular active or resisted extension and abduction of the thumb is painful, with resistance of the former regarded as the result of the hitchhiker's thumb test.[8] Supination is reported to be more painful than pronation. The patient may feel weakness and may demonstrate diminished grip and pinch strength. Since the radial styloid forms the proximal wall of the snuffbox, tenderness is elicited just proximal to the radial styloid. The area of the extensor sheath may also appear or feel thickened. Triggering of the thumb, not to be confused with trigger finger of the flexor sheath, secondary to increased involvement of the first dorsal compartment has been reported.[6] Fine crepitus may result from excessive overuse and resultant tenosynovitis.[5]

7. How is concomitant inflammation of the tendon of the third dorsal compartment evaluated?

Sometimes involvement of the extensor pollicis longus is found to accompany inflammation of the first dorsal compartment and is evaluated by testing the resisted thumb extension while stabilizing the proximal and distal joints. Discomfort with selective tension dictates rest and immobilization of this tendon.[10]

8. What other conditions must be ruled out upon eliciting pain and tenderness at the snuffbox?

Although excruciating pain in the area of the radial styloid is helpful in diagnosis, it is not pathognomonic of de Quervain's disease. Other causes must be ruled out and include the following:

- *Scaphoid fracture.* Since the scaphoid lies at the base of the anatomic snuffbox, pain in the hollow just distal to the radial styloid is characteristic of scaphoid fracture when followed by a history of falling forward on outstretched hands. When the hand is laid palm down against a flat surface, the bony resting points on the heel of the hand are the scaphoid tubercle radially and the pisiform tubercle ulnarly. When one falls on an outstretched arm and an extended wrist, the scaphoid tubercle is more vulnerable to fracture than the pisiform because the scaphoid is trapped against the distal end of the radius whereas the pisiform is free to move and usually escapes injury (see Fig. 5-2 and p. 37).
- *Radial nerve neuritis.* The superficial radial nerve (SRN) is purely sensory and supplies cutaneous innervation to the dorsoradial aspect of the thumb and thenar eminence, as well as the dorsum of the index, long, and ring fingers as far as the proximal interpha-

langeal joints. This nerve branches off the radial nerve at the level of the lateral epicondyle and travels under cover of the brachioradialis to emerge distally in the distal third of the forearm between the extensor carpi radialis longus and brachioradialis tendons where it becomes subcutaneous. Entrapment of the SRN may occur when the forearm is pronated, compressing the nerve by the scissors-like action of the two tendons.[7] Patients may complain of dysesthesia, numbness, and tingling in the radial nerve distribution, possibly with pain radiating proximally to the elbow or shoulder. A positive Tinel's sign may be elicited over the radial nerve and the junction of the middle and distal forearm. Wrist flexion, ulnar deviation, and forearm supination will increase symptoms because these positions place traction on the nerve.

Compressive neuritis may also occur from a tight-fitting wristwatch, bangle, or handcuff, or from a tight cast.[6] Finkelstein's test will be positive. SRN neuritis is differentiated from de Quervain's disease by a maneuver that tenses the radial nerve. Beginning distally with thumb flexion, wrist ulnar deviation, and forearm pronation, one subjects the proximal upper extremity to the following sequence of postures: elbow flexion, shoulder depression, medial rotation, abduction, or extension as well as cervical lateral flexion.[2] Regardless of the cause of nerve damage, an electrophysiologic test with diminished amplitude of the sensory action potentials confirms the suspected diagnosis. Compression of the radial nerve secondary to de Quervain's disease is unlikely. Carpal tunnel syndrome in which the median nerve is compressed may occur secondary to acute and chronic flexor tenosynovitis.

- *Basal joint arthritis.* The carpometacarpal (CMC) joint of the thumb is the articulation of trapezium and the first metacarpal. Osteoarthritis has a predilection for the CMC joint of the thumb and is known as basal (or CMC) joint arthritis. This condition may yield painful thumb motion and a positive Finkelstein's test with pain not at the snuffbox but at the involved joint. Basal joint arthritis may be further distinguished from de Quervain's disease by a *positive axial compression test* (such as passive grinding and rotation of the metacarpal against the trapezium), resulting in pain, tenderness, and swelling over the site of the CMC joint. Unlike true de Quervain's disease, pain is not elicited on resisted thumb extension and abduction. Nor is pain experienced in that position that places the tendons and sheath on stretch (that is, ulnar wrist deviation while the thumb is fixed in flexion). Additionally, joint play movements at the CMC joint will be painful and restricted. Basal joint arthritis may be viewed on an x-ray film. Involvement of the interphalangeal joint of the thumb is more common in rheumatoid and psoriatic arthritis.

- There is a syndrome involving tenosynovitis of the tendons of the second dorsal compartment as that compartment is crossed over by the muscle bellies of the abductor pollicis longus (APL) and the extensor pollicis brevis (EPB) of the first dorsal compartment (Fig. 3-3). The significance of the term "outcropping muscles" describing the muscles of the first dorsal compartment is that although they lie within the deep layer of the forearm their tendons rise to the surface by "outcropping" so as to allow the extensor carpi radialis longus and brevis of the second dorsal compartment to pass through. The tendons of the second dorsal compartment may be stressed to elicit pain, swelling, and crepitus on wrist movement more proximal to that of de Quervain's disease. These tendons become palpable when the fist is clenched. This syndrome goes by many names such as *tenosynovitis crepitans, intersection syndrome, peritendinitis crepitans,* and *abductor pollicis longus bursitis.*

- *Double-crush phenomenon.* The double-crush phenomenon in which proximal disorders ranging from tennis elbow, shoulder capsulitis, or cervical spondylosis frequently coexist with de Quervain's disease (see p. 31.)

9. Which metabolic abnormalities, though not causative, are associated with this condition?

Metabolic abnormalities, though not demonstrated to be causative, are at times associated with de Quervain's disease and include diabetes, hyperuricemia, hypothyroidism, rheumatoid arthritis, and gonococcal arthritis. De Quervain's disease may also, as in carpal tunnel syndrome, occur during pregnancy and may occasionally persist until nursing is terminated.[20] Patients who do not respond to simple therapeutic measures should be suspected of secondary medical conditions and be ruled out as causative factors.

10. What medical management is typical for this patient, and what, if any, are deleterious effects of this management?

Several steroidal injections are made directly into the fibrous sheath of the first dorsal compartment. The problems of steroids are well documented and may

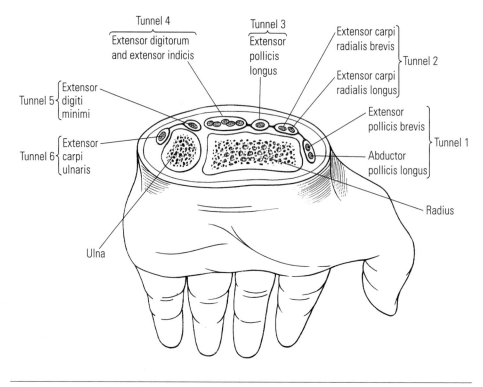

FIG. 3-3 The six tunnels on the dorsum of the wrist that transport the extensor tendons to the hand.

cause subcutaneous fat atrophy, tendon deterioration, and skin depigmentation.

11. What surgical management is appropriate for this patient, and what complications are associated with surgery?

If the second or third steroidal injection provides no relief, surgical decompression may be considered. De Quervain's tenosynovectomy involves slitting open the tendon's fibrous sheath of the first dorsal compartment by a transverse incision; this is favored over the longitudinal incision because it minimizes scar and keloid formation.[12,16] This is then followed by a longitudinal incision of the overlying retinaculum. After surgery the thumb is immobilized in a spica splint applied with the wrist in slight extension for 3 to 5 days, after which early mobilization is begun. Some surgeons prescribe immediate early active range of motion without mobilization.[16]

Complications after surgery primarily include superficial radial nerve injury either from direct nerve laceration, vigorous retraction of the superficial radial nerve when the surgical field is exposed, or neu-

roma from scar hypertrophy. These problems may be caused when surgeons are unaccustomed to the anatomy of the region.[6] These complications may not result in sensory loss but, rather, in extremely painful paresthesias such that some sensitive patients may not even tolerate anything touching their skin. This may be accompanied by reflex sympathetic dystrophy.[15] Another complication is tendon subluxation from overaggressive incision of too extensive a portion of the retinaculum overlying the first compartment structures.

12. What therapeutic intervention will best rehabilitate this patient?

Ninety percent of nonsevere cases of de Quervain's disease may expect relief with conservative management. Treatment may be divided into two phases.

PHASE I (WEEKS 1 TO 4)

- Rest.
- Iontophoresis or phonophoresis of antiinflammatory agents into area of first dorsal compartment.

- Ice massage, with avoidance of prominences, for a maximum duration of 5 minutes.
- Nonsteroidal antiinflammatory medication.
- Thumb spica splint is a forearm-based splint fabricated from a volar or radial approach; its design immobilizes the wrist, carpometacarpal, and metacarpophalangeal joints of the thumb and serves to rest both the radial wrist extensors and the proximal thumb. The following positions are prescribed: wrist in a 15° extension, carpometacarpal joint in a 40° to 50° palmar abduction, and the metacarpophalangeal joints in 5° to 10° of flexion to allow for light prehensile and opposition activities. The interphalangeal joint is left free to perform active motion unless the pollicis longus extensor is involved. It is very important to ensure that the superficial radial nerve and ulnar digital nerve of the thumb are not compromised. The splint is worn at all times except for removal for hygiene and exercise. Upon removal of the splint the patient is reminded not to exacerbate symptoms by "testing out his hand."
- Gentle active range of motion exercises for short periods lasting 10 to 20 minutes within the pain-free range are performed to prevent joint stiffness and adhesion formation between tendons and sheath, enhance circulation, and minimize protective posturing.
- Performing overhead finger pumping every few hours and encouraging the patient to elevate the involved hand above the heart as much as possible.
- Hygienic activities of daily living should be performed by gentle stabilization of the thumb against the lateral aspect of the index finger.
- Towel gathering and unfolding with the thumb initially actively splinted against the index finger and becoming actively involved as treatment progresses.
- Grasp and release of small objects emphasizing a wide variety of prehensile patterns that avoid overuse of first dorsal compartment tendons.[10]

PHASE II (WEEKS 4 TO 12)

In this stage the patient is gradually weaned from the protective splint during daylight hours but still wears it at night.

- Incorporate adaptive equipment, such as built-up handles for writing, or the use of a hammer and a bent handle.
- After beginning strengthening with isometric exercises, because this involves little or no tendon excursion, by pushing a dowel through putty with the thumb initially stabilized laterally on the proximal phalanx of the index finger, the patient then progresses to placing the thumb around (such as medial to) the dowel and finally atop the dowel. Frequency is 5 minutes for three times per day. The patient is progressed to the subsequent position when multiple repetitions are pain free.
- Patient then progresses to isotonic strengthening by (1) moving the thumb up and down the length of a pencil while the fingers are wrapped transversely around the length of the pencil to provide graded resistance, (2) syringe use, (3) link belt fabrication, and (4) putty pinching.
- Isokinetic strengthening of thumb in liquid, as during daily bath.[10]

REFERENCES

1. Boyes JH: *Bunnel's surgery of the hand,* Philadelphia, 1970, Lippincott.
2. Butler D: *Mobilization of the nervous system,* Melbourne, 1991, Churchill Livingstone.
3. Calliet R: *Hand pain and impairment,* Philadelphia, 1982, FA Davis.
4. Conklin JE, White WL: Stenosing tenosynovitis, *Surg Clin North Am* 40(2):531, 1960.
5. Cyriax J: *Textbook of orthopedic medicine,* vol 2, London, 1987, Bailliere-Tindall.
6. Dawson DM, Hallet M, Millender LH: *Entrapment neuropathies,* ed 2, Boston, 1990, Little, Brown.
7. Dellon AL, Mackinnon SE: Susceptibility of the superficial sensory range of the radial nerve to form painful neuromas, *J Hand Surg* 9B:42-45, 1984.
8. Goldberg S: *Clinical anatomy made ridiculously simple,* Miami, 1988, MedMaster.
9. Hall CL: Chronic stenosing tenovaginitis of the wrist, *J Int College Surg* 14(1):48, 1950.
10. Hunter JM, Schneider LH, Mackin EJ, et al, editors: *Rehabilitation of the hand: surgery and therapy,* ed 3, St Louis, 1990, Mosby.
11. Hymovich L, Lindholm M: Hand, wrist and forearm injuries, *J Occup Med* 8(11):573, 1966.
12. Keon-Cohn B: de Quervain's disease, *J Bone Surg* 33B(1):96, 1951.
13. Kilgore E, Graham W: *The hand: surgical and non-surgical management,* Philadelphia, 1977, Lea & Febiger.
14. Leaao L: De Quervain's disease, *J Bone Joint Surg* 40A(5):1063, 1958.
15. Lee VH: The painful hand. In Moran C, editor: *Hand rehabilitation,* New York, 1986, Churchill Livingstone.
16. Muckart RD: Stenosing tenovaginitis of abductor pollicis longus and extensor pollicis brevis at the radial styloid (de Quervain's disease), *Clin Orthop* 33:201, 1964.
17. Netter FH: *The CIBA collection of medical illustrations, vol 8: musculoskeletal system,* part 2, Summit, NJ, 1990, CIBA-Geigy.

18. Poole B: Cumulative trauma disorder of the upper extremity from occupational stress, *J Hand Ther* 1(4):172, 1988.
19. Salter RB: *Textbook of disorders and injuries of the musculoskeletal system,* ed 2, Baltimore, 1987, Williams & Wilkins.
20. Schumacher HR, Bomalski JS: *Case studies in rheumatology,* Philadelphia, 1990, Williams & Wilkins.
21. Strandell G: Variations of the anatomy in stenosing tenosynovitis at the radial styloid process, *Acta Chir Scand* 113:234, 1957.
22. Viegas SF: Trigger thumb of de Quervain's disease, *J Hand Surg* 11A(2):235, 1986.

RECOMMENDED READING

Armstrong TJ, Fine LJ, Goldstein SA, et al: Ergonomics consideration in hand and wrist tendinitis, *J Hand Surg* [AM] 12A(5):830-837, 1987.

Conklin JE, White WL: Stenosing tenosynovitis, *Surg Clin North Am* 40:531, 1960.
Hunter JM, Schneider LH, Mackin EJ, et al, editors: *Rehabilitation of the hand: surgery and therapy,* ed 3, St Louis, 1990, Mosby.
Pick RY: de Quervain's disease: a clinical trial, *Clin Orthop* 143:165, 1979.
Saplys R, Mackinnon SE, Dellon AL: The relationship between nerve entrapment versus neuroma complications and the misdiagnosis of de Quervain's disease, *Contemp Orthop* 15:51-57, 1987.

4

Nocturnal Wringing of Painful Tingling Right Hand

A 51-year-old female pianist complains of annoying nighttime numbness of 6 weeks in duration to her entire right hand that is relieved by placing her hand under cold running water for 5 minutes. The patient is ambidextrous and admits to having recently performed intense calligraphy of some 300 invitations in preparation for her daughter's wedding with her left hand, which, she admits, "also feels funny." Numbness and tingling are prominent to her right index finger when driving her automobile or playing piano. She states that she had entered menopause 3 years previously. When asked, the patient also reveals that she is a non-insulin dependent diabetic of 6 years in duration but denies any paresthesias to the feet, loss of balance, history of injury, or any neck and shoulder pain.

OBSERVATION   No swelling, trophic changes, atrophy, or deformity observed.

PALPATION   No tenderness or swelling are present at hand, wrist, or cubital fossa; there is good capillary refilling.

RANGE OF MOTION   Within functional limits to both hands.

MOTOR TESTS   Good minus muscle strength in thumb opposition and abduction in right hand compared to a normal grade for left hand.

SENSATION   Normal to light touch, two-point discrimination and vibration to all fingertips except for the thumb.

SELECTIVE TENSION   Resisted pronation and supination, as well as all other resistive tests are negative.

SPECIAL TESTS   Negative Allen test, positive Phalen's test, negative Tinel's sign, negative axial compression test of the spine, and negative hyperabduction test.

CLUE   Nerve conduction velocities are as follows:

	Right	Left	Normal
Sensory latency across wrist	3.7	3.6	<3.5 msec
Motor latency across wrist	4.5	4.4	<4.5 msec

? **Q**uestions

1. What is most likely causing this woman's symptoms?
2. What is the cause of carpal tunnel syndrome (CTS)?
3. What anatomy is relevant to understanding this disorder?
4. What are the functions of the flexor retinaculum?
5. What is the clinical presentation?
6. What is the clinical course of the disorder?
7. What is the differential diagnosis?
8. What is anterior interosseous syndrome?
9. What are the electrophysiologic findings in CTS?
10. What other pathologic conditions are associated with CTS?
11. How is motor function best tested?
12. Which provocative tests elicit symptoms?
13. What disorders of the workplace are implicated as possible causes of CTS?
14. What chronic, rheumatologic, or metabolic disorders are associated with CTS?
15. What is the double-crush phenomenon?
16. What nonsurgical treatment or treatments are appropriate before surgical decompression?
17. What are indications for surgery, and what does surgery involve?
18. What is postsurgical management?
19. What sequelae may follow surgery?

1. What is most likely causing this woman's symptoms?

Carpal tunnel syndrome (CTS) is one of the most common, best defined, and most carefully studied entrapment neuropathies. CTS commonly affects middle-aged females between 40 and 60 years of age,[6] that is, menopausal women, a characteristic suggestive of a hormonal aberration as a cause in the development of this disorder.[16] The most common cause of CTS is an idiopathic nonspecific flexor tenosynovitis[6] that may simply arise from chronic repetitive occupational stress.[16] CTS may occur acutely after lunate bone dislocation or from a Colles fracture and requires immediate medical attention so as to prevent acute nerve ischemia.[6]

2. What is the cause of carpal tunnel syndrome (CTS)?

The causes of CTS may be subdivided into one of four categories:

1. An increase in volume or tunnel contents secondary to nonspecific tenosynovitis of the flexor tendons within the carpal tunnel.
2. Thickening (fibrosis) of the transverse carpal ligament.
3. Alteration of the osseous margins of the carpus caused by fractures, dislocations, or arthritic joint changes.
4. Tumor or systemic disease.

3. What anatomy is relevant to understanding this disorder?

The median nerve enters the hand through an osseofibrous carpal tunnel that is bounded dorsally and laterally by the convex bony carpus and volarly by the thick transverse carpal ligament, otherwise known as the *flexor retinaculum*.[6] The corners of this tunnel are the pisiform, hamate, scaphoid tubercle, and trapezium tubercle.[17] The transverse carpal ligament spans between the scaphoid tubercle radially and the hamate bone ulnarly. The median nerve shares the tunnel with nine other flexor tendons, each of which is covered with two layers of synovium (Fig. 4-1). The radial and ulnar arteries, the ulnar nerve, and flexor palmaris longus do not pass through the carpal tunnel and are referred to as extracarpal structures. After its passage through the carpal tunnel, the median nerve divides into five digital branches,[6] the most radial of which supplies the thenar musculature and the latter two finger lumbricales; the other four (ulnar) branches supply sensation to the palmer aspect of the lateral (that is, radial) three and a half digits and their dorsal fingertips. The palm itself is spared of sensory loss in CTS because the palmer cutaneous sensory branch takes leave of the median nerve before that nerve enters the carpal tunnel.[5] This cutaneous branching occurs approximately 3 cm proximal[6] to the transverse carpal ligament between the tendons of the

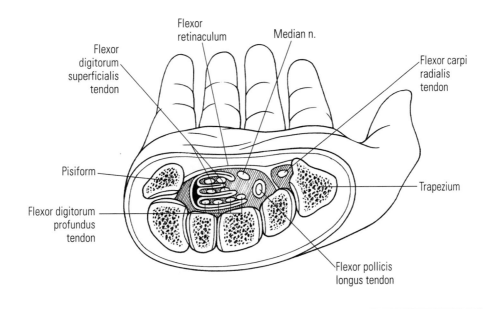

Flexor retinaculum

Flexor digitorum superficialis tendon

Median n.

Flexor carpi radialis tendon

Pisiform

Flexor digitorum profundus tendon

Trapezium

Flexor pollicis longus tendon

FIG. 4-1 Cross-sectional view of the carpal tunnel and its contents. The median nerve lies adjacent to the tendons of the flexor digitorum superficialis tendons.

palmaris longus and flexor carpi radialis muscles, beyond which the nerve travels superficially toward the palm (Fig. 4-2). The essential concept is that there is little if any spare space within the carpal tunnel, and so anything that decreases volume within the tunnel such as swollen tendons will occupy more space and will do so at the expense of the median nerve suffering ischemia.

4. What are the functions of the flexor retinaculum?

Forming the roof of the carpal tunnel, the stout transverse carpal ligament offers attachment for the thenar and hypothenar muscles, helps maintain the transverse carpal arch of the hand, prevents bowstringing of the extrinsic flexor tendons, and offers protection to the median nerve.

5. What is the clinical presentation?

Some patients will merely complain of numbness *(hypoesthesia)*, without much pain, in the median nerve distribution.[16] Many patients complain of nocturnal pain that may occur from the flexed position the body's extremities assume during sleep. Patients may be awakened by tingling *(paresthesia)* or burning[16] pain and will wring or fling the hand up and down in an attempt to alleviate symptoms. Because of variable in-

nervation of the median nerve as well as subjective difficulty interpreting symptoms while half asleep, some patients will complain of dysesthesia of the entire hand and not of just the thumb, index, middle, and radial half of the fourth digit.[17] The patient often returns to sleep by hanging the affected limb over the edge of the bed[11] in the loose-packed position. During the day, functional activities such as driving, sewing, or hammering precipitate symptoms. As this condition progresses, symptoms may spread above the wrist to the forearm and, less commonly, to the upper arm. Sensory testing may demonstrate diminishment or absence of tactile sensation *(anesthesia)*.* Motor symptoms, that is, loss of thumb opposition and abduction, as well as thenar atrophy generally appear late in the course of CTS.[11] Bilateral upper extremity CTS is common.[16] In long-standing cases the thumb metacarpal bone may become fixed in supination because of muscle imbalance.

6. What is the clinical course of the disorder?

Patients with CTS can be grouped into three categories (or stages outlined by Sunderland) convenient not only for diagnosis but also as a guide to treatment and prognosis. These groupings may be said to correspond to

*Moore KL: *Clinically oriented anatomy,* ed 2, Baltimore, 1984, Williams & Wilkins.

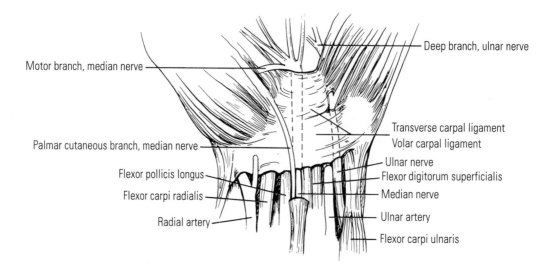

Motor branch, median nerve

Deep branch, ulnar nerve

Palmar cutaneous branch, median nerve

Transverse carpal ligament
Volar carpal ligament

Flexor pollicis longus

Ulnar nerve
Flexor digitorum superficialis

Flexor carpi radialis

Median nerve

Radial artery

Ulnar artery

Flexor carpi ulnaris

FIG. 4-2 Anterior view of the wrist and palm showing extracarpal course of the palmar cutaneous branch of the median nerve. (Redrawn from The American Society for Surgery of the Hand: *Regional review course in hand surgery,* Aurora, Colo., 1985.)

neuropraxia, axonotmesis, and neurotmesis, respectively. It is helpful to bear the following two items in mind before reading on:

- The median nerve has both sensory and motor branches. During median nerve compression at the carpal tunnel sensory abnormalities usually occur first[17] only to progress to motor involvement as the pathology evolves.
- Clinical findings are proportional to the degree of nerve damage, which in turn is related to the severity of compression and not to the duration of compression.[6]

Group I presents with the mildest symptoms of weakness or clumsiness brought on by drawing, holding a newspaper, or performing manual labor. Symptoms are initially sporadic only to increase in frequency over time. No abnormal findings may occur during the initial examination. Physiologic changes include progressive obstruction of venous return resulting in circulatory slowing, hence impaired nutrition to the nerve fibers.

Group II is characterized by pain, often of a burning quality, and is often a major complaint during this stage, with some thenar weakness or atrophy, skin changes, sensory loss, realization of clumsiness, loss of pinch, and loss of dexterity. The patient requires longer periods of hand wringing, rubbing, or placing of the hand under running water so as to help alleviate

symptoms. There may be a positive Phalen's test or Tinel's sign.[6] Pain may be referred as proximally as the shoulder. Physiologic changes include slowing of capillary circulation so severely that anoxia damages the endoneurium.

Group III is characterized by pronounced thenar wasting and sensory loss, skin atrophy, and significant loss of dexterity; there is often loss of two-point discrimination and significant functional impairment. Pain may have either subsided or become severe. Here the prognosis is very poor regardless of treatment[6] because the compressed nerve has become a fibrotic cord.

7. What is the differential diagnosis?

- C6 radiculopathy caused by *cervical spondylosis* most commonly occurs in middle-aged or elderly patients and is the root with the greatest degree of nearly identical symptoms to those of median nerve pathosis.[6] Patients with CTS may complain of some mild to moderate diffuse aching pain in the forearm or arm, whereas neck and shoulder pain are distinctly unusual. Pain with coughing, sneezing, or when bearing down (Valsalva maneuver) during a bowel movement are not commonly associated with radiculopathy but are highly specific when reported; these do not occur with CTS. Similarly, pain radiating posteriorly along the medial scapular border is characteristic

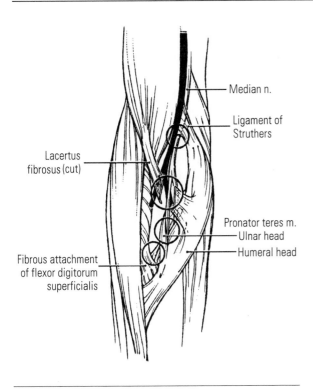

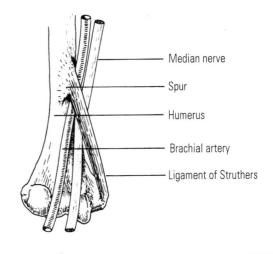

FIG. 4-4 Median nerve compression by the anomalous ligament of Struthers. (From Magee DJ: *Orthopaedic physical assessment,* Philadelphia, 1987, Saunders.)

FIG. 4-3 Sites of median nerve compression in pronator syndrome. (From Chabon SJ: *Physician Assistant,* Sept 1990.)

of radiculopathy. Relief from pain by massaging, shaking, or immersing one's hand in water are common evasive maneuvers in CTS, whereas patients suffering from radiculopathy often find that use of the hand and arm makes the pain even worse. Additionally, patients suffering from cervical root irritation from cervical spondylosis tend to have a quiet night's sleep only to experience morning pain upon awakening, or daytime pain with arm usage, whereas patients with CTS usually experience pain at night.

If the sixth cervical nerve is affected, there may be weakness of elbow flexion and wrist extension, the biceps reflex may be lost or reduced, and electromyographic (EMG) studies will show denervation out of median nerve territory if the cause of the disorder is nerve root damage;[6] sensory loss of the sixth cervical dermatome differs topographically from that of the median nerve distribution.

Diminished biceps and brachioradialis (C5, C6) reflexes with increased triceps reflex (C7) is known as the *inverted radial reflex* and is a clinical clue to spondylosis causing C6 nerve root compression. The idea here is that excess tone may be recircuited so as to manifest briskly in nerve roots supplying other deep tendon reflexes (DTR) further distally along the spinal cord, in this case the next immediate DTR.[8]

- With CNS lesions, an intermittent condition affecting one cerebral hemisphere such as a *focal motor seizure* or *transient vascular episode* in the carotid distribution may mimic CTS. Complaints can be surprisingly restricted in their territory, with reports of numbness, tingling, or weakness of one or two fingers of one hand with episodes lasting several minutes, hours, or even permanently in the event of infarction. Absence of pain is a characteristic of such CNS lesions.[6]

    Lesions of the spinal cord such as tumors, *syringomyelia,* and *multiple sclerosis* do not usually yield transient or intermittent symptoms that vary from one hour to the next.[6]

- *Pronator syndrome* (Fig. 4-3) refers to compression of the median nerve (1) by pronator muscle as it passes through the heads of that muscle and (2) to a lesser extent by fibrous bands[16] near the origin of the deep flexor muscles,[16] known as the lacertus fibrosus and flexor digitorum superficialis arcade,[2] and (3) even less commonly by the ligament of Struthers (Fig. 4-4), an anomalous structure found in about 1% of the population.[18] This ligament runs from an abnormal bone spur located on the medial aspect of the distal humerus to the medial humeral epicondyle. This syndrome commonly occurs in patients whose jobs require repetitive pronation-supination motions, or in those who have sustained trauma to the proximal volar part of the forearm.[7,19]

Although the pronator syndrome may also be expressed with median nerve paresthesias mimicking those of CTS, it differs in several aspects. Night pain, symptoms brought on by wrist movement, intrinsic weakness of opponens and abduction movements, as well as positive Phalen and Tinel wrist signs are not common to this condition. The pronator syndrome is distinguished by exacerbation attributable to resisted pronation and passive supination activities, positive Tinel's sign at the proximal forearm overlying the median nerve, tenderness and paresthesias in the median nerve distribution on direct compression over pronator muscle, and pain and median nerve paresthesias with forced pronation, as well as passive supination at the limit of full extension. Like anterior osseous syndrome, there is also difficulty with pincer movement involving the thumb to the index finger. Nerve conduction velocity (NCV) and EMG studies show slowed conduction velocity across the forearm and denervation potentials of flexor pollicis longus and abductor pollicis brevis. Treatment includes stretching exercises to both pronator and supinator muscles; surgical decompression is appropriate when conservative treatment is ineffective.[4]

- In *Raynaud's phenomenon,* the symptoms caused by local vasospasm are differentiated from CTS in the sense that Raynaud's phenomenon does not involve any distinction between the fingers, with all the fingers and palm being equally affected. This relationship to cold is not observed in patients with CTS.[6]
- *Reflex sympathetic dystrophy* (RSD) (see Chapter 6) is similar to CTS in the sense that pain, paresthesias, trophic changes, puffy hands, and decreased function of flexor tendons are features of both pathoses. In addition, both conditions can show sympathetic abnormalities. However, in patients with true RSD there is more trophic change, redness, cyanosis and atrophy of fingertips, and pronounced variation in color with dependence of the limb.[6]
- *Diabetic neuropathy* can manifest as an asymmetric condition reflecting partial or complete infarction of nerves or nerve trunks, usually occurring in relationship to the lumbosacral plexus or to the sciatic or femoral nerves. The result is sudden onset and often painful asymmetric loss of function with prominent weakness and little sensory loss. The median nerve is rarely affected.[6]

8. What is anterior interosseous syndrome?

The anterior interosseous nerve arises from the median nerve 5 to 8 cm distal to the lateral epicondyle and moves distally to the anterior interosseous membrane. It is the last major tributary branch off the median nerve.[6] Purely a *motor nerve,*[17] the anterior interosseous nerve innervates the flexor pollicis longus, the flexor digitorum profundus to the index and long digits, and the pronator quadratus.

The cause of *anterior interosseous syndrome* is controversial and may be ascribed to one of several causes that include a tendinous origin of the deep head of the pronator teres muscle (Fig. 4-5) or of the flexor digitorum superficialis of the long finger, or from accessory muscles and tendons from the latter muscle, or from the flexor pollicis longus, as well as aberrant ves-

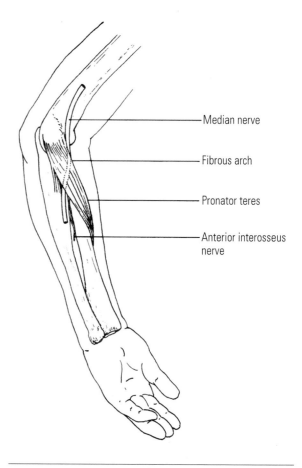

Median nerve

Fibrous arch

Pronator teres

Anterior interosseus nerve

FIG. 4-5 The anterior interosseus nerve, which is a branch of the median nerve, may become entrapped as it passes between the two heads of the pronator teres. (From Magee DJ: *Orthopaedic physical assessment,* Philadelphia, 1987, Saunders.)

sels, or thrombosed collateral vessels.[6] Spontaneous anterior interosseous nerve paralysis may result from minimal trauma only in the presence of one of the aforementioned preexisting anomalous conditions. Specifically, motions such as excessive and repetitive elbow flexion and pronation are seen in butchers, carpenters, or leather cutters.[15] Strenuous exercise and lifting heavy weights have also provoked this syndrome.[10,12] Provocation of this syndrome may occur directly and not as a function of overuse, in fractures, gunshot wounds, and lacerations, and from drug injections by addicts.[6] Extrinsic pressure causes include wearing a cast and carrying a handbag.

Clinical features of spontaneous anterior interosseous syndrome include acute pain prodrome in the proximal forearm lasting hours to days. There may be a recent history of heavy muscular exertion or local trauma. With the onset of paresis, patients may notice a loss of dexterity and discover that their pinching is impaired. Physical examination shows characteristic difficulty in flexing the distal interphalangeal joints of the thumb and index finger to form a pincer movement because of weakness (Fig. 4-6). Paralysis of the pronator quadratus is tested with the elbow in flexion to block the contraction from the humeral head of the pronator teres.[6] There may be elbow pain on resisted pronation or while one stretches the pronator quadratus in extreme supination.

Treatment of this relatively common condition[6] includes a 6-month conservative trial of therapy that includes avoidance of movements or the occupation that exacerbates symptoms. An ergonomic analysis of the workplace is appropriate and suggestions should be offered how to perform one's occupation in a nonprovoking manner. Therapy also includes rest, nonsteroidal antiinflammatory medications, and immobilization of the forearm in partial supination to relieve pressure on the pronator teres. The physician may inject a steroid in the region of the pronator teres.[6]

9. What are the electrophysiologic findings in CTS?

Electrophysiologic studies are indicated when the clinical diagnosis is uncertain. The first step is to examine the sensory action across the wrist so as to rule out generalized neuropathy. The second step involves motor-conduction studies in the hope of finding a prolonged distal motor latency or, even better, a prolonged residual latency and normal conduction velocity in the forearm that would confirm focality of the lesion. The third step is electromyography, which is mainly useful to rule out coexisting radiculopathy although this test may prove normal in as much as one fourth of patients suffering from CTS.[14]

10. What other pathologic conditions are associated with CTS?

Patients with CTS may have other forms of tendon pathoses such as de Quervain's disease, rotator cuff tendinitis, or trigger finger. CTS is a common complication of chronic renal failure treated by hemodialysis; beta 2-microglobulin-derived amyloid can be found deposited in the transverse carpal ligament.[17] Although not a pathologic condition, some women who experience pregnancy may succumb to CTS, with typical time of onset at the sixth month.[6] It may be that changes in hormonal levels or weight gain somehow influence fluid retention.

11. How is motor function best tested?

The *abductor pollicis brevis* is the easiest of the thenar muscles to be tested. The thumb is brought up perpendicularly to the palm, and the patient resists pressure directed against the distal phalanx (Fig. 4-7). However, the clinician must be on guard against tricky substitution by the abductor pollicis longus, which is innervated by the radial nerve and abducts the thumb radially. Alternatively the patient may flex the thumb across the palm using the long flexor, which is innervated by the median nerve proximal to the forearm. Either substitution will not yield true 90° abduction.[6]

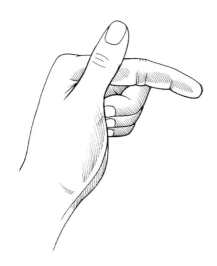

FIG. 4-6 Hand posture associated with anterior interosseous nerve palsy.

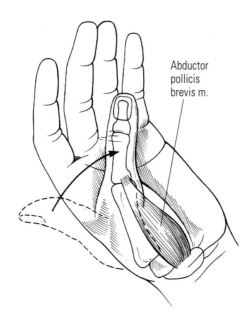

Abductor
pollicis
brevis m.

FIG. 4-7 Manual abductor policis brevis testing for median nerve injury. Weakness manifests as a decreased ability to abduct the thumb, making it difficult to grasp a large object. Eventually an adduction deformity of the thumb may result (ape hand)

The significance in choosing to test this muscle becomes apparent when we consider how the other muscles supplied by the median nerve either have dual innervation or may be compensated for by the long forearm muscles.[13] One can best test opposition by requesting the patient to place the tips of the thumb and fifth finger together and resist the examiner's attempt to break this pinch. It is helpful to remember that the dominant hand is normally 10% stronger than the nondominant hand.

12. Which provocative tests elicit symptoms?

In *Phalen's test* or *Tinel's sign* (Fig. 4-8), the median nerve is easily depolarized when mechanically stimulated by direct tapping over the palmaris longus tendon over the flexor retinaculum. However, positive findings occur only in approximately 45% of all cases.[14] Intercarpal pressure is greatest at 90° wrist flexion superimposed on ulnar deviation.

13. What disorders of the workplace are implicated as possible causes of CTS?

Repeated overuse, whether at work or in recreation, will result in swelling of the tendons or of the synovia

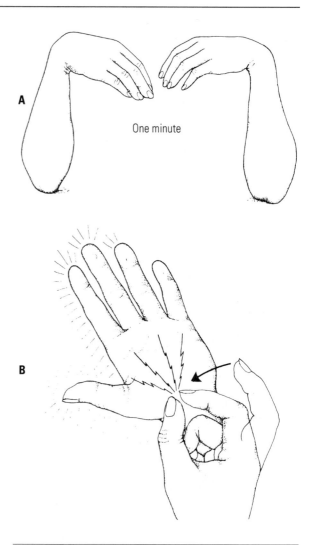

A

One minute

B

FIG. 4-8 A, Phalen's test: The patient is asked to report any sensory changes in the median nerve–innervated area after holding his wrists flexed for 1 minute. **B,** Tinel's sign: The examiner taps the hand from the fingertips proximally to the palm. The patient is asked to report any "electric shocks" or tingling when percussed. (From The American Society for Surgery of the Hand: *The hand examination and diagnosis,* New York, 1983, Churchill Livingstone.)

surrounding those tendons. Occupational variants predisposing CTS may include carpentry, secretarial work, keyboard operators, and jackhammer operators.

14. What chronic, rheumatologic, or metabolic disorders are associated with CTS?

Chronic disorders associated with CTS include trauma, obesity, pregnancy, local tumors, and infection. Rheumatic disorders associated with CTS include rheumatoid arthritis, systemic lupus erythematosus, gout, and pseudogout. Metabolic disorders associated with CTS include hypothyroidism, diabetes mellitus, acromegaly, myxedema, eosinophilic fasciitis, dysproteinemia, amyloidosis, and mucopolysaccharidoses.[17]

15. What is the double-crush phenomenon?

A nerve may be compressed at more than one site (Fig. 4-9), a condition known as *double-crush syndrome*. Since nerve tissue is extremely sensitive to ischemia, pressure on the nerve at the neck, at the thoracic outlet, or at the elbow will make the nerve even more susceptible to even mild pressure in the carpal tunnel. By tautening the nerve along its proximal and distal length in a specific sequence a clinician may confirm a suspected double-crush. This sequence of postures tenses the brachial plexus, particularly the median nerve trunk, and includes shoulder depression and abduction, elbow extension, forearm supination, wrist extension, and lateral cervical flexion.[3] The idea here is that the nerve tract is susceptible to mechanical injury because of either tethering at the intervertebral foramen or proximity to unyielding bone or simply because branching at an abrupt angle compromises the nerve's gliding mechanisms.[3] Suspicion of a second crush site of the median nerve at a more proximal site may be confirmed if one superimposes a series of upper limb postures that tauten the nerve along its length. Shoulder depression, abduction, elbow extension, forearm supination, and wrist extension may elicit provocation of symptoms and confirm the presence of a suspected additional proximal lesion. Thus, in those patients with new onset of symptoms after surgical release, attention ought to be directed to more proximal sites of possible compression rather than reattempting surgery. Conservative treatment may more likely have positive results, especially when patients readily report relief of hand symptoms after proximal stretching techniques, massage of the upper trapezius area, or other therapeutic modality.

16. What nonsurgical treatment or treatments are appropriate before surgical decompression?

Nonsurgical treatment is advised for patients with mild or intermittent symptoms and includes the following:
- Rest.
- Modification of work condition and habits, wrist posture, and tool design.
- Cock-up volar splint with wrist in loose-packed position (10° to 30° dorsiflexion) to be worn at night as

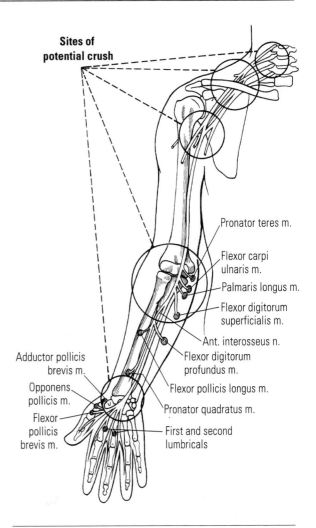

Sites of potential crush

Pronator teres m.

Flexor carpi ulnaris m.

Palmaris longus m.

Flexor digitorum superficialis m.

Ant. interosseus n.

Flexor digitorum profundus m.

Flexor pollicis longus m.

Pronator quadratus m.

First and second lumbricals

Adductor pollicis brevis m.

Opponens pollicis m.

Flexor pollicis brevis m.

FIG. 4-9 Double-crush phenomenon. After an initial "crush," the involved nerve presumably becomes sensitized and thereby more vulnerable to ischemic injury elsewhere along its length. A second "crush" site may occur proximally where the median nerve exits the spine at the intervertebral foramen, between the first rib and the clavicle (costoclavicular space), or at any of the nerve's multiple branchings in the vicinity of the cubital region.

well as by day continually for 4 to 6 weeks and with gradually decreasing splint use over the subsequent 4 weeks.[9]
- A short course of nonsteroidal antiinflammatory medication or oral steroids.
- A trial of diuretics, especially when symptoms are perimenstrual.
- Avoidance of certain wrist and hand postures and repetitive wrist motions such as gripping or pinching

objects while flexing the wrist and performing repetitive wrist flexion-extension exercise motions.

- One hundred to 200 mg of vitamin B6 per day is sometimes added to the diet despite inconclusive evidence that pyroxidine is beneficial.*

- Local steroid injection proximal to the transverse carpal ligament and into the perineurium but not into the nerve itself, since the latter is quite painful and dangerous. Injection should not be performed if significant swelling is present because the presence of additional volume only exacerbates the symptoms. Relief occurs within 1 to 3 days. If there is no change in symptoms, the second injection is not indicated. Repeated injections carry the danger of tendon attrition and rupture as well as permanent median nerve injury; a total of 3 or 4 injections are the maximum allowable number before one should insist on surgical release. Greater than 4 injections are considered only in a patient with a poor surgical risk or in an elderly patient.

- It is imperative to evaluate the work environment and to suggest alternatives such as an ergonomically designed keyboard for a secretary or a bent handle on a hammer for a carpenter.

- *Tendon-gliding exercises* facilitate isolated excursion of each of the two flexor tendons to each finger passing through the carpal tunnel. Each exercise is initiated from a position of full finger and wrist extension. To obtain maximum differential gliding of profundus with respect to superficialis excursion, the patient assumes a hooked-fist position. To obtain maximum flexor digitorum superficialis excursion, the patient is instructed to flex the metacarpophalangeal joints and the proximal interphalangeal joints while maintaining the distal interphalangeal joints in extension. A full fist exercise completes the series of tendon-gliding exercises and provides maximum profundus tendon excursion. These exercises are performed five times each, five times daily.

- For some patients experiencing transient episodes of CTS (as in pregnancy), reassurance and explanation are often all that is needed.

17. What are indications for surgery, and what does surgery involve?

Absolute surgical indications include failure of nonoperative treatment or clinical evidence of thenar atrophy. A relative indication for surgery is the patient with persistent sensory loss, especially if long standing.[6] De-

Merck Manual, Rahway, NJ.

compression, by way of division of the flexor retinaculum, often provides gratifying results[16] with dramatic immediate relief and has a good long-term prognosis in the treatment of CTS.

Before surgery, electrophysiologic studies are performed so as to provide a baseline value in determining the postoperative state of the nerve should surgery fail to relieve the patient of his or her symptoms.[6] Surgery is performed under local anesthesia with sedation, or regional intravenous anesthesia. The most accepted surgical incision is a curved interthenar incision along the bisected line through the fourth digit. Complications reported from using the older transverse incision at the wrist crease involving blind release of the flexor retinaculum include injury to the superficial palmar arch and laceration of the sensory branch of the median nerve.[6]

18. What is postsurgical management?

Postoperatively, because pressure on the median nerve increases with wrist motion, a bulky hand dressing and wrist splint are applied for 1 week after surgery. If the patient is allowed to remove the cast before 1 week, wrist motion may result in prolonged hypersensitivity and early digital motion is encouraged. One week after surgery the volar cast is removed and a volar wrist extension splint is fabricated, positioning the wrist in some 10° to 20° of wrist extension. This splint is worn at night during sleep and during strenuous exercise.[6]

Depending on the preoperative severity of symptoms as well as response to surgery, patients may require few or no therapy sessions, moderate intervention (3 to 8 weeks), whereas others require a comprehensive rehabilitation program (8 to 16 weeks).

The goals of therapy during the first 3 weeks after surgery are edema control, maintaining range of motion, preventing adhesion formation, and protected hand use. This is accomplished by instructing the patient to elevate the involved hand constantly and to do retrograde massage, three sets of 10 repetitions of tendon-gliding exercises and thumb flexion, extension, and opposition exercises, as well as shoulder and elbow exercises.[1]

Therapeutic goals during weeks 3 to 8 include edema reduction, scar modeling, reduction of hypersensitivity, and increasing strength and functional use. If thick hypertrophic scar develops along the incision site, elastomer is applied to the palmar scar to model it. Active and passive exercises are initiated for the digits and wrist if the patient lacks full motion. If edema persists, the patient may be instructed to perform overhead bilateral fisting exercises, one set of 20 repetitions per hour. String wrapping may also be helpful, as are elevated prehension activities, such as macramé, that recruit gravity to assist in edema reduction. *Nerve-gliding exercises* (Fig. 4-10) are initiated to ensure that the median nerve glides through the carpal tunnel and adjacent thenar and hypothenar eminences. Passive stretching of the thumb is necessary to prevent adhesion formation along the palmar cutaneous and motor branch of the median nerve. These exercises are performed for three sets of 10 repetitions daily.[1]

At the eighth week after surgery, graded isometric as well as isotonic strengthening exercises for the hand and wrist are initiated. The patient is cautioned against overexercise that might result in tenosynovitis. Work hardening is initiated at 8 to 12 weeks. Return to sedentary or clerical work is reasonable at this time, as is

NERVE GLIDING PROGRAM
For Median Nerve Decomposition at the Wrist

Exercises to be done _____ times each, _____ times a day.
Hold position to a count of _____.

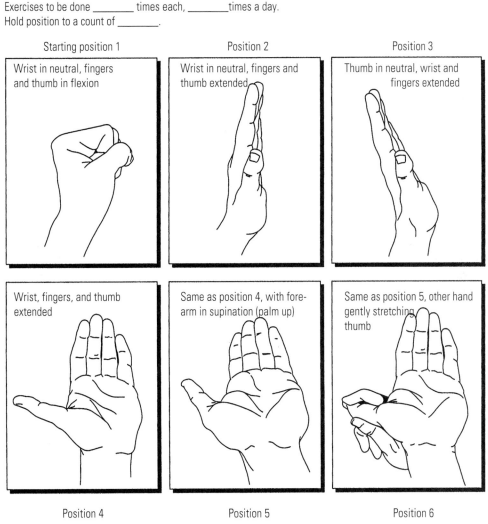

Starting position 1 — Wrist in neutral, fingers and thumb in flexion

Position 2 — Wrist in neutral, fingers and thumb extended

Position 3 — Thumb in neutral, wrist and fingers extended

Position 4 — Wrist, fingers, and thumb extended

Position 5 — Same as position 4, with forearm in supination (palm up)

Position 6 — Same as position 5, other hand gently stretching thumb

FIG. 4-10 Nerve-gliding exercises permit mobilization of the median nerve. (From Hunter JM, Schneider LH, Mackin EJ et al, editors: *Rehabilitation of the hand: surgery and therapy,* ed 3, St. Louis, 1990, Mosby. Exercises developed by Dr. James Hunter; home program designed by Julie Belkin, OTR.)

light house repair and housecleaning chores, but any strenuous activity is best preceded by a work-tolerance program. Premature return to heavy work can cause local pain, tenosynovitis, painful scarring, and local arthritis.[1]

Raynaud's phenomenon may be present in association with CTS and may be related to disordered neurovascular hand function after median nerve decompression.[16]

19. What sequelae may follow surgery?

Reflex sympathetic dystrophy (Chapter 6) can often be forestalled and staved off by being especially on guard for the anxious patient with low pain tolerance who will not actively flex the digits after surgery.

REFERENCES

1. Baxter-Petralia PL: Therapist's management of carpal tunnel syndrome. In Hunter JM, Schneider LH, Mackin EJ, et al, editors: *Rehabilitation of the hand: surgery and therapy,* ed 3, St Louis, 1990, Mosby.
2. Beaton LE, Anson BJ: The relation of the median nerve to the pronator teres muscle, *Anat Rec* 75:23, 1939.
3. Butler D: *Mobilisation of the nervous system,* Melbourne, 1991, Churchill Livingstone.
4. Chabon SJ: Uncommon compressive neuropathies of the forearm, *Physician Assist* 19(9):57, 1990.
5. Dandy DJ: *Essential orthopaedics and trauma,* Edinburgh, 1989, Churchill Livingstone.
6. Dawson DM, Hallet M, Millender LH: *Entrapment neuropathies,* ed 2, Boston, 1990, Little, Brown.
7. Gessini L, Jandolo B: The pronator teres syndrome: clinical and electrophysiologic features in six surgically verified cases, *J Neurosurg Sci* 31:1-5, 1987.
8. Hauser SL, Levitt LP, Weiner HL: *Case studies in neurology for the house officer,* Baltimore, 1986, Williams & Wilkins.
9. Lillegard WA, Rucker KS: *Handbook of sports medicine: a symptom-oriented approach,* Boston, 1993, Andover Medical Publishers.
10. Nakano KK, Ludergen C, Okihiro MM: Anterior interosseous nerve syndromes, *Arch Neurol* 34:477, 1977.
11. Netter FH: *The CIBA collection of medical illustrations, vol 1: nervous system. Part 2. Neurologic and neuromuscular disorders,* West Caldwell, NJ, 1986, CIBA-Geigy.
12. O'Brien MD, Upton ARM: Anterior interosseous nerve syndrome: a case report with neurophysiological investigations, *J Neurol Neurosurg Psychiatry* 35:531, 1972.
13. Patton J: *Neurological differential diagnosis,* ed 2, London, 1996, Springer-Verlag.
14. Pianka G, Hershman EB: Neurovascular injuries. In Nicholas JA, Hershman EB, editors: *The upper extremity in sports medicine,* St Louis, 1990, Mosby.
15. Rask MR: Anterior interosseous nerve entrapment (Kiloh-Nevin syndrome), *Clin Orthop* 142:176, 1979.
16. Rodman GP, Schumacher HR: *Primer on the rheumatic diseases,* ed 8, Atlanta, 1983, Arthritis Foundation.
17. Schumacher RH, Bomalski JS: *Case studies in rheumatology for the house officer,* Baltimore, 1990, Williams & Wilkins.
18. Spinner M, Spencer PS: Nerve compression lesions of the upper extremity: a clinical and experimental review, *Clin Orthop Rel Res* 104:46, 1974.
19. Werner CO, Rosen I, Thorngren K: Clinical and neurophysiological characteristics of the pronator syndrome, *Clin Orthop* 197:231-236, 1985.

RECOMMENDED READING

Baxter-Petralia PL: Therapist's management of carpal tunnel syndrome. In Hunter JM, Schneider LH, Mackin EJ et al, editors: *Rehabilitation of the hand: surgery and therapy,* ed 3, St Louis, 1990, Mosby.

Butler D: *Mobilisation of the nervous system,* Melbourne, 1991, Churchill Livingstone.

Dawson DM, Hallet M, Millender LH: *Entrapment neuropathies,* ed 2, Boston 1990, Little, Brown.

Phalen GS: The carpal-tunnel syndrome: 17 years' experience in diagnosis and treatment of 654 cases, *J Bone Joint Surg* 48A:211-228, 1966.

Schumacher RH, Bomalski JS: *Case studies in rheumatology for the house officer,* Baltimore, 1990, Williams & Wilkins.

5

Fall Resulting in Wrist Deformity

A 58-year-old white female fractured her wrist after falling and slipping on ice in front of her home and now appears in your office 1 day after cast removal. There is a slight dinner-fork deformity observed. Her skin appears flaky and looks somewhat smaller than the contralateral limb. There is no history of congestive heart failure. Your associate, the orthopod, saw this patient several weeks ago, administered a local anesthetic, and with your help manipulated the wrist and forearm so as to disimpact the fracture and appose the fragment ends. The patient is now referred to your practice for rehabilitation.

? Questions

1. What is a Colles' fracture, and how does it occur?
2. What is the mechanism of injury, the resulting pattern of deformity, and why?
3. What requisite kinesiology of wrist biomechanics is necessary to fully appreciate the ramifications of a Colles' fracture?
4. What are the three different kinds of Colles' fractures?
5. Why does deformity tend to recur after setting and immobilization of a displaced Colles' fracture?
6. When is external fixation appropriate?
7. What other disorders may occur from a similar or near-similar mechanism of injury?

8. How may a Colles' fracture be confused with a Galeazzi fracture-dislocation?
9. Describe the important role of the pronator teres in radial fractures and how this determines fragment splinting.
10. What are some sequelae of a Colles' fracture?
11. What potential loss of range of motion may occur from typical bone setting of a Colles' fracture in pronation and wrist flexion, and why?
12. What rehabilitative therapy is appropriate after cast removal?

1. What is a Colles fracture, and how does it occur?

A *Colles' fracture* is a dorsally angulated fracture of the distal end of the radius with or without accompanying ulnar fracture and was described by the Irish surgeon Abraham Colles in 1814 in the only article he ever wrote.[8] The Colles' fracture is the commonest fracture in adults over 50 years of age and more common in white females than in other groups. This fracture has the same sex and age incidence as a femoral neck fracture has and for the same reason: a combination of senile and postmenopausal osteoporosis.[12] There are several components to a Colles' fracture:

- Backward (dorsal) angulation of the distal fragment.
- Backward displacement of the distal fragment.
- Radial deviation.
- Transverse fracture pattern with main fracture line within distal 2 cm of the radius. This occurs because the lunate acts as a wedge to shear the distal 2 cm of the radius off in a dorsal direction.[3]
- Comminution of the thin cortex, especially in osteoporotic bone of the elderly. A cross section of the radius can show how the thick cortical bone of the shaft thins out to form only a thin layer over the cancellous bone at the distal end. This anatomic design flaw is compounded by the presence of osteoporosis.[6]
- Proximal impaction caused by the jagged ends of bone having been driven one into the other and further causing the distal ends of the radius and ulna to be level,[9] instead of the normal relationship between those two bones in which the radius extends slightly beyond the distal end of the ulna.

- It may be associated with sprain of the ulnar collateral ligament and avulsion fracture of the ulnar styloid. The latter occurs secondarily to displacement of the distal end of the radius because of the concomitant pull of the biconcave articular disk connecting the distal ends of the radius and ulna.[9]
- Subluxation or partial dislocation of the distal radioulnar joint.
- Supination. Since the fracture occurs in conjunction with a supination moment, supination is preserved in the deformity.
- When the pronated arm is laid upon the examining table, its profile resembles a dinner fork lying horizontally with the tines pointing downward, so that the base of the tines forms an upward curve[2] (Fig. 5-1).

2. What is the mechanism of injury, the resulting pattern of deformity, and why?

Typically a patient either slips or trips and attempts to break his or her fall by means of a parachute reflex, landing on the outstretched volar surface of the hand with the forearm pronated.[12] The intended outcome is dissipation of force that is transmitted along the length of the upper extremity, which, unfortunately, does not always occur. Two mechanisms contribute to fracture at the distal end of the radius, as follows:

- In the attempt to break a fall, the hand moves into physiologic extension while the proximal carpal row moves palmarly, locking the radius against the scaphoid and lunate bones (Fig. 5-2). While the hand stops moving once it contacts the ground, that distal end of the arm will continue to move toward the ground,

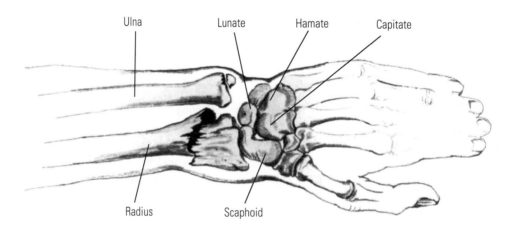

Ulna   Lunate   Hamate   Capitate

Radius   Scaphoid

FIG. 5-1 Profile of a Colles fracture. (From Peterson L, Renström P: *Sports injuries; their prevention and treatment,* London, 1986, Martin Dunitz, Ltd.)

causing a shearing of the distal end of the radius off the main body of bone.[3]

- A supination moment is created by the pronator quadratus and brachioradialis muscles. The latter muscle is a better supinator than the pronator because of the sudden reflexive stretching in the pronator direction, causing maximal stress at the junction of cortical and cancellous bone in the distal radial metaphysis.[5]

3. What requisite kinesiology of wrist biomechanics is necessary to fully appreciate the ramifications of a Colles' fracture?

- At the wrist, the radius is the principal bone in the sense that it and not the ulna articulates with joint of the carpal bones (that is, the radiocarpals). The ulna has no direct contact with the carpus. The wrist is stabilized by the radial and ulnar collateral ligaments.[7]
- The hand moves along with the radius as it pivots about the ulna. The ulna cannot rotate at all because of the nature of the humeroulnar joint. Thus pronation and supination are more the function of the radius than of the ulna and occurs at the proximal and distal radioulnar joints. It is during pronation that the radius rotates and crosses the ulna. In supination both bones lie parallel with each other (see Fig. 5-10).

- With motions of the wrist the (convex) proximal row of carpal bones slides in the direction opposite the physiologic motion of the hand.
- There is an oblique axis between the distal ends of the radius and ulna, much the same as in the distal ends of the tibia and fibula in the lower extremity. In the same way ankle inversion has a greater range of motion than eversion because the fibular malleolus extends more distally, ulnar deviation has slightly greater range than radial deviation, since the radial styloid extends more distally.
- Since the advent of *Homo erectus* the interosseus membrane between the radius and ulna no longer has been needed to prevent splaying, just as the same structure (that is, the tibiofibular syndesmosis) functions in the lower extremity. Rather, the interosseous membrane provides additional surface area for muscle and tendon attachment.
- The principal supinators are the biceps brachii and supinator muscles. The former supinates by virtue of its distal attachment to the posterior radial tuberosity. When the biceps contracts, not only is the forearm flexed, but also the radius unwinds as its tuberosity is anteriorly rotated (that is, forearm supination). The biceps's twin function is best remembered as the twisting of a corkscrew into a bottle (supination) and

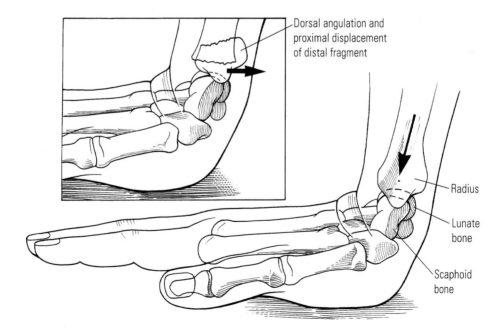

Dorsal angulation and proximal displacement of distal fragment

Radius

Lunate bone

Scaphoid bone

FIG. 5-2 Mechanism of a Colles fracture.

then a pulling out of the cork (flexion) (see Fig. 8-3). The chief pronators are the pronator teres and the pronator quadratus.

4. What are the three different kinds of Colles' fractures?

The three kinds of Colles' fractures are as follows:
- Undisplaced fractures, which are uncommon and require immobilization in a below-elbow cast for 4 weeks.
- Displaced fractures, having one main transverse fracture with little cortical comminution.
- Unstable fractures, having gross comminution of cortical bone and pronounced crushing of softer cancellous bone.

The latter two categories may be radiographically differentiated.[12]

5. Why does deformity tend to recur after setting and immobilization of a displaced Colles' fracture?

Perfect anatomic alignment is often impossible without the use of skeletal fixation (such as an external bar, intramedullary pin, or bone graft to fill in the defect at the distal part of the radius). Despite successful manipulation and alignment with immobilization, the deformity, in a displaced Colles' fracture, tends to recur for two reasons:
- Whereas before the fracture occurred the ulna projected distally slightly less than the radius did, after a fracture the distal parts of the radius and ulna are aligned one with the other. Because the crushed cancellous bone of the distal radial fragment does not return to stay at its proper location on reduction, a cavity is created, and the distal comminuted cortical shell is internally unsupported. Normally, forces arising from muscle pull will produce further shortening with angulation of the distal fragment so that the wrist, particularly in the elderly, will yield a characteristic hump resembling a dinner fork *(dinner-fork deformity)*. Since the blood supply to the distal end of the radius is excellent, bony malunion may occur. The surgeon's competence is often called into question despite the resultant good hand function in the patient. As such, patients must be warned of the possible cosmetic deformity caused by closed reduction and plaster immobilization.
- If painful restriction occurs with deformity, excision of the distal end of the ulna will relieve pain, and improve the range of motion and cosmesis, as it recreates the original anatomic alignment.

- Many patients will have bony resorption at the fracture site that, over time, translates into shortening of the radius.

6. When is external fixation appropriate?

External fixators such as the Hoffman frame or the Roger-Anderson frame have two pins proximally through the radius and two pins distally in the second and third metacarpals and are used as anchors because they are immobile. External fixation is appropriate in the extremely comminuted (hence unstable) Colles' fracture, particularly in persons under 60 years of age or in those having careers such as modeling where a premium is placed on the aesthetic of near perfect and permanent anatomic alignment. External fixation is also important in persons who must use their hands and cannot wear a cast, such as professional piano players. Other approaches may include percutaneous pinning, or open reduction with internal fixation to achieve the desired result.[12]

7. What other disorders may occur from a similar or near-similar mechanism of injury?

In the years after Colles's description of this fracture an eponym war erupted over other, slightly different fracture patterns at the distal radius. Today the trend is to lump them all as distal radius fractures and simply describe the exact pattern of fracture lines. Listed below are some of the more well-known fractures.[8]
- R.W. Smith succeeded Colles as professor of surgery at Dublin, Ireland, and described the reverse Colles' fracture, or *Smith's fracture* (Fig. 5-3), which occurs after a fall onto a flexed wrist. The resulting fracture pattern, like the mechanism of injury, is reverse from that of a Colles' fracture in that the distal fragment is forward (palmar) versus backward (Fig. 5-3). The fracture line is usually obliquely upward and forward. Upon presentation it is observed as a reverse dinner-fork deformity with the tines pointing upward, or more imaginatively as a garden-spade deformity. Pressure applied during traction is the reverse of that of a Colles' fracture.[2]
- John R. Barton of Philadelphia, the founding father of American orthopedic surgery, described a fracture in which the fracture line of the distal end of the radius enters the radiocarpal joint and forces (that is, subluxes) the carpal bones upward and backward, causing a fracture dislocation. The resulting deformity, a *Barton's fracture,* also presents as the typical dinner-fork deformity but differs from a Colles' fracture in

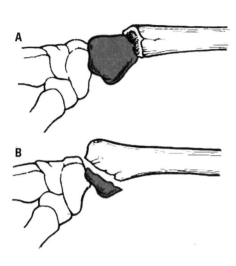

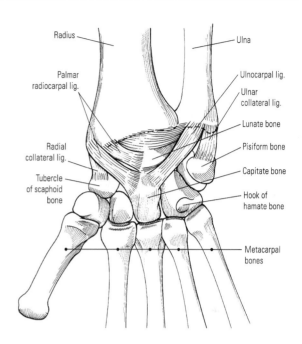

FIG. 5-3 A, Smith's fracture. **B,** Barton's fracture, which enters the joint. (From Dandy DJ: *Essential orthopaedics and trauma,* Edinburgh, 1989, Churchill Livingstone.)

FIG. 5-4 Ligaments of the volar aspect of the wrist with the transverse carpal ligament removed.

two ways: (1) the anterior and posterior prominences are at a lower level and (2) the radial styloid can be palpated in its normal position. Displacement is corrected with local or general anesthesia and is then casted for 4 to 5 weeks.[1]

- A *wrist sprain* may occur from landing on outstretched hands as well as from hyperflexion and torsion and may damage either one of the ligaments stabilizing the wrist (that is, the radial and ulnar collateral ligaments) as well as the lunate capitate ligament dorsally and the radiocarpal ligament palmarly[6] (Fig. 5-4). Localized swelling after a wrist injury almost never accompanies an isolated ligamentous injury. Every sprain should be radiographed in all views to rule out fracture or dislocation. Pain on radial deviation with tenderness over the scaphoid area implicates the ulnar collateral ligament, whereas pain on ulnar deviation is suggestive of a radial collateral ligament involvement. Pain provocation of the dorsal lunocapitate and palmar radiolunate ligaments are often reproduced when the patient places his or her hand on the examining table and places his or her body weight over the wrist by leaning forward. Passive and active movements may be painless. Resisted movement may be strong and painless. Dorsal palmar glide of the capitate on the lunate and the lunate on the radius may produce pain.

When in doubt regarding a suspect radial collateral ligament sprain, one should cast the arm for 3 weeks suspecting potential scaphoid fracture. If no tenderness is present in conjunction with normal radiographs, wrist sprain is implicated by the process of elimination.[1] For a lateral collateral ligament injury, follow the same protocol as with any sprain. If pain is severe, immobilization in a cast from the palmar crease to the midforearm area is appropriate, otherwise an elastic bandage may suffice.[1] Management of a sprain to the lunate-capitate and radiocarpal ligaments is by rest and by friction massage to increase mobility of the collagen fibers without longitudinal stressing of the ligament. Ultrasound may be used as an adjunct in the resolution of chronic inflammatory exudates.[6]

- Isolated *fracture of the ulnar styloid* is rare and occurs when one lands on the ulnar side of the radially deviated hand. Although there is little swelling, there is considerable pain. Treatment is by wrist immobilization in ulnar deviation for 3 to 4 weeks. If nonunion occurs, the fragment should be removed.

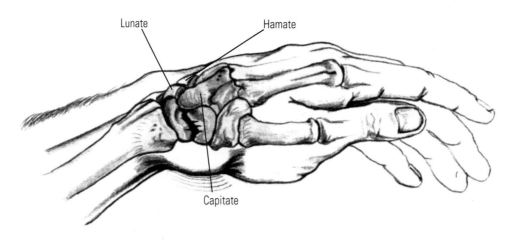

Lunate

Hamate

Capitate

FIG. 5-5 Fracture of the scaphoid. (From Peterson L, Renström P: *Sports injuries: their prevention and treatment,* London, 1986, Martin Dunitz, Ltd.)

- *Triquetral fractures* may occur from either one of two possible mechanisms: (1) falling onto a flexed wrist held in radial deviation resulting in an avulsion fracture of the dorsal surface of the bone, or less commonly (2) compression fracture from falling onto a hyperextended wrist. Radial deviation and wrist flexion are painful, with acute tenderness localized over the dorsal surface of the wrist just distal to the ulna. Treatment is by immobilization only until clinical symptoms subside.[4]
- Colles' fractures in children do not occur for one simple reason. Despite an obvious dinner-fork deformity, damage is either in the form of a greenstick fracture (alias buckle or torus fracture) or one of five general patterns of radial epiphyseal growth plate injuries. The reason is that the cartilaginous epiphyseal plate is stronger than bone whereas bone is relatively more supple in children. It is a clinical error to consider children as miniature models of adults. Generally children's bone structure is more resilient and adaptable, whereas their muscles, tendons, and ligaments are relatively stronger and more elastic than those of adults.[2]
- *Scaphoid fractures* (Fig. 5-5) are the most common of carpal bone fractures,[5] are often misdiagnosed as a sprained wrist or thumb, and occur when one falls onto a hyperextended and radially deviated wrist. Ironically, despite their relative frequency, they are the most commonly missed fractures of the upper limb.[10] Often, they are passed off as simply a wrist sprain.[12] In this injury the scaphoid bone bears the brunt of injury because, locked between the radius and the capitate, it is the only bony link between the forearm and the hand.[12] Fracture will most likely occur in the middle of the scaphoid (Fig. 5-6). Avascular necrosis and nonunion are a complication of this injury that may occur because the scaphoid is usually supplied by two nutrient arteries, one to the proximal half and then one to the distal half. However both vessels supply the distal segment in most persons, which is the same as saying that the proximal pole is supplied by way of the distal pole. A fracture through the wrist will subsequently cause devitalization of the proximal pole.[4] An oblique radiograph is needed for diagnosis since standard radiographs may miss this fracture. Positive radiographic findings may demonstrate cyst formation at the fracture site as well as sclerosis of fracture surfaces. Continued movement will contribute to nonunion of bone fragments. Thus, even if no fracture is visualized, a scaphoid cast should be applied for several weeks.[11] This below-elbow cast should include the proximal phalanx of the thumb while holding it roughly opposite the ring finger and not in wide abduction, since that interferes with function and may displace fracture fragments.

Minimal immobilization with the wrist in 20° dorsiflexion and slight radial deviation is for 6 weeks but may require several months in the event that no union has occurred. Healing is characteristically slow because the relative absence of periosteal bone covering places the burden of healing on endosteal callus

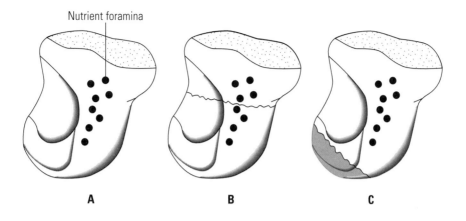

Nutrient foramina

A   **B**   **C**

FIG. 5-6 Blood supply of the scaphoid. **A,** Blood enters the bone principally in its distal half. **B,** Fracture through the waist of the scaphoid. Vessels to the proximal scaphoid are preserved. **C,** Fracture near the proximal pole of the scaphoid. In this case there are no vessels supplying the proximal fragment, and aseptic necrosis of bone is therefore inevitable. (From Ellis H: *Clinical anatomy,* ed 7, Oxford, 1983, Blackwell Scientific Publications.)

formation. In cases of suspected fracture, scaphoid radiographs should be repeated 10 days after the injury, since a fracture line may more easily be seen because of decalcification (that is, bone resorption) along its length and partly because of the slight separation of fragments. Operative treatment for nonunion varies according to the presence of traumatic arthritis. The clinical signs of scaphoid fracture are tenderness and swelling in the anatomic snuffbox or on the anterior aspect of the wrist over the scaphoid tubercle.[12]

- *Lunate dislocation* may also occur when one falls onto a hyperextended hand, which may push the carpus off the back of the radius, except for the lunate, which remains attached to the radius by the palmar radiocarpal ligament through which it derives its blood supply. Dislocation is easily missed on the anteroposterior radiograph but is obvious on the lateral view. The typical deformity observed is an anterior bulge or swelling just proximal to the volar wrist crease. Wrist flexion is limited and painful. Shortly afterward, dislocation pressure on the median nerve may provoke an acute carpal tunnel syndrome necessitating immediate closed reduction. The lunate bone is relocated under general anesthesia and must be immobilized for at least 4 weeks in 20° of wrist flexion, occasionally in a bivalved cast to allow for swelling. With an early reduction, prognosis is excellent; however, if neglected, closed reduction may be impossible and may necessitate open reduction.[1]

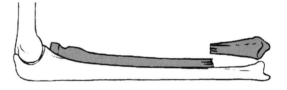

FIG. 5-7 Galeazzi fracture. (From Dandy DJ: *Essential orthopaedics and trauma,* Edinburgh, 1989, Churchill Livingstone.)

8. How may a Colles' fracture be confused with a Galeazzi fracture-dislocation?

A *Galeazzi fracture* (Fig. 5-7) is similar to a Colles' fracture in that the radius will fracture, yield deformity, and be accompanied by disturbance of the distal radioulnar joint. It differs, however, in several respects:

- Fracture of the shaft of the radius occurs more proximal than that of a Colles' fracture.
- There is more striking clinical deformity, having a wrenched look.
- There is complete disruption and even dislocation of the distal radioulnar joint.
- It usually occurs in young adults.[12]

Like its mirror image, the *Monteggia fracture* (fractured one half of the ulna and dislocated proximal radioulnar joint, Fig. 5-8) requires internal fixation. The reason is that the strong pull of forearm muscles will cause either angulation or longitudinal torsion of

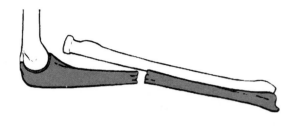

FIG. 5-8 Monteggia fracture. (From Dandy DJ: *Essential orthopaedics and trauma,* Edinburgh, 1989, Churchill Livingstone.)

fragments and will result in a considerable loss of pronation and supination. Thus a Galeazzi fracture is not treated with a short forearm cast as if it were a Colles fracture.[12]

9. Describe the important role of pronator teres in radial fractures and how this determines fragment splinting.

The important role of the pronator teres in radial fractures is clarified when we consider Fig. 5-9. In proximal fractures (Fig. 5-9, *A*) above the insertion of the pronator teres, the distal fragment is pronated. Such a fracture must be splinted in the supinated position. When the fracture is distal to the pronator teres insertion (Fig. 5-9, *B*), the action of this muscle on the proximal fragment is cancelled by the supinator action of the biceps. This fracture is therefore held reduced in the neutral position, midway between pronation and supination.

10. What are some sequelae of a Colles' fracture?

Most persons with a Colles' fracture are left with some albeit minor residual dysfunction. Complications after a Colles' fracture abound and include the following:

- Malunion occurs because of either imperfect reduction or inadequate immobilization. Malunion secondary to crushed cancellous bone and comminuted cortical bone may be anticipated. Associated with malunion is painful subluxation of the distal radioulnar joint with limitation of wrist motion.

Operations for malunion include the following:

- For the elderly patient, simple excision of the distal ulna improves appearance but may disturb wrist stability.
- Corrective osteotomy of the radius with or without distal ulna excision may be required if the main problem is backward angulation of the radius.
- With Baldwin's procedure a 2 cm long segment of the ulna is excised along with its periosteum while leav-

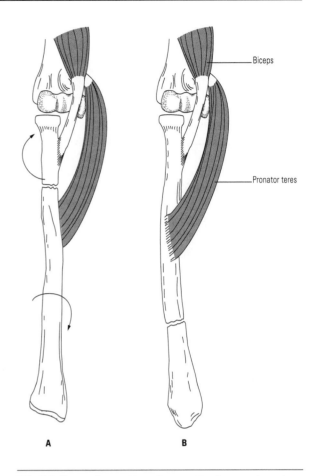

FIG. 5-9 The casting position after a radius fracture depends on whether the fracture occurs proximally, **A,** or distally, **B,** to the insertion of the pronator teres on the radius. (From Ellis H: *Clinical anatomy,* ed 7, Oxford, 1983, Blackwell Scientific Publications.)

ing the ulnar styloid intact so that the ulnar head is allowed to move.

- With late rupture of the extensor pollicis longus (EPL) tendon, the EPL moves distally to the hand through the third dorsal tunnel, acting as a simple pulley located at the ulnar side of the radial (that is, Listers) tubercle. In the event of this tubercle's disturbance by a fracture, the EPL tendon will undergo fraying and eventual rupture because of friction against a roughened or sharp shard of bone. This usually develops 1 to 2 months after the fracture and suddenly manifests by the patient's inability to extend the thumb. Surgical repair is ineffective though tendon transfer may be contemplated.
- In median nerve compression and ischemia, the nerve may be compressed by initial bleeding around it or by

later bleeding after the cast is removed when the nerve catches against the callus while the wrist moves.

- The sensory branch of the radial nerve supplying the dorsal hand may be stretched or torn. Anesthesias and paresthesias usually resolve after several weeks.

- The extensor carpi ulnaris runs through the sixth dorsal tunnel and is most palpable when the wrist simultaneously ulnarly deviated with wrist extension. If the distal ulnar styloid is fractured during a Colles fracture, the dorsal carpal ligament may tear, resulting in dislocation of the extensor tendon during pronation, and is accompanied by an audible snap with or without pain.

- Residual finger stiffness may be forestalled by encouragement of active range of motion exercises and elevation of the fingers during immobilization.

- In Sudeck's atrophy anesthetic block of the inferior cervical or stellate ganglion will often relieve this condition if more conservative measures are unsuccessful.

- Nonunion is not considered a complication, since the blood supply to the distal end of the radius is excellent.[2]

11. What potential loss of range of motion may occur from a typical bone setting of a Colles' fracture in pronation and wrist flexion, and why?

There is clinical significance to describing the radius and ulna as two bones that have a bow inherent to their anatomic features (Fig. 5-10). When the forearm is pronated, the distance between the two bows is lessened, and the convexity of each bow may be said to face each other (Fig. 5-10, *A*). However, when the forearm is supinated, the transverse distance between the two bones is greatest, and so the bones face away from each other (Fig. 5-10, *B*). The problem with casting in pronation is that any soft tissue spanning from the radius to the ulna will develop a contracture, which leads to difficulty in regaining premorbid forearm supination.

12. What rehabilitative therapy is appropriate after cast removal?

Provided that the bone or bones are well healed:

- During immobilization in a cast it is important to stress full range of motion of the noninvolved joint and muscle groups of the shoulder, elbow, thumb, and other fingers.

- Regular forearm isometric exercises within a cast will stave off muscle atrophy and edema.

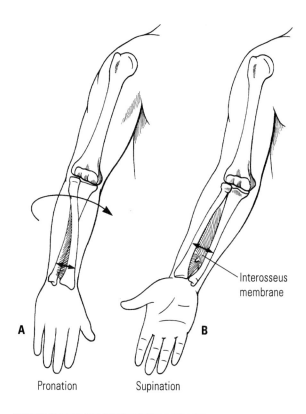

FIG. 5-10 A, The attachments of the interosseous membrane are approximated when the forearm is pronated. **B,** When the forearm is supinated, the distance between the radius and the ulna is greatest. Casting the forearm in any position other than supination will predispose shortening of the interosseous membrane, which may limit joint motion once the cast is removed.

- Retrograde massage helps decrease edema once the cast is removed.

- Progressive exercises begin with passive ones and progress to active and resistive exercises, which include the following:
  1. Approximation of thumb pad to each of the finger pads.
  2. Finger flexion, extension, abduction, and adduction.
  3. Wrist flexion and extension.
  4. Wrist radial and ulnar deviation.
  5. Circular wrist motions in clockwise and counterclockwise directions.
  6. Passive, active, and resistive pronation/supination exercises in sequential progression.

- If the skin is dry and flaky, use of a whirlpool is appropriate unless the patient has edema as well, in which case a hot whirlpool with the hand in a dependent position will only exacerbate the edema.

- Gentle dorsal and ventral glide (joint mobilization) of distal ends of radius and ulna, respectively, one relative to the other in pronation and especially in the supinated position.
- Dorsal and ventral glides of the radiocarpal joint to facilitate wrist flexion and extension.
- Shoulder and elbow abduction and adduction range of motion to prevent stiffness.
- Encouragement of the patient to use the wrist and hand in daily living activities so as to stave off neglect of the involved extremity.

REFERENCES

1. Conwell HE: Injuries to the wrist, *Clin Symp* 22(1):14, 1982.
2. Dandy DJ: *Essential orthopaedics and trauma,* Edinburgh, 1989, Churchill Livingstone.
3. De Palma F: *The management of fractures and dislocations: an atlas,* ed 2, Philadelphia, 1990, Saunders.
4. Ellis H: *Clinical anatomy,* ed 7, Oxford, 1983, Blackwell Scientific Publishers.
5. Gould JA III: *Orthopaedic and sports physical therapy,* ed 2, St Louis, 1990, Mosby.
6. Hertling D, Kessler RM: *Management of common musculoskeletal disorders,* ed 2, Philadelphia, 1990, Lippincott.
7. Kapit W, Elson LM: *The anatomy coloring book,* New York, 1977, Harper & Row.
8. Meals RA: *One hundred orthopaedic conditions every doctor should understand,* St Louis, 1992, Quality Medical Publishing.
9. Moore KL: *Clinically oriented anatomy,* ed 2, Baltimore, 1985, Williams & Wilkins.
10. Netter F: *The CIBA collection of medical illustrations, vol 8: Musculoskeletal system,* part 3, Summit, NJ, 1993, CIBA-Geigy.
11. Peterson L, Renström P: *Sports injuries: their prevention and treatment,* London, 1986, Martin Dunitz.

RECOMMENDED READING

Dandy DJ: *Essential orthopaedics and trauma,* Edinburgh, 1989, Churchill Livingstone.

Gould JA III: *Orthopaedic and sports physical therapy,* ed 2, St Louis, 1990, Mosby.

Meals RA: *One hundred orthopaedic conditions every doctor should understand,* St Louis, 1992, Quality Medical.

Peterson L, Renström P: *Sports injuries: their prevention and treatment,* London, 1986, Martin Dunitz, (distributor in USA: Mosby, St Louis).

Netter F: *The CIBA collection of medical illustrations, vol 8: Musculoskeletal system,* part 3, Summit, NJ, 1993, CIBA-Geigy.

PART II

ELBOW AND FOREARM

6

Burning Pain, Swelling, and Trophic Changes in Hand, Wrist, and Forearm out of Proportion to a 2-Week-Old Negligible Injury

A 29-year-old woman of average height and ruddy cheeks presents with a constant burning pain of her right hand, wrist, and distal forearm that, she reports, has spread proximally over the preceding 2 weeks. She complains of loss of use of her right extremity, which at times feels alternately cold and hot.

The patient recalls being stung in the right foot by a stingray some 4 months previously while snorkeling in the Caribbean. Subsequently, she developed severe cellulitis in that extremity for which she was hospitalized for a short period until the infection resolved. Upon returning home, she subsequently sustained a deep gash over her right anatomical snuff-box, which necessitated three stitches.

Her physician reveals to you his suspicions regarding the source of her malady over the telephone and mentions that all radiographic and MRI data for the neck, shoulder, and lungs were negative. He also ruled out scleroderma, venous obstruction, and angioedema. Radiographs of the hand demonstrate patchy osteopenia.

The patient offers that she has been seeing a psychologist for counseling over the past 2 years for occasional attacks of anxiety. When inquiring about her occupation, you learn that she is an aspiring actress with a leading role in an off-Broadway play of a patient who feigns a hysterical conversion disorder. There is no history of rheumatoid arthritis.

OBSERVATION   There is moderate swelling to the right hand, the wrist, as well as slight fusiform swelling to the fingers of the right hand. Light moisture appears to cover the whole right hand as if it were perspiring. When compared to the contralateral hand, the involved hand appears shiny.

PALPATION   Even a slight touch causes the patient to cringe and pull away; the involved hand feels warm. The contralateral palm feels moist. The patient mentions that she has always had sweaty palms.

RANGE OF MOTION   There is mild to moderate stiffness of the right wrist and fingers, with the fingers in slight flexion, and flattening of the palmar crease lines over the interphalangeal and metacarpophalangeal joints.

MUSCLE STRENGTH   Untested secondary to pain and tenderness.

SPECIAL TESTS   Negative compression/distraction tests to the cervical spine.

SENSATION   Paresthesia in a glove-and-stocking type of distribution over the distal right extremity.

? **Q**uestions

1. What is most likely afflicting this woman?
2. What is the normal sympathetic reflex?
3. What is the course of nerve-impulse transmission generated by the normal reflex sympathetic arc?
4. What is the abnormal reflex sympathetic arc?
5. What are the five clinical types of reflex sympathetic dystrophy (RSD)?
6. What is minor causalgia?
7. What are the three most common nerves injured whose sequelae include minor causalgia?
8. What is minor traumatic dystrophy?
9. What is the shoulder-hand syndrome?
10. What is major traumatic dystrophy?
11. What is major causalgia?
12. What are the signs and symptoms common to RSD?
13. What are the stages of RSD?
14. What factor does diathesis play in the development of RSD in certain individuals?
15. What is the differential diagnosis of RSD?
16. What medical intervention is appropriate to management of RSD?
17. What are the cardinal and secondary signs and symptoms of RSD, and how does their presence justify trial sympathetic block?
18. What therapeutic intervention is appropriate to management of RSD?

1. What is most likely afflicting this woman?

Reflex sympathetic dystrophy (RSD) is a well known but poorly understood condition of the extremities[1] that was first clearly described by the American Civil War neurologist Silas Mitchell in the last year of that war (1864).[4] Most cases of RSD occur after major or minor trauma to the extremity in question or may also stem from visceral sources of injury such as myocardial infarction, stroke, stomach ulcer, or Pancoast's tumor to the apex of the lung.[3] RSD is now understood to be generated by an abnormal sympathetic reflex that encompasses painful states ranging from mildly uncomfortable vasomotor disorders to the full-blown classic Mitchell type of causalgia. Pain is the outstanding feature of the various clinical types of RSD and is grossly out of proportion to that expected from an injury or surgical insult.[1] The sympathetic nervous system has, of late, been implicated as an important mediator of this disorder,[5] though the exact cause and pathogenesis of RSD remain unknown.[3] Females more commonly suffer from RSD.[3]

2. What is the normal sympathetic reflex?

The normal *sympathetic reflex arc* is the body's reactive mechanism to trauma or disease that works by negative feedback to return the abnormal deranged state to that of normalcy (homeostasis).[3]

3. What is the course of nerve-impulse transmission generated by the normal reflex sympathetic arc?

After trauma, afferent nerve fibers transmit a pain message from the extremity and synapse in the posterior root ganglion projecting to the posterior horn and finally to the lateral horn where the pain message is communicated to the sympathetic nerve cell bodies. The sympathetic reflex (Fig. 6-1) is activated when efferent sympathetic impulses are sent out the anterior horn through the anterior root to sympathetic chains. This reflex is then communicated through the white ramus in the sympathetic ganglion, where a synapse occurs. The postganglionic sympathetic fiber then leaves the ganglia through the gray ramus where it enters the peripheral nerve and travels distally along with it to the extremity to produce small-vessel vasoconstriction. This *vasoconstrictive reflex,* or *sympathetic pain reflex,* is believed to be a protective mechanism necessary to prevent excessive bleeding within injured tissue; this reparative process gives way to vasodilatation after a few hours as part of an orderly stepwise progression culminating in the return to homeostasis.[3]

4. What is the abnormal reflex sympathetic arc?

Occasionally the normal sympathetic reflex arc does not shut down at the appropriate time for unknown rea-

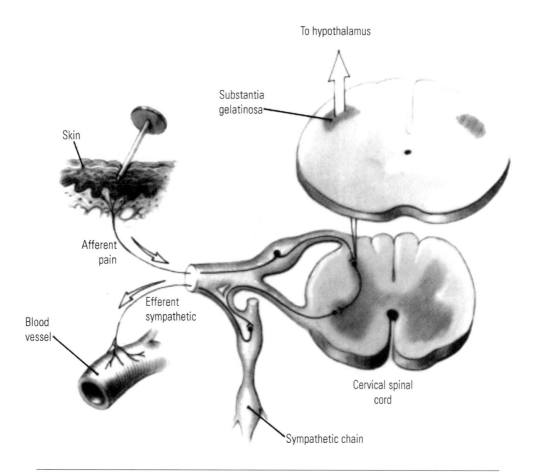

To hypothalamus

Substantia
gelatinosa

Skin

Afferent
pain

Efferent
sympathetic

Blood
vessel

Cervical spinal
cord

Sympathetic chain

FIG. 6-1 A normal sympathetic nerve reflex arc is set into motion with any painful stimulus; it results in a temporary vasoconstrictive action of the small vessels. However, if this normal sympathetic reflex arc fails to shut down at the appropriate time, an abnormal sympathetic reflex may develop, thus producing one of the etiologic factors of reflex sympathetic dystrophy. (From Lankford LL, Thompson JE: *Reflex sympathetic dystrophy, upper and lower extremity: diagnosis and management.* In American Academy of Orthopaedic Surgeons: Instructional course lectures, vol 26, St. Louis, 1977, Mosby.)

sons. Rather, the reflex continues on in an accelerated fashion, and will ultimately produce an intense degree of sympathetic activity (Fig. 6-2). The increased and persistent vasoconstriction leads to tissue ischemia, which is painful and causes increased afferent pain impulses to be sent centrally. Hence there is initiated a vicious cycle (Fig. 6-3) in which the sympathetic reflex arc is repeatedly propagated resulting in maintenance of sympathetic nerve activity, which, with time, manifests as reflex sympathetic dystrophy. The precise cause of malfunction in the shutdown mechanism of the sympathetic reflex arc is not known.[3]

5. What are the five clinical types of reflex sympathetic dystrophy (RSD)?

Because of its varied vasomotor manifestations, RSD has been described by various nomenclature. However, the common denominator to all forms of RSD is that all share a common mechanism of pathosis: the abnormal reflex arc. Because of this, all forms of this disorder fall under the nomenclature heading of reflex sympathetic dystrophy. These varied manifestations may be reduced to five clinical types: (1) minor causalgia, (2) minor traumatic dystrophy, (3) shoulder-hand syndrome, (4) minor traumatic dystrophy, and (5) major causalgia.

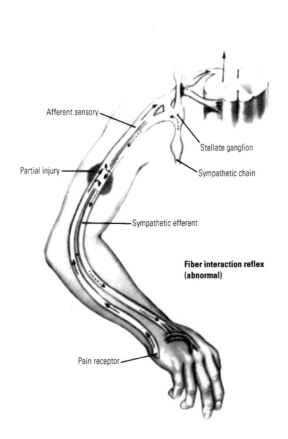

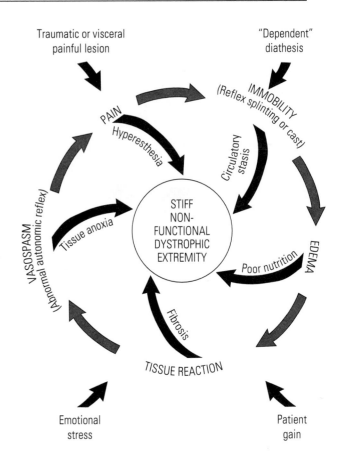

FIG. 6-2 Doupe described a physiologic breakdown of myelin sheath in an area of partial nerve injury that produced a "fiber interaction" of efferent and afferent impulses, which results in increased sympathetic nerve activity and increased pain. (From Lankford LL, Thompson JE: *Reflex sympathetic dystrophy, upper and lower extremity: diagnosis and management.* In American Academy of Orthopaedic Surgeons: Instructional course lectures, vol 26, St. Louis, 1977, Mosby.)

FIG. 6-3 Vicious circle is produced when tissue ischemia produces greater tissue reaction and pain caused by vasoconstrictive action of increased sympathetic nerve activity, resulting in a painful, stiff, swollen, and dystrophic extremity, as seen in reflex sympathetic dystrophy. (From Lankford LL, Thompson JE: *Reflex sympathetic dystrophy, upper and lower extremity: diagnosis and management.* In American Academy of Orthopaedic Surgeons: Instructional course lectures, vol 26, St. Louis, 1977, Mosby.)

6. What is minor causalgia?

Minor causalgia (Kausos: burning heat; algia: pain) is a type of RSD caused by injury to a peripheral nerve, most commonly in the distal part of the extremity. Symptoms and signs may be limited to only one or two fingers and are relatively less noxious. Whether the nerve became injured and scarred and underwent repair or the nerve was even cut through, as may occur during amputation, a neuroma may develop. Nerve fibers will sprout from the cut or lacerated nerve into nowhere in particular and are, not surprisingly, abnormally sensitive to pressure, movement, squeezing, or stretching. Many are also sensitive to

norepinephrine (noradrenaline), which is emitted all around them by the accompanying sympathetic nerve fiber. Over time these nerve fibers very commonly bind down to surrounding fixed structures with adhesions so that any movement, such as wrist flexion, will produce a painful stretching of the nerve. This stretching, in turn, generates fibrous tissue proliferation (scar tissue), which serves only to further enmesh the nerve. The result of this process is a painful *neuroma,* with additional pain impulses being fired off to the spinal cord after subsequent provocation.[3] The pain of minor causalgia is constant, and other features of RSD such as pain on motion, swelling, stiffness, and osteoporosis are much greater than would be expected from simple neuroma.[3]

7. What are the three most common nerves injured whose sequelae include minor causalgia?

The nerve most commonly injured is the *dorsal superficial sensory branch of the radial nerve*[3] overlying the radial styloid area of the wrist. It may have iatrogenic sequelae to de Quervain's tenosynovectomy, after bone grafting for the carpal scaphoid, or from intravenous lines or shunts for hemodialysis. De Quervain's tenosynovectomy is considered to be minor surgery but is occasionally performed by physicians unaccustomed to the anatomy of that region.[1]

The next most common site of nerve injury is the *palmar cutaneous branch of the median nerve.* This branch takes leave of the median nerve 3 cm proximal to the transverse carpal ligament and enters the hand superficially through the wrist. This nerve offshoot may be inadvertently injured by a surgeon employing the frowned-upon transverse incision of the flexor retinaculum at the volar side of the wrist in the treatment of carpal tunnel syndrome.[1,3]

The next most common sites of nerve injury include the *dorsal superficial sensory branches of the ulnar nerve,* especially over the dorsal ulnar aspect of the wrist and hand, and the common digital and proper digital branches of the median and ulnar nerves.[3]

8. What is minor traumatic dystrophy?

Minor traumatic dystrophy is the most common clinical type of RSD because minor traumas are more common and also because injuries more often do not involve a specific nerve. This type of RSD is also the *most frequently overlooked form,* since it is not common knowledge that RSD can involve only a small segment of the hand. The inciting factor is a minor injury such as a fracture, dislocation, sprain, or even a penetrating wound that does not involve injury to a nerve. Signs and symptoms vary and the degree of involvement may encompass only one or two fingers rather than the entire hand. Redness is characteristically found over the dorsum of the metacarpophalangeal joints and interphalangeal joints as well as over the collateral ligaments. A mild degree of palmar fasciitis may also be present. The digits are usually stiffened in flexion.[3]

9. What is the shoulder-hand syndrome?

The *shoulder-hand syndrome* is incited by a proximal insult, whether external or internal, and typically occurs in patients between 45 and 55 years of age and more commonly affects females than any other form of RSD. Shoulder-hand syndrome usually starts with considerable pain and stiffness in the shoulder, spreads to the distal part of the extremity, and produces moderate to pronounced swelling of the wrist, hand, and sometimes the upper arm. There is often a fusiform swelling of the fingers that are stiffened in extension rather than flexion. Palmar fasciitis with nodules are more commonly found. Redness, when present, is diffuse, and the hand is usually warmer and dryer than normal.[3]

10. What is major traumatic dystrophy?

Major traumatic dystrophy may occur after a major trauma such as a crushed hand, Colles' fracture, or a severe fracture dislocation of the wrist. This form of RSD yields the greatest degree of pain, stiffness, swelling, and dysfunction in the non-nerve injury type of RSD. Flexion contractures of the digits are more frequent than extension contractures. Wrist motion is usually severely limited, and flexion deformities may be present. There is often accompanying limitation of rotary forearm motion, especially in pronation.[3]

11. What is major causalgia?

Major causalgia is the classic Mitchell causalgia. It causes the greatest degree of pain and devastation to the patient. The median nerve is most commonly involved in the upper extremity, whereas the sciatic nerve is most commonly involved in the lower extremity. These two nerves possess a greater sympathetic nerve distribution as compared with other nerves of the extremities. Pain is characteristically described as "burning," which may become exacerbated by a light touch of the skin, by becoming emotionally upset, or even by auditory stimulation such as hearing a squeaky noise. Pain may become so severe at times that a patient might consider amputation of the part. The vibration from riding in an automobile or even from another person walking across the floor may aggravate the pain. The patient may seek relief by wrapping his or her hand or extremity in wet towels. At first, pain is confined to the distribution of the injured nerve, but it soon spreads to the hand and entire extremity. Early stages of this form of RSD find the extremity almost always pale or cyanotic in color with sweating and coolness a prominent feature. Flexion contractures of the fingers occur, and, although stiffness is extreme, the degree of contracture is often not so great as in major traumatic dystrophy.[3]

12. What are the signs and symptoms common to RSD?

- *Pain,* characteristically described as having a burning quality, is the most prominent symptom of RSD. Although most forms of trauma and disease states produce pain that eventually abates over time, the distinguishing feature of RSD is that the pain experienced is entirely out of proportion to the original injury and in fact worsens with time and so what began as a burning sensation will intensify into pressure, crushing, binding, searing, cutting, cramping, or aching superimposed on the initial pain. The pain is constant and is aggravated by active or passive attempts at motion, making examination difficult because the patient will often withdraw from the examiner. Initially, pain is limited to a small area, such as the area of distribution of a given nerve at the site of injury, only to soon spread to encompass the entire extremity. In many cases pain may not begin until after a cast to treat a fracture is removed. Tenderness is quite pronounced, especially around the interphalangeal joints of the fingers.[3]

- *Swelling,* usually the first physical sign, occurs initially in the involved area and then slowly spreads to encompass the entire extremity in some cases. Finger swelling, which at first has a fusiform appearance, gradually leads to circumarticular thickening at the joints. At first, the swelling manifests as a soft edema but over time becomes a hard and brawny edema that almost certainly contributes to loss of motion.[3]

- *Stiffness,* like pain, is distinctive in that it increases over time—unlike trauma without the presence of RSD in which stiffness abates as the wound heals. The initial lack of motion is attributable to enforced immobility so as to escape further aggravation of pain. Subsequently, stiffness is attributed to fibrosis of the ligamentous structures and adhesion formation around tendons that causes the adjacent gliding structures to stick to one another. The result is that all fibrous joint structures become thickened, hard, and inelastic. Accompanying palmar fasciitis only serves to add to the severity of flexion contractures in the joints.[3]

- *Discoloration* is an ever-present sign that initially manifests as redness (rubor) and is most commonly located over the dorsum of the metacarpophalangeal and interphalangeal joints of the fingers or may at times diffusely involve the entire hand. Redness occurs as a function of vasodilatation of both the arterial and venous systems. As the disease progresses, the hand may become pale, whereas at other times turn pale to cyanotic. Pallor results from simultaneous vasoconstriction of both sides of the vascular tree, whereas blueness occurs from vasoconstriction of the venous system. Purplish discoloration may often be seen in the flexor creases of the fingers and palm, especially if palmar fasciitis has developed. Although redness and vasodilatation occur initially in the disease process, vasoconstriction may be present in the very early stages of RSD.[3]

- *Osteoporosis.* Initial demineralization occurs in the carpal bones producing punched-out areas as well as in the polar regions of the long bones of the metacarpals and phalanges. This spotty involvement evolves, in the untreated condition, to become a diffuse osteoporosis. Demineralization primarily occurs from increased blood flow to the joints and secondarily from immobilization.[2]

- *Sudomotor changes.* Excessive moisture (hyperhidrosis) is more often present in the early stages of RSD. At times the diaphoresis is so great that beads of sweat are observed to drop from the hand. In the later stages of RSD, dryness is the rule.[3]

- *Temperature.* In the early stages of RSD when redness is present, the temperature is more commonly elevated (hyperthermia), whereas when pallor or cyanosis is present, as it commonly is toward the severe stage of the disease, the temperature is nearly always diminished. In some instances there may be simultaneous increased temperature over the reddened joints and diminished temperature in between the joints where pallor is observed.

- *Palmar fasciitis.* Palmar fasciitis with acute nodules and thickening of the longitudinal bands of palmar fascia in the fingers and hand may be seen in several clinical types of RSD.

- *Vasomotor instability.* Prolonged capillary refill time, indicative of vasoconstriction, is commonly found in RSD and is generally found with pallor, cyanosis, or excessive sweating. In contrast, rapid capillary refill may be seen in the reddened hand, and this is indicative of vasodilatation.

- *Trophic changes.* The characteristic glossy, often shiny skin appearance in RSD is initially attributable to swelling and ironing out of skin wrinkles secondary to lack of joint motion. The skin feels quite tight to the patient. Later on, nutritional (trophic) changes occur resulting in a glossy, shiny skin surface as a result of subcutaneous tissue atrophy. Fingertips may take on a "pencil-pointing" appearance because of atrophy of the finger fat pad or pads and concomitant downward curving of the fingernail or fingernails.[3]

13. What are the stages of RSD?

The course of RSD is usually divided into three stages:

STAGE I

Stage I has an average duration of 3 months. Signs and symptoms include painful paresthesia to light touch, pitted swelling over the dorsum of the hand, observed skin tightness, decreased motion in the fingers and wrist, vasoconstriction or peripheral vasospasm resulting in paleness or cyanosis, and increased sweating and coolness. Near the end of stage I pain becomes aggravated by attempts at motion, and redness as well as dryness may manifest. Osteoporosis may be seen by the fifth week.[3]

STAGE II

Pain is the most prominent feature in stage II, and swelling changes from that of a soft nature to a brawny, hard edema. It is difficult to reduce swelling by elevation and other standard means during this stage; subsequently, stiffness continues to increase. Additionally, redness, increased heat, and decreased sweating are most commonly observed during this stage. Increasing demineralization appears as a more widespread homogeneous radiographic appearance. The shiny, glossy-looking skin is maintained during this stage and may intensify. The duration of stage II commonly progresses through the ninth month.

STAGE III

In stage III the severity of pain has peaked and either remains constant for several months or just slowly improves. In many cases, however, pain continues for up to 2 years and indefinitely in some cases. Swelling changes from brawny edema to periarticular thickening of the joints. The hand becomes pale, dry, and cool, and the glossy appearance peaks at this stage. Skin and subcutaneous tissue atrophy results in "pencil-pointing" of the fingertips. Osteoporosis is profound, and the hand is severely dysfunctional.[3]

14. What factor does diathesis play in the development of RSD in certain individuals?

Diathesis is defined as individual disposition that causes susceptibility to given disease. Two different types of diathesis are recognized in RSD though neither is mutually exclusive of the other.
1. The first diathesis tends to occur in those individuals possessing an increased sympathetic nerve activity that is evidenced by a history of sweaty palms (hyperhidrosis), pallor, or excessive coolness of fingers and toes when exposed to colder temperatures. On physical examination the clinician finds evidence of peripheral vasoconstriction and poor capillary refill of the uninvolved extremity. There may be historical evidence of vasomotor dysfunction such as fainting spells, excessive flushing or blanching, or even migraine headaches.
2. The second diathesis has to do with the psychologic makeup of the individual, which is considerably more difficult to discern than the aforementioned hypersympathetic factor. Psychiatrists have described several psychologic traits present in many RSD patients that include fearful, suspicious, emotionally labile, or inadequate personality; a chronic complainer; a dependent personality, and an insecure and unstable personality. Patients who develop RSD also tend to have a very low pain threshold, in contrast to the stoic or spartan type of individual. The patient may ask a multitude of irrelevant questions, try to control his or her own treatment, display lack of cooperation, may think up excuses for not doing what he or she is told, seek to place blame for the condition upon others, and try to control and manipulate the treatment. It is important to realize that the patient cannot control this diathesis and therefore cannot willfully cause this to happen to his or her self.[3]

There is speculation that RSD may in fact be a hysterical conversion disorder, highlighting the strong relationship that exists between mind and body. It would seem that patients would probably not benefit greatly from concurrent psychologic counseling, since they would tend to resist the implication that anything might be wrong with them emotionally.[3]

15. What is the differential diagnosis of RSD?

Differential diagnoses of RSD include rheumatoid arthritis, scleroderma, angioedema, and venous obstruction. The last condition may produce hand edema but usually causes more proximal swelling and does not tend to be so painful.[5]

16. What medical intervention is appropriate to management of RSD?

The old axiom that early diagnosis and early treatment produce the best results has never been more correct than in the case of RSD.

Stellate ganglion block is both diagnostic of RSD as well as an effective treatment for RSD because it interrupts the abnormal sympathetic reflex by blockade of all sympathetic efferent impulses to the extremity without anesthesia or paralysis. The stellate ganglion is composed of the fusion of the superior and middle cervical ganglia. Confirmation of successful blockade is provided by an immediate accompanying Horner's sign, though effective sympathectomy may occur without the presence of this sign. Patients often react in amazement at the immediate change in the condition of their hands as well as a very prompt and distinct improvement of pain and generalized feeling of well being. Benefit may last from 1 to 3 days before reassertion of sympathetic nerve hyperactivity and regeneration of the abnormal sympathetic reflex. Because of potential tissue irritation, not more than one or two blocks are administered per week unless the patient is in very severe distress. The usual number of blocks often necessary for the abolition of the abnormal sympathetic reflex is either four or five.

With very severe cases of RSD or if stellate ganglion blocks have not been started early enough, it may not be possible to break adequately the abnormal sympathetic reflex cycle. If definite improvement has accrued from several blocks, although relief is of short duration, surgical sympathectomy involving removal of the first four thoracic sympathetic ganglia may be considered.[3]

17. What are the cardinal and secondary signs and symptoms of RSD, and how does their presence justify trial sympathetic block?

Cardinal signs and symptoms include (1) pain, (2) swelling, (3) stiffness, and (4) discoloration. *Secondary signs and symptoms* are often present, though not inevitable, and include (1) osseous demineralization, (2) sudomotor changes, (3) trophic changes, (4) temperature changes, (5) vasomotor instability, and (6) palmar fibromatosis.

If all four of the cardinal signs and symptoms are present and at least several of the secondary signs and symptoms are found, a presumptive diagnosis of RSD is made. Actual confirmation comes after interruption of the sympathetic nerve reflex. At least three or four blocks with completely negative effects are administered so that one can completely rule out RSD.[3]

18. What therapeutic intervention is appropriate to management of RSD?

- Treatment of RSD requires early aggressive therapy *within and not to or beyond* the limits of pain. The overzealous therapist who ignores this warning is more likely to worsen the patient's condition rather than to improve it. The old adage of pain is gain certainly does not hold true here. Exercise is an impor-

tant part of the treatment of RSD but only when the protective umbrella of sympathetic blockade has been provided.[3]

- The patient, in many cases, may have a poor self-image and may have given up hope and experienced a psychologic amputation of the limb.[3]
- The patient is administered a highly structured but simplified program of therapy. The therapist must attempt to instill motivation in the patient and communicate that he or she has the power to improve his or her condition.
- Establish a baseline value of perceived pain using a scale for assessing pain before initiating a pain management program.[3]
- Volumetric evaluations before and after treatment modalities for hand and wrist circumference reading are appropriate only when one or two digits are involved.[6]
- Initially, *gentle active exercises* without reaching the point of pain, performed frequently and for short periods, as well as *light massage.*
- TENS (transcutaneous electrical nerve stimulation) treatment sends sensations of light touch, pressure, and proprioception by way of the faster-transmitting, larger-diameter, myelinated, and afferent nerve fibers to bypass pain transmitting C fibers. Thus the normal-sensation impulses flood the sensorium and become a vocal majority that outshout the pain message by virtue of arriving at the T cells in the substantia gelitanosa faster and en masse and thus close the gate to the pain impulse (the gate-control theory of pain).[3] TENS treatment is best performed frequently, and a change of electrode position facilitates maximum benefit.
- *Stress-loading program* of the affected extremity for pain relief and desensitization. This treatment may be instituted as an early intervention strategy when RSD is suspected, whereas invasive techniques cannot.
  1. *Scrub:* The patient is positioned in quadruped on the floor. With a coarse bristled scrub brush in the affected hand the patient is instructed to lean on the arm with the shoulder directly over the hand for maximum pressure. The patient is then instructed to "scrub" a plywood board using a back and forth motion beginning with three-minute sessions of steady scrubbing three times per day. The program is increased to 7 minutes after 2 weeks; alternatively, a 10-minute session twice a day may be substituted if tolerated by the patient.
  2. *Carry:* The patient loads the extremity by carrying a weight with the affected arm in elbow and wrist extension. The amount of weight is

determined at the first session, generally ranging from 1 to 5 pounds (a purse or briefcase). The weight should be carried throughout the day whenever the patient is standing or walking. The amount of weight carried is recorded daily on a record sheet. Increases in the amount of weight are incremental.[6]

- *Thermotherapy* is by way of hot packs or a paraffin bath to relax muscles and soften scar tissue to facilitate improved range of motion. *Fluidotherapy* is ideal for desensitization of the limb affected by RSD as well as for softening of scar tissue. Heat is often helpful if coupled with elevation.[3]

- Jobst *intermittent compression treatment* is most effective in patients demonstrating pitting edema. The treatment lasts 45 minutes to 1 hour with compression set at 60 to 90 mm Hg while the affected limb is elevated. If the Jobst unit is used to increase passive interphalangeal flexion, compression must be reduced to a range of 30 to 60 mm Hg, and the fingers should be positioned alternately in flexion and extension. After compression treatment, gentle *retrograde massage* for 10 minutes with lanolin-based cream as a lubricant to decrease edema, desensitize the extremity, soften scar tissue, and facilitate further gain in range of motion.

- Use a pressure wrap or a thermoelastic compression glove after Jobst treatment and massage.

- Use gentle joint mobilization to facilitate gain in range of motion and softening of tightened joint capsules.

- *Ice treatment* for 20 minutes in contrast baths may decrease edema, though this, similar to other edema-reducing modalities, is often not well tolerated in RSD patients because it may cause painful vasoconstriction.[3]

- Advise patients to stop smoking so as to avoid tissue ischemia from vasoconstriction.

- The use of a *hot* whirlpool bath is *contraindicated*[3] because heat applied with the extremity in a dependent position will cause stagnation of the lymphatic and venous system and result in increased swelling.

- *Splinting* to relieve pain on motion and relieve muscle spasm has been proposed. The goal of splinting is to, by means of exerting passive motion on the joint, return the hand to the "resting-hand" position of 45° wrist extension, slight ulnar wrist deviation, 70° metacarpophalangeal joint flexion, and 30° proximal interphalangeal joint flexion. The value of this position is that it is that range in which the least number of deforming forces act upon the joints of the hand. The key to splinting at the wrist is to understand that

one cannot expect to reduce extensor contractures of the PIP joints without first getting the wrist into extension. This is accomplished by a volar thermoelastic splint with Velcro straps customized with as much wrist extension as the patient can comfortably tolerate. The splint is periodically reheated to accommodate increasing wrist extension. Vigorous contracture reduction of the flexed PIP joints and the extended MP joints may be attempted after reduction of the wrist flexion contracture. The former reductions are facilitated by use of dynamic splints in the form of a dorsal thermoplastic splint with an outrigger and rubber-band slings that produce a gentle extension force over the IP joints; this, however, may be achieved only if an equal or greater force is exerted on flexing of the MP joints. This is accomplished by use of a lumbrical bar that pushes down on the dorsum of the proximal segments of the fingers (so as to yield MP joint flexion) with the same or greater force than is used to extend the IP joints. This setup may also be achieved by the use of flexion rubber bands and slings affixed to a wristlet band, thus providing a respectable flexion force applied to the MP joints. The passive forces applied to the joints will be detrimental if the patient experiences pain from an ill fitting or too tightly adjusted dynamic splint. Although the splints ought to be worn the majority of the time, they may be removed every 30 minutes for the duration of the exercise program.[3]

- Skateboard exercises for the shoulder and elbow (Fig. 6-4).

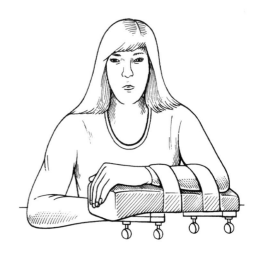

FIG. 6-4 Skateboard exercises for the shoulder and elbow.

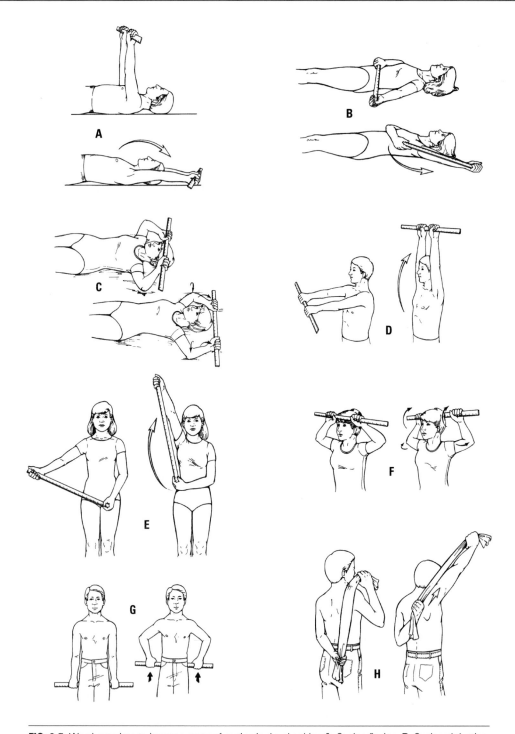

FIG. 6-5 Wand exercises to increase range of motion in the shoulder. **A,** Supine flexion, **B,** Supine abduction. **C,** Supine external rotation. **D,** Standing flexion. **E,** Standing abduction. **F,** Standing external rotation. **G,** Standing internal rotation. **H,** Standing internal rotation with towel. (From Saunders HD: *Evaluation treatment and prevention of musculoskeletal disorders,* Bloomington, Minn., 1985, Education Opportunities.)

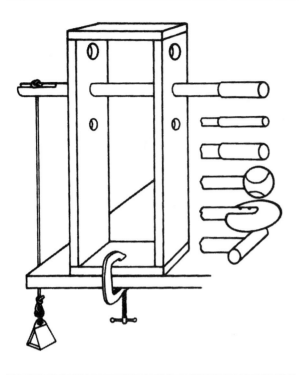

FIG. 6-6 Weight well exercise device with interchangeable handles for wrist and hand exercises. (From Hunter JM, Schneider LH, Mackin EJ, Callahan AD, editors: *Rehabilitation of the hand: surgery and therapy,* ed 3, St. Louis, 1990, Mosby.)

overstretching the muscle by increasing muscle contractions gradually against resistance. This system employs a series of 10 contractions against 100% of maximum weight.[7]

- *Weight well exercises,* (Fig. 6-6), in addition to active strengthening, elevate the hand to decrease edema and assist venous flow through the pumping action of the forearm and hand musculature.[7]

- Activities of daily living and craft activities are extremely important with patients suffering from RSD, since these patients typically avoid using the upper extremity. Through simple accomplishments in craft projects, the patient is made aware that his or her hand is functional and, as such, will begin to use it once again. Simple rote crafts such as linking a belt, stacking blocks, or placing wooden rings over round pegs reincorporate the spontaneous use of the injured hand into their lives. This is accomplished because the patient has no set expectations about a craft activity never before attempted but is often unwilling to accept substandard performance of self-feeding and other forms of activities of daily living. The therapist should try to be one step ahead of the patient in the setting of goals, with appropriate adulation expressed that will psychologically boost the patient and spur him or her on to new levels of accomplishment.[3] Eventually the therapist should guide the patient into performing the kind of functional activities that simulate the kind of work the patient will perform when he or she will return to employment.

- Begin gentle exercises distally in the fingers and progress proximally with time. Initially, very gentle passive motion is administered as far as possible without coming to the point of pain, followed by active assistive movement to the limit of painless motion and maintenance of this position for 10 seconds. These exercises are performed in both flexion and extension, with selective isolation of each joint of each finger while providing proximal stability. Similar exercises are performed in finger adduction and abduction as well as for the wrist in all planes of motion. This entire regimen should be ideally repeated once every 30 minutes.[3]

- Active dowel or wand exercises to increase shoulder, elbow, and forearm range of motion and strength (Fig. 6-5). A Velcro cuff weight may eventually be added for resistance.[7]

- Progressive resistive exercises by means of the *treppe* (German for "staircase") *method* gradually warming up the muscle for maximum exertion without risk of

REFERENCES

1. Dawson DM, Hallet M, Millender LH: *Entrapment neuropathies,* ed 2, Boston, 1990, Little, Brown.
2. Genant HK, Kozin F, Bekerman C, et al: The reflex sympathetic dystrophy syndrome, *Radiology* 117:28, 1975.
3. Lankford LL: Reflex sympathetic dystrophy. In Hunter JM, Schneider LH, Mackin EJ, et al, editors: *Rehabilitation of the hand: surgery and therapy,* ed 3, St Louis, 1990, Mosby.
4. Mitchell SW, Morehouse GR, Keen WW: *Gunshot wounds and other injuries of nerves,* Philadelphia, 1864, Lippincott.
5. Schumacher HR, Bomalski JS: *Case studies in rheumatology for the house officer,* Baltimore, 1990, Williams & Wilkins.
6. Watson HK, Carlson L: Treatment of reflex sympathetic dystrophy of the hand with an active "stress loading program," *J Hand Surg* 12A(5)(part 1):779, 1987.
7. Waylett-Rendall J: Therapist's management of reflex sympathetic dystrophy. In Hunter JM, Schneider LH, Mackin EJ, et al, editors: *Rehabilitation of the hand: surgery and therapy,* ed 3, St Louis, 1990, Mosby.

RECOMMENDED READING

Lankford LL: Reflex sympathetic dystrophy. In Hunter JM, Schneider LH, Mackin EJ, et al, editors: *Rehabilitation of the hand: surgery and therapy,* ed 3, St Louis, 1990, Mosby.

Patt RB, Balter K: Posttraumatic reflex sympathetic dystrophy: mechanisms and medical management, *J Occup Rehab* 1(1), 1991.

Waylett-Rendall J: Therapist's management of reflex sympathetic dystrophy. In Hunter JM, Schneider LH, Mackin EJ, et al, editors: *Rehabilitation of the hand: surgery and therapy,* ed 3, St Louis, 1990, Mosby.

Bilateral Epicondylar Elbow Pain

A middle-aged man enters your office with complaints of both right and left elbow pain. The gentleman underwent his second divorce 2 months previously and spends most of his time away from the office avidly playing golf. The gentleman is right handed and leads his golf stroke with his left elbow. He does not play tennis. He reports that daily high doses of aspirin are helping him. There is no history of injury or injection to either elbow, nor is there any history of gout.

OBSERVATION   Both elbows appear normal; there is neither swelling nor redness.

PALPATION   yields point tenderness immediately anterior, medial, and distal to the left lateral epicondyle, directly over the extensor brevis, and distally 1 to 2 inches along the course of pronator teres and flexor carpi radialis, as well as the right medial epicondyle; there is no tenderness over the olecranon process. Both epicondyles feel slightly warm.

ACTIVE RANGE OF MOTION   Full and painless with no evidence of contracture.

MUSCLE STRENGTH   There is good minus strength in the extensor-supinator muscle group in the left arm, as well as in the flexor-pronator muscle group in the right arm as compared to the contralateral arm.

JOINT PLAY   Movements are full and painless.

SPECIAL TESTS   No pain to left elbow below outer epicondyle after a varus stress test, and no pain to right elbow below inner epicondyle after valgus stress test. Normal compression and distraction test results of the cervical spine.

CLUE   Selective tension reveals the following patterns for the left and right elbows:

Left elbow. *Resisted* wrist extension (with elbow extended) and radial deviation, forced passive wrist flexion and ulnar deviation, and forearm pronation (with elbow extension) reproduce pain in the vicinity of the lateral epicondyle.

Right elbow. Pain elicited on *resisted* wrist flexion (with the elbow straight) and pronation, as well as extremes of passive wrist extension with forearm supination (and elbow extension) and ulnar deviation, all mimic pain at the medial epicondyle.

? Questions

1. What is the cause of this man's pain?
2. What is the sequential progression of this disorder?
3. Which vocations or avocations are commonly associated with lateral epicondylitis?
4. What are the three types of tennis elbow?
5. Why does lateral tennis elbow most commonly present as a chronic disorder?
6. What is the histologic basis for this disorder?
7. What are radiographic findings?
8. What is pitcher's elbow?
9. What may account for the lesser incidence of medial epicondylitis?
10. What adjacent ligamentous disorder may pitchers incur from excessive valgus stress at the elbow?
11. What is the epidemiology of tennis elbow?
12. What factors contribute to lateral epicondylitis in tennis players?
13. What is the significance of provocative testing with the elbow in extension?
14. What is the differential diagnosis for tennis elbow?
15. What is radial tunnel syndrome?
16. Why is lateral tennis elbow a persistent disorder that does not tend to resolve spontaneously?
17. What therapeutic management best serves the patient?
18. At what point does surgery become a treatment option?

1. What is the cause of this man's pain?

This gentleman has lateral epicondylitis of the left elbow and medial epicondylitis of the right elbow (Fig. 7-1). The most common contractile lesions occurring in the elbow region involve the proximal attachments of the wrist extensors and flexors.[10] Both are an overuse syndrome involving strain and inflammation of a common tendon and share a common mechanism of disorder: the pull of many muscles on a small origin creates a high load per unit area.[20] However, both disorders are quite different in several ways. *Lateral epicondylitis,* or *(lateral) tennis elbow,* is a disorder deriving from a faulty backhand stroke (Fig. 7-2) and involves the lateral humeral epicondyle serving as the origin of the superficial layer of forearm wrist and finger extensors by way of a common extensor tendon. Provocation occurs by resistive wrist extension, radial deviation, and passive stretching of the wrist flexors, ulnar deviators, and forearm pronators. In contrast, *medial epicondylitis,* otherwise known as *golfer's elbow* (or *medial tennis elbow*), is a less common disorder that may result from a faulty forehand tennis stroke.[8] This involves a disorder of the medial humeral epicondyle, which serves as a proximal attachment for all the middle and superficial layer wrist flexors and extrinsic finger flexors by way of the common flexor tendon. Provocation of this disorder occurs by means of resisted

wrist flexion and forearm pronation as well as wrist extension with passive supination and ulnar deviation. Tennis is by no means the only cause of tennis elbow; here, a right-handed golf player succumbed to left-sided tennis elbow. Both disorders affect those who play neither tennis nor golf.

2. What is the sequential progression of this disorder?

GRADE I

Generalized elbow soreness with activity is an early warning signal that most players ignore.[17] A vicious cycle of irritation, inflammation, inadequate healing, pain, and weakness is initiated and gains full expression in subsequent grades of injury.

GRADE II

Playing or working through the soreness may increase pain, which becomes localized at the lateral condyle or radial head[22] and persists after activity. The lateral aspect of the elbow becomes tender to touch and may become swollen and warm. Pain will interfere with his or her game and the player may find that he or she can no longer take a backhand stroke. As the condition persists, pain may radiate down the extensor surface of the

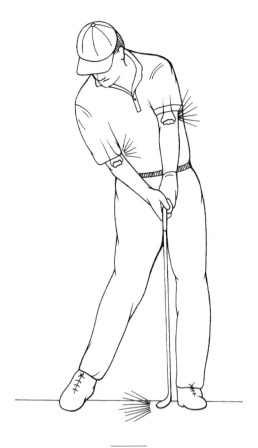

FIG. 7-1

forearm toward the wrist or it may extend into the upper arm and shoulder.[9]

GRADE III

As the condition progresses, even simple activities of daily life such as shaking hands, turning a doorknob, holding a pen or pencil, or lifting a cup (positive *coffee-cup sign*) may become difficult or painful. There may occur sudden twinges that render the grip momentarily powerless so that the patient may even drop the teacup or racket he holds.[8] Continued playing can cause secondary problems such as rotator cuff tendinitis, biceps tendinitis, and low back pain as other joints attempt to compensate and help attenuate stresses. The result is the alteration of normal biomechanics of the upper extremity and trunk. If playing continues and pain is ignored, arthritic changes in the proximal radioulnar joint may eventually occur.

3. Which vocations or avocations are commonly associated with lateral epicondylitis?

Carpentry, gardening, dentistry, politicians (from handshaking), racquetball players, squash players, golfers, bowlers, baseball players, javelin throwers, needlework,[20] or scouring pots[8] all involve repetitive forearm use while gripping an object. The common denominator of the aforementioned repetitive tasks involve wrist ulnar deviation combined with wrist extension or forearm pronation contributing to excessive tensile stress on the extensor-supinator muscle mass, passed along the flattened common extensor tendon and delivered to the lateral epicondyle.

4. What are the three types of tennis elbow?

- *Lateral tennis elbow* commonly involves the origin of the extensor-supinator muscle mass in the following descending order: extensor carpi radialis brevis, extensor digitorum communis, extensor carpi radialis longus, extensor carpi ulnaris, and supinator. The extensor carpi radialis is most commonly involved probably because the positions of wrist flexion, elbow extension, and forearm pronation stretch the tendon over the prominence of the radial head. The most common cause of lateral epicondylitis in almost 90% of afflicted tennis players is technique related, particularly an incorrect backhand technique.[17] By incorrectly leading with the elbow on the backhand stroke, the racket head will lag behind the elbow only to accelerate faster than the elbow as it moves in to meet the ball. At impact the racket immediately decelerates, resulting in transmission of impact forces along the upper extremity to the lateral epicondyle.
- *Medial tennis elbow* (synonym: golfer's elbow) is medial epicondylitis[20] and involves the flexor-pronator muscle mass: the pronator teres, the flexor carpi radialis, and occasionally the palmaris longus, flexor carpi ulnaris, and flexor digitorum superficialis. Golfer's elbow may occur in recreational tennis players using a faulty forehand technique[20] or in top-level players who use a serving action during which the wrist is flexed and radially deviated at the same time the forearm is pronated. It may also occur in players who excessively pronate while hitting an exaggerated top spin, in swimmers after they make pull-through strokes, or in baseball pitchers.
- *Posterior tennis elbow* involves a sudden severe strain to the triceps tendon as the arm is fully extended and can result from a twisted serve in competitive players.[20] This rare condition occurs from intrinsic over-

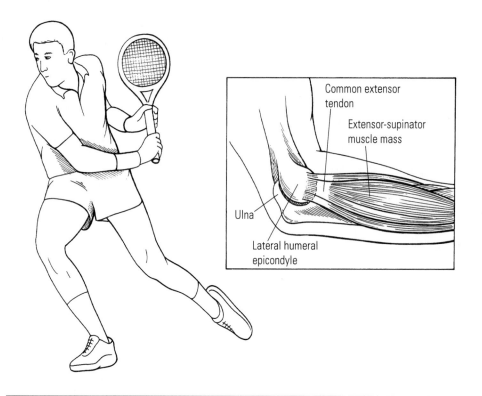

FIG. 7-2 A faulty backhand technique is implicated as the mechanism in classic tennis elbow disorder. Excessive stress is transmitted through the extensor-supinator muscle mass, particularly the extensor carpi radialis brevis, to the lateral epicondyle.

load of the triceps tendon in activities that require a sudden snapping of the elbow into extension, as in javelin throwing.[6] Pain is reproduced by fully resisting elbow extension while the patient stands with the elbow flexed and the forearm fully supinated.[12]

5. Why does lateral tennis elbow most commonly present as a chronic disorder?

Lateral tennis elbow is more commonly a chronic disorder related to a degenerative process. The majority of patients presenting with this disorder are 35 years of age or older. Except in sports clinics where the majority of patients present with the acute form of tennis elbow, the majority of patients do not relate the onset or aggravation of the disorder to playing tennis. In contradistinction to the acute presentation, most patients with lateral epicondylitis relate the onset of symptoms as being gradual and usually appearing after an activity.

With aging, the loss of mucopolysaccharide chondroitin sulfate results in decreased tendon extensibility. If activities are not modified or curtailed as se-

nescence advances, the energy of tensile loading must be absorbed as internal strain of the collagen fibers rather than temporary deformation of the tendon. This decrease in the tensile modulus may result in fatigue and microfractures of the collagenous fibers composing the tendon. An inflammatory response occurs as an attempt at tissue healing by the laying down of immature collagen.[12]

6. What is the histologic basis for this disorder?

There seems to be controversy whether lateral epicondylitis and medial epicondylitis are primarily a disorder of the musculotendinous junction (MTJ)[4,13,24] or of the tenoperiosteal junction (TPJ).[8] In the former, scar tissue fills in the space between torn fibers that, over time, reduces the widened gap between the two edges. Eventually, enough scar tissue fills the gap so that the two edges lie in apposition and any tension on the scar ceases. Periosteum is a layer of connective tissue that invests most bone; tendons attach to bone by means of the periosteum. In the latter scenario, a periosteal avulsion, a cleft, forms between the cortical bone below and the periosteum above. The body treats this insult like a fracture and lays bone down in the cleft forming an exostosis. Without rest this bone spur will grow and result in more inflammation as soft tissues rub against it.

7. What are radiographic findings?

Radiographs of the elbow joint can be unremarkable[1] and are important to rule out other pathoses. However, there may be evidence of dystrophic calcific deposits[14] in the area of degeneration in the extensor muscle origin[23] as well as evidence of traumatic arthritis in the form of bone spurring.[14]

8. What is pitcher's elbow?

Pitcher's elbow is medial epicondylitis incurred when a curve ball is imparted a spin by rapid acceleration (that is, whipping) of the elbow into the extremes of extension, forearm supination, and ulnar deviation. This motion focuses considerable traction on the pronator-flexor muscle mass and their common origin by way of the common flexor tendon. It is essential to realize that the movement into this range occurs by concentric and eccentric contraction of the pronator-flexor muscle group. Baseball pitchers are better off using a tissue-sparing pitch such as a knuckle ball.

9. What may account for the lesser incidence of medial epicondylitis?

Because the medial epicondyle is somewhat larger than the outer epicondyle,[11] the pressure, defined as force per unit area, delivered through the common flexor tendon is more widely dissipated. In addition, pressure is further dissipated by virtue of the forearm flexor muscles having more bulk. Both factors may account for the statistic that medial epicondylitis is approximately 10 times less common than lateral epicondylitis.

10. What adjacent ligamentous disorder may pitchers incur from excessive valgus stress at the elbow?

Repetitive valgus stress to the medial epicondyle may result in a strain of the ulnar collateral ligament (Fig. 7-3). The pitcher most commonly presents with a vague medial elbow pain that worsens during activity. Upon evaluation, the patient presents with palpable tenderness just inferior to the medial epicondyle, along the anterosuperior portion of the ligament. Pain or instability provocation on valgus stress testing the elbow at 30° (Fig. 7-4) confirms the diagnosis. Radiographs may

show traction spurs and loose bodies. Additionally there may also be heterotrophic ossification of the ulnar ligament. Ulnar collateral ligament strain generally responds to conservative treatment such as rest, ice, nonsteroidal antiinflammatory medication, and modification of the sport technique.[14]

11. What is the epidemiology of tennis elbow?

Almost one third of today's 32 million regular tennis players suffer from lateral epicondylitis at some point in their game, and the risk is even greater among those who play tennis for more than 2 hours per week, with an estimated 45% developing tennis elbow.[5] Lateral epicondylitis is a form of nonarticular rheumatism, most commonly occurring in the dominant elbow, though it occurs in bilateral elbows some 60% of the time. Patient age averages between 40 and 50 years.[20] Because of this, age is implicated as a causative factor possibly related to tendon degeneration. Prevalence is equal for men and women.

12. What factors contribute to lateral epicondylitis in tennis players?

- *Improperly sized racket grip.* A grip that is too small can increase muscle fatigue and make it more difficult to stabilize the wrist at impact.
- *A hard court surface* such as concrete will cause the ball to travel faster, thereby increasing the impact force against the racket.
- *Heavy tennis balls*—wet or dead balls—require a greater force to stop as well as to propel forward than normal balls.
- *High string tension* increases the impact, which means that the racket can absorb less shock, which subsequently is transmitted to the arm.
- *A small racket size* reduces the sweet spot available for optimal force contact. A sweet spot is the mathematical center of percussion located in the racket face where minimal torsion occurs on impact. Striking the ball outside the perimeter of this spot produces a moment arm about which the force of the ball may create a high pronatory torque. If the player's wrist extensors are weak, the wrist may be forced into flexion. The combined effects of active and passive tension created in the extensor-supinator muscle mass result in high loading of the extensor tendons. These combined sources of tension are reproduced during provocative tennis elbow testing (Fig. 7-5).
- *Increased racket stiffness,* that is, using metal rackets, which vibrate at impact.

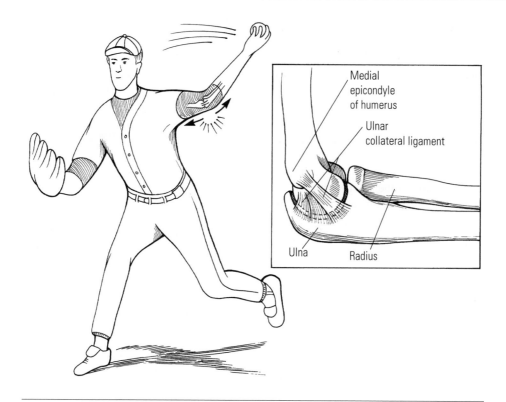

FIG. 7-3 Excessive valgus stress to the elbow during the acceleration phase of pitching or other throwing activities may sprain the ulnar collateral ligament.

• *Wrong racket size.* A casual player should best use a light racket because a heavier one may cause greater load.[20]

13. What is the significance of provocative testing with the elbow in extension?

Because the soft tissues implicated span more than one joint, placing them on stretch will more clearly reveal presence of a disorder by provoking the inflamed portion of the tissue. Otherwise, a false-negative result may be obtained. In lateral tennis elbow pain is reproduced when one asks the patient to make a fist and extend the wrist. Sudden, severe pain is elicited at the lateral epicondyle when the examiner forcefully extends the patient's wrist (Fig. 7-5).

14. What is the differential diagnosis for tennis elbow?

Radiographs of the radiohumeral joint are important when another pathologic condition is suspected. The radiograph may confirm suspicions by showing only soft-tissue swelling. Tennis elbow should not produce swelling at the elbow joint.

• *Cervical spine disease.* Pain from impingement of a cervical nerve may radiate to the elbow and be mistaken for tennis elbow.
• *Radiohumeral joint inflammation* and swelling may occur from rheumatoid arthritis, gout, or infectious arthritis, especially in the last if there has been a history of injections to this area, such as repeated steroid injections for recalcitrant tennis elbow; swelling, if present, will occur between the lateral epicondyle and the olecranon process below.[25] Fluid extraction with examination for crystals as well as fluid cultures for aerobic and anaerobic bacteria, mycobacteria, fungi, and other organisms are appropriate; if these studies have normal results, a synovial biopsy is performed with biopsy material cultured and examined histologically.[25]

15. What is radial tunnel syndrome?

Radial tunnel syndrome may occur concomitantly with lateral epicondylitis, is a common cause of treatment-resistant cases, and should be considered suspect when tennis elbow fails to respond to conservative treatment. The radial nerve runs down the medial posterior hu-

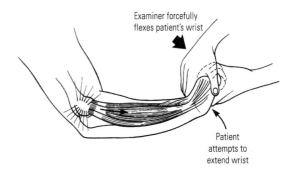

Examiner forcefully flexes patient's wrist

Patient attempts to extend wrist

FIG. 7-5 Provocation test for lateral tennis elbow generates active and passive tension delivered to the lateral epicondyle. With the forearm in pronation the patient attempts to make a fist and to extend the wrist, as the therapist forcefully overcomes the patient by flexing the wrist.

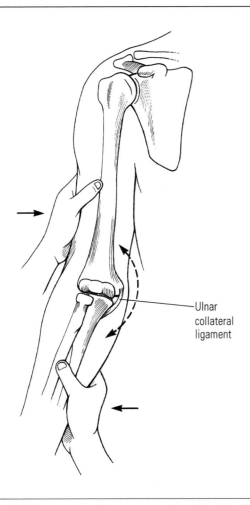

Ulnar collateral ligament

FIG. 7-4 Valgus stress test for assessment of stability of the integrity of the ulnar collateral ligament at the elbow.

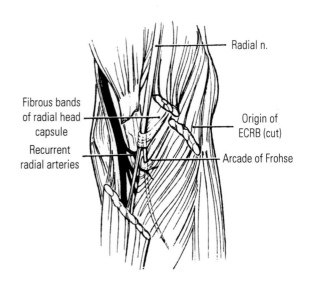

Radial n.

Fibrous bands of radial head capsule

Origin of ECRB (cut)

Recurrent radial arteries

Arcade of Frohse

FIG. 7-6 Common sites of compression in radial tunnel syndrome. ECRB, Extensor carpi radialis brevis. (From Chabon SJ: Uncommon compressive neuropathies of the forearm. *Physician Assistant*, p 60, Sept 1990.)

meral wall en route to the forearm and is transmitted laterally through the musculospiral groove in the distal third of the humerus. The nerve does not cross the antecubital fossa but rather runs laterally to it in a cleft between the brachioradialis muscle and the biceps brachii. As soon as it leaves that cleft, it crosses directly over the supinator and splits into two major branches; a deep motor branch supplies the dorsal musculature whereas a sensory branch supplies the dorsal forearm and radial dorsum of the hand.

The radial nerve is susceptible to compression at four different sites (Fig. 7-6) listed here in proximal to distal order: (1) the fibrous bands surrounding the radial head and joint capsule; (2) the recurrent radial arteries; (3) the arcade of Frohse[15]—a fibrous arcade overlying the deep radial nerve as it enters the supinator; and finally (4) the most common site of compression the fi-

brous edge of the origin of the extensor carpi radialis brevis.[21] Although patients suffering from radial tunnel syndrome often present with complaints resembling that of lateral epicondylitis, the former contrasts the clinical presentation of the latter in the following manner: pain over the proximal dorsal forearm, maximal tenderness at the site of the radial tunnel (that is, 4 cm distal to the lateral epicondyle) over the posterior interosseous nerve, radial nerve paresthesia heightened by direct compression over the radial tunnel, weakness of the extensor digitorum communis, and pain localized to the radial tunnel upon resisted supination, will all be characteristic of the radial tunnel syndrome and not of lateral epicondylitis.[3] The therapist may tension-test the radial nerve tract to further confirm a suspicion of involvement of that deep radial nerve known as the *posterior interosseous nerve.* This may be performed by superimposition of the following sequence of limb postures upon the upper extremity: shoulder depression (that is, adducted close to the side), medial rotation, extension or abduction forearm pronation, elbow extension, wrist flexion, and ulnar deviation, together with lateral head flexion away from the involved side.[2] Several months of nonoperative treatment should be taken before surgical consideration.

16. Why is lateral tennis elbow a persistent disorder that does not tend to resolve spontaneously?

A dilemma arises when we consider an appropriate treatment strategy for lateral tennis elbow. If total rest is imposed upon the patient, there may not be adequate stress to the new collagen to stimulate maturation. In this case, the immature collagen composing the scar may break down after resumption of activities. On the other hand, if the patient continues to perform activities that aggravate the condition, the immature collagen produced by an attempted repair is broken down before it has a chance to mature and the chronic inflammatory process continues. Because of this, lateral epicondylitis tends to persist chronically in many individuals.[12]

17. What therapeutic management best serves the patient?

- *Selective rest.* Preferably avoid stressful activity until the pain has subsided; however pain-free movement is encouraged.[24] Excessive activity or early return to activity may direct excessive stress to healing scar tissue. Activities that involve strong, repetitive grasping, such as hammering or tennis playing, should be restricted until there is minimal pain on resisted isometric wrist extension and little or no pain when the tendon is passively stretched.
- *Ice massage* for 20 minutes, three times a day in the acute stage and the use of heat during acute or subacute stages. Elevation and compression are not necessary because appreciable swelling does not occur.
- In the acute state, total rest is achieved by immobilization of the wrist, hand, and fingers in a resting *splint.* The splint may be removed several times a

day, so that the patient can gently and slowly actively move the wrist into flexion, the forearm into pronation, and the elbow into extension to maintain muscle and tendon extensibility.[12]

- *Gentle cross-fiber massage* within tolerance to the site of lesion to mechanically influence tissue maturation so that immature collagen becomes oriented along the lines of stress. Transverse friction massage is essentially intentional stress that is limited to helping toward maturation of new collagen and permits resolution of the healing process. In this fashion the defect heals with a maximum degree of tissue extensibility and is less likely to be overstressed as activity is resumed.
- *Ultrasound* provides a deep heating effect that may enhance increased blood flow and resolution of inflammatory exudates including lysosomal enzymes and other cellular "debris."[12]
- *Lateral counterforce brace.* A 4-inch strap[1] worn tightly around the forearm just distal to the elbow splints the area and alters the biomechanics such that the origin of the wrist extensors is transferred more proximally. This shift ensures that forces delivered to this area are absorbed by the bulk of muscle bellies, which presumably withstand greater forces than the tendon can.[26] This tennis elbow splint is applied when the arm is relaxed and should be worn until the rehabilitation period is completed[20] as well as during a graduated return to sports activity. The patient should be gradually weaned from brace use as strength, mobility, and painless function increase. This device may also be applied to the forearm flexors for medial tennis elbow. Cybex testing and biomechanical studies have confirmed the clinical validity of this treatment adjunct.[18,19]
- *Strengthening.* Gradual concentric as well as eccentric strengthening (Fig. 7-7) is important, as different authorities ascribe, since each of these modes of contraction is culpable in the development of a pathosis.[7,16] Since the common extensor tendons suffer a loss of tensile adaptation with age and the mechanism of injury involves tensile overloading of those tendons, a logical strategy would emphasize eccentric work, since this in large part is the nature of the force producing the injury. Increased muscle bulk by way of hypertrophy helps attenuate stress because there is more soft tissue to dissipate disruptive forces. Exercises should include strengthening of the ipsilateral shoulder. All exercises of the extensor-supinator group should be started with the elbow in flexion.[24] Wall pulleys may be used to simulate tennis swings (Fig. 7-8).

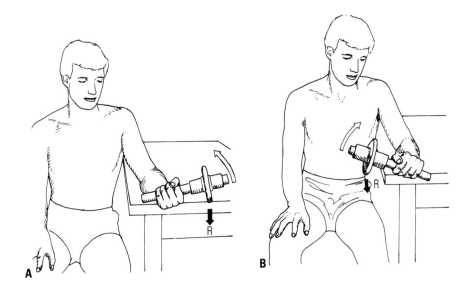

FIG. 7-7 Mechanical resistance exercise using a small bar with asymmetrically placed weight for strengthening forearm pronators, **A,** and supinators, **B.** (From Kisner, C, Colby LA: *Therapeutic exercise: foundations and techniques,* ed 2, Philadelphia, 1990, FA Davis Co.)

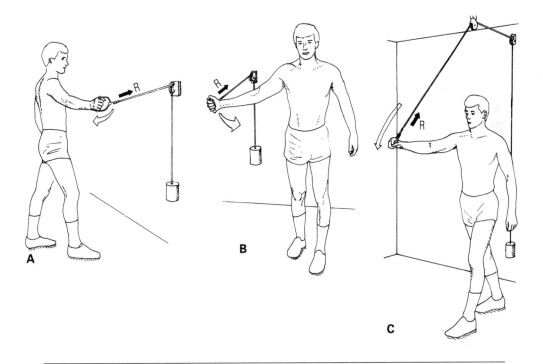

FIG. 7-8 Mechanical resistance exercise using wall pulleys to simulate tennis swings; backhand stroke, **A;** forehand stroke, **B;** and serve, **C.** (From Kisner, C, Colby LA: *Therapeutic exercise: foundations and techniques,* ed 2, Philadelphia, 1990, FA Davis Co.)

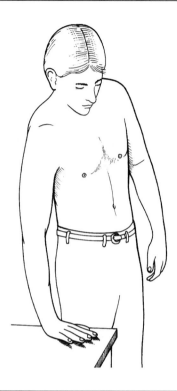

FIG. 7-9 Technique to stretch the flexor palm muscles.

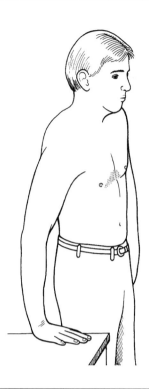

FIG. 7-10 Technique to stretch the wrist flexors.

- *Stretching regimen.* Gaining length in the extensor-supinator muscle mass will take up some of the pull placed on the origin of those muscles. Stretching of the entire hand, forearm, and shoulder complex should be performed emphasizing normal muscle balance. This may be especially helpful after ultrasound and friction massage. Teaching the patient to self-stretch is very helpful as part of the home exercise program. Self-stretching exercises include the following three:
- To stretch the *flexor palm muscles,* hold the hand flat on a table with the elbow extended and the wrist extended to 90° Gently pull up on your fingers, stretching the flexor muscles of the palm. Hold for 10 seconds and repeat twice (Fig. 7-9).
- To stretch the *wrist flexors,* keep your hand flat on the table and gently lean forward over your hand stretching the flexor muscles in your forearm. Hold for 10 seconds and repeat twice (Fig. 7-10).
- To stretch the *wrist extensors,* place the back of your hand flat on the table while keeping your elbow straight. Gently lean back over your palm stretching the extensors in your forearm. Hold for 10 seconds and repeat twice (Fig. 7-11).

- *Proper equipment.* A fiberglass, graphite, or wood racket is more flexible than a metal one. A large sweet spot is preferable. Gut strings give more resilience and less vibration than nylon ones do. The strings should ideally be strung to a range of 52 to 55 pounds of tension. If nylon is used, 16-gauge strings are preferred. Increasing the racket handle diameter helps the player with relatively weak wrist extensors from incurring a passive pronatory torque when the ball is struck outside the sweet spot. Modifying the playing surface is also helpful. The common denominator in all equipment modifications is a reduction of tensile force applied to the lateral epicondyle.
- *Proper technique.* An emphasis should be made on recruiting the whole of the shoulder and trunk in hitting the ball so as to dissipate forces as widely as possible. With a correct backhand stroke the elbow is held straight and the stress of the ball's impact is transmitted up along the arm and shoulder musculature. Additionally it is imperative to hit strokes with a firm wrist and not to return the ball by the use of wrist movements. The wearing of an elastic wrist splint may help. Use of a two-handed backhand may be helpful to some. Players with poor technique

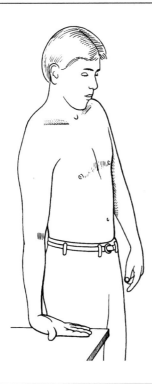

FIG. 7-11 Technique to stretch the wrist extensors.

should consider obtaining a lesson to identify areas where technique can be improved upon. It is helpful to learn to strike the ball with the center point of the strings while avoiding the periphery.

- *High-voltage galvanic stimulation*[14] has been found helpful in relieving pain and inflammation.
- *Gradual return to activity* is predicated upon normal restoration of strength and return of normal range of motion without pain.
- *Antiinflammatory medication* as prescribed by a physician may help relieve pain and inflammation.
- *Local antiinflammatory treatment, although often resulting in dramatic relief of symptoms,* **has no lasting benefit** *because it does not influence the cause of the pathologic process.* **Often, the patient misinterprets sudden relief as license to play tennis with all the vigor he or she can muster only to return soon to treatment because of relapse.** *Local antiinflammatory treatment, at best, is used as an adjunct management of the acute state.*
- *Iontophoresis* or *phonophoresis* with hydrocortisone cream and lidocaine (Xylocaine) or dexamethasone (Decadron).[24]

- *Steroid injections* are not to exceed two or three and are administered with the intent of providing pain relief only to allow progression of rehabilitation effort; healing occurs through rehabilitation not from steroid injection.[14]

18. At what point does surgery become a treatment option?

The prognosis for tennis elbow is generally good. On rare occasions operative treatment is warranted only after a trial of quality rehabilitation of some 3 to 4 months.[14] Surgery involves division and distal retraction of the fascial attachment of the extensor muscles to the lateral epicondyle.[23] After surgery, an interval of 8 to 11 weeks should elapse before tennis playing is resumed.[20]

REFERENCES

1. Berkow R: *The Merck manual of diagnosis and therapy,* Rahway, NJ, 1987, Merck, Sharp & Dohme Research Laboratories.
2. Butler D: *Mobilisation of the nervous system,* Melbourne, 1991, Churchill Livingstone.
3. Chabon SJ: Uncommon compressive neuropathies of the forearm, *Physician Assistant* 14(9):65, 1990.
4. Chusid J, McDonald J: *Correlative neuroanatomy and functional neurology,* ed 17, Los Altos, Calif, 1979, Lang Medical Publications.
5. Constable G, editor: *Restoring the body: treating aches and injuries,* Alexandria, Va, 1987, Time-Life.
6. Corrigan B, Maitland GD: *Practical orthopaedic medicine,* Stoneham, Mass, 1985, Bitterworth.
7. Curwin S, Standish WD: *Tendinitis: its etiology and treatment,* Lexington, Mass, 1984, Collamore Press.
8. Cyriax J: *Textbook of orthopaedic medicine, vol 1: Diagnosis of soft tissue lesions,* Philadelphia, 1982, Bailliere-Tindall.
9. Ellison MD et al, editors: *Athletic training and sports medicine,* Chicago, 1985, American Academy of Orthopedic Surgeons.
10. Gould JA: *Orthopaedic and sports physical surgery,* ed 2, St Louis, 1990, Mosby.
11. Gray H: *Anatomy, descriptive and surgical,* ed 15, New York, 1977, Bounty Books.
12. Hertling D, Kessler RM: *Management of musculoskeletal disorders,* ed 2, Philadelphia, 1990, Lippincott.
13. Kapjandi IA: *The physiology of the joints,* vol 1, Edinburgh, 1970, Churchill Livingstone.
14. Lillegard WA, Rucker KS: *Handbook of sports medicine—a symptom oriented approach,* Boston, 1993, Andover Medical Publishers.
15. Moss SH, Switzer H: Radial tunnel syndrome: a spectrum of clinical presentations, *J Hand Surg* 4:414-419, 1983.
16. Nirschl RP: Tennis elbow, *Orthop Clin North Am* 4:787-800, 1973.

17. Nirschl RP: The etiology and treatment of tennis elbow, _Am J Sports Med_ 2:308-319, 1974.

18. Nirschl RP: Medial tennis elbow: the surgical treatment. Presented at the annual meeting of the American Academy of Orthopaedic Surgeons, Atlanta, March 1, 1980.

19. Nirschl RP: Muscle and tendon trauma: tennis elbow. In Morrey BF, editor: _The elbow and its disorders,_ Philadelphia, 1985, Saunders.

20. Peterson L, Renström P: _Sports injuries: their prevention and treatment,_ London, 1986, Martin Dunitz (distributor in U.S.: Mosby, St Louis).

21. Ritts G, Wood M, Linshield R: Radial-tunnel syndrome: a ten-year surgical experience, _Clin Orthop_ 219:201-205, 1987.

22. Rodman GP, Schumacher HR: _Primer on rheumatic diseases,_ ed 8, Atlanta, 1983, Arthritis Foundation.

23. Salter RB: _Textbook of disorders and injuries of the musculoskeletal system,_ ed 2, Baltimore, 1983, Williams & Wilkins.

24. Saunders HD: _Evaluation, treatment, and prevention of musculoskeletal disorders,_ Bloomington, Minn, 1985, Educational Opportunities.

25. Schumacher HR, Bomalski JS: _Case studies in rheumatology for the house officer,_ Baltimore, 1990, Williams & Wilkins.

26. Wadsworth PT et al: Effects of the counterforce armband on wrist extensor and grip strength and pain in subjects with tennis elbow, _Orthop Sports Phys Ther_ 11:192-197, 1989.

RECOMMENDED READING

Hertling D, Kessler RM: _Management of common musculoskeletal disorders,_ ed 2, Philadelphia, 1990, Lippincott.

Peterson L, Renström P: _Sports injuries: their prevention and treatment,_ London, 1986, Martin Dunitz (distributor in U.S.: Mosby, St Louis).

PART III

SHOULDER

8

Persistent Pinpoint Tenderness over Bicipital Groove Despite Shoulder Rotation and Painful Arc during Resistive Supination and Elevation

A 51-year-old electrician spends most of his professional time installing ceiling light fixtures for several lighting stores in his area. He complains of right anterior shoulder pain. There is full range of motion with painful arc present on elevation and depression at approximately 50° on both the upswing and the downswing. There is no observed muscle wasting. Palpation yields tenderness over the bicipital groove. There is no cuff wasting, and the patient admits to a history of cuff impingement and suspected tear of his right shoulder of several years' duration that was operated on last year. His history also includes generalized arthritis and occasional bouts of gout since age 28, though there is no exacerbation at present. Muscle strength is good throughout, except for right forearm supination, which is decreased to good minus; elbow flexion is graded as good. Shoulder abduction in either direction of glenohumeral rotation is painful. Resisted flexion with the forearm fully pronated is mildly uncomfortable, whereas resisted flexion and supination is most definitely painful. Placement of the biceps muscle in passive insufficiency caused by simultaneous passive shoulder depression, elbow extension, and forearm pronation yields pain in the vicinity of the anterior deltoid. Flexibility testing also reveals tightness in the latissimus and pectoral muscle groups. There is normal joint play present in all joints of both shoulder girdles except for tightness of the posterior glenohumeral joint capsules of both shoulders. The patient takes no medications for his pain.

SPECIAL TESTS Negative Yergason's test, negative drop-arm test, negative Ludington's test, positive impingement sign, positive sawing test, positive Speed's test, positive deAnquin's test, positive Hueter's sign, negative Lippman's test, negative axial compression/distraction.

? Questions

1. What most likely accounts for this individual's anterior shoulder pain?
2. What anatomy is relevant to understanding biceps brachii disorders?
3. What is the kinesiology of the biceps brachii?
4. What effect if any does the long biceps brachii tendon have in contributing to humeral head depression?
5. What other function does the long head of the biceps brachii share with the rotator cuff?
6. What is the most important restraint of the long tendon of the biceps brachii as it courses down the arm?
7. What osseous anatomy is relevant to understanding biceps brachii tendon disorders?
8. What unique functional relationship exists between the long tendon of the biceps brachii and the proximal humerus?
9. What is the function of the bicipital aponeurosis?
10. What happens to the tendon of the long head of the biceps brachii during rotator cuff attrition and tear?
11. What is the most common form of proximal biceps brachii tendinitis?
12. What comparative anatomy studies may shed light on the origin of biceps brachii tendinitis and rotator cuff disorders?
13. What are the clinical signs of proximal bicipital tendinitis within the glenohumeral joint?
14. Describe five provocative tests implicating lesions of the biceps brachii tendon.
15. What accounts for painful nocturnal exacerbation in many painful shoulder conditions?
16. What is primary biceps brachii tendinitis?
17. Which sports are associated with proximal biceps brachii tendinitis and subluxation?
18. What happens to the long tendon of the biceps brachii during subluxation or dislocation?
19. How is the bicipital groove best palpated?
20. What forms of imaging are appropriate in detecting biceps brachii lesions?
21. What is the clinical sign of strain of the long head of the biceps brachii at its glenoid origin?
22. At which sites does the biceps brachii tendon most likely rupture, and who is most vulnerable?
23. What is the presentation of sudden proximal tendon rupture?
24. What is the mechanism for distal tendon avulsion?
25. What is bicipital tenosynovitis at the lower arm?
26. What is bicipital tendinitis of the lower arm?
27. How is a brachialis muscle disorder differentiated from a lesion of the biceps brachialis?
28. What is the differential diagnosis?
29. What rehabilitative treatment is most appropriate for proximal biceps brachii tendinitis, and when is surgery appropriate?
30. What postoperative care is appropriate to patients having undergone surgery for a proximal biceps brachii lesion?

1. What most likely accounts for this individual's anterior shoulder pain?

Bicipital tendinitis within the glenohumeral joint.

2. What anatomy is relevant to understanding biceps brachii disorders?

The biceps brachii, a long fusiform muscle that arises by two heads, has no direct connection with the humerus as it originates above the shoulder and inserts below the elbow joint. As such it can be moved about, when grasped, more easily than muscles that take their origin on the humerus. The tensile strength of the biceps tendon has been measured at between 150 and 200 lb.[6,12]

The tendon of the long head of the biceps arises from the supraglenoid tubercle and arches obliquely across the top of the humeral head within the capsule of the shoulder joint. This biceps tendon is intraarticular but extrasynovial. Imperative to understanding the pathology of the long tendon is that the tendon penetrates the rotator cuff between the subscapularis and the supraspinatus tendons. The tendon then begins its descent superficially along the anterior humeral shaft via the bi-

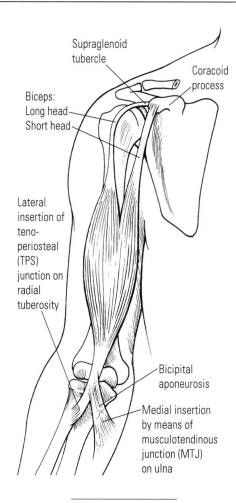

Supraglenoid
tubercle

Coracoid
process

Biceps:
Long head
Short head

Lateral
insertion of
teno-
periosteal
(TPS)
junction on
radial
tuberosity

Bicipital
aponeurosis

Medial insertion
by means of
musculotendinous
junction (MTJ)
on ulna

FIG. 8-1 Biceps brachii.

cipital groove (intertubercular sulcus) located in the anterior proximal humerus.

The short head of the biceps arises with the coracobrachialis from the scapula's coracoid process and runs down the medial side of the long head of the biceps. The two bellies join as a common distal tendon shortly above the elbow joint as a flattened tendon, only to separate into two distal insertions. Although the lateral insertion on the radial tuberosity is a *tenoperiosteal junction,* the main medial insertion attaches to the ulna as a *musculotendinous junction* by means of the bicipital aponeurosis, a triangular flat sheet running medially from the main tendon through the arm's deep fascia into the ulna (Fig. 8-1).

3. What is the kinesiology of the biceps brachii?

The significance of the two different origins and insertions of the biceps muscle as well as the humeral length

that it traverses make the biceps a jack of all trades but master of none in relation to the shoulder joint, the elbow joint, and even the distal wrist joint.

Aside from being a major forearm flexor by means of its ulnar insertion, the biceps is also a powerful supinator when the forearm is flexed by its radial insertion. During contraction, in addition to forearm flexion, there is concomitant radial unwinding as the tuberosity is rotated anteriorly (Fig. 8-2).

This second function, performed routinely when one opens a corkscrew or turns a screw into hardwood, is best performed in flexion (Fig. 8-3) because this position places the biceps muscle at its ideal length and optimum mechanical advantage.

4. What effect if any does the long biceps brachii tendon have in contributing to humeral head depression?

Electromyographic studies show that the biceps tendon does have a weak active head depressor effect. Based on its anatomic saddling of the humeral head it, at the very least, serves as a static checkrein preventing cephalad humeral excursion (Fig. 8-4). In the event of medial subluxation of the biceps tendon, this checkrein effect is lost.[2]

5. What other function does the long head of the biceps brachii share with the rotator cuff?

Another function that the long head of the biceps shares with the adjacent supraspinatus tendon is shoulder *abduction.* In the absence of deltoid strength, for example, from posterior joint dislocation with resultant axillary nerve injury, the biceps may be recruited to abduct the shoulder 50° in the context of the following substitution pattern: by externally rotating the shoulder, the biceps has a line of pull that is placed parallel with the coronal plane, making the biceps an abductor. Elevation above 50° is not possible as a function of a fixed lever arm secondary to a tethering of the tendon by the bicipital retinaculum. The biceps is also a shoulder flexor to 50° but only when the shoulder is in neutral with respect to rotation.

6. What is the most important restraint of the long tendon of the biceps brachii as it courses down the arm?

The gliding of the long tendon of the biceps is guided by the *coracohumeral ligament* (Fig. 8-5). This ligament runs through the interval between the subscapularis and supraspinatus tendons known as the *rotator interval* and serves to reinforce the glenohumeral

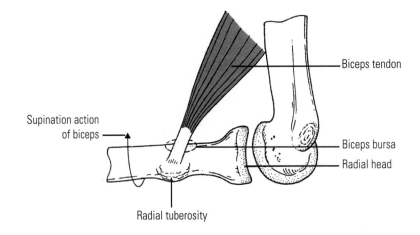

Supination action of biceps

Biceps tendon

Biceps bursa

Radial head

Radial tuberosity

FIG. 8-2 When the biceps supinates the forearm, the radius is uncrossed relative to the ulna and lies parallel with that bone. Supination is most powerful when the elbow is flexed at the right angle. (From Ellis H: *Clinical anatomy*, ed 7, Oxford, 1983, Blackwell Scientific Publications.)

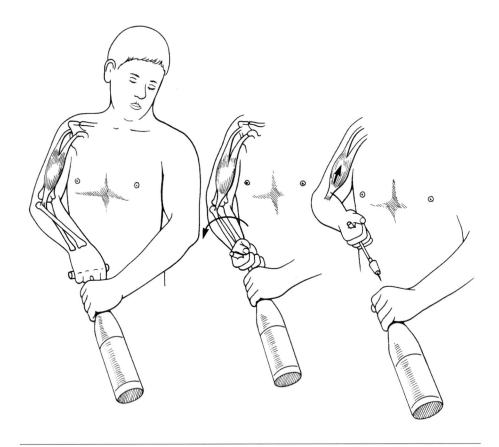

FIG. 8-3 The elbow flexion and forearm supination function of the biceps brachii illustrated by uncorking a bottle.

joint capsule at that locale. Additionally, this ligament together with the edges of the subscapularis and supraspinatus tendons thicken and reinforce that portion of the capsule so as to stabilize the tendon within the intertubercular groove. This portion of reinforced

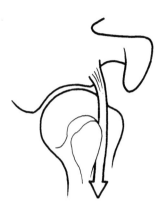

FIG. 8-4 Electromyographic analysis shows the long biceps tendon to be an active head depressor, albeit a weak one. Given its line of pull and the resultant vector, the biceps tendon is certainly at very least a static head depressor. (From Habermeyer P, Kaiser E, Knappe M et al: *Unfallchirurg* 90[7]:319-329, 1987.)

capsule serves as the principle obstacle to medial tendon dislocation. In cases of dislocation this ligament may become torn or stretched.

7. What osseous anatomy is relevant to understanding biceps brachii tendon disorders?

The bicipital groove is located between the lesser and greater tuberosities. Although the medial wall of this sulcus is formed by the lesser tuberosity, the lateral wall is formed by the edge of the greater tuberosity. The intertubercular sulcus is measured according to its width, depth, and medial wall angle (Fig. 8-6); medial wall angles in humans are unique among primates in that they vary widely between 15° and 90° but with the majority of the population falling between 60° and 75° (Fig. 8-7). Groove variations, whether too wide and shallow or excessively deep, may lead to problems. A positive correlation exists between lower medial wall angles (that is, shallower grooves) and subluxation or dislocation of the biceps tendon. Excessively deep grooves tend to be too narrow and may compress the tendon.[4,5] Furthermore, a bony anomaly, known as the *supratubercular ridge* (Fig. 8-8), extending from the lesser tuberosity is present in some people; when it is, the ridge decreases sulcus depth and diminishes the

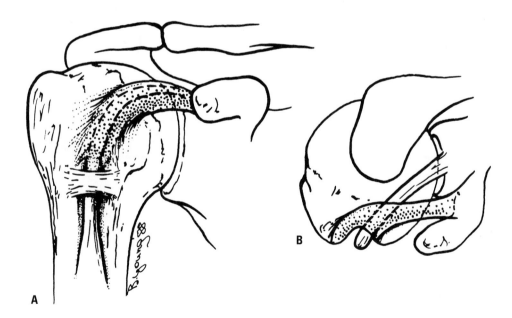

FIG. 8-5 The coracohumeral ligament thickens the rotator interval, inserts on either side of the bicipital groove, and is an important stabilizer of the biceps tendon. **A,** anterior view, **B,** superior view. (Modified from Paavolainen P, Slatis P, Aalto K: Surgical pathology in chronic shoulder pain. In Bateman JE, Welsh RP, editors: *Surgery of the shoulder,* St. Louis, 1984, Mosby.)

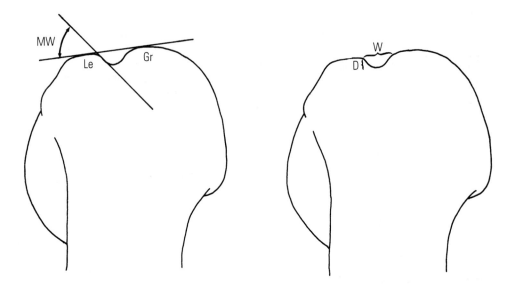

FIG. 8-6 Measurements taken by Cone and associates, including the medial wall angle as well as the width and depth of the bicipital groove. _D,_ depth of groove; _Gr,_ greater tuberosity; _Le,_ lesser tuberosity; _MW,_ medial wall angle; _W,_ width of groove. (From Cone RO, Danzig L, Resnick D, Goldman AB: _Am J Roentgenol_ 41:781-788, 1983.)

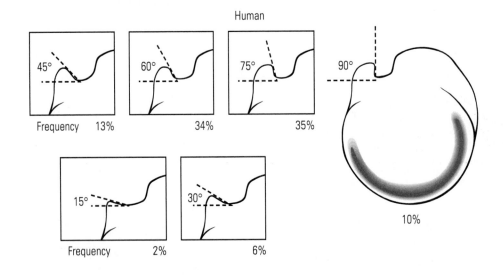

FIG. 8-7 Humans are unique among primates in exhibiting variations in bicipital groove characteristics, including depth, width, and hence medial wall angle. The average medial wall angle varies between 60°-75° throughout in the majority of people. Groove characteristics in all other primates are constant within the species. (Modified from Hitchcock HH, Bechtol CO: Painful shoulder: Observations in the role of the tendon of the long head of the biceps brachii in its causation. _J Bone Joint Surg_ 30 A:263-273, 1948.)

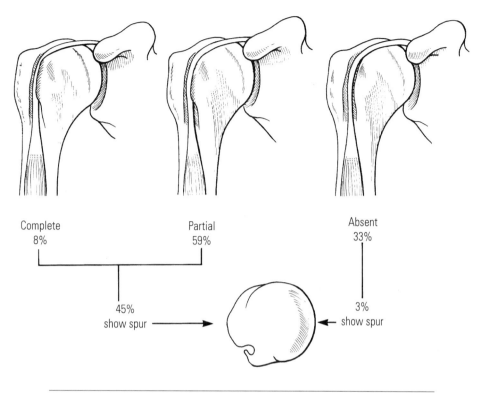

FIG. 8-8 Medial wall spurs are more common in individuals with supratubercular ridges.

effectiveness of the tuberosity as a pulley. Medial wall spurs are much more common in individuals with supratubercular ridges.[13]

8. What unique functional relationship exists between the long tendon of the biceps brachii and the proximal humerus?

It is important to understand that, unlike most tendons, the long head of the biceps moves on a fixed area of bone (that is, the superior glenoid rim during shoulder motion). From vertical adduction and depression to complete shoulder elevation the bicipital groove moves along the tethered long tendon of the biceps for a distance of as much as 6-8 cm. Motion of the long tendon in its groove occurs with motion of the shoulder joint. At any given point, a different amount of biceps tendon is found within the joint (Fig. 8-9). For example, on abduction and flexion, the intraarticular portion of this tendon is only a few centimeters long, whereas on adduction or extension this length increases to 4 cm. To facilitate ease of motion, the synovial pouch of the glenohumeral joint extends distally to line the greater extent of the bicipital groove.

9. What is the function of the bicipital aponeurosis?

The *bicipital retinaculum* (Fig. 8-10) serves to hold the tendon of the long head of biceps against the proximal humerus within the bicipital groove. The functional significance of this becomes apparent during shoulder elevation, which limits biceps contribution to either flexion or abduction by tethering of the long tendon within the bicipital groove. By way of analogy, the humerus travels on the biceps tendon like a monorail on its track.[2] The retinaculum prevents the biceps from deflecting away from the humerus during contraction by keeping it straddled between the two tuberosities, thus limiting its leverage as a significant elevator.

10. What happens to the tendon of the long head of the biceps brachii during rotator cuff attrition and tear?

The triad of proximal bicipital impingement, tendinitis, and tearing must be viewed against the backdrop of that tendon's intimate association with the rotator cuff. The biceps tendon is well situated to produce humeral head depression in partnership with the cuff and thus bears additional load when the rotator cuff ruptures. In many

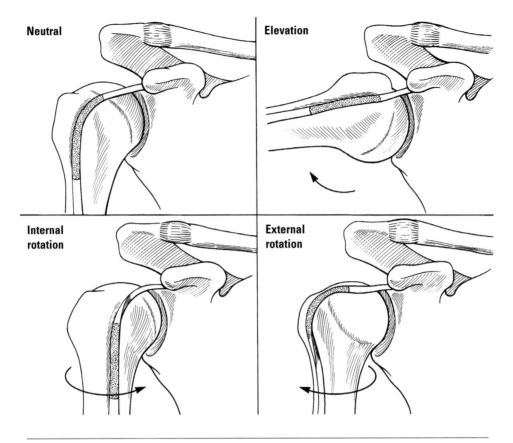

Neutral

Elevation

Internal rotation

External rotation

FIG. 8-9 A different amount and portion of biceps tendon is located with the glenohumeral joint, depending on the plane of shoulder movement. Tendon excursion occurs because the biceps tendon is tethered against the bone. Movement occurs when the humerus moves on the tendon. Tendon excursion is greatest during shoulder elevation, particularly in abduction.

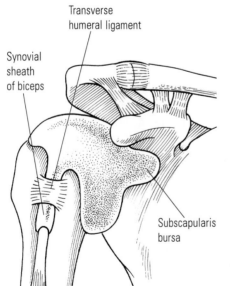

Transverse humeral ligament

Synovial sheath of biceps

Subscapularis bursa

FIG. 8-10 Transverse humeral ligament.

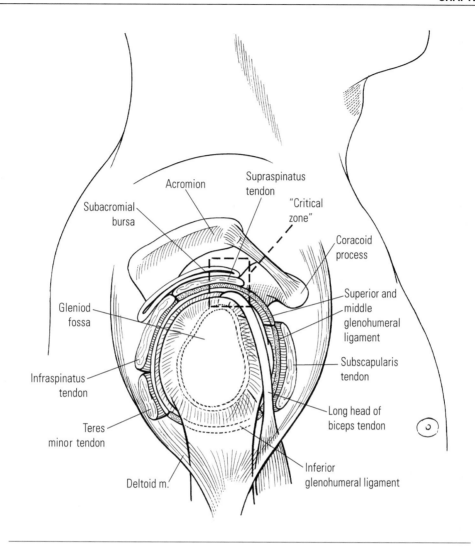

FIG. 8-11 Right shoulder. Orientation of tendinous origins of supraspinatus and the long tendon of the biceps brachii in relation to the "critical zone" vis-à-vis the subacromial arch.

cases of surgical exposure the biceps is revealed to be hypertrophied and flattened to the contour of the humeral head almost as if it were trying to become a substitute cuff. The missing downward force by the cuff results in upward displacement of the humeral head causing greater impingement of the coracoacromial arch on the biceps tendon. *Because of the intimate relationship of the biceps tendon with the rotator cuff, whenever one considers the diagnosis of a biceps long tendon disorder, one should also consider impingement of the rotator cuff.* A complete tear of the biceps tendon will usually produce no shoulder pain; thus, the patient with a rupture of the long tendon of the biceps may also be suspected of having a cuff tear.[2] Rotator cuff rupture increases exposure of the long biceps tendon to com-

pression from the acromion above and the humeral head below. As with the rotator cuff, impingement may progress to tendinitis.

11. What is the most common form of proximal biceps brachii tendinitis?

The most common cause (95% to 98%) of bicipital tendinitis actually results as a secondary involvement of the biceps after primary impingement or tearing of the rotator cuff (Fig. 8-11). This is more easily imagined when we appreciate that the biceps tendon passes directly under the critical zone of the supraspinatus tendon. In fact, the intracapsular portion of the biceps tendon has its own *critical zone* of avascularity caused by a "wringing-out" phenomenon when the arm is abducted.[18] In fact, the close functional relationship between the rotator cuff and the biceps long tendon is emphasized by the frequency with which tears of these two structures coincide.

Bicipital tendinitis may also occur secondary to an intraarticular problem such as rheumatoid or osteoarthritis.

12. What comparative anatomy studies may shed light on the origin of biceps brachii tendinitis and rotator cuff disorders?

When we look comparatively at the progressive changes in the relationship between the scapula and the bicipital groove, we notice a pronounced shift in the transition from quadruped mammals such as the opossum to that of biped primates. The human arm is essentially derived from the foreleg of a quadruped with a principal function of weight bearing. Subsequently, when locomotion evolved from quadruped to biped, the upper limb, no longer operating in a closed kinetic chain, moved away from the body to enable the arm to operate in a wide range of circumduction.

This modification was accomplished by (1) a progressive anteroposterior flattening of the thorax (Fig. 8-12) resulting in an increased angle formed between the scapula and the thorax as well as a relative lateral scapular displacement; (2) a shortened forearm that, along with changes in scapular position, necessitates a greater medial humeral rotation for the hand to reach

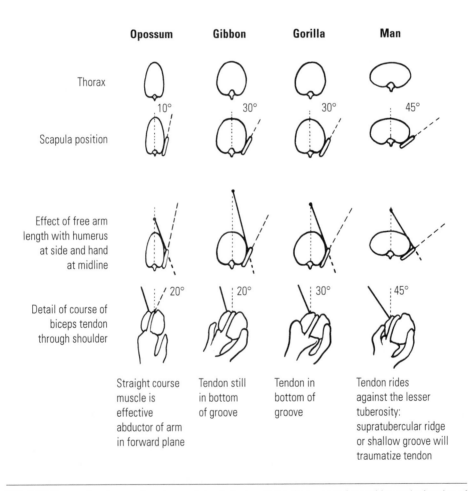

FIG. 8-12 Progressive changes in anteroposterior flattening of the thorax scapular position and migration of the biceps tendon from the quadruped to the biped. (Modified from Hitchcock HH, and Bechtol CO: Painful shoulder: Observations on the role of the tendon of the long head of the biceps brachii in its causation. *J Bone Joint Surg* 30 A:263-272, 1948.)

midline. These two changes were incompletely compensated for by torsion of the humerus.

In the opossum, for example, the biceps tendon runs a *straight* course through the bicipital groove and is therefore an effective shoulder elevator. In humans, however, by virtue of an approximately 35° retroversion, the biceps tendon is left behind on the anterior aspect of the shoulder joint straddled by the tuberosities as the distal tendon courses *obliquely* over the glenohumeral joint.[2]

The idea has been advanced[1] that the human embryo, during the course of its growth, metamorphoses through many stages of its evolutionary advancement; thus, the genetic code that guides the growing human neonate is expressed as an evolutionary metamorphisication of the various stages of man's vertebral ancestry that includes fish, amphibians, reptiles, and mammals.[15a] An example of ontogeny recapitulating phylogeny is how gill slits actually develop early on, only to mature into lungs as the neonate grows; similarly, the tail bud is resorbed into the coccyx, which is hidden by no more than a pronounced skin dimple. In the same vein upper limb rotation occurs at the elbow and is reflected at the elbow as humeral retroversion during the ninth week of gestation.

Thus, with the advent of *Homo erectus,* the biceps tendon became lodged against the lesser tuberosity (see Fig. 8-7), where the presence of either a medial supratubercular ridge or a shallow groove created a milieu for increased likelihood of a pathologic condition. This was further disadvantaged by the shortened forearms (and hence power arms) that no longer needed to be of equidistant height with the hind legs and most often worked resistively against the weight of held objects in an open kinetic chain. In this unfavorable mechanical situation the short lever arm is forced to work against a longer lever arm (that is, the object held), and this situation focuses undue excessive disruptive force, which may lead to tendinitis of the biceps or the rotator cuff. As such, bicipital tendinitis is yet another one of those disorders that are heir to the legacy of mankind's evolutionary advancement.

13. What are the clinical signs of proximal bicipital tendinitis within the glenohumeral joint?

Proximal biceps tendinitis is evidenced by proximal anterior shoulder pain and possibly a painful arc[16,20] during shoulder flexion and extension while the biceps is tensed *(sawing test)* and by tenderness in the bicipital groove on palpation. Pain may radiate distally to the

muscle belly or proximally, like pain from cuff impingement, radiate to the deltoid insertion. There is no radiation into the neck or distally beyond the biceps muscle belly. The patient is typically young or middle aged with a history of overhead repetitive arm use. Pain is less intense during rest and worse with use. Nighttime exacerbation is common. Active or passive internal rotation with abduction is often painful because the long tendon works against the medial wall of the groove and thereby tenses that tendon. Similarly, abduction with external rotation is also painful when the long tendon occupies the floor of the groove and is again made taut when that tendon pulls downward on the humeral head. Resisted forward flexion may be painful.

14. Describe five provocative tests implicating lesions of the biceps brachii tendon.

See the provocative tests implicating lesions of the biceps tendon (Fig. 8-13).

15. What accounts for painful nocturnal exacerbation in many painful shoulder conditions?

Painful conditions of the shoulder are made worse at night for the following reasons:
- The supine position places the shoulder at or below the level of the heart.
- Rolling over the involved shoulder further increases the problem by decreasing the venous return from the upper extremity.
- Compression loading.[2]

16. What is primary biceps brachii tendinitis?

Primary bicipital tendinitis is uncommon as an isolated entity. However, this condition often accompanies cuff impingement and contributes to anterior shoulder pain. It involves changes in the tendon and enveloping synovial membrane within the bicipital groove; as such, it may be referred to as *bicipital tenosynovitis* of the upper arm. Tendinitis also goes by the name of *palm-up pain syndrome,* since symptoms are elicited during the supination portion of Yergason's maneuver. Pathologic changes are akin to other disease entities involving the passage of tendons through a fibroosseous tunnel, such as de Quervain's tenosynovitis in the wrist region. Synovial reaction includes edema, intense erythema, thickening of the transverse humeral ligament, as well as tendon narrowing and attrition beneath the sheath. A bony spur may develop, causing stenosis and attrition

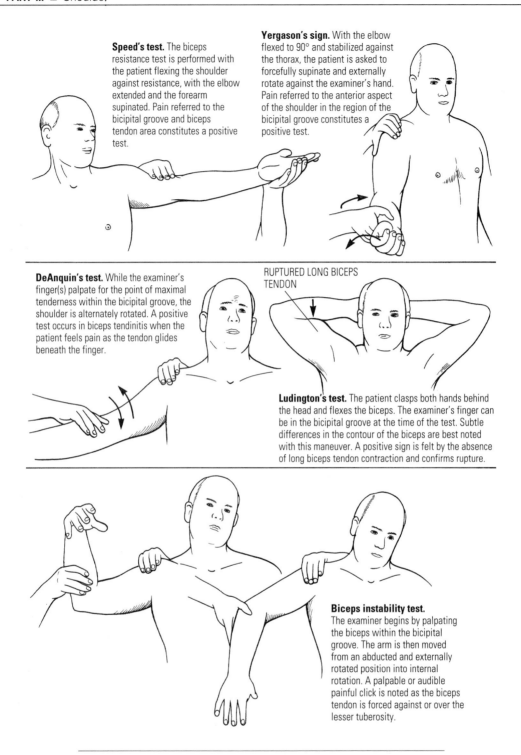

Speed's test. The biceps resistance test is performed with the patient flexing the shoulder against resistance, with the elbow extended and the forearm supinated. Pain referred to the bicipital groove and biceps tendon area constitutes a positive test.

Yergason's sign. With the elbow flexed to 90° and stabilized against the thorax, the patient is asked to forcefully supinate and externally rotate against the examiner's hand. Pain referred to the anterior aspect of the shoulder in the region of the bicipital groove constitutes a positive test.

DeAnquin's test. While the examiner's finger(s) palpate for the point of maximal tenderness within the bicipital groove, the shoulder is alternately rotated. A positive test occurs in biceps tendinitis when the patient feels pain as the tendon glides beneath the finger.

RUPTURED LONG BICEPS TENDON

Ludington's test. The patient clasps both hands behind the head and flexes the biceps. The examiner's finger can be in the bicipital groove at the time of the test. Subtle differences in the contour of the biceps are best noted with this maneuver. A positive sign is felt by the absence of long biceps tendon contraction and confirms rupture.

Biceps instability test. The examiner begins by palpating the biceps within the bicipital groove. The arm is then moved from an abducted and externally rotated position into internal rotation. A palpable or audible painful click is noted as the biceps tendon is forced against or over the lesser tuberosity.

FIG. 8-13 Provative tests implicating long bicipital tendinitis, rupture, and instability.

of the long tendon of the biceps. This type of bicipital tendinitis (attrition tendinitis, see fig. 8-19) may be very painful and contributes to complete tendon rupture.[2] Treatment is by local rest with an arm sling, and one or more steroid injections may be required. Occasionally symptoms are so severe as to warrant operative treatment in which the degenerated tendon is divided and the distal stump is sutured to the bicipital groove.

17. Which sports are associated with proximal biceps brachii tendinitis and subluxation?

Degenerative processes are common in football quarterbacks because of the weight of the ball and the need for additional pushing action in softball pitchers because of forceful supinator strain with the arm and forearm in flexion.[11,17] Bicipital tendinitis is frequently seen in patients who participate in golf, tennis, swimming, pitching, or other throwing sports. The common denominator here is that humeral rotation at or above the level of the horizontal approximates the tuberosities, the intervening groove, the biceps tendon, and rotator cuff in direct contact with the anterior acromion or coracoacromial ligament.[2]

18. What happens to the long tendon of the biceps brachii during subluxation or dislocation?

Subluxation of the tendon of the long head may be isolated and result from attrition but is often concomitant with moderate to massive tears extending into the anterior portion of the cuff. A fully displaced bicipital tendon lies in the sling of the ruptured cuff and may, in the early phase of this lesion, slip in and out of the groove. As the sulcus gradually fills with scar tissue, the groove becomes shallower, and so finally the tendon remains in a medially dislocated position[2] (Fig. 8-14).

When an excessive load is applied to the arm in the position of abduction and external rotation, the line of pull of the long bicipital tendon is placed in the coronal plane and presses against the medial wall of the groove but is restrained from bowstringing by the lesser tuberosity acting as a simple pulley. In the event of a shallow groove or excessive force the tendon is restrained by the coracohumeral ligament as well as the restraining aponeurosis but may nonetheless luxate medially out of the groove and over the lesser medial tuberosity in one of two patterns: (1) rupture of the transverse ligament and subluxation of the biceps tendon out of the groove, with the tendon lying anterior to the subscapularis muscle, or (2) tendon subluxation beneath the subscapularis muscle belly (Fig. 8-15). The long tendon

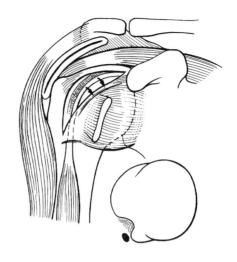

FIG. 8-14 Subluxation of the biceps. A tear in the medial portion of the coracohumeral ligament causes subluxation and medial displacement of the tendon out of the bicipital groove. (Redrawn from Paavolainen P, Slatis P, Aalto K: Surgical pathology in chronic shoulder pain. In Bateman JE, Welsh RP, editors: *Surgery of the shoulder,* St. Louis, 1984, Mosby.)

will then return of its own accord back into the groove once the upper arm is rotated medially and then laterally while the forearm is flexed at the elbow[14] as in the provocative test of Yergason (Fig. 8-16). A positive test reproduces pain, and the examiner may feel the tendon snapping in and out of the groove. Motion is often accompanied by a palpable snap or pop. This may be attributable to actual subluxation of the biceps tendon but is more likely caused by the roughened edges of the cuff tendons catching against the anterior edge of the acromion and coracoacromial ligament. Pain is felt at the front of the shoulder, and one may reproduce it by simply raising the upper arm to 90°.

19. How is the bicipital groove best palpated?

Pinpoint tenderness in the biceps groove is best localized with the humerus in about a 10° of internal rotation, placing the long tendon to face directly anteriorly and located 6 cm below the acromion (Fig. 8-17). This point tenderness should move with rotation of the arm and often disappears as the lesser tuberosity and groove rotate internally under the short head of the biceps and the coracoid. This "tenderness in motion" is likely the most specific sign implicating bicipital lesions. It does not, however, differentiate biceps tendinitis from long

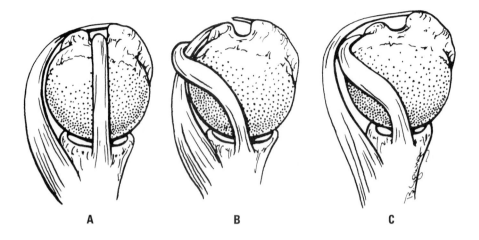

A **B** **C**

FIG. 8-15 A, The normal relationship of the biceps tendon in the groove by the transverse humeral ligament. **B,** Rupture of the transverse ligament and subluxation of the biceps tendon out of the groove with the tendon lying anterior to the subscapularis muscle. **C,** Intratendinous disruption of the subscapularis commonly occurs in which the subscapularis insertion degenerates and the tendon subluxates beneath the muscle tendon belly. The subscapularis tendon may be attached to the greater tuberosity through the coracohumeral and transverse ligaments. (Modified from Petersson CJ: *Aeta Orthop Scand* 54:277-283, 1983.)

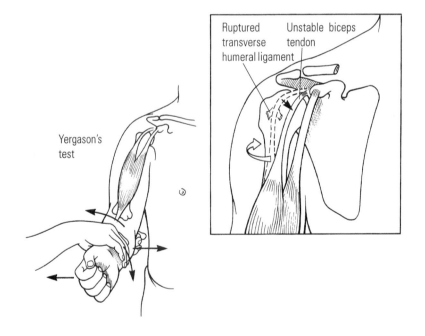

Yergason's test

Ruptured transverse humeral ligament

Unstable biceps tendon

FIG. 8-16 Yergason's test for long biceps tendon stability. The examiner resists supination as the patient simultaneously externally rotates the shoulder against resistance.

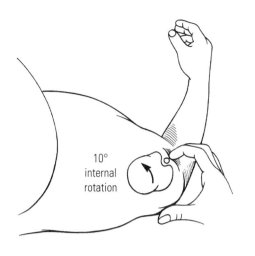

FIG. 8-17 The biceps tendon may be palpated directly anteriorly with the arm in 10° of internal rotation.

biceps tendon instability. Although some authorities claim that the long tendon can actually be felt subluxating in and out of the groove, it is in reality difficult to discern whether what one is feeling is actually a subluxating tendon or deltoid muscle bundles rolling up against the humerus by the examiner's hand pressed against the humerus; this is especially so in a well-muscled individual.[2]

20. What forms of imaging are appropriate in detecting biceps brachii lesions?

Because routine plain radiographs of the shoulder appear normal with proximal biceps tendinitis, special views are indicated when biceps involvement is suspected. The bicipital groove view determines medial wall angle; the width, presence, or absence of bicipital groove spurs; coexisting degenerative changes in the greater or lesser tuberosity; and the presence or absence of a supratubercular ridge. In addition, a caudal tilt view may reveal the degree of anterior acromial prominence or spurring, which would implicate a commonly missed source of proximal biceps tendon lesions: coracoacromial arch impingement syndrome.[2]

Shoulder arthrography may also provide information on the state of the biceps tendon; for example, whether a shallow groove appearing on a plain radiograph is associated with a dislocation of the long tendon. Arthrography in patients with biceps tendinitis shows an intact rotator cuff but with the biceps poorly outlined, having a thickened sheath, or elevated at its origin.

The long tendon as well as the bicipital groove can also be assessed with computerized tomographic arthrography.

21. What is the clinical sign of strain of the long head of the biceps brachii at its glenoid origin?

Localized pain is felt at the acromioclavicular joint. All passive and resistive movements of the shoulder and elbow, including pronation and supination, are painless. Only resisted adduction is painful, and only when the elbow is kept extended. This characteristic is suggestive of the constant-length phenomenon and implicates the long tendon of biceps.[4] Treatment is by steroid injection.[3]

22. At which sites does the biceps brachii tendon most likely rupture, and who is most vulnerable?

Rupture of the biceps most commonly occurs in the long head at one of three locations: (1) in the shoulder joint, (2) at the bicipital groove, or (3) distally at the musculotendinous junction on the ulna. A fourth location, the origin of the long tendon on the supraglenoid tubercle, may also occur.[15] Ruptures most commonly affect middle-aged individuals, most likely as a result of attritional and degenerative changes in the tendon. Rupture may occur spontaneously or as the result of muscular strain as from lifting a heavy load.

23. What is the presentation of sudden proximal tendon rupture?

During sudden tendon rupture the patient experiences immediate sharp pain[15] at the time of rupture, a feeling that something has snapped[5] or "given way."[9] There is sometimes an audible pop in the shoulder. Mild swelling and ecchymosis of the upper anterior arm[15] as well as a change of contour of the biceps muscle occurs over the next several days because of subcutaneous bleeding.[5] Weakness of the forearm supinators and elbow flexors also develop. With time, swelling and bruising will subside and the muscle fibers comprising the long head may still contract, albeit unrestrained proximally. This takes the appearance of a firm ball of muscle[5] that is more distal than normally expected and is palpable as a soft hump when the elbow is flexed or the forearm is supinated,[15] especially against resistance. This deformity will persist and is sometimes called the *Popeye sign* after the well-known cartoon sailorman (Fig. 8-18). The short head of the biceps continues to function and may even hypertrophy. There is little loss of power because of the contractile[5] contributions of the

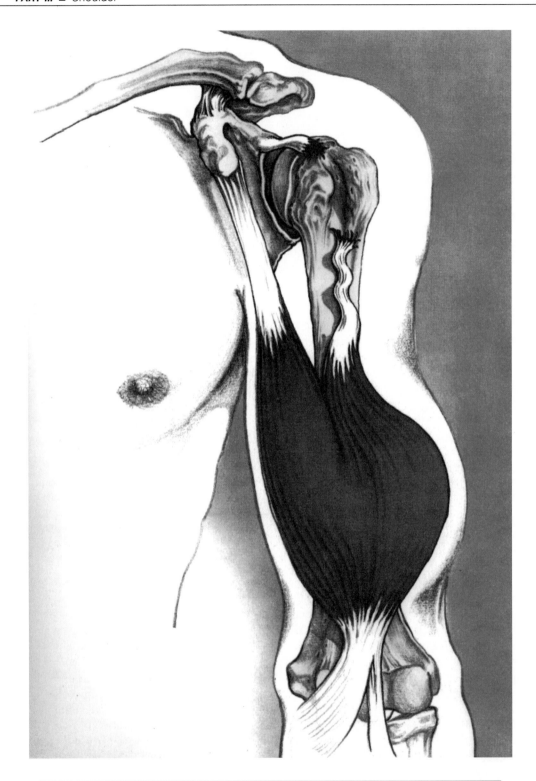

FIG. 8-18 Proximal long tendon biceps rupture with retraction of torn tendon ends. (From Peterson L, Renström P: *Sport injuries: their prevention and treatment,* London, 1986, Martin Dunitz, Ltd.)

short biceps head and brachialis and brachioradialis muscles.[15] Movement of the shoulder is little affected.[15] Surgical repair is not necessary, since the resulting disability is mild and is indicated only for individuals involved in strong physical work that requires strong elbow flexion, as well as for cosmesis. Surgery is therefore appropriate in young or athletic patients and in those individuals performing heavy physical labor.[15]

24. What is the mechanism for distal tendon avulsion?

Avulsion or rupture of the distal tendon off the ulna is uncommon and is caused by sudden forceful flexion of the elbow against resistance.[15] There may be a history of heavy exertion against a major resistance[7] that may have, in times past, initiated degenerative changes in the tendon or at its insertion at the radial tuberosity.[15] Pain is sudden and profound[5] and is accompanied by pronounced swelling. Forearm supination is considerably weakened, whereas elbow flexion strength has a good muscle grade because of substitution of other muscles. Unlike with proximal tendon rupture, there is minimal upward retraction deformity because of the yet-intact second distal attachment at the radial tuberosity. Long-term symptoms of moderate aching and supination weakness are sometimes permanent and lead to moderate disability of the arm. Surgical repair consisting of reattaching the tendon to the radial tuberosity is usually indicated but not mandatory unless the bicipital aponeurosis is also ruptured. Results of surgery are generally good.[15]

25. What is bicipital tenosynovitis at the lower arm?

This disorder usually occurs in athletes who engage in repetitive activities such as weight lifting, bowling, and gymnastics. Symptoms include elbow pain and weakness, with the former exacerbated by direct palpation of the distal end of the tendon and provoked by resisted flexion and supination,[7] just as full passive pronation does at the elbow joint. This exacerbation is especially noted when the elbow is held flexed because this position presses the radial tuberosity against the ulna.[3] Pain may radiate down the anterior forearm as far distally as the wrist. X-ray findings are unremarkable. Treatment includes rest, ice, elevation, compression, NSAID modalities, deep friction massage, iontophoresis, and modification of training errors.[7] Deep transverse friction massage is performed by application of the tip of the thumb to the top of the radial tuberosity anteriorly while the therapist's other hand alternately pronates and

supinates the forearm while grasping the patient's hand.[4] Therapeutic exercises should focus on increasing flexibility of the flexor mechanism as well as muscle strength.[7] Steroid injection may be performed but is best avoided because of the risk of tendon rupture.

26. What is bicipital tendinitis of the lower arm?

With bicipital tendinitis of the lower arm, pain is confirmed by palpation over the distal musculotendinous junction into the ulna and is confirmed by local anesthesia. Treatment includes deep friction massage,[4] stretching, strengthening, and NSAIDs.

27. How is a brachialis muscle disorder differentiated from a lesion of the biceps brachialis?

Pain elicited on resisted flexion with the forearm fully pronated is produced only by the brachioradialis, whereas pain on flexion with supination implicates the biceps as well as the brachialis. The position of the forearm does not affect brachialis function, since this muscle is recruited under all conditions of flexion. The biceps is recruited to assist the brachialis if heavy resistance is required in supination or to move very quickly.

28. What is the differential diagnosis?

Differential diagnosis includes the following:
- *Anterior shoulder instability* caused by glenohumeral joint dislocation has several features in common with dislocation of the long biceps tendon. Pain is present in the anterior shoulder, is episodic in nature, and is, like the biceps lesion, associated with a palpable and audible clunk. Indeed the mechanism of injury described for both of these conditions is very similar in that they most commonly occur with forced abduction and external rotation. The differential diagnosis can be even more confusing in the event that anterior shoulder instability and impingement syndrome coexist. The differences between these two pathologic conditions are quite noticeable, and so the examiner need not confuse one with the other. In anterior shoulder instability, aside from there often being an obvious swelling within the patient's armpit, the maximum point of apprehension and clicking should be at 90° abduction and maximum external rotation (that is, a positive apprehension sign). Whereas in the patient with a medially subluxating biceps tendon, pain is not maximal until the arm is brought down from the position of maximum abduction and external rotation

and the click occurs as the examiner begins to internally rotate the arm *(biceps instability test)*. Yergason's and Speed's signs should not be present in patients with anterior shoulder instability. In addition to provocative testing, roentgenographic shoulder views clarify the diagnosis. Computerized tomography (CT) is helpful in demonstrating both the biceps tendon within the groove as well as lesions of the anterior cartilaginous labrum in patients with instability. If, after the above studies, the diagnosis still remains unclear, glenohumeral arthroscopy may be performed and allows direct visualization of the anterior labrum as well as the intraarticular portion of the biceps tendon, the aperture of the sulcus, and the surrounding cuff tissue.[2]

- *Glenoid labrum tears without instability,* such as those that occur in the superior one third of the labrum adjacent to the biceps origin, may demonstrate symptoms similar to those of biceps tendon subluxation and rotator cuff tear. Superior labrum tears occur in athletes who throw, such as baseball players, and result in an audible or palpable clunk occurring as the tear flips in and out of the joint, impinging on normal humeral head excursion during rotation above the horizontal plane. When encountering a throwing athlete with shoulder pain, one finds that patients may report more pain on ball release because of the deceleration effect of the biceps pulling on the torn labrum. Computerized tomography may occasionally not reveal this lesion, and the best way to differentiate this disorder from that of a subluxating biceps tendon may be by glenohumeral arthroscopy.[2]

- The *coracoid impingement syndrome* shares similar symptoms to biceps tendinitis and instability. The normal coracoid-to-humeral distance is calculated at 8.6 mm and is noted to be decreased to some 6.7 mm in patients with coracoid impingement syndrome. Thus this condition is associated with patients who have excessively long or laterally placed coracoid processes, or in those individuals who have undergone bone block or osteotomy procedures for instability. Symptoms of coracoid impingement include dull pain in the front of the shoulder with referral to the front and upper arm and occasionally extending into the forearm. Symptoms are consistently provoked by forward flexion and internal rotation or abduction and internal rotation, and it differs from the more common type of impingement syndrome by being most painful on forward flexion between the un-usual ranges of 120° to 130°. Suspicion of this condition is confirmed by obliteration of the patient's pain by a subcoracoid injection.[2]

- The tenderness of *cuff impingement* is often diffuse, is located more proximally, and is accompanied by tenderness in the arm, anterior acromion, coracoacromial ligament, coracoid process, and supraspinatus insertion. Additionally, pain does not move with rotation of the arm. Primary biceps tendinitis rarely exists as an isolated entity and occurs secondarily to cuff impingement syndrome. If one is in doubt, selective injection with a local anesthetic is an indispensable part of the physician's evaluation. Patients suffering from either primary or secondary bicipital tendinitis, unlike those with rotator cuff tendinitis, find no relief from lidocaine injection into the subacromial space. Injection is performed at the lateral or posterolateral corner of the acromion into the subacromial space so as to avoid inadvertent injection into the groove. It is important to remember that the subdeltoid bursa, which extends to the groove, is continuous with the subacromial bursa, and so inadvertent injection into the groove area will anesthetize the subacromial bursa. If an isolated biceps injection relieves all pain and restores 100% of motion, a diagnosis of primary biceps tendinitis is justified.[2]

- Tenderness of *subdeltoid bursitis* is generally more diffuse and should not change with arm rotation.[2]

- Early *glenohumeral joint arthritis* frequently presents as anterior shoulder pain with limited range of motion. Because the long biceps tendon is an intra-articular structure, it may become involved with any process within the joint. Thus inflammatory changes occur in the synovia of the biceps recess just as they do in the subscapular and axillary recess. Plain radiographs may show bone spurring of the proximal humerus with a ring osteophyte and flattening of the glenoid. Double-contrast arthrography may reveal thinning of the articular cartilage before the development of obvious osseous spur formation.[2]

- *Brachial neuritis* (syndrome of Parsonage and Turner) is an extremely painful condition that frequently presents as anterior shoulder pain. The early course of this condition, usually preceded by viral illness, manifests as pain exceeding neurologic findings, and the examiner may be fooled into thinking that he or she is dealing with an acute calcific tendinitis. Later, numbness and weakness with obvious atrophy become prominent. This condition occurs mainly in young men and produces supraclavicular pain, weakness, and diminished reflexes in the distribution of the brachial plexus as well as minor sensory abnormalities. The rostral plexus and thus proximal musculature become involved in two thirds of all cases. Profound weakness may occur within a day to a week of onset, only to regress over the subsequent 3 months. The cause is unknown, though viral or immunologic inflammatory processes are suspected. The course is variable.[2]

- *Thoracic outlet syndrome* (see Chapter 18) is ruled out when provocative tests such as Wright's maneuver, Adson's test, or Roo's overhead grip test score positive with negative or equivocal findings in Yergason's, Speed's, and impingement tests. Subacromial and bicipital injections should not completely alleviate pain.[2]

- *Frozen shoulder* (see Chapter 13) is differentiated from biceps lesions by the presence of severely diminished joint play in the former. Additionally, when the physician injects and infiltrates the biceps tendon sheath with 2 to 3 ml of lidocaine and the patient's pain is obliterated but there is no appreciable change in motion, adhesive capsulitis is suspected.[2]

- *Cervical radiculopathy,* especially at the level of C5-C6, may also mimic primary shoulder lesions. Similarly, *peripheral nerve entrapment* caused by carpal tunnel syndrome (see Chapter 4) ulnar neuritis, or posterior interosseous nerve entrapment may refer pain proximally to the shoulder. These pathologic conditions may be a source of differential confusion in the patient with proximal bicipital tendinitis. These entities however are distinguished from biceps disorders by careful neurologic examination, provocative testing, and electromyograph and nerve conduction velocity testing when in doubt.[2]

- In patients with persistent anterior shoulder pain in whom a work-up for a primary shoulder disorder shows normal results and neurologic examination is unrevealing, a tumor may be suspected.[2]

29. What rehabilitative treatment is most appropriate for proximal biceps brachii tendinitis, and when is surgery appropriate?

The treatment of the varied lesions of the biceps tendon, except for acute traumatic rupture in the young patient or in association with massive cuff tear in an active patient, is best managed with conservative care and repeated evaluation. The guiding criterion is that, as long as the patient is making gradual improvement, surgical intervention is not recommended. Surgery is indicated only after a minimum of 6 consecutive months of conservative care. This is especially so in patients over 65 years of age.[2]

In the case of proximal biceps *impingement tendinitis,* treatment initially closely follows that of rotator cuff impingement and tendinitis (see pp. 113-118, and 133-135). In the event of a failed conservative treatment outcome, surgical treatment primarily focuses on repair of the rotator cuff and decompression of the subacromial arch (acromioplasty procedure). Biceps tenodesis is appropriate only in the event that the tendon is extremely frayed as from severe attrition wear, such that rupture appears to be imminent, or in the event that reconstruction of the fibrous roof of the arch is impossible.

No attempt is usually made to repair chronic ruptures (greater than 6 weeks) of the long biceps tendon; here, surgery involves only removal of the intraarticular portion of the tendon. The patient is informed preoperatively that he or she will continue to have a bulge in the lower portion of the arm.

Surgical treatment of *biceps instability* is often recommend in patients under 50 years of age, especially if the injury is acute. *Once dislocation of the biceps tendon is clinically suspect and then confirmed by sonography, one may also assume concomitant rupture of a portion of the rotator cuff. This concomitance depends on the intimate relationship the biceps tendon shares with the rotator cuff tendons just proximal to the groove, where the latter serve as a significant medial restraint to the long tendon of the biceps. The idea here is that if the long tendon restraint is compromised the probability of medial subluxation is greatly increased because of loss of the cuff's dynamic checkrein preventing subluxation and dislocation.* Indeed, surgically proved biceps instability is virtually always related to a degenerative process in the cuff, restraining capsule, and coracohumeral ligament in the proximal portion of the groove. As such, confirmed instability warrants open tendon reduction and reconstruction of the rotator cuff and subacromial decompression.[2]

Patients who suffer from *attrition tendinitis* (Fig. 8-19) best respond to judicious use of rest, NSAIDs, moist heat, and gentle exercises. Judicious use of corticosteroid injection may also be helpful; however, it is absolutely imperative that injection be into the bicipital

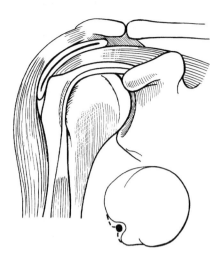

FIG. 8-19 The cuff is exposed to show the constriction of the biceps tendon within the groove. Local formation of new bone and connective tissue causes stenosis of the bicipital groove, leading to attrition of the tendon of the long head of the biceps. (Modified from Paavolainen P, Slatis P, Aalto K: Surgical pathology in chronic shoulder pain. In Bateman JE, Welsh RP, editors: *Surgery of the shoulder,* St. Louis, 1984, Mosby.)

sheath and not into the tendon so as not to cause collagen necrosis. There may be as much as a 35% loss of tendon strength immediately after injection, and such a loss reverses after approximately 2 weeks. However, ultrastructural changes within the tendon do not completely revert for 6 weeks. Because of this, patients should avoid any strenuous activity for 3 weeks. These injections frequently make the patient more comfortable quickly and shorten the course of the illness. Although injection has been shown to be equally efficacious to the use of indomethacin (Indocin), some patients unfortunately cannot tolerate a nonsteroidal antiinflammatory agent in the doses required. Surgery is recommended only if the patient fails to respond to conservative care over a 6 to 12-month period.[2]

30. What postoperative care is appropriate to patients having undergone surgery for a proximal biceps brachii lesion?

During the first 3 postoperative weeks a Velcro elastic immobilizer is often utilized, and the patient is encouraged to take his or her elbow out of the immobilizer and gently flex and extend it passively with the opposite hand. Gentle pendulum exercises are initiated on the first postoperative day, and passive elbow flexion is initiated on the second postoperative day. Pulley exercises should be avoided during the immediate postoperative period, since holding onto a pulley handle requires some active contraction of biceps; instead, passive shoulder flexion and external rotation are appropriate. At 1 month, a pulley may safely be introduced and gentle, active elbow flexion started. Strengthening of the repaired cuff, deltoid, and biceps generally begins at 2 months and becomes more vigorous at 3 months. Jobs that require lifting should be avoided until approximately 6 months postoperatively.[2]

REFERENCES

1. Asimov I: *The human body,* New York, 1992, NAL-Dutton.
2. Burkhead WZ: The biceps tendon. In Rockwood CA, Matsen FA, editors: *The shoulder,* vol 2, Philadelphia, 1990, Saunders.
3. Cyriax J: *Textbook of orthopaedic medicine, vol 1: diagnosis of soft tissue lesions,* ed 8, London, 1982, Bailliere-Tindall.
4. Cyriax J: *Textbook of orthopaedic medicine,* vol 2, ed 11, London, 1984, Bailliere-Tindall.
5. Dandy DJ: *Essential orthopaedics and trauma,* Edinburgh, 1989, Churchill Livingstone.
6. Gilcreest EL: Rupture of muscles and tendons, particularly subcutaneous rupture of the biceps flexor cubiti, *JAMA* 84:1819-1822, 1925.
7. Lillegard WA, Rucker KS: *Handbook of sports medicine: a symptom-oriented approach,* Andover, Mass, 1993, Butterworth-Heinemann.
8. Lippman RK: Frozen shoulder, periarthritis, bicipital tenosynovitis, *Arch Surg* 47:283-296, 1943.
9. Lippman RK: Bicipital tenosynovitis, *NY State J Med* 44:2235-2240, 1944.
10. Magee DJ: *Orthopaedic physical assessment,* Philadelphia, 1989, Saunders.
11. McCue FC III, Zarins B, Andrews JR, et al: Throwing injuries to the shoulder. In Zarins B, Andrews JR, Carson WG, editors: *Injuries to the throwing arm,* Philadelphia, 1985, Saunders.
12. Mercer A: Partial dislocations: consecutive and muscular affectations of the shoulder joint, *Buffalo Med Surg* J 4:645-652, 1959.
13. Meyer AW: Spolia anatomica: absence of the tendon of the long head of the biceps, *J Anat* 48:133-135, 1913-1914.
14. Moore KL: *Clinically oriented anatomy,* ed 2, Baltimore, 1985, Williams & Wilkins.
15. Netter FH: *The CIBA collection of medical illustrations, Musculoskeletal system,* part II, vol 8, Summit, NJ, 1990, CIBA-Geigy.
15a. Netter F: *The CIBA collection of medical illustrations,* vol 8, part I.
16. Neviaser RJ: Painful conditions affecting the shoulder, *Clin Orthop* 173:63-69, 1983.
17. O'Donohue D: Subluxating biceps tendon in the athlete, *Clin Orthop* 164:26, 1982.

18. Rathbun JB, McNab I: The microvascular pattern of the rotator cuff, *J Bone Joint Surg* 52B:540-553, 1970.

19. Salter RB: *Textbook of disorders and injuries of the musculoskeletal system,* ed 2, Baltimore, 1983, Williams & Wilkins.

20. Simon WH: Soft tissue disorders of the shoulder: frozen shoulder, calcific tendinitis, and bicipital tendinitis, *Orthop Clin North Am* 6:521-539, 1975.

RECOMMENDED READING

Burkhead WZ: The biceps tendon. In Rockwood CA, Matsen FA, editors: *The shoulder,* vol 2, Philadelphia, 1990, Saunders.

Lillegard WA, Rucker KS: *Handbook of sports medicine: a symptom-oriented approach,* Andover, 1993, Butterworth-Heinemann.

Peterson L, Renström P: *Sport injuries: their prevention and treatment,* London, 1986, Martin Dunitz, Ltd.

9

Loss of Active Right Shoulder Elevation after Injury without Painful Arc

A 43-year-old male house painter spent the past 21 years of his working life engaged in the vocation of ceiling painting as his specialty. He reports having a history of bilateral shoulder tendinitis with "clicking" while raising his arms overhead. About 2 weeks ago he reports how half a can of paint fell onto his right shoulder. Since that time he complains of not quite being able to use his shoulder the same as before and feels stiff and weak when attempting to elevate his right arm overhead. When asked to elevate actively, he does so with the following bizarre substitution: by placing his hand on the outer side of his ipsilateral thigh and then twitching his hip outwardly while bending his trunk over to the opposite side. There is no report of pain anywhere along the active range; nor is there any painful arc of passive range, though passive movement seems guarded after 110° of elevation. When asked to elevate without substitution, he attempts what appears to be an overexaggerated right shoulder shrug that manages to elevate to some 40° momentarily before flopping down to his side (positive Mosely test).

OBSERVATION   There is no ecchymosis observed at the shoulder.

PALPATION   Mild tenderness is elicited over the right proximal humeral tuberosities and bicipital groove.

RANGE OF MOTION   There is full active as well as passive medial and lateral rotation of the right shoulder joint, though some pain is reported through these ranges.

MUSCLE STRENGTH   The muscle strength was not clearly tested with secondary guarding in various ranges; nevertheless, external right shoulder rotation appears to show decreased strength by at least one entire muscle grade. Otherwise normal.

SELECTIVE TENSION   Symptoms of pain and guarding as well as apprehension are elicited on passive right shoulder internal rotation. Resistive external rotation yields similar results. Otherwise normal.

SPECIAL TESTS   Negative Ludington's test, negative Yergason's test, negative Allen test, negative impingement sign, positive drop arm test, negative Speed's test, negative Adson's maneuver.

SENSATION   Normal.

DEEP TENDON REFLEXES   Normal.

After referring the patient for a radiographic series of both shoulders, the radiologist confirms your suspicion.

CLUE:

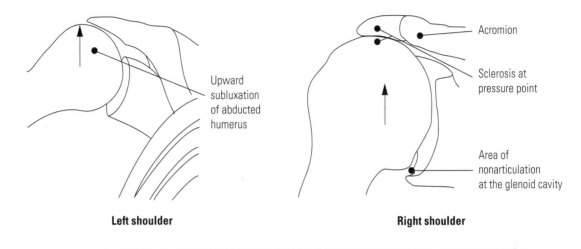

Xeroradiograph schematic of right and left shoulder. (From Dieppe PA, Bamji AN, Watt I: *Atlas of clinical rheumatology,* Baltimore, 1980, Lea & Febiger.)

❓ Questions

1. What is most likely wrong with this painter's shoulder?
2. What is the mechanism of injury?
3. What four stages successively occur during the evolution of rotator cuff disorders?
4. What area of the cuff tendon or tendons is most susceptible to involvement of rotator cuff injury?
5. What occurs during fiber failure, and what are the adverse effects, if any?
6. What is the likelihood for self-repair after cuff tear?
7. How do the cuff tendons contribute to humeral head elevation after cuff tear?
8. Is there an age-related epidemiologic correlation associated with rotator cuff tears?
9. What is the classification of injury in rotator cuff tendon disorders?
10. What is the differential diagnosis?
11. Is the presence of painful arc on passive or active elevation clinically revealing?
12. Can diagnosis of cuff tears be reliably made from the patient's history and physical examination alone?
13. What imaging techniques are best suited for confirmation of cuff tear?
14. What conservative treatment is appropriate in the stage I lesion?
15. What rehabilitative therapy is appropriate for the stage II and chronic stage III shoulders?
16. When is surgery appropriate?
17. What is the most commonly used surgical technique?
18. What factors account for decreased likelihood of success after surgical attempt at cuff repair?
19. What rehabilitation is appropriate after surgery?
20. How are partial- and full-thickness cuff tears managed in the elderly?

1. What is most likely wrong with this painter's shoulder?

Full-thickness tear of the right rotator cuff (Fig. 9-1), and partial-thickness tear of the left rotator cuff tendons. The former is obviated when viewing radiographs of the right shoulder showing cephalic humeral head subluxation and compression lesion at the head of the acromion.[8a]

2. What is the mechanism of injury?

The proposed causes of cuff tendon failure have included trauma,[4] attrition,[8] ischemia,[18] impingement,[23] and steroid injection.[19] Age-related changes in the rotator cuff include diminution of tendon vascularity, diminution of fibrocartilage at the cuff insertion, fragmentation of the tendon with loss of cellularity, disruption of the attachment to bone via Sharpey's fibers,[2] and eventually tendon infarct.[26] Let us assume that the normal cuff starts life out well vascularized and with a full complement of fibers; throughout its active life the cuff is subjected to repeated adverse exposure the likes of which include traction, contusion, impingement, inflammation, injections, and age-related degeneration, each of which place the cuff tendons at jeopardy for increased risk of injury[19] (Fig. 9-2). It is perhaps a wonder then that pathologic states do not occur more commonly than they do.

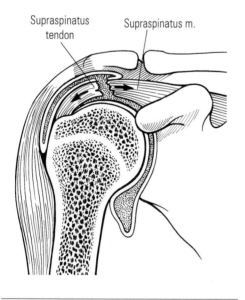

Supraspinatus tendon

Supraspinatus m.

FIG. 9-1 Full-thickness tear of the rotator cuff tendons.

3. What four stages successively occur during the evolution of rotator cuff disorders?

STAGE I

Edema and hemorrhage[11] initiated by repeated microtrauma and presenting as a toothache-like discomfort felt after activity that is aggravated by provocative movements such as forced flexion at end range (impingement sign), forced internal rotation with the arm horizontally adducted and the shoulder at a 90° elevation, and a painful arc at around a 90° abduction. The supraspinatus tendon will be painful to palpation because of[11] impingement in this stage I disorder. Similarly the adjacent biceps tendon may also be tender at its bicipital groove exit in the event that it impinged under the subacromial arch. This *subacute stage*[11] is most often present in patients under 25 years of age,[24] but onset may occur at virtually any age. Stage I is *reversible* and may be viewed as a setting stage for the next level of disorder along the continuum of rotator cuff pathosis: tendinitis.

STAGE II

Tendinitis is characterized by thickening and fibrosis of the tendons and bursae because of a vicious cyclic reinforcement of impingement vis-à-vis inflammation-edema–increased tendon volume with decreased suprahumeral space whose end result is further aggravation and impingement that eventually results in tendon infarct[11] and scarring. This stage most commonly occurs in the 25 to 40 year age group[23] and presents as a toothache-like pain most frequently experienced at night or after athletic activity.[23] The range of motion begins to decrease because of fibrosis and thickening of soft tissue. Rest, though important, is of limited value in that it can no longer reverse the pathologic process. Some stiffness may be reported.[11] All the previously mentioned signs applicable to the preceding impingement stage also apply here, including the presence of an impingement sign.

STAGE III

Partial-thickness tear caused by further tendon degeneration with toothache-like pain usually severe enough to cause a limitation of activity and loss of sleep occurs, and there may also be weakness reported and greater stiffness than before.[11] There is usually a history of tendinitis.[11] The patient can begin abduction but experiences pain or a painful arc during the attempt. Active abduction becomes more comfortable after injection of a local anesthetic, and this feature helps differentiate tendinitis or partial tear from a complete tear of the rotator cuff, since the patient with a large tear does not regain strength (i.e., active range of motion) after the subacromial space is anesthetized. If ignored, cuff tears, like a rip in nylon, tend to propagate themselves.[19]

STAGE IV

Full-thickness tear of the rotator cuff occurs as the final stage of a degenerative process in which the provoked tendon succumbs to something as trivial as opening up a stuck window or more seriously after sustaining a fall on the shoulder[28] or on an outstretched adducted arm.[11] A complete tear may also occur after greater humeral tuberosity fractures, or from shoulder dislocations. The patient, usually a man over 60 years of age, cannot initiate abduction and merely shrugs the shoulder on attempting to do so;[28] there is also weakness on flexion and external rotation.[19] Thus, while he exhibits a lack of active range, his passive range is not severely limited unless chronic or painful.[11] The synchronized force couple between deltoid and the rotator cuff muscle is lost, and the deltoid, acting unopposed, causes upward humeral migration that is visible on a radiograph and an observed altered glenohumeral rhythm. Altered biomechanics adversely influence the length-tension relationships of the remaining intact cuff musculature by placing them at a mechanical disadvantage, thus

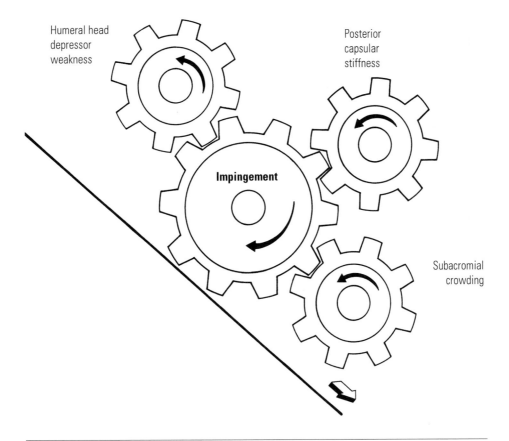

FIG. 9-2 Normal shoulder function is dependent on normal function of the humeral head depressors, normal capsular laxity, and adequate subacromial space. Some of the effects of impingement (weakness of the humeral head depressors, stiffness of the posterior capsule, and crowding of the subacromial space with thickened bursa) may further intensify impingement, producing a self-perpetuating process. (From Rockwood CA, Matsen FA, editors: *The shoulder,* ed 2, vol 1, Philadelphia, 1990, Saunders.)

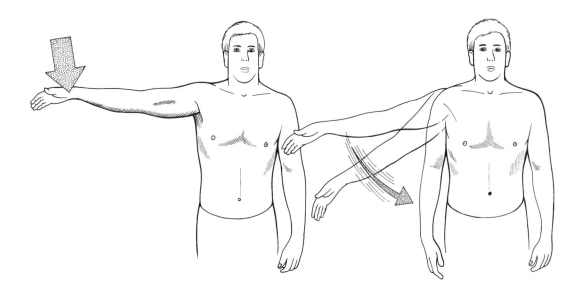

FIG. 9-3 A full-thickness tear of the rotator cuff is verified by a positive *drop-arm test*. The patient is unable to lower his arm slowly to the side in the presence of a torn cuff.

predisposing atrophy and wasting of these muscles. In long-standing cases, muscle wasting may be observed. If the arm is passively abducted to 90°, the patient is capable of maintaining this position by means of the deltoid muscle;[28] the drop-arm test scores as positive[11] (Fig. 9-3).

Many patients with full-thickness cuff tears have palpable cuff defects, as well as mild tenderness over the proximal humeral tuberosities, bicipital groove,[19] and anterior acromion and usually over the acromioclavicular joint.[13] Muscle wasting in the suprascapular and infrascapular fossae may occur, especially when the condition is long standing.[13] A large tear will preclude active shoulder abduction even when local anesthesia is administered to block pain perception.[20] After complete tear the proximal portion of the tendon will retract, allowing the glenohumeral joint to freely communicate with the subacromial bursa. Thus arthrography provides confirmation of the suspected full-thickness tear when injected radiopaque dye into the glenohumeral joint spreads into the bursae.

4. What area of the cuff tendon or tendons is most susceptible to involvement of rotator cuff injury?

Tears of the rotator cuff are usually *longitudinal* but may be transverse and occur in a *critical zone* (see Fig. 8-10) situated at the anterior portion of the cuff located within the subacromial space between the supraspinatus tendon and the coracohumeral ligament.

5. What occurs during fiber failure, and what are the adverse effects, if any?

Cuff tendon ruptures clinically present as soft-tissue disruption both at the tendon insertion as well as at its midsubstance. Fibers fail when the applied load (whether repetitive or abrupt, compressive or tensile) exceed tendon strength and may fail a few at a time or en masse (known as an acute tear or acute extension). Because fibers are under a load even with the arm at rest, they will retract after rupturing. Each instance of fiber failure has, at the very least, three adverse effects: (1) it increases the load on the neighboring soft tissue because there are now fewer fibers to share the load; (2) it detaches muscle fibers from bone and therefore diminishes the force the cuff can deliver; (3) it risks the anastomotic vascular elements in proximity by distorting their anatomic features.[19]

6. What is the likelihood for self-repair after cuff tear?

Although some tendons such as the Achilles tendon have a remarkable propensity to heal after rupture, rotator cuff tendons lack a similar resiliency since the intraarticular environment does not favor the rebuilding of new fibers. The reason is that cuff ruptures com-

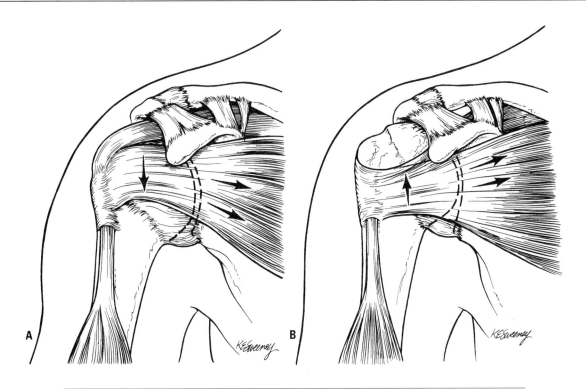

FIG. 9-4 A, In addition to the supraspinatus, the anterior and posterior rotator cuff muscles and the long head of the biceps tendon depress the humeral head and balance the upward-directed forces applied by the deltoid muscle. **B,** Major cuff fiber failure and retraction allow the humeral head to protrude upward through the cuff defect, creating *boutonniere lesion.* When the remaining cuff tendons slip below the equator of the head, their action is converted from humeral head depression to humeral head elevation. (From Rockwood CA, Matsen FA, editors: *The shoulder,* vol 1, ed 2, Philadelphia, 1990, Saunders.)

municate with joint and bursal fluid, which removes any hematoma that might contribute to cuff healing.[19] Additionally the tear itself compromises the cuff tendon blood supply,[19] and even if the tendon could heal with a scar, scar tissue lacks the normal resilience of tendon and is therefore under increased risk for failure with subsequent loading.[19] Finally, rupture itself is accompanied by retraction of the torn ends of the tendon. The cumulative effect of these factors considerably diminish the cuff's ability to repair itself effectively.

7. How do the cuff tendons contribute to humeral head elevation after cuff tear?

One of the major functions of the rotator cuff is humeral head depression though this function is progressively compromised during the evolution of rotator cuff disorder. With progressive loss of the depressor mechanism the humeral head rises higher and higher because of the unrelenting upward pull of the deltoid. In the event of a major defect in the rotator cuff after rupture, the humeral head can now migrate even further proximally by protruding through the defect. Eventually, the relationship of the cuff tendons to the humeral head is such that the tendons slip below the equator of the humeral head. The biomechanics are changed to such an extent that the action of the intact tendons are converted from depression to that of humeral head elevation. This *boutonniere deformity,* just like that in the finger, victimizes the buttonholed cuff by changing its line of pull so as to convert balancing forces into unbalancing forces[19] (Fig. 9-4).

8. Is there an age-related epidemiologic correlation associated with rotator cuff tears?

Yes. Patients with rotator cuff tears are almost always over 40 years of age.[25] The supraspinatus does not often rupture in young people because their tendons are so strong that they rather will avulse the tip of the greater tubercle of the humerus than rupture the tendon.[22]

9. What is the classification of injury in rotator cuff tendon disorders?

Many terms have been used to classify cuff tendon failure, such as partial- and full-thickness tears, acute and chronic tears, and traumatic and degenerative tears.

Full-thickness tear refers to when the tendon deficit extends all the way through the articular surface to the bursal surface of the rotator cuff. *Partial-thickness tear* refers to when the tendon defect involves only the deep surface, midsubstance, or superficial surface of the tendon; these tears occur twice as often as full-thickness tears.

Chronic tears are those that have existed 3 months or more; they may be insidious in onset and are degenerative in nature. *Acute tears* occur suddenly, usually the result of a definitive injury such as a fall. An already chronic tear is at risk for an *acute extension*—the sudden failure of additional fibers with the production of acute symptoms superimposed on those of a chronic tear.

Cuff tears are also characterized according to the length of detachment from the humerus, the specific tendons involved, and the state of the detached tendon or tendons, such as retracted, atrophic, or absent. It is important to realize that cuff failure is always almost peripheral, near the tenoperiosteal junctions on the tuberosities, and nearly always on the supraspinatus tendon because that tendon runs adjacent to the biceps tendon.[19]

10. What is the differential diagnosis?

Differential diagnosis includes the following:
- *Cuff tendinitis* and *bursitis* are differentiated from cuff tears through arthrography or ultrasonography.
- Whereas partial-thickness cuff defects may demonstrate motion restriction, patients with full-thickness defects usually have a good range of passive motion but may be limited in strength or active range of motion.
- Although *cervical spondylosis* at C5 or C6 may produce pain and weakness in a pattern similar to rotator cuff involvement, radiculopathy is also inclusive of sensory, motor, and reflex abnormalities as additional diagnostic findings and furthermore as abnormal electromyographic findings, as well as pain often elicited on neck extension or when the chin is turned to the affected side.[19]
- *Suprascapular neuropathy* is characterized by dull pain over the shoulder exacerbated by shoulder movement, weakness in overhead activities, weakness of external rotators, spinal wasting, and normal radiographic evaluation, ultrasonography, and arthrography. Suprascapular neuropathy may arise from one of three causes: (1) *traction* injury to the suprascapular nerve as in an Erb's palsy type of injury, (2) *stenosis* at the suprascapular notch causing suprascapular nerve entrapment and resulting in chronic recurrent pain and weakness aggravated by shoulder use, (3) *brachial neuritis,* such as acute brachial neuropathy of unknown causes characterized by spontaneous onset of rather intense shoulder pain lasting several weeks with onset of weakness noted as pain subsides; atrophy and weakness occur chiefly in the rotator cuff, deltoid, and triceps as well as in muscles not supplied by the brachial plexus (that is, serratus anterior, trapezius, and the diaphragm); additionally there is occasionally minor sensory deficiency mainly affecting the axillary nerve distribution. The diagnosis of brachial neuritis is based on this observed pattern, recorded by electromyography, and occurring only in those individuals with no history of trauma.[32]
- A *snapping scapula* may produce shoulder pain on elevation and a catching sensation reminiscent of a rotator cuff tear. However, whereas the latter is usually elicited regardless of whether the scapula is stabilized or is allowed to rotate freely, scapular snaps arise from the superomedial scapular corner with just mere shoulder shrugging and without the presence of glenohumeral joint motion.[19]
- A superior sulcus *(Pancoast's) tumor*[19] (see p. 195).

11. Is the presence of painful arc on passive or active elevation clinically revealing?

Most probably yes. Cyriax maintained that active elevation yielding painful arc is indicative of tendinitis only, whereas a positive test for painful arc on passive elevation indicates rupture of supraspinatus.[7] Other authorities do not differentiate between active or passive pain-provoking movement possibly because of clinical evidence of full active range of motion in many cases of supraspinatus rupture.

12. Can diagnosis of cuff tears be reliably made from the patient's history and physical examination alone?

No. Imaging evaluation is necessary because cuff tears are not always symptomatic.[19] Patients with full-thickness and certainly partial-thickness tears have been known to exhibit strong active shoulder elevation, possibly attributable to substitution by other intact shoulder elevators.

13. What imaging techniques are best suited for confirmation of cuff tear?

Plain radiographs are usually normal in small cuff tears, except for some sclerosis on the acromial undersurface, but demonstrate upward humeral head displacement (that is, *subluxation*) with respect to both glenoid and acromion in partial tears because of loss of the tendons interposed between the humerus and acromion; this feature is better viewed by external rotation of the arm as the patient attempts isometric abduction. Plain radiographs of full-thickness tears are additionally characterized by several outstanding features: (1) appearance of a narrowed interval or even articulation between the humeral head and the acromion; this *acromiohumeral interval* normally measures between 7 and 14 mm; (2) concomitant widening or even nonarticulation of the inferior aspect of the humeral head with the inferior glenoid fossa; and (3) frequent sclerosis and osteophyte formation on the anteroinferior acromion and possibly on the greater tuberosity[13] as well.

Diagnostic ultrasonography reliably demonstrates the location and extent of cuff tears greater than 1 cm,[19] has the advantage of speed and safety, and is usually half the cost of an arthrogram and one eighth the cost of a magnetic resonance imaging (MRI) scan, all this despite the fact that ultrasonography does not detect small full-thickness tears and partial-thickness defects.[19] Arthrography shows intravasation of dye into the subacromial space (bursa) after injection and vigorous exercise that extends beyond the normal cuff attachment at the greater tuberosity, as well as a *geyser sign,* that is, dye leakage into the acromioclavicular joint. Arthrography is particularly effective in revealing suspected partial-thickness tears as well as larger tears but cannot reveal midsubstance or superior-surface tears. Shoulder MRI suffers from problems of image resolution.[19]

14. What conservative treatment is appropriate in the stage I lesion?

(See pp. 118-120 for a hypothetical treatment strategy of supraspinatus impingement syndrome.)

Stage I treatment: Because stage I is reversible, the primary thrust of treatment must be prevention of the underlying process causing injury. This is accomplished by vocational or athletic activity modification so as to permit noninjurious and biomechanically efficient motion. By educating the patient, coach, and trainer to understand how, for example, internal shoulder rotation during elevation may cause impingement vis-à-vis the subacromial arch, the patient may learn to substitute his or her motions with noninjurious movement patterns. This aspect of treatment cannot be overemphasized because treating the inflammation will do little good if the precipitating source of injury is still operative.

- Pain-limited *stretching* into external rotation in several positions of abduction is initiated because external rotation provides clearance, allowing the greater humeral tuberosity to swing back freely under the anterior acromion during active shoulder abduction; otherwise impingement will serve only to further exacerbate the injury.[11]

- Isolated *strengthening* of the supraspinatus, infraspinatus, and teres minor muscles while deemphasizing the deltoid muscle group serves to centralize the humeral head within the glenoid fossa and works to counter the tendency toward superior humeral invasion of the suprahumeral space.[11] The rotator cuff muscles are isolated for strengthening by the positions of (1) internal and external rotation in the neutral position, (2) external rotation at 90° of abduction,[16] and (3) shoulder abducted to 90° only, with the arm in slight forward flexed 30° to 45° and in full internal rotation[1] (Fig. 9-5). Electromyographic output of the supraspinatus is greatest in this last exercise.[16]

Shoulder elevation above 90° should be initiated with a D1F (flexion–adduction–external rotation) proprioceptive neuromuscular (PNF) pattern before one advances to a D2F (flexion–abduction–external rotation) pattern.[29]

A light weight ought to be used (up to 5 lb), and the patient must remain in the pain-free range. Shoulder rotation exercises may initially be performed with the patient in side-lying position because the supraspinatus and subacromial bursae are unlikely to become irritated in this position. Also, this position is more likely to prevent reflex inhibition of muscles (Fig. 9-6).

The use of rubber tubing (Fig. 9-7) is especially helpful because the slow return of the limb to the rest position delivers an eccentric contraction to the muscles antagonistic to the desired direction of strengthening. Concentric and eccentric exercises may also be performed using wall weights (Fig. 9-8).

- *Selective strengthening* of the serratus anterior and other scapular rotators is essential. The scapula functions as a floating origin for the rotator cuff muscles, and its movement must be in synchrony with the demands of glenohumeral joint motion. By ensuring that the scapular muscles work in time with the demands of shoulder elevation, one can also ensure that

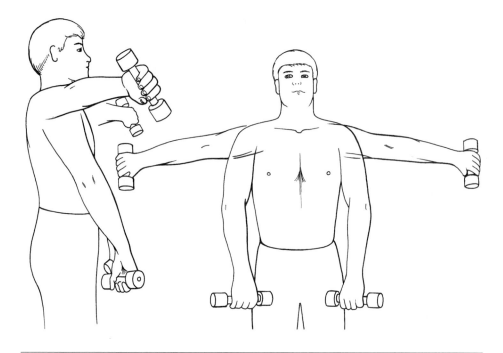

FIG. 9-5 Selective strengthening of the supraspinatus muscle. The patient should stand with the arm at the side and internally rotate the shoulder so as to pronate the forearm. The patient then starts elevation by moving diagonally toward abduction and arrives at 90° of abduction at 30° to 45° in front of the coronal position.

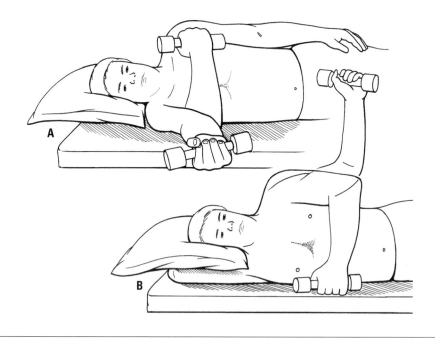

FIG. 9-6 Internal and external rotator-strengthening exercises using free weights. **A,** Internal rotator strengthening. **B,** External rotator strengthening.

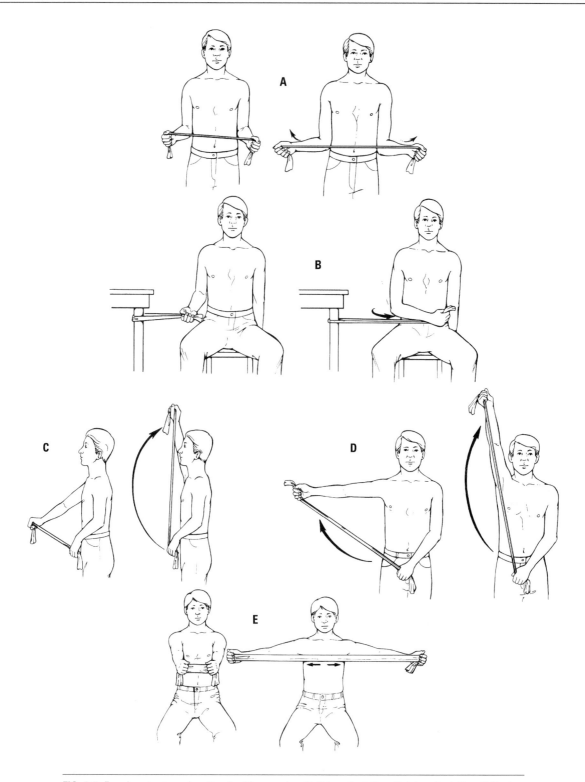

FIG. 9-7 Exercises to strengthen the shoulder muscles. **A,** External rotation. **B,** Internal rotation. **C,** Flexion. **D,** Abduction. **E,** Horizontal abduction. (From Saunders HD: *Evaluation, treatment and prevention of musculo-skeletal disorders,* Bloomington, Minn., 1985, Educational Opportunities.)

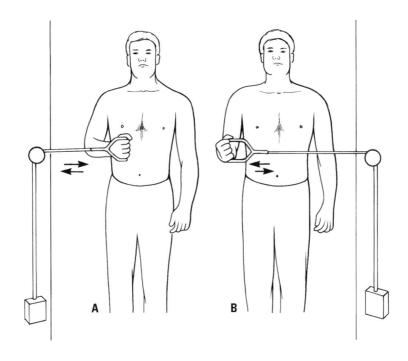

FIG. 9-8 External and internal rotator concentric and eccentric strengthening using wall weights.

the muscles and tendons of the rotator cuff will operate close to an ideal length and tension and are less likely to suffer fatigue and undergo attrition. Furthermore, kinesiologically sound scapular protraction permits timely elevation of the coracoid process allowing it to rotate clear of the abducting humerus.[17] Two exercises that help strengthen the upper trapezius and the serratus anterior are shoulder shrugs and push-ups with the arm abducted to 90°.[3]

• *Selective flexibility* of tightened shoulder girdle muscles. The affected muscles are slowly stretched while antagonistic isometric contraction is performed. After isometric contraction, the muscles relax, and further stretching may be applied (contract-relax technique). Contraction of the antagonist produces reciprocal relaxation of the agonist, permitting more effective stretching.[34] Stretching activities are recommended after a hot bath, as well as before and after aerobic exercise.[36]

Stretching activities may be performed in supine with a two to five pound cuff weight wrapped around the waist. Three important stretches are: (1) 90° shoulder abduction and elbow flexion, with as much external rotation as possible will stretch the anterior shoulder capsule and soft tissues; (2) 135° shoulder flexion with

external rotation to stretch the anteroinferior capsule and soft tissues; and (3) reaching as far overhead as possible, with the palm toward the ceiling and the elbow extended will stretch the most inferior portion of the shoulder capsule[44] (Fig. 9-9).

• A valuable treatment in the management of a stage I lesion is the application of light to deep *transverse friction massage* to the supraspinatus tendon. Pressure is applied just proximal to the tendon insertion on the greater tubercle. Friction is applied in a direction perpendicular to the normal orientation of the tendon.[14]

• Selective total *rest*. Selective rest does not mean complete inactivity but rather an alternative motion that will permit the shoulder to achieve the movement objective. For example, a pitcher may resort to the use of a different pitching style while time is allowed for healing of the rotator cuff. However, some authorities maintain that pain sufficient to affect performance is an indication for total rest from the aggravating activity.

Rest should extend beyond the activity, whether vocational or avocational, that precipitated impingement. It is important to emphasize to the patient the responsibility of elevating the arm in ways that avoid im-

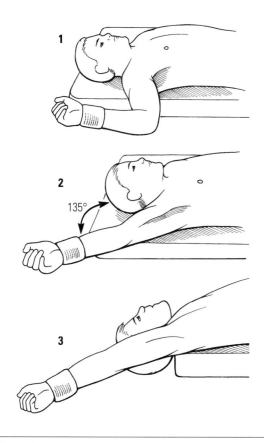

FIG. 9-9 Stretching of the rotator cuff muscles and glenohumeral shoulder capsule. Position 1 stretches the medial rotators and anterior shoulder capsule. Position 2 stretches the anterioinferior capsule. Position 3 stretches the inferior capsule.

pingement in all his or her activities of daily living. This is very important during this potentially reversible stage.

- *Cryotherapy* for approximately 10 minutes after workouts[10] using an ice cup, slush bag, ice pack, or refreezable gel pack.
- *Therapeutic ultrasound* increases blood flow and increases permeability of cell membranes, resulting in improved exchange of metabolic products.[12] The ultrasound dosage to the treatment of the supraspinatus and bicep tendons vary according to the amount of interposing tissue. The more superficial biceps tendon requires between 0.8 and 1.2 watts/cm for 5 minutes daily for 10 days, whereas the supraspinatus tendon requires 1.2 watts/cm for 5 minutes daily for 10 days.[13] The use of ultrasound is controversial because being a deep-heat modality it may occasionally exacerbate symptoms.

- *Transcutaneous electrical nerve stimulation*[30] helps decrease pain. Electrotherapy may promote organization of collagen alignment because of a piezoelectric effect within the tendon during the healing phase.[6]
- An upper-arm *counterforce brace* may be placed high on the arm directly over the biceps tendon. It is theorized that the strap has a tenodesis effect on the biceps, making it a more effective humeral head depressor.[17]
- Emphasis on *prevention* cannot be stated enough at this still-reversible stage. Time therefore is an important ally in treatment. Warm-up routines should involve flexibility exercises and isometric contractions or light isotonic activities. The purpose of warm-up activities is to increase body temperature, particularly for muscles. As such, it is important to avoid fatiguing the shoulder with these preliminary exercises. Cooldowns after exercise are also important.
- *Massage* of shoulder muscles promotes increased circulation and relaxation and may be helpful before workouts.[13]
- Steroid injection into the adjacent subacromial bursa[11] is losing popularity because of catabolic effects to local metabolism. A less-invasive and more-benign form of relief provided by delivery corticosteroids is by *phonophoresis* or *iontophoresis*.[27]
- Pendulum exercises with[5] or without[9] weights may be performed during the acute phase.
- Orally administered *nonsteroidal antiinflammatory medications*.

The advanced phase of rehabilitation concentrates on the progressive return to normal function. The patient may progress from the use of free weights to resistive activities performed on an exercise machine.

15. What rehabilitative therapy is appropriate for the stage II and chronic stage III shoulders?

A nonoperative trial of conservative therapy is attempted. The patient is forewarned that it may take up to 6 weeks to yield improvement and is admonished not to abandon therapy just because the shoulder is not better in a few days! Treatment includes all exercises of the previous stage except for the use of surgical tubing, which is contraindicated because it tends to overload the rotator cuff.[31]

- Rest.
- Nonsteroidal antiinflammatory medication.
- Avoidance of precipitating activities.
- Steroid injections.[24]

- Gentle stretching activities to the rotator cuff muscles in all areas of tightness.
- Gentle internal and external rotation-strengthening exercises beginning with isometrics and progressing to rotation against resistance using rubber bands or light weights with instruction to the patient not to overdo exercise lest the cuff becomes further aggravated. A useful guide to the patient is that any soreness from exercises must subside within a few minutes after finishing the workout. Strengthening with the shoulder above 60° of elevation is avoided so as to prevent excessive tendon loading as well as tendon wear under the coracoacromial arch.
- Greater emphasis should be placed on range-of-motion activities to prevent adhesive capsulitis.

16. When is surgery appropriate?

If at the end of a 6-week conservative treatment regimen cuff imaging indicates an intact rotator cuff, patients are advised to continue working on their program for an additional 6 weeks. Patients with persistent symptoms are examined frequently and should not be lost to follow-up study; otherwise they may come back a year or so later with an irreparable cuff tear.[19] Criteria for operative treatment includes (1) a patient is younger than 60 years of age, (2) failure to improve after a nonoperative treatment regimen of not less than 6 weeks, (3) presence of a full-thickness tear, either clinically or by imaging techniques, (4) the patient's need to use the involved shoulder in a vocation or an avocation, (5) full passive range of motion that must be present to warrant operative treatment, (6) the patient's own willingness to forego loss of some active abduction in exchange for decreased pain and increased strength of external rotation, and (7) the ability and willingness of the patient to cooperate.[19] In addition, acute tears are best repaired within 3 weeks of initial injury before retraction, scarring, tendon-edge degeneration, and muscle atrophy occur to a substantial degree.

17. What is the most commonly used surgical technique?

Open acromioplasty (partial acromionectomy) accompanied by connective tissue reconstruction and surgical reattachment of the torn tendon complex into a bony trough created on the greater tuberosity.[11] However, when major amounts of cuff tissue have been lost, repair is not possible.[13]

18. What factors account for decreased likelihood of success after surgical attempt at cuff repair?

- An insidious, atraumatic onset of rotator cuff disorder
- Grade 3 or less of external shoulder rotation strength
- Age greater than 60 years
- Upward humeral head displacement relative to the glenoid and acromion
- History of multiple steroid injections

The surgeon may, in fact, find that the cuff tendons have all the strength of wet Kleenex.[19] This is the situation in which a neglected rotator cuff tear remains untreated and the lesion progresses to what is known as *rotator cuff arthropathy,* a term that denotes destruction of the humeral articulating surface occurring after a neglected massive cuff tear that is distinctly different from changes such as osteoarthritis, rheumatoid arthritis, and avascular necrosis of the humeral head. Whatever remains of these severely weakened cuff tendons are prone to failure after any attempted cuff repairs.

19. What rehabilitation is appropriate after surgery?

Postoperatively the patient's shoulder is immobilized in a position of abduction for 3 weeks[28] by an abduction bolster to protect against early tension on the repaired tendon from the adducted position. Horizontal adduction and internal rotation are also to be avoided. As early as the second postoperative day passive range of motion exercises with the splint in place are performed within the limits of comfort in the direction of forward flexion and external rotation so as to avoid adhesions and disuse atrophy.[13] Abduction with the shoulder in external rotation is also permitted this early but only if the patient is relaxed in a supine position because the sitting position increases the risk that the patient will assist in an antigravity movement,[11] which is not yet permitted.

The repair is likely to be weakest at 3 weeks when the healing process is underway but no enhancement of tensile strength has yet occurred.[19] During the first 3 postoperative months the cuff repair will not be stronger than it was immediately after surgery.[13]

Active range of motion, including active abduction, may begin at 6 weeks after operation, progressing from gravity-eliminated to gravity-resisted positions. Resistance training is begun at 7 to 8 weeks after operation beginning with 1 lb and focusing on isolated strengthening to each of the cuff muscles.[11] Challenging the repair with large loads should be avoided 6 months to a year.[19]

20. How are partial- and full-thickness cuff tears managed in the elderly?

In the elderly, the best treatment after injury is with simple active exercises as soon as possible with the strategy of preventing shoulder stiffness and palliative measures as well as to reduce pain. Once the possibility of adhesive capsulitis is reduced, rest may eventually permit regain of some active range of motion as the small tear scars over.

Another school of thought advocates placement of the shoulder in a position that most closely approximates the ends of torn fibers while eliminating any movement that may elongate the cuff. This immobilization strategy continues for anywhere between 3 to 8 weeks and promotes the smallest span of scar tissue between the frayed tendon ends while avoiding abduction, forward flexion, and external rotation. Joint mobilization of those shoulder girdle joints not immobilized is imperative to minimize onset of adhesive capsulitis.[21]

REFERENCES

1. Anderson TE: Rehabilitation of common shoulder injuries in athletes, *J Musculoskeletal Med,* p 17, Dec 1988.
2. Brewer BJ: Aging of the rotator cuff, *Am J Sports Med* 7(2):102-110, 1979.
3. Brewster CE, Shields CL, Seto JL, et al: Rehabilitation of the upper extremity. In Shields CL, editor: *Manual of sports surgery,* New York, 1987, Springer-Verlag.
4. Codman EA: Complete rupture of the supraspinatus tendon: operative treatment with report of two successful cases, *Boston Med Surg J* 164:708-710, 1911.
5. Cuillo J: Swimmer's shoulder, *Clin Sports Med* 5:115-136, 1984.
6. Curwin S, Stanish W: *Tendinitis: its etiology and treatment,* Lexington, Mass, 1984, Collamore Press.
7. Cyriax J: *Textbook of orthopaedic medicine, vol 1: Diagnosis of soft tissue lesions,* ed 8, London, 1982, Bailliere-Tindall.
8. DePalma AF, Gallery G, Bennet CA: Variational anatomy and degenerative lesions of the shoulder joint, *Instr Course Lect* 6:255-281, 1949.
8a. Dieppe PA, Banjami AN, Watt I: *Atlas of clinical rheumatology,* Baltimore, 1980, Lea & Febiger.
9. Flicker P: The painful shoulder, *Prim Care* 7:271-285, 1990.
10. Gordon EJ: Diagnosis and treatment of common shoulder disorders, *Med Trial Tech Q* 28:25-73, 1981.
11. Gould JA III: *Orthopaedic and sports physical therapy,* ed 2, St Louis, 1990, Mosby.
12. Hawkins RJ, Kennedy JC: Impingement syndrome in athletes, *Am J Sports Med* 8:57, 1980.
13. Hawkins RJ, Hobeika PE: Impingement syndrome in the athletic shoulder, *Clin Sports Med* 2(2):390, 1983.
14. Hertling D, Kessler RM: *Management of common musculoskeletal disorders,* ed 2, Philadelphia, 1990, Lippincott.
15. Holt LE: *Scientific stretching for sports,* Halifax, Nova Scotia, 1973, Dalhousie University.
16. Jobe F, Moynes D: Delineation of diagnostic criteria and rehabilitation program for rotator cuff injuries, *Am J Sports Med* 10:336-339, 1982.
17. Johnson J, Sim F, Scott S: Musculoskeletal injuries in competitive swimmers, *Mayo Clin Proc* 62:289-304, 1987.
18. Lindblom K: Arthrography and roentgenography in ruptures of the tendon of the shoulder joint, *Acta Radiol* 20:548, 1939.
19. Matsen FA, Arntz CT: Rotator cuff failure. In Rockwood CA, Matsen FA, editors: *The shoulder,* vol 1, Philadelphia, 1990, Saunders.
20. Meals RA: *One hundred orthopaedic conditions every doctor should understand,* St Louis, 1992, Quality Medical Publishing.
21. Moffat M: *Musculoskeletal therapeutic exercise,* New York University Department of Physical Therapy Lecture, Nov. 1990.
22. Moore KL: *Clinically oriented anatomy,* ed 2, Baltimore, 1985, Williams & Wilkins.
23. Neer CS II: Anterior acromioplasty for the chronic impingement syndrome in the shoulder: a preliminary report, *J Bone Joint Surg* 54A:41-50, 1972.
24. Neer CS II: Impingement lesions, *Clin Orthop* 173:70-77, 1983.
25. Neer CS II, Flatow EL, Lech O: *Tears of the rotator cuff: long term results of anterior acromioplasty and repair.* Paper presented at the American Shoulder and Elbow Surgeons, fourth meeting, Atlanta, Feb 1988.
26. Nirsche RP, Pettrone F: Tennis elbow: the surgical treatment of lateral epicondylitis, *J Bone Joint Surg* 61A:8332, 1979.
27. Richardson A: Overuse syndromes in baseball, tennis, gymnastics and swimming, *Clin Sports Med* 2:379-389, 1983.
28. Salter RB: *Textbook of disorders and injuries of the musculoskeletal system,* ed 2, Baltimore, 1983, Williams & Wilkins.
29. Sullivan PE, Markos PD, Minor MA: *An integrated approach to therapeutic exercise: theory and clinical application,* Reston, Va., 1982, Reston Publications.
30. Sunderstrom WR: Painful shoulders: diagnosis and management, *Geriatrics* 38:77-92, 1983.
31. Thein LA: Impingement syndrome and its conservative management, *J Orthop Sports Phys Ther* 11:189, 1989.
32. Weaver HL: Isolated suprascapular nerve lesions, *Br J Accident Surg* 15:117-126, 1983.

RECOMMENDED READING

Blackburn TA: The off-season program for the throwing arm. In Zarins B, Andrews JR, Carson WG, editors: *Injuries to the throwing arm,* Philadelphia, 1985, Saunders.
Cofield RH: Current concepts review: rotator cuff disease of the shoulder, *J Bone Joint Surg* 67A:974-979, 1985.
Hawkins RJ, Hobeika PE: Impingement syndrome in the athletic shoulder, *Clin Sports Med* 2:394, 1983.
Moynes DR: Prevention of injury to the shoulder through exercises and therapy, *Clin Sports Med* 2(2):413-422, 1983.

10

Chronic Right Shoulder Pain and Crepitus during Elevation, Swimming, or Carrying a Briefcase

A 23-year-old female complains of pain when elevating her right shoulder and when carrying her briefcase in either hand to and from work. She has worked as a lifeguard specializing in swim instruction of the crawl and butterfly strokes for the past four summers at an all-girls summer camp. She appears to be in excellent physical condition and, when questioned, admits to swimming 200 laps a day during the three summer months for several years. She also complains of a slight "grinding" or "crunching" sensation when actively elevating her right shoulder. She admits that her left shoulder bothers her as well, though not as much as her right shoulder. There is no history of injury.

OBSERVATION   There is no apparent muscle wasting of the suprascapular or infrascapular fossae. She has prominent pectoralis and anterior deltoid muscles because of hypertrophy.

PALPATION   There is mild pinpoint tenderness slightly inferior to the anterior border of the acromion while the shoulder is passively extended. In addition, there is a slight sensation of crepitus felt upon active elevation.

RANGE OF MOTION   Within functional limits but with a positive upward painful arc at 80° to 120°.

STRENGTH   Normal.

FLEXIBILITY   Normal.

JOINT PLAY   There is mild posterior capsular tightness of the right glenohumeral joint.

SELECTIVE TENSION   Presence of painful resisted external rotation and abduction as well as during passive internal rotation while the shoulder is elevated to 80°.

SPECIAL TESTS   Negative drop-arm test, positive impingement sign, negative Speed's test, negative Adson maneuver.

? QUESTIONS

1. What is the most likely cause of this woman's pain?
2. What is "impingement syndrome"?
3. What are the subacromial arch and its components?
4. What osseous variations in acromial architecture predispose to a rotator cuff disorder?
5. What synergic relationship exists between deltoid and supraspinatus that is imperative to successful shoulder elevation?
6. Can elevation occur if either supraspinatus or deltoid is weak or paralyzed?
7. What is the pathokinesiology accounting for painful arc symptoms?
8. What accounts for the painful arc experienced at elevation end range in patients whose impingement has progressed to tendinitis?
9. What is the clinical presentation?
10. What provocative tests serve as important clinical confirmation?
11. Which pattern of capsular tightness of the glenohumeral joint is commonly found with the impingement syndrome?
12. What effect does an immobilized scapula have on the impingement syndrome?
13. What is the proposed mechanism of the pathologic condition in the young athletic population?
14. What accounts for the greater percentage of impingement syndrome in butterfly swimmers?
15. How do weight lifters become prone to supraspinatus tendinitis?
16. How do tennis players become vulnerable to supraspinatus tendinitis?
17. What is the proposed degenerative mechanism of the pathologic condition in the older population?
18. Are the subacromial arch disorders clinically differentiable?
19. Is there any single model that explains the mechanism of impingement?
20. Which occupations are particularly prone to development of impingement syndrome?
21. What cuff-imaging techniques are available to help diagnose this condition?
22. What therapeutic management is most appropriate to patients suffering from impingement syndrome?
23. Describe a hypothetical treatment sequence for this patient.
24. When is surgery appropriate?
25. What are the three surgical options?
26. What is the postoperative surgical program?
27. What is the success rate for returning athletes to competition after surgery?

1. What is the most likely cause of this woman's pain?

Impingement of the right supraspinatus tendon (Fig. 10-1).

2. What is "impingement syndrome"?

The term "impingement syndrome" was popularized by Charles Neer in 1972.[18,20] Neer ascribed a unity to the range of pathologic conditions plaguing the shoulder by introducing the concept of a continuum of shoulder disorders that may begin with supraspinatus impingement and may eventually progress to partial or even complete tears of the rotator cuff. He also pointed out that physical as well as plain radiographic findings are often inadequate and unreliable in differentiating between chronic bursitis and partial-thickness tears versus full-thickness cuff tears.[19] Presumably the structures involved are quite small (as when compared to the larger soft-tissue structures of the lower extremity) and are packaged together so tightly that provocative movement of one structure, whether by active, passive, or resistive movement, may elicit pain in an adjacent structure by virtue of being in tight proximity. "Impingement" of the supraspinatus or other cuff tendons within the narrow confines of the subacromial arch is not simply another way of saying rotator cuff tendinitis. Rather, impingement may be thought of as the predecessor of that next and worsened level of injury along

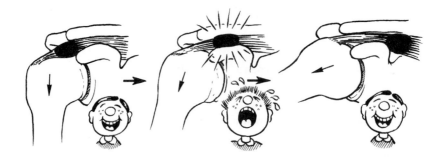

FIG. 10-1 Painful impingement of the right supraspinatus tendon. (From Dandy DJ: *Essential orthopaedics and trauma,* New York, 1989, Churchill Livingstone.)

the continuum of rotator cuff disorders known as *supraspinatus tendinitis* (see pp. 107-108).

3. What are the subacromial arch and its components?

The coracoacromial (synonym: subacromial) arch is a tunnel whose walls are formed by two scapular processes—the acromion located posteriorly and laterally and the coracoid processes located anteriorly and medially. The coracoacromial ligament connects these two processes and does so perforce by means of an oblique orientation of span. Finally the superior rim of the glenoid fossa (scapula) serves as the floor of the arch (Fig. 10-2).

The arch transmits the supraspinatus tendon, the tendon of the long head of the biceps, the subacromial (subdeltoid) bursa, and the coracohumeral ligament. These encased structures are subject to a potential lesion as a function of the arch's fixed volume because of increased pressure secondary to overactivity of the tendons, inflammation, bleeding, or edema.

4. What osseous variations in acromial architecture predispose to a rotator cuff disorder?

Variations in acromial shape are commonly observed in patients with impingement and rotator cuff tears[2] (Fig. 10-3). Three types of acromion are identified: type I (flat), type II (curved), and type III (hooked). The acromion, defining the posterolateral aspect of the subacromial arch, projects anteriorly from the lateral scapular spine. With type III acromia the anteriormost acromial projection is angled inferiorly. There appears to be a strong association between cuff tears and type III acromia.[17] Additionally, degenerative spurs on the anterior

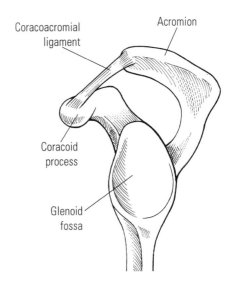

FIG. 10-2 Components of the subacromial arch.

surface of the anterior acromial process[18] may further decrease the volume of the subacromial arch and predispose impingement.

5. What synergic relationship exists between deltoid and supraspinatus that is imperative to successful shoulder elevation?

The kinesiology of shoulder elevation with respect to the subacromial arch is characterized by precise concerted action of the deltoid and supraspinatus muscles. These muscles respectively yield compressive and rotational force components to synergistically facilitate successful shoulder elevation. While the deltoid muscle exerts a compressive force that lifts the shaft of the hu-

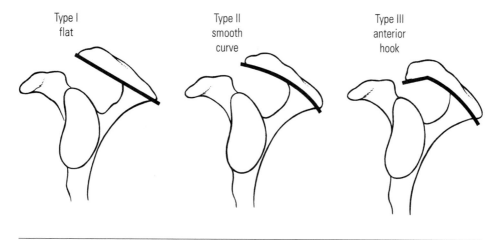

Type I	Type II	Type III
flat	smooth	anterior
	curve	hook

FIG. 10-3 Variations in human acromial posture. (From Rockwood CA, Matsen FA, editors: *The shoulder,* Philadelphia, 1990, Saunders.)

merus into the subacromial space, the supraspinatus, accompanied by the other cuff muscles, pulls the humeral head inferiorly on the glenoid fossa.[23] Without this coupled action, lack of clearance of the greater tuberosity beneath the acromion results in upward ramming of the greater tuberosity against the arch and impingement of the interposing cuff tendon or tendons.

6. Can elevation occur if either supraspinatus or deltoid is weak or paralyzed?

Substitution of adjacent muscles compensates for lack of function of either supraspinatus or deltoid muscles so as to facilitate elevation.

- In the absence of strength or as a result of deltoid weakness, the long head of the biceps brachii may partially assume the deltoid's role when the humerus is externally rotated 90° permitting partial abduction; this may occur though the elevation strength is greatly decreased to some 50% of normal power.[24]
- In the case of a paralyzed supraspinatus, partial active abduction may be achieved by the three remaining and functioning rotator cuff muscles. Initiation of abduction occurs at about 80% of normal power but is rapidly lost as the 90° mark is approached, and so the arm barely resists the pull of gravity.[7] This rationale serves as the basis of the *positive drop-arm test* (see Fig. 9-3) for detection of tears in the rotator cuff, principally of the supraspinatus tendon.[10] Here the substituting musculature lacks sufficient torque to maintain resistance against gravity or the downward push of the examiner's hand.

7. What is the pathokinesiology accounting for painful arc symptoms?

The deltoid muscle is hinged at its origin and therefore exerts a shear force that forces the humerus upward on the glenoid labrum at 0° abduction.[1] As elevation commences and proceeds to 90°, the deltoid's shear forces are converted to a compressive force that vertically forces the humerus more directly into the glenoid cavity[7] (Fig. 10-4). In the event of a weak or damaged supraspinatus tendon, the loss of the rotational force component results in painful impingement attributable to the imbalance of forces (Fig. 10-5).[7] Toward the end of the range of motion, the deltoid's shear forces translate the humeral head on the glenoid labrum,[7] albeit in a downward direction and corresponding to cessation of pain.

8. What accounts for the painful arc experienced at elevation end range in patients whose impingement has progressed to tendinitis?

The 50° to 130° of shoulder range associated with painful arc may be associated with an ischemic wringing out of the less vascular portion of the supraspinatus tendon.[14] Cyriax[6] hypothesized a rationale to explain away *both* the painful arc phenomenon that often occurs as the elevation commences between the 50° to 130° of range and the pain elicited at the very end range of abduction or flexion. Whereas active or passive painful arc is caused by rubbing of the underside of the acromion against a lesion or scar located superficially in the tendon, pain elicited at the end of the range of elevation

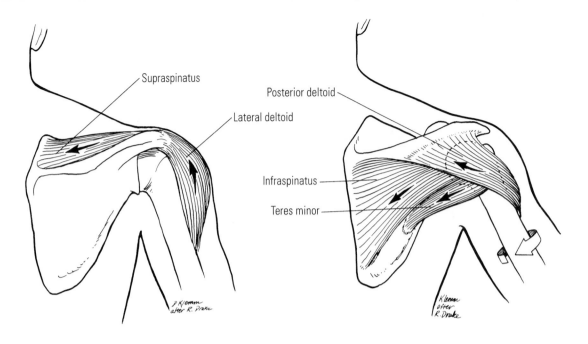

FIG. 10-4 The rotator cuff and deltoid muscle forces at the onset of abduction (0°) and with the arm elevated 90°. The deltoid force changed from a shear to a compressive force. Thus a damaged or weakened supraspinatus muscle causes loss of counterbalance and allows the vertical force of the deltoid muscle to compress the tissue more. (From Bogumill GP: Functional anatomy of the shoulder and elbow. In GIN: Pettrone FA, editor: In *AAOS Symposium on upper extremity injuries in athletes,* St. Louis, 1986, Mosby.)

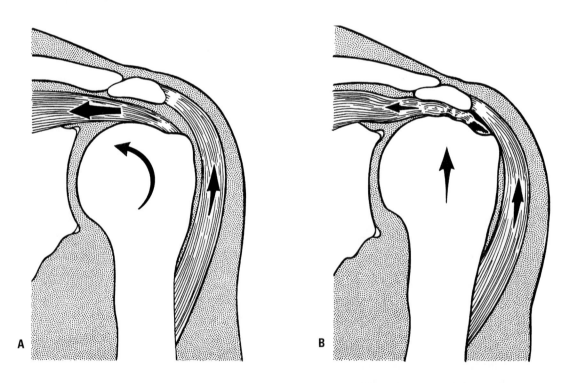

FIG. 10-5 Supraspinatus, exerting a rotational force component, works in synergy with deltoid, which yields a compressive force. Working together, **A,** both muscles facilitate shoulder elevation. **B,** Deep surface tearing of the supraspinatus weakens the cuff's ability to hold the humeral head down and away from the underside of the acromion, resulting in impingement. (From Rockwood CA, Matsen FA, editors: *The shoulder,* Philadelphia, 1990, Saunders.)

is caused by passive stretching of a deep distal scar (Fig. 10-6).

- Fig. 10-6, *A,* shows a superficially located lesion at the tenoperiosteal junction; this will elicit a painful arc during active shoulder elevation due to tensile distraction of the superficial tendon lesion.
- Fig. 10-6, *B,* shows a deeply located lesion at the tenoperiosteal junction; this will elicit pain on full passive elevation since the lesion will be pinched between the greater tuberosity and glenoid rim.
- Fig. 10-6, *C,* shows a lesion that has eroded the entire substance of the distal tendon, that is, at the tenoperiosteal junction as well as proximally throughout the entire tendon; this elicits both passive and active painful arc as well as pain from stretching during full passive elevation.
- Fig. 10-6, *D,* shows a lesion located more proximally at the musculotendinous junction, yielding neither a painful arc nor pain on passive elevation.

9. What is the clinical presentation?

Patients with impingement syndrome usually do not present themselves to the therapist or physician acutely but only after their shoulder symptoms have failed to resolve with time, rest, and trying to "work it out." Patients usually complain of functional losses attributable to pain, stiffness, weakness, and "catching" when the arm is used in the flexed and internally rotated position. Symptoms may also include difficulties in sleeping on the affected side and while carrying out routine activities, such as taking a container of milk from the refrigerator. Pain is often felt down the lateral aspect of the upper arm near the deltoid insertion, over the anterior proximal humerus, or in the periacromial area.[16]

Inspection of the shoulder may reveal deltoid or cuff atrophy, particularly if the condition has been chronic. Palpation usually reveals little if any tenderness, which is in considerable contrast to the sharply localized tenderness characteristic of acute calcific tendinitis. The range of motion is often limited, particularly internal rotation and horizontal adduction, affirming some degree of posterior capsule tightness. Passive motion through the 60° to 90° arc of flexion may be accompanied by pain and crepitus, accentuated as the shoulder is moved in and out of internal rotation. Active elevation of the shoulder is usually more uncomfortable than passive elevation. Strength testing of the shoulder may reveal weakness of flexion and external rotation, which may be either the result of disuse or tendon damage. Pain on resisted abduction or external rotation may

also indicate that the integrity of the cuff tendons has been compromised.[16]

10. What provocative tests serve as important clinical confirmation?

1. *Neer test,* or *positive impingement sign,* is a sign popularized by Neer and Walsh and reproduces pain and concomitant facial grimace when the arm is forcibly flexed forward by the examiner, jamming the greater tuberosity against the anteroinferior acromial surface (Fig. 10-7).
2. The *Hawkins test* consists of flexing the humerus to 90° and forcefully internally rotating the shoulder driving the greater tuberosity farther under the coracoacromial ligament. This test is less reliable than Neer's test[8] (Fig. 10-8).

In both maneuvers injection of 10 ml of lidocaine into the subacromial space followed by pain relief helps confirm the diagnosis and rules out other causes of shoulder pain such as acromioclavicular joint sprain and adhesive capsulitis, which are not relieved by injection.[14]

11. Which pattern of capsular tightness of the glenohumeral joint is commonly found with the impingement syndrome?

Commonly associated with the other signs of impingement is stiffness of the posterior glenohumeral joint capsule[16] resulting in limited forward flexion, internal rotation, and horizontal shoulder adduction.[16] With normal shoulder motion, the humeral head remains centered on the glenoid, whereas with a tightened posterior capsule the humeral head is forced upward against the anteroinferior acromion during forward flexion[16] (Fig. 10-9). Thus the impingement process is a self-perpetuating[16] one that is viciously fed by an increasingly failing humeral head depressor mechanism, a tightened posterior capsule that facilitates encroachment, as well as a limited subacromial volume that is decreased by edematous inflammation.

12. What effect does an immobilized scapula have on the impingement syndrome?

The scapula serves as a floating origin for the cuff muscles, maintaining optimum length-tension ratio of those muscles spanning from scapula to humerus throughout the wide range of shoulder movement. A scapula that does not glide freely over the thoracic wall will adversely affect the length-tension ratios, resulting in impaired cuff function, hence impaired proximal hu-

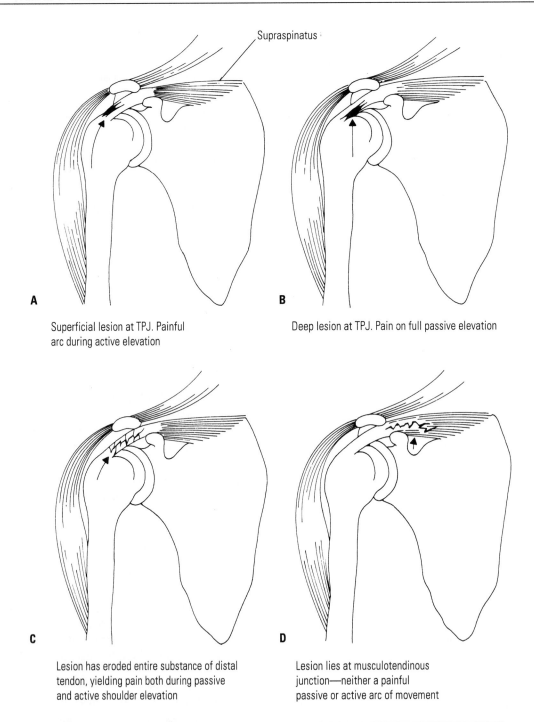

Supraspinatus

A

Superficial lesion at TPJ. Painful
arc during active elevation

B

Deep lesion at TPJ. Pain on full passive elevation

C

Lesion has eroded entire substance of distal
tendon, yielding pain both during passive
and active shoulder elevation

D

Lesion lies at musculotendinous
junction—neither a painful
passive or active arc of movement

FIG. 10-6 The relationship between the site of lesion, range during which pain is perceived, and whether symptoms occur during passive or active provocation. (From Scully RM, Barnes MR, editors: *Physical therapy,* Philadelphia, 1989, Lippincott.)

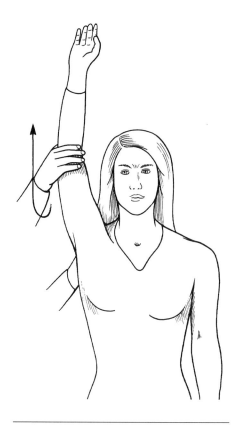

FIG. 10-7 Neer test or positive impingement sign.

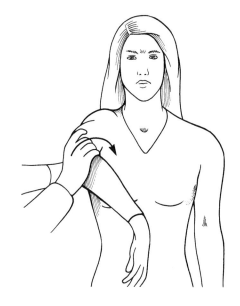

FIG. 10-8 Hawkins test.

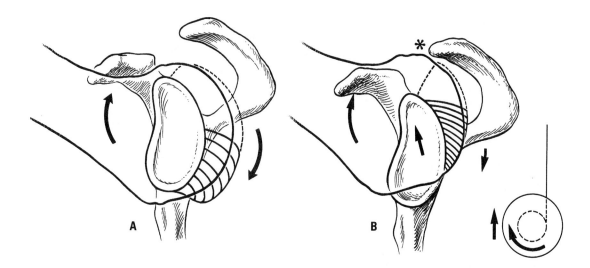

FIG. 10-9 Stiffness of the posterior glenohumeral capsule is commonly associated with signs of impingement. **A,** Normally lax posterior capsule allows the humeral head to remain centered in the glenoid with shoulder flexion. **B,** Stiffness of the posterior joint capsule will aggravate the impingement process by forcing the humeral head upward against the anteroinferior acromion as the shoulder is flexed. This upward transition in association with rotation is analogous to the action of a spinning Yo-Yo climbing a string. (From Rockwood CA, Matsen FA, editors: *The shoulder,* vol 1, Philadelphia, 1990, Saunders.)

meral head depression function. Furthermore, the acromion being both the roof of the arch and a part of the scapula will not be able to elevate high enough to allow optimal clearance of the greater humeral tuberosity.

13. What is the proposed mechanism of the pathologic condition in the young athletic population?

Repetitive microtrauma to the soft tissues housed in the subacromial arch is often attributable to elevation of the glenohumeral joint performed above 80°[7] during sport activities. Classified as an *overuse syndrome,* impingement is most notable with internal humeral rotation[14] during an overhand tennis stroke, the butterfly or crawl swimming strokes, or throwing motion sports. The common traumatic denominator is the proximation of the greater tuberosity to the thick and sharp coracoclavicular ligament.[7]

14. What accounts for the greater percentage of impingement syndrome in butterfly swimmers?

The mechanics of the butterfly stroke, freestyle stroke (Fig. 10-10), and backstroke are similar because they share repeated abduction and internal rotation during the recovery phase. The average competitive swimmer subjects his or her shoulders to approximately 16,000 revolutions per week as compared to the 1000 rev/wk of the professional tennis or baseball player.[11] During the butterfly stroke the humerus is internally rotated during the critical 70° to 120° range of elevation. With pitching, however, the humerus is externally rotated during the windup. This relative external rotation helps clear the greater tuberosity by allowing space for clearance as the humeral head rides beneath the subacromial arch.[7] Additionally, repetitive flexion and internal rotation during swimming may strengthen the pectoralis and the anterior deltoid to the point of hypertrophy. With the passage of time, this may pull the humeral head more anteriorly and only serves to further approximate the humerus to the acromion.

15. How do weight lifters become prone to supraspinatus tendinitis?

The disadvantage of overdevelopment of the deltoid and pectoralis muscles, though esthetically pleasing to some, is an altered biomechanics that contributes to pathologic states. Overdevelopment of the anterior

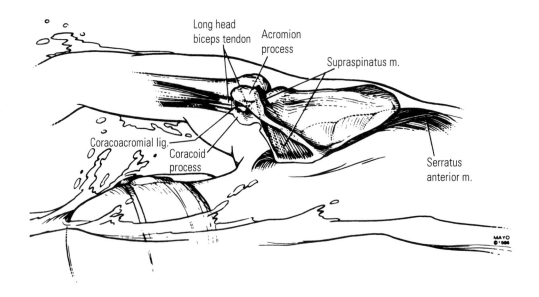

FIG. 10-10 Impingement of supraspinatus and biceps tendons between humeral head and coracoacromial arch can occur with abduction and internal rotation of humerus, as in recovery phase of freestyle stroke. Notice how serratus anterior muscle rotates scapula into abduction as humerus is abducted to allow a greater range of shoulder motion. Scapular rotation also delays impingement of greater tuberosity under coracoacromial arch until humerus is maximally abducted to near 180°. With fatigue or underdevelopment of serratus, humeral impingement may occur at an earlier point in recovery stroke at a lower angle of shoulder abduction. (From Johnson JE, Sim FH, Scott SG: *Mayo Clin Proc* 62:289-304, 1987.)

chest causes an excessively protracted scapula, which alters normal biomechanics by requiring greater external humeral rotation when one is attempting to position the hand overhead. A tightened pectoralis may cause excessive bicipital tendon tracking against the medial border of the bicipital groove.[7] In addition, excessive deltoid hypertrophy may upset the force couple it shares with the cuff muscles and cause upward pulling of the humeral shaft, infringing on the suprahumeral space.[7] Weight lifters must be reminded not to forget strengthening the cuff musculature, coupled with stretching of tight internal rotators.

16. How do tennis players become vulnerable to supraspinatus tendinitis?

Tennis players (see Chapter 7) can irritate their rotator cuff during the follow-through of an overhead shot, allowing the racket to twist their shoulder into internal rotation and extension lateral to their hip. A more correct movement would be letting the racket finish the overhead stroke across the front of the body. Also, a proper toss during the serve may also greatly decrease the faulty mechanics associated with rotator cuff tendinitis.[7]

17. What is the proposed degenerative mechanism of the pathologic condition in the older population?

One of the many important functions of the rotator cuff is depression of the humeral head so as to prevent upward humeral migration. Depression is paramount to ensuring enough clearance during that all-important 70° to 120° elevation range.[14] It is in this range that the perhaps already avascular or swollen portion of cuff tendon barely clears the roof of the arch, if not actually colliding against it.

With the passage of time, age-related changes in the rotator cuff, whether attributable to ischemic or to other changes, result in eventual cuff failure. This process may be accelerated in athletes such as pitchers and swimmers, who place heavy demands upon their shoulders. With progressive loss of the depressor mechanism, the humeral head migrates ever higher because of the overpowering upward pull of the deltoid. The end stage of this process is one in which protrusion of the humeral head occurs through the cuff muscles as a shoulder equivalent of a *boutonniere lesion*. Here, the cuff tendons have slipped below the equator of the humeral head, resulting in an altered biomechanic pattern in which the action of the rotator cuff

is redirected from that of humeral head depression to one of humeral head elevation. Just as in the boutonniere of the finger, the buttonholed cuff is victimized by the conversion of balancing forces into imbalancing forces[16] (see Fig. 9-4).

18. Are the subacromial arch disorders clinically differentiable?

If we understand that the emerging clinical picture is shared by many pathologic states along the continuum of rotator cuff disorders, it is easy to appreciate the great variability of signs and symptoms. However, these finding are not always distinguishable, since tears of the rotator cuff may produce signs and symptoms identical to those found with impingement without rotator cuff tear.[12] Additionally the structures involved are quite small (as compared to the larger soft-tissue structures of the lower extremity) and are packaged tightly together within the subacromial arch, such that provocative movement of one structure, whether active, passive, or resistive, may elicit pain in an adjacent structure by virtue of being in tight proximity.

19. Is there any single model that explains the mechanism of impingement?

Normal shoulder function is dependent on normal function of the humeral head depressors, normal capsular laxity, and adequate subacromial space. There are several models that attempt to explain the basis of impingement. Whatever the mechanism, whether it is Neer's mechanical model, the Pappas et al theory of proximal humeral migration caused by cuff weakness, architectural variations of the acromion that predispose to susceptibility, or the microvascular model offered by Rathbun and MacNab, these theories may be complementary and interdependent in accounting for impingement in an anatomically confined area.[16]

20. Which occupations are particularly prone to development of impingement syndrome?

Painting, carpentry, warehousing, nursing, longshoring, grocery checking, fruit picking, and tree pruning.[15]

21. What cuff-imaging techniques are available to help diagnose this condition?

Many authorities believe that standard radiographs are of little value and even useless in the assessment of rotator cuff impingement.[27] Nevertheless, radiographs may reveal evidence of some of the conditions associated with impingement syndrome, such as acromioclavicular arthritis, chronic calcific tendinitis, and unfused acromial apophyses before age 21.[5] The last refers to the fact that the acromion arises from three separate centers of ossification—preacromion, mesoacromion, and metacromion[3]—that unite by 22 years of age.[22] When these centers fail to unite, impingement may arise from both downward hinging of the acromion as well as from soft spurs or soft-tissue proliferation at the nonunion site.[18]

Plain radiographs may also show subacromial sclerosis from chronic overloading of the acromial undersurface, known as the *"sourcil,"* or *"eyebrow,"* sign. Corresponding sclerosis or cystic changes involving the greater tuberosity may also occur.

Since partial-thickness tears of the rotator cuff may yield an identical clinical picture compared with impingement syndrome, arthrography is a valuable adjunct in the complete evaluation of patients with suspected impingement problems.[4]

Although both shoulder arthrography and arthroscopy may reveal rotator cuff defects involving the deep surface, there is not, as yet, a nonsurgical technique demonstrating midsurface tears of the cuff.[16]

22. What therapeutic management is most appropriate to patients suffering from impingement syndrome?

See pp. 101-105 for an in-depth treatment strategy of stage I rotator cuff lesions.)

The mainstay of *rehabilitative therapy* includes the following:

- Stretching of the posterior glenohumeral joint capsule by mobilization techniques[16]
- Strengthening of humeral depressors
- Maintenance of normal range of motion so as to avoid the onset of adhesive capsulitis[26]
- Strengthening external rotators, extensors, shoulder retractors, and horizontal abductors in swimmers
- Scapulothoracic mobilization
- Emphasizing to patient the importance of consciously externally rotating while elevating the upper extremity
- Resting from activity
- Modifying activities
- Nonsteroidal antiinflammatory medication
- Modality use to relieve symptoms
- Functional electrical stimulation (FES) to suprascapular fossa to strengthen supraspinatus and other cuff muscle bellies

23. Describe a hypothetical treatment sequence for this patient.

- *Range of motion* activities beginning with passive range of motion and progressing to active range of motion were performed in supine position through the range that elicited pain in the erect posture. Thus abduction, flexion, horizontal adduction, and external rotation were performed above the 120° range.
- *Manual traction* to the glenohumeral joint was applied throughout the range of abduction and external rotation to help reduce any painful catching experienced by the patient. After several weeks, traction was required only in the 90° to 110° range. Upper extremity weight bearing on a Swiss ball also helped through the patient's painful range of motion.
- Grade I and Grade II *joint mobilization* were applied to the glenohumeral joint to stretch the tightened posterior capsule. Gains in the extensibility of this portion of the capsule manifested in improved range of motion and a decrease in the perceived painful arc.
- *Moist heat* was applied to the right shoulder and cervical regions for 10 to 15 minutes at the beginning of each treatment. This was performed to increase tissue extensibility of the region and to prime the glenohumeral joint capsule for mobilization.
- Soft-tissue *massage* to the right upper trapezius, levator scapulae, and deltoid regions are helpful before exercise to facilitate tissue extensibility and promote increased circulation and relaxation.
- *Strengthening* of the force couples of the shoulder and scapula was performed by proprioceptive neuromuscular facilitation principles. Diagonal patterns were initially performed isometrically. The patient then progressed to isotonic exercises using three-pound weights. D1F pattern preceded the D2F pattern particularly when the patient is elevating the shoulder above 90°.

Selective strengthening of serratus anterior progressed from wall push-ups to counter push-ups, with the arm abducted to 90°. At the end range of elbow extension, an additional push was encouraged to stress the serratus anterior and thereby enhance protraction. Upper trapezius strengthening progressed from 5 to 8 pounds.

Exercises for shoulder external and internal rotation, flexion, abduction, and extension progressed from isometrics to Thera-Band (see Fig. 9-7) and finally to weights (see Figs. 9-6 and 9-8). Selective strengthening of the rotator cuff was performed with progressively increasing weights (see Fig. 9-5). An Airdyne bicycle was used for shoulder endurance, and strength training progressed from moderate use of the right upper extremity to active propulsion from 5 to 15 minutes.

- *Stretching* of the rotator cuff musculature (see Fig. 9-9) was emphasized as well as the upper and lower fibers of the hypertrophied pectoralis major muscle (Fig. 10-11). Contract-relax techniques proved helpful. The posterior shoulder capsule was stretched by placing the arm in 90° elevation while using the opposite hand to pull the shoulder into horizontal adduction. The inferior capsule may be stretched in the standing position by elevating the arm overhead as far as possible with the elbow flexed and pulling the arm behind the head as far as possible.

- After treatment, *ice* was used for 15 minutes to help retain gains in soft-tissue extensibility. This was terminated after 3 weeks once the patient demonstrated significant gain in painless range of motion and no longer experienced any posttreatment shoulder irritation.[25]

- Application of light *transverse friction* massage just proximal to the insertion of the greater tubercle. Transverse friction disrupts scar tissue and interfibrillary adhesions within the substance of the tendon by forcible broadening of the tendon at its insertion into bone.[6] The induced hyperemia is particularly important here, since hypovascularity may contribute to a rotator cuff tendon disorder.[9] Friction was applied perpendicularly to the span of tendon for 1 to 2 minutes until tenderness subsided, after which pressure was slightly increased for an additional 2 minutes of friction massage. Friction was applied rhythmically at two cycles per second.[9] With successive treatments, pressure and time were gradually increased to 10 minutes. Treatment continued for 10 sessions until the patient reported a decrease in pain.

- The patient was taught *voluntary humeral depression.* The patient was asked to attempt to push her arm caudally, while the therapist provided slight resistance against her elbow for proprioceptive feedback (there was also some scapular depression). The therapist provided verbal reinforcement when the patient suc-

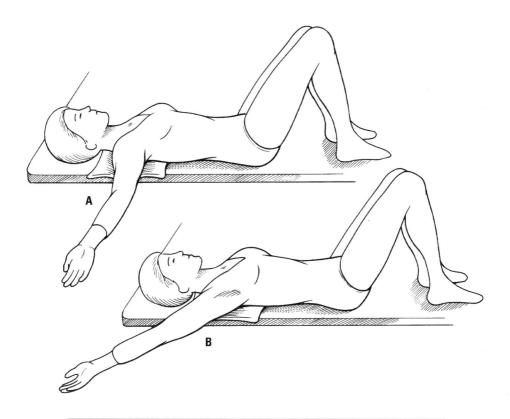

FIG. 10-11 Stretching of, **A,** the upper and **B,** the lower fibers of the pectoralis major.

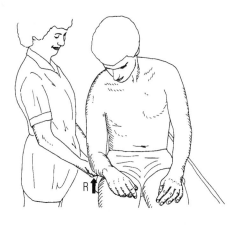

FIG. 10-12 Resistive humeral depression. (From Kisner C, Colby LA: *Therapeutic exercise: foundations and techniques,* ed 2, Philadelphia, 1990, FA Davis.)

cessfully performed caudal glide (Fig. 10-12). The patient then progressed to performing caudal glide upon active abduction.[13]

- *Neuromuscular reeducation* was used to decrease impingement and to facilitate normal shoulder biomechanics. The patient was educated regarding proper warm-ups and cooldowns before and after sport activity.
- A comprehensive individualized *home exercise program* was developed for this patient to help maintain the gains made in the clinic and to prevent recurrence of impingement. This program consisted in progressive stretching and strengthening exercises as well as self-mobilization of the posterior glenohumeral capsule (see Fig. 13-6). All home activities were observed by the therapist to ensure proper form.

After 7 weeks of 21 treatment sessions the patient reported a decrease in pain from 5/10 to 1/10 when carrying her briefcase. She has switched to carrying her briefcase to her left shoulder and has lightened her load by carrying only what is absolutely necessary. She is able to perform overhead activities without pain and demonstrates normal muscle length of her pectoralis major muscle. There is no longer a positive impingement sign. Selective tension is positively painful on external rotation 2/10 from 5/10 at the initial evaluation. She swims frequently and has taken several lessons to modify her stroke. She will continue to perform her home exercise program for both shoulders as well as warm-ups and cooldowns as prevention against future

impingement. The patient was extremely pleased with the results of therapy.

24. When is surgery appropriate?

Surgery is considered only in those patients who, after having undergone a conservative regimen for a minimum of 6 months,[25] and having explored vocational rehabilitation, continue to experience substantial impingement symptoms.[16] In addition, there must be complete active or passive range of motion in the shoulder joint.[21]

25. What are the three surgical options?

All attempts at surgical treatment of impingement syndrome share the common goal of eliminating the arch of the subacromial tunnel. Surgical procedures in order of increasing severity include the following three:

- Resection of the coracoacromial ligament through a deltoid split.[8]
- Partial acromionectomy (open acromioplasty) involves resection of the anteroinferior acromion with most of the coracoacromial ligament removed. Here, the deltoid undergoes a T-shaped incision that permits inspection of the rotator cuff as well as repair of tears, which are later repaired with sutures or wires. The arm is distracted, so that the subacromial space can be visualized, and a bald spot on the humeral head indicates a rotator cuff tear.[21] After surgery, the arm is placed in a sling and passive range of motion exercise is begun on the fourth day. At 8 postoperative weeks strengthening exercises may be initiated. Other surgeons may prefer active assisted range of motion exercise to be performed immediately the same day as surgery as well as internal and external rotation strengthening also begun immediately. Unless there is concern for the strength of the deltoid reattachment the patient is allowed active shoulder range of motion exercise within the range of comfort. Full recovery may take as long as 4 to 6 months.[21] A radical acromionectomy procedure may worsen a patient's condition and compromise shoulder function.[16]
- With arthroscopic acromioplasty the same amount of bone is removed from the anteroinferior acromion as with an open acromioplasty. Afterwards the arm is placed in a sling for 3 to 8 days followed by range of motion exercise initially and progressing to cuff-strengthening exercises over time. The rehabilitation period takes up to 3 months.[21]

26. What is the postoperative surgical program?

Rehabilitation usually begins within the first postoperative week,[7] and on the very day of surgery according to some,[16] with passive range of motion below 80° of flexion and abduction. Passive elevation above 80° is delayed for 2 weeks according to the amount of shoulder inflammation present. Active range of motion exercise begins at 2 postoperative weeks so as not to stress the deltoid. Progressive strengthening with minimum resistance followed by isolation of the rotator cuff muscles so as to promote humeral head centralization while the impingement range of 80° to 120° is avoided. Full external rotation range must be gained before overhand activity is attempted so that clearance and not impingement will occur in the suprahumeral space.[7]

27. What is the success rate for returning athletes to competition after surgery?

The low success rate in returning athletes to competition after surgical decompression[27] tends to reinforce the importance of nonoperative management in this population. Strengthening, stretching, and technique modification are the most effective methods for managing impingement in the athlete.[16]

REFERENCES

1. Bechtro CO: Biomechanics of the shoulder, *Clin Orthop* 146:37, 1980.
2. Bigliani LU, Norris TR, Fischer J, et al: The relationship between the unfused acromial epiphysis and subacromial impingement lesion, *Orthop Trans* 7(1):138, 1983.
3. Chung SMK, Nissenbaum MM: Congenital and developmental defects of the shoulder, *Orthop Clin North Am* 6:382, 1975.
4. Cofield RH, Simonet WT: Symposium on sports medicine: part 2, The shoulder in sports, *Mayo Clin Proc* 59:157-164, 1984.
5. Cuillo J: Swimmer's shoulder, *Clin Sports Med* 5:115-136, 1984.
6. Cyriax J: *Textbook of orthopaedic medicine,* vol 2, ed 11, London, 1987, Bailliere-Tindall.
7. Gould JA III: *Orthopaedic and sports physical therapy,* ed 2, St Louis, 1990, Mosby.
8. Hawkins RJ, Hobeika PE: Impingement syndrome in the athletic shoulder, *Clin Sports Med* 2(2):394, 1988.
9. Hertling D, Kessler RM: *Management of common musculoskeletal disorders,* ed 2, Philadelphia, 1990, Lippincott.
10. Hoppenfeld S: *Physical examination of the spine and extremities,* Norwalk, Conn, 1976, Appleton-Century-Crofts.
11. Johnson D: In swimming, shoulder the burden, *Sports Care and Fitness* 1(2):24-30, 1988.
12. Kennedy J, Hawkins R, Krissoff W: Orthopaedic manifestations of swimming, *Am J Sports Med* 6:309-322, 1978.
13. Kisner C, Colby LA: *Therapeutic exercise: foundations and techniques,* ed 2, Philadelphia, 1990, FA Davis.
14. Lillegard WA, Rucker KS: *Handbook of sports medicine: a symptom-oriented approach,* Boston, 1993, Andover Medical Publishers.
15. Luopajarvi T, Kuorinka I, Virolainen M, et al: Prevalence of tenosynovitis and other injuries of the upper extremities in repetitive work, *Scand J Work Environ Health,* 5(3):48-55, 1979.
16. Matsen FA, Arnitz CT: Subacromial impingement. In Rockwood CA, Matsen FA, editors: *The shoulder,* ed 2, Philadelphia, 1990, Saunders.
17. Morrison DS, Bigliani LU: The clinical significance of variations in acromial morphology. Paper presented at the American Shoulder and Elbow Surgeons, third meeting, San Francisco, 1987.
18. Neer CS II: Anterior acromioplasty for the chronic impingement syndrome in the shoulder: a preliminary report, *J Bone Joint Surg* 54A:41-50, 1972.
19. Neer CS II, Bigliani LU, Hawking RJ: Rupture of the long head of the biceps related to subacromial impingement, *Orthop Trans* 1:111, 1977.
20. Neer CS II: Impingement lesions, *Clin Orthop* 173:70-77, 1983.
21. Netter FH: *The CIBA collection of medical illustrations,* vol 1, Summit, NJ, 1986, CIBA-Geigy.
22. Petterrson G: Rupture of the tendon aponeurosis of the shoulder joint in antero-inferior dislocation, *Acta Chir Scand* 77(suppl):1-187, 1942.
23. Saunders HD: *Evaluation, treatment and prevention of musculoskeletal disorders,* Minneapolis, 1985, Viking Press.
24. Staples OS, Watkins AO: Full active abduction in traumatic paralysis of the deltoid, *J Bone Joint Surg (Am)* 25:85, 1934.
25. Stroh S: Shoulder impingement, *J Manual and Manipulative Ther* 3(2):59-64, 1995.
26. Thein LA: Impingement syndrome and its conservative management, *J Orthop Sports Phys* Ther 11:189, 1989.
27. Tibone J, Jobe F, Kerlan R, et al: Shoulder impingement syndrome in athletes treated by anterior acromioplasty, *Clin Orthop* 198:134-140, 1985.

RECOMMENDED READING

Hawkins RJ, Hobeika PE: Impingement syndrome in the athletic shoulder, *Clin Sports Med* 2(2):391-405, 1983.

Hertling D, Kessler RM: *Management of common musculoskeletal disorders,* ed 2, Philadelphia, 1990, Lippincott.

Kisner C, Colby LA: *Therapeutic exercise: foundations and techniques,* ed 2, Philadelphia, 1990, FA Davis.

Matsen FA, Arnitz CT: Subacromial impingement. In Rockwood CA, Matsen FA, editors: *The shoulder,* Philadelphia, 1990, Saunders.

Stroh S: Shoulder impingement, *J Manual and Manipulative Ther* 3(2):59-64, 1995.

Thein LA: Impingement syndrome and its conservative management, *J Orthop Sports Phys Ther* 11:189, 1989.

11

Chronic Shoulder Discomfort That Progressed to Acute Unrelenting Pain over 4-Month Period

A 46-year-old female homemaker enters your office holding her right upper extremity in a guarded posture with a complaint of acute and worsening throbbing pain of 3 days' duration in her right shoulder that is unrelieved by rest. When questioned, the patient admits to mild pain and tenderness that began 4 months ago, with tenderness over the deltoid muscle and pain elicited when rolling over onto the right shoulder while sleeping. Also there was initially a loss of range of motion as well as a catching and painful sensation whenever the right arm was elevated between 75° to 100°. The patient states that high doses of aspirin have helped ease her pain. She reports a new onset of non-insulin dependent diabetes for 1 year and reports no history of trauma to either shoulder.

CLUE:

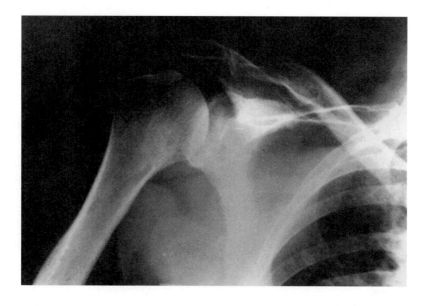

FIG. 11-1 (From Nicholas JA, Hershman EB: *The upper extremity in sports medicine,* ed 2, St. Louis, 1995, Mosby.)

OBSERVATION   No redness or sign of atrophy of spinatus muscle bellies.

PALPATION   Warmth and extreme tenderness over anterior deltoid area just superior to greater humeral tuberosity.

RANGE OF MOTION   Unassessed as patient refuses to move her shoulder.

MUSCLE STRENGTH   Untested.

SELECTIVE TENSION   Untested.

JOINT PLAY   Attempts to assess arthrokinematic motion are met with resistance caused by pain.

UPPER QUADRANT SCREENING   Negative results to compression or distraction of the cervical spine.

SENSATION   Normal.

? Questions

1. What is most likely wrong with this woman?
2. What is the cause of this disorder?
3. What is the incidence of calcified tendinitis?
4. What is the pathogenesis of calcific tendinitis?
5. What is the clinical presentation?
6. What radiologic views are necessary, and how are apparent calcifications classified?
7. How do arthritic changes of this region differ radiologically from calcified tendinitis?
8. What is the radiologic appearance of calcific rupture into an adjacent bursa?
9. What is the differential diagnosis?
10. What rehabilitative therapy is appropriate during the subacute phase?
11. What is the appropriate management during the acute phase?

1. What is most likely wrong with this woman?

Fig. 11-1 shows calcification of the insertion of the supraspinatus tendon. *Calcific tendinitis* of the rotator cuff is a common disorder that demonstrates a cyclic nature of calcium deposition and eventual resorption as the tendons heal. While calcium is deposited, the patient suffers only mild to moderate discomfort, whereas during the later resorption phase the shoulder becomes acutely painful.[17] Many pathologic conditions are characterized by a sequential evolution from an acute to a chronic disease state; however, calcific tendinitis does not fit this clinical picture, and these descriptions are perhaps inappropriate in describing this condition. Instead, what we have here is the opposite progression, that is, the patient's subjective report of chronic symptoms preceding acute symptoms. Calcifying tendinitis constitutes a disease entity in its own right[18] and is not related to generalized systemic disease despite the in-creased frequency of HLA-A1 antigen present in many patients, implying a genetic component to this condition.[15] An association with diabetes mellitus or gout is suspected[5] but has never been proved.[17] Most authors agree that no relationship exists between calcifying tendinitis and external trauma.[17]

2. What is the cause of this disorder?

The cause of calcific tendinitis is unknown, but it is believed that tissue hypoxia is the primary etiologic factor.

Approximately one-half inch proximal to the insertion of the supraspinatus[2] is an area of tendon, dubbed the *"critical zone,"*[10] that corresponds to the area of anastomoses between the osseous and muscular vessels.[11] The vascularity of this area is questioned because certain positions of the upper extremity have a "wringing out" effect resulting from pressure of the humeral head on the tendon when the arm is held in the resting position of adduction and neutral rotation.[13] Additionally there may be an inherent anatomic hypovascularity of the deep substance of the supraspinatus insertion as compared with its superficial aspect.[16] Regardless of which factor is the cause of the disorder, the result is hypoperfusion and tissue hypoxia that leads to a sequence of degeneration, necrosis, and reactive calcification.[17]

3. What is the incidence of calcified tendinitis?

The epidemiology of this disorder varies greatly. Females are more often affected than males, and the right shoulder is usually more often affected than the left.[17] However, cuff tendons of the dominant arm show no greater incidence of involvement than those from the contralateral shoulder.[12] Occupation seems to play some role in the development of this disorder though exactly how is uncertain. Close to 50% of patients in some studies were housewives or persons having clerical jobs. The incidence of calcific tendinitis peaks between 40 and 50 years of age, and bilateral involvement does occur in 15% of patients affected with this disorder.[14] In the athletic population, calcific tendinitis is generally seen in middle-aged athletes.[1]

4. What is the pathogenesis of calcific tendinitis?

Codman and other investigators believe that degeneration of tendon fibers precedes calcification[2] and occurs as a function of the wear-and-tear effect of aging. This hypothesis is supported by the fact that calcific tendinitis seldom affects persons before the fourth decade.[17] On the other hand, there is no evidence that a worker engaged in heavy manual labor will develop calcific tendinitis over time.[17] The tendons of the supraspinatus and the infraspinatus, in fact, undergo an alteration in structure during the middle years,[12] possibly related to chronic trauma, causing the normally orderly parallel collagen bundles composing the tendon to become thin, frayed, irregular, split, ischemic, and necrotic. Eventually the tendons undergo calcification,[17] succumbing to a process that is reminiscent of myositis ossificans. As such, calcific tendinitis is viewed as one possible intermediate pathologic stage along the continuum of cuff tendinopathies that begin with impingement syndrome and terminate with full-thickness rupture of one or more cuff tendons.

On the other hand, the self-healing nature of calcifying tendinitis is not characteristic of a degenerative disease but is rather an evolution of three stages of disease: (1) precalcific, (2) calcific, and (3) postcalcific.[17] Thus, rather than understanding this pathologic condition as two unrelated degenerative disease processes that include both an acute and a chronic calcific tendinitis, we can understand it as a disease cycle (Fig. 11-2) that is inclusive of both manifestations of a singular disease entity.

1. In the initial *precalcific* stage, the predilected area of tendon undergoes histologic change (such as fibro-

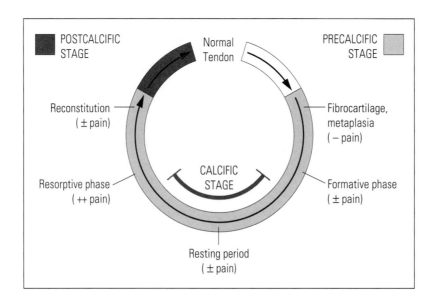

FIG. 11-2 Cycle of pain and inflammation with calcific tendinitis.

cartilaginous transformation, presumably triggered by tissue hypoxia). This stage is characterized by two phases and incorporates both the acute and subacute and the chronic stages of this disease.

- *Formative phase.* This phase is the reactive deposition of calcium crystals as the body's reaction to the chronic trauma, possibly in combination with senescence, that follows tendon degeneration, ischemia, and necrosis. If the patient undergoes surgery at this stage, the deposit appears hard and chalklike. This initial state of deposit formation lacks vascular and cellular reaction.
- *Resorptive phase.* This phase occurs after a relative period of inactivity of the disease process and is characterized by increased vascularization at the periphery of the deposit that ushers in macrophages, which phagocytose and remove calcium. This combination of vascular proliferation and cell exudation causes pain by raising the intratendinous pressure. This in turn may be further exacerbated by increased tendon volume within the unyielding subacromial arch. Lavage performed at this phase yields a thick, white cream-like or toothpastelike exudate.[17]

2. In the *postcalcific* stage there is remodeling of collagen in alignment with the longitudinal axis of the tendon in the space previously occupied by calcium by fibroblasts and newly developed vascular channels.[17]

5. What is the clinical presentation?

There is a tendency to believe that this disorder begins with acute symptoms and progresses to a chronic state. On the contrary, calcification is often symptomless, or at most just moderately uncomfortable at the beginning, whereas the disappearance of calcification is associated with pain.

Chronic signs and symptoms include pain or tenderness. The most frequent site of pain is referred to the insertion of the deltoid. Patients cannot sleep on the affected shoulder and complain of increased night pain. Decreased range of motion, a painful arc between 70° and 110°,[8] and a sensation of catching when going through an arc of motion are often reported. Supraspinatus muscle belly atrophy is a sign of long-standing calcifying tendinitis.

During the acute resorptive stage pain is so severe that patients refuse to move their shoulders. Pain is described as "throbbing" and is unrelieved by rest. Any attempt at mobilization of the glenohumeral joint will be resisted by the patient who will hold her or his upper extremity close to the body. Symptoms may last up to 2 weeks when acute, 3 to 8 weeks when subacute, and 3 months or more when chronic.

6. What radiologic views are necessary, and how are apparent calcifications classified?

In cases of suspected tendon calcification a radiograph must be taken and should include anteroposterior films in neutral as well as medial and lateral rotation. Supraspinatus deposits are readily visible in neutral rotation, whereas deposits on infraspinatus and teres minor are best seen in internal rotation. Subscapularis tendon calcification is rare and only clearly viewed on radiographs taken with the shoulder in external rotation. Scapular views are helpful in determining whether calcification has caused impingement. A positive finding confirms, at the very least, the presence of an intact cuff and rules out rupture of cuff tendons.[17]

There are two different radiologic appearances of calcific tendinitis, corresponding to the chronic and acute phases of this disease:[17]

- Corresponding to the *formative phase* in which the patient experiences mild or moderate discomfort (that is, chronic or subacute), the deposit appears dense, homogeneous, and with well-defined borders.
- Corresponding to the *resorptive phase* in which the patient experiences acute symptoms, the deposit appears fluffy, fleecy, or cloudlike, with ill-defined borders that are often barely visible (that is, with decreased density) and may extend into the adjacent bursa.[3,4]

7. How do arthritic changes of this region differ radiologically from calcified tendinitis?

Whereas deposits in calcific tendinitis are for the most part localized inside the tendon and may extend into the bursa, calcification seen in arthropathy is in continuity with or extending into the bone. Moreover, the latter are small and stippled in appearance, overlie the greater tuberosity, and are often accompanied by degenerative or articular changes characteristic of osteoarthritis. In addition, the acromiohumeral (that is, subacromial) space may be narrowed.[17]

8. What is the radiologic appearance of calcific rupture into the adjacent bursa?

Ruptures into the bursa appear as a crescentlike shadow overlying the actual calcification, extending over the greater tuberosity, and outlining the extent of the bursa.[9] This appearance may be viewed during the acute stage, corresponding to the resorptive phase of this disease cycle.

9. What is the differential diagnosis?

Differential diagnosis includes the following:

- Dystrophic calcifications are viewed as small stippled deposits seen around the torn edges of the tendon but especially sitting over the greater tuberosity after a complete tear of the supraspinatus or other cuff tendons. This tear appears as narrowing of the interval between the humeral head and the acromion. In contradistinction, calcific tendinitis deposits are situated inside the tendon without contacting the bone.
- Massive calcification as is seen in the Milwaukee shoulder.[6]
- Osteoarthritis.[17]

10. What rehabilitative therapy is appropriate during the subacute phase?

Therapeutic intervention is based on severity of symptoms and radiologic assessement. Patients with subacute symptoms are classified as belonging to the formative phase, unless radiographs show signs of resorption. The goals of therapy in this stage include maintenance of range of motion and strength. The degenerative changes of the rotator cuff that may result in calcific tendinitis are similar to those responsible for rotator cuff tear. As such, it is imperative that management strategy address prophylaxis and treatment so as to prevent recurrence of the rotator cuff disorder (see pp. 113-118).

Rehabilitative therapy during the subacute formative stage may include the following:

- Acetic acid iontophoresis for calcific deposits with the negative electrode over the site of lesion. The positive electrode may be placed on the ipsilateral forearm. The acetate radical replaces the carbonate radical in the insoluble calcium carbonate deposit, forming soluble calcium acetate.[7]
- Ultrasound so as to facilitate mobilization of calcium crystals.
- Phonophoresis with hydrocortisone.
- Corticosteroid injection with lidocaine to inhibit vascular proliferation, local hyperemia, and macrophage activity.
- Maintaining the shoulder in the position of abduction as often as possible. This position may be achieved by placement of the arm on the backrest of a chair or on a seat beside the patient. When supine, a pillow may be placed in the axilla.

- Moist heat.
- Rest.
- Transcutaneous electrical stimulation.
- Pendulum exercises.
- Exercises to increase range of motion, though it is important to avoid exercises that might cause upward humeral migration.
- Superficial heat such as diathermy in a chronic condition before exercises.

11. What is the appropriate management during the acute phase?

Calcific tendinitis may resolve spontaneously, requiring only nonsteroidal antiinflammatory medications for a week to 10 days during the acute phase of the disease. It is essential for the therapist to prevent the development of frozen shoulder during this phase (see pp. 140-143). Local ice application may be of help before pendulum exercises or glenohumeral joint mobilization. Iontophoresis to decrease pain, using hydrocortisone or lidocaine, may help relieve pain. However, the physician may attempt lavage during the resorptive phase. Here, symptoms are often acute, with radiographs confirming resorption. If lavage is unsuccessful, the needling usually helps relieve symptoms by decreasing intratendinous pressure and is followed by an intrabursal corticosteroid injection. The site of pain is then treated with ice massage and pendulum exercises, as well as nonsteroidal antiinflammatory medications. Once symptoms have decreased, range of motion activities and strengthening may begin.

Surgical removal is the exception and resorted to only when conservative treatment has failed and symptoms interfere with activities of daily living.

REFERENCES

1. Anderson TE: Rehabilitation of common shoulder injuries in athletes, *J Musculoskeletal Med*, p 24, Dec 1988.
2. Codman EA: *The shoulder*, Boston, 1934, Thomas Todd.
3. DePalma AF, Druper JS: Long term study of shoulder joints afflicted with and treated for calcific tendinitis, *Clin Orthop* 20:61-72, 1961.
4. De Seze S, Welfling J: Tendinites calcificantes, *Rhumatologie* 22:5-14, 1970.
5. Gschwend N, Scherer M, Lohr J: Die tendinitis calcarea des Schultergelenks, *Orthopäde* 10:196-205, 1981.
6. Halverson PB, McCarty DJ, Cheung HS, et al: Milwaukee shoulder syndrome, *Ann Rheum Dis* 43:734-741, 1989.
7. Kahn J: *Principles and practice of electrotherapy*, ed 2, New York, 1991, Churchill Livingstone.
8. Kessel L, Watson M: The painful arc syndrome, *J Bone Joint Surg* 59B:166-172, 1977.

9. Milone FP, Copeland MM: Calcific tendinitis of the shoulder joint, *AJR* 85:901-913, 1961.

10. Moseley HF, Goldie I: The arterial pattern of the rotator cuff of the shoulder, *J Bone Joint Surg* 45B:780-789, 1963.

11. Nixon JE, DiStefano V: Ruptures of the rotator cuff, *Orthop Clin North Am* 6:423-447, 1975.

12. Olsson O: Degenerative changes of the shoulder and their connection with shoulder pain, *Acta Chir Scand* 181 (suppl):1-110, 1953.

13. Rathbun JB, Macnab I: The microvascular pattern of the rotator cuff, *J Bone Joint Surg (Br)* 52(3):540-553, 1970.

14. Rodnan GP, Schumacher HR: *Primer on the rheumatic diseases,* ed 8, Atlanta, 1983, Arthritis Foundation.

15. Thompson LL: *The electromyographer's handbook,* Boston, 1981, Little, Brown.

16. Uhthoff HK, Loehr J, Sarkar K: The pathogenesis of rotator cuff tears. *Proc Third International Conference on Surgery of the Shoulder,* Fukuoka, Japan, Oct 27, 1986.

17. Uhthoff HK, Sarkar K: Calcifying tendinitis. In Rockwood CA, Matsen FA, editors: *The shoulder,* vol 1, Philadelphia, 1990, Saunders.

18. Welting J, Kahn MF, Desroy M, et al: Les calcifications de l'épaule, II. La maladie des calcifications tendineuses multiples, *Rev Rhum* 32:325-334, 1965.

RECOMMENDED READING

Brewer BJ: Aging of the rotator cuff, *Am J Sports Med* 7:102-110, 1979.

Griffin EJ, Kavselis TC: Physical agents for physical therapists. In *Ultrasonic energy,* ed 2, Springfield, Ill, 1982, Charles C Thomas.

Uhthoff HK, Sarkar K: Calcifying tendinitis. In Rockwood CA, Matsen FA, editors: *The shoulder,* vol 1, Philadelphia, 1990, Saunders.

12

Acute and Excruciating Shoulder Pain after Intense Bout of Exercise and Relieved by Rest

A 55-year-old male presents himself at your office with sudden pain and loss of function of the right shoulder 5 days ago. Symptoms actually began a week ago and were preceded by spending an intense Sunday afternoon helping his wife do her annual spring cleaning during which he performed lots of overhead activity with his dominant right arm. Pain has increased since 5 days ago and now is severe. The shoulder is held away from the body in 30° to 40° abduction. The patient points to the anterolateral arm over the areas of the middle and upper deltoid muscle bellies as the source of his pain. There is a positive history of prior cuff tendinitis some 4 years ago contralaterally, gout in the right hallux 12 years ago, and a history of mild generalized arthritis. The patient recalls no injury and admits to taking six aspirin per day for the past 3 days, which he reports helps alleviate pain. He has no history of any stomach ulcers.

OBSERVATION   There is no redness.

PALPATION   The shoulder is only mildly warm. There is tenderness over the bicipital groove, over the cuff tendons, but particularly beneath the right acromion process.

RANGE OF MOTION   Active and passive elevation is painful at 50° and yields an empty end feel (that is, the patient refuses to let you, the examiner, move the limb any further along the normal range) because the patient begs you to desist from further elevation, despite the fact that you feel that more movement is possible.[5] Rotation in either extreme is painless and is demonstrated at the end of allowable elevation range; hence a noncapsular pattern is observed. Abduction is noted to be more limited than forward flexion.

MUSCLE STRENGTH   Appears to be at least in the fair plus range.

SELECTIVE TENSION   Painless resisted motion at a specified range that becomes painful only when one is testing through the 50° to 130° range.

SPECIAL TESTS   Negative drop arm test, positive impingement sign.

? Questions

1. What is most likely the matter with this gentleman?
2. What requisite anatomy is essential to understanding this disorder?
3. Is subacromial bursitis a primary or a secondary disorder?
4. How many bursae exist in the shoulder, and what are their locations?
5. What are the specifics of the mechanism in the evolution of this condition?
6. What are the signs and symptoms of this condition?

7. How are the subdeltoid and subacromial bursae best palpated?
8. What do radiographs reveal about this condition?
9. How does the migration of calcification from the cuff tendon to the adjacent bursae facilitate beneficial resolution of the disorder?
10. How is calcified cuff tendinitis differentiated from bursitis?
11. What is the differential diagnosis of shoulder bursitis?
12. What rehabilitative therapy is helpful in the treatment and resolution of this pathologic condition?

1. What is most likely the matter with this gentleman?

Subacromial bursitis of the right shoulder.

2. What requisite anatomy is essential to understanding this disorder?

The *coracoacromial arch* is composed of two scapular processes—the coracoid and the acromion. These scapular components are connected by the roof of the arch—the coracoacromial ligament. Passage of the cuff tendons under this unyielding arch is managed by the presence of the *subacromial bursa*[12] and its extension the *subdeltoid bursa*.[3] These two soft tissues are actually two serosal surfaces (one on the underside of the acromion and deltoid, and the other *over* the cuff tendons) lubricated by synovial fluid so that they may intimately slide over each other.[12] The analogy is one of two fluid-inflated balloons pressed against each other and moving relative to each other during shoulder movement. When normally inflated, as during the inflammatory process, the bursa may enlarge to about the size of a golf ball.[11] These membranes are lined with a synovial membrane that can increase or decrease the amount of synovial fluid available on minimal stimulation.[2]

3. Is subacromial bursitis a primary or a secondary disorder?

Although subacromial bursitis may occur as a primary disorder after a blow to the shoulder,[11] it most frequently occurs secondarily to degenerative lesions of the rotator cuff and is part of the continuum of the many rotator cuff disorders.[15] Additionally bursitis may also be viewed as a separate yet related pathologic condition to calcific tendinitis. That is, although bursitis may evolve as a distinct clinical entity in its own right, it may also evolve secondarily to acute tendon calcification.

4. How many bursae exist in the shoulder, and what are their locations?

Most of the body's bursae exist in or around the shoulder complex,[1] and Codman lists up to 12. However, the most commonly present bursa locations include the following (Fig. 12-1):
1. Subacromial and subdeltoid
2. Between the coracoid and the glenohumeral joint capsule
3. Summit of the acromion
4. Between the infraspinatus and the joint capsule
5. Between the teres major and the long head of the biceps
6. Between the subscapularis and the joint capsule
7. Anterior to and posterior to the tendinous insertion of the latissimus dorsi
8. Behind the coracobrachialis muscle[9]

5. What are the specifics of the mechanism in the evolution of this condition?

Shoulder bursitis is a function of the intimate relationship between the supraspinatus tendon and the adjacent bursa within the coracoacromial arch. The disorder may

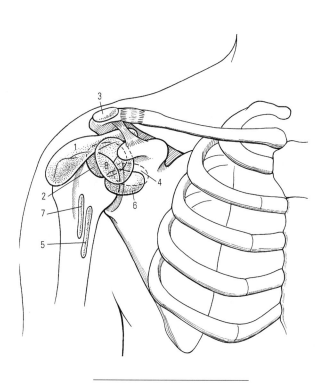

FIG. 12-1 Common shoulder bursae.

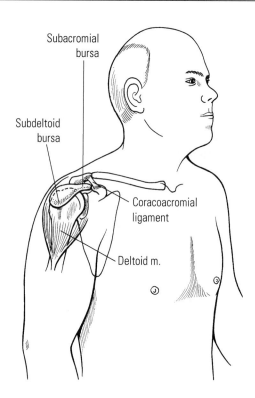

FIG. 12-2 The subdeltoid and subacromial bursae are really one but are separately named according to their adjacent anatomic structures.

often evolve in the following manner. Repetitive shoulder movements cause a reactive accumulation of fluid within the bursa in the attempt to attenuate friction. If shoulder movement continues excessively, bursal effusion will maximize, causing tissue tension and pain in the shoulder.[11] Alternately or even simultaneously, bursitis is initiated or worsened in the event that a supraspinatus impingement disorder is already present. Inflammation soon follows and cramps the contents of the subacromial space because of edema accumulation and fibrosis of the tendon. Over time, these changes will spread to include the bursae, which also undergo hypertrophy (proliferative lining) and fibrosis (that is, thickened) so as to interfere with their normal lubrication. The cumulative effect of these changes is to contribute to increasing rather than decreasing friction within the subacromial space.[4]

6. What are the signs and symptoms of this condition?

Bursitis will have a swift onset[15] of extremely severe shoulder pain[14] with dramatic tenderness[16] localized to the insertion of the deltoid at the upper middle third of the anterolateral proximal arm.[15] This is in contrast to

the more diffuse involvement found with impingement of the supraspinatus or biceps tendon or pain found adjacent to the coracoid process at the medial aspect of the shoulder in subcoracoid bursitis.[16] The patient, usually a man of middle age or older who has done an unusual bout of exercise,[14] experiences a sudden and unprovoked onset of extreme pain within a few days[5] that causes him to seek immediate relief. There is often a history of previous attacks.[9] A *noncapsular end feel* at the end of the range of passive motion with free rotation in either direction is *diagnostic for this disorder.* The clinician may also detect an *empty end feel* with passive movement.[15] If the bursitis is primary and thus not involving the cuff tendons, resistive movement would register painless,[5] implicating a noncontractile structure as the source of pain. This is not the case for resistance testing throughout the range, especially between the 50° to 130° range, where the contracting tendon may compress the inflamed bursa lying between the undersurface of the acromion and the supraspinatus tendon.[15]

The patient maintains the shoulder in an adducted position, which keeps the painful lesion away from the

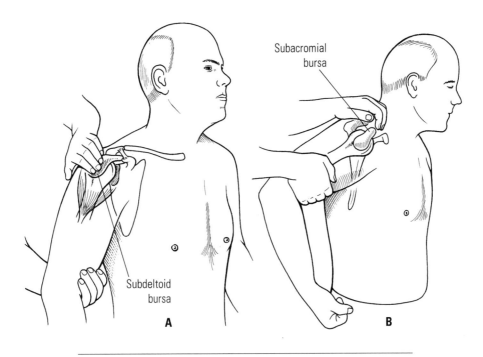

FIG. 12-3 Palpation of the bursa. **A,** Subdeltoid bursa. **B,** Subacromial bursa.

acromial undersurface. Elevation is hindered, abduction more so than forward flexion, and a painful arc between 50° and 130° is present whether movement is active or passive.[14] On palpation there is exquisite local tenderness over the subacromial bursa, which may feel thickened[6] as compared to the contralateral shoulder. Tenderness may also extend as far down as the bicipital groove.[6] Tests for supraspinatus tendinitis and impingement will be positive in this condition.[8]

7. How are the subdeltoid and subacromial bursae best palpated?

The subdeltoid bursa is easily palpated beneath the deltoid muscle (Fig. 12-2). The subacromial bursa is brought within the examiner's reach by moving the shoulder into passive extension, thus rotating both the cuff tendons and the superficial bursa out from under the acromion[6] (Fig. 12-3).

8. What do radiographs reveal about this condition?

Calcific subacromial bursitis and calcific supraspinatus tendinitis may be indistinguishable both radiographically as well as clinically.[1] However, once rupture of calcific material into the bursa has occurred, radiographic study shows a diffuse, lacy, amorphous pattern characteristic of spreading of the calcified mass throughout the bursal cavity.[13]

9. How does the migration of calcification from the cuff tendon to the adjacent bursae facilitate beneficial resolution of the disorder?

During the evolution of a calcific supraspinatus disorder, the calcium expands throughout the substance of the tendon to adhere[10] and irritate[14] the undersurface of the subacromial bursa. This new source of pain serves only to magnify the patient's already throbbing and excruciating pain that is unrelieved by rest.[14] Treatment involves aspiration, under local anesthesia, accompanied by hydrocortisone injection. Although aspiration may not yield calcium, it does, by virtue of multiple punctures, have the effect of allowing the calcium to become dispersed into the bursa where it can be resorbed. On the other hand, if calcific migration is allowed to continue through the bursal membrane, the calcium will eventually rupture the bursa. This *chemical bursitis* is actually beneficial, since the bursa, having a good blood supply, will gradually absorb the calcium, thus allowing symptoms to subside[14] (Fig. 12-4).

10. How is calcified cuff tendinitis differentiated from bursitis?

Although the locale of pain in calcified cuff tendinitis is often indistinguishable from shoulder bursitis because of the proximity of these structures as well as the relat-

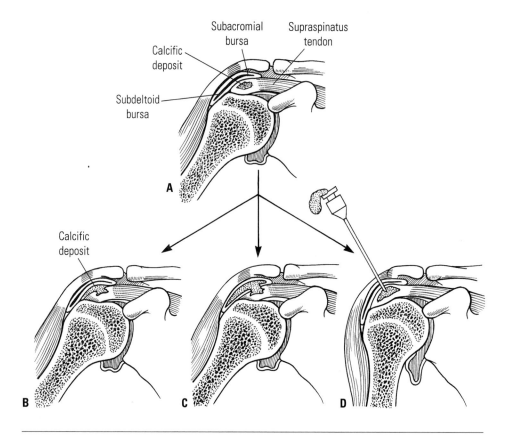

FIG. 12-4 A, Calcific deposit in the tendon creates increased cramping within the subacromial space, which further aggravates inflammation and pain. Symptomatic relief when space-occupying calcium no longer concentrates within the subacromial space may occur in one of three ways; **B,** spontaneous upward rupture of the deposit beneath the floor of the bursae; **C,** spontaneous downward rupture of the deposit into the bursa where it may be resorbed; **D,** needle rupture and deposit removal.

edness of these disorders, the former is distinguishable from the latter by pain unrelieved by rest. Moreover, with shoulder bursitis the patient experiences relatively less pain and will permit evaluation of some shoulder movement.

11. What is the differential diagnosis of shoulder bursitis?

Differential diagnosis includes the following:
- Infection caused by pus producing (pyogenic) organisms, particularly *Staphylococcus aureus.* Infection is suspected in the event of particularly red, warm, and painful swellings.[1]
- Rheumatoid arthritis
- Gout
- Inflammatory arthritis

12. What rehabilitative therapy is helpful in the treatment and resolution of this pathologic condition?

Because shoulder bursitis frequently occurs secondarily to lesions of the rotator cuff, it may be viewed along the continuum of rotator cuff disorders. Because of this, shoulder bursitis may be heir to many of the same limitations inherent to rotator cuff lesions, and management will closely follow treatment of rotator cuff disorder. For a more complete discussion of treatment see pp. 101-105 and 118-120.
- *Rest.*
- *Ice* to reduce spasm, pain, and inflammation.
- *Phonophoresis* (pulsed ultrasound so as to avoid heat) with hydrocortisone ointment as a coupling agent.

- Codman's *pendulum* and gravity-eliminated rotation exercises in the pain-free range to maintain joint capsule mobility; weights should not be used in the acute stage.[15]
- *Nonsteroidal antiinflammatory medication* in high doses, such as indomethacin, naproxen, or ibuprophen.[1]
- As the acute condition subsides, either *ice or heat* may be used, and a *selective strengthening program* of the rotator cuff muscles is appropriate in short arcs of motion so as to circumvent pain felt at the end of the range of motion. Rotation exercises are best done with the shoulder in approximately 30° to 40° abduction so as to avoid wringing out the supraspinatus tendon.[15]
- Gentle grade I or grade II *joint mobilization* to the glenohumeral joint[7] and shoulder girdle joints so as to stave off the effects of stiffening.
- Sparing *steroid injection* after aspiration in those patients experiencing intensely severe and disabling pain.[14] However, a trial of therapeutic management with nonsteroidal antiinflammatory medication is attempted before injection, since multiple injections have been shown to cause weakening of myotendinous structures and, at best, are treating only inflammation as often evidenced by short-term relief that is followed by gradual return of the disorder. In any event, if pain relief is gained, a serious isolated rotator cuff strengthening program must be launched, as well as appropriate capsular and soft-tissue stretching, with the strategy of treating the aforesaid disorder at its origin, such as the altered biomechanics at the shoulder.[15]
- *Surgical exploration,* excision of calcific deposit, and possibly subtotal acromionectomy are indicated in the occasional completely refractory patient.[13]

REFERENCES

1. Berkow R: *The Merck manual of diagnosis and therapy,* ed 15, Rahway, NJ, 1987, Merck, Sharp & Dohme Research Laboratories.
2. Bland JD, Merrit JA, Boushey DR: The painful shoulder, *Semin Arthritis Rheum* 7(1):21, 1977.
3. Codman EA: *The shoulder,* Boston, 1934, Thomas Todd.
4. Cuillo J: Swimmer's shoulder, *Clin Sports Med* 5:115-136, 1984.
5. Cyriax J: *Textbook of orthopaedic medicine, vol 1: diagnosis of soft tissue lesions,* London, 1982, Bailliere-Tindall.
6. Hoppenfeld S: *Physical examination of the spine and extremities,* Norwalk, Conn, 1976, Appleton-Century-Crofts.
7. Kisner C, Colby LA: *Therapeutic exercise: foundation and techniques,* ed 2, Philadelphia, 1990, FA Davis.
8. Lillegard WA, Rucher KS: *Handbook of sports medicine: a symptom-oriented approach,* Boston, 1993, Andover Medical Publishers.
9. Moffat M: Lecture and handout series on musculoskeletal therapeutic exercise, New York, Fall 1989, New York University Department of Physical Therapy.
10. Moore KL: *Clinically oriented anatomy,* ed 2, Baltimore, 1985, Williams & Wilkins.
11. Peterson L, Renström P: *Sports injuries: their prevention and treatment,* London, 1986, Martin Dunitz.
12. Rockwood CA, Matsen FA, editors: *The shoulder,* vol 2, Philadelphia, 1990, Saunders.
13. Rodman GP, Schumacher HR: *Primer on the rheumatic diseases,* ed 8, Atlanta, 1983, Arthritis Foundation.
14. Salter RB: *Textbook of disorders of the musculoskeletal system,* ed 2, Baltimore, 1983, Williams & Wilkins.
15. Saunders ED: *Evaluation, treatment and prevention of musculoskeletal disorders,* Minneapolis, 1985, Viking Press.
16. Schumacher HR, Bomalaski JS: *Case studies in rheumatology for the house officer,* Baltimore, 1990, Williams & Wilkins.

RECOMMENDED READING

Rodman GP, Schumacher HR: *Primer on the rheumatic diseases,* ed 8, Atlanta, 1985, Arthritis Foundation.
Salter RB: *Textbook of disorders of the musculoskeletal system,* ed 2, Baltimore, 1983, Williams & Wilkins.
Saunders ED: *Evaluation, treatment and prevention of musculoskeletal disorders,* Minneapolis, 1985, Viking Press.

13

Stiff and Painful Shoulder

A 64-year-old white female presents with a history of a left fractured rib 8 weeks ago while she was sleeping. She reports a history of osteoporosis as well as insulin-dependent diabetes. Her side no longer hurts, yet she complains of a diffuse aching left shoulder pain by day that wakes her at night, especially when she rolls onto the shoulder. When asked, she reports that she is unable to sleep on her left side. Pain is vaguely reported over the area of the deltoid muscle. Dressing and grooming have become nearly impossible because of the pain. There is no complaint of pain to the neck, upper back, elbow, or hand. She complains that she can no longer unbuckle her brassiere from behind, though she can perform most functional activities with her right dominant upper extremity.

OBSERVATION   Her left arm appears close against her body in the position of shoulder internal rotation, adduction, and elbow flexion. When she is asked to elevate her left shoulder, she appears to hike her shoulder upward to approximately 40°. There is slight muscle wasting observed over the bellies of the musculocutaneous cuff musculature.

PALPATION   There is point tenderness present over the bicipital groove.

ACTIVE AND PASSIVE MOVEMENTS   An empty end feel is appreciated. Specific ranges are difficult to measure because of gross limitation of left shoulder movement in virtually all ranges. Approximate ranges are as follows:

External rotation (ER):	45°
Abduction:	80°
Internal rotation (IR):	70°

The following pattern emerges: ER is more limited than abduction which, in turn, is more limited than medial rotation.

JOINT PLAY   Anterior and inferior glide are particularly limited, as is lateral distraction. The scapulothoracic (ST) joint feels partially bound because retraction and protraction are grossly limited to one half of their normal range as compared to the contralateral scapula.

RESISTIVE TESTING   Left shoulder yields pain when reaching the end range but no pain at midrange.

SENSATION   Normal.

REFLEXES Normal.

CLUE An arthrogram of the left shoulder showed a reduced volume of the left glenohumeral joint capsule as well as inapparent axillary fold and biceps brachii sheath.

? Questions

1. What disorder is most likely affecting this woman?
2. How is frozen shoulder (FS) classified?
3. What is the mechanism of contracture formation at the tissue level in secondary FS?
4. What anatomy is requisite to understanding the FS disorder?
5. What is the result in the clinical course of either type of FS?
6. What are the epidemiologic characteristics of FS?
7. What is the clinical presentation of FS?

8. What are the signs and symptoms of FS?
9. What is meant by reverse scapulothoracic rhythm?
10. What accounts for pinpoint tenderness over the bicipital groove?
11. What is the differential diagnosis?
12. How revealing are laboratory investigations?
13. What rehabilitative therapy is appropriate to treating this condition?
14. What does manipulation or surgery involve, and when is it appropriate?

1. What disorder is most likely affecting this woman?

Adhesive capsulitis, or *frozen shoulder* (FS), is a distinct clinical syndrome[33] associated with pain and restricted range of active and passive glenohumeral motion.[24] In the majority of cases, frozen shoulder is a self-limiting disorder that resolves with time though leaving some residual loss of motion in up to 70% of all patients.[2] Because of functional loss in 10% to 15% of patients[2] and because there is no consistently effective treatment, a strong case exists for prevention through avoidance of immobilization after trauma or other pathologic state in the shoulder.[16]

2. How is frozen shoulder (FS) classified?

PRIMARY FS

Patients having no positive findings in their history, clinical examination, or radiographic review that could explain their pain and a decrease in shoulder motion are classified as having primary FS.[19] These primary idiopathic cases are the most common forms of FS and result from an unknown stimulus that produces profound histologic changes in the capsule that are substantially different from changes produced by simple immobilization.[32] An autoimmune theory has been proposed as

the pathomechanics of primary FS, but no conclusive evidence has been found.[5b,37a]

SECONDARY FS

In contrast to the former, secondary FS develops after a variety of antecedent episodes such as accidental injury, surgery of the breast or upper limb, upper limb immobilization, rib fracture, primary cancer or infection, myocardial infarction, cervical disc disease, arthritis, or lengthy duration of intravenous infusion.[18] In most cases, the common denominator is disuse of the upper extremity with the shoulder typically held in internal rotation (IR) and in adduction and with the elbow in flexion. Disuse of the limb in this position places the anteroinferior portion of the glenohumeral (GH) joint such that the capsular attachments approximate and foreshorten with time as adhesions develop.[34]

3. What is the mechanism of contracture formation at the tissue level in secondary FS?

Histologically the GH joint capsule is composed of bundles of type I collagen aligned with the axis of tensile strength of the capsule. In secondary FS restriction is caused by thickening and tightening of the capsule by

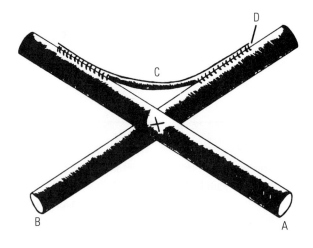

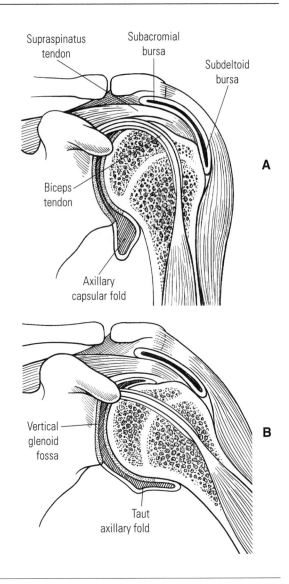

FIG. 13-1 Mechanism of contracture formation at the tissue level. Collagen fibrils, *A* and *B*, come into close contact at point ✕ because of loss of spacing-ground substance. New collagen fibrils, *C*, become fixed by cross-linking, *D*, to inhibit normal gliding. (From Akeson WH, Amiel D, Woo SL-Y: *Biorheology* 17:95-110, 1980.)

binding and proliferation of individual collagen fibers (Fig. 13-1).

4. What anatomy is requisite to understanding the FS disorder?

The GH joint is statically supported by secondary thickenings of the GH joint capsule. The tendons of the rotator cuff adjacent to the joint capsule thicken and support the capsule anteriorly, superiorly, and posteriorly, but not inferiorly (Fig. 13-2, *A*). It is this hiatus that is responsible for the disorder of anteroinferior (that is, subglenoid) shoulder dislocation. In the normal resting position with the arm at the side, it is the oblique orientation of the glenoid fossa that provides a resting shelf for the humeral head. As elevation commences and progresses, the fossa's orientation becomes increasingly vertical as the humeral glides, by analogy, along its runway toward the infraglenoid tubercle. At peak elevation the humeral head is held against an almost vertical fossa as a function of scapular protraction and is prevented from being dislocated inferiorly by the *inferior capsule*—that redundant (double) *axillary fold* of now-tautened ligamentous tissue forming the inferior recess. This inferior capsular ligament will collapse into a lax, pouchlike fold when the arm hangs down in adduction, the slack of which is quickly taken up during elevation because of tautening of this inferior capsule (Fig. 13-2, *B*).

FIG. 13-2 A, Coronal section of a left glenohumeral joint showing the inferior capsule unsupported by dynamic constraints. This inferior recess makes a redundant fold with the arm at the side. **B,** As the shoulder is elevated the redundant axillary fold is tautened, providing static support and preventing excessive inferior excursion of the glenohumeral head.

5. What is the result in the clinical course of either type of FS?

A low-grade inflammatory response may develop involving the capsule, synovial membrane (synovitis), and musculocutaneous cuff.[24] As a result, adhesions form between all these structures as the normal capsular folds, pouches, and joint cavity become obliterated. The contracted and thickened joint capsule is drawn

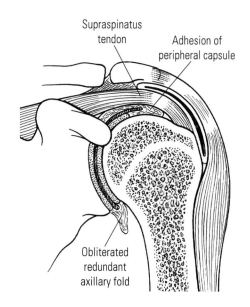

Supraspinatus tendon

Adhesion of peripheral capsule

Obliterated redundant axillary fold

FIG. 13-3 Cross-sectional view of left shoulder shows adhesion development obliterating the redundant axillary fold.

tightly around the humeral head[25] to eventually become fixed to the bone,[27] and the musculocutaneous cuff muscle bellies become contracted, fixed, and inelastic[22] (Fig. 13-3).

6. What are the epidemiologic characteristics of FS?

Occurring twice as often in females as in males,[24] FS is rarely seen in patients less than 40 and over 70 years of age,[5] except for diabetic patients. Frozen shoulder is more common in the nondominant arm,[14] and about 12% of all patients develop the condition bilaterally.[32] There is a higher than normal association between FS and diabetes mellitus. The incidence of FS in the general population ranges from 2% to 5% whereas among diabetics, 10% to 20%.[4] Insulin-dependent diabetics have an even higher incidence (36%) of FS as well as a considerably increased frequency of bilateral shoulder involvement (42%).[6]

7. What is the clinical presentation of FS?

Frozen shoulder is a self-limiting disorder lasting 12 to 18 months[10] that classically presents as a cycle of three distinct stages:[33] freezing, frozen, and thawing.[30] These stages are neatly packaged in literature as spanning 6 months each but may actually last shorter or longer because they vary from individual to individual. In pa-

tients with secondary FS, these three phases may not always be recognizable.

STAGE 1

The *freezing,* or *painful inflammatory, phase* is characterized by acute constant shoulder pain and muscle spasm that restricts movement in all directions, particularly in a *capsular pattern.* The onset is gradual and is experienced as diffuse shoulder pain which the patient has difficulty in localizing anatomically.[33] It is often difficult to obtain a history of any precipitating event. Patients often describe a progressive onset of pain lasting for weeks and months before seeking orthopedic consultation. Pain is usually worse at night and is exacerbated when the patient lies on the affected side. It is during this initial phase that patients are most anxious. As the patient uses the arm less and less, there is usually less discomfort, with the patient taking false satisfaction that he or she is doing the best thing for the shoulder. The duration of this phase is variable, lasting anywhere from 2 to 9 months.[30] The pain during this phase is even elicited during the midrange of movement.

STAGE 2

The *frozen,* or *stiff, phase* is characterized by subsiding pain[16] and progressive loss of shoulder movement in a capsular pattern. When elicited, pain is not felt during midrange but rather at end range, such that suddenly reaching out to grab a swinging door or to catch a falling object is vividly described by the patient as being sharply painful. In this stage pain during rest subsides, and discomfort in the form of a dull ache[33] occurs during movement.[16] Functional restrictions increase as immobility sets in, and patients often seek out the clinician[14] at this stage because they are alarmed by their inability to reach out for a telephone, remove a wallet from a back pocket, reach for an object in the back seat of a car, or swing a golf club or tennis racket.[33] The duration of this phase may last anywhere between 4 to 12 months.[30]

STAGE 3

The *thawing phase* is characterized by gradual regaining of shoulder movement, as the shrunken and adherent capsule becomes separated from the humeral head. As motion slowly increases, there is a progressive lessening of discomfort, which comes as a great relief to the patient.[33] This occurs when a patient regains functional stages, such as being able to tuck one's shirt or blouse behind the back, wash one's hair, or achieve a more natural golf swing.[2] The time for regaining of shoulder motion is variable and unpredictable. For some this may require a 4- to 6-week period to resolve, whereas for others this may take up to 6 or even 9 months.[33]

8. What are the signs and symptoms of FS?

Limitation of shoulder motion and its imposition on function is usually the symptom that prods the patient to seek initial attention.[14] Motion is guarded with protective muscle spasm as a common feature that accounts for the arm held against the body in shoulder adduction and medial rotation. Because of pain and guarding, the patient often refuses to allow the joint to be moved to where resistance is felt by the examiner (that is, an *empty end feel*). Later on, after pain has subsided and only decreased motion persists, a capsular end feel is imparted by capsular structures limiting the range.[35]

The limitation of passive range of motion found in FS is characteristic of a capsular pattern. Lateral rotation is more limited than abduction, which in turn is more limited than medial rotation. During maximal capsular restriction, glenohumeral (GH) joint measurements average approximately 45° ER, less than 80° of abduction, and less than 70° of medial rotation.[18] Testing for accessory GH joint movements demonstrates tightness (that is, physiologic loss of motion) in the anterior and inferior aspects of the GH joint capsule, correlating to osteokinematic loss of lateral rotation and abduction respectively (capsular pattern); lateral distraction is also limited.[36] There may also be decreased scapulothoracic range because of secondary adhesions developing within that joint.

The pain of FS is present during both activity and rest, with patients frequently complaining of pain at night and being unable to sleep on the affected side.[14] As the condition progresses, pain during rest subsides, and discomfort occurs only during movement. Eventually pain will abate, whereas restriction of motion will persist.[16] There is usually no painful arc of motion.[36]

Pain may vary from a mild to a severe ache and is vaguely distributed over the deltoid muscle area, with *point tenderness at the bicipital groove.*[29] Pain may radiate distally throughout the C5 dermatome or more

proximally to the upper back and neck, a symptom probably attributable to compensatory overuse of shoulder girdle muscles such as the trapezius, rather than to referred pain from the shoulder.[29] Disuse atrophy may be evident in the rotator cuff, deltoid, biceps brachii, and triceps brachii muscles.[36] Sensory and reflex testing show normal results.[36]

Resisted movements in the midrange of motion during the early painful stage is usually asymptomatic and leads the examiner to conclude that contractile tissues (such as the bicipital and cuff tendons) are uninvolved.[36] In contradistinction, these (capsular) contractile structures are unlikely to elicit pain on passive movement, whereas inelastic (capsular) soft-tissue structures may produce such pain.

9. What is meant by reverse scapulothoracic rhythm?

In healthy individuals approximately 120° elevation is attributable to the glenohumeral joint, and the remaining motion occurs at the scapulothoracic joint in a 2:1 ratio. There is considerable individual deviation[33] from this 2:1 (GH:ST) ratio among the general populace, with differences varying from person to person. With FS, limitation at the GH joint leads to compensatory movement at the ST joint[29] during attempted elevation resulting in an altered or *reverse scapulothoracic rhythm* or ratio. This is observed as a shoulder-hike[20] or girdle-hunching maneuver[36] (Fig. 13-4).

10. What accounts for pinpoint tenderness over the bicipital groove?

The joint capsule of the GH joint bridges the gap between the lesser and greater tuberosities,[17] known as the *transverse humeral ligament* or bicipital aponeurosis (see Fig. 8-9). The synovial membrane that lines the GH joint capsule invests the tendon of the long head of the biceps as that tendon passes deep to the transverse humeral ligament within the bicipital groove. In fact, this synovial sheath may extend for a distance of 5 cm beyond the transverse ligament inferior to the bicipital groove, especially when the arm is in abduction (such as the position where the least amount of biceps tendon lies within the GH joint; see Fig. 8-9).[23] Thus the synovitis within the GH joint during FS is exposed outside the GH joint at the bicipital groove and is available for provocation during palpation. This may also account for why the biceps tendon sheath is outlined arthrographically in the majority of cases of adhesive capsulitis.

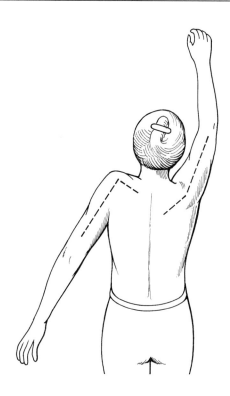

FIG. 13-4 Reverse scapulothoracic rhythm. Broken lines indicate the position of the scapular spine and humeral axis on each side, showing little or no movement in the left shoulder. This "shoulder-hiking" attempt at abduction elevates rather than depresses the humeral head.

11. What is the differential diagnosis?

Because FS is a symptom complex rather than a specific diagnostic entity, several causative factors are presented:

- *Posterior shoulder dislocation* presents as blocked external rotation and an overall limitation of shoulder motion that is superficially likened to FS. Appropriate history and radiographs, specifically an axillary view, conclusively determines whether the humeral head articulates with the glenoid.[33]
- In cases of *acute tendinitis* or *bursitis* restrictions of both active and passive movements of the GH joint may mimic that of FS. The history of onset should raise suspicion as to the correct diagnosis. Furthermore, although injection of the subacromial bursa will greatly improve passive range of motion (PROM) with the tendinitis-bursitis type of disorder, it will have little or no effect improving the range of motion (ROM) of the FS patient.[33] In addition, resistive muscle testing in midrange will be painless with

FS but painfully implicates the biceps brachii or rotator cuff tendons.[8] Furthermore, whereas in FS there is initially painful restriction in every direction, supraspinatus tendinitis is characterized by pain elicited during active movement through a specific arc of movement.[36]

- A large *calcific deposit* may occasionally block active and passive shoulder motion. Shoulder radiographs taken to display the subacromial space, with the humerus in internal and external rotation, should detect such a calcification.[19]
- A painful acromioclavicular (AC) joint may also mimic FS and is suspected when clinical findings reveal localized tenderness over the AC joint. Lidocaine into the AC joint should relieve all symptoms in a primary *AC joint disorder* such as arthritis. In the event of partial pain relief, but without improvement in ROM, the clinician must look beyond the AC joint for the cause of symptoms.[33] AC joint sprain is characterized by a large lump over the lateral end of the clavicle.
- *Osteochondromatosis* or other causes of intra-articular loose bodies may present as a painful stiff shoulder and are identified by the typical locking or catching of the GH joint. Loose bodies may appear on the radiograph.[33]
- Primary or secondary *malignancy* must be ruled out in most patients in their sixth decade or older who present with localized skeletal pain. Radiographic imaging of soft tissues, radionuclide bone scanning, and blood screening are indicated. A biopsy may be considered once a specific lesion is identified.[33]

12. How revealing are laboratory investigations?

Arthrography is the standard diagnostic test for FS.[27] This technique reveals at least a 50% reduction of shoulder joint volume (such as, 5 to 10 ml compared to approximately 20 to 30 ml in healthy shoulders).[32] Other findings include irregular joint outline,[26] tight and thickened capsule,[27] loss of axillary fold, and biceps brachii tendon sheath not evident[24] because of dye absence.[10] Arthrographic findings do not indicate the type of onset (primary or secondary) or the rate and extent of recovery.[3] No abnormality is detected on plain radiographs except mild to moderate bone demineralization (osteopenia)[31] caused by disuse[24] in those patients who have had a prolonged period of disuse.[31] Decreased space between the acromion and the humeral head[32] may also be apparent. Radionuclide bone scanning often slows an increased uptake of contrast material in patients with FS.[37] Hematologic investigations reveal an association between HLA-B27 histocompatibility antigen and patients suffering from FS.[5a]

13. What rehabilitative therapy is appropriate to treating this condition?

The treatment objective in the early stage of FS is to interrupt the cycle of pain and inflammation and facilitate an early "thaw" of the frozen joint. Improvement tends to be characterized by spurts and plateaus.[34] Initially, treatment modalities include:

- *Salicylate analgesics* with or without codeine[33] to allow movement into the painful range.
- *Pendulum* swing and circular swing exercises for 2 to 3 minutes every 1 to 2 hours to be performed into the painful range.[33] Moving tissues engorged with blood and inflammatory exudate stimulates circulation and resorption of cellular debris.[36] Pendulum exercises with attached cuff weights at the wrist permit some range of motion with passive distraction of the glenohumeral joint.
- *Passive range of motion exercise* facilitates improved motion,[21] but may also reduce pain because of a neuromodulation effect on joint mechanoreceptors.[1] The therapist may assist in depressing the humeral head as the patient attempts to elevate, to prevent pinching of subacromial tissue.
- *Iontophoresis* or *phonophoresis* using ions with analgesic and antiinflammatory properties.
- *Transcutaneous electrical stimulation* to relieve pain.

    If after approximately 2 weeks pain continues, an injection of corticosteroid with lidocaine may give significant pain relief.

    As the pain subsides, the following therapeutic modalities may be added to the treatment regimen:

- *Active range of motion* in forward elevation with either internal or external rotation into the painful end range so as to prevent adhesion formation.[34] The therapist may passively assist during the end range of movement as he or she may guide the limb further into the range without eliciting spasm or a stretch reflex that accompanies muscle guarding. Initially, active abduction is best carried out while the therapist passively depresses the humeral head so as to avoid pinching subacromial tissue.
- *Strengthening exercises* are very important, since FS often leads to muscle shortening, weakness, and atrophy. Strengthening begins as the range of GH motion returns, and is most effective as short arc exercises using an elastic band within the *pain-free* range.[34]

Exercises may initially be isometric because attempts at isotonic activity may be thwarted by reflex inhibition and pain.

- *Joint mobilization* (grades I or II) even into *painful* physiologic range is appropriate because this is not harmful and simply facilitates increased capsular mobility[34] by stretching and breaking adhesions. Good mobilization strategy would include stretching the predominantly tight portions of the capsule that limit motion in a capsular pattern, that is, to stretch the anterior and medioinferior portions of the capsule so as to facilitate increased range in external rotation and abduction respectively. Mobilization must seek to localize stretch to specific portions of the joint capsule and then gradually to increase intensity without eliciting protective muscle contraction.

    Inferior glide is comfortable for patients and very helpful in relieving muscle spasm. Achieving this movement is particularly important, since spasm, present in the acute stage, interferes with normal joint mechanics by causing the humeral head to move superiorly. Inferior glide may be performed with the patient lying prone and with the arm hanging freely off the side of the plinth.[12]

- Gentle self-mobilization exercises may be incorporated in the subacute stage as the patient begins to tolerate capsular stretching. Moving the body in relation to a stabilized humerus is safer for the joint and less painful for the patient to perform[15] (Fig. 13-5, *A*).
- *Moist heat*[33] before mobilization and stretching exercises, provided that inflammation is reduced, is helpful to increasing tissue extensibility. Gains in reclaiming range of motion may be preserved by ice packing with the shoulder supported in the position of maximum abduction and external rotation.[34]
- *Ultrasound* provides a deep heating effect precisely to the muscle-bone interface and is best applied at the anteroinferior capsule with the arm stretched into abduction and ER. Ultrasound also breaks down molecular binding that causes criss-crossed collagen fibers in the joint capsule to adhere to one another.[11] By increasing tissue extensibility, ultrasound is especially useful when used before manual techniques stretching the glenohumeral joint capsule.
- *Stretching* activities include using the good extremity to assist the affected arm up the back progressively achieving greater range of IR. A towel in the opposite hand passed over the opposite shoulder pulling the affected hand up the back may accomplish the same effect. IR stretching may be initiated when one

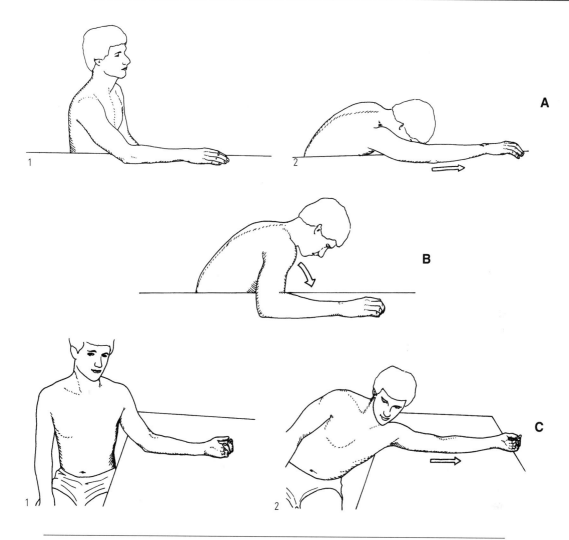

FIG. 13-5 A, Beginning, *1,* and end, *2,* positions for self-stretching to increase shoulder flexion with elevation. **B,** End position for self-stretching to increase shoulder external rotation. **C,** Beginning, *1,* and end, *2,* positions for self-stretching to increase shoulder abduction with elevation.   *Continued*

stretches into extension using a stick behind the back. Forward elevation stretch may be performed by assisted elevation of the arm so as to reach up to a solid object just beyond one's reach. Patients stand on tiptoes and then lower themselves and sustain a moderate stretch adjusted to tolerance for 20 to 30 seconds. This stretching is repeated 5 times, and then the arm is assisted down by use of the opposite arm, since freefall from the new upper limit of forward elevation can be very painful.[33] It may be necessary to achieve stretching of the joint capsule before one performs stretches into specific ranges.

- *Wand exercises* to increase range of motion and strength to the shoulder. A Velcro cuff may eventually be added for resistance. (See Fig. 6-5.)
- *Muscular reeducation* to minimize the substitution pattern of left shoulder elevation by means of a right shoulder shrug and right trunk lean. Once normal range is regained, the patient is instructed to palpate the left upper trapezius for muscular activity while performing left shoulder elevation before a mirror. This allows incorporation of visual feedback of trapezius activity and avoidance of right-sided trunk bending.

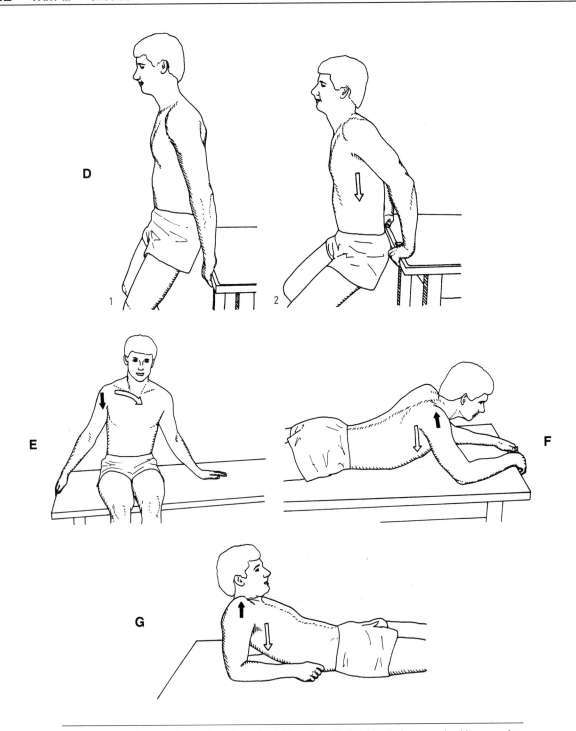

FIG. 13-5, cont'd. D, Beginning, *1,* and end *2,* positions for self-stretching to increase shoulder extension. **E,** Self-mobilization; caudal glide of the humerus occurs as the person leans away from the fixed arm. **F,** Self-mobilization; posterior glide of the humerus occurs as the person shifts his body weight downward between the fixed arms. **G,** Self-mobilization; anterior glide of the humerus occurs as the person leans between the fixed arms. (From Kisner C, Colby LA: *Therapeutic exercise: foundations and techniques,* ed 2, Philadelphia, 1990, FA Davis.)

- *Prevention.* A strong case for prevention may be made because no treatment is consistently effective for management of FS.[16] Many patients receive little or no advice from the emergency room or orthopedic physician regarding the need for early motion. The classic example is of a patient sent home from the doctor wearing a shoulder sling cradling the upper extremity after a finger or wrist fracture.

14. What does manipulation or surgery involve, and when is it appropriate?

Manipulation under anesthesia as treatment of FS is a source of much controversy in orthopedic circles[9] because of complications such as fracture, dislocation, brachial plexus injury, and gross tearing of soft tissue causing further scarring.[35] When it is performed, an assistant stabilizes the scapula while the humerus is abducted until the capsule tears. Some surgeons also perform forced lateral and medial manipulations after abduction, whereas others consider these manipulations too risky because of potential fracture.[10] After injection of corticosteroids, patients begin gentle range of motion exercise in forward elevation, external rotation, and use of a pulley for stretching on the very same day as manipulation.[33] To prevent the ruptured tissues from healing in their former state of retraction, the arm must be abducted at least 90° for 1 to 2 weeks while the patient is recumbent.[27]

Surgery is usually a last resort in those patients who have not responded to conservative treatment or for whom manipulation is contraindicated because of a history of osteoporosis, dislocation, or fracture.[27] The use of systemic steroids has inherent risks for potential systemic complications.[7]

Because there are no serious medical complications of FS, a judgment to accept restricted motion rather than undertake manipulation or surgical release is acceptable. Many patients can learn to function quite well with a moderately restricted range of shoulder motion.[33]

REFERENCES

1. Barak T, Rosen ER, Sufer R: Mobility: passive orthopaedic manual therapy. In Gould JA, Davies GJ, editors: *Orthopaedic and sports physical therapy,* St Louis, 1985, Mosby.
2. Binder AI, Bulgen DY, Hazleman BL, et al: Frozen shoulder: a long-term prospective study, *Ann Rheum Dis* 43:361-364, 1984.
3. Binder AI, Bulgen DY, Hazleman BL, et al: Frozen shoulder: an arthrographic and radionuclear scan assessment, *Ann Rheum Dis* 43:365-369, 1984.
4. Bridgman JF: Panarthritis of the shoulder and diabetes mellitus, *Ann Rheum Dis* 31:69-71, 1972.
5. Bruckner FE, Nye CJS: A prospective study of adhesive capsulitis of the shoulder ("frozen shoulder") in a high risk population, *Q J Med* 198:191-204, 1981.
5a. Bulgen DY, Hazleman BL: Letter, *Lancet* 2:760, 1981.
5b. Bulgen DY, Binder A, Hazleman BL, et al: Immunological studies in frozen shoulder, *J Rheumatol* 9(6):893-898, 1982.
6. Conti V: Arthroscopy in rehabilitation, *Orthop Clin North Am* 10(3):709-711, 1979.
7. Cruess RL: Corticosteroid-induced osteonecrosis of the humeral head, *Orthop Clin North Am* 16(4):789-796, 1985.
8. Dandy DJ: *Essential orthopaedics and trauma,* London, 1989, Churchill Livingstone.
9. De Seze S: Les épaules douloureuses et les épaules bloquées, *Concours Med* 96(36):5329-5357, 1974.
10. Grey RG: The natural history of idiopathic frozen shoulder, *J Bone Joint Surg* 60:564, 1978.
11. Griffin J: Physiological effects of ultrasonic energy as it is used clinically, *Phys Ther* 46:18-23, 1966.
12. Hertling D, Kessler RM: *Management of common musculoskeletal disorders,* ed 2, Philadelphia, 1990, Lippincott.
13. Kaltenborn F: Course notes, Kent, Ohio, April 1931.
14. Kessel L, Bayley I, Young A: The upper limb: the frozen shoulder, *Br J Hosp Med* 25:334, 336-337, 339, 1981.
15. Kisner C, Colby LA: *Therapeutic exercise: foundations and techniques,* ed 2, Philadelphia, 1990, FA Davis.
16. Kuzin F: Two unique shoulder disorders: adhesive capsulitis and reflex sympathetic dystrophy syndrome, *Postgrad Med* 73:207-210, 214-216, 1983.
17. Last RJ: *Anatomy, regional and applied,* ed 5, London, 1972, Churchill Livingstone.
18. Loyd JA, Loyd HM: Adhesive capsulitis of the shoulder: arthrographic diagnosis and treatment, *South Med J* 76:879-883, 1983.
19. Lundberg BJ: The frozen shoulder, *Acta Orthop Scand* 119(suppl):1-59, 1969.
20. Magee DJ: *Orthopaedic physical assessment,* Philadelphia, 1989, Saunders.
21. Maitland GO: Treatment of the glenohumeral joint by passive movement, *Physiotherapy* 69:3-7, 1983.
22. McLaughlin HL: On the frozen shoulder, *Bull Hosp Joint Dis* 12:383-393, 1951.
23. Moseley HF: *Shoulder lesions,* Springfield, Ill, 1945, Charles C Thomas.
24. Netter FM: *The CIBA collection of medical illustrations, vol 8: Musculoskeletal system,* part 2, Summit, NJ, 1990, CIBA-Geigy.
25. Neviaser JS: Adhesive capsulitis of the shoulder, *J Bone Joint Surg* 27:211-222, 1945.
26. Neviaser JS: Arthrography of the shoulder joint, *J Bone Joint Surg* 44:1321-1330, 1962.
27. Neviaser JS: Adhesive capsulitis and the stiff and painful shoulder, *Orthop Clin North Am* 11:327-333, 1980.
28. Nicholson GG: The effects of passive joint mobilization on pain and hypomobility associated with adhesive capsulitis of the shoulder, *Orthop Sports Phys Ther* 6:238-246, 1985.
29. Post M, editor: *The shoulder: surgical and nonsurgical management,* Philadelphia, 1978, Lea & Febiger.

30. Reeves B: The natural history of the frozen shoulder syndrome, *Scand J Rheumatol* 4:193-196, 1975.

31. Resnick D: Shoulder pain, *Orthop Clin North Am* 14(1):81-97, 1983.

32. Rizk TE, Pinals RS: Frozen shoulder, *Semin Arthritis Rheum* 11:440-452, 1982.

33. Rockwood CA, Matsen FA, editors: *The shoulder,* vol 2, Philadelphia, 1990, Saunders.

34. Saunders HD: *Evaluation, treatment and prevention of musculoskeletal disorders,* Bloomingdale, Minn, 1985, Educational Opportunities.

35. Simon WH: Soft tissue disorders of the shoulder: frozen shoulder, calcific tendinitis, and bicipital tendinitis, *Orthop Clin North Am* 6:521-539, 1975.

36. Wadsworth CT: Frozen shoulder, *Phys Ther* 66(12):1878-1883, 1986.

37. Wright MG, Richards AJ, Clarke MB: Letter: *99mTc-pertechnetate scanning in capsulitis,* Lancet 2:1265-1296, 1975.

37a. Young A: Immunological studies in the frozen shoulder. In Bailey J, Kessel L, editors: *Shoulder surgery,* Berlin-Heidelberg, 1982, Springer-Verlag.

RECOMMENDED READING

Grey RG: The natural history of idiopathic frozen shoulder, *J Bone Joint Surg* 60:564, 1978.

Rockwood CA, Matsen FA, editors: *The shoulder,* vol 2, Philadelphia, 1990, Saunders, pp. 837-862.

Wadsworth CT: Frozen shoulder, *Phys Ther* 66(12):1878-1883, 1986.

14

Painful Bump over Distal End of Clavicle

A 31-year-old father presents with immediate pain and a bump over the left distal end of the clavicle, which happened yesterday when he tried to demonstrate a cartwheel to his 4-year-old son. When asked, he reports that he fell onto his shoulder. The patient volunteers that attempting to touch his right shoulder with his left hand and trying to elevate his shoulder are most painful.

CLUE:

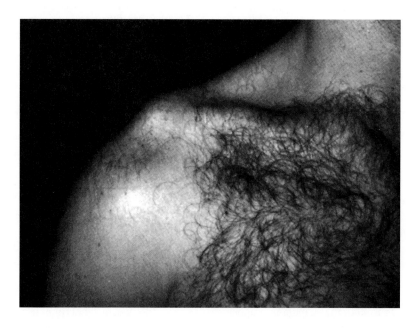

(From Nicholas JA, Hershman EB, editors: *The upper extremity in sports medicine,* ed 2, St Louis, 1995, Mosby.)

PALPATION   There is pain and tenderness, with protruding bump felt over left distal end of clavicle.

PASSIVE RANGE OF MOTION   Painful at extremes of motion.

ACTIVE RANGE OF MOTION   Full and painful, though left shoulder abduction to 90° and horizontal abduction elicited increased pain. Left shoulder shrugging is also painful.

MUSCLE STRENGTH   Left shoulder flexion and abduction to 90° are weakened to good minus.

SELECTIVE TENSION   Resistive horizontal adduction is painful.

? Questions

1. What is most likely to have happened?
2. What is the anatomy of the acromioclavicular (AC) joint?
3. What are four bony variations of the AC joint in decreasing order of incidence?
4. Is there a disk or meniscus interposed between the articulating ends of the clavicle and the acromion?
5. What is the kinesiology of the AC joint?
6. What are the pathomechanics of injury?
7. What is the clinical presentation?
8. What is the classification of injury?
9. What therapeutic management is appropriate for first- and second-degree AC joint sprains?
10. What is the recommended treatment for third-degree AC joint sprain?

1. What is most likely to have happened?

A shoulder disarticulation referred to as a shoulder separation involving the acromioclavicular joint. When untreated, the injury may result in permanent residual deformity, weakened shoulder abduction,[7] and eventual traumatic arthritis.

2. What is the anatomy of the acromioclavicular (AC) joint?

The AC joint is a planar (that is, gliding) synovial joint. The flat lateral flare of the scapular spine known as the "acromion process" articulates with the lateral end of the convex clavicle. Stability of this joint is primarily provided by the *AC joint capsule and ligament complex*. Providing *anteroposterior stability* of the AC joint, this complex is the first structure to absorb an impact in the event of injury. A *secondary static stabilizer* is the *coracoclavicular ligament*, consisting of a *medial conoid band and a lateral trapezoid portion* (Fig. 14-1), which together provide *vertical plane stability*. These latter two ligaments, by virtue of the orientation of span, enable the clavicle to hold the scapula and upper limb[6] in what is colloquially described as a "broad shoulder." The third source of stability to the AC joint is the dynamic contribution of the trapezius and deltoid attachments to the superior aspect of the AC ligaments.

3. What are four bony variations of the AC joint in decreasing order of incidence?

Bony variations of the AC joint are presented according to their increased frequency within the population.
- Distal end is oblique and overrides a congruous obliquity of the acromion.
- Articular surfaces are vertical and congruous.
- Articular surfaces are incongruous.
- Distal surface is oblique and underrides a congruous acromial articular surface.[5]

4. Is there a disk or meniscus interposed between the articulating ends of the clavicle and the acromion?

The wedge-shaped intraarticular disk (Fig. 14-2) has been found to be missing in approximately 80% of the population. Before 20 years of age, segments of human population possess menisci or an intraarticular disk interposed between the acromion and the clavicle. After 30 years of age, many people show degenerative changes of these structures.[5]

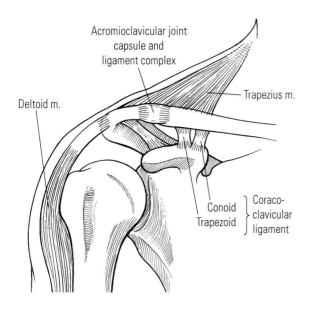

FIG. 14-1 Acromioclavicular joint stability provided by primary, secondary, and tertiary joint stabilizers.

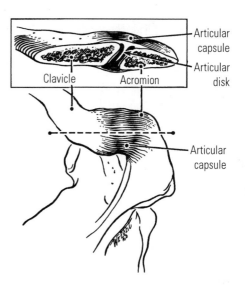

FIG. 14-2 Superior view of the right acromioclavicular joint. *Inset,* Coronal section of the joint showing a wedge-shaped intraarticular disk. (From Moore KL: *Clinically oriented anatomy,* ed 2, Baltimore, 1985, Williams & Wilkins.)

5. What is the kinesiology of the AC joint?

The kinesiologic function of the AC joint must be understood in the context of clavicle function. The clavicle undergoes long axis rotation between both the AC and the sternoclavicular (SC) joints. Because of its gentle "S" shape the clavicle acts as a mechanical crank. What this means is that motion at one end will cause a reverse motion at the other end. During shoulder elevation, there is cephalad glide of the clavicle with anterior rotation at the acromial end, and caudal glide (depression) with posterior rotation at the sternal end of the clavicle. The opposite motions occur during shoulder depression. This may be confirmed by simultaneous palpation and observation of both the medial and lateral ends of the clavicle while the shoulder is moved through its range of flexion and depression (Fig. 14-3).

6. What are the pathomechanics of injury?

This injury is common in contact sports resulting from a hard fall onto the point of the shoulder (Fig. 14-4) as when a hockey player is "driven into the boards." This is the same mechanism as that involving injury to the upper brachial plexus that rends the shoulder and neck apart because of a great force of impact. The caudalward force drives down the acromion, though the clavicle does not descend along with it because it is strongly anchored in place by the trapezius and sternomastoid muscles; instead the stabilizing ligaments are tensed and may sprain if the force of injury exceeds their inherent strength.

7. What is the clinical presentation?

The patient presents with a large lump over the lateral end of the clavicle that is tender and severely painful at the exact site of the joint.[13] The observed protuberance occurs because the shoulder falls away from the clavicle unsupported by the weight of the upper limb so that the acromion passes inferior to the lateral end of the clavicle. In addition, the clavicle is pulled upward by the unopposed action of the trapezius and sternomastoid muscles.[7] The result is a *stair-step deformity*[3] (see p. 145) best viewed when the arm is allowed to hang at the side. Although resistive motions, except for horizontal adduction, do not hurt, passive movements, especially at the extremes of motion are quite painful. The most painful movement is passive adduction across the front of the upper thorax; active horizontal adduction is also painful.[3] Active motion above 90° of shoulder motion will cause pain. The clavicle hangs freely, and the precise and interrelated components of shoulder function are altered so that abduction will be compro-

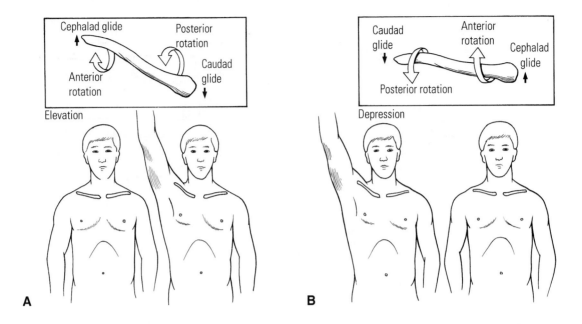

FIG. 14-3 Medial and lateral clavicular movements corresponding to shoulder elevation and depression. **A,** Shoulder elevation is accompanied by the latter end of the clavicle undergoing elevation and anterior rotation; the opposite motions occur at the medial end. **B,** Reverse motion sequence occurs. Thus, the two ends of the clavicle move vertically, albeit inversely to each other, like a mechanical crank. This, as well as inverse rotations on either end, occur as a direct function of the crank-like shape of the clavicle.

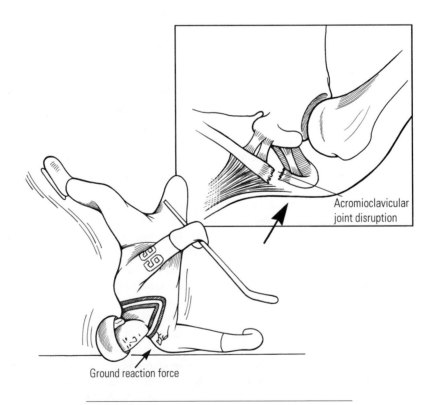

FIG. 14-4 Acromioclavicular joint sprain. Mechanism of injury.

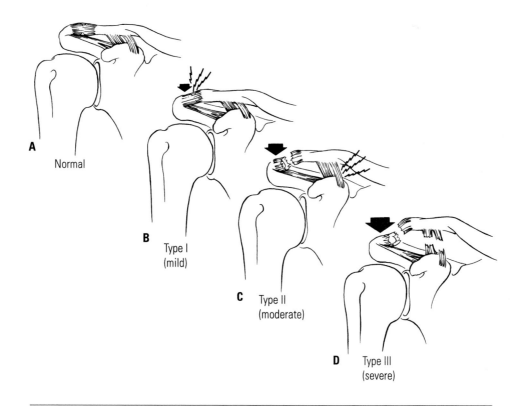

A
Normal

B
Type I
(mild)

C
Type II
(moderate)

D
Type III
(severe)

FIG. 14-5 These schematic drawings illustrate the ligamentous injuries that occur to the acromioclavicular joint. **A,** Normal anatomic relationships. **B,** In type I injury, a mild force is applied to the point of the shoulder, which stretches only the acromioclavicular articulation but does not disrupt the fibers of that joint. **C,** In type II injury, a moderate force applied to the point of the shoulder displaces the acromion process distally, disrupts the acromioclavicular ligaments, and may partially stretch the coracoclavicular ligaments. **D,** In type III injury, the severe force applied to the point of the shoulder drives the acromion and accompanying coracoid process downward, disrupting both the acromioclavicular ligaments. (From Pettrone FA, editor: *AAOS symposium on upper extremity injuries in athletes,* St Louis, 1986, Mosby; modified from Allman FL: *J Bone Joint Surg* 49A:774, 1967. In Rockwood CA, Green OP, editors: *Fractures in adults,* ed 2, Philadelphia, 1984, Lippincott.)

mised. Pain is in fact attributable to injury to the deltoid muscle, especially on abduction, where the free end of the lateral clavicle rams up painfully into the interior of the deltoid.

8. What is the classification of injury (Fig. 14-5)?

TYPE I, FIRST DEGREE, MILD INJURY

A mild force stretches the AC joint capsule and ligament complex but does not disrupt the fibers of the joint. There is no palpable instability here.

TYPE II, SECOND DEGREE, MODERATE INJURY

A moderate force disrupts the AC joint capsule and ligament complex fibers and may partially stretch or tear the coracoclavicular ligament complex. Moderate

anteroposterior (A-P) instability and possible mild vertical plane instability is referred to as subluxation of the AC joint. Here the characteristic "step" becomes obvious and is made even more visible if the patient is given a weight to hold in each hand.

TYPE III, THIRD DEGREE, SEVERE INJURY

A severe force drives the scapula and its two processes downward, disrupting both the acromioclavicular and the coracoclavicular ligaments. The muscular attachments may have also been compromised. Pronounced A-P instability with vertical-plane instability is termed *dislocation,* since the AC joint surfaces have lost all contact. A gap may be viewed on a stress A-P radiograph and is emphasized if the patient stands while a weight is suspended from the wrist.[3]

9. What therapeutic management is appropriate for first- and second-degree AC joint sprains?

GRADE I

No immobilization is needed in a first-degree sprain and treatment may be with ice massage and progressive active range of motion as pain allows. Strengthening exercises should begin as the pain decreases[3] and should emphasize trapezius and deltoid strengthening to help stabilize the AC joint. Unrestricted activity is usually permitted some 7 to 10 days after the injury.[5]

GRADE II

- Immobilization using an immobilizer that holds the humerus superiorly and the clavicle inferiorly[3] so as to approximate the torn ends. This position permits approximation of scar tissue so as to provide maximum stability once healing is complete.
- Cross-fiber massage to the capsule or ligaments to organize scar-tissue alignment.[4]
- Mobilization to the glenohumeral (GH), scapulothoracic (ST), and sternoclavicular (SC) joints to forestall the effects of stiffening.
- Intermittent ice.
- Gentle range of motion begun early on[3] within pain-free limits.
- As the pain decreases, wean patient off immobilization and increase activity.
- Nonpainful strengthening exercises, especially to deltoid and trapezius muscles.
- Unrestricted activity is usually achieved 2 to 3 weeks after the injury.

After a moderate sprain, some degree of residual subluxation of the AC joint may occur,[3] and may become evident when the patient later feels difficulty when working with the arms in front of the body (as when writing on a blackboard, operating a keyboard, or carrying a tray).[2]

10. What is the recommended treatment for third-degree AC joint sprain?

Treatment of type III injury is controversial and has two approaches:

CONSERVATIVE APPROACH

Kenny-Howard sling halter[1] for 4 to 6 weeks,[3] ice, and isometrics to tolerance. Range of motion exercises after immobilizer is removed and progressive strengthening when mobilization is permitted are indicated. The deltoid and trapezius work should not be emphasized because this may apply disruptive force to the AC joint capsule and ligament complex.

SURGICAL APPROACH

1. Open reduction, capsular repair, and *internal fixation* by insertion of a threaded wire through the acromion, across the AC joint, and well into the clavicle. The wire is removed after 6 weeks.[7] After surgery, isometrics are performed as pain permits, while active range of motion exercise begins 2 to 4 weeks after the operation, followed by progressing to active strengthening 4 to 6 weeks after the operation.[3]
2. Open reduction by *screw fixation* of the clavicle to the coracoid process and transfer of the tip of the coracoid and attached pectoralis minor muscle to the clavicle.[3] The arm is then immobilized in a sling with early gentle active range of motion exercises and isometrics followed by AROM exercises to 90°, usually after 7 to 10 days. Progressive strengthening begins 4 to 6 weeks after the operation.[7]

REFERENCES

1. Cyriax J: *Textbook of orthopaedic medicine, vol 1: diagnosis of soft tissue lesions,* London, 1982, Bailliere-Tindall.
2. Dandy DJ: *Essential orthopaedics and trauma,* Edinburgh, 1989, Churchill Livingstone.
3. Gould JA III: *Orthopaedic and sports physical therapy,* ed 2, St Louis, 1990, Mosby.
4. Kisner C, Colby LA: *Therapeutic exercise: foundations and techniques,* ed 2, Philadelphia, 1990, FA Davis.
5. Moffat M: Lecture and handout series on musculoskeletal therapeutic exercise, Fall 1989, New York University Department of Physical Therapy, New York University Medical Book Store.
6. Moore KL: *Clinically oriented anatomy,* ed 2, Baltimore, 1985, Williams & Wilkins.
7. Salter RB: *Textbook of disorders of the musculoskeletal system,* ed 2, Baltimore, 1983, Williams & Wilkins.

RECOMMENDED READING

Bearden JM, Hughston JC, Wheatley GS: Acromioclavicular dislocation: method of treatment, *J Sports Med* (4):5-17, 1973.
Bowers KD: Treatment of acromioclavicular sprains in athletes, *The physician and sports medicine* 2(1):79-89, 1983.
Malone T, McPoil T, Nitz AJ: *Orthopaedic and sports physical therapy,* ed 3, St Louis, 1996, Mosby.
Moffat M: Lecture and handout series on musculoskeletal therapeutic exercise, Fall 1989, New York University Department of Physical Therapy, New York University Medical Book Store.
Rockwood, CA, Young DC: Disorders of the acromioclavicular joint. In Rockwood CA, Matsen FA: *The shoulder,* ed 2, vol 1, Philadelphia, 1990, Saunders.

15

Fall on Point of Shoulder, Causing Sagging of Upper Extremity, Loss of Shoulder Function, and Much Pain on Movement

A 34-year-old adult male was riding his dirtbike over a mountain trail when the front wheel of his bike dipped suddenly into a gully, causing the rider to pitch forward over the handlebars to land on the point of his right shoulder. The patient acutely presented the following appearance (Fig. 15-1).

The patient now presents himself to you 3 weeks later in a swathe-and-sling binder with a prescription from the local orthopod for "therapy." The patient informs you that he works in a heavy industry plant that requires him to hoist heavy objects and to pull down on large heavy machine levers.

 Questions

1. What is most likely to have occurred to this man's shoulder?
2. How is the clavicle embryologically unique as compared to other long bones?
3. What is the biomechanical significance of the strutlike design of the collarbone?
4. What is the most common pattern of clavicle fracture?
5. What is the mechanism involved in fracture of the middle third of the clavicle?
6. What is the classification of clavicle fractures?
7. What is the typically observed deformity after fracture of the clavicle?
8. What concomitant internal injuries may accompany fractures of the medial third of the clavicle?
9. What kind of pulmonary insult may occur to the lung or lungs during fracture of the medial clavicular section?
10. What type of nerve injury is suspected after fracture of the medial third of the clavicle?
11. What major vascular injury may concurrently occur with fractures of the medial third of the clavicle?
12. What other skeletal injuries may accompany clavicle fracture?
13. What mechanism accounts for clavicle fracture in newborns?
14. What is the clinical presentation of birth fracture of the clavicle?

15. **What mechanism most often accounts for clavicle fractures in children?**

16. **What radiography is appropriate when one suspects clavicular fracture?**

17. **What is the medical management of clavicle fracture?**

18. **How long does the clavicle require to heal after fracture?**

19. **How soon after clavicle fracture may active and resistive activity commence?**

---

1. What is most likely to have occurred to this man's shoulder (Fig. 15-1)?

Clavicle fracture.

2. How is the clavicle embryologically unique as compared to other long bones?

The clavicle is embryologically unique in being the first bone in the body to ossify and the only long bone to ossify by intramembranous ossification without going through a cartilaginous stage.[10] Cosmetically, the crank-shaped clavicle bespeaks grace yet conveys strength in its slender swanlike appearance. Its name is derived from the Latin word *clavis* 'key,' the diminutive of which is *clavicula*.[17] Although appearing nearly straight when viewed from the front, it actually appears as an "S-shaped" or *crank-shaped* bone when viewed from above (Fig. 15-2).

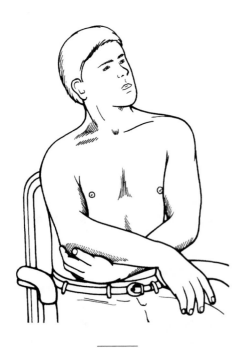

FIG. 15-1

3. What is the biomechanical significance of the strutlike design of the collarbone?

The clavicle is the sole bony strut linking the trunk to the shoulder girdle and arm. The significance of this is twofold:

- In the domestic cat, the clavicle, unlike in man, is free at both ends and perforce does not link the sternum and humerus (Fig. 15-3). Uniquely adapted to land on its forelegs, the cat will therefore not fracture its clavicle since its clavicle absorbs the impact energy of landing by moving to a limit set by restraining soft tissue.

   Man's clavicle, however, is adapted for carrying weights because of its firm attachment to the sternum medially and the acromion and coracoid processes laterally by ligaments (Fig. 15-4), the tensile strength of which exceeds that of bone.[7] The impact absorbed by a fall onto an outstretched arm is thus transmitted up the length of the clavicle to either dissipate or cause fracture at that bone's weakest point, the middle third.

- The clavicle is mechanically analogous to the cantilever (Fig. 15-5). A cantilever is a beam supported only at one end while projecting freely at the other end. The mechanical advantage gained by this lever system is the ability to carry loads significantly greater than its own weight. Airplane wings, for example, that have no props or struts to brace them are examples of cantilevers that tolerate considerable forces of air lift. A cantilever bridge has two towers on opposite sides of the river, and each tower supports beams that meet in the middle of that bridge. If half of the bridge were dismantled, say, by an explosive, the other half could still carry as much weight, in the form of trucks, trains, and automobiles, as before.

   By linking the arm to the axial skeleton by a cantilever system, the weight of the body serves as a counterweight that permits the carrying of loads greater than the weight of the arm itself.[7] This capability is diminished or made impossible when the clavicle becomes fractured, since the length of the le-

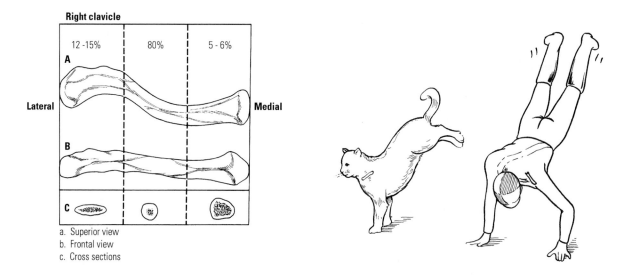

Right clavicle

12 -15%   80%   5 - 6%

A

Lateral   Medial

B

C

a. Superior view
b. Frontal view
c. Cross sections

FIG. 15-2 The clavicle appears as an S-shaped double curve when viewed from above, *a.* It appears nearly straight when viewed from in front, *b.* The outer end of the clavicle is flat in cross-section but becomes more tubular in the medial aspect, *c.* (From Craig EV: Fractures of the clavicle. In Rockwood CA, Matsen FA, editors: *The shoulder*, vol 1, Philadelphia, 1990, Saunders.)

FIG. 15-3 Falls on the outstretched arms. The cat, unlike man, does not fracture its clavicle because it does not link the sternum and humerus as in man. (From Dandy DJ: *Essential orthopaedics and trauma*, Edinburgh, 1989, Churchill Livingstone.)

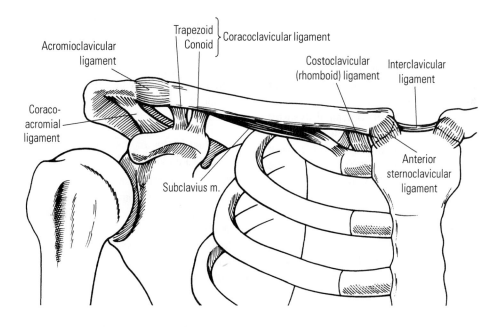

Acromioclavicular ligament

Trapezoid
Conoid } Coracoclavicular ligament

Costoclavicular (rhomboid) ligament

Interclavicular ligament

Coraco-acromial ligament

Subclavius m.

Anterior sternoclavicular ligament

FIG. 15-4 The clavicle is securely bound by ligaments at both the sternoclavicular and the acromioclavicular joints. It is the only bony strut from the torso to the upper extremity.

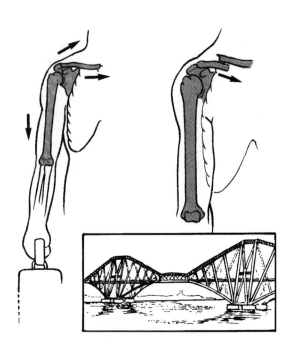

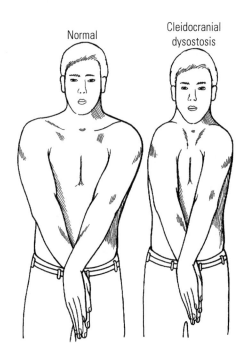

FIG. 15-5 Cantilever action of the clavicle. When the clavicle is broken, the shoulder is not supported and moves downwards and medially. Inset: *Cantilever bridge.* (From Dandy DJ: *Essential orthopaedics and trauma*, Edinburgh, 1989, Churchill Livingstone.)

FIG. 15-6 Cleidocranial dysostosis.

ver arm is subsequently decreased. Muscle spasm pulls the outer fragment beneath the inner one, further diminishing its length. In light of this it then becomes obvious why individuals with cleidocranial dysostosis (congenital absence of the clavicle, Fig. 15-6) may exhibit weakness when supporting overhead loads; it is precisely the overhead position that calls upon the leverlike function of the clavicle to prop weighted objects away from the body.

4. What is the most common pattern of clavicle fracture?

Group I clavicle fracture refers to a break of the middle third of that bone and is the most common pattern of fracture (80%)[18,20] in both adults and children.[8] Aside from stability imparted to the proximal and medial ends of the clavicle by ligamentous and muscular attachments, the cross-sectional diameter of the clavicle differs along the length of its shaft such that the middle third of that bone is most vulnerable to injury. Whereas the flat outer third of the clavicle is ideally suited to the myriad attachments of muscles and liga-

ments, the tubular medial third has a cross section that best protects those branches of the brachial plexus lying behind the clavicle. The vulnerable central section, however, is not just free of any stabilizing attachments but is also in fact the thinnest cross section of that bone and perforce the weakest, especially to axial loading.[15]

5. What is the mechanism involved in fracture of the middle third of the clavicle?

The classic mechanism of fracture to the middle third of the clavicle is from a fall onto an outstretched arm and is best understood by the counterpoint idea of the three-point force system. The *indirect force* travels up along the shaft of the humerus until it encounters two counterpoints: one at the glenohumeral joint and one at the sternoclavicular joint (Fig. 15-7). Force dispersal will then, one would hope, occur along the length of the shaft of the clavicle but will result in a *spiral fracture* of the middle third in the event that disruptive forces exceed intrinsic bone strength.[8] Injury may also occur from a *direct force* as occurs from a blow directly over the middle third of the clavicle, resulting in a fracture (Fig. 15-8). Injury may also occur from a direct fall onto the point of the shoulder,

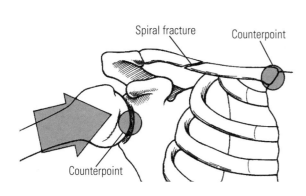

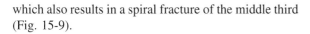

FIG. 15-7 An indirect force encounters counterpoints at the gleno-humeral and sternoclavicular joints causing a spiral fracture at the middle third of the clavicle. (Modified from DePalma AF: *Surgery of the shoulder,* ed 3, Philadelphia, 1983, Lippincott.)

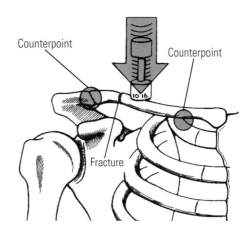

FIG. 15-8 A direct force applied over the middle third of the clavicle causing a fracture to occur at the juncture of the middle and outer thirds. (Modified from DePalma AF: *Surgery of the shoulder,* ed 3, Philadelphia, 1983, Lippincott.)

which also results in a spiral fracture of the middle third (Fig. 15-9).

6. What is the classification of clavicle fractures?

Although fractures of the clavicle have in the past been classified according to fracture configurations (that is, greenstick, oblique, transverse, and comminuted),[24] the common classification is now according to the location of fracture. This approach is more reflective of a comprehensive view, if one takes into consideration the mechanism of injury, clinical presentation, and alternative treatment methods.[4]

Both group II and group III fractures refer to breakage at the distal and medial thirds of the clavicle respectively. These groupings are further subdivided according to the integrity of ligamentous structures supporting the clavicle at the sternoclavicular joint medially and the acromioclavicular joint laterally. With children, these injuries are often epiphyseal fractures. With adults, these injuries often have sequelae of degenerative joint changes and associated posttraumatic arthritis.

7. What is the typically observed deformity after fracture of the clavicle?

The deformity of a fractured clavicle has the following observable presentation: the (distal fragment of the) affected shoulder appears lower and droops forward and inward, whereas the proximal fragment is displaced up-

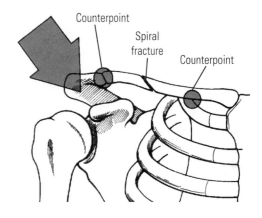

FIG. 15-9 A direct force applied onto the point of the shoulder forcing the clavicle downward against the first rib and resulting in a spiral fracture of the middle third. (Modified from DePalma AF: *Surgery of the shoulder,* ed 3, Philadelphia, 1983, Lippincott.)

ward and backward, causing a tent-like tautening of the overlying skin. This displacement of segments occurs as a function of the specific muscle attachments on different portions of the clavicle. Attaching to the distal third of the clavicle, the upper trapezius cannot bear the weight of the upper extremity unconnected to the axillary skeleton after fracture, and so gravity causes sagging of the entire upper extremity and the outer fragment as a unit. Additionally, the lateral fragment is adducted by the pectoralis major; this adduction causes the lateral fragment to override the medial fragment and gives the appearance of a shortened clavicle. The inner fragment is elevated by the sternocleidomastoid muscle (Fig. 15-10).

The head and chin are tilted away from the fracture site to relax the pull of the sternocleidomastoid. Or the patient may angle his or her head toward the injury, attempting to relax the pull of the trapezius on the outer fragment. The patient may often splint the sagging arm against the body while holding the affected elbow with the other hand.[4]

8. What concomitant internal injuries may accompany fractures of the medial third of the clavicle?

Injuries to the lungs, brachial plexus, or subclavian and axillary vessels may occur from accompanying fractures of the first rib or of the medial third of the

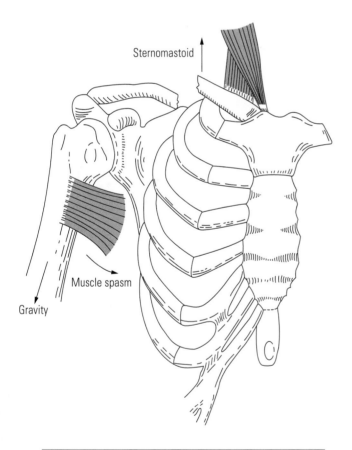

FIG. 15-10 Deformity accompanying a clavicle fracture. (From Ellis H: *Clinical anatomy,* ed 7, Oxford, 1983, Blackwell Scientific Publications.)

clavicle. Although the usual adult clavicular shaft fracture is oblique in nature, excessive forces may instead cause a dangerous comminuted fracture. If the middle spike projects from superior to inferior, the clinician must be alerted to the potential for associated pulmonary or neurovascular injuries. Generally, manipulation of fracture fragments, regardless of fracture pattern, is inadvisable without x-ray studies of the position of those fragments.[27]

9. What kind of pulmonary insult may occur to the lung or lungs during fracture of the medial clavicular section?

Because the apical pleura and lobes of the upper lung lie adjacent to the clavicle, a shard from a severely displaced fracture may puncture the pleura and result in pneumothorax or hemothorax.[20] As such, the anteroposterior radiographic view should include the upper lung fields taken in the upright position with particularly close attention paid to the lung outline. It is essential to auscultate for asymmetry as well as the decrease of breath sounds to rule out pneumothorax.

10. What type of nerve injury is suspected after fracture of the medial third of the clavicle?

The neurovascular bundle emerges from the thoracic outlet under the clavicle atop the first rib.[19] The portion of the medial cord of the brachial plexus that gives rise to the ulnar nerve crosses the first rib directly under the medial third of the clavicle, and is at risk for injury.[4] The other two cords of the plexus are too far laterally and posteriorly to be injured after fracture.

11. What major vascular injury may concurrently occur with fractures of the medial third of the clavicle?

The subclavius muscle and the thick cervical fascia act as a barrier to direct injury of the vessels. If initial displacement of fracture fragments has not injured the vasculature, they are unlikely to become further injured, since their migration (secondary to muscle spasm) often pulls them out of harm's way.[4]

The anterior curve of the medial two thirds of the clavicle provides a rigid arch beneath which the great vessels pass as they move from the thoracic outlet down toward the axilla.[25] Fracture of the medial third of the clavicle may result in one of the following four severe vascular phenomena:

- A laceration resulting in life-threatening hemorrhage is suggested by an upper limb that is cold, pulseless, and pale and by the presence of a bruit[26] or a difference in pressure[29] between both arms.

- Arterial thrombus and occlusion may lead to distal ischemia.
- Damage to the arterial wall may lead to aneurysm formation and late embolic phenomena.
- Venous thrombosis may lead to late pulmonary embolism.[4]

If a major vessel injury is suspected, an arteriogram should be performed.[29] In the rare event of a tear of a large vessel, surgical exploration is required.[4]

12. What other skeletal injuries may accompany clavicle fracture?

Associated skeletal injuries may include sternoclavicular or acromioclavicular separations or fracture dislocations through these joints.[3,13,]

13. What mechanism accounts for clavicle fracture in newborns?

Several factors account for clavicular fracture at birth, the most significant being presentation of the infant. In cephalic presentation of the vaginally delivered newborn, compression of the leading clavicle against the maternal symphysis pubis occurs.[16] With breech delivery, direct traction may occur as the obstetrician, trying to depress the shoulders and free the arm in the delivery of the head, inadvertently fractures the clavicle.[23] No incidence of fracture is reported in babies delivered by cesarean section.[1] Other contributing factors causing clavicular fractures in newborns include size (>52 cm),[11] birth weight (3800 to 4000 g), inexperience of the physician, and midforceps deliveries.

The infant's mother might notice that her baby cries after being picked up and appears to be hurt.[2] The baby does not seem to use his or her arm naturally and cries if the arm is moved during activities such as dressing. The mother may notice swelling or crepitus or take the baby to the pediatrician because of the "sudden appearance of a lump;"[6] this lump is caused by fracture callus and typically appears 7 to 11 days after fracture.[5] On palpation, one may feel a tender, uneven border of the clavicle, which is asymmetrical when compared to the contralateral side.

14. What is the clinical presentation of birth fracture of the clavicle?

Clinical presentations of the clavicle are twofold:

- The fracture may be clinically inapparent, and a crack may or may not be heard during delivery.[2] Close examination may reveal an asymmetry of the clavicle contour or a shortening of the neck line.[4]
- The fracture may be clinically apparent (pseudoparalysis) as a form in which the child exhibits some degree of unilateral upper extremity paresis on attempted volitional movement or during elicitation of the Moro reflex.[9,22] Here, clavicular fracture must be differentiated from the following conditions: Erb's palsy, separation of the proximal humeral epiphysis, and acute osteomyelitis of the clavicle or proximal humerus. A clavicle fracture may coexist with brachial plexus injury.[23]

15. What mechanism most often accounts for clavicle fractures in children?

The mechanism of injury for clavicle fractures in children is identical to that of adults and may occur from a fall onto the point of the shoulder or upon an outstretched hand from a changing table, high chair, or bunk bed. Unlike the adult, trauma often results in a greenstick or incomplete fracture rather than a displaced fracture. As with other fractures of long bones, clavicular fractures may be a sign of trauma in the physically abused child.[4]

16. What radiography is appropriate when one suspects clavicular fracture?

Radiographic evaluation of the shaft of the clavicle is best viewed in two projections:

- An anteroposterior view that typically reveals the upward displacement of the proximal fragment as well as caudal displacement of the distal fragment secondary to muscle spasm.
- A 45° cephalic tilt view permits more accurate assessment of the anteroposterior relationships of the two fragments.[4]

Fractures of the distal third of the clavicle are easily missed with the above-mentioned views and are easily passed off as acromioclavicular sprains. The reason is that the standard exposure overexposes the distal end of the clavicle. When suspect, fractures of the distal third are confirmed by employment of one third of the exposure used for the shoulder joint.

Often the novice clinician will not know that these views should be ordered and misdiagnose the injury as an AC sprain based on abnormal standard views as well as the absence of a classic presentation, which may be absent in distal fractures of the clavicle. However, the presence of pain and tenderness on movement some 10 to 14 days after the injury is cause for suspicion of fracture. Standard radiographs at this time will reveal either a line of bony absorption along the clavicular shaft or callus formation at the site of fracture.

17. What is the medical management of clavicle fracture?

With adolescents and adults, provided that no displacement of fracture fragments has occurred, treatment is by supporting the weight of the arm in a broad sling or a posterior figure-of-eight bandage[4] (Fig. 15-11) for 3 weeks.[6] Lack of consistent immobilization may contribute to increasing the likelihood of nonunion; thus immobilization must continue, at the very least, until clinical union has occurred and, there is doubt, even beyond that time. The principle behind this bandage is to raise the distal fragment and depress the inner fragment while simultaneously enabling the ipsilateral elbow and hand to be used in activities of daily living, thus helping stave off adhesion development and loss of range in that extremity.[4]

When there is displacement and overriding of fracture ends, an attempt must be made to reduce the fracture and restore the normal length of the clavicle; local anesthesia may be required. Then, with the fracture reduced, a posterior figure-of-eight bandage with plaster reinforcement or even full-shoulder immobilization in a spica cast is appropriate.[4]

Treatment for newborns consists in simply immobilizing the arm to the infant's trunk for 2 weeks, after which the fracture is sufficiently healed to permit painless volitional movement.[4]

18. How long does the clavicle require to heal after fracture?

The healing period for fracture of the middle third of the clavicle is as follows: infants heal within 2 weeks, children within 3 weeks, young adults heal within 4 to 6 weeks, and adults usually require 6 weeks or longer.[20] Although the fracture site may clinically unite as early as 3 weeks in the adult, radiologic union may not appear until 12 weeks or longer. Nonunion of unoperated clavicle shaft fracture, defined as failure to show radiographic progression of healing for 4 to 6 months, is rare.[4]

19. How soon after clavicle fracture may active and resistive activity commence?

The clinically relevant question for the therapist treating a patient with a 3- to 4-week-old clavicular fracture is: Will active or resistive exercises serve to stress the fracture site? This question is especially relevant to the 90° to 180° range of shoulder elevation when the clavicle is maximally stressed vis-à-vis its cantilever function.

The guidelines are as follows: During the period of clinical union active range of motion is permitted up to 90° for shoulder elevation as well as passive range of motion above 90°, provided that there is absence of any motion of fragments or tenderness at the fracture site. Glenohumeral joint and scapular mobilization and also shoulder shrugging for the purpose of decreasing the dangers of immobilization are appropriate. After radiologic union, an active range of motion greater than 90° is permitted with the gentle introduction of resistance exercises.

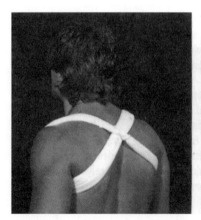 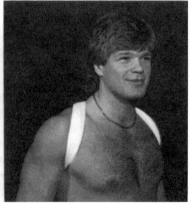

FIG. 15-11 Figure-of-eight bandage. (From Peterson L, Renström P: *Sports injuries: their prevention and treatment,* London, 1986, Martin Dunitz, Ltd.)

REFERENCES

1. Balata A, Olzai MG, Porcu A, et al: Fractures of the clavicle in the newborn, *Pediatr Med Chir* 6:125-129, 1984. Article in Italian also available in *Riv Ital Pediatr.*

2. Batemen JE: *The shoulder and neck,* Philadelphia, 1978, Saunders.

3. Butterworth RD, Kirk AA: Fracture dislocation of sterno-clavicular joint: case report, *Virginia Med Month* 79:98-100, 1952.

4. Craig EV: Fractures of the clavicle. In Rockwood CA, Matsen FA, editors: *The shoulder,* vol 1, Philadelphia, 1990, Saunders.

5. Cummings WA: Neonatal skeletal fractures: birth trauma or child abuse? *J Can Assoc Radiol* 30:30-33, 1979.

6. Dameron TB Jr, Rockwood CA: Fractures of the shaft of the clavicle. In Rockwood CA, Wilkins KE, King RE, editors: *Fractures in children,* Philadelphia, 1984, Lippincott.

7. Dandy DJ: *Essential orthopaedics and trauma,* Edinburgh, 1989, Churchill Livingstone.

8. DePalma AF: *Surgery of the shoulder,* ed 3, Philadelphia, 1983, Lippincott.

9. Freedman M, Gamble J, Lewis C: Intrauterine fracture simulating a unilateral clavicular pseudoarthrosis, *J Assoc Radiol* 33(1):37-38, 1982.

10. Gardner E: The embryology of the clavicle, *Clin Orthop* 59:9-16, 1968.

11. Gitsch VG, Schatten C: Frequenz und potentielle Faktoren in der *Genese der geburtstraumatisch bedingten Klavicula Fraktur, Zentralbl Gynäkol.*

12. Javid H: Vascular injuries of the neck, *Clin Orthop* 28:70-78, 1963.

13. Kanoksikarin S, Wearne WN: Fracture and retrosternal dislocation of the clavicle, *Aust NZ J Surg* 48:95-96, 1978.

14. Klier I, Maayor PB: Laceration of the innominate internal jugular venous junction: rare complication of fracture of the clavicle, *Orthop Rev* 10:81-82, 1981.

15. Ljunggren AE: Clavicular function, *Acta Orthop Scand* 50:261-268, 1979.

16. Madsen ET: Fractures of the extremities in the newborn, *Acta Obstet Gynecol Scand* 34:41-74, 1955.

17. Mosely HF: The clavicle: its anatomy and function, *Clin Orthop* 58:17-27, 1968.

18. Neer CS II: Fractures of the clavicle. In Rockwood CA, Green DP, editors: *Fractures in adults,* Philadelphia, 1984, Lippincott.

19. Reid J, Kennedy J: Direct fracture of the clavicle with symptoms simulating a cervical rib, *Br Med J* 2:608-609, 1925.

20. Rowe CR: An atlas of anatomy and treatment of mid-clavicular fractures, *Clin Orthop* 58:29-42, 1968.

21. Salter RB: *Textbook of disorders and injuries of the musculoskeletal system,* ed 2, Baltimore, 1983, Williams & Wilkins.

22. Sanford HN: The Moro reflex as a diagnostic aid in fracture of the clavicle in the newborn infant, *Am J Dis Child* 41:1304-1306, 1931.

23. Tancher S, Kolishev K, Tanches P, et al: Etiology of a clavicle fracture due to the birth process, *Akush Ginekol* 24(2):39-43, 1985.

24. Taylor AR: Nonunion of fractures of the clavicle: a review of 31 cases, Proc British Orthopaedic Association, *J Bone Joint Surg* 51B:568-569, 1969.

25. Telford ED, Mottershead S: Pressure at the cervicobrachial junction: an operative and an anatomical study, *J Bone Joint Surg* 30B:249, 1948.

26. Tse DHW, Slabaugh PB, Carlson PA: Injury to the axillary artery by a closed fracture of the clavicle, *J Bone Joint Surg* 62A:1372-1373, 1980.

27. Van Vlack HG: Comminuted fracture of the clavicle with pressure on brachial plexus: report of a case, *J Bone Joint Surg* 22A:446-447, 1940.

28. Widner LA, Riddervold HO: The value of lordotic view in diagnosis of fractured clavicle, *Rev Interam Radiol* 5:69-70, 1980.

29. Yates DW: Complications of fractures of the clavicle, *Injury* 7(3):189-193, 1976.

RECOMMENDED READING

Craig EV: Fractures of the clavicle. In Rockwood CA, Matsen FA, editors: *The shoulder,* vol 1, Philadelphia, 1990, WB Saunders.

Peterson L, Renström P: *Sports injuries: their prevention and treatment,* London, 1986, Martin Dunitz.

16

Painful Bump over Proximal Section of Clavicle

A 21-year-old well-built broad-shouldered man presents with acute pain over his right medial clavicle after a football tackle during which eight other men piled on top of him at a preseason training game. Your friend, an athletic trainer by profession, immediately examines this person, and the following clinical picture emerges. The player cradles his right arm with his left upper extremity and tilts his head toward his right side. He complains of considerable pain.

CLUE:

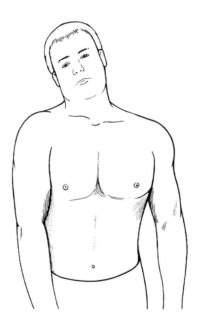

OBSERVATION   Prominence over the medial end of the clavicle is noticed. The right shoulder appears to be shortened and thrust forward when compared to the uninvolved side. The clavicle appears less prominent than on the left side.

PALPATION   There is a palpable anteriorly projecting bump over the middle of the clavicle that is tender and feels warm to the dorsum of the examiner's hand.

RANGE OF MOTION   Appears to be limited, but exactly how much is masked by muscle guarding in all directions.

MUSCLE STRENGTH   Difficult to test secondary to pain.

PULSES   Normal as is color to distal end of right extremity.

NOTE   Discomfort increases when the patient is placed in supine and refuses to lie back entirely; thus his right scapula is slightly lifted off the grass.

? Questions

1. What is most likely to have occurred in this athlete?
2. What requisite anatomy is relevant to fully understanding this injury?
3. Describe sternoclavicular (SC) joint incongruity.
4. Describe the ligamentous stability of the SC joint.
5. What is the first line of ligamentous defense against SC joint disruption?
6. What are the functions of the intraarticular disk ligament and the interclavicular ligament?
7. Describe the costoclavicular and SC ligaments and their function.
8. What is the kinesiology of the SC joint?
9. What is the range of motion of the SC joint?
10. What direct force mechanisms cause posterior SC joint injury?
11. What indirect force mechanisms cause anterior SC joint injury?
12. What is the classification of SC joint injury?
13. Why is diagnosis predicated on clinical evidence rather than on radiologic evidence?
14. What is the medical treatment of subluxation or dislocation when not life threatening?
15. What therapeutic intervention and advice is appropriate?

1. What is most likely to have occurred in this young athlete?

Anterior dislocation *separation* of the sternoclavicular (SC) joint is an uncommon injury that may occur after a blow or fall to the front of the shoulder that drives the medial inner end of the clavicle forward and the lateral outer end backward.[10] Excessive forces are transmitted along the long axis of the clavicle (serving as a first line of defense), where they may dissipate or fracture the clavicle near the junction of that bone's middle or lateral third.[6] If the clavicle fails to transmit or absorb these forces, injury may then occur more medially at the SC joint.

2. What requisite anatomy is relevant to fully understanding this injury?

When thinking about the SC joint, it is important to realize that the entire mass of the shoulder girdle, including the scapula, attaches to the axial skeleton at the SC joint. This linkage sequence begins from sternum to clavicle and from clavicle to scapula by way of the coracoid and acromion and from scapula to humerus by way of the ligamentous connections of the coracoid process. This *coracohumeral ligament,* an anterior medial structure that anastomoses with the hoodlike tendons of the cuff muscles, affords checking against excessive external rotation together with the *glenohu-*

meral ligament. Additionally, the joint cavity of the SC joint is oblique and contains a meniscus, or disk of sorts.[8] The most common causes of SC dislocation are vehicular accidents and sport injuries in that order.[7]

3. Describe sternoclavicular (SC) joint incongruity.

The SC joint is a diarthrodial joint composed of a large medial concave surface from front to back and as a convex surface vertically on its clavicular end that articulates with the curved notch of the manubrium of the sternum.[3] The joint is of a saddle variety the joint surfaces of which are so incongruent as to give the SC joint the distinction of having the least amount of bony stability of all major body joints.[9]

4. Describe the ligamentous stability of the SC joint.

Because of considerable joint incongruity, integrity at the SC joint is principally afforded by surrounding ligaments. These ligaments include the capsular ligament, the intraarticular disk ligament, costoclavicular (rhomboid) ligament, sternoclavicular ligament, and interclavicular ligament, all of which contribute toward maintenance of normal shoulder poise (Fig. 16-1).

5. What is the first line of ligamentous defense against SC joint disruption?

The *capsular ligament,* covering the anterosuperior and posterior aspects of the SC joint, represents thickenings of the joint capsule that are more prominent anteriorly.[9] These thickenings serve as a first line of defense, since they are the most important structures preventing me- dial upward displacement caused by downward disruptive force upon the distal end of the clavicle.[1]

6. What are the functions of the intraarticular disk ligament and the interclavicular ligament?

The *intraarticular disk ligament* passes through the SC joint while going from the first rib to the sternum and, as such, divides the joint into two separate joint spaces. This ligament acts as a checkrein against medial displacement of the inner clavicle. The interclavicular ligament connects the superomedial aspects of each clavicle with the capsular ligaments and upper sternum.[9] This band, homologous to the wishbone in birds,[3] assists in maintenance of shoulder poise (such as holding up the shoulder).[9]

7. Describe the costoclavicular and SC ligaments and their function.

The *costoclavicular ligament,* together with the *sternoclavicular ligament,* strongly anchor the medial end of the clavicle to the sternum. The former ligament is short and strong, consisting of an anterior and a posterior fasciculus with a bursa interposed between the two fasciculi.[1] The fibers composing these two fascicular components cross and have a twisted (cruciate) appearance.[4] The anterior fascicular fibers rising from the anterior medial surface of the first rib are directed upward and laterally[9] so that their kinesiologic function is to resist excessive upward clavicular rotation.[1] In contrast, the posterior fascicular fibers are shorter in span and arise just lateral to the anterior fibers on the first rib and are directed upward and

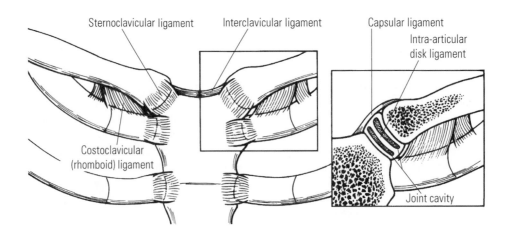

FIG. 16-1 Ligamentous stabilizers of the sternoclavicular joint.

medially[9] so as to check excessive downward clavicular rotation.[1] Thus the costoclavicular ligaments, analogous to the knee cruciate ligaments, provide stability to the SC joint during clavicular rotation (such as shoulder elevation and depression). Additionally, this two-part ligament is in many ways similar to the two-part configuration of the coracoclavicular ligament stabilizing the acromioclavicular joint on the lateral end of the clavicle.[9]

8. What is the kinesiology of the SC joint?

The costoclavicular ligament acts as a pivot for the clavicle, which seesaws about this fixed point[2] as the outer end of the clavicle elevates and depresses with shoulder flexion/abduction and extension/adduction. This motion and the importance of the various supporting ligaments are illustrated by the following thought experiment[9] (Fig. 16-2).

9. What is the range of motion of the SC joint?

The SC joint, like the saddle joint in the thumb, is freely movable with motions in almost all planes, including rotation. During normal shoulder rotation the clavicle and therefore the medial articulation of that long bone, such as the sternoclavicular joint, are capable of 30° to 35° of elevation or depression, 35° of combined forward and backward movement, and 45° to 50° of long-axis rotation[9] (Fig. 16-3).

10. What direct force mechanisms cause posterior SC joint injury?

Force applied to the anteromedial aspect of the clavicle causes the clavicle to become pushed posteriorly behind the sternum and into the mediastinum.[9] Posterior (retrosternal) dislocation (Figs. 16-4 and 16-5) is rare and dangerous,[10] and if it is suspected, both airways and peripheral pulses must be assessed, since the posterior protruding clavicle may compress both the trachea and the great vessels behind it.[5] Ways in which this injury may occur include a head-on vehicular collision in which the steering wheel pushes directly on the sternum and the heart, a kick delivered to the front of the middle of the clavicle, action of a person being run over by a vehicle, action of a person being pinned between a vehicle and a wall, and compression when an athlete lying on the ground is jumped upon. The jumper's knee lands directly over the medial third of the clavicle. Because of our anatomy, barring a javelin or some other projectile entering through the back and leaving anteriorly, it would be most unusual for a direct force to produce an anterior SC dislocation.[9]

11. What indirect force mechanisms cause anterior SC joint injury?

The most common mechanism of injury causing SC dislocation by indirect force occurs by anterior SC dislocation[9] (Figs. 16-6 and 16-7). An indirect force occurs when the shoulder is laterally compressed while simultaneously rolled backward, resulting in ipsilateral anterior dislocation. If the shoulder, however, is rolled forward, ipsilateral posterior dislocation will occur. A football pile-on in which the player falls to the ground and lands on the lateral area of his shoulder commonly results in indirect forces contributing to a pathologic condition. Before the player can get out of the way, several other players pile on top of both of his shoulders, applying significant compressive force on the clavicle down toward the sternum in one of two patterns. If during the compression the landed lateral part of the shoulder is rolled backward, the clavicle will lever backward producing an anterior dislocation medially, where the clavicle meets the SC joint; whereas, if the shoulder is rolled forward, the force directed down onto the clavicle yields a posterior dislocation of the SC joint. Other types of indirect forces causing SC joint dislocation include a cave-in on a ditch digger with lateral shoulder compression by falling dirt; lateral compressive forces on the shoulder when an individual becomes pinned between a vehicle and a wall; and a person's falling onto an outstretched abducted arm, which serves to drive the shoulder medially in the same manner as lateral compression of the shoulder does.[9]

12. What is the classification of SC joint injury?

MILD SPRAIN

All the ligaments are intact, and the joint is stable. There is mild to moderate pain, particularly on upper extremity movement. Although the joint may be slightly swollen and tender, there is no instability noted.[9]

MODERATE SPRAIN

There is anterior or posterior subluxation of the SC joint because of partial disrupture or severe stretch of the capsule, intraarticular disk, and costoclavicular ligament. Swelling is noted and pain is intense, especially with any arm movement.[9]

SEVERE SPRAIN

There is complete disruption of the SC ligaments with dislocation being either anterior or posterior. Severe

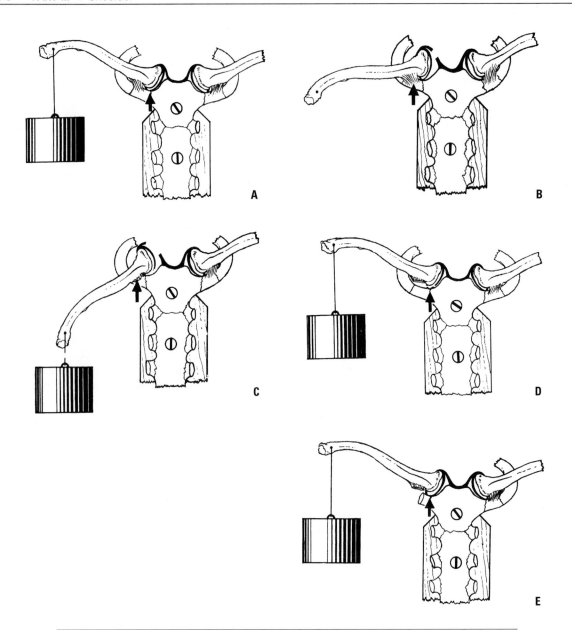

FIG. 16-2 Thought experiment demonstrating the importance of the various ligaments around the sternoclavicular joint in maintaining normal shoulder poise. **A,** The lateral portion of the clavicle is maintained in an elevated position through the sternoclavicular ligaments. The *arrow* indicates the fulcrum. **B,** When the capsule is completely divided, the lateral portion of the clavicle descends under its own weight without any loading. The clavicle will seem to be supported by the intra-articular disk ligament. **C,** After division of the capsular ligament, it was determined that a weight of less than 5 pounds was enough to tear the intra-articular disk ligament from its attachment on the costal cartilage junction of the first rib. The fulcrum was transferred laterally so that the medial third of the clavicle hinged over the first rib in the vicinity of the costoclavicular ligament. **D,** After division of the costoclavicular ligament and the intra-articular disc ligament, the lateral end of the clavicle could not be depressed as long as the capsular ligament was intact. **E,** After resection of the first medial costal cartilage along with the costoclavicular ligament, there is no effect on the poise of the lateral end of the clavicle as long as the capsular ligament remains intact. (From Bearne JG: *J Anat* 101:159-170, 1967.)

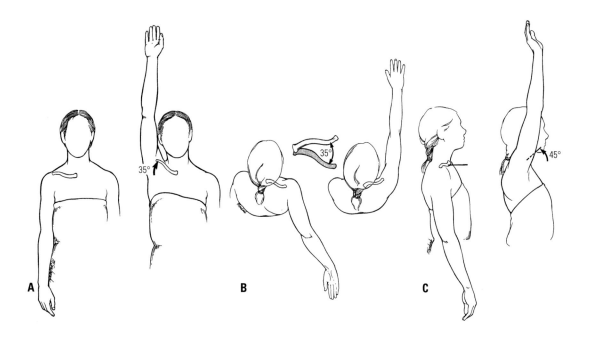

FIG. 16-3 Motions of the clavicle and the sternoclavicular joint. **A,** With full overhead elevation the clavicle elevates as far as 35°. **B,** With adduction and extension the clavicle is displaced anteriorly and posteriorly by 35°. **C,** The clavicle rotates on its long axis over a range of 45° as the arm is elevated to the full overhead position. (From Rockwood CA, Matsen FA, editors: *The shoulder*, vol 1, Philadelphia, 1990, Saunders.)

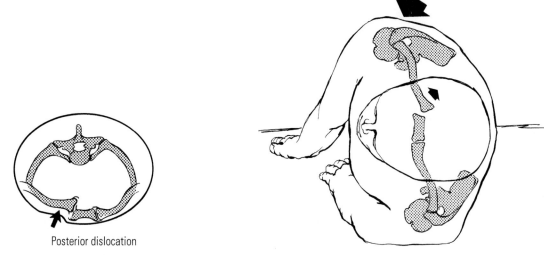

Posterior dislocation

FIG. 16-4 Posterior dislocation of the sternoclavicular joint. A cross-sectional view through the thorax. (From Rockwood CA, Greene DP, editors: *Fractures*, ed 2, Philadelphia, 1984, Lippincott.)

FIG. 16-5 Mechanisms that produce anterior or posterior dislocations of the sternoclavicular joint. If the patient is lying on the ground and a compression force is applied to the posterior lateral aspect of the shoulder, the medial third of the clavicle will be displaced posteriorly. (From Rockwood CA, Greene DP, editors: *Fractures*, ed 3, Philadelphia, 1984, Lippincott.)

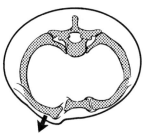

Anterior dislocation

FIG. 16-6 Anterior dislocation of the sternoclavicular joint. A cross-sectional view through the thorax. (From Rockwood CA, Greene DP, editors: *Fractures,* ed 3, Philadelphia, 1984, Lippincott.)

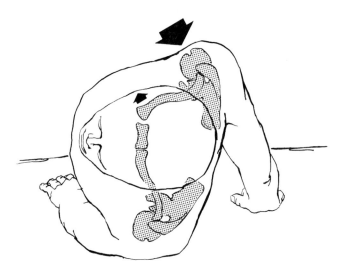

FIG. 16-7 When the lateral compression force is directed from the anterior position, the medial third of the clavicle is dislocated posteriorly. (From Rockwood CA, Greene DP, editors: *Fractures,* ed 2, Philadelphia, 1984, Lippincott.)

pain is present and is increased by any arm movement, though especially when the shoulders are laterally pressed together. Discomfort is increased when the patient is placed in the supine position; it will be noted that in this position the involved shoulder will not lie back flat on the table. The patient will usually support the injured arm across the trunk with the uninvolved arm. The affected shoulder appears to be shortened and thrust forward when compared with the normal shoulder. In addition, the head may be tilted toward the side of the dislocated joint.[9] Whereas an anterior SC joint injury shows a visibly prominent medial clavicle that

can be palpated anterior to the sternum, the anterosuperior fullness of the chest normally imparted by the superior outline of the clavicle is less prominent and visible with posterior SC joint dislocation. Additionally, with posterior dislocation the corner of the sternum becomes more easily palpated as compared with the normal contralateral SC joint. There is greater pain experienced with posterior dislocation, and the patient may complain of shortness of breath, experience a choking sensation, feel tightness of the throat, experience decreased circulation of the ipsilateral arm, be in a state of shock, or possibly have a pneumothorax.[9]

13. Why is diagnosis predicated on clinical evidence rather than on radiologic evidence?

Aside from a history of injury, this condition is more readily diagnosed clinically by local tenderness and prominence of the medial third of the clavicle than by radiographic determination. The reason is that even with specially recommended oblique views distortion may occur from clavicles being superimposed one over the other.[9]

14. What is the medical treatment of subluxation or dislocation when not life threatening?

Dislocation, if present, may be reduced by local pressure over the dislocated end of the clavicle,[10] and the reduction can be maintained by immobilization of a figure-of-eight bandage.[5] In the event of moderate sprain with subluxation, reduction is achieved by the physician drawing the patient's shoulders backward as if reducing and holding a clavicular fracture, followed by a clavicle strap or figure-of-eight strap to hold the reduction in place.[9]

15. What therapeutic intervention and advice is appropriate?

In the event of a *mild sprain,* application of ice for the first 12 to 24 hours, followed by heat, has proved to be helpful. The upper extremity is immobilized for 3 to 4 days in a sling with gradual return to everyday activities thereafter. With *moderate sprains,* ice is appropriate for the first 12 hours, followed by heat for 24 to 48 hours, as well as immobilization. For both mild and moderate sprains nonsteroidal antiinflammatory medications and rest are appropriate.[5] Selective strengthening of coracoclavicular-ligament dynamic synergists (that is, the pectoralis minor and subclavius muscles) is a treatment strategy that, by virtue of increased tone and hypertrophy, diminish disruptive forces and further strain to the already frayed fibers of the SC ligamentous supports. When only mild to moderate sprain has occurred, the injured athlete can resume sporting activity relatively early, even if pain and other symptoms remain for several months.[8]

REFERENCES

1. Bearn JG: Direct observations of the function of the capsule of the sternoclavicular joint in clavicular support, *J Anat* 101(1):159-170, 1967.
2. Dandy DJ: *Essential orthopaedics and trauma,* Edinburgh, 1989, Churchill Livingstone.
3. Grant JCB: *Method of anatomy,* ed 7, Baltimore, 1965, Williams & Wilkins.
4. Gray H: *Anatomy of the human body,* ed 28 (CM Guss, editor), Philadelphia, 1966, Lea & Febiger.
5. Lillegard WA, Rucker KS: *Handbook of sports medicine: a symptom-oriented approach,* Boston, 1993, Andover Medical Publishers.
6. Moore KL: *Clinical oriented anatomy,* ed 2, Baltimore, 1985, Williams & Wilkins.
7. Nettles JL, Linscheid R: Sternoclavicular dislocations, *J Trauma* 8(2):158-164, 1968.
8. Peterson L, Renström P: *Sports injuries: their prevention and treatment,* London, 1986, Martin Dunitz.
9. Rockwood CA, Matsen FA, editors: *The shoulder,* vol 1, Philadelphia, 1990, WB Saunders.
10. Salter RB: *Textbook of disorders of the musculoskeletal system,* ed 2, Baltimore, 1983, Williams & Wilkins.

RECOMMENDED READING

Rockwood CA: Disorders of the sternoclavicular joint. In Rockwood CA, Matsen FA, editors: *The shoulder,* vol 1, Philadelphia, 1990, WB Saunders.

17

Diver Accident with Acute Pain and Deformity in Shoulder

A 50-year-old man jumped head first off a high diving board, with arms overhead, landing in deep water directly on upturned palms. The swimmer immediately felt something "out of place" in his left shoulder and could not use that shoulder because of pain. He yelled for help and treaded to safety where he was assisted out of the pool and then cradled his left upper extremity with his right arm, sling style.

CLUE:

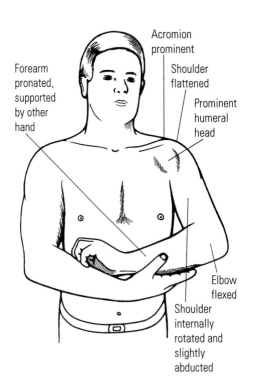

Acromion
prominent

Shoulder
flattened

Prominent
humeral
head

Forearm
pronated,
supported
by other
hand

Elbow
flexed

Shoulder
internally
rotated and
slightly
abducted

1. What is most likely to have occurred in this man's shoulder?
2. How do we understand the role of the glenohumeral joint in terms of kinesiologic stability and mobility?
3. What osseous anatomy is relevant to an understanding of shoulder dislocation?
4. How does size, shape, and tilt of the glenoid fossa affect glenohumeral joint stability?
5. What contribution does atmospheric pressure have on glenohumeral joint stability?
6. What are the dynamic glenohumeral joint stabilizers?
7. What are ligamentous and capsular restraints that contribute to glenohumeral stability?
8. What predisposing motion causes this injury?
9. What neural, vascular, tendinous, or skeletal structures might be damaged along with this injury?
10. What other joints or bones could be damaged by a fall onto an outstretched hand and pronated forearm?
11. What are the four kinds of anterior dislocation?
12. What is the clinical presentation of anterior dislocation?
13. What special tests are appropriate?
14. What are the three kinds of posterior dislocation?
15. What is the mechanism of posterior dislocation, and how is this managed?
16. Why is posterior dislocation more likely than anterior dislocation after electric shock?
17. What is the clinical presentation of posterior dislocation?
18. What radiographs are appropriate in detecting dislocation?
19. What medical treatment is appropriate in the treatment of anterior dislocation?
20. What are some common forms of reduction?
21. What is the postreduction management?
22. What is the difficulty in managing chronic anterior traumatic dislocations?
23. What accounts for the high incidence of recurrent dislocation?
24. What is the mechanism of recurrent dislocation?
25. What is "apprehension shoulder"?
26. What is recurrent instability with an atraumatic onset?
27. How is recurrent instability categorized, and how is it managed?
28. What nonoperative management is appropriate after shoulder dislocation?
29. What is surgical management in those patients for whom operative treatment is advisable?
30. What postoperative therapeutic management is appropriate?

1. What is most likely to have occurred in this man's shoulder?

Anterior (subcoracoid) glenohumeral joint dislocation (Fig. 17-1) is the most common (>90%)[16] of all four[17] possible glenohumeral (GH) dislocations. The shoulder joint is the most commonly dislocated major body joint.[17]

2. How do we understand the role of the glenohumeral joint in terms of kinesiologic stability and mobility?

It is important to understand that with every joint system there is a unique trade-off between stability versus mobility. For example, the hip joint sacrifices mobility, that is, circumduction in lieu of stability, whereas the GH joint sacrifices stability for mobility, hence the greater likelihood of GH joint dislocation. The glenohumeral joint evolved from being an essentially weight-bearing joint of a foreleg into a limb that functions mostly in an open kinetic chain and exhibits a wide range of movement capabilities. Thus the GH joint is better suited for mobility and is an example of yet another adaptive change that, despite the price of lost proximal stability, opened the door to unparalleled distal prehensile dexterity. The carpometacarpal joint of the human thumb is the virtuoso of prehension that per-

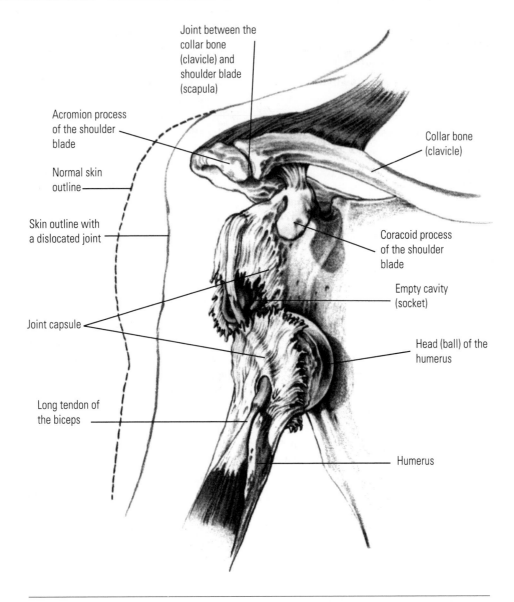

Joint between the collar bone (clavicle) and shoulder blade (scapula)

Acromion process of the shoulder blade

Normal skin outline

Skin outline with a dislocated joint

Joint capsule

Long tendon of the biceps

Collar bone (clavicle)

Coracoid process of the shoulder blade

Empty cavity (socket)

Head (ball) of the humerus

Humerus

FIG. 17-1 Subcoracoid (anterioinferior) dislocation of the glenohumeral joint with tear of the glenoid labrum and joint capsule. (From Peterson L. Renström P: *Sports injuries: their prevention and treatment,* London, 1986, Martin Dunitz, Ltd.)

mitted an opposition capability virtually unparalleled in primates. Ironically, once freed of the quadruped posture, the upright posture enabled man to develop from the most defenseless of all creatures into the most powerful of creatures as a direct function of man's ability to fashion and use weapons and tools.*

---

*Interestingly, manipulations of the thumb are represented by a larger portion of the cerebral motor homunculus than in the total control of the chest and abdomen.

3. What osseous anatomy is relevant to an understanding of shoulder dislocation?

The small and shallow glenoid fossa of the scapula articulates with the relatively large spherical head of the humerus but provides little coverage for the head, especially when the shoulder is (1) adducted, flexed, and internally rotated; (2) abducted and elevated; or (3) adducted at the side with the scapula rotated downward.[4,29,35] Despite this relative lack of coverage, the normal shoulder kinesiology precisely constrains the head to within 1 mm of the center of the glenoid cavity throughout its wide arc of movement.[12,24] Whether the arm resists the gravitational pull of the limb for long periods of time by just hanging at the side, lifting large resistive loads, or even a professional baseball pitcher's ability to throw a ball at speeds approaching 100 miles per hour, the shoulder incredibly holds together. It is curious then that shoulder instability is not more common than it really is. The reason for this is that glenohumeral joint stability results from a hierarchy of passive and *active stabilizing mechanisms*. Minimal loads such as the gravitational pull of the upper limb are resisted by passive mechanisms such as concavity of the glenoid and labrum, finite joint volume, and surface tension provided by joint fluid (synovia). Larger loads such as serving a tennis ball or picking up a child are facilitated by the action of various shoulder muscles.[17]

4. How does size, shape, and tilt of the glenoid fossa affect glenohumeral joint stability?

There is considerable variation in the radii of curvature of the glenoid fossa. The glenoid (acting as a shelf) faces anteriorly at an angle of about 45° to the coronal plane, which places it behind the humeral head for most uses of the shoulder.[17] Obviously, GH joint stability is directly affected by the size, shape, and tilt of the glenoid fossa. The depth and hence stability of this bony fossa are enhanced by contributions of the articular cartilage and glenoid labrum (a thickened capsular attachment to the glenoid rim). Together, they provide an element of plasticity that serves to enhance the quality of GH coupling, similar to the "feathered" edge of a contact lens.[17]

5. What contribution does atmospheric pressure have on glenohumeral joint stability?

The normal shoulder joint is sealed by a joint capsule that prevents outside fluid from entering. There is minimal free fluid[17] (less than 1 ml) with the GH joint that is imbued with a slightly negative pressure of −4.0 mm Hg.[33] An analogy may be drawn when one attempts to pull up the plunger of a plugged syringe that is held upside down; a relative vacuum is created, and it resists upward displacement of the plunger. Similarly the shoulder joint is stabilized by a limited joint volume, and as long as that volume remains in a closed space with minimal free fluid, the joint surfaces cannot be easily distracted or subluxed. Small translations of the humerus on the glenoid (that is, joint play) are permitted as they are balanced by fluid flow in the opposite direction.[17]

When the gap between the articular surfaces becomes very small, intermolecular forces of surface tension, cohesion, and adhesion provide continued coupling of the humerus to the glenoid.[17] *Surface tension* refers to the tendency of the surface of a liquid to contract its surface area so that as little energy is expended as possible to maintain that shape. This is clarified when we consider liquid drops, whether they be molten metal, plain water, or drops of oil; all these examples, like an inflated balloon, assume that configuration having the least surface per given volume: the sphere. The familiar example of two wet microscope slides pressed together illustrates these forces; the two slides readily slide on each other but cannot easily be pulled apart by forces applied at right angles to their flat surfaces. "Tension" refers to the elastic quality of a liquid surface that resembles a membrane under tension. It is surface tension that permits razor blades or sewing needles to "float" when placed on a water surface and permits water bugs to move across the surface of the water.

Adhesion refers to the attraction between unlike substances (liquid to solid, such as joint fluid to bone), whereas *cohesion* refers to the attraction of like substances (joint fluid to joint fluid). These intermolecular forces account for capillary action responsible for bringing water to the roots of plants, for the flow of blood through capillary vessels, for the oil to rise in a lamp wick, or for causing water in a dipped corner of a sugar cube to quickly spread throughout the entire lump.

The addition of excess fluid into the GH joint works to nullify both the joint volume effect and the intermolecular effect. For example, the addition of blood into the joint due to an intracapsular fracture may result in inferior subluxation.[17] Thus we may venture that in the unopened state of the joint, the weight of the limb is almost entirely borne by atmospheric pressure.[14]

Interarticular forces may also be overwhelmed by the application of traction, as for example in the cracking sound of the metacarpophalangeal joint as that joint cavitates. Subatmospheric pressure within the joint releases gas (80% CO_2) from joint solution, and that release is accompanied by a sudden jump of the finger caused by joint separation. The finger does not fall away because the finger is relatively light and does not overwhelm the restraining soft tissue, which keeps it attached to the hand. Once a joint has been cracked it will not do so until about 20 minutes later when all the gas has been reabsorbed.[26,36]

6. What are the dynamic glenohumeral joint stabilizers?

Dynamic GH joint stability is provided by a cowl of muscles[3] composed of the rotator cuff. By virtue of these tendons blending with the GH capsule and ligaments, selective contraction of these muscles adjust the tension of those static structures, producing "dynamic" ligaments.[2] Second, by contracting simultaneously, these muscles press the humeral head into the glenoid socket, securing it into the center of that fossa.[24] Third, by way of selective contraction so as to resist displacing forces, as when the lateral deltoid initiates shoulder abduction, supraspinatus (primarily) and the long biceps tendon actively resist upward displacement of the humeral head relative to the fossa.[21,34] When the pectoralis major and the anterior deltoid elevate and flex the shoulder, they tend to push the humeral head posteriorly out the back of the fossa. This displacement is selectively resisted by the combined contractile efforts of subscapularis, infraspinatus, and teres minor muscles.[17]

Additionally, the glenoid fossa has an upward, lateral, and forward orientation that serves as a seat or shelf for the humeral head. This bony source of stability is provided by the normal muscle tone of the shoulder protractors, the serratus anterior and upper trapezius. In the event of decreased tone, as may occur after a stroke, dynamic stability is lost, and the humeral head simply slides down and off the now almost vertical fossa.

7. What are ligamentous and capsular restraints that contribute to glenohumeral stability?

There are five scapulohumeral ligaments (Fig. 17-2) serving as important static shoulder stabilizers when they are under tension. These ligaments provide a passive *checkrein* function that serve as the last guardian of shoulder stability after all other passive and dynamic mechanisms have been overwhelmed.[17] The anteromedial and anteroinferior glenohumeral ligaments serve to restrain the humeral head during abduction[22] and external rotation[35] of the shoulder respectively, whereas the posteroinferior and posterosuperior capsule serve to restrain the humeral head from posterior dislocation.[32] Inferior to the GH joint, at the axilla, these ligaments manifest as redundant and crenated ligaments that help hold the humeral head against the glenoid. Considerable variation exists in the size of these ligaments, which may explain why certain shoulders appear more unstable.

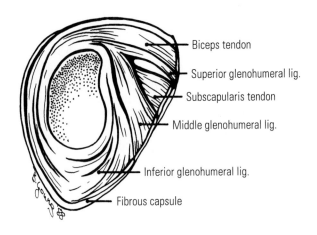

FIG. 17-2 Scapulohumeral ligaments. The coracohumeral and posteroinferior glenohumeral ligaments are not shown. (From Rockwood CA, Matsen FA, editors: *The shoulder*, vol 1, 1990, Philadelphia, Saunders.)

8. What predisposing motion causes this injury?

The intrinsic instability of the shoulder is increased when shoulder abduction is superimposed on external rotation and extension.[31] These movements yield forces that challenge the anterior capsular ligaments, the glenoid rim, and rotator cuff mechanism and, if sufficient in magnitude, propel the humeral head along a path of least resistance toward the inferior glenoid where it may subluxate. As a result, the fibrous ligamentous capsule may be partially torn (sprained), the glenoid labrum may become partially or completely detached from the glenoid (Bankart lesion),[31] or the rotator cuff[15] is damaged. The last may occur because the tendons of the rotator cuff blend in with the capsule as they insert onto the humeral tuberosities.[17] The most common mechanism of injury occurs after a forward fall in which our protective extension response protects our head at the expense of injury elsewhere. Had our swimmer positioned his hand forward instead of upward in extension, he would have provided himself a more streamlined shape and would have avoided landing on the volar surfaces of his hand. In the elderly, this same mechanism of injury fractures the humeral neck rather than dislocates the joint because the bones, having become brittle, are weaker than the ligaments.[3] Anterior dislocation is common in downhill skiing injuries,[1a] in grand mal seizures, and after racket sports when the arm is quickly brought back to meet an oncoming ball, and it may also occur from a ball or blow directly onto the posterolateral aspect of the shoulder.

9. What neural, vascular, tendinous, or skeletal structures might be damaged along with this injury?

Complications of traumatic anterior dislocation include the following:

- Compression *fractures* of the humeral head (Hill-Sachs lesion), fractures of the anterior glenoid lip, and fractures of the acromion or of the coracoid processes associated with superior shoulder dislocation after an extreme forward and upward force on the adducted arm.[17] The greater humeral tuberosity may avulse in tandem with anterior dislocation, especially when the patient lands on outstretched arms, or from a blow or fall onto the shoulder, particularly in older patients. Although the fragment readily unites in good position, the supraspinatus tendon may pull it away. The healed fragment may then wedge in the subacromial arch and obstruct elevation.[3]

- *Cuff tears* may accompany anterior and inferior GH dislocation, especially if the mechanism of injury was a fall onto the lateral aspect of the shoulder.[10] The frequency of this complication increases with age, and its incidence exceeds 30% in patients greater than 30 years of age and is over 80% in patients older than 60. Rotator cuff tears may present as pain or weakness on testing of external rotation or abduction.[17]

- *Vascular injuries* most frequently occur in elderly patients with stiffer, more fragile vessels.[17] Injury may occur in the axillary artery, the axillary vein, or the branches of the axillary artery (Fig. 17-3) and most often occur after inferior dislocation. This complication most commonly occurs during closed reduction of an old anterior dislocation mistaken for an acute injury.[17] The vessel is brittle and cannot tolerate the required traction involved in reduction. The radial pulse should be checked and its presence recorded after every reduction, whether chronic or acute. The patient must be closely monitored because this dangerous situation may require emergency surgery.[17]

- *Neural injuries.* The brachial plexus and axillary artery lie immediately anterior, inferior, and medial to the GH joint.[9] The axillary nerve originates at the posterior cord of the brachial plexus, and the anterior branch of this nerve (that is, the circumflex humeral) wraps directly around the humeral wall in the area of the surgical neck.[3] Thus this nerve has no padding and is predisposed to injury from a hard blow to the area, from a fracture of the upper humerus, or after anterior shoulder dislocation. Anterior dislocation may cause traction strain to this nerve in that portion

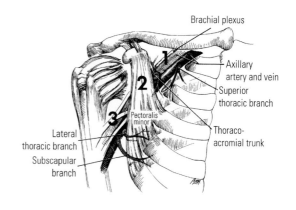

FIG. 17-3 The axillary artery is divided into three parts by the pectoralis minor muscle; the second part is behind it, and the third part is lateral to it. (From Rockwood CA, Green DP, editors: *Fractures,* ed 2, Philadelphia, 1984, Lippincott.)

of nerve lying in close relation to the underside of the GH joint articular capsule[20] (Fig. 17-4). Injury most commonly causes a traction neurapraxia resulting in partial or complete paralysis of the deltoid muscles.[17] Although there is usually complete recovery, the nerve should undergo electromyographic studies after injury and then 3 weeks later.[3] Since the deltoid muscle cannot be adequately assessed, it is not enough to simply rely on testing the sensory area over the middle of the deltoid because this method is unreliable.[20] Sensation may also be compromised in the distribution of the musculocutaneous nerve (lateral antebrachial cutaneous nerve) supplying the lateral surface of the forearm. Subsequently, if no change has occurred between the two examinations, the nerve is explored and repaired.[3] Lower brachial plexus injuries may also occur and should be suspected if there has been a concomitant violent abduction strain.

10. What other joints or bones could be damaged by a fall onto an outstretched hand and pronated forearm?

Other types of injury occurring after a fall onto an outstretched hand with the forearm pronated include posterior GH joint dislocation, clavicular fracture, humeral head fractures in senescent adults, supracondylar fractures in children or anterior elbow dislocation in adults, dislocated radial head, fractures of the radial head, fractures of the capitellum, Colles' fracture, scaphoid fracture, and lunate dislocation.[30] This list highlights the

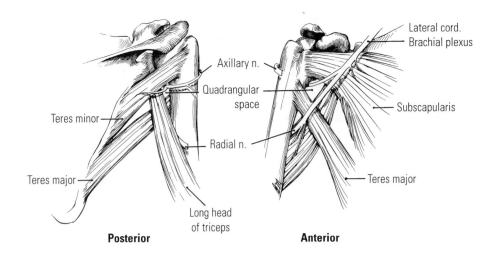

FIG. 17-4 Relations of the axillary nerve to the subscapularis muscle, the quadrangular space, and the humeral neck. With anterior dislocations the subscapularis is displaced forward, and such displacement creates a traction injury to the axillary nerve. The nerve cannot move out of the way because it is held above by the brachial plexus and below where it wraps around behind the neck of the humerus. (From Rockwood CA, Green DP, editors: *Fractures,* ed 2, Philadelphia, 1984, Lippincott.)

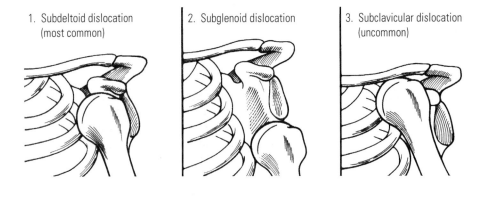

FIG. 17-5 Anterior glenohumeral joint dislocation. *1,* Subcoracoid dislocation is the most common. *2,* Subglenoid dislocation. *3,* Subclavicular dislocation is uncommon.

orthopedic principle in which the same injury mechanism produces age-specific injuries.[19]

11. What are the four kinds of anterior dislocation?

CLASSIFICATION OF ANTERIOR DISLOCATION
(Fig. 17-5):

- *Subcoracoid.* The humeral head is displaced anteriorly with respect to the glenoid and is inferior to the coracoid process. This is the most common type of anterior dislocation.

- *Subglenoid.* The humeral head lies anterior and below the glenoid fossa.
- *Subclavicular.* The humeral head lies medial to the coracoid process, just inferior to the lower border of the clavicle.
- *Intrathoracic.* The humeral head lies between the ribs and thoracic cavity.
- *Subclavicular* dislocation is uncommon, whereas intrathoracic dislocation is rare. These two forms of dislocation are usually associated with severe trauma.[17]

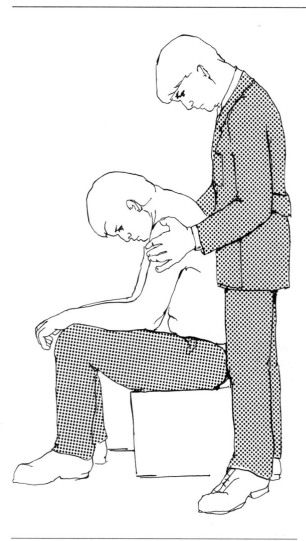

FIG. 17-6 Visualization of the anterior and posterior aspects of the shoulders may best be accomplished by having the patient sit on a low stool, with the therapist standing behind him. The injured shoulder may then be easily compared with the uninjured one. (From Rockwood CA, Green DP, editors: *Fractures,* ed 2, Philadelphia, 1984, Lippincott.)

12. What is the clinical presentation of anterior dislocation?

The acute anteriorly dislocated shoulder is very painful (that is, sharp stabbing pain), and muscles are in spasm in the attempt to stabilize the joint. The dislocated humeral head may be palpable anteriorly or inferiorly in the armpit.[5] In the posterior part of the shoulder, a cavity may be palpated below the acromion where the humeral head usually resides. The arm is held in slight ab-

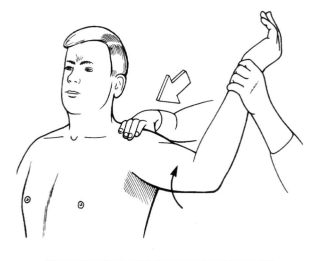

FIG. 17-7 Apprehension test for anterior dislocation.

duction and external rotation. Anterior dislocation usually yields a shoulder that is incapable of complete internal rotation and abduction.[17]

The characteristic profile (on p. 168) presents as a flat lateral shoulder contour that produces a straight drop in line of the shoulder from the tip of the acromion[5] to the lateral humeral epicondyle, known as the *positive Hamilton's ruler test.*[3] A square shoulder[31] with apparent indentation beneath the acromion is apparent. Although a similar flat contour is also seen in patients with either wasted deltoid muscles or displaced surgical neck fractures, these latter patients score negative on the ruler test, since the humeral head is still in its normal position.[3] If the distance between the acromion process to the lateral humeral epicondyle on the involved side is not slightly greater than on the uninvolved side, a fracture of the proximal end of the humerus should be suspected.

13. What special tests are appropriate?

Crank, or apprehension, test (Fig. 17-7), sulcus test, and fulcrum test are for anterior instability; jerk test and posterior apprehension test (Fig. 17-8) are for posterior instability.[17]

APPREHENSION TEST

With the patient sitting or standing, the examiner stands behind and raises the patient's arm to 90° of abduction and begins to rotate the shoulder externally. While one hand pulls back on the patient's wrist, the other is placed

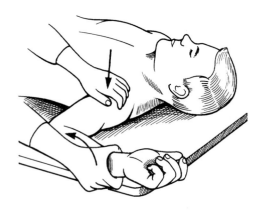

FIG. 17-8 Posterior apprehension test for posterior glenohumeral dislocation. The examiner abducts and medially rotates the patient's shoulder, followed by a posterior force applied on the proximal end of the patient's humerus. Resistance by the patient or apprehension observed on his or her face scores positive for this test.

over the humeral head with the thumb pushing posteriorly for extra leverage. The other fingers are placed anteriorly to monitor any sudden instability that may occur.

FULCRUM TEST

The fulcrum test is a variation of the apprehension test that is performed with the patient supine for the purpose of using body weight to immobilize the scapula. Here the body acts as a counterweight. The table surface (or edge) or the examiner's hand under the glenohumeral joint acts as a fulcrum, and the patient's arm acts as a lever. With maintenance of gentle external rotation for 1 minute, the subscapularis is fatigued; apprehension will occur soon because the capsule then is challenged to maintain stability. This test isolates movement of the glenohumeral joint and allows a clear assessment of anterior translation. Also the range of external rotation causing apprehension will decrease as the patient recovers and therefore serves as an objective measure of improvement.

14. What are the three kinds of posterior dislocation?

Classification of posterior dislocation
- *Subacromial (most common).* Head lies behind the glenoid and beneath the acromion (Fig. 17-9).
- *Subglenoid.* Head behind and beneath the glenoid.
- *Subspinous.* Head medial to the acromion and beneath the scapular spine.[14]

15. What is the mechanism of posterior dislocation, and how is this managed?

Posterior dislocation tends to happen in the elderly.[16] The following are classic examples: when a purse is snatched from behind an owner who refuses to let go; from a blow to the front of the shoulder; or from a fall onto an outstretched upper extremity. Dislocation will occur from a combination of sudden forceful internal rotation, adduction, and flexion. Lesser tuberosity fractures are common and often cause the humeral head to become locked in the dislocated position. Reduction is accomplished by longitudinal forward traction on the arm with the elbow bent, accompanied by anterior pressure on the humeral head; the arm is then adducted, externally rotated, and then internally rotated to reduce the humeral head back into the glenoid cavity (Fig. 17-10). Immobilization in the elderly is only for 2 to 3 weeks in a handshake cast applied with the shoulder in neutral rotation and slight extension after confirmation of closed reduction by radiographs. Ice and nonsteroidal antiinflammatory agents may bring relief. External rotation and posterior deltoid strengthening are emphasized during rehabilitation. Push-ups and bench-press exercises are to be avoided.[17]

16. Why is posterior dislocation more likely than anterior dislocation after electric shock?

Although convulsive seizures, accidental electric shock, or electric shock therapy may cause anterior dislocation, dislocation is usually posterior because the strong internal rotators simply overpower the relatively weaker external rotators. The reason is that the combined strength of the latissimus dorsi, pectoralis major, and subscapularis muscles overwhelms the infraspinatus and teres minor muscles by virtue of greater muscle bulk represented as a force vector of greater magnitude.[17]

17. What is the clinical presentation of posterior dislocation?

Recognition of posterior shoulder dislocation may be hampered by a lack of striking deformity as well as by the fact that any observed anomaly is masked by the shoulder being held in the traditional sling position of adduction and internal rotation.[17] Diagnosis may be missed because posterior dislocations are so rare (1%). In the initial interval before diagnosis of posterior dislocation is declared, the injury may be misdiagnosed as frozen shoulder, for which vigorous therapy may mis-

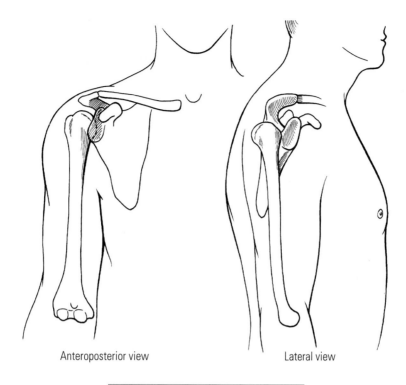

Anteroposterior view   Lateral view

FIG. 17-9 Posterior (subacromial) dislocation.

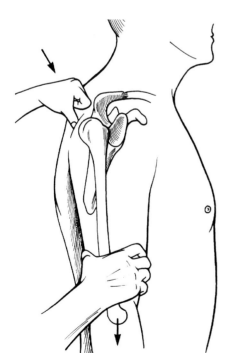

FIG. 17-10 Closed reduction of posterior glenohumeral joint dislocation.

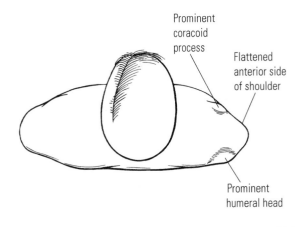

Prominent coracoid process

Flattened anterior side of shoulder

Prominent humeral head

FIG. 17-11 Profile of posterior glenohumeral shoulder dislocation.

takenly be initiated in an attempt to restore range of motion.[11] A proper history is therefore absolutely necessary during the examination.

The classic clinical features of posterior dislocation include the following:

- Limited external rotation of the shoulder (often to less than 0°) and limited shoulder elevation (often to less than 90°) because of the humeral head becoming fixed or even impaled on the posterior glenoid rim by muscle forces. The shoulder appears fixed in abduction. Over time, the posterior rim of the glenoid may become further impacted into the fracture of the humeral head and produce a deep hatchet-like defect or V-shaped compression fracture of the lesser tuberosity, which engages the head and locks it even more securely in the position of posterior dislocation.
- Flattening of the anterior aspect of the shoulder and posterior prominence of the humeral head is best appreciated when one views the shoulders from above while standing behind the patient. The coracoid process may be prominent[17] (Fig. 17-11).

After confirmation of closed reduction by radiographs a handshake cast is applied in neutral shoulder rotation and slight extension for 3 weeks.

18. What radiographs are appropriate in detecting dislocation?

Anteroposterior views in the plane of the body are often deceptive and may lead the clinician into a diagnostic trap.[18] Rather, a series of radiographs in the plane of the scapula (that is, anteroposterior, scapular lateral, and axillary) are appropriate for all types of suspected dislocation.[17]

Humeral head defects confirming previous anterior dislocation in the case of posteromedial head defects and posterior dislocations in the event of anterolateral head defects are identified with special radiographic views.

19. What medical treatment is appropriate in the treatment of anterior dislocation?

Initial treatment includes the application of ice and the use of a sling. Although spasm occurs within a few minutes after dislocation, reduction should not be attempted until the shoulder is radiologically examined, regardless of how obvious the diagnosis may be. Reduction attempts are ill advised and may be dangerous if there is an associated fracture.[3] Acute GH joint dislocation should be reduced as quickly and gently as possible because early relocation quickly reduces stretch and compression of neurovascular structures, minimizes the degree of muscle spasm that must be overcome to reduce the joint, and prevents progressive enlargement of the humeral head defect in locked dislocations.[17]

20. What are some common forms of reduction?

There are two different principles used in the reduction (Fig. 17-12) of anterior shoulder dislocation: *traction* (or countertraction) and *leverage*. Leverage, however, involves the application of great force and may result in damage to the capsule, axillary vessels, or brachial plexus;[17] a simple and perhaps less painful reduction technique.

21. What is the postreduction management?

Postreduction treatment focuses on optimizing shoulder stability as well as muscle rehabilitation (that is, strengthening the rotator cuff and long biceps muscle) to impose a normal biomechanic pattern on a disrupted shoulder kinesiologic character.[17] Cryotherapy and nonsteroidal antiinflammatory agents are appropriate when needed for either age group.

Controversy exists regarding the length of the immobilization period.[15] Because recurrent dislocation is common in patients less than 20 years old (90%) and may result from movements as trivial as raising one's hand behind the head, using the backstroke while swimming, or reaching into the back seat of a car, stability is essential to proper management. Thus, in young patients, immobilization should be approximately 3 weeks, while bearing in mind that young people are much less vulnerable to the effects of joint

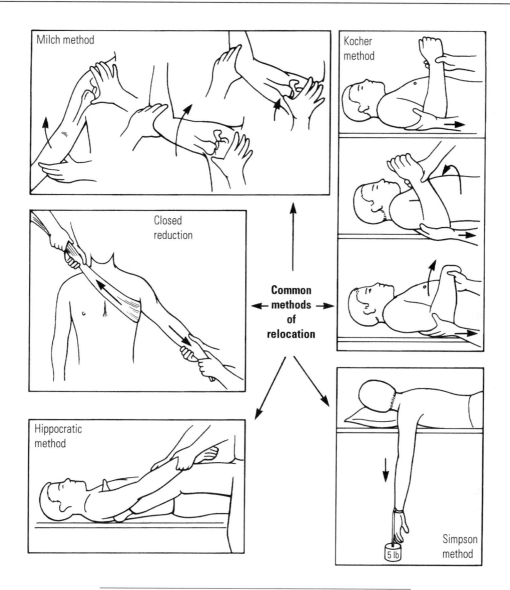

FIG. 17-12 Various methods of reduction of anterior shoulder dislocation.

stiffness and the development of adhesions. However, once dislocation has occurred a second time in this age group, the chance of frequent recurrence is almost 100% and is therefore usually indication for open shoulder reconstruction.[10]

In patients older than 30 years of age, the chances of recurrence are lower because as one gets older the collagen composing the static shoulder restraints becomes stiffer and hence less elastic. In such patients, immobilization should not exceed approximately 1 week because the position of the immobilization sets the anteroinferior shoulder capsule in such a way that

the capsular attachments may approximate and foreshorten (that is, adhesive capsulitis; Chapter 13).

22. What is the difficulty in managing chronic anterior traumatic dislocations?

A GH joint that has been dislocated for several days is a *chronic dislocation*. As the chronicity of dislocation persists, so do the complications of reduction. There are no established rules of management here because the age of the patient, length of time from dislocation, degree of symptoms, range of motion, radiographic findings, and general stability of the patient may vary greatly. When one encounters an elderly patient with shoulder pain and anterior dislocation on radiographs, a very careful history is mandatory to determine whether the injury occurred acutely or a week to several months earlier. The problem here is that by 2 to 3 weeks after dislocation the humeral head is so firmly impaled on the anterior glenoid and there is so much soft-tissue contracture and interposition that it is impossible to perform a gentle closed reduction.

If no more than 2 to 3 weeks have elapsed since the dislocation, a gentle closed reduction may be performed with minimal traction, without leverage, and with total muscle relaxation under general anesthesia. If this fails, a choice is made either to simply leave it alone, or to consider an open procedure. An open procedure can be very difficult because of the distorted anatomy of the axillary artery and nerves and because the structures are tight and "scarred" down.[17]

23. What accounts for the high incidence of recurrent dislocation?

In order to understand why it is that anterior shoulder dislocation is associated with a high incidence of recurrent dislocation, it is helpful to study Fig. 17-13.

In the normal shoulder, the motion of external rotation results in lateral rotation of the humeral head and stretching of the anterior capsule. In the absence of an intact anterior capsule glenoid labrum, as often occurs after anterior dislocation, there is a loss of balance of the static support of the glenoid rim. Subsequently, during attempted external shoulder rotation, arthrokinematic joint rotation is substituted by anteroinferior translation, resulting in redislocation. It is for this reason that chronic instability is obviated during external rotation of the shoulder. Instability is compounded when an indentation fracture is created by impaling of the humeral head on the anterior margin of the glenoid

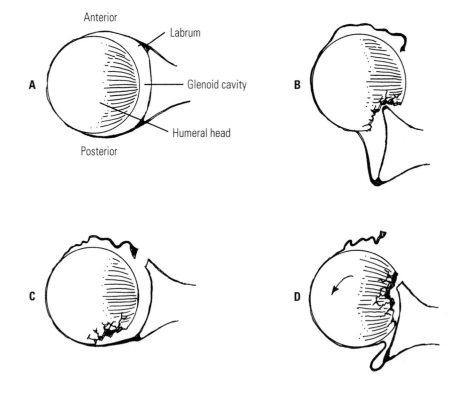

FIG. 17-13 Stages in the formation of a Hill-Sachs lesion with diagram of a left GH joint. **A,** Glenohumeral joint stability is enhanced by an intact labrium, a fibrous rim that deepens the glenoid cavity. **B,** Anterior dislocation with anterior glenoid rim indenting the posterolateral part of the humeral head. **C,** Reduction after anterior dislocation. **D,** After reduction there is chronic instability in external rotation, *arrow.* This tends to reinforce the head defect. (From Meals RA: *One hundred orthopaedic conditions every doctor should understand,* St. Louis, 1992, Quality Medical Publishing.)

rim (Hill-Sachs lesion). A reverse lesion may occur on the anteromedial portion of the humeral head after posterior dislocation (reverse Hill-Sachs lesion).

24. What is the mechanism of recurrent dislocation?

In most cases of recurrent traumatic anterior instability, injury recurs from forced abduction and external shoulder rotation. This injury may occur from a fall onto an outstretched arm or after a blow delivered to the shoulder. A classic example is of a football player who tries to make an arm tackle on a ball carrier only to wind up having his own arm pulled back into extension, abduction, and external rotation. Similarly, a kayaker may have his arm pulled back over his head while bracing himself in white water, or a skier may fall onto an abducted arm. These movements yield a sharp and stabbing shoulder pain. Reduction may occur spontaneously or may require medical intervention. Subsequently the shoulder may demonstrate the "dead-arm syndrome,"[27] that is, recurrent dislocation,[25] or even frank dislocation when the arm assumes the positions of external rotation, abduction, and shoulder rotation.[17]

25. What is "apprehension shoulder"?

Apprehension shoulder is an overuse injury in swimmers, occurring most frequently during the backstroke, when the athlete enters the flip turn. At this instant the shoulder, in full abduction and external rotation, undergoes momentary anterior luxation onto the rim of the glenoid fossa as the swimmer's arm pushes off forcefully from the pool wall (Fig. 17-14).

26. What is recurrent instability with an atraumatic onset?

Recurrent instability may also have an atraumatic onset, that is, without a major injury the humeral head begins to slide out of its normal position. This instability may be anterior, posterior, inferior, or multidirectional. Careful questioning usually reveals that the original injury was minor in nature and occurred with actions such as lifting up a garage door, swinging a baseball bat, taking an overhead swing at a tennis ball, or having a minor fall on the shoulder. There are several important clues that hint at a diagnosis of atraumatic subluxation or dislocation: the original injury was minor and not usually associated with significant pain; the patient returned to his or her activities without much pain or difficulty; the subluxation or dislocation spontaneously reduced itself; or the patient has generalized ligamentous laxity.

In the event that one encounters a patient who can dislocate his or her shoulder voluntarily, the examiner must endeavor to determine whether voluntary instability, that is, the patient's desire to dislocate, is the underlying problem, in which case surgical stabilization is unlikely to succeed. However, surgery is appropriate if the patient's shoulder just happens to be able to be susceptible to dislocating itself. The patient with voluntary

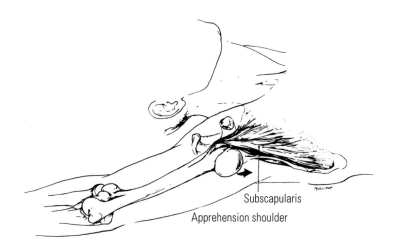

Subscapularis
Apprehension shoulder

FIG. 17-14 Apprehension shoulder with vulnerable position of full abduction and external rotation as found in the backstroke turn. (From Kennedy JC, Hawkins R, Krissoff WB: *Am J Sports Med* 6:309, 1987.)

instability usually has no history of injury but has memories stretching back to childhood of the ability to slip one or both shoulders out of place with minimal discomfort. In the late teens or early twenties the patient may note how the shoulder begins to slip out of place when stress is placed on it.

27. How is recurrent instability categorized, and how is it managed?

It is helpful to categorize patients with recurrent shoulder instability into one of two groupings: the shoulder that goes out because it has suffered a major injury is different from one that goes out because it is constitutionally loose.[17]

The first of these categories, known as a *Bankart lesion,* is characterized by a history of definite trauma, as may occur to an 18-year-old skier whose recurrent anterior instability began with a fall on an abducted externally rotated arm. These shoulders have definite structural damage, particularly avulsion of the GH ligaments at their glenoid attachments, causing *unidirectional instability.* These shoulders frequently require surgery to reachieve stability.[17]

The second group of patients have no history of significant trauma, and instability hence is termed atraumatic. These patients are much more prone to *multidirectional instability.* Rehabilitation, particularly rotator cuff strengthening and flexibility exercises are the first line of management. In this situation the typical patient is a 16-year-old swimmer whose shoulders are becoming painful and on examination are found to be loose in all directions.[17]

28. What nonoperative management is appropriate after shoulder dislocation?

Although any form of GH joint instability may benefit from conservative rehabilitation, nonoperative management is particularly indicated in patients with atraumatic, multidirectional, bilateral instability.[17] Physical therapy is also appropriate for patients with voluntary instability or posterior GH joint instability and for those patients requiring a supranormal range of motion, such as baseball pitchers, swimmers, and gymnasts. These latter patients have looser GH joint capsules and a relatively greater dependence of the dynamic stabilizing mechanism and are not good candidates for surgical management because it does not permit return to a competitive level of function.

The mainstay of therapeutic rehabilitation for anterior GH joint instability is *strengthening* of the rotator cuff musculature. Both internal and external rotator strengthening contribute to anterior and posterior stability respectively, by serving as a buttress to hold the humerus in the glenoid and resist potentially displacing forces. Activation of the infraspinatus tendon and teres minor draw the humeral head posteriorly and thus unload stress on the damaged anterior capsule; an analogy may be made here to strengthening strategy of the hamstrings after anterior cruciate injury in the knee. A similar thesis may be advanced regarding the effects of internal rotation in the late treatment of posterior shoulder dislocation, similar to quadriceps strengthening after posterior cruciate knee injury.

MANAGEMENT OF ANTERIOR DISLOCATION

- *Rotator cuff strengthening exercises* (see pp. 101-104) are most effectively performed when one keeps the humerus close to the body in adduction and internally rotates the arm in the following progression: isometrics, isotonics, resistance, and eccentric strengthening. Strengthening of the internal rotators and adductors is appropriate, since increased tone in these antagonistic muscles serve to limit external rotation and abduction. Isolated external rotation is not an appropriate treatment modality at this early time. Additionally, contraction of the internal shoulder rotators causes the humeral head to migrate posteriorly, away from the anterior locus of instability.

Pain-free isometrics are begun early on so as to prevent atrophy with avoidance of the combined motions of external rotation and abduction. At 2 to 4 weeks after injury, the patient may progress to isotonics and isokinetics as well as rubber tubing (resistive) exercises, spring exercises, or weights in the sidelying position as pain permits, while avoiding the aforementioned positions. Eccentric lengthening contractions are a velocity-decreasing strategy that slow things down during high-velocity movements; as such, they match the functional demands on these muscles when they are recruited to resist forced abducted and external rotation.

At 4 to 6 weeks strengthening may be performed, if pain permits, with the shoulder no longer adducted to the patient's side. Only now may external rotation strengthening be added to facilitate centralization of the humeral head inside the glenoid fossa, which is possible only when all the cuff muscles are working harmoniously together. Abduction and adduction may now be performed to 90° of elevation while the shoulder is maintained in neutral rotation. Overhead flexion and shoulder extension is also permitted. This position is followed by the allowance of three different positions of internal and external rotation: 0° of abduction, 45° of abduction, and 90° of forward flexion. Strengthening of the scapular stabilizers is helpful and best performed if one begins with a modified push-up and progresses to standard push-ups. Push-ups should be performed with the arms somewhat adducted. Rubber Therabands and hand weights are to be used as part of a home exercise program, with emphasis on high repetition and low weight to improve endurance as well as low repetition and high weight to improve strength. Exercising the upper body in shoulder flexion and extension with an ergometer is appropriate at this phase of rehabilitation.[6]

- D2 proprioceptive neuromuscular facilitation (PNF) muscle strengthening. D1 extension is not recommended, since it involves posterior glenoid activity, hence anterior humeral head migration. (D, Diagonal pattern of movement.)

- Posterior GH joint *mobilization* to facilitate shoulder flexion that may have lessened during the 2- to 3-week period of immobilization in adduction and internal rotation.

- Use of single-channel electromyographic *biofeedback,* to centralize the humeral head, with emphasis on control rather than on strength and with electrode placement below the scapular spine for the purpose of learning to consciously contract and strengthen the rotator cuff musculature with the arm in neutral and slowly progressing through various levels and speeds of elevation. The basis of this treatment protocol derives from electromyographic studies showing the external rotators, particularly the infraspinatus, to be the primary dynamic shoulder stabilizers in abduction and overhead motion.[23] One performs this by tightening the rotator cuff muscles in the neutral position in order to glide and hold the humeral head posteriorly. Treatment should be performed for 10 sets of 10 repetitions before one progresses to active movement. By electronic monitoring and amplification of external rotation activity during an apprehensive motion, immediate visual and auditory feedback is provided to the patient. Performance is changed when muscle control is emphasized as an important adjunct to muscle strengthening. Movement progressions occur as the patient masters each level and include (1) forward flexion with a straight elbow, (2) forward flexion with increasing external rotation, (3) abduction with flexion, progressing to elbow extension, (4) abduction with elbow extension with increasing external rotation, (5) abduction from flexion, (6) abduction

from flexion with increasing external rotation, and (7) reaching for objects behind the back or overhead. Electrode placement over the posterior deltoid is contraindicated because increased activity in this muscle drives the humeral head anteriorly.[28]

- Educate patients to avoid forced or high-velocity movement of external rotation, abduction, and hyperextension.

- Educate patients with voluntary shoulder instability by carefully explaining the importance of avoiding intentional GH joint subluxation and dislocation, stressing that each time they perform this maneuver they make their shoulder looser and more prone to unpredictable instability.

- Advise the patient to avoid following the standard Nautilus arm cross exercises on the double chest machine, regardless of position, latissimus pulldowns, behind the head military press, wide grip press, and lowering the bench press excessively into horizontal extension.

MANAGEMENT OF POSTERIOR DISLOCATION

Posterior dislocations are infrequent, but when they do occur, they are at risk for redislocating when the shoulder is internally rotated. Thus external shoulder rotation and posterior deltoid strengthening are emphasized during rehabilitation so as to limit internal rotation and adduction, with push-ups and bench press exercises being avoided. Initially, passive range of motion and pendulum exercises are started after several days of complete immobilization in a reverse sling or spica cast to hold the shoulder in external rotation. It is essentially to avoid excessive forward flexion and internal rotation during passive range of motion exercises. Later on, as dynamic strengthening ensues, it is important not to begin strengthening the external rotators in the position of full internal rotation. Similarly, as shoulder function improves, it is important to point out to the patient the importance of avoiding activities that would place the shoulder at the limits of shoulder flexion, internal rotation, or horizontal adduction so as not to redislocate.[6]

29. What is surgical management in those patients for whom operative treatment is advisable?

The *Bankart procedure* involves suturing of the anterior capsule and labrum to the anterior glenoid rim. Many shoulder surgeons consider this the procedure of choice in management of traumatic unidirectional instability. This procedure requires a healthy capsule and most probably results in the best postoperative shoulder range of motion but is technically a more difficult operation to perform. Popularity of this procedure is attributable to the work of Bankart who first performed the operation in 1923 on one of his former house surgeons. Patients generally have their shoulder immobilized after surgery in the position of internal rotation and adduction by wearing a sling or a commercially available shoulder immobilizer. Immobilization is for 2 to 3 weeks after surgery and then only at night during the subsequent 3 to 6 weeks.[6]

With *staple capsulorrhaphy* (Fig. 17-15) the detached anterior capsule and labrum are secured back onto the glenoid by use of staples. This can be performed either as an open repair or arthroscopically. The advantage of this procedure is that range exercises, such as Codman's pendulum, may begin within the first week after surgery.

Putti-Platt procedure is an example of one of the subscapularis muscle procedures, first used by Sir Harry Platt of England and Vittorio Putti of Italy in the 1920s. Muscle transfers are considered to be *indirect repairs* and are designed to effect repair by altering the biomechanics extrinsic to the GH joint; this is to be distinguished from *direct repairs,* as are the Bankart and staple capsulorrhaphy procedures, which attempt to restore normal anatomy.

The results of surgery are often successful from the point of view of whether dislocation recurs. Clearly such dislocation does not recur. However this simply cannot be equated with an excellent result, since the patient now has 45° of external rotation and can no longer throw with that shoulder. The goal of postsurgical therapy is to ideally attempt to regain as much external rotation and elevation as possible if one bears in mind

that one inevitably falls short of meeting that goal. It is important to bear in mind that the patient must not place his or her shoulder at the limits of external rotation, abduction, or hyperextension during overenthusiastic exercise or activities of daily living because these ranges may potentially cause recurrence of dislocation. Patients need to have this explained to them.[17]

30. What postoperative therapeutic management is appropriate?

Surgery involving direct repairs may begin with submaximal isometrics during the first several weeks after the operation, since contractile tissues were not cut during surgery. With Bankart repairs, from 3 to 6 weeks after surgery, active abduction is permitted to 90°, whereas external rotation is limited to neutral. After these 6 weeks abduction and external rotation are slowly increased as pain and active motion permits. These exercises include progressive isometrics, isotonics, eccentric activities. A home program is instituted using rubber tubing and hand weights for isolated cuff, deltoid, and pectoralis strengthening and multiple plane strengthening, such as patterns of proprioceptive neuromuscular facilitation, to be later incorporated into a well-balanced program. Although attention is focused on the internal and external rotators and adductors, it is done at the expense of neglecting other prime movers of the GH joint. If motion is slow to return, more aggressive range of motion is initiated no earlier than 7 to 8 weeks after surgery. Functional activities may be performed from 8 to 12 weeks after surgery.[6] With staple capsulorrhaphy, the patient is usually kept in a sling for 1 week, followed by active assistive range of motion permitted within pain tolerance during the second week. Progression to active

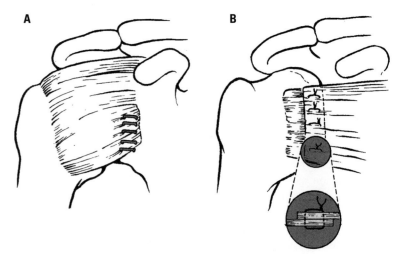

FIG. 17-15 Operations for recurrent anterior shoulder dislocation. **A,** Staple capsulorrhaphy involves reattachment of the inferior border of the capsule and labrum onto the glenoid using staples. **B,** Shortening of the subscapularis tendon. (From Dandy DJ: *Essential orthopaedics and trauma,* Edinburgh, 1989, Churchill Livingstone.)

range of motion then occurs at the beginning of week 3, as well as light resistance initiated from weeks 3 to 6. Rehabilitation of postsurgical Putti-Platt repairs differs in that the patient is usually kept wearing the sling for 2 to 4 weeks. Active range of motion to pain tolerance is encouraged for 3 to 6 weeks, at which time passive range of motion and strengthening exercises are initiated. Maximal internal rotation effort is usually delayed until 8 weeks after the operation, though some 10 to 15 repetitions may begin at 6 weeks.[8]

REFERENCES

1. Blom S, Dahlback LO: Nerve injuries in dislocations of the shoulder joint and fractures of the neck of the humerus, *Acta Chir Scand* 136:461-466, 1970.

1a. Bracker MD: New treatment for dislocated shoulders. In *The Physician and Sports Medicine* 12(7): July 1984.

2. Cleland J: On the actions of muscles passing over more than one joint, *J Anat Physiol* 1:85-93, l866.

3. Dandy DJ: *Essential orthopaedics and trauma,* Edinburgh, 1989, Churchill Livingstone.

4. Das SP, Roy GS, Saha AK: Observations on the tilt of the glenoid cavity of scapula, *J Anat Soc India* 15:114, 1966.

5. Duckworth T: *Lecture notes on orthopaedics and fractures,* ed 2, Oxford, 1984, Blackwell Scientific Publications.

6. Gould JA III: *Orthopaedic and sports physical therapy,* ed 2, St Louis, 1990, Mosby.

7. Gowen I, Jobe F, Tibone J, et al: A comparative electromyographic analysis of the shoulder during pitching, *Am J Sports Med* 15:586-599, 1987.

8. Grana WA, Holder S, Schelberg-Karnes E: How I manage acute anterior shoulder dislocations, *Phys Sports Med* 15(4):88-93, 1987.

9. Grant JCB: *Grant's atlas of anatomy,* ed 6, Baltimore, 1972, Williams & Wilkins.

10. Henry JH: "How I manage dislocated shoulder," *The Physician and Sports Medicine* 12(9):66, 1984.

11. Hill NA, McLaughlin HL: Locked posterior dislocation simulating a "frozen shoulder," *J Trauma* 3:225-234, 1963.

12. Howell SM, Galinat BJ, Renzi AJ, et al: Normal and abnormal mechanics of the glenohumeral joint in the horizontal plane, *J Bone Joint Surg* 70A(2):227-232, 1988.

13. Jobe F, Tibone J, Perry J, et al: An EM analysis of the shoulder in throwing and pitching, *Am J Sports Med* 11:3-5, 1983.

14. Kumar VP, Balasubramaniam P: The role of atmospheric pressure in stabilising the shoulder: an experimental study, *J Bone Joint Surg* (Br) 67(5):719-721, 1985.

15. Lillegard WA, Rucker KS: *Handbook of sports medicine: a symptom-oriented approach,* Boston, 1993, Andover Medical Publishers.

16. Mallon B: *Orthopaedics for the house officer,* Baltimore, 1990, Williams & Wilkins.

17. Matsen FA, Thomas SC, Rockwood CA: Anterior glenohumeral joint instability. In Rockwood CA, Matsen FA: *The shoulder,* vol 1, Philadelphia, 1990, WB Saunders.

18. McLaughlin HL: Posterior dislocation of the shoulder, *J Bone Joint Surg* 34A:584, 1952.

19. Meals RA: *One hundred orthopaedic conditions every doctor should understand,* St Louis, 1992, Quality Medical Publishing.

20. Moore KL: *Clinically oriented anatomy,* ed 2, Baltimore, 1985, Williams & Wilkins.

21. Moseley HF, Overgaard B: The anterior capsular mechanism in recurrent anterior dislocation of the shoulder, *J Bone Joint Surg* 44B:913-927, 1962.

22. Ovesen J, Nielson S: Stability of the shoulder joint: cadaver study and stabilizing structures, *Acta Orthop Scand* 56:149-151, 1985.

23. Perry J: Anatomy and biomechanics of the shoulder in throwing, swimming, gymnastics, and tennis, *Clin Sports Med* 2(2):247-270, 1983.

24. Poppen NK, Walker PS: Normal and abnormal motion of the shoulder, *J Bone Joint Surg* 58A:195, 1976.

25. Rockwood CA Jr, Burkhead WZ Jr, Brna J: Subluxation for the glenohumeral joint: response to rehabilitative exercise in traumatic vs. atraumatic instability. Presented at second open meeting of American Shoulder and Elbow Surgeons, New Orleans, 1986.

26. Roston JB, Haines RW: Cracking in the metacarpophalangeal joint, *J Anat* 81:165-173, 1947.

27. Rowe CR, Zarins B: Chronic unreduced dislocations of the shoulder, *J Bone Joint Surg* 64A:494-505, 1982.

28. Saboe L, Chepeha J, Reid D, et al: *The unstable shoulder: electromyography: applications in physical therapy.* Protocol from The Glen Sather Sports Medicine Clinic and Division of Orthopaedics at the University of Alberta, Thought Technology, Ltd, Edmonton, Alberta, 1990.

29. Saha AK: Dynamic stability of the glenohumeral joint, *Acta Orthop Scand* 42:491-505, 1971.

30. Saidoff DC: Diving accident results in acute pain and deformity in shoulder, *Advance for Physical Therapists* 3(9):12, 1992.

31. Salter RB: *Textbook of disorders and injuries of the musculoskeletal system,* ed 2, Baltimore, 1983, Williams & Wilkins.

32. Schwartz RR, O'Brien SJ, Patterson RF: Unrecognized dislocations of the shoulder, *J Trauma* 9:1009-1023, 1969.

33. Simkin PA: Structure and function of joints. In Schumacher HR, editor: *Primer on the rheumatic diseases,* ed 9, Atlanta, Ga, 1988, Arthritis Foundation.

34. Symeonides PP: The significance of the subscapularis muscle in the pathogenesis of recurrent anterior dislocation of the shoulder, *J Bone Joint Surg* 54B:476-483, 1972.

35. Turkel SJ, Panio MW, Marshall JL, Girgis FG: Stabilizing mechanisms preventing anterior dislocation of the glenohumeral joint, *J Bone Joint Surg* 70A(2):227-232, 1988.

36. Unsworth A, Dowson D, Wright V: "Cracking joints": a bioengineering study of cavitation in the metacarpophalangeal joint, *Ann Rheum Dis* 30:348, 1971.

RECOMMENDED READING

Malone TR, McPoil T, Nitz A: *Orthopedic and sports physical therapy,* ed 3, St Louis, 1997, Mosby.

Matsen FA, Thomas SC, Rockwood CA: Anterior glenohumeral joint instability. In Rockwood CA, Matsen FA, editors: *The shoulder,* vol 1, Philadelphia, 1990, WB Saunders.

Perry J: Anatomy and biomechanics of the shoulder in throwing, swimming, gymnastics, and tennis, *Clin Sports Med* 2(2):247-270, 1983.

PART IV

BRACHIAL PLEXUS, THORACIC OUTLET, AND SHOULDER GIRDLE

18

Pain, Dysesthesia, and Paresthesia in Ulnar Three Digits Caused by Proximal Lesion

A 41-year-old violin virtuoso belonging to the Metropolitan Opera orchestra complains to you of numbness, paresthesia, dysesthesia, pain, and clumsiness in his right ulnar three digits toward the end of long operas that significantly compromise his performance. He occasionally complains of nocturnal pain that abates if he sits up in bed. His pain coincides with the three nights per week during which he follows a disciplined regimen of weight lifting to stay in shape and strengthen his shoulder girdle. Symptoms also appear when he blowdries his hair. The gentleman, a bachelor, spends his time reading despite his severe myopia and admits to being a long-time heavy smoker. Upon calling the referring physician you learn that recent apical chest radiographs are clear and there is no evidence of the presence of a cervical rib or abnormally long C7 transverse process. Nor is there any sign of cervical spine disease. Electrolytes are at normal levels. An electromyogram and a nerve conduction velocity test proved negative. The patient denies any color changes, hyperhidrosis, swelling, trauma, joint pain, dry eyes, dry mouth, or photophobia. His past medical history is normal, as is his family history.

OBSERVATION   Forward neck posture with rounded shoulders; minor atrophy of right interossei and thenar and hypothenar eminences, and proximal and middle portions of the medial forearm. There is apparent hypertrophy of pectoralis major, pectoralis minor, and all the anterolateral neck muscles, which seem to stand out strongly. There is noted hypertrophy of bilateral scalene muscles. Upon observing the patient's breathing pattern, you notice that his chest moves up and down with each breath without any apparent accompanying diaphragmatic component.

PALPATION   No point tenderness over neck or upper extremity; there is no redness or warmth anywhere.

RANGE OF MOTION   Full painless range present in bilateral upper extremities.

MUSCLE STRENGTH   Normal to bilateral upper extremities.

SELECTIVE TENSION   Resistive testing at midrange demonstrates no pathologic condition.

JOINT PLAY   Hypermobility is noted in the lower cervical spine, and hypomobility is present in the sternoclavicular joint, particularly anterior and inferior glide.

SENSATION   Decreased to light touch to proximal and middle portions of the medial area of the forearm.

REFLEXES   C5, C6, and C7 are normal.

VITAL SIGNS   Normal, with clear breath sounds.

SPECIAL TESTS   Negative compression and distraction of the cervical spine; negative Tinel sign at the ulnar groove adjacent to the medial epicondyle; negative Adson's maneuver, negative costoclavicular maneuver; positive hyperabduction test though no bruit is auscultated over the supraclavicular fossa; radial pulse pressure is less pronounced with contralateral neck flexion and rotation.

? | Questions

1. What disorder is most likely the cause of this man's symptoms?
2. What relevant anatomy is requisite to understanding this disorder?
3. What are the three categories of risk factors in the development of thoracic outlet syndrome (TOS)?
4. What congenital factors directly cause or predispose for TOS?
5. How do forms of local and distal trauma alter the local anatomy of the thoracic outlet?
6. What is the relationship between posture and TOS?
7. What anatomic sex differences might account for a higher incidence of TOS in certain females?
8. What is the relationship between affective depression and the thoracic outlet?
9. What is the typical presentation of the postural variety of TOS?
10. What are the clinical signs and symptoms?
11. What is the differential diagnosis?
12. How common is vascular compromise in TOS?
13. What problems are there with many of the time-honored clinical tests used to diagnose TOS?
14. Describe the Hunter's test and Elvey's upper extremity tension test.
15. Are electrodiagnostic tests helpful in confirming the presence of TOS?
16. What rehabilitative therapy is appropriate in the treatment of TOS?
17. What is the prognosis of TOS?
18. What surgical options are available after a failed conservative regimen of treatment?

1. What disorder is most likely the cause of this man's symptoms?

The *thoracic outlet syndrome* (TOS) complex refers to a series of neurovascular compression syndromes in the shoulder region. The plethora of specific nomenclature for this pathologic condition include cervical rib syndrome, scalenus anticus syndrome, subcoracoid pectoralis minor syndrome, costoclavicular compression syndrome,[17] scalenus medius syndrome, first thoracic rib syndrome, hyperabduction syndrome, Paget-Schroetter syndrome, and droopy shoulder syndrome.[25] Each syndrome name may be said to reflect a shift in thinking as to the origin of the disorder in question. Over time, disenchantment of given nomenclature gave way to a new theory and treatment of the symptoms and

that in turn fell into disfavor because treatment of that entity did not conclusively cause abatement of symptoms. Today, TOS is recognized as an entrapment compression vasculopathy of the subclavian vessels but more commonly involving the lower trunk or medial cord of the brachial plexus at any one of four sites[20] (Fig. 18-1).

2. What relevant anatomy is requisite to understanding this disorder?

The *thoracic outlet* is bounded by the anterior scalene muscle anteriorly, medial scalene muscle posteriorly, clavicle superiorly, and first rib inferiorly[25] (Fig. 18-2). The uniting of the ventral primary rami of the 5 cervical through the first thoracic roots to form the superior,

A. Sternocostovertebral space

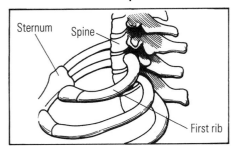

B. Scalene triangle

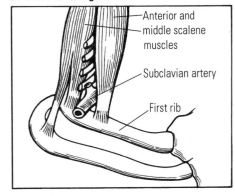

C. Costoclavicular space

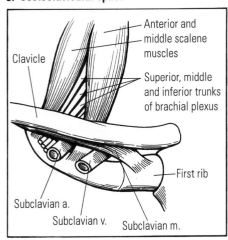

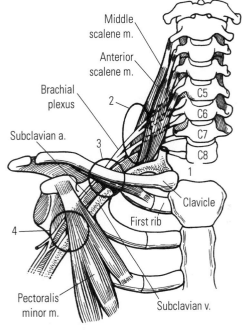

D. Coracopectoral space

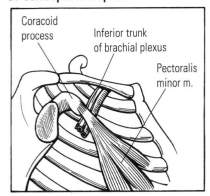

FIG. 18-1 The thoracic outlet has four sections. **A,** *Sternocostovertebral space.* Pancoast tumors present at this locale. **B,** The *scalene triangle* is narrower in many patients with thoracic outlet syndrome resulting in emergence of the neurovascular bundle from the apex of that triangle.* This may cause excessive rubbing of the neurovascular bundle against adjacent structures. Additionally, nerve adhesion to muscle may occur at this site. **C,** The *costoclavicular space* contains all the structures of the scalene triangle and the subclavian vein. **D,** The *coracopectoral space* contains the inferior trunk of the brachial plexus. (From Sanders RJ, Roos DB: The surgical anatomy of the scalene triangle. *Contemporary Surgery,* 1989, 35:11-16.)

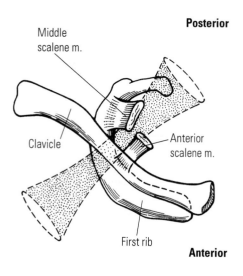

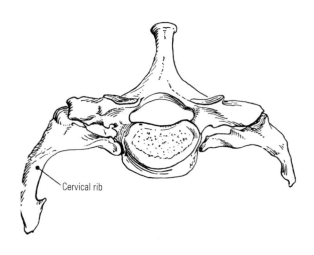

FIG. 18-2 Superior view of the dimensions of the thoracic outlet.

FIG. 18-3 Cervical rib. (From Moore KL: *Clinically oriented anatomy,* ed 2, Baltimore, 1985, Williams & Wilkins.)

middle, and inferior trunks of the brachial plexus occurs supraclavicularly in that part of the neck known as the posterior triangle.[14] The brachial plexus travels away from the spinal cord by passing between the cleft of the scalenus anticus and medius muscles into the supraclavicular region.[14] Here the ventral primary rami unite to form the superior, middle, and inferior trunks.[14] The ventral rami of C8 and T1 unite to form the inferior trunk, which exits the neck to enter the axilla by crossing between the first rib[14] and the clavicle (costoclavicular space)[20] on its way to the upper extremity. After leaving the costoclavicular space those nerve fibers composing the inferior trunk pass infraclavicularly underneath the muscular fibers of pectoralis minor en route to their distal destination by way of the coracopectoral space. Upper plexus involvement may occur after spasm of the scalenus muscles, whereas lower plexus involvement may occur in the costoclavicular space or underneath the pectoralis minor.[20]

The thoracic outlet has four sections: (1) The *sternocostovertebral space.* Pancoast tumors present themselves here. (2) The *scalene triangle* is narrower in many patients with TOS resulting in the emergence and rubbing of the neurovascular bundle against the apex of this triangle. Additionally, nerve adhesion to muscle may occur at this site. (3) The *costoclavicular space* contains all the structures of the scalene triangle plus

the subclavian vein. (4) The *coracopectoral space* containing the inferior trunk of the brachial plexus (see Fig. 18-1).

3. What are the three categories of risk factors in the development of thoracic outlet syndrome (TOS)?

- Congenital-structural anomaly
- Traumatic-structural alterations in the size of the thoracic outlet
- Postural alteration in the size of the thoracic outlet.[25]

4. What congenital factors directly cause or predispose for TOS?

Anatomic anomalies include the presence of a *cervical rib* (Fig. 18-3), unusually *long transverse processes* of the seventh cervical vertebrae, or soft tissue in the form of an *anomalous fibrous band.* This band is located near the cervical rib and may cause as much trouble as a bony rib though it is radiographically undetected because it is not ossified.[4] The presence of this band is suggested when the seventh cervical transverse process projects as far as the thoracic rib instead of being 1 cm shorter.[4] Cervical ribs, which articulate with the seventh cervical vertebra (Fig. 18-4), are present in 1% of the population, where they extend into the neck where their anterior end may either be free or attach to the first rib or sternum.[14] Although the presence of these varia-

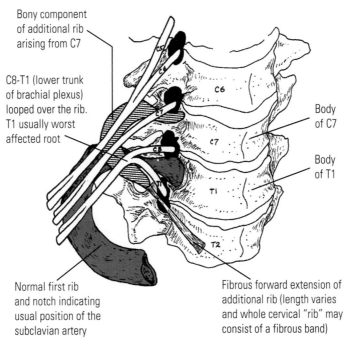

Bony component
of additional rib
arising from C7

C8-T1 (lower trunk
of brachial plexus)
looped over the rib.
T1 usually worst
affected root

Body
of C7

Body
of T1

Normal first rib
and notch indicating
usual position of the
subclavian artery

Fibrous forward extension of
additional rib (length varies
and whole cervical "rib" may
consist of a fibrous band)

Subclavian artery lies anterior to roots. Stenosis
and poststenotic dilation at this point may be
more significant than root stretching (see text)

FIG. 18-4 Relation of the cervical rib to its surrounding structures. (From Patten J: *Neurological differential diagnosis,* ed 2, London, 1996, Springer-Verlag.)

tions may cause little or no trouble under normal circumstances, after injury and loss of normal posture they represent a risk factor in the development of TOS.[25]

5. How do forms of local and distant trauma alter the *local* anatomy of the thoracic outlet?

Posttraumatic alterations of local anatomy may be caused by a malunited clavicle fracture resulting in exuberant callus formation and significantly diminishing the space between the clavicle and the first rib.[25] Another common example of local trauma is whiplash tears to the scalene muscle, which often result in protective spasm. Increased scalene muscle tone will excessively elevate the first rib and reduce the thoracic outlet aperture.[25] A delayed onset of local trauma would be whiplash-caused tears of the scalene muscle. The resultant tear fills in with scar tissue that, over time, undergoes contractures and fibrosis,[25] strangling that portion of the plexus that travels through its substance. Compression within the interscalene space may occur

after reflex muscle spasm of the scalenes, cervical spondylosis because of facet joint inflammation attributable to degenerative disk disease or cervical radiculopathy, overhead work postures, or heavy lifting.[1]

Distant trauma refers to painful lesions of the upper extremity that occur distal to the thoracic outlet. For example, a painful lesion of the hand, such as a neuroma, results in an involuntary guarding posture of the entire upper extremity. Although an abnormal posture protects the injured part from potential mechanical stimulation, it does so at the expense of altering the carriage of the shoulder girdle and hence potentially decreasing the size of the thoracic outlet. This decreased size may cause direct compression of the brachial plexus, especially in the presence of extra ribs or aberrant fibrous bands. The latter is an example of how postural abnormality can exacerbate a previously asymptomatic congenital factor. The involuntary maintenance of an abnormal posture causes compression, which is worsened by a vicious cycle of muscle spasm.[25]

6. What is the relationship between posture and TOS?

Loss of correct posture of the shoulder girdle is highly significant in the development of thoracic outlet syndrome and is explained in the following manner. During embryologic development, the forelimb buds must rotate 270° to produce the human upper extremity. Rotation occurs at the thoracic outlet level, and the nerves of the brachial plexus are twisted (circumducted) and positioned precariously at the center of rotation between the clavicle anterosuperiorly and the first rib posteroinferiorly.[25] Thus the descending neurovascular bundle exits the upper thorax by way of a bony aperture with limited diameter. This outlet may be thought of as a dynamic tunnel that changes diameter as a direct function of postural alteration. What we have here is the creation of a unique situation in which the diameter of aperture of this tunnel-like outlet is maintained by soft tissue attaching onto the scapula.*

Descent, or *ptosis,* of the scapula[13] manifests with age, especially with the advent of middle age,[4] because of gravity. As such, TOS is yet another example of a malady caused by forcing an anatomy designed for the quadruped position to tolerate the erect posture. In light of the above, we may state that alteration of the scapular posture will alter the thoracic outlet and may cause symptoms of TOS.[13] Nearly all humans may experience compromise of the thoracic outlet since the human shoulder is itself a risk factor.[25]

7. What anatomic sex differences might account for a higher incidence of TOS in certain females?

The upper margin of the sternum is level with the lower part of the second dorsal vertebra in males and on the lower part of the third dorsal vertebra in females. In the female, the medial third of the clavicle is lower than that in the male and thereby decreases the available space between the clavicle and the first rib (costoclavicular space). In addition, scapular ptosis may be greater in females with large breasts. Attaching to the pectoralis major muscle, the breasts exert a downward pull of the superior proximal attachment off the sternal half of the clavicle and thus further reduce the thoracic outlet aperture. This problem, referred to as *droopy shoulder syndrome,* may be accelerated by increased pressure from a narrow brassiere strap.

---

*Wearing a backpack or scuba tank may result in an acute postural alteration that may precipitate neurovascular compression at the thoracic outlet.

8. What is the relationship between affective depression and the thoracic outlet?

The distal attachment of the upper fibers of the trapezius insert onto the lateral third of the superior border of the clavicle and unilaterally act as a dynamic sling. The normal tone of these upper fibers elevates the clavicle while simultaneously preventing the shoulder girdle from sagging down on the chest. The individual who feels defeated by life will not hold his or her head up high because of "loss of face." Instead there are slumped shoulders in the absence of this normally acting dynamic sling. Thus, emotional depression may be physically expressed as scapular ptosis.[13]

9. What is the typical presentation of the postural variety of TOS?

The patient, nearly always a middle-aged woman, succumbs to inferior trunk compression by day resulting from stooped posture, which often accompanies middle age. Complaining of waking up anytime at night from severe "pins and needles" in one or both hands, the patient finds relief by letting her arms hang over the edge of the bed or by sitting or standing up. She then falls back asleep only to be awakened several hours later with recurrence of symptoms, or she may sleep uninterrupted until morning. On waking, the hands may feel numb for half an hour and exhibit clumsiness during small motions such as turning on the light or holding a toothbrush. The nocturnal symptoms may be a release phenomenon representing ischemic recovery of the nerve trunk, manifesting during sleep when the day's constant downward strain is relieved by the recumbent position. Thus the lower brachial plexus trunk moves upward and out of contact with the first rib in the gravity-eliminated, recumbent position. By day the patient is little troubled unless he or she wears a heavy overcoat, carries a heavy weight, or simply holds the arm in a dependent position for any length of time. The patient may eventually come to realize that the more she exerts herself physically by day the more pain she is likely to experience that night. Moreover, nocturnal symptoms may entirely abate after a bout of influenza causing the patient to remain essentially bed bound for several days or even after a "lazy holiday."[4]

10. What are the clinical signs and symptoms?

Thoracic outlet syndrome is an affectation of the brachial plexus and not of the cervical nerve roots. Consequently the patient will not experience symptoms at the base of the neck (supraclavicular fossa) where the lesion lies but rather distally along the upper limb.[4] The cutaneous distributions affected are those of the ulnar nerve and the medial cutaneous nerve of the forearm corresponding to the ulnar distribution in the hand and medial aspect of the forearm.[7,12] These two nerves represent the last two adjacent branches off the medial cord of the brachial plexus before that cord joins with the lateral cord to form the median nerve.

Paresthesias may later be accompanied by aching pain that is either poorly localized or over the whole arm. Paresthesia is often confined to the medial area of the forearm as well as hypothenar region of the hand. Either symptom may be exacerbated by such use of the arm as lifting and carrying heavy objects such as a container of milk or a suitcase or just standing about or walking. The patient may aggravate symptoms by merely reading[30] (think posture!), and the clinician may observe unequal shoulder heights and guarded posture.[25]

Motor deficits are not usually pronounced with TOS[25] and, when present, consist of a sense of weakness and clumsiness in the fingers. The patient may state that his or her grip or pinch strength is reduced. Atrophy, reflective of long-term TOS, will affect all the intrinsic hand muscles, since the involved plexus fibers are derived from the C8 and T1 roots, which furnish intrinsic hand innervation. Atrophy may also manifest in either the thenar[5] or hypothenar eminences.[25] Tendon reflexes remain normal.[5]

11. What is the differential diagnosis?

The major problem of diagnosis stems from the lack of a good definitive objective test to confirm the presence of TOS.[25] Because of this the diagnosis is a clinical one that is largely reached by exclusion.[20]

- *Ulnar nerve entrapment* is also suggested by nocturnal numbness, but these patients never have sensory loss in the proximal or middle portions of the forearm.[5] In addition, patients with ulnar nerve entrapment should have no atrophy of the intrinsic muscles innervated by the median nerve in the thenar eminence.[5]
- *Carpal tunnel syndrome* may also cause thenar atrophy, but the sensory loss, if present, manifests in the first two digits. The former is additionally differentiated from TOS by electrophysiologic studies indicating distal and not proximal compression.
- In *C8 cervical radiculopathy* there is compression with an almost identical pattern of T1 nerve fibers as in TOS. However, TOS may also involve the subtrac-

tion of some T1 and even C8 fibers that do not travel in the medial cord of the plexus. Cervical spondylosis rarely involves the C8 root emerging from the C7 to T1 interspace but should be suspected if there is obvious involvement of several other roots as well. Neck pain, triceps weakness, reduced triceps reflex, and weakness of finger extensors furnish a clue toward involvement of the C8 nerve root.[5]

- *Intramedullary or extramedullary spinal cord processes* such as syringomyelia, glioma of the spinal cord, extramedullary cervical tumor, infarction of the spinal cord, or meningioma in the foramen magnum may mimic TOS. The following signs direct attention away from the thoracic outlet: long tract signs such as brisk reflexes or extensor plantar response, loss of tendon reflexes in the arms, Horner's syndrome, or weakness of the upper arm or shoulder.[5]
- *Pancoast tumor*, also known as pulmonary superior sulcus tumor, is accompanied by rapid and severe weakness of all the small muscles of the hand and, in advanced cases, results in radiographically visible cancerous erosion of the first and second ribs, as well as possible hoarseness attributable to paralysis of one vocal cord.[4] A regular anteroposterior radiograph may yield a false-negative result, whereas apical views or computerized tomography is more definitive.[20] The apical lung tumors ought to be especially suspect in patients who have a history of smoking.[13]
- *Pronator teres syndrome* (see p. 27 and Fig. 4-3) shares many of the same symptoms as TOS. In TOS pain generally arises in the shoulder and the proximal area of the arm with radiation into the ulnar aspect of the hand with numbness experienced in the fifth digit and along the ulnar aspect of the forearm. With pronator teres syndrome symptoms are primarily at the elbow with radiation into the radial aspect of the hand and numbness that extends into the median nerve distribution. With the passage of time, atrophy of the thenar musculature will occur. The different provocative maneuvers eliciting the symptoms of each respective disorder as well as the absence or presence of Tinel's sign should additionally help differentiate the two conditions.[5]

12. How common is vascular compromise in TOS?

Most patients with TOS do not have vascular symptoms and therefore do not require arteriography. When symptoms do occur, they include distal edema,[3] coldness, muscle ache, and loss of strength on continued use, which are more typical of vascular compromise than of neural compression.[17] The patient may notice that his or her hand grip gives out while carrying a heavy suitcase. In addition, the hand may turn pale and cyanotic similar to Raynaud's phenomenon though most authorities agree that the full set of changes typical to Raynaud's phenomenon are not a component of TOS. Gangrene of the fingertips or trophic skin and nail changes may occur secondary to arterial insufficiency.[5] When evidence of vascular insufficiency presents, arteriography should be done and the lesion promptly repaired, since the lesion is progressive and delay will only exacerbate it.[5]

13. What problems are there with many of the time-honored clinical tests used to diagnose TOS?

The Adson, hyperabduction, and costoclavicular maneuvers are provocative movements and postures that attempt to reproduce pain, paresthesias, a change in radial pulse, or a supraclavicular bruit. The reliability of these tests has never been established, and it is now apparent that positive findings occur in many normal people who have no arm symptoms whatsoever.[24] Nevertheless, judgment of the clinical significance of a positive result may be made when one considers the speed of onset and the severity of symptoms during examination.[25] Cyriax advocates lifting the lower trunk of the brachial plexus off the first rib by having the patient lie supine with the arm passively resting over the head for 10 minutes, resulting in a positive sign of relief and abatement of symptoms. All this, against the backdrop of suggestive history and differential exclusion, enable a firm diagnosis to be made.[4]

14. Describe Hunter's test and Elvey's upper extremity tension test.

HUNTER'S TEST

Hunter's test is begun with the shoulder abducted to 90° and the elbow flexed to 90°. The arm is then straightened. A positive sign results in a painful shooting sensation down the arm in the distribution of the involved nerves presumably from sudden traction of the tethered medial cord of the brachial plexus.[25] Similar tension tests may be performed to stretch the ulnar and radial nerve tracts. The appropriate limb postures may be extrapolated when one studies Fig. 24-20 and positions the various joints of the upper extremity so as to stretch each tract by considering its relation to the axis of the joints it crosses. A proximal-to-distal sequence of me-

dial shoulder rotation and depression, forearm pronation, elbow extension, wrist flexion, and ulnar deviation may isolate the radial nerve. An ulnar-nerve stretch bias may be performed by wrist extension and radial deviation, forearm supination, elbow flexion, shoulder depression, and abduction.[2]

ELVEY'S UPPER EXTREMITY TENSION TEST

Elvey's upper extremity tension test (UETT) determines the mobility of the brachial plexus and nerve root, particularly the median nerve. Similar to the straight leg raise test in the lower extremities, this test may determine if any restrictions of the nerve roots or plexus have occurred in those structures stretched by a sequence of upper extremity movements. The three superimposed component movements include (1) shoulder abduction, lateral rotation, and extension behind the coronal plane; (2) forearm supination and elbow extension; and (3) wrist and finger extension[6,11] (Fig. 18-5).

Similar tension tests may be performed to stretch the ulnar and radial nerves. Provocative upper limb postures may be extrapolated from a study of Fig. 24-20. Limb postures that tension-bias certain nerves may be inferred by reflecting upon the course of given nerve in relation to axis of the joint it crosses. A proximodistal sequence of imposed upper limb postures in the following order tenses the *radial nerve:* shoulder depression and medial rotation, elbow extension, forearm pronation, wrist flexion, and ulnar deviation. An *ulnar nerve* bias is provoked by the following sequence: shoulder depression and abduction, elbow flexion, forearm supination, wrist extension, and radial deviation.[2]

15. Are electrodiagnostic tests helpful in confirming the presence of TOS?

Electrophysiologic testing for TOS is controversial[5] because consistent electromyographic (EMG) criteria are often not met, thus calling into question the existence of the diagnosis or even of the syndrome itself.[25] Nevertheless, testing should include EMG and measurement of ulnar nerve sensory action potential as well as ulnar motor conduction at the elbow, the latter to rule out an elbow (ulnar nerve) lesion.[5] A ruled-out ulnar nerve lesion may suggest a proximal compromise of the thoracic outlet. Characteristic electrodiagnostic changes include but are not limited to prolonged latency of the ulnar F wave and reduced amplitude of the ulnar sensory evoked amplitude.

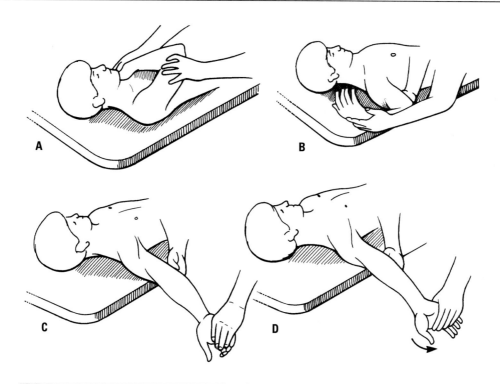

FIG. 18-5 Elvey's upper extremity tension test is a provocative sequence of motions that determines mobility (that is, gliding) of the nerve tract including the brachial plexus and nerve root. This particular test biases the *median nerve* and the anterior interosseous nerve for tension by way of mechanical stretch. **A,** First the arm and scapula are placed in a resting position. **B,** Next the arm is placed in the position of 90° shoulder abduction, lateral rotation, and elbow flexion with the forearm pronated. **C,** The elbow and forearm are then extended and supinated. **D,** The wrist is then extended to reproduce symptoms. Cervical lateral flexion to the left or right may then be added. It is essential for the examiner to maintain each posture before superimposing the next position in this sequence.

16. What rehabilitative therapy is appropriate in the treatment of TOS?

REHABILITATIVE THERAPY

- The treatment strategy is to facilitate more balance in the shoulder girdle so as to effect permanent lifting of the lower trunk of the brachial plexus off the first rib or to reduce pressure from the pectoralis over the nerve or nerves coursing beneath. This strategy is accomplished by a threefold approach of (1) postural reeducation, (2) selective muscle strengthening, and (3) selective soft-tissue stretching. This program must be introduced gently so as to avoid provocation of symptoms.[18] The therapist must be in close contact with the patient so that the program may be closely monitored. If a particular exercise causes pain, it must be modified or eliminated. Simply admonishing a patient to "stand straight like a West Pointer and get the shoulders back" is likely to result in frustration rather than relief. The time limit for this program should be 3 to 4 months.[13]

  The goals of therapy include (1) control of symptoms, (2) restoration of foreshortened tissues to normal length, (3) restoration of muscle balance, (4) improvement in posture, (5) development of stress-management techniques, and (6) prevention of recurrence of symptoms.[8]

- The use of *modalities* such as heat, cold, ultrasound, electrical stimulation (of high-frequency), diathermy, laser, and electroacupuncture have been used in providing temporary pain relief.[1]

- Careful *positioning* of the upper extremity such that the brachial plexus is neither compressed nor stretched (Fig. 18-6). This rest position is with the scapula in abduction and elevation and the shoulder in internal rotation and adduction (that is, the hand is placed on the contralateral shoulder). The patient must be warned, however, that maintaining this position for long periods will only inhibit progress, since the plexus will tend to become adhered to the underlying tissue and further motion may be lost.[1]

- *Stretching* of tightened soft tissue such as the levator scapula,[3] pectoralis major (see Fig. 10-2) and pectoralis minor, and all neck musculature.[19] Cervical spine exercises restore normal muscle length to the scalenes. Exercises include cervical retraction (Fig. 18-7), side flexions, and cervical flexion and extension. Patients should begin from either the position of minimal or absent pain, and proceed to the point of discomfort or

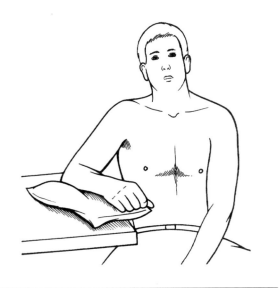

FIG. 18-6 Sitting rest position using a pillow to support the arm.

strain without pushing through their pain. If there is no pain or strain felt, the patient or therapist may apply gentle overpressure.[1] Targeting tight structures is a major facet of the evaluation and treatment of this condition. Restoration of normal length of adaptively shortened tissue is paramount to successful treatment. Foreshortened tissue may either compress or prevent normal movement of the brachial plexus. Lengthening of such tissue, provided that inflammation has receded, is imperative to a successful treatment regimen. Pain-reducing modalities may need to be used before or during lengthening to offset the inflammatory response.[1] Slow leaning into a corner with both hands on each wall at shoulder level, inhaling as the body leans forward, and exhaling as the body leans back is a particularly good stretch.[18]

- A self-stretching program of 5 to 10 repetitions every 2 to 4 hours throughout the day. Each repetition ought to be performed from a position of rest or neutral to the point where pain or strain is felt. The patient is warned not to push through the pain because doing so may lead to more inflammation and hinder progress. As treatment progresses, the point at which pain or strain is perceived is progressed further into that range. Between exercises, the patient may use the arm within tolerable limits or maintain the arm in the rest position.[1]

- Gentle *brachial plexus gliding exercises* (Fig. 18-8) to maintain free excursion of the plexus within the upper extremity. Free excursion is necessary, since inflammation of the plexus may cause adhesive binding of the plexus to surrounding tissue. Gliding may be accomplished by use of the UETT as an exercise.

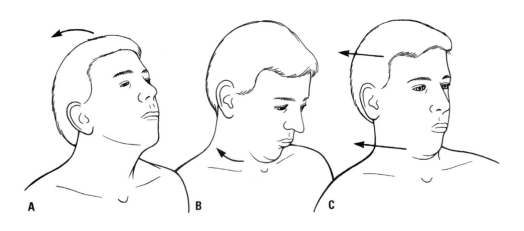

FIG. 18-7 Cervical retraction exercises. **A,** Poor technique—elevated chin. **B,** Poor technique—depressed chin. **C,** Good technique.

Each repetition should proceed from an area of minimal or no discomfort to the point at which discomfort starts and back to the rest position. As the restriction diminishes, more shoulder abduction and external rotation may be incorporated into the exercise. During the later stages of treatment, wrist extension and contralateral cervical side flexion may be added to produce further stretch. These gliding exercises are not appropriate to the acutely inflamed thoracic outlet condition.[1]

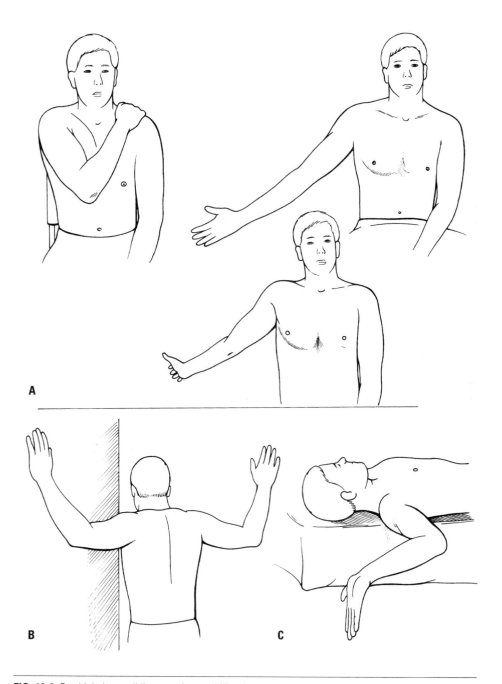

FIG. 18-8 Brachial plexus gliding exercises mobilize the nerves and may help prevent adhesions. **A,** Brachial plexus stretch while sitting. **B,** Brachial plexus stretch while leaning into a corner. **C,** Brachial plexus stretch in supine position using wrist extension and external rotation at 90° abduction.

- *Strengthening* of muscles antagonistic to tightened muscle groups.[18] An appropriate strengthening and stretching strategy focuses on strengthening the protractors and scapula elevators (serratus anterior and upper trapezius) while stretching the scapula retractors and depressors (rhomboids and middle and lower trapezius).
- *Postural reeducation* is a major facet of conservative treatment.[13] Exercises to make the trapezius repeatedly contract and relax altogether miss the point, since these muscles are already strong in most people. The patient must learn to keep his or her shoulders very slightly shrugged most of the time, that is, to maintain a slight constant postural tone in the trapezii because this habit can be inculcated.[4]
- Use of a figure-of-eight *harness strap* to pull the shoulders back out of their forward round-shoulder posture.
- *Joint mobilization* of the sternoclavicular joint[19] emphasizing anterior and inferior glide as well as scapular mobilization.[18] Mobilization of the first and second rib articulations are indicated to facilitate increased thoracic cage flexibility.
- Emphasize *diaphragmatic breathing*. When the patient works with his hands at or above chest level, as in the case of a violin player, the scalene and sternomastoid muscles, secondary respiratory muscles, are recruited and may eventually hypertrophy because of continued use. The diaphragm actively contracts and descends during normal quiet breathing. Ascent against gravity occurs during exhalation and is synergistically assisted by the recoiling properties of the lung and expiratory chest muscles. During quiet breathing diaphragmatic mobility is about 1 to 3 cm and is responsible for approximately two thirds of pulmonary ventilation, with the remaining third accomplished by other respiratory muscles. Breathing facilitated by the use of secondary respiratory muscles may gradually result in a weakened diaphragm and alter this 1:3 respiratory muscle ratio. The diaphragm may be strengthened by abdominal breathing (Fig. 18-9) exercises. The patient lies on his or her back with the legs drawn up with one hand on the chest and the thumb of the other just below the navel. During inhalation the chest remains stationary while the abdomen protrudes. Instruct the patient to exhale through pursed lips while manually assisting the abdomen to draw inward. The exercise may be performed for 3 minutes for two or three times per day and may be done without the use of hands once

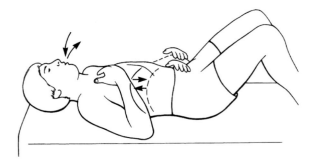

FIG. 18-9 Abdominal breathing exercises.

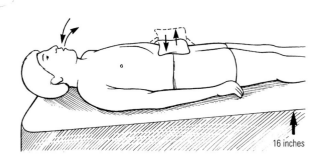

16 inches

FIG. 18-10 Abdominal weight exercises.

mastery is achieved. Abdominal weight exercises (Fig. 18-10) are performed with the foot of the bed raised approximately 16 inches and use of a one-pound weight (that is, a sandbag, book, or hot water bottle). Breathing is performed as during the latter exercise though the patient lies supine. This may be performed for 5 to 10 minutes twice per day and with addition of one-half pound every third day to a total of 5 pounds. This exercise may be prolonged up to 10 minutes as the patient progresses. Teach the patient to make use of primary respiratory muscles so that a therapist placing his hands over the patient's chest will move out and inward.[19]

- *Weight reduction* when the patient is obese.[13] The use of an underwire brassiere with wider straps may be helpful.
- Emotional depression may negatively affect TOS because it can be physically expressed in scapular ptosis and should be appropriately dealt with either by the help of a mental health professional or by the use of antidepressants.[13]

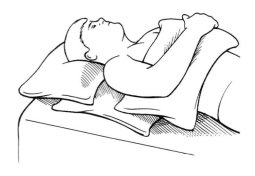

FIG. 18-11 Rest position in supine. Pillows or use of a triangle foam wedge should be used to support the thoracic spine, scapula, and arm.

- Scrutinize daily living activities as well as the patient's work conditions so that appropriate adjustments may be made.[13]
- Avoid wearing a heavy coat. Down coats are preferable. Avoid carrying heavy weights.
- Patients with nocturnal pain should sleep with their affected arm supported and in a neutral position. The pillow should not lift the shoulders off the bed[19] (Fig. 18-11).
- While one is sitting, arm supports such as those provided by an armchair are a must[19] because they unload the weight of the upper limb through the forearms so that the scapula is supported without effort. Use of a lumbar support during sitting may be helpful.
- Sitting each evening for one-half hour in an armchair before one goes to bed allows the nerve trunk to recover, as evidenced by the reappearance of familiar symptoms during sitting and eventual abatement after several minutes. The patient may then sleep, free from fear of being awakened.[4]
- Relaxation exercises to relax the upper thorax.[3]
- Massage of the trapezius and surrounding musculature.

17. What is the prognosis of TOS?

Fifty to ninety percent of sufferers of TOS respond rapidly and favorably to a conservative treatment program[3,9] and regain normal pain-free function of the upper extremity. The remainder may require surgery or a more extensive program that requires psychologic counseling as well as more involved rehabilitative intervention. Patients who do not respond to either conservative or surgical intervention often suffer from a host of physical and psychologic problems and should be referred to chronic pain centers, which are designed to address these problems.[10]

18. What surgical options are available after a failed conservative regimen of treatment?

The criteria for surgical treatment that demonstrate failure of conservative treatment include (1) signs of muscle wasting, (2) intermittent paresthesias being replaced by sensory loss, and (3) pain becoming incapacitating.[16] Surgery performed by most shoulder surgeons[13] includes depression of the scalene muscles and resetting of the first rib, removal of the cervical rib if present, removal of the clavicle, severing of the pectoralis minor muscle, and trisection of the subclavius muscle above the coracoid ligament.[19] Eighty percent of surgical candidates respond favorably after surgery, and a period of rehabilitation emphasizing maintenance of full range of motion so as to reduce adhesions of the brachial plexus by scar tissue as well as postural correction is indicated.[21]

REFERENCES

1. Barabis J: Therapist's management of thoracic outlet syndrome. In Hunter JM, Schneider LH, Mackin EJ, et al, editors: *Rehabilitation of the hand: surgery and therapy,* ed 3, St Louis, 1990, Mosby.
2. Butler D: *Mobilisation of the nervous system,* Melbourne, 1991, Churchill Livingstone.
3. Kisner C, Colby LA: *Therapeutic exercise: foundations and techniques,* ed 2, Philadelphia, 1990, FA Davis.
4. Cyriax J: *Textbook of orthopaedic medicine, vol 1: Diagnosis of soft tissue lesions,* ed 8, London, 1982, Bailliere-Tindall.
5. Dawson DM, Hallet M, Millender LH: *Entrapment neuropathies,* ed 2, Boston, 1990, Little, Brown.
6. Elvey R: Brachial plexus tension tests and the pathoanatomical origin of arm pain. In Glascon E et al, editors: *Aspects of manipulative therapy,* ed 2, New York, 1985, Churchill Livingstone.
7. Gilliatt RW, LeQuesne PM, Ligue V, et al: Wasting of the hand associated with a cervical rib or band, *J Neurol Neurosurg Psychiatry* 33:615, 1970.
8. Hawkes C: Neurosurgical considerations in thoracic outlet syndrome, *Clin Orthop* 207:24, 1980.
9. Hoffman J: Electrodiagnostic techniques for and conservative treatment of thoracic outlet syndrome, *Clin Orthop* 207:21, 1986.
10. Jaeger S, Read R, Smullens SM, Breme P: Thoracic outlet diagnosis and treatment. In Hunter JM, Schneider LH, Mackin EJ, Callahan AD, editors: *Rehabilitation of the hand,* St Louis, 1984, Mosby.
11. Kenneally M, et al: The upper arm tension test: the SLR of the arm. In Grant R, editor: *Physical therapy of the cervical and thoracic spine,* New York, 1988, Churchill Livingstone.

12. Lascelled RG, Mohr PD, Neary D, et al: The thoracic outlet syndrome, *Brain* 100:501, 1977.

13. Leffert RD: Neurological problems. In Rockwood CA, Matsen FA, editors: *The shoulder,* vol 1, Philadelphia, 1990, WB Saunders.

14. Moore KL: *Clinically oriented anatomy,* ed 2, Baltimore, 1983, Williams & Wilkins.

15. Netter FH: *The CIBA collection of medical illustrations, vol 7: Respiratory system,* Ardsley, NY, 1980, CIBA-Geigy.

16. Pang D, Wessel H: Thoracic outlet syndrome, *Neurosurgery* 22:105, 1988.

17. Peet RM, Hendriksen JD, Anderson TP, et al: Thoracic outlet syndrome: evaluation of a therapeutic exercise program, *Staff Meet Mayo Clin* 31:281, 1956.

18. Peet RM, Hendriksen JD, Anderson TP, et al: Thoracic-outlet syndrome: evaluation of a therapeutic exercise program, *Proc Mayo Clin* 3:265, 1956.

19. Pronsati MP: Treatment of thoracic outlet syndrome comes under scrutiny, *Advance for physical therapists,* p 14-15, Sept 9, 1991.

20. Schumacher HR, Bomalski JS: *Case studies in rheumatology for the house officer,* Baltimore, 1990, Williams & Wilkins.

21. Sunderland S: *Nerves and nerve injuries,* ed 2, London, 1978, Churchill Livingstone.

22. Swift TR, Nichols FT: The droopy shoulder syndrome, *Neurology* 34:212, 1984.

23. Swift TR, Roos DB: TOS or just droopy shoulders, *Aches Pains* 6:813, 1984.

24. Telford ED, Mottershead S: Pressure at the cervico-brachial junction: an operative and anatomical study, *J Bone Joint Surg* 30:2490, 1948.

25. Whitenack SH, Hunter JM, Jaeger SH, et al: Thoracic outlet syndrome complex: diagnoses and treatment. In Hunter JM, Schneider LH, Mackin EJ, et al, editors: *Rehabilitation of the hand: surgery and therapy,* ed 3, St Louis, 1990, Mosby.

RECOMMENDED READING

Barbis J: Therapist's management of thoracic outlet syndrome. In Hunter JM, Schneider LH, Mackin EJ, et al, editors: *Rehabilitation of the hand: surgery and therapy,* ed 3, St Louis, 1990, Mosby.

Butler D: *Mobilisation of the nervous system,* Melbourne, 1991, Churchill Livingstone.

Peet RM, et al: Thoracic outlet syndrome: evaluation of a therapeutic exercise program, *Staff Meetings Mayo Clin,* p 281, 1956.

Sanders RJ, Haug CE: *Thoracic outlet syndrome: A common sequelae of neck injuries,* Philadelphia, 1991, JB Lippincott.

Whitenack SH, Hunter JM, Jaeger SH, Read RL: Thoracic outlet syndrome complex: diagnosis and treatment. In Hunter JM, Schneider LH, Mackin EJ, editors: *Rehabilitation of the hand: surgery and therapy,* ed 3, St Louis, 1990, Mosby.

19

Large and Broad-Shouldered Infant with Monoparetic Arm after Breech Delivery

While working at the community hospital outpatient clinic 3 days a week, you are referred a case in the neonatal nursery. The infant, only 2 days old, presented with a breech delivery and appears to limply hang her left lower extremity adducted to her side with the forearm held in pronation. The baby weighed 9 pounds at birth, scored 6 on the Apgar test initially and then 7 five minutes later, and appears to have well-defined, almost broad shoulders. The infant is a first born. Radiographs have ruled out any clavicle or shoulder fracture.

CLUE:

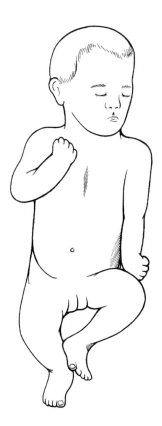

? Questions

1. What is most likely afflicting the infant?
2. What is the mechanism involved in brachial plexus injury?
3. How does brachial plexus injury most commonly occur in the neonate?
4. How does brachial plexus injury most commonly occur in the adult?
5. What is the anatomy of the brachial plexus?
6. How does architectural design of the brachial plexus serve as a force distributor?
7. What are the clinically observed patterns of injury?
8. What is the range of severity of injury?
9. What other conditions are associated with brachial plexus injury after birth trauma?
10. What abnormal respiratory function may occur with Erb's palsy?
11. What primary soft-tissue deformities occur after upper root paralysis?
12. What secondary contractures and osseous deformity occur after upper plexus injury?
13. What osseous deformities occur over time after upper root paralysis?
14. What radiographic changes eventually occur in the newborn after upper brachial plexus injury?
15. What is the difference between a preganglionic and a postganglionic nerve lesion?
16. Describe avulsion pain after preganglionic root avulsions.
17. What electrodiagnostic tests are appropriate?
18. What is the differential diagnosis of Erb's palsy?
19. What is the prognosis for recovery?
20. What is the prognosis after root avulsions?
21. How do evaluations of motor function differ when one is assessing a flail arm?
22. What operative management is appropriate in adults after brachial plexus injury?
23. What surgery is appropriate to improving elbow biomechanics?
24. What operative management is appropriate in infants or children after brachial plexus injury?
25. What are the goals of nonoperative management after brachial plexus injury?
26. How is the passive range of motion modality best administered?
27. How is the active range of motion modality best administered?
28. What is the role of electromyography in rehabilitative management?
29. How is the modality of stretching exercises most appropriately administered?
30. What positioning is appropriate in the infant after brachial plexus injury?
31. What is the role of electrical stimulation in the conservative treatment of plexus injury?
32. How is pain managed?
33. Is splinting appropriate in the management of brachial plexus injury?
34. What is a flail arm splint?

---

1. What is most likely afflicting the infant?

Upper *brachial plexus* injury known as Erb's palsy.

2. What is the mechanism involved in brachial plexus injury?

After the elimination of poliomyelitis as a serious cause of paralysis in the industrial world, brachial plexus injury has become the most common cause of shoulder paralysis. The brachial plexus is attached by fascia to the first rib medially and to the coracoid process laterally, so that lateral head movement with simultaneous shoulder depression will both stretch the upper plexus and compress it against the first rib. This upper brachial plexus injury, known as *Erb's palsy,* is the most common type of shoulder paralysis and occurs after violent excessive separation of the shoulder from the neck (Fig. 19-1). Lower brachial plexus injury occurs from excessive, often violent hyperabduction of the shoulder attributable to upward arm traction causing stretch to the lower plexus and simultaneous compression by the underside of the coracoid process.[20]

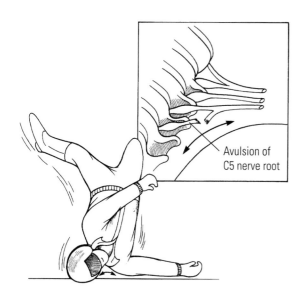

Avulsion of
C5 nerve root

FIG. 19-1 Avulsion of C5 nerve root after a motorcycle accident.

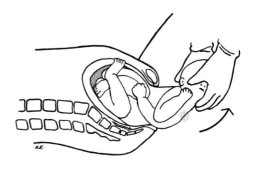

FIG. 19-2 Mechanism of upper brachial plexus birth injury. Excessive traction and lateral flexion of head and neck during delivery. (From Moore KL: *Clinically oriented anatomy*, ed 2, Baltimore, 1985, Williams & Wilkins.)

3. How does brachial plexus injury most commonly occur in the neonate?

Obstetrical Erb's palsy commonly occurs during the last phase of vaginal delivery, especially when the infant has disproportionately large shoulders (fetal dystocia) in which the obstetrician facilitates delivery by way of traction and lateral flexion (Fig. 19-2); this is complicated by the presence of a narrow (that is, android) maternal pelvis. Other birth risk factors include midforceps delivery, vacuum extraction, and low forceps delivery in decreasing order of incidence. Other significant factors, regardless of method of delivery, include high birth weight (macrosomia), that is, greater than 3500 g, pregnant mothers succumbing to glucose intolerance (gestational diabetes), use of oxytocin, vertex and breech deliveries, occipitoposterior or transverse presentations, rotation of the head in cephalic presentation, and first pregnancies. Additionally, infants with such injury often have lower Apgar scores and are more commonly delivered after spinal or epidural anesthesia after a prolonged second stage of labor.[8,14,16,18]

Overall incidence of brachial plexus injury has shown epidemiologic variation according to the quality of prenatal care and neonatal care during delivery. The incidence is approximately one in 1000 births.[16] Although the likelihood of such injury after cesarean delivery is extremely unlikely, it may occasionally occur because of either a failed attempt at forceful vaginal delivery or an imperfect extraction during cesarean surgery.[18]

William Heinrich Erb, a professor at the University of Heidelberg and the first neurologist to utilize a reflex hammer,[17] demonstrated with electrical studies (1874) that pressure at the junction of the fifth and sixth brachial nerve roots, that is, *Erb's point*, located 2 to 3 cm above the clavicle and just behind the posterior edge of the sternomastoid muscle,[18] yields the characteristic type of muscle paresis. In 1884, Augusta Dejerine-Klumpke described a paralytic lesion of the lower brachial plexus that was subsequently named after her. Erb-Duchenne-Klumpke's palsy (C5-T1) represents the second most common brachial plexus injury. Pure Klumpke's palsy (C5-T1) represents the second most common brachial plexus injury. Pure Klumpke's palsy (C8-T1) occurs very infrequently.[22]

4. How does brachial plexus injury most commonly occur in the adult?

The majority of upper brachial plexus injuries in the adult population result from high-velocity motorcycle accidents during which the driver is thrown forward and lands on the point of the shoulder, resulting in excessive separation of the neck and shoulder. This may also occur after a bicycle injury, after a pedestrian is struck and thrown by an automobile, or after a hard blow to the lateral area of the head, as by a baseball bat while the ipsilateral shoulder is simultaneously depressed. Patients are usually young males in their late teens or early twenties, often unskilled or beginning manual occupations.[12]

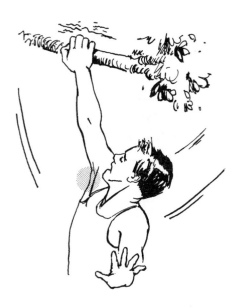

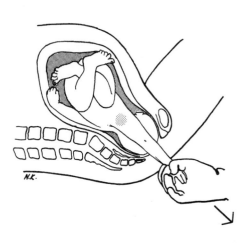

FIG. 19-3 Mechanism of injury in lower brachial plexus injury involves excessive, sudden, and forceful hyperabduction of the upper extremity. (From Moore KL: *Clinically oriented anatomy,* ed 2, Baltimore, 1985, Williams & Wilkins.)

FIG. 19-4 Mechanism of lower brachial plexus injury incurred during birth. Forceful pull of the upper limb during birth into hyperabduction. (From Moore KL: *Clinically oriented anatomy,* ed 2, Baltimore, 1985, Williams & Wilkins.)

A common mechanism of lower brachial plexus injury is that of *excessive hyperabduction* as may occur after free fall in which an individual attempts to break his fall by attempting to grasp an object such as a tree limb[15] (Fig. 19-3). In the newborn, injury may have been incurred during attempted extraction of the upper limb by way of hyperabduction (Fig. 19-4). The plexus may also suffer injury from heroin injection, delayed reaction to radiation treatment, serum injection, apical lung tumors (such as Pancoast's tumor), or during an operation on the axilla; the last two may cause lower brachial plexus injury.

Postanesthetic upper brachial plexus palsy may occur from malposition of the head, neck, or arm during general anesthesia and surgery. This is not permanent, and the prognosis for full recovery is excellent.[12]

5. What is the anatomy of the brachial plexus?

That interlacing of nerve fibers composing the brachial plexus (Fig. 19-5) is fascinating, complex, and yet frustrating because although one might memorize a textbook diagram of the plexus it would not be adequate for application to a significant number of clinical situations because of the significant variations in plexuses. Generally the "classic" brachial plexus is composed of the distal distribution of the anterior primary rami of C5 to

T1 *spinal roots* (or nerves). The brachial plexus has contributions from C4 (cervical plexus) in a significant number of patients and is said to be "prefixed." Similarly, T2 contributions, occurring in a very small proportion of the population, lend the designation of "postfixed plexus."

The roots continue distally to form *trunks.* The fifth and sixth cervical roots merge into the *upper trunk,* the seventh root continues to become the *middle trunk,* whereas the eighth cervical and first thoracic roots form the *lower trunk.* Each trunk then separates into anterior and posterior divisions (relative to the axillary artery). The anterior divisions of the upper and middle trunks unite to form the *lateral cord,* whereas the anterior division of the lower trunk forms the *medial cord.* The posterior divisions of each trunk unite and together form the *posterior cord* of the plexus. Although individual nerves such as the dorsal scapular nerve to the rhomboids and levator scapulae muscles come directly off the fifth cervical root before the upper trunk is formed, the aforementioned cords give off the largest number of terminal nerves. There is then a further subdivision in which the lateral and medial cords subdivide into branches, two of which fuse to become the median nerve. The remaining branches of the medial and lateral cords continue distally and respectively give rise to the

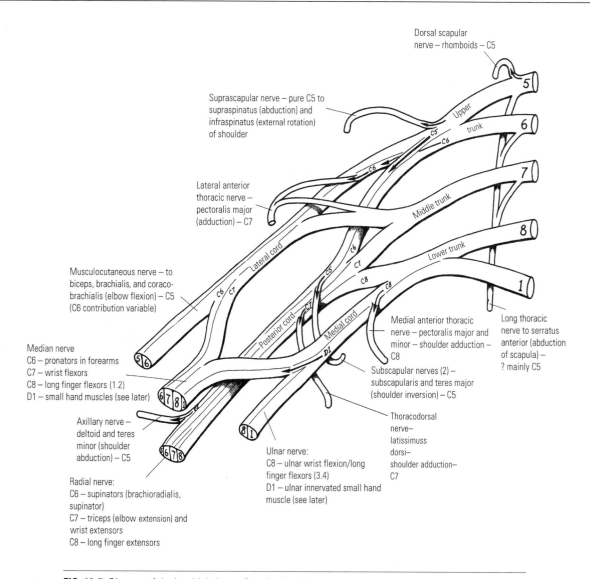

Dorsal scapular
nerve – rhomboids – C5

Suprascapular nerve – pure C5 to
supraspinatus (abduction) and
infraspinatus (external rotation)
of shoulder

Upper trunk

Middle trunk

Lower trunk

Lateral anterior
thoracic nerve –
pectoralis major
(adduction) – C7

Lateral cord

Musculocutaneous nerve – to
biceps, brachialis, and coracobrachialis (elbow flexion) – C5
(C6 contribution variable)

Posterior cord

Medial cord

Median nerve
C6 – pronators in forearms
C7 – wrist flexors
C8 – long finger flexors (1.2)
D1 – small hand muscles (see later)

Axillary nerve –
deltoid and teres
minor (shoulder
abduction) – C5

Radial nerve:
C6 – supinators (brachioradialis,
supinator)
C7 – triceps (elbow extension) and
wrist extensors
C8 – long finger extensors

Medial anterior thoracic
nerve – pectoralis major and
minor – shoulder adduction –
C8

Subscapular nerves (2) –
subscapularis and teres major
(shoulder inversion) – C5

Ulnar nerve:
C8 – ulnar wrist flexion/long
finger flexors (3.4)
D1 – ulnar innervated small hand
muscle (see later)

Thoracodorsal
nerve –
latissimuss
dorsi –
shoulder adduction –
C7

Long thoracic
nerve to serratus
anterior (abduction
of scapula) –
? mainly C5

FIG. 19-5 Diagram of the brachial plexus. Contributions from each root are shown in the cross section of each cord as well as the median, ulnar, radial, and musculocutaneous nerves. (From Patten J: *Neurological differential diagnosis,* ed 2, London, 1996, Springer-Verlag.)

medial cutaneous nerve to the upper arm, forearm, and the musculocutaneous nerve; the latter is the physical continuation of the lateral cord. Additionally the medial and lateral pectoral nerves derive from the medial and lateral cords respectively.

6. How does architectural design of the brachial plexus serve as a force distributor?

In the course of phylogenetic changes of the human upper extremity from closed kinetic chain (weight-bearing) function to that of open kinetic chain function, there occurred changes in plexus design to reflect this divergence of function. The architectural zigzag mesh composing the brachial plexus (Fig. 19-6), by virtue of design, is more capable of dissipating force by means of elongation, so that tension delivered to one trunk is distributed throughout the whole plexus.[22]

This *force-distributing strategy* is absent in the lumbosacral plexus, since destabilizing traction to the lower extremity is less likely, given the relatively greater stability present at the hip joint. Again we appreciate the price paid in terms of increased likelihood of upper extremity disorder in lieu of stability exchanged for mobility as mankind evolved from the

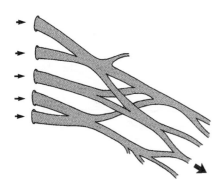

FIG. 19-6 The brachial plexus as a force distributor. Tension on one trunk will be distributed throughout the entire plexus. The angulation inherent to this design strategy enhances rather than minimizes the plexus reaction to the disruptive stretch by means of elongation and distribution of stress. (From Butler D: *Mobilisation of the nervous system*, Melbourne, 1991, Churchill Livingstone.)

quadruped to the biped posture. It is significant to note that the brachial nerves have spiral bands enabling them to stretch a full 16% without damage; this accommodating elasticity is absent in the lumbosacral plexus[2] (Fig. 19-7).

7. What are the clinically observed patterns of injury?

Patterns of muscle dysfunction include the following:

C5-C6 LESION

Muscle weakness and paralysis manifest in the rhomboids, levator scapulae, serratus anterior (that is, the scapular movers), supraspinatus and infraspinatus (lateral humeral rotators), the deltoid muscle, biceps brachii, brachioradialis, and supinator (the elbow flexors and forearm supinators), which accounts for the forearm becoming contracted in pronation. The wrist extensors may or may not be paralyzed, and, if they are, patients may still be able to dorsiflex the wrist if the

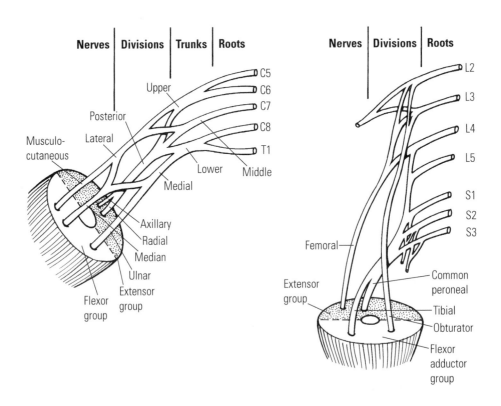

FIG. 19-7 Comparative architecture of plexus design. Although the brachial plexus is suited to dissipate tension by means of distribution of force throughout the plexus, the lumbosacral plexus lacks this design method.

finger extensors are preserved. Functional deficits include an inability to control shoulder movement, which can neither be forward flexed nor abducted. Although the elbow may be extended, it cannot be actively flexed. Active hand motion is infrequently affected. Sensory loss, which is difficult to distinguish, is often absent and when present may show variable deficits along the outer surface of the upper arm, forearm, thumb, and index finger.

The upper extremity will assume a characteristic *waiter's tip posture*[15] (Fig. 19-8) with the shoulder held in internal rotation and adduction next to the trunk. The elbow is extended, the forearm pronated, and the hand held in flexion. This is the posture, conceivably, that one would assume while accepting a tip or bribe without letting the giver have the satisfaction of seeing the receiver's face, while scouting the periphery to ensure that no one was looking. After brachial plexus injury, this posture is accounted for when one considers how the normal magnitude of tonal output is shunted to the remnant undamaged nerves and hence expressed as excess tone in the antagonistic muscles: the adjacent C7-C8-T1 level muscles. This clinical presentation makes the diagnosis obvious. Whether accompanied with a history of injury in the adult patient, or after birth trauma in an infant, the patient essentially fails to move the shoulder, which is held limp against the trunk with only some active wrist and finger flexion. In the neonate, an asymmetric Moro reflex[16] confirms the diagno-sis. Erb's palsy is commonly diagnosed within 24 hours after birth.[17]

C5-C6-C7 LESION

The C5 to C7 lesion includes all the deficits of the previous group with the addition of loss of active elbow, wrist, and finger extension. It is as if a radial nerve palsy were superimposed upon a C5-C6 lesion. As a result, there is a slightly wider area of sensory loss, that is, one involving the middle finger.

C7-C8-T1 LESION

The uncommon C7 to T1 lesion essentially presents as a combined median and ulnar nerve palsy of the hand as well as some radial nerve deficit manifesting as partial weakness in wrist extension, since the radial nerve receives some fibers from C8 and T1. Denervation of flexor muscles in the wrist and hand manifests as loss of active finger flexion and extension and as loss of all intrinsic hand function without producing a clawhand deformity[12] in some patients. A *clawhand* deformity (Fig. 19-9) occurs from loss of intrinsic hand function and from overpull of the extrinsic extensor muscles (that is, innervated by the radial nerve) of the proximal phalanx of the fingers. Thus the metacarpophalangeal joints become hyperextended while the proximal and distal interphalangeal joints become flexed. Therefore, if radial

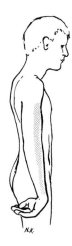

FIG. 19-8 Characteristic waiter's tip posture associated with upper brachial plexus injury. (From Moore KL: *Clinically oriented anatomy,* ed 2, Baltimore, 1985, Williams & Wilkins.)

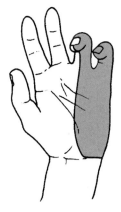

FIG. 19-9 Ulnar nerve palsy resulting in *main en griffe,* or clawhand. (From Ellis H: *Clinical anatomy,* ed 7, Oxford, 1983, Blackwell Scientific Publications.)

innervation is preserved, a clawhand deformity will manifest; otherwise it will not.

Sensory loss is usually confined to the little and ring fingers as well as to the ulnar border of the hand and inner forearm; however, if C7 dermatome is involved, the middle finger will lose sensation as well. The former two fingers are hyperextended at the metacarpophalangeal joints because the medial two lumbrical muscles are paralyzed and the extensor digitorum is unopposed.[15] Proximal function of the upper arm and shoulder are preserved with this lesion, though triceps function may be compromised. Horner's syndrome may be present because of involvement of sympathetic nerve fibers from T1. In the neonate, an absent grasp reflex is the most prominent clinical feature.[16] Infants and children may unwittingly, because of sensory loss, traumatize their fingertips even to the point of occasionally losing a fingertip.

C5 TO T1 LESION

Trauma to the entire plexus is unfortunately the second most common type of brachial plexus injury.[12] This disastrous injury is accompanied by profound motor weakness and total loss of sensation resulting in flail-anesthetic limb. Prognosis for spontaneous recovery is extremely poor.

8. What is the range of severity of injury?

Stretching of the nerve roots or trunks of the plexus beyond the elastic limit of that nerve may result in one of several types of injuries. The range of injuries includes (1) minimal stretch causing mild edema, which may in turn damage more myelin with subsequent blocking of nerve impulses, (2) hemorrhage and subsequent scar formation within the nerve, (3) axonal rupture (tearing) of the nerve with or without wide separation of segments[4] or, at the very worst, (4) intraspinal root avulsion off the spinal cord. Considerable variation also exists in the number of levels affected, ranging from the mildest stretch and subsequent edema of only one or two roots to avulsion of the entire plexus.

9. What other conditions are associated with brachial plexus injury after birth trauma?

The most commonly associated condition of obstetrical brachial plexus injury is *facial nerve paralysis* resulting from difficult delivery that necessitated forceps use. There is also significant occurrence of ipsilateral idiopathic infantile muscular *torticollis* in breech-

presentation infants. *Spasticity* occurs in those neonates afflicted with more severely involved root avulsions, since this results in focal hemorrhage up and down as well as in the vicinity of the cervical and thoracic spinal cord. *Fractures* of the clavicle, proximal humerus, and humeral shaft occur in that order of decreasing frequency. Other nerve injuries may include sympathetic nerve function associated with the first thoracic root producing ipsilateral *Horner's syndrome*. Additionally, involvement of the fourth cervical root may produce phrenic nerve injury[18] and subsequent paralysis of the diaphragm.

10. What abnormal respiratory function may occur with Erb's palsy?

More commonly occurring in those individuals with a prefixed plexus, injury to the upper brachial plexus may be accompanied by phrenic nerve disruption and hence hemidiaphragmatic paralysis. This is often observed by asymmetric thoracic and abdominal movement upon unilateral diaphragmatic observation. Phrenic nerve paralysis may result in respiratory distress and cyanosis and may mimic diaphragmatic hernia.[19] Examination of diaphragmatic function by electromyograph and fluoroscopy is not routinely carried out for infants with upper or whole types of paralysis, since ultrasound may yield accurate information in a noninvasive fashion. If the lesion is only a temporary neurapraxia, it is important to prevent respiratory problems such as atelectasis until recovery occurs. Positioning with the paralyzed side underneath is to be avoided. Prevention of secretion retention in relatively immobile portions of lungs is facilitated by postural drainage in the prone position at a 45° angle in the home several times a day. Respiration may be aided by oxygen and continuous positive airway pressure or continuous negative pressure[22] in severe cases.

11. What primary soft-tissue deformities occur after upper root paralysis?

After upper brachial plexus injury and resultant paresis or paralysis of the shoulder abductors and flexors as well as the scapular protractors and retractors, excess tone expressed to the intact neuromuscular junctions postures the shoulder in adduction, internal rotation, and slight forward flexion (Fig. 19-10). The summation of these unbalanced forces disturbs the synchronized and exquisitely balanced force couples that maintain normal kinesiologic function. Proximal muscle imbalance favors the shoulder adductors and medial

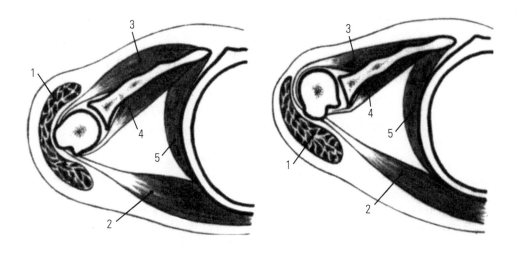

FIG. 19-10 Resulting muscle imbalance after upper brachial plexus injury results in shoulder deformity. Horizontal section comparing the normal shoulder *(left)* with the shoulder affected with an upper root lesion *(right)*. *1,* Deltoid, *2,* pectoralis major; *3,* infraspinatus; *4,* subscapularis; *5,* serratus anterior. Such imbalance postures the shoulder in adduction, internal rotation, and slight forward flexion. (From Scaglietti O: *Surg Gynecol Obstet* 66:868-877, 1938.)

rotators with soft-tissue contractures into the extremes of these latter ranges because those muscles adaptively foreshorten.

The scapula too is affected because both the serratus anterior and the rhomboids are weakened or nonfunctional. As a result, those muscles linking the humerus to the scapula (subscapularis, teres minor, latissimus dorsi) now cause the scapula to adhere to the humerus. This in turn upsets the normal 6:1 scapular-humeral rhythm during the first 30° of movement, and so any shoulder elevation, if any, is accompanied by a 1:1 ratio instead.[22]

The functional result of muscle imbalance is abnormal movement or abnormal combinations of movement that most commonly manifest as compensatory shoulder abduction with elbow flexion while one is attempting to reach out. This apparent disorganization of movement is actually the patient's attempt to reach in the most biomechanically advantageous manner, given the preservation of some muscle group as well as newly adapted muscle length. This substitution pattern, termed *Erb's engram,*[10] is a reasonably effective attempt at reaching, given the unfortunate state of affairs. A *visuokinesthetic motor engram*[8a] is a movement formula for the organization and execution of action.[13] When this movement substitution is practiced by the infant, it becomes learned to the extent of becoming

"engrammed" on the motor cortex and eventually becomes automatic and dominant despite apparent substantial recovery.

At the elbow joint, the elbow flexors and anterior capsule become contractured over time because of weakness of the biceps brachialis and supinator. This also accounts for the forearm becoming contracted in pronation.[21] There may be only partial weakness of the triceps because that muscle receives most of its innervation from the C7 dermatome.

12. What secondary contractures and osseous deformity occur after upper plexus injury?

Secondary soft-tissue contractures include atrophy of the posterior deltoid, contracture of the subscapularis as well as the pectoralis major, and lengthening and atrophy of the infraspinatus contributing to posterior capsular insufficiency. Because of incessant and unbalanced internal shoulder rotation, the humeral head eventually suffers posterior subluxation. Additionally the anterior shoulder joint capsule becomes tight while the posterior capsule stretches. Secondary bony changes may also occur in the acromion, which bends forward and downward to hook over the front of the posteriorly subluxed humeral head. This hooking increases with age and varies directly with the degree of posterior subluxation. The coracoid process may become greatly elongated because of the pull of the now contracted coracobrachialis muscle. The clavicle becomes shorter because of its becoming slowly curved more acutely than on the opposite side secondary to the unopposed weight of the upper extremity and from the vector sum of unbalanced muscular forces.

13. What osseous deformities occur over time after upper root paralysis?

Because of muscle imbalance in favor of those muscles (that is, the middle and lower root levels) antagonistic to a given level of injury, accompanying bony deformities will eventually occur. Over time the humeral head will become retroverted, and persistent unbalanced internal shoulder rotation will cause flattening of the medial aspect of the humeral head. Additionally the glenoid fossa will in turn become hypoplastic and sclerotic and may even form a "saddle" type of joint with the depressed humeral head.[6]

14. What radiographic changes eventually occur in the newborn after upper brachial plexus injury?

Radiographic changes include the following: In the newborn the proximal humerus will lie more distant to the glenoid, and development of the proximal epiphyseal ossification center is retarded. This epiphyseal center is lateral to that of the greater tuberosity as ossification occurs because of the internally rotated humerus. The humeral head succumbs to posterior subluxation, the coracoid process becomes elongated,

and the acromion is elongated, hooked, and flared on its end. The clavicle and glenoid are undeveloped. The diaphragm may be elevated if there is phrenic nerve paralysis.[7]

15. What is the difference between a preganglionic and a postganglionic nerve lesion?

Preganglionic lesions (that is, root avulsions) are characterized by the following signs, symptoms, and history: (1) a high-speed impact injury, (2) a period of loss of consciousness, (3) associated injuries such as multiple fractures, (3) a head injury, (4) vascular injury, (5) positive Horner's sign, (6) presence of sensory action potentials, (7) presence of meningoceles on a myelogram (which indicates avulsion), and (8) pain in the anesthetic limb.

Postganglionic lesions (that is, distal ruptures) are characterized by the following signs, symptoms, and history: (1) slow-speed impact injury, (2) no loss of consciousness, (3) no associated injuries, (4) negative Horner sign, (5) negative sensory action potentials, (6) normal myelogram, (7) positive Tinel's, or neuroma, sign, and (8) no pain[5] (Fig. 19-11).

16. Describe avulsion pain after preganglionic root avulsions.

Preganglionic avulsion pain is not usually immediate but occurs 2 to 3 weeks after injury. Patients describe the pain as a constant, burning, or crushing sensation akin to the hand being crushed in a vice. Pain may

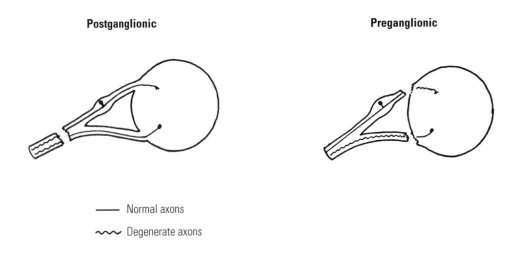

Postganglionic   **Preganglionic**

—— Normal axons

〜〜 Degenerate axons

FIG. 19-11 Site of lesion may be preganglionic or postganglionic, each of which manifests a different clinical presentation. (From Bonney G: *Brain* 77:588-609, 1954.)

manifest as sudden, sharp, electric, or shooting paroxysms of pain that crescendo for several seconds to 1 minute and gradually recede to a constant burning. The pain may be so intense that the patient may stop talking as pain literally takes his breath away as he grips his arm during the peak of discomfort. The pain does not vary with external stimuli. Patients may experience difficulty falling asleep but, once asleep, are not usually awakened by pain. This incessant pain is accounted for by a lack of central inhibition and hence unsuppressed firing of the cells of the dorsal horn.[24] This lack of central inhibition originates in sudden deafferentation of the spinal cord at the time of injury. Pain is frequently felt in the dermatome of the root that has been avulsed. This is curious, since no pathways remain between that dermatome in the arm and the spinal cord.

Preganglionic and postganglionic lesions respectively score positive and negative to histamine and cold vasodilatation response.[1] These data are useful in evaluating preoperative nerve repair in adults with accidental brachial plexus injury.[18]

17. What electrodiagnostic tests are appropriate?

Needle electromyograph of the paraspinal muscles is appropriate in determining whether root avulsion has occurred (Fig. 19-12). The reason is that the posterior cervical musculature is serially innervated by the posterior primary rami of the same-level spinal nerves innervating the anterior primary rami that make up the plexus. For example, if the limb musculature is denervated but the erector spinae muscles corresponding to that level are functioning normally, we have confirmation that the posterior rami at that level are intact. We may then make the following deduction: given that the posterior primary rami are given off immediately after the spinal nerves as they exit the intervertebral foramen, the lesion must be farther distally (that is, postganglionic rupture) somewhere along the course of the trunk, cord, or nerve branch and not proximally (that is, preganglionic avulsion). If, on the other hand, both sets of muscles are denervated, we may assume that an avulsion has occurred. Furthermore, the site of lesion can often be defined from the distribution of fibrillation

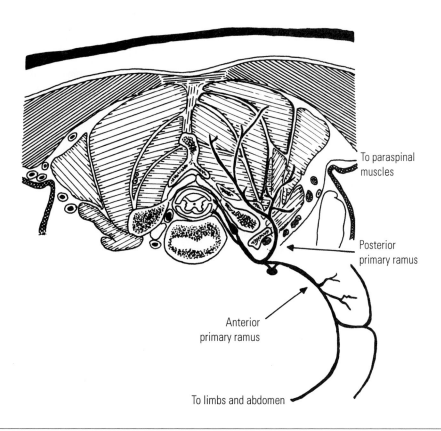

To paraspinal muscles

Posterior primary ramus

Anterior primary ramus

To limbs and abdomen

FIG. 19-12 Anterior and posterior primary rami. (From Hunter JM, Schneider LH, Mackin EJ, Callahan AD, editors: *Rehabilitation of the hand: surgery and therapy,* ed 3, St. Louis, 1990, Mosby.)

activity.[12] Absence of fibrillation activity several weeks after nerve insult is suggestive of a good prognosis, since most of the axons are probably intact.

Nerve conduction velocity (NCV) studies can also distinguish between distal ruptures and root avulsions. The latter will manifest as preservation of sensory conduction only, without a value recorded for motor conduction velocity, since the axon is separated from the anterior horn cell in the spinal cord. Sensory conduction is preserved however, since the dorsal root ganglion remains in continuity with the axon or dendrite.[12]

Electromyographic studies (EMGs) are very difficult to perform with small infants. Rather than determining the site of lesion, they are more useful in determining the extent of injury and the presence or absence of recovery.[18]

18. What is the differential diagnosis of Erb's palsy?

Fractures of the humerus or clavicle are differentiated from brachial plexus injury by voluntary elbow motion elicited by forearm or hand stimulation. With spastic hemiplegia, the ipsilateral lower extremity is involuted as well and may be accompanied by persistent Babinski's sign and sustained ankle clonus.

19. What is the prognosis for recovery?

Most cases of brachial nerve injury have a favorable prognosis.[23] If only a small segment of the axon is stretched but not ruptured, quick self-repair and recovery are likely. Temporary blockage of nerve impulses from swelling will resolve as edema subsides as long as no axon damage has occurred. However, if the axon is interrupted, reinnervation may take a long time, if one considers the slow rate of axonal growth in the peripheral nervous system (about 1 mm a day).[16] Although Erb's palsy is generally reported as having the best prognosis of all types of brachial plexus injuries, if no deltoid or biceps recovery has occurred by the third month, the result is often poor. Prognosis for full recovery is poor in Klumpke's palsy, and complete axon rupture is unlikely to recover regardless of level of injury. Similarly, a whole-plexus type of injury has an extremely poor prognosis for recovery. If recovery occurs, reinnervation will generally be complete in 4 to 5 months with Erb's palsy and anywhere between 7 months to 2 years in total plexus injury.[4]

20. What is the prognosis after root avulsions?

For plexus lesions determined to be of the root avulsion type, prognosis for spontaneous recovery is very poor. Given our present level of technology it is impossible to replant a spinal nerve that has been avulsed from the cord. However, if there is sufficient nerve length available distal to the intervertebral foramen, surgical repair may be attempted.[12] The results are often unsatisfactory.

21. How do evaluations of motor function differ when one is assessing a flail arm?

Motor functional assessment of a *flail arm* is approached differently from that of ordinary muscle testing. The examiner attempts to identify flickers of movement (as in the rhomboids) that would indicate sparing of the C5 nerve root from rupture. Bear in mind that a trace muscle grade of the upper pectoralis major (that is, clavicular) fibers implies sparing or recovery of the mainly upper trunk, whereas such a grade or greater observed in the lower pectoralis major fibers (sternal fibers) would indicate lower trunk recovery. A muscle gradation of trace flicker (that is, grade 1) means that there is evidence of slight contractility on observation or palpation, without observable joint motion.[5]

22. What operative management is appropriate in adults after brachial plexus injury?

In adults with brachial plexus injury, surgery is most often considered only when no evidence of either electromyographic or clinical recovery has occurred within the first 6 months after injury, since the outlook for spontaneous recovery is poor. The time in which surgery holds most promise for reinnervation is within the first 6 to 9 months after injury. A lapse of more than 1 year makes it hardly worthwhile considering. Neural reconstruction by microsurgery is accomplished by use of an autograft, usually the sural nerve and occasionally the medial cutaneous nerve of the forearm.[12] Surgery is considered successful if the interval between surgical repair and onset of observable recovery of elbow flexion is between 1 year and 18 months.[12] Results of repair for elbow restitution are significantly better than that for shoulder function, and about three fourths of these patients regain the ability to flex the elbow against gravity and resistance. With regard to the shoulder, success is often no better than the ability to shrug one's shoulder or overcome inferior shoulder joint subluxation. In all cases it is absolutely vital that the suprascapular nerve be repaired or else the all-important lateral rotary stability will be lacking. Most patients will not be able to raise their arms overhead after surgical reinnervation of shoulder musculature. Repair is rarely performed in the lower trunk of the plexus, since intrinsic muscle fibrosis will have occurred in the hand by the time nerve growth is complete.

It is because of the often poor functional result of neural reconstruction that many authorities consider secondary peripheral reconstruction the mainstay of surgical intervention. Surgery attempts correction of secondary osseous and soft-tissue deformities that have developed as a result of muscle imbalance. Reinforcement of weak or paralyzed muscles may be addressed by the use of tendon transplants, whereas osseous deformities may be addressed by humeral derotation osteotomy or shoulder arthrodesis. With the latter procedures, it is imperative that the trapezius and the serratus anterior function normally, since this is the minimal operating muscle pattern that will allow good postoperative function. In the event of flail glenohumeral joint, arthrodesis overcomes painful joint subluxation and will permit the patient to utilize the upper limb functionally. Limitation of abduction and rotation make it impossible to move the involved arm passively with the healthy hand in some activities of daily life such as dressing and combing one's hair.[3]

23. What surgery is appropriate to improving elbow biomechanics?

After brachial plexus injury, lack of full elbow flexion is not considered to be a significant disability, whereas the latter coupled with a fixed supination deformity is considered significant because this permits only limited hand function. Hand function is limited because this forearm deformity places the palm of the hand in a position useless for anything more than carrying objects. A weakened hand is much more useful if the forearm is partially pronated, since the functional portion of the hand faces the working surface of a desk or table. Correction is most simply performed by forearm osteotomy[18] or by correcting the excessive internal rotation at the shoulder (Fig. 19-13). Although effective, elbow flexorplasty, such as pectoralis major or latissimus dorsi transfer, may result in a conspicuous scar. Procedures to improve hand and wrist use are often individualized according to the given pattern of dysfunction.

24. What operative management is appropriate in infants or children after brachial plexus injury?

Microsurgery is generally not performed during infancy and is indicated only in the event of (1) a completely flail arm with Horner's syndrome after 1 month or (2) absence of biceps function after 3 months. Postoperative immobilization involves a body jacket for 3 weeks. The prognosis for recovery after pediatric surgery is more favorable than surgery in the adult brachial plexus injury. In the older child (such as 5 or 6 years of age) surgery to stabilize the joints, tendon transplant, and soft-tissue elongation may be performed because patients may benefit from regained improvement in function.[12]

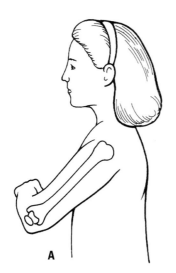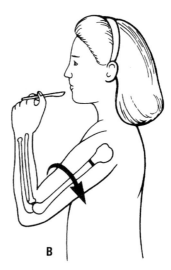

FIG. 19-13 Rotational osteotomy at the shoulder may improve function. (Redrawn from Rockwood FA, Matsen CA, editors: *The shoulder,* vol 2, ed 2, Philadelphia, 1990, Saunders.)

25. What are the goals of nonoperative management after brachial plexus injury?

The cornerstone of initial treatment in all cases of brachial plexus injury is nonoperative management.[9] Unfortunately, in some instances ignorance, inexperience, or lack of financial resources stymies success of an early nonoperative treatment approach. Goals of management include prevention of (1) soft-tissue contracture, (2) neglect, (3) substitution patterns, (4) injury to insensate parts, (4) and prevention of subluxation. Of paramount importance is appropriate psychologic support to control anxiety and fears of the future, address the injury to the patient's body schema, and discuss issues of vocation and depression.

26. How is the passive range of motion modality best administered?

Passive range of motion (PROM). Initially the infant is passively supported in a swing or swathe together with a collar or cuff to support the shoulder so as to prevent subluxation. No passive range of motion is to be performed for the first several days so as to permit early traumatic neuritis to subside.[18] This also avoids tension on the irritated plexus and allows resolution of hemorrhage and edema.[22] PROM of the shoulder girdle should then commence in those planes in which loss of active muscle contraction occurs in external shoulder rotation and abduction, forearm supination, wrist extension, finger extension, and thumb abduction. These exercises serve to stretch the weakened or paralyzed muscles. All movements must be performed gently so as not to damage the shoulder. The infant should not cry as a result of these movements. Additionally the normal scapulohumeral relationship should be manually mimicked during shoulder joint elevation. The scapula should not be manually restrained once the humerus rises above the $30°$[20] elevation mark. The reason is that elevation unaccompanied by scapular rotation (or lateral humeral rotation) results in potential impingement within the subacromial arch beyond 30°. Particular effort should be taken to teach the infant's parents how to perform passive movements appropriately. An overzealous parent can severely injure an infant's arm and must be carefully impressed with the importance of keeping within the normal range.

In the adult, the hand often tends to conform to the contour of the abdomen against which it rests, resulting in eventual ankylosis of the metacarpophalangeal joints in full extension, with the thumb in the plane of the hand and therefore useless even if motor control returns. PROM taught to the adult ought to be simple and few in quantity because the more complex and numerous, the less likely the patient is to perform them regularly.[12]

27. How is the active range of motion modality best administered?

Active range of motion (AROM). The therapist must not simply stimulate movement. Rather he or she must perform *motor training,* that is, stimulation of movement while minimizing and preventing disorganized limb movement, that is, habituated substitution patterns. To facilitate this, the therapist uses manual guidance of the limb during elevation together with verbal praise to the infant, such as appropriate cooing and wooing, to ensure that the infant moves as normally as possible. Abnormal tone dominates the limb, and, given the sheer limits or practicality, the infant's nervous system may, despite well-intentioned therapy, engram a substitution movement pattern. It is for this reason that motor training must involve *intense* training of the limb in specific planes of movement. For example, in training the deltoid and external rotators to contract and elevate the shoulder, the exercise is first done on the child's side where gravity is eliminated. The therapist then slowly progresses the child to gravity-resisted movements in the supine position while simultaneously deemphasizing unwanted substitutions. Objects of grasp used to stimulate should be irresistible in form and color so as to motivate the child. Verbal feedback and positive reinforcement in the form of tone and smile are a must, and part and parcel of the repertoire of skills the therapist cultivates while treating such children. Additionally, the object of attraction (such as a bright fishing lure without its hook) is best kept 5 to 7 inches away from the child's face because this range includes the infant's acute field of vision.[22] Objects will also be more easily detected if they move rather than if they are simply held stationary. AROM is performed, at the very least, with each diaper change.

When the child is old enough to interact with adults and to obey simple commands, play activities are initiated. The therapist must be very imaginative, so that games are performed and nursery rhymes may be sung with each exercise so as to stretch contracted muscles or strengthen weakened muscles.

28. What is the role of electromyography in rehabilitative management?

Serial electromyographic (EMG) studies ought to be begun within the first few weeks after birth and repeated at 6- to 8-week intervals for as long as indicated. EMG signs of return such as decreased denervation potentials and the appearance of reinnervation potentials often predate clinically apparent return by several weeks. Potential recovery is maximized when the appearance of these EMG findings is immediately followed by intense therapy to stimulate activity in affiliated muscle groups. Although excessive fatigue is to be avoided, specific motor training at this juncture may be crucial to actualizing potential neural recovery. Thus EMG is used as a guide to the motor training program.[20,22]

29. How is the modality of stretching exercises most appropriately administered?

Stretching activities of the active musculature are appropriate, since the excess tone delivered to the unopposed muscles causes them to shorten more quickly. Muscles that require regular stretching include wrist and finger flexors, elbow extensors, forearm pronators, shoulder adductors, and internal rotators.

30. What positioning is appropriate in the infant after brachial plexus injury?

Positioning. When placed in supine or prone positions, infants should have their arm placed with the shoulder in midrange of abduction and external rotation and with the elbow in flexion. This position somewhat approximates a natural neonate posture, avoids excessive joint stretch, and reinforces the goals of range of motion exercises. Propped and sidelying on the sound side is a position that permits the involved arm to be free for play and permits encouragement of midline orientation as well as hand-to-hand or hand-to-mouth activity; however, the affected arm is relatively nonfunctional secondary to paralysis. Occasional sidelying on the affected side is permitted with appropriate protection from undue compression achieved by propping of the infant in a well-supported position, with the trunk slightly rolled back toward supine to reduce body weight on the arm. A small pillow or folded baby blanket is tucked under the infant's head so as to achieve a neutral alignment of the neck along the body axis. This position allows the baby to play with the sound arm, which is less influenced by gravity.[20]

31. What is the role of electrical stimulation in the conservative treatment of plexus injury?

Electrical stimulation is appropriate in most kinds of brachial plexus injury, including those in infants. The goal of electrical stimulation is to prevent muscle atrophy and fibrosis from setting into denervated muscle.[13]

Here, the reference electrode is placed on the baby's ipsilateral forearm or leg while the active electrode is attached to the dorsum of the therapist's hand. In this fashion the therapist feels everything that the infant does and can thus monitor the magnitude of stimulation directly. Pinpoint stimulation is then provided by way of the therapist's fingers, for example, by placement of the tip of each finger on the motor points of shoulder force-coupled muscles. Treatment should be minimized in the pediatric population to no longer than several minutes at a time.[11]

32. How is pain managed?

Pain treatment. A significantly high percentage of patients with traction injuries to the brachial plexus suffer pain that may initially be very severe; this is particularly true after an avulsion of the nerve root. Fortunately, discomfort usually diminishes with time. In the interim, however, pain may be managed with transcutaneous electric stimulation (TENS) or acupuncture. The deafferentation of the spinal cord after an avulsion injury leads to changes in the firing of the dorsal horn cells in the spinal cord. One might argue that TENS artificially restores the afferent input to the spinal cord by allowing completion of the disrupted circuit. Thus, if TENS is to work by this mechanism, electrodes ought to be placed proximally to the level of the lesion (Fig. 19-14). Single-channel units are usually adequate, though large pads are preferable so as to facilitate as large an afferent input as possible.

Electrode placement involves one large pad placed over the appropriate damaged dermatome (providing that there is some residual afferent input), whereas the other pad is placed over the nerve trunk of the appropriate root level of damage. Electrodes may be placed more distally in the event of some residual arm sensation. Pads may also be applied over the impaired area of sensation, provided that the area is not anesthetic, since this arrangement would provide no afferent pathway along which the electrical stimulus could pass to the spinal cord. A minimum duration of treatment of 8 hours a day for 3 weeks is recommended.[5] TENS treatment is contraindicated in infants.

The treatment of pain with narcotics on a long-term basis is contraindicated, since this is chronic, "benign" pain. Once the patient is started on the use of narcotic medication by well-meaning physicians, the result is often considerable difficulty in weaning patients from these drugs. Cordotomy, rhizotomy, or sympathectomy as sources of pain relief are not considered appropriate by some authorities. Indeed, the problem of pain occur-

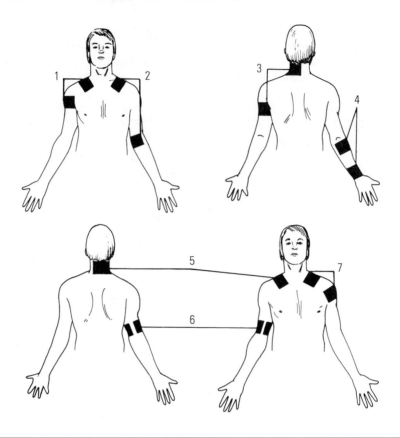

FIG. 19-14 Transcutaneous electric stimulation (TENS) electrode placements *1* to *7* for brachial plexus patients with avulsion pain. (From Hunter JM, Schneider LH, Mackin EJ, Callahan AD, editors: *Rehabilitation of the hand: surgery and therapy,* ed 3, St. Louis, 1990, Mosby.)

ring after brachial plexus injury continues to be a difficult one for which no clearly dependable solution exists.[12]

33. Is splinting appropriate in the management of brachial plexus injury?

Continuous *splinting* of the extremity after a brachial plexus injury is a controversial topic and is no longer routinely employed as a treatment modality. A once commonly used splint is the "Statue of Liberty" position designed to immobilize the shoulder in the corrected position, but it may eventually cause hypermobility and even anterior glenohumeral dislocation. Pinning the sleeve to a pillow or mattress with the shoulder in 90° abduction and external rotation essentially does the same thing and is inappropriate. Intermittent positional splinting is appropriate during those times when active intervention with the infant is not possible, provided that

it is not substituted for regular active range of motion activities. Elbow splints have also been known to cause a pathologic condition such as elbow flexion contracture, dislocation and flattening of the radial head, and bowing of the proximal end of the ulna.

Resting hand splints are often appropriate to prevent flexion contractures of the fingers and to stabilize the thumb and fingers in good functional alignment. Dynamic splints to reinforce and reeducate wrist and finger extensors have been used with infants sustaining C7 injury.[20]

34. What is a flail arm splint?

Flail anesthetic limb is defined as total loss of limb sensitivity compounded with profound motor weakness; it has an extremely poor prognosis for spontaneous recovery. The adult with a flail arm should never be splinted because of the rapidity with which contractures

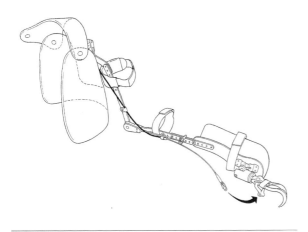

FIG. 19-15 Flail arm splint. (From Robinson C: *Br J Occup Ther* 49[10]:1986.)

set in. However, wearing a functional *flail arm splint* is appropriate in providing the patient with bilateral upper extremity function while he or she waits for recovery to occur. It is up to the rehabilitation team or the patient's therapist to discern whether a given patient is appropriate for this splint. The reason is that the patient who is not truly motivated or suitable for a flail arm splint may well cause a lot of time to be wasted by both therapist and patient.

The *flail arm splint* (Fig. 19-15) is a lightweight modular splint that is actually a skeleton of an upper limb prosthesis that fits over the paralyzed arm. This orthosis provides the necessary shoulder support to allow for some shoulder abduction while preventing subluxation. An elbow lock device permits alternative positions for elbow flexion as well as being a forearm-to-wrist support trough having a platform on the volar aspect, onto which standard artificial limb appliances may be fitted. The splint is operated in the same manner as a prosthesis, that is, by a cable running from the terminal appliance to a shoulder strap on the opposite shoulder. The flail arm splint can be fitted in 1½ to 2 hours, functions as a tool for use at work as well as for hobbies, and can be taken off when not in use. When compared to an upper extremity prosthetic, its advantage over a prosthetic is a cosmetic one that allows the patient to retain his or her limb after and hence the psychologic benefit of maintaining his or her sense of body schema, which is lost after amputation. Amputation is uncommon because paralysis of the shoulder girdle muscles in most brachial plexus injuries precludes good operation of the artificial limb.[5]

REFERENCES

1. Bonney G: The value of axon responses in determining the site of lesion in traction injuries of the brachial plexus, *Brain* 77:588-609, 1954.
2. Bonney G: Prognosis in traction lesions of the brachial plexus, *J Bone Joint Surg* 41B:4, 1959.
2a. Butler D: *Mobilisation of the nervous system,* Melbourne, 1991, Churchill Livingstone.
3. Comtet JJ, Sedel L, Fredenucci JF, et al: Duchenne-Erb palsy: experience with direct surgery, *Clin Orthop* (237):17-23, Dec 1988.
4. Eng GD, Koch B, Smokvina MD: Brachial plexus palsy in neonates and children, *Arch Phys Med Rehabil* 59:458, 1978.
5. Frampton YM: Therapist's management of brachial plexus injuries. In Hunter JM, Schneider LH, Mackin EJ, et al, editors: *Rehabilitation of the hand: surgery and therapy,* ed 3, St Louis, 1990, Mosby.
6. Goddard NJ, Fixsen JA: Rotation osteotomy of the humerus for birth injuries of the brachial plexus, *J Bone Joint Surg* 66B:257-259, 1984.
7. Gorden M, Rich F, Deutschberger J, et al: The immediate and long term outcome of obstetric birth trauma. 1. Brachial plexus paralysis, *Am J Gynecol* 117:5-56, 1973.
8. Griffen PP: *Orthopedics in the newborn: neonatology, pathophysiology and management of the newborn,* ed 2, edited by GB Avery, Philadelphia, 1981, Lippincott.
8a. Heilman KM, Rothi LJG: Apraxia. In Heilman KM, Valenstein E, editors: *Clinical neuropsychology,* ed 2, Oxford, 1985, Oxford University Press.
9. Jackson ST, Hoffer MM, Parrish N: Brachial plexus palsy in the newborn, *J Bone Joint Surg* 70A(8):1217-1220, 1988.
10. Johnson EW, Alexander MA, Koenig WE: Infantile Erb's palsy (Smellie's palsy), *Arch Phys Med Rehabil* 58:175, 1977.
11. Kahn J: *Principles and practice of electrotherapy,* ed 2, New York, 1991, Churchill Livingstone.
12. Leffert RD: Rehabilitation of the patient with an injury to the brachial plexus. In Hunter JM, Schneider LH, Mackin EJ, et al, editors: *Rehabilitation of the hand: surgery and therapy,* ed 3, St Louis, 1990, Mosby.
13. Liberson WT, Terzis JK: Some novel techniques of clinical electrophysiology applied to the management of brachial plexus palsy, *Electromyogr Clin Neurophysiol* 27:371, 1987.
13a. Leipmann H: *Drei Aufsätze aus dem Apraxiegebiet,* Berlin, 1908, Karger.
14. McFarland LV, Raskin M, Daling JR, et al: Erb/Duchenne's palsy: a consequence of fetal macrosomia and method of delivery, *Obstet Gynecol* 68(6):784-788, 1986.
15. Moore KL: *Clinically oriented anatomy,* ed 2, Baltimore, 1985, Williams & Wilkins.
16. Netter FH: *The CIBA collection of medical illustrations, vol 1: Nervous system,* part 2, Summit, NJ, 1986, CIBA-Geigy.
17. *Phys Ther Forum* 1x(12):1, 1990.
18. Rockwood CA, Matsen FA, editors: *The shoulder,* vol 2, Philadelphia, 1990, WB Saunders.
19. Rose FC, editor: *Paediatric neurology,* Oxford, 1979, Blackwell Scientific Publishers.
20. Semmer CJ, Hunter JG: *Early occupation therapy intervention: neonates to three years,* Gaithersburg, Md, 1990, Aspen Publications.

21. Sever JW: Obstetric paralysis: a report of 470 cases, *Am J Dis Child* 12:541-578, 1916.
22. Shepherd RB, Campbell SK: Brachial plexus injury. In Campbell, SK, editor: *Pediatric neurologic physical therapy,* ed 2, New York, 1991, Churchill Livingstone.
23. Sjöberg I, Erichs K, Bjerre I: Cause and effect of obstetric (neonatal) brachial plexus palsy, *Acta Paediatr Scand* 77:357, 1988.
24. Wells PE, Frampton VM, Bawsher D: *Pain management in physical therapy,* vol 1, East Norwalk, Conn, 1988, Appleton & Lange.

RECOMMENDED READING

Frampton YM: Therapist's management of brachial plexus injuries. In Hunter JM, Schneider LH, Mackin EJ, et al, editors: *Rehabilitation of the hand: surgery and therapy,* ed 3, St Louis, 1990, Mosby.

Leffert RD: Rehabilitation of the patient with an injury to the brachial plexus. In Hunter JM, Schneider LH, Mackin EJ, et al, editors: *Rehabilitation of the hand: surgery and therapy,* ed 3, St. Louis, 1990, Mosby.

Shepherd RB: Brachial plexus injury. In Campbell SK, editor: *Clinics in physical therapy: pediatric neurologic physical therapy,* ed 2, New York, 1991, Churchill Livingstone.

Semmer CJ, Hunter JG: *Early occupation therapy intervention: neonates to three years,* Gaithersburg, Md, 1990, Aspen Publications.

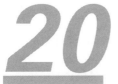

20

Exquisite Pinpoint Muscle Pain and Taut Bands within Muscle Substance and Remote Referral to a Locale within the Same Myotome

A 38-year-old fireman fell through the roof of a burning building and sustained a superficial laceration of the right dorsal wrist and right dorsoproximal forearm. Several weeks later he was referred for physical therapy because of persistent paresthesia along the ulnar aspect of the right hand. He has been unable to return to work.

PALPATION   Elicited stabbing wrist pains on ulnar or radial deviation as well as dorsal numbness in digits four and five of his right hand.

MOTION AND STRENGTH ARE DECREASED AS SHOWN:

	Left	Right
Wrist flexion:	85°	75°
Wrist extension:	62°	30°
Radial deviation:	20°	20°
Ulnar deviation:	45°	15°
Grip strength:	31 kg	6 kg
Lateral pinch:	5.8 kg	4 kg
Pulp pinch:	6.2 kg	5 kg

SENSATION   There is decreased sensation to touch and pinprick along the ulnar distribution of the hand.

SPECIAL TESTS   The patient tested negative for all clinical neurologic and electrodiagnostic testing.

? Questions

1. What is myofascial pain syndrome (MFP)?
2. What historical overview is necessary to an understanding of the development of MFP?
3. What is a trigger point?
4. What triggers a muscle to develop an active trigger point?
5. Is there a relationship between loss of range of motion and the presence of trigger points?
6. What is the cause of trigger points?
7. What is the relationship between the trigger point and the referred pain?
8. How are trigger points quantitatively measured?

221

9. What steps are involved in an MFP evaluation?

10. What palpation technique is employed when one is searching a length of muscle for trigger points?

11. What is the rationale for the referral of pain several segmental levels caudad or cephalad?

12. With MFP, is the precipitating injury chronic or acute?

13. What therapeutic intervention is appropriate in the treatment of MFP?

14. What is the spray and stretch treatment?

15. What is injection treatment, and is there a less invasive alternative in the treatment of MFP?

16. What forms of electrotherapy are appropriate in the treatment of MFP?

17. What connective-tissue techniques are appropriate in the treatment of MFP?

18. What is the ischemic-pressure technique in the treatment of MFP?

19. What cold modalities may be used in the treatment of MFP?

20. What role does static splinting play in the treatment of MFP?

21. What exercises are helpful in the treatment of MFP?

22. Describe a hypothetical treatment sequence for the injured fireman's hand.

1. What is myofascial pain syndrome (MFP)?

Myofascial pain (MFP) is defined as a local irritation mainly in muscle and possibly fascia, tendon, or ligament that exhibits local tenderness, specific pain patterns, and autonomic symptoms that are easily reproducible and specific to that tissue. Myofascial pain is essentially a single-muscle syndrome that may combine to form single myotome or dermatome patterns of involvement. Detection and management of this condition follow established parameters. Terms such as *trigger point, referred pain,* and *locus of pain* are concepts characteristic of MFP symptoms.

2. What historical overview is necessary to an understanding of the development of MFP?

Myofascial pain is not a new concept but is rather an evolving clarification that slowly emerged after a legacy of confusion regarding this disorder.

A confusing series of names has alternately been used in describing MFP and includes muscular rheumatism, nonarticular rheumatism, myalgia spots, idiopathic myalgia, fibrositis, rheumatic myalgia, and rheumatic myopathy. The nomenclature describing myofascial pain is understood in the historical context of the evolution of this condition. In the early twentieth century the term *muscular rheumatism* was commonly employed to describe generalized musculoskeletal pain of unknown cause. With time, this appellation was criticized as serving as a diagnostic scrap box for painful ailments that could not be otherwise classified. In response, Sir William Gowers, the English neurologist, in 1904 renamed this condition *fibrositis* and thus implied a proposed cause of inflammation of fibrous or connective tissue.[9]

Half a century and many scientific books and papers later, Janet Travell, M.D., began in 1952 to promote the terminology *myofascial pain* and *myofascial syndrome.* Travell was the first female physician for the White House, serving as President Kennedy's personal physician and friend. She treated Kennedy's trigger points in his back and prescribed his famous rocking chair as part of his treatment program.[24]

Notwithstanding, MFP continued to be a controversial topic and was considered to be a wastebasket term in need of redefinition. It was not until the 1986 Symposium on Fibrositis/Fibromyalgia debate that MFP came into its own with the understanding and clarification of clinical presentation and management.

3. What is a trigger point?

Central to an understanding of MFP is the idea of the trigger point. *Trigger points* are described as small hypersensitive areas in muscle, ligament, or fascia, which, when stimulated, give rise to referred pain.[25] This is a consistent feature of the trigger point. Trigger points are classified as either *latent or active.*

Latent trigger points evoke pain and tenderness in those same locales as active trigger points do, and they can be made to refer pain remotely by palpation. Additionally, latent trigger points may be present in individuals without a diagnosis of MFP and are differentiated from active trigger points by the following circumstance: When the individual is asked whether he or she has ever felt this pain at any time other than palpation of the given area, the answer is no; in other words, the latent trigger point is only painful when provoked.[17] Without perpetuating factors, an active trigger point tends to revert to and persist as a latent trigger point.[21]

An acute strain caused by sudden overload of muscle can produce an active trigger point that causes referred pain. Chronic repetitive strain of a muscle may also yield an active trigger point. If the demands of the muscle are reduced, the referred pain may spontaneously subside within several days or weeks. However, in the event that the provoking stimulus continues incessantly, an acute MFP syndrome may persist or even become chronic. With time, MFP may even propagate to other muscles within the same or nearby myotomes as secondary and satellite trigger points.[21]

Interestingly, studies have shown that up to 71% of trigger points have been found to have identical locations with acupuncture points.[16] This, however, could be coincidental, since there are some 1000 acupuncture points identified in the literature on that topic.[22]

4. What triggers a muscle to develop an active trigger point?

A variety of situations can incite a muscle to develop a trigger point. These include direct trauma, stress, overuse, fatigue, posture, stressful sleeping, and work postures. Two common findings characteristic of trigger points are (1) the local twitch response elicited by snapping palpation of the trigger point and (2) reproduction of the patient's pain by sustained pressure applied to that area.

5. Is there a relationship between loss of range of motion and the presence of trigger points?

The shoulder musculature frequently contains an abundance of trigger points, though the diagnosis is often mistaken as a bursitis or tendinitis. Typically, when the patient fails to respond to conventional treatment, he or she is told to simply "live with it." However, on closer examination the clinician will often discover a limitation of joint motion produced by adaptive or reflexive shortening of the structure containing the trigger point that crosses that joint.[2,18,23] Similarly the involved muscle may produce pain when stretched. For example, if the trigger point is found to be located in the substance of the infraspinatus muscle, the resultant limitation of motion will be at the glenohumeral joint in external rotation and horizontal abduction.[17]

6. What is the cause of trigger points?

Various attempts to explain the existence of trigger points in physiologic, anatomic, or neurophysiologic terms have proved frustrating. Proposed causes include inflammatory, anatomic, ischemic, neurophysiologic; altered autonomic nervous system; and connective tissue irritation. Interestingly, when viewed under the electron microscope, trigger points have a moth-eaten ragged appearance similar to that of overused muscle.[2]

Trigger points develop most commonly in antigravity muscles such as trapezius, the erector spinae, or gastrocnemius because of the unrelenting burden of contraction these muscles experience in the erect posture. For example, the trapezius, along with other muscles, bears the task of supporting the head in normal posture. This burden possibly taxes the ability of muscles to disburse concentrations of lactic acid, which aggregates at specific areas known as trigger points. Having developed trigger points, a muscle is more likely to become fatigued. Hence a vicious cycle is established in which continued contraction sustains and perhaps fortifies the cycle.

7. What is the relationship between the trigger point and the referred pain?

Trigger points often *refer* pain remotely but consistently to specific areas, such as the interosseous muscles of the hand. So consistent are these remote referrals of pain that mappings demonstrate a relationship that appears remarkably consistent with dermatome or myotome patterns[10] (Fig. 20-1).

Thus the *locus of pain* refers to the origin of pain resulting in remote and often distal, referral sites. This relationship between the trigger point and the reference area of pain emphasizes the following emergent principle of management: patients with MFP must be treated according to the locus of their pain and not necessarily the presentation site.

8. How are trigger points quantitatively measured?

The tissue compliance meter (TCM) is a hand-held instrument that, unlike other devices that measure the presence of trigger points, offers the advantage of being objective, since measurements are not dependent on a patient's reaction or cooperation. This device offers an immediate and simple reading of the depth of penetration of a rubber disk at a known pressure, the relation of which expresses tissue compliance. The TCM objectively documents compliance for trigger points, taut

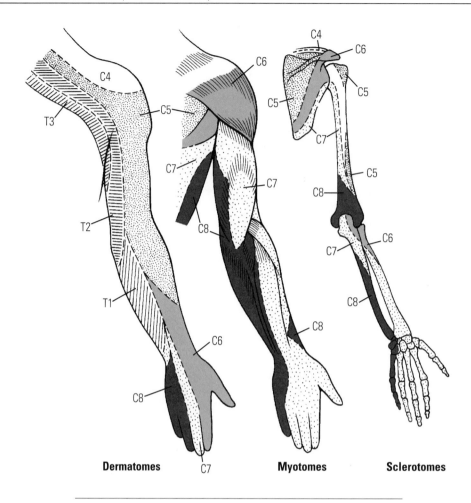

Dermatomes   **Myotomes**   **Sclerotomes**

FIG. 20-1 Dermatomes, myotomes, and sclerotomes of the upper extremity.

bands, scar tissue, fibrositic nodules, edema, and spasm and thus provides an early objective indication of either healing or resolution in the soft-tissue disorder.

The universal clinical dynamometer is a pocket-sized, hand-held device that is used in quantitative measurement of muscle strength. Thermography documents trigger points that appear as areas that are discoid. Thermography also measures the presence of muscle spasm.[6]

9. What steps are involved in an MFP evaluation?

Once all conventional pathologic conditions have been ruled out, the clinician explores the possibility of the myofascial component as the source of pain. MFP is a diagnosis of exclusion, and laboratory and imaging studies are helpful only to rule out other diseases. The MFP evaluation follows a sequence of gathering information regarding the patient's subjective complaints as well as objective measurements taken before one searches for the source of pain. Diagnosis is accomplished when one takes a history and a physical examination.

The patient's history may reveal a direct or indirect trauma precipitating the pain. The chief complaint may be local, referred, or both, and may be colored in by the patient on a body chart. The diagram is then reviewed with the patient, who goes over additional factors such as the date of onset, nature of the pain (that is, dull, sharp, or a deep ache), and precipitating factors. The patient may initially have a limitation in the range of motion, experience autonomic changes, and frequently complain of weakness and stiffness. Pain intensity is preferably recorded on an analog pain scale. If the patient complains of numbness, as many do, then

Semmes-Weinstein monofilaments and a vibrometer may be used.[17]

The "hands-on" portion of the evaluation commences with the clinician seeking a myofascial component in the form of positively identified trigger points that reproduce the patient's pain. Two findings that greatly help to make the diagnosis are the presence of exquisite spot tenderness at the trigger point and a palpable band of taut muscle fibers running through the trigger point. Once the source of pain is discovered, it is confirmed by pain on active contraction or passive stretching of the structure. It is important to note that palpation of the entire length of the identified muscle ought to be performed by the therapist. In the event that no source is found, an investigation of the muscles innervated by, at the very least, one spinal segment above or below should commence. A successful MFP evaluation cannot be limited to examining the muscles innervated by the same level of the pain presentation.

Remotely referred pain is most often perceived distally to the source of pain and is mapped out carefully with the therapist screening for a pattern following a dermatomal or myotomal distribution. However, Travell and Simons identified the following muscles in the upper quadrant that typically refer pain proximally: sternocleidomastoid, biceps brachii, the long head of triceps, supinator, brachioradialis, and adductor pollicis. Palpation continues so as to identify any pain elicited in muscles innervated by the same level of dermatome or myotome of the pain presentation.[17]

10. What palpation technique is employed when one is searching a length of muscle for trigger points?

Palpation of muscle for the presence of trigger points is similar to the palpation for tendinitis. The purpose of evaluation is twofold: (1) reproduction of pain and (2) tissue turgor.

The examiner applies firm pressure with the pulp of the thumb across the entire span of the muscle, from origin to insertion. The patient is asked to inform the therapist if he or she feels pain and, if so, whether the pain is his or her pain. At times the patient may literally jump and exclaim, "That is my pain," in what is known as a *positive jump sign.*[7]

Tissue turgor evaluation may be accomplished by the following two methods of palpation: (1) *Skin rolling* (Fig. 20-2) involves lifting the skin off the muscles, opposing the index finger and thumb, and then rolling the skin in all directions for the purpose of eliciting pain

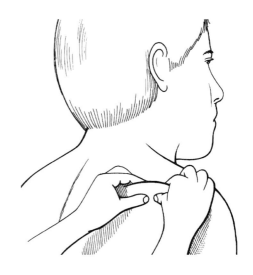

FIG. 20-2 Skin rolling is a connective tissue technique used for evaluation and treatment.

over the trigger point. (2) *Light palpation* is accomplished by use of the index finger pulp with the middle finger lying atop the index fingernail. This latter technique is employed to sense the depth of the trigger point as well as to detect for palpable bands, that is, rope-like structures lying parallel with the muscle fibers.[17] These palpable bands may undergo a local twitch response when the trigger point is stimulated with a snapping palpation.[11,21]

11. What is the rationale for the referral of pain several segmental levels caudad or cephalad?

The neuroanatomic pathway that can be traced from the trigger point to the spinal cord provides a possible rationale for referred pain several segments caudad or cephalad to the actual level of the culprit muscle. When noxious stimuli from trigger points are strong enough, action potentials will propagate along the axon to synapse in the spinal cord. The fibers bifurcate, with most remaining in the same spinal level but some spreading cephalocaudal in the lateral section of dorsal white matter, including Lissauer's tract. A spread of only two or three segments is believed to occur in man.[13]

12. With MFP, is the precipitating injury chronic or acute?

The precipitating injury inciting the onset of MFP may be either acute or chronic in nature,[21] and the patient's presentation may be quite diverse. This malady may occur in patients as diverse as a dental hygienist referred for treatment of a wrist tendinitis, to a middle aged man referred with a diagnosis of hand arthritis and who sustained a hyperextension wrist injury in an automobile accident 3 months earlier, or to a 24-year-old individual referred with a diagnosis of reflex sympathetic dystrophy after a closed forearm crush involving no fractures some 2½ years previously.

13. What therapeutic intervention is appropriate in the treatment of MFP?

Myofascial pain patients offer an exciting challenge to the clinician. The key to successfully treating the patient with MFP is to realize that simply treating the painful area will not correct the patient's condition. Physical therapy must be directed to the locus of the patient's pain. It is recommended that the therapist refer to dermatome and myotome charts and to *Travell's Trigger Point Manual*. One then solves the emerging clinical puzzle one piece at a time by palpating those muscles that have the potential for referring pain, given the clinical presentation. Therapy may be directed at more than one source when the evaluation includes all those muscles innervated by the same level as the myotome and dermatome of the pain presentation or several spinal levels above or below that level.

Treatments directed at the loci of pain include spray and stretch, phonophoresis and iontophoresis, heat modalities, electrotherapy, ultrasound, connective tissue technique, ischemic pressure technique, splinting, and exercise. Medical management may also include injection and dry needling. Selection of treatment is based on tissue response to given treatment (such as changes in trigger point irritability). If the treatment does not relieve the patient's pain, then reidentification of the pain locus or a change in the treatment technique is necessary. Treatment frequency is dependent on the patient's response, since resolution of the trigger point or movement of referred pain proximally is proof of a successful treatment.

Confirmation of treatment success is accomplished by the patient completing another body chart and the therapist comparing initial findings to subsequent findings. More conventional methods include quantitative passive and active range of motion exercises as well as muscle strength grading. Treatment in the chronic case of MFP must not be directed only toward alleviating the trigger point irritability but also toward strengthening the involved muscles so that joint balance and posture may be reestablished. Without these important factors being addressed, trigger point activation may recur.

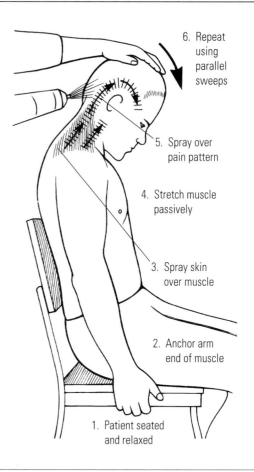

6. Repeat using parallel sweeps

5. Spray over pain pattern

4. Stretch muscle passively

3. Spray skin over muscle

2. Anchor arm end of muscle

1. Patient seated and relaxed

FIG. 20-3 Application scheme of use of vapor coolant spray followed by stretch of involved muscle. (Redrawn from Hunter JM, Schneider LH, Mackin EJ, Callahan AD, editors: *Rehabilitation of the hand: surgery and therapy*, ed 3, St. Louis, 1990, Mosby.)

14. What is the spray and stretch treatment?

Spray and stretch refers to the use of vapor coolant spray, typically Fluori-Methane, over the muscle's referred zone of pain. The spray is administered at least 18 inches away from the skin surface parallel to the involved muscle fibers (Fig. 20-3). The vapor coolant provides a barrage of cutaneous impulses over the irritated muscle and the referred zone that reflexively inhibits the muscle, thus permitting the therapist to stretch the muscle to its normal length.[17] The barrage of skin impulses block the pain impulses from the trigger point[8,25] within the muscle that would prevent stretching under normal circumstances. This is followed by application of a hot pack for 5 to 10 minutes and then active exercises.[17]

15. What is injection treatment, and is there a less invasive alternative in the treatment of MFP?

Trigger point injection with either procaine, xylocaine, or corticosteroid is a common treatment for trigger point pain in MFP. This treatment has proved to be effective in both acute and chronic cases of MFP.

Phonophoresis or *iontophoresis* may be used in the delivery of corticosteroids and analgesics in lieu of injection,[1,10,11] and are more comfortable for the patient. After iontophoresis, the trigger point may be massaged or receive heat to facilitate disbursement of the medication. Phonophoresis treatment interfaces well with ischemic pressure technique and interferential current.[17]

16. What forms of electrotherapy are appropriate in the treatment of MFP?

Several forms of *electrotherapy* have been advocated in the treatment of MFP and include high volt electrical stimulation, transcutaneous electrical stimulation (TENS), interferential current, and electroacupuncture.[12,14-16,19,20] Interferential current is applied by use of both channels so that channel crossing occurs at the trigger point; the mode may be *fixed or sweep*. With TENS, electrodes are sized appropriately when one is treating the trigger points (TrPs) of the small hand muscles. Use of a probe is also helpful in such cases. TENS electrodes ought to bracket the TrP so that stretching of the involved muscle may occur during treatment without irritating the TrP.[17]

17. What connective-tissue techniques are appropriate in the treatment of MFP?

Deep transverse friction technique introduced by Cyriax involves constant application of heavy pressure across the trigger point for the purpose of breaking up adhesions[4,5] (Fig. 20-4).

Skin rolling is a painful technique that involves release of fascia from underlying muscle or overlying skin. Employed by the therapist both during the evaluation (see Fig. 20-2) as well as during treatment, this technique is applied during the latter for approximately 5 or 10 minutes in chronic cases of MFP. Reassessment with palpation follows and identifies those trigger points that are still irritable, which may be treated with ultrasound or interferential current.

Knuckling (Fig. 20-5) is a soft-tissue stretching technique in which the therapist applies stress parallel to muscle fiber. This technique is appropriate with chronic cases where there is adaptive shortening of soft tissue, but it should not be used with the acute patient.

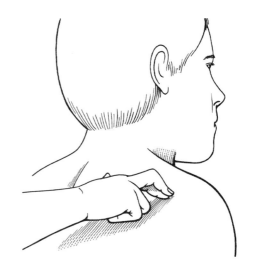

FIG. 20-4 Disruption of trigger point irritation by way of friction massage technique.

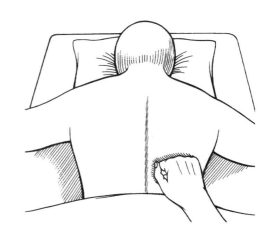

FIG. 20-5 Knuckling is performed parallel to the fibers of the restricted muscle.

During stretching, the therapist uses his or her knuckles to stress, hence stretch, the connective tissue enveloping the muscle fibers.[17]

18. What is the ischemic-pressure technique in the treatment of MFP?

Travell described an *ischemic-pressure technique* in which graded pressure over the trigger point is applied for up to 60 seconds to provide reflex inhibition of the trigger point.[25] The key to this technique is a gentle, graded pressure (Fig. 20-6). When pressure is applied,

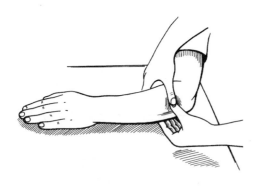

FIG. 20-6 Ischemic pressure technique involves slow and constant application of pressure for the disruption of trigger point irritation.

the patient will report a graded decrease and resolution of his or her pain during the 60-second interval. An increase of pressure is not applied until the patient feels a decrease in pain. This treatment may be used before TENS or ultrasound treatment.[17]

19. What cold modalities may be used in the treatment of MFP?

Cold modalities aside from the use of vapor coolant spray may aggravate the condition of MFP. The exception to this rule is the use of quick icing for pain relief and the maintenance of hard-won gains in the tissue length in the patient with the chronic disorder. Because these patients require vigorous soft-tissue techniques and multiple treatments, which can yield local erythema and swelling, the application of a plastic bag of slush ice and alcohol may be applied for 5 minutes with a paper towel interposed between the skin and the bag. Slush may be formed by the mixing of one part of alcohol with three parts of water. Longer application involves chilling to excess, which is a causative factor in MFP.[17]

20. What role does static splinting play in the treatment of MFP?

Splinting use is appropriate during the early stage of treatment when the movement of involved muscles reactivate the trigger point or points before that muscle regains full length and strength. Most commonly, the thumb (adductor pollicis muscle trigger point) and the wrist (wrist flexor and extensor muscle trigger points) are splinted until the trigger point is completely resolved. As the patient begins strengthening, the patient is gradually weaned from usage of the splint.

21. What exercises are helpful in the treatment of MFP?

In many cases the patient's posture at work or leisure provoked the onset of MFP. For example, the glenohumeral joint of the ipsilateral upper extremity is often positioned in a protracted posture. It is important to identify any such alternations in muscle imbalance and restore soft-tissue imbalance about joints by stretching contracted areas and strengthening overstretched muscle. Addressing muscular imbalances is imperative to the prevention of reactivation of trigger points.[17]

22. Describe a hypothetical treatment sequence for the injured fireman's hand.

The initial treatment was addressed toward scar remodeling and not MFP techniques because it was the scar adherence that was provoking the trigger points. Heat, scar massage, and wrist curls were performed while TENS bracketed the scar. The TENS served to dampen the effects of the trigger points during conventional treatment.

During the second visit the patient was able to tolerate an increase of the weight during wrist curls, using approximately 1 kg because of a significant decrease in the pain. An Otoform pad (Alimed, Deedham, Mass.) was fabricated for scar remodeling. Treatment visits 3 and 4 focused on ultrasound and friction massage to both trigger points, followed by ice.

On the sixth visit, TENS bracketed the trigger points while low-resistance work simulation was begun. For the subsequent eighth session, our patient continued to undergo an MFP regimen of friction massage, TENS, and ice while the magnitude of his work simulation was increased. By the twelfth session his trigger points had resolved and work hardening commenced for an additional six sessions. At the end of the work-hardening sequence he was discharged and returned to work full time.

REFERENCES

1. Antich T: Phonophoresis: the principles of the ultrasonic driving force and efficacy in treatment of common orthopaedic diagnoses, *J Orthop Sports Phys Ther* 4:99, 1982.
2. Bengtsson A, Hendriksson KG, Larsson J: Muscle biopsy in primary fibromyalgia: light microscope and histochemical findings, *Scand J Rheumatol* 15:1, 1986.
3. Bonica J: Management of myofascial pain syndromes in general practice, *JAMA* 164:732, 1957.
4. Chamberlain GJ: Cyriax's friction massage: a review, *J Orthop Sports Phys Ther* 4:16, 1982.

5. Cyriax J: *Textbook of orthopaedic medicine: diagnosis of soft tissue lesions,* vol 1, ed 6, Baltimore, 1975, Williams & Wilkins.

6. Fischer AA: Documentation of myofascial trigger points, *Arch Phys Med Rehabil* 69:286-291, 1988.

7. Good M: Objective diagnosis and curability of non-articular rheumatism, *Br J Phys Med* 14:1, 1951.

8. Gordon EE, Hass A: A surface analgesic in treatment of musculoskeletal affections, *Ind Med Surg* 28:217, 1959.

9. Gowers W: Lumbago: its lessons and analogies, *Br J Phys Med* 1:117, 1904.

10. Harris P: Iontophoresis: clinical research in musculoskeletal inflammatory conditions, *J Orthop Sports Phys Ther* 4:109, 1982.

11. Kraft G, Johnson E, Laban M: The fibrositis syndrome, *Arch Phys Med Rehabil* 49:155, 1968.

12. Kraus H: Trigger points and acupuncture, *Acupunct Electrother Res* 2:323, 1977.

13. Lamotte C: Distribution of the tract of Lissauer and the dorsal root fibers in the primate spinal cork, *J Comp Neur* 172:529, 1977.

14. Melzack R: Prolonged relief of pain by brief, intense transcutaneous somatic stimulation, *Pain* 1:357, 1975.

15. Melzack R: Myofascial trigger points: relation to acupuncture and mechanisms of pain, *Arch Phys Med Rehabil* 62:114, 1981.

16. Melzack R, Stillwell K, Fox E: Trigger points and acupuncture points for pain: correlations and implications, *Pain* 3:3, 1977.

17. Moran CA, Saunders SR, Tribuzi SM: Myofascial pain in the upper extremity. In Hunter JM, Schneider LH, Mackin EJ, et al, editors: *Rehabilitation of the hand: surgery and therapy,* ed 3, St Louis, 1990, Mosby.

18. Nielson AJ: Case study: myofascial pain of the posterior shoulder relieved by spray and stretch, *J Orthop Sports Phys Ther* 3:21, 1981.

19. Omura Y: Electro-acupuncture: its electrophysiological basis and criteria of effectiveness and safety, part 1, *Acupunct Electrother Res* 1:157, 1975.

20. Procacce P, Zoppi M, Maresca M: Transcutaneous electrical stimulation in low back pain: a critical evaluation, *Acupunct Electrother Res* 7:1, 1982.

21. Simons DG: Myofascial pain syndromes: Where are we? Where are we going? *Arch Phys Med Rehabil* 69:208, 1988.

22. Smith G, Covino B: *Acute pain,* Stoneham, Mass, 1985, Butterworth Publs.

23. Travell J, Rinzler SH: The myofascial genesis of pain, *Postgrad Med* 11:425, 1952.

24. Travell J: *Office hours day and night,* New York, 1968, World Publishing.

25. Travell J, Simons DG: *Myofascial pain and dysfunction of the trigger point manual,* Baltimore, 1983, Williams & Wilkins.

RECOMMENDED READING

Moran CA, Saunders SR, Tribuzi SM: Myofascial pain in the upper extremity. In Hunter JM, Schneider LH, Mackin EJ, et al, editors: *Rehabilitation of the hand: surgery and therapy,* ed 3, St Louis, 1990, Mosby.

Nielson AJ: Case study: myofascial pain of the posterior shoulder relieved by spray and stretch, *J Orthop Sports Phys Ther* 3:21, 1981.

Simons DG: Myofascial pain syndromes: Where are we? Where are we going? *Arch Phys Med Rehabil,* 69:208, 1988.

Travell J, Simons DG: *Myofascial pain and dysfunction of the trigger point manual,* Baltimore, 1983, Williams & Wilkins.

Wolfe F: Fibrositis, fibromyalgia, and musculoskeletal disease: The current status of the fibrositis syndrome, *Archives of Phys Med Rehabil,* 69:527-531, 1988.

21

Chronic and Generalized Aches, Pains, Stiffness at Three Anatomic Sites and Multiple Tender Points as Well as Insomnia and Headache of at Least 3 Months in Duration

A 45-year-old female assistant bank manager presents a prescription from her rheumatologist that reads: "Primary fibromyalgia syndrome—therapy as needed." The patient offers her hand and offers you a limp handshake. It is the winter season.

OBSERVATION The patient is a well-dressed, groomed, and slightly graying individual who conveys the impression of seriousness. She holds herself in a ramrod straight, military type of posture.

SUBJECTIVE The patient complains of a history of diffuse aching pain in her shoulders, hips, and low back lasting for 2 years. Recently, symptoms have become increasingly severe in the early morning and late afternoon. She reports sensitivity to bright lights and loud noises and confided that she was concerned about what she viewed as decreased work productivity, since the onset of her condition. She often wakes up after a night's sleep feeling unrefreshed and often experiences ill-defined headaches in the morning hours. She admits to not having taken a vacation for the past 4 years or taking time out to exercise or relax. She further complains of occasional vague numbness in her fingers, which she could not relate to any particular position or activity. As of late she finds that she needs to urinate quite frequently and has been experiencing a loose bowel more often as well. She does not drink, smoke, or bite her nails.

PALPATION The patient jumps and cries out during palpation over the upper trapezius and low back areas. There is no tenderness in any of her joints.

RANGE OF MOTION Grossly within functional limits.

STRENGTH Grossly within normal limits relative to her age.

FLEXIBILITY Gross tightness is observed in the upper back and shoulders as well as in the lower extremities (manifesting as tight hamstrings, quadriceps, and triceps surae muscle groups).

SENSATION Normal to light touch and pinprick in both upper extremities.

? Questions

1. What is primary fibromyalgia syndrome (PFS)?
2. What is the clinical presentation of PFS?
3. What is the cause of PFS?
4. What are the most common sites of tenderness?
5. What is the differential diagnosis of fibromyalgia?

6. What is the difference between myofascial pain and fibromyalgia (fibrositis)?
7. What therapeutic intervention is appropriate for PFS?

1. What is primary fibromyalgia syndrome (PFS)?

Fibromyalgia is a nonarticular rheumatic disorder that affects approximately 6 million Americans.[5] Of the many forms of nonarticular rheumatic disorders, fibromyalgia is specific to the fibrous white connective tissue[1] components of muscle, tendons, ligaments, and other "white" connective tissue in the large muscles of the shoulders, back, and hips; hence, an appropriate synonym for fibromyalgia is *muscular rheumatism*.[1,3] Women constitute 70% to 90% of all afflicted patients, and the most common age of diagnosis is between 35 and 55 years;[2,8,10] this condition, however, does occur among juveniles and the elderly.[9] Fibromyalgia may be the same disorder as chronic fatigue syndrome, though the etiologic role the Epstein-Barr virus has not been established with either disorder.[5] The term "fibrositis" has historically been associated with fibromyalgia but is actually a misnomer, since no inflammation is present with PFS. Moreover, fibrositis has been also used to describe myofascial pain, and so, because fibrositis means different things to different people, it has been appropriately suggested that this term be abandoned.[1,9]

2. What is the clinical presentation of PFS?

The clinical presentation of PFS includes pain that is widely[4] and even vaguely distributed, an amplified sensation (such as hypersensitivity of pain, weather, cold, humidity,[9] bright lights, and loud noises; stiffness; generalized fatigue or tiredness and exhaustion; and disturbed or nonrestorative sleep). Patients often wake up unrefreshed and more exhausted than the night before with chronic and diffuse headaches, irritable bowel, subjective swelling or numbness, urinary frequency caused by an enhanced perception of bladder fullness,[4] and paresthesia such as numbness that is ill defined over variable areas, implying neurologic disease; however, confirmation of objective neurologic findings in the latter complaint are absent.[5]

Some patients have significant anxiety and stress,[9] are typically hard driving, and are demanding both of themselves and of others. Patients may be emotionally trying but are often very effective at work because of their dedication. Patients may dislike alcohol, drugs, or other emotional or psychologic crutches.[4]

During the examination patients with PFS may give the impression that they are not making a full effort. During palpation, tenderness is not simply reported but may be demonstrated by dramatic twisting leaps. Grip strength (which may be evaluated by shaking the patient's hands) is reduced and poorly sustained. The evaluative encounter is often exhausting for the examiner and the patient and is indicative of the interactive stresses generated between such patients and others.[4]

3. What is the cause of PFS?

The cause of PFS as a system complex is unknown because there is no specific histologic abnormality suggestive of cellular inflammation.[1] Psychologic factors are present in one fourth of all patients. Interestingly the EEG wave patterns during non-rapid eye movement sleep in patients with fibromyalgia are quite similar to non-REM wave patterns of healthy individuals during delta-wave sleep deprivation.[2]

Primary fibromyalgia syndrome may be induced or intensified by physical or mental stress, poor sleep, trauma, or exposure to dampness and cold. A viral infection or toxemia from bacterial infection may also precipitate this syndrome in an otherwise predisposed host.[1] Symptoms may also be exacerbated by emotional stress or by the clinician who does not give proper credence to the patient's concerns and discharges the matter as being "all in your head."

An association between PFS and primary dysmenorrhea, as well as Raynaud's phenomenon, has been established.[9] There may be a constitutional predisposition to this condition.[9]

4. What are the most common sites of tenderness?

Tender points are largely unknown to patients and often not even central to their areas of pain.[4] Areas of point tenderness (Fig. 21-1) include:

- The upper scapular area, particularly the midpoint of the upper trapezius.
- The middle or lower part of the sternocleidomastoid muscle.
- The lateral portion of the pectoralis major muscle, or the second costochondral junction.
- The midsubstance of the supraspinatus muscle located in the suprascapular fossa.
- The middle to upper and outer quadrant of the buttock at the iliac crest.
- Just distal to the medial or lateral epicondyles of the elbow.
- The medial fat pad at the knee.
- Just posterior to the hip trochanters.[9]

5. What is the differential diagnosis of fibromyalgia?

Fibromyalgia is characterized by chronic generalized aches, pains, and stiffness involving at least three anatomic sites as well as multiple tender points at characteristic locations; persistence of these criteria for at least 3 months must occur, without any other underlying cause or disease to account for pain, before a diagnosis of PFS is confirmed.[5] Additionally, three of the 10 minor criteria must also be met, including variation of symptoms according to weather, physical activities, aggravation of symptoms by stress or anxiety, general fatigue, poor sleep, chronic headache, subjective swelling and numbness, and irritable bowel syndrome.[6]

Whereas PFS specifically refers to signs and symptoms not caused by any underlying disease,[9] secondary fibromyalgia may result from hypothyroidism, polymyalgia rheumatica,[9] systemic lupus erythematosus,[1] early

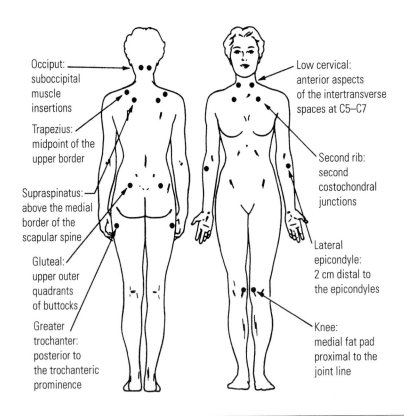

Occiput: suboccipital muscle insertions

Trapezius: midpoint of the upper border

Supraspinatus: above the medial border of the scapular spine

Gluteal: upper outer quadrants of buttocks

Greater trochanter: posterior to the trochanteric prominence

Low cervical: anterior aspects of the intertransverse spaces at C5–C7

Second rib: second costochondral junctions

Lateral epicondyle: 2 cm distal to the epicondyles

Knee: medial fat pad proximal to the joint line

FIG. 21-1 Location of 14 typical sites of deep tenderness in fibromyalgia. (From the Bulletin on the rheumatic diseases, located in Rodan GP, Schumacher HR: *Primer on rheumatic diseases,* ed 8, Atlanta, 1983, The Arthritis Foundation.)

onset of rheumatoid arthritis,[1] depression, anemia, and myopathy.

6. What is the difference between myofascial pain and fibromyalgia (fibrositis)?

Although there appears to be a blurred distinction between the somewhat similar sounding names of myofascial pain and primary fibromyalgia syndrome (PFS), it is erroneous to equate these two conditions. It is essential that practitioners recognize and understand the clear distinction between the two maladies. A lack of differentiation between these two conditions greatly influences the choice of management and thus makes an enormous difference to the patient.

The similarities of PFS and myofascial pain syndrome (MPS) include muscle pain, muscle tenderness on palpation, and the fact that both are very common maladies. However, with MPS, pain may be acute or chronic; there is a referred pain pattern specific to each involved muscle; nonmusculoskeletal symptoms are unusual; myofascial trigger points (TrPs) are found only in muscle, and radiate pain remotely, that is, beyond the site of palpation to a referred zone of pain, whereas the number of trigger points may be confined to one or more; muscles containing trigger points frequently contain taut bands; the twitch response of culprit muscle is present; the psychologic status of patient is usually not a factor; and poor sleep may result from the pain.[9]

On the other hand, the clinical presentation of PFS includes pain that is chronic; there is diffuse pain involving many muscles, ligaments, or bones; nonmusculoskeletal symptoms are common; fibromyalgic tender points (TePs) are found in muscle and other sites such as tendon insertions, fat pads, and bony prominences; TePs do not refer pain remotely on application of pressure; the presence of twitch response taut bands are unusual; TePs are usually more than four within some 14 specified sites; disturbed sleep is a factor in most cases; and psychologic factors are important in about 25% of patients.[9]

There is, however, some speculation as to whether myofascial pain and primary fibromyalgia syndrome are two separate disease entities or somewhat related pathologic conditions. This uncertainty is prompted by the clinical encounter of patients who occasionally present a confusing array of signs and symptoms from both conditions. One cannot help but wonder whether these two conditions are actually related along a range of a similar disease process seen from different points of view. Resolution of this question remains to be discovered.[7]

7. What therapeutic intervention is appropriate for PFS?

Since many patients suffering from PFS are sedentary, symptoms of this malady are frequently relieved by a major effort at physical reconditioning. The following activities and modalities have been found therapeutically beneficial toward relief of the symptoms of PFS: local heat, stretching exercises, strengthening exercises, massage, relaxation techniques, restful sleep, nonsteroidal antiinflammatory medication, moderate activity, warm, dry weather, posture instruction and exercises, swimming exercises, aerobic prescription of exercise, and a low dosage of tricyclic agents at bedtime to promote deeper sleep.[1,5] Patients should be reassured that they do not have a dangerous, life-threatening illness and PFS does not cause degenerative or deforming illness.[19] The prognosis for PFS is favorable with a comprehensive and supportive program.

REFERENCES

1. Berkow R: *The Merck manual of diagnosis and therapy,* Rahway, NJ, 1987, Merck, Sharp & Dohme Research Laboratories.
2. Moldofsky H, Scarisbrick P, England R, et al: Musculoskeletal symptoms of non-REM sleep disturbance in patients with "fibrositis syndrome" and healthy subjects, *Psychosom Med* 37:341-351, 1975.
3. Netter F: *The CIBA collection of medical illustrations, vol 8: Musculoskeletal system,* part 2, Summit, NJ, 1990, CIBA-Geigy.
4. Rodan GP, Schumacher HR: *Primer on rheumatic diseases,* ed 8, Atlanta, 1983, The Arthritis Foundation.
5. Schumacher HR, Bomalski JS: *Case studies in rheumatology for the house officer,* Baltimore, 1990, Williams & Wilkins.
6. Simons DG: Myofascial pain syndromes: Where are we? Where are we going? *Arch Phys Med Rehabil* 69:209, 1988.
7. Skootsky S: Incidence of myofacial pain in an internal medical group practice. Presented to the American Pain Society, Washington, D.C., Nov 6-9, 1986.
8. Wolfe F, Hawly DJ, Cathey MA, et al: Fibrositis: symptom frequency and criteria for diagnosis: evaluation of 291 rheumatic disease patients and 58 normal individuals, *J Rheumatol* 12:1159-1163, 1985.
9. Yunus MB, Kalyan-Raman UP, Kalyan-Raman K: Primary fibromyalgia syndrome and myofascial pain syndrome: clinical features and muscle pathology, *Arch Phys Med Rehabil* 69:451-454, 1988.
10. Yunus MB, Masi AT, Calabro JJ, et al: Primary fibromyalgia (fibrositis): clinical study of 50 patients with matched normal controls, *Semin Arthritis Rheum* 11:151-171, 1981.

RECOMMENDED READING

Goldenberg DL: Fibromyalgia syndrome: an emerging but controversial condition, *JAMA* 257:2782-2787, 1987.

Simons DG: Myofascial pain syndromes: Where are we? Where are we going? *Arch Phys Med Rehabil* 69:209, 1988.

Smythe HA: Fibrositis syndrome. In Conn HF, editor: *Current therapy,* ed 27, Philadelphia, 1975, Saunders.

Starlanye D, Copeland ME: *Fibromyalgia and chronic myofascial pain syndrome: a survival manual,* Oakland, Calif, 1996, New Harbringer Publications.

Yunus MB, Kalyan-Raman UP, Kalyan-Raman K: Primary fibromyalgia syndrome and myofascial pain syndrome: clinical features and muscle pathology, *Arch Phys Med Rehabil* 69:451-454, 1988.

22

Neonate Presenting with Leftward Head Tilt and Rightward Facial Flattening

Your clinic receives overflow from the local managed care center and in walks a mother with her infant, presenting a prescription that states "WRYNECK - therapy: TIW for 9 weeks." The baby is male, 7 weeks old, and presents with a slight rightward head tilt and slight leftward facial flattening. There is a history of breech presentation and an initial Apgar score of 8 and then 9, minutes later.

OBSERVATION   Both femurs and tibiae appear to be of equal length when viewed from above as well as from the side.

PALPATION   There is a firm fusiform swelling in the distal aspect of the right sternocleidomastoid muscle.

RANGE OF MOTION   Rightward neck rotation is limited, as is leftward neck tilt. Bilateral hip motion demonstrates greater than 60° of abduction.

MUSCLE STRENGTH   Head extension while in prone position to approximately 30°.

SPECIAL TESTS   Negative Barlow's and Ortoloni's signs. There is no measurable leg-length discrepancy.

CLUE:

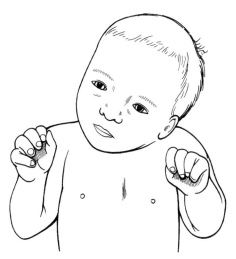

? Questions

1. What is wryneck?
2. What anatomy is prerequisite to understanding this disorder?
3. What are the kinesiologic characteristics of the interesting sternocleidomastoid (sternomastoid) muscle?
4. What is the evolution of this disorder, and what is the clinical presentation?
5. What are the cause and pathologic features of this condition?
6. What are associated conditions, if any?
7. What is the differential diagnosis?
8. What acute conditions may be confused with congenital muscular torticollis?
9. What osseous lesions are to be ruled out?
10. What inflammatory disorders are to be ruled out?
11. What neurologic disorders are to be ruled out?
12. What is ocular torticollis?
13. What trauma may result in torticollis?
14. What miscellaneous disorders may be confused with congenital muscular torticollis?
15. What cosmetic deformities of the face and skull may result in the untreated condition of this disorder?
16. What therapeutic intervention is appropriate in the treatment of this condition?
17. What are the criteria for operative management?
18. What therapeutic intervention is appropriate after surgery?

1. What is wryneck?

Wryneck deformity, in this child, is classified as *congenital* or *infantile muscular torticollis.* Wryneck is actually a composite of both *torticollis* and *anterocollis*[1] and is immortalized in the statue of Alexander the Great located in the British Museum, without, however, the accompanying facial distortion.[3] The former designation derives from two Latin words, that is, *tortus,* which means "twisted", and *collum,* meaning the "neck"; in effect, *rotation.* Anterocollis refers to the tilt component of this disfigurement. This condition is relatively common, since the incidence of the pathologic condition ranges from 0.3% to 0.5% of the general population.[6] Contracture typically occurs on the right side.[2]

2. What anatomy is prerequisite to understanding this disorder?

The *sternocleidomastoid (sternomastoid) muscle* is composed of two major divisions known as the sternal and clavicular heads, each of which has its own subdivisions. Although each division possesses a separate head of origin distally, all subdivisions merge to insert proximally as a composite head (Fig. 22-1). The proper or full name of this interesting muscle, that is, the sternocleidomastoid, bespeaks the two distal origins of that muscle, namely, the sternum and the clavicle, as well as the proximal insertion located at the tip of the mastoid process. The main motor supply is from the spinal accessory nerve, which itself is composed of the vagus nerve and segments of the upper five cervical nerves.

3. What are the kinesiologic characteristics of the interesting sternocleidomastoid (sternomastoid) muscle?

Contraction of one side of the sternomastoid turns the head to the opposite side; this is equivalent to saying that turning one's head to the right is accomplished by contraction of the left sternomastoid muscle. Simultaneous contraction of both muscles extends the head on the neck. In both instances, this superficial muscle boldly stands out, clearly defining the neck's contour. Unilateral sternomastoid contraction is opposed by contralateral trapezius activity, so that rightward head turning is opposed by the left trapezius. If both muscles contract, the face and head will extend on the cervical spine. Sternocleidomastoid secondarily aids respiration by virtue of elevating the thoracic cage.

4. What is the evolution of this disorder, and what is the clinical presentation?

Although minimal at birth, wryneck deformity is usually discovered in the first 6 to 8 weeks of life[4] as a unilateral, firm, nontender, and enlarging swelling, eventually reaching the size of the distal phalanx of the adult thumb. The site of this mass is just beneath the skin and is attached to or embedded within the

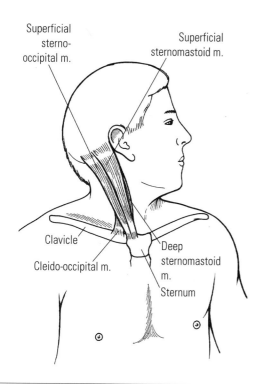

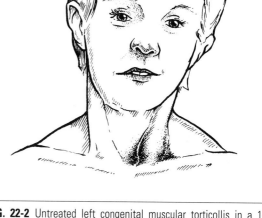

FIG. 22-1 External view of right sternocleidomastoid muscle. Unilateral contraction of this muscle permits ipsilateral lateral cervical flexion and contralateral head rotation. Bilateral sternomastoid contraction permits neck flexion. (Redrawn from Rockwood CA, Matsen FA, editors: *The shoulder*, vol 2, ed 2, Philadelphia, 1990, Saunders.)

FIG. 22-2 Untreated left congenital muscular torticollis in a 14-year-old boy. Notice the asymmetry of the face. On the affected side the face is shortened from above downwards. The levels of the eyes and ears are asymmetrical. (From Dandy DJ: *Essential orthopaedics and trauma*, Edinburgh, 1989, Churchill Livingstone.)

body of the sternomastoid muscle.[2] This mass attains maximum size within the first month of life and then gradually regresses over a subsequent period of 6 to 12 weeks.[2]

The temporary growth and regression of this mass interferes with unilateral longitudinal muscular growth, thus leaving in its wake an imbalance between the neck's two sternomastoid muscles. Contracture follows and is accompanied by head tilt toward the affected side with rotation of the chin contralaterally (Fig. 22-2). As a result, rotation of the neck to the side of the deformity is limited, as is lateral tilt to the opposite side. If untreated, craniofacial disfigurement will ensue during the first year.[2]

5. What are the cause and pathologic features of this condition?

The pathologic characteristic of this condition is simply the replacement of muscle with fibrous tissue. The exact cause of fibrosis is unknown. A multifactorial theory is postulated attributing the fibrotic mass to ischemia of the sternomastoid muscle,[6] particularly the sternal head, because of intrauterine malposition or increased pressure otherwise resulting during passage through the birth canal.[2]

6. What are associated conditions, if any?

As many as 20%[2] of all infants who have congenital muscular torticollis also have congenital dysplasia, that is, dislocation of one or both hips.[4] As such, a high index of suspicion is appropriate to justify clinical examination for hip dislocation.[6] Additionally the hips of suspected infants must therefore be imaged by ultrasound or a single anteroposterior pelvic radiograph even if the clinical exam is normal (Fig. 22-3). Bear in mind that the radiograph is not a reliable image until 10 weeks when the hip has completely ossified.[5] The aforementioned epidemiology supports the hypothesis that both wryneck and hip dysplasia are related to intrauterine malposition or presentation.[5]

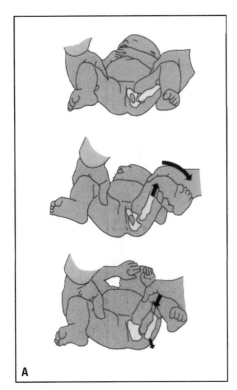
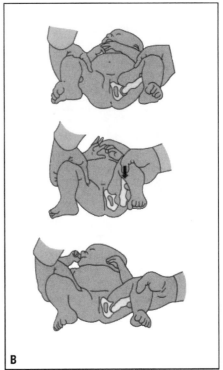

FIG. 22-3 A, Barlow's sign. Hip instability is demonstrated when one attempts to gently displace the hip out of the socket over the posterior acetabular rim. **B,** Ortolani's sign. The hip is first adducted and the thigh is depressed to subluxate or dislocate the hip. The thigh is then abducted. The reduction of the displaced hip causes a palpable "cluck" as the femoral head reenters the socket. (From Staheli LT: *Fundamentals of pediatric orthopedics,* New York, 1993, Raven Press.)

7. What is the differential diagnosis?

The differential diagnoses of congenital muscular torticollis may be divided into seven categories: acute torticollis, osseous causes, inflammatory causes, neurologic disorders, ocular torticollis, trauma, and miscellaneous.

8. What acute conditions may be confused with congenital muscular torticollis?

Acute calcification of the intervertebral cervical disk of unknown cause that produces neck pain and spasm often results in torticollis postures. This rare and idiopathic condition[5] most commonly involves the C6-C7 disk space. Calcification occurs only after an abrupt onset of symptoms that include fever (in about one fourth of all patients),[2] neck pain and stiffness, and torticollis. Management includes rest, use of a cervical collar, and nonsteroidal antiinflammatory medication.[5] Two thirds

of afflicted children are symptom free within 3 weeks of onset, whereas others may require up to 6 months.[2]

Acute rotary displacement of the atlantoaxial joint, either from acute rotational injury or from upper respiratory infection[2] (such as acute pharyngitis), may cause fixed head tilt. In this case there is a characteristic radiographic appearance of the dens in relation to the lateral masses. Both these conditions occur in the older child and are very rare in the infant.

9. What osseous lesions are to be ruled out?

Every patient should have radiographs of the cervical site to exclude congenital bony anomalies. *Osseous lesions* manifest in two types:

Hemivertebra in the cervical spine is confirmed by radiographs and is technically defined as a pure lateral tilt without a rotary component. Essentially a lateral

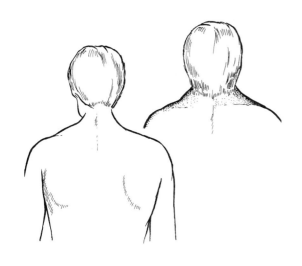

FIG. 22-4 Klippel-Feil syndrome. A short webbed neck with a low hairline. (From Dandy DJ: *Essential orthopaedics and trauma,* Edinburgh, 1989, Churchill Livingstone.)

kink in the spine, a hemivertebra causes compensatory scoliosis above and below, which may cause root irritation and strain the small joints of the spine. When occurring in the cervical region of the spine, the caudal compensation may manifest as torticollis.

Klippel-Feil syndrome is an uncorrectable bony neck malformation attributable to congenital fusion of two or more cervical vertebrae.[2] The characteristic appearance in severe cases is that of a short, broad, "webbed" neck, low posterior hairline, thoracic kyphosis deformity, and gross restriction of motion[5] (Fig. 22-4). Because of natural cervical fusions, motion is often concentrated at one or more levels and is frequently associated with instability, thus placing the cervical cord at risk for injury. For this reason, children with this syndrome should not participate in activities such as diving, contact sports, gymnastics, or use of the trampoline. Renal ultrasound is essential to rule out internal congenital defects. Despite its being unsightly, the concomitant deformity is not amenable to correction.[5]

10. What inflammatory disorders are to be ruled out?

INFLAMMATORY CAUSES

- *Cervical pharyngitis.* A major cause of torticollis in older children is *bacterial or viral pharyngitis* of the cervical nodes. Children typically between 5 and 10 years of age may suddenly develop a painless, stiff, and torticollis neck after a sore throat. Resisted neck

movements may be slightly painful but are not weak. This condition most probably results from a swollen gland lying under and therefore irritating the sternomastoid muscle; resolution is approximately within 2 weeks from onset.

- *Juvenile rheumatoid arthritis,* causing erosion of the waist of the dens in those patients with systemic or polyarticular onset during the first 1 or 2 years after onset; this predisposes the odontoid to becoming more susceptible to fracture and displacement.

- *Cervical adenitis,* caused by retrophalangeal or tonsil infection that often appears as a conspicuous unilateral upper palate bulge on the same side as the torticollis.

- Tuberculosis

11. What neurologic disorders are to be ruled out?

NEUROLOGIC CAUSES

- *Paroxysmal torticollis* is seen in infants 2 to 8 months of age and manifests as recurrent attacks of head tilt lasting from a few hours to a few days. This occurs as a result of a variety of neurologic causes including drug intoxication.[2]

- *Dystonia musculorum deformans* is a rare progressive syndrome usually beginning in childhood and is characterized by dystonic movements that result in sustained and often bizarre postures. Symptoms usually begin with torticollis, or inversion and plantar flexion of the foot while walking. Two hereditary patterns are described for this condition: autosomal dominant in families of northern European extraction and recessive in some Ashkenazi Jewish families. In advanced stages the body may become twisted "like a pretzel." Mentation is usually preserved, and treatment is usually unsatisfactory.

- *Cerebellar tumors* may result in torticollis, though onset is gradual; other peripheral neurologic signs are usually present.

- *Cervical spinal cord tumor*

- *Syringomyelia*

12. What is ocular torticollis?

Ocular torticollis, such as *rotary strabismus,* is usually the result of an imbalance of either the superior or inferior oblique eye muscles, or occurring after fourth cranial nerve dysfunction. Torticollis does not begin to manifest until 4 to 6 months of age, that is, when the infant begins to focus on objects. This form differs from muscular torticollis in two ways: (1) there is full neck range of motion, and (2) with muscular torticollis the face is turned *away* from the side of the head tilt and angled upwards, whereas with the ocular type the face is slightly turned *toward* the side of the head tilt.[6]

13. What trauma may result in torticollis?

Torticollis commonly occurs after an injury to the C1-C2 articulation, or fracture or dislocation of the dens (C2). Similarly, children with Down's syndrome, Morquio's syndrome, skeletal dysplasia, and spondylo-epiphyseal dysplasia commonly suffer from C1-C2 instability and accompanying torticollis.[2]

14. What miscellaneous disorders may be confused with congenital muscular torticollis?

- *Sandifer's syndrome* is sudden posturing of the neck and trunk because of esophagitis caused by gastroesophageal reflux with or without hiatal hernia that may not always be accompanied by vomiting. Abnormal posturing is believed to be attributable to the discomfort felt by reflux.
- *Fibrodysplasia ossificans progressiva* is enlargement of the sternocleidomastoid and other neck muscles that is accompanied by areas of soft-tissue calcification in the cervical musculature.
- *Surgery of the upper pharynx*, such as *tonsillectomy*, may result in inflammation and local edema, which in turn causes local ligamentous laxity; as a result of this, a greater motion of C1 on C2 than normal is allowed and may precipitate rotary subluxation.[2]

15. What cosmetic deformities of the face and skull may result in the untreated condition of this disorder?

Muscle contracture prevents bilateral even longitudinal muscle growth and therefore, as the spine grows, the involved muscle and soft tissue fail to keep pace and their relative shortness is reinforced.[6] If the contracture is left untreated, secondary deformities of the face and skull (plagiocephaly) can develop in the first year. Flattening of the face or back of the head occurs as a function of the sleeping posture[2] while one is afflicted with this condition. Children who sleep prone will be more comfortable with the affected side down; ergo, that ipsilateral side of the face becomes distorted. In children who sleep supine, reverse modeling of the contralateral posterior skull may occur.

If the condition continues to remain untreated during the years of skeletal growth, considerable cosmetic deformity will commence. The relative levels of the eyes and ears change but may be compensated for and made less noticeable when the head is slightly tilted to one side but made more obvious when the head and neck are straight in midline. Eye strain may result from an ocular imbalance, whereas a lower cervical–upper dorsal scoliosis with concavity toward the affected side may develop. As growth proceeds, the soft tissue on the affected side, including the scalenus anterior and scalenus medius muscles, and the carotid vessel and adjacent soft tissue undergo adaptive shortening. Thick, fibrotic, and tendon-like bands eventually replace the sternomastoid muscle, which, along with the thickened and contracted deep cervical fascia, make the head appear to be tethered to the clavicle.[2]

16. What therapeutic intervention is appropriate in the treatment of this condition?

Eighty-five to ninety percent of patients yield good results after conservative intervention of range-of-motion and stretching exercises.[2] Intensive[4] therapy is essential and ought to begin as soon as possible for a duration of at least 1 year.[1] From a practical standpoint, however, it is very difficult to perform adequate stretching on an infant more than six months of age because of resistance. Because of this, aggressive yet gentle stretching is appropriately initiated early on and continued for as long as the child will tolerate it or until the condition resolves.

- Give gentle, nonsudden, slow, and passive stretching of contracted muscle and related soft tissue, such as tilting of the head so that the higher ear approximates or touches its adjacent shoulder. This is followed by rotation of the head so that the chin approaches or touches the shoulder on the side of the affected muscle (Fig. 22-5).
- When adequate stretching has been obtained with head in neutral, these maneuvers should be repeated with the head in hyperextension, while countertraction is applied when the ipsilateral shoulder and chest are held. Gravity assists when the infant is positioned supine in the mother's lap with the head lolling in hyperextension.
- Conscientiously stretch at least 3 or 4 times per day for 10 times per session and hold the involved muscle in the stretched position for a count of 10 seconds.
- Position the crib so that the infant's affected side is to the wall, so that he or she will rotate his head toward the uninvolved side when his attention is distracted. The infant will then actively stretch the involved soft tissue when reaching and grasping for toys.
- Massage[1] to the contracted sternomastoid muscle while taking care to avoid the area over the carotid artery.

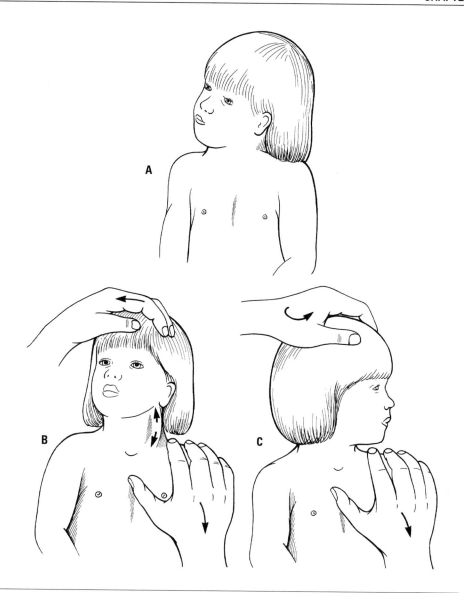

FIG. 22-5 Sequence of passive stretching exercises to the contracted left sternomastoid muscle in congenital muscular torticollis.

- Teach appropriate range-of-motion and stretching techniques to parents, while stressing the need for consistent adherence to the treatment regimen. Parents must be cautioned not to use excessive force or speed in their desire to "get better quicker."

17. What are the criteria for operative management?

In those children who go untreated during the early months of life, the developing deformity becomes progressively resistant to stretching.[4] Established facial asymmetry and limitation of normal motion beyond 30° usually precludes a good result. In this patient population and approximately 10% to 15% of cases resistant to conservative treatment, surgical release of the contracted muscle is appropriate. Removal of the mass in early infancy is inappropriate.

18. What therapeutic intervention is appropriate after surgery?

A postoperative therapeutic regimen includes passive stretching exercises of the same kind performed preoperatively and should begin as soon as the patient can tolerate handling of the neck. The patient, with time, is eventually progressed to active exercises. The surgeon may prescribe a head cast, brace, or helmet to position the head in an overcorrected position for 6 weeks after surgery.[5]

REFERENCES

1. Berkow R: *The Merck manual of diagnosis and therapy,* ed 15, Rahway, NJ, 1987, Merck, Sharp & Dohme Research Laboratories.
2. Netter FH: The *CIBA collection of medical illustrations: vol 8: Musculoskeletal system,* part 2, Summit, NJ, 1990, CIBA-Geigy.
3. Pineyro JR, Yoel J, Rocco M: Congenital torticollis, *J Int Coll Surg* 34:495-505, 1960.
4. Salter RB: *Textbook of disorders and injuries of the musculoskeletal system,* ed 2, Baltimore, 1983, Williams & Wilkins.
5. Staheli LT: *Fundamentals of pediatric orthopedics,* New York, 1992, Raven Press.
6. Wilkins KE: Special problems with the child's shoulder. In Rockwood CA, Matsen FA, editors: *The shoulder,* vol 2, Philadelphia, 1990, WB Saunders.

RECOMMENDED READING

Staheli LT: *Fundamentals of pediatric orthopedics,* New York, 1992, Raven Press.
Wilkins KE: Special problems with the child's shoulder. In Rockwood CA, Matsen FA, editors: *The shoulder,* vol 2, Philadelphia, 1990, WB Saunders.

PART V

NERVE AND MUSCLE LESIONS

23

Acute Hemiparalysis of All Facial Muscles after Cold Exposure

A 32-year-old female participated in a human rights protest during a cold evening that brought on the first frost of the winter season. A candlelight vigil was held until the wee hours of the morning during which the wind intensified the cold. She wore no scarf or ear-muffs. At dawn she went home to sleep for 5 hours and woke up with a pain in her left cheek. Upon looking in the mirror she was horrified to view her face grossly misshapen on one side. She immediately went to the emergency room at the local hospital. The neurologist on staff diagnosed her as having Bell's palsy and referred her to therapy. When asked, the patient admits to waking up in the morning and finding her pillow wet from saliva having drooled out of the left side of her mouth during sleep. Obvious facial asymmetry is observed, and the ipsilateral forehead appears flattened and lacking normal skin creases. Muscle testing revealed less than fair strength in the following muscles: occipitofrontalis, frontalis, orbicularis oculi, zygomaticus major, corrugator, buccinator, mentalis, and platysma. Sensory testing revealed loss of sweet and salty taste in the anterior two thirds of the tongue. There is a positive Bell's sign.

CLUE:

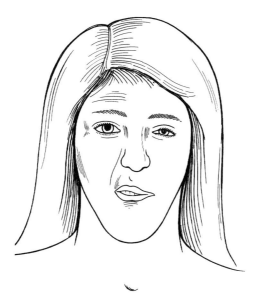

? Questions

1. What is acute idiopathic facial palsy?
2. What relevant microbiology is appropriate to an understanding of the herpes simplex virus?
3. What method of entry do viruses employ when entering the human nervous system?
4. Is there a relationship between the acute onset of Bell's palsy and exposure to cold?
5. What are the signs and symptoms at clinical presentation?
6. What is the anatomy of the facial nerve?
7. What is the topographic paradigm in understanding facial palsy?
8. How does a lesion at the internal auditory meatus manifest?
9. How does a lesion proximal to the geniculate ganglion manifest?
10. How does a lesion of the geniculate ganglion manifest?
11. What is the manifestation of a high facial canal lesion?
12. What is the function of the stapedius muscle?
13. What is the manifestation of a more distal facial canal lesion?
14. What is the manifestation of a lesion at the stylomastoid foramen?
15. How does facial palsy of the upper motor neuron type differ from Bell's palsy, which is of the lower motor neuron type?
16. What is the corneal blink test?
17. What is the differential diagnosis?
18. What is the prognosis for recovery?
19. What is the medical management of Bell's palsy?
20. What is the traditional therapeutic management of Bell's palsy?
21. Why are nonspecific gross facial exercises inadequate to the management repertoire of Bell's palsy?
22. What are the psychologic ramifications to the patient's being afflicted with facial palsy?
23. What neuromuscular training (NMR) techniques are available to the patient after facial paralysis?
24. What is the premise of NMR, and for what population is it appropriate?
25. What is the role of therapy in NMR?
26. What is the role of the home exercise program in NMR?
27. When is NMR management not appropriate?
28. What is the optimal time for referral?
29. What are the essential components to neuromuscular retraining?
30. What is the method of NMR?
31. What are the two categories of motor disturbance that facial paralysis is classified into?
32. What NMR treatment strategy addresses the patient with flaccid paralysis or paresis?
33. What NMR treatment strategy addresses the patient with synkinesis or mass action?
34. What is the rationale behind electrical stimulation as a treatment modality?
35. When is surgery appropriate?

1. What is acute idiopathic facial palsy?

Clinical, epidemiologic, and laboratory data suggest that what was once referred to as *idiopathic facial palsy,* better known as *Bell's palsy,* is actually an acute, benign, cranial polyneuritis that is most likely caused by the *herpes simplex virus.*[1] Named after the Scottish anatomist and surgeon John Bell, Bell's palsy occurs unilaterally and with *sudden onset,* often overnight, and reaches peak flaccidity with resultant paresis or paralysis within a few hours. For all its shocking and horrible insult to its victim, this malady is a nonprogressive,

non–life threatening, and often spontaneously remitting process. A large proportion of sufferers experience a premonitory symptom, referred to as a *prodrome,* which is actually a symptom indicating that onset of this pathologic condition is imminent. Similar to carpal tunnel syndrome, there is an increased incidence of Bell's palsy during pregnancy,[17] as well as an increased incidence of diabetes mellitus in patients afflicted with Bell's palsy. Some evidence exists for a genetic predisposition to Bell's palsy. The incidence of Bell's palsy has been estimated at between 15 to 40 cases per

100,000 population with no age, sex type, or racial predilections.[24]

2. What relevant microbiology is appropriate to an understanding of the herpes simplex virus?

Although nearly 80 known Herpesviridae infest animals, only six of these are known to infect humans. Three of the more famous of these include the herpes simplex virus, the Epstein-Barr virus, and the varicella-zoster virus, which causes herpes zoster, which is responsible for chickenpox during a primary infection and for shingles neuralgia in the aged after a period of dormancy and reactivation. Herpesviruses are ubiquitous in the sense of their having worldwide distribution, since few humans escape becoming infected by them during their lifetime. Because herpesviruses are fragile and do not survive long periods in the environment, transmission is principally through direct contact by bodily secretions at susceptible sites, such as oral, ocular, genital, or anal mucosa, the tympanic membrane, the bloodstream by injection, or the respiratory tract by someone else's sneeze. The virus does not penetrate keratinized skin.[26]

Herpes simplex viruses (HSV) are among the most common troublesome and annoying maladies affecting humans. Occasionally, they may be life threatening, as when they progress to herpes simplex encephalitis, in which the cerebrospinal fluid is bloody in the absence of any trauma. Known as the most common sporadic disease of the brain in the United States today, this pathogen carries a 70% mortality.[26]

Herpes simplex virus is subdivided into HSV-1, commonly known as oral herpes, and HSV-2, or genital herpes. Whereas the former infection spreads by oral secretions and is identified as the occupational hazard of dentists, dental hygienists, respiratory care unit personnel, and wrestlers, the latter infection is spread through sexual contact. With both herpes strains, recurrent infections occur frequently by reactivation of the endogenous virus, despite the presence of circulating antiviral antibodies. Precipitating factors include emotional stress, menstruation, fever, sunlight, and other factors. Thus all herpes viruses induce a lifelong latent infection in their natural hosts.[26]

3. What method of entry do viruses employ when entering the human nervous system?

Viruses enter the nervous system by either one of two routes: (1) through blood, or (2) directly through the nervous system. In the latter, the virus requires a specific receptor to interface with to gain access. For example, the poliovirus enters via the anterior horn cell, whereas the viruses causing viral meningitis interface upon a specific receptor on the meninges of the nervous system. The herpes simplex virus, as in rabies, gains entry through a peripheral nerve or nerves and moves proximally to the central nervous system by retrograde axoplasmic flow.[26]

Transmission and primary infection by herpes simplex is similar to that of all herpesvirus infections, except for herpes zoster, in that all are mostly asymptomatic. As the patient recovers from the primary infection, HSV travels up the sensory nerve pathways to reside latently in sensory cranial nerve ganglia such as the trigeminal, vagal, and perhaps the facial nuclei as well.[1]

4. Is there a relationship between the acute onset of Bell's palsy and exposure to cold?

The virus is somehow reactivated and replicates within the ganglion cells where it is protected from circulating antibodies. Reactivation may be related to cold exposure, since circumstantial evidence seems to link the onset of Bell's palsy after recent exposure to cold. Proximal damage is caused by the virus traveling up the nerve to the brainstem where it may induce a localized meningoencephalitis (as evidenced by increased protein in the cerebrospinal fluid). Distally the virus travels down the axon or axons to induce a radiculitis of the facial nucleus nerve cells, manifesting the signs and symptoms of Bell's palsy. This radiculitis is in fact caused by autoimmune demyelinization[1] rather than ischemic compression of the facial nucleus nerve cells. Inflammation (neuritis) and concomitant edema leading to ischemic constriction of the nerve axon may play a contributory role within the narrow unyielding bony confines of the more distal facial canal, located in the vicinity of the middle ear cavity within the temporal bone.[1]

5. What are the signs and symptoms at clinical presentation?

Some but not necessarily all of the following characteristics are present in typical Bell's palsy (Fig. 23-1):

- Ipsilateral muscle sagging with ironed-out appearance of normal folds and lines about the lips, nose, eyes (crow's feet), and forehead; there is a widened palpebral fissure present.
- Inability to fully or even partially puff cheeks, whistle, or wrinkle one's forehead.
- Miosis (of the eyelid).

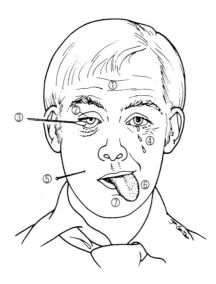

FIG. 23-1 Some common neurologic signs in patients diagnosed with Bell's palsy: *1,* flattening of the ipsilateral forehead; *2,* miosis; *3,* loss of corneal sensation; *4,* normal tearing on the uninvolved side only; *5,* diminished nasolabial fold, ipsilateral facial laxity, and dropping of the ipsilateral mouth; *6,* tongue deviation if unilateral hypoglossal paralysis is also suspected; *7,* loss of taste papillae on the anterior two thirds of the tongue. (From May M: *The facial nerve,* New York, 1986, Thieme-Stratton.)

- Ipsilateral numbness or pain of ear, face, neck, or tongue, occurs in approximately half of all patients.
- When asked to squeeze one's eyes tightly shut, the patient, in attempting to comply, demonstrates a positive Bell's sign: the eyeball rolls upward and inward, exposing the white sclera (Fig. 23-2). This movement on attempted closure is an involuntary synkinetic movement that usually but not invariably occurs when we close our eyes or sleep. With Bell's palsy, this movement may now be viewed because the levator superioris palpebrae (cranial nerve III) is unopposed by the orbicularis oculi (cranial nerve VII). This inability to close the eyelid is called *lagophthalmos.*
- The patient will report in the affirmative when asked about food becoming lodged between his or her teeth and cheek because of paralysis of the buccinator muscle, saliva and drink dribbling out of the mouth, or noticing upon his or her waking from sleep how the pillow had become wet from saliva.
- Diminished submandibular salivary flow or ipsilateral tearing.

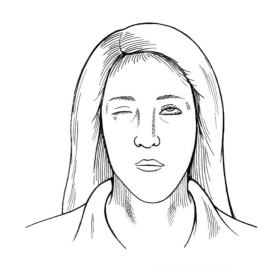

FIG. 23-2 Positive Bell's sign of left eye.

- Speech, particularly labial sounds, are affected.
- Decrease in or loss of ipsilateral stapes reflex.
- An absent ipsilateral blink reflex.
- When the patient attempts to smile or bare teeth, the lower facial muscles are pulled to the opposite side by the intact contralateral muscles, giving the impression of a sneer. Normally, this would not occur because the facial muscles, akin to many muscles elsewhere on the body, are arranged so that a balance exists and provides for symmetry of expression. This imbalance may lead to facial muscle contracture on the normal side, with muscle lengthening or stretching on the flaccid side.
- Loss of (sweet, sour, and salty) taste in the anterior two thirds of the tongue and decreased salivation on the affected side. Taste alterations may also occur with trauma or tumors.
- Hyperacusis caused by affectation of the nerve branch supplying the stapedius muscle; the patient may complain of holding the telephone away from the ear.
- Examination may show an area of decreased pinprick sensation along the distribution of Arnold's nerve behind the involved ear.
- Red appearance of the chorda tympani nerve in somewhat less than half of all patients evaluated within the first 10 days after onset in whom this nerve could be visualized.

6. What is the anatomy of the facial nerve?

The facial nerve is a mixed nerve consisting of motor, sensory, and autonomic fibers. The motor and sensory roots of the facial nerve emerge from a small fissure in the posterior area of the skull to enter the *internal auditory meatus* located in the petrous portion of the temporal bone (which also contains the middle and inner ear).

Having emerged from the meatus, the two roots, now called the "facial nerve" because they are now encased within the facial canal, proceed distally, to the vicinity of the inner ear, where the sensory nerves synapse with the cell bodies of the sensory neurons of the facial nerve collectively known as the *geniculate ganglion.* Beyond this point, axons responsible for different functions are routed either anterior (autonomic and sensory components) or posterior (motor) to the ganglion, the latter coursing toward the stylomastoid foramen.

Once emerging from the stylomastoid foramen behind the earlobe, the facial nerve (with its motor component) enters the parotid salivary gland to bifurcate into two main divisions (Fig. 23-3). The upper division divides into temporal and zygomatic branches, whereas the lower division gives rise to the buccal, mandibular, and cervical branches. These branches have been listed in cephalic to caudal order and serve to innervate the muscles of facial expression and those of the scalp and neck; additionally, two muscles at the floor of the mouth, namely, the stylohyoid and the posterior belly of the digastric muscle, are also innervated by the facial nerve. The muscles of the jaw not supplied by the facial nerve are the masseter, temporalis, and pterygoid muscles, which are innervated by the trigeminal nerve (V).

The *occipitofrontalis* controls the muscles of the scalp, the frontal belly of the *epicranius* raises the eyebrows and wrinkles the forehead as in surprise or fright, the *corrugator supercilii* draws the eyebrows together "tightly knit" and is associated with frowning, the *orbicularis oculi* controls the sphincter muscles of the eyelids, the *buccinator* controls the muscles of the cheek, nose, and mouth. One can test the latter by asking the patient to "pull back the corners of your mouth." The alar position of the *nasalis* permits nostril flaring, the transverse portion of the *nasalis* permits narrowing of the nostrils, the *procerus* allows scrunching up of the face, as may occur when smelling something offensive, the orbicularis oris puckers the lips as in whistling, the

mentalis scrunches up the chin and protrudes the lower lip as in pouting, whereas the *pterygoideus medialis* and *pterygoideus lateralis* permit protrusion of the lower jaw that occurs when one bares the lower teeth. Additionally, the *zygomaticus major* is the principal muscle used in laughing, whereas the *risorius* permits that facial expression associated with a nongenuine, lame, or half-attempted smile. The *platysma* is tested when one asks the patient to "wrinkle up the skin on your neck" or "pull down the corners of your mouth."

7. What is the topographic paradigm in understanding facial palsy?

The topographic paradigm in diagnosis of facial paralysis is classic in the otolaryngologic study of Bell's palsy. This idea is based on the idea that loss of function has a one-to-one correspondence with given portions of nerve that have undergone disorder. There is nothing mystifying about this. An analogy may be made of the median nerve of the upper extremity. The median nerve courses down along the shaft of the humerus and, at the cubital fossa, branches off to supply the majority of muscles of the flexor compartment of the forearm. In the event of a knife or bullet wound immediately before that branch supplying the flexor carpi radialis, preservation of function to the pronator teres would be maintained, and partial or total loss of function would manifest distal to that location.

In the same manner, a focal lesion to the facial nerve anywhere along its route would spare sensory and motor function up until but not beyond that point (Fig. 23-4). The questions that follow present the sites of lesions and their manifestations in an order that begins with the proximal and hence more severe manifestations of facial palsy and work their way to less severe manifestations as the lesion site manifests more distally.

8. How does a lesion at the internal auditory meatus manifest?

Having passed only a short distance through the posterior cranial fossa, the motor and sensory roots of the facial nerve, accompanied by the vestibulocochlearis nerve (VIII), enter the internal auditory meatus. A lesion at the entrance to the internal auditory meatus may occur from tumor of the vestibulocochlearis nerve or its nerve sheath and manifests in a full-blown facial palsy that is accompanied by deafness and possibly balance problems.[27]

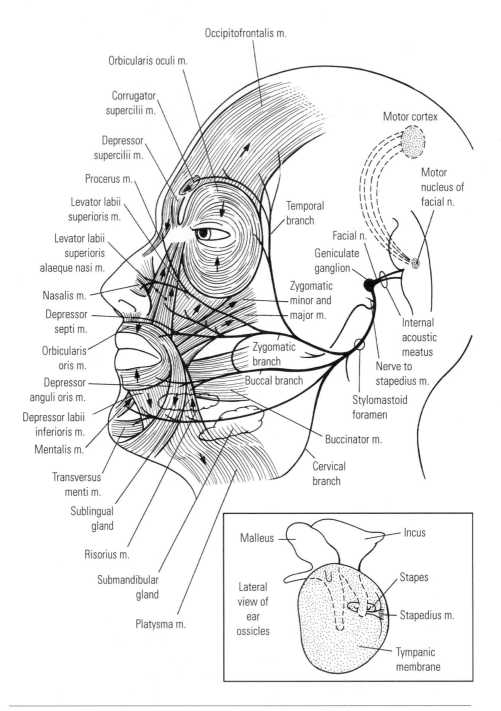

FIG. 23-3 Course and distribution of the facial nerve. *Arrows* demonstrate direction and angle of pull for respective muscles.

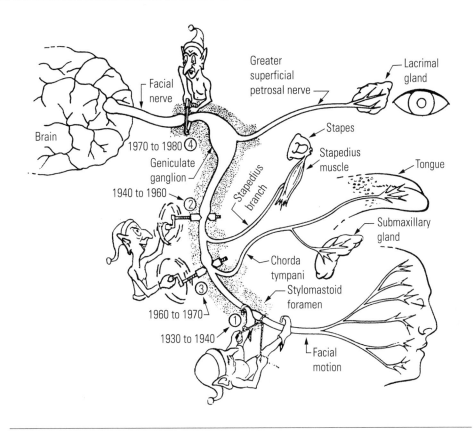

FIG. 23-4 This illustration portrays the decades-old controversy between otolaryngologists and head and neck surgeons. The latter have maintained that idiopathic facial palsy was attributable to inflammation resulting in ischemic *compression,* whereas the former correctly maintained that the operative mechanism was *auto-immune demyelinization.* Over time, head and neck surgeons slowly capitulated but nevertheless maintained that decompression was the appropriate management as specific sites were abandoned and other sites more proximal were targeted for surgery. Currently, the stalemate centers about the locale of the internal auditory meatus. This illustration may be conveniently referred to as charting the sites of lesion locales. (From Adour KK: *Otolaryngol Clin North Am* 24(3):664, 1991.)

9. How does a lesion proximal to the geniculate ganglion manifest?

A lesion proximal to the geniculate ganglion will result in diminished or lack of tear secretion and consequent eye drying, since the greater superficial petrosal nerve is blocked from transmitting parasympathetic impulses to the spinopalatine ganglion. The net result is a full-blown facial palsy accompanied by dry, red, and swollen eye.

10. How does a lesion of the geniculate ganglion manifest?

A lesion at the geniculate ganglion results in a full-blown facial palsy but with normal tear secretion, since the lacrimal fibers have been spared. In fact, it

may appear as if there is an overproduction of tears, though this is actually not the case. The eye may still dry out because of weakness of the orbicularis oris. Weakness of this muscle causes the lacrimal puncta to no longer contact the glove to collect tears into the conjunctival sac. These wasted tears will then uselessly pour over the cheek rather than bathe the eye. Additionally, pain is often felt behind the ear.[27]

11. What is the manifestation of a high facial canal lesion?

A lesion high up in the facial canal refers to that area just distally beyond the geniculate ganglion and manifests with *hyperacusia* (that is, normal sounds heard abnormally loud) because of the effect of ischemia to that nerve branch supplying the stapedius muscle. Full-blown facial palsy will occur without the preceding manifestations of more proximal lesions. On examination, a decrease in or loss of the ipsilateral stapes reflex will manifest.

12. What is the function of the stapedius muscle?

The middle ear chamber is a cavity within the skull that contains the smallest bones in the body, the malleus (hammer), incus (anvil), and stapes (stirrup). These bones are suspended within the cavity by ligaments in a mechanically significant order: the distal malleus, rigidly attached to the eardrum, covers greater than one half the drum area, but the footplate of the stirrup covers the oval window, the entrance to the inner ear. These auditory ossicles form a mechanical linkage that interestingly perform a twofold antagonistic function:

- The ossicles together function as a lever mechanism to amplify pressure from sound waves imparted to the eardrum and deliver them to the oval window and are amplified considerably. This lever system enables us to hear sounds the energies of which are some 1,000 times weaker than we would otherwise hear.
- The middle ear's second function engages this same ossicle linkage to protect the inner ear from excessively loud sounds. Sound-intensity dampening is accomplished by two small muscles; one, the tensor tympani (cranial nerve V), is connected to the eardrum, the other, the *stapedius* (cranial nerve VII), inserts on the stapes (see Fig. 23-3). In the event of an intensely loud sound, these muscles contract and, in doing so, momentarily dismantle this amplifying system by drawing in the eardrum and drawing the stapes away from the oval window. Unfortunately, because this protective mechanism does not work instantaneously, sudden, intensely loud sounds can wreak permanent damage in the form of hearing loss.

13. What is the manifestation of a more distal facial canal lesion?

A lower facial canal lesion will spare the nerve to the stapedius muscle but will involve the chorda tympani, thereby causing interruption of fibers that permit normal salivation and normal taste in the anterior two thirds of the tongue. This will result in a dry mouth and an unpleasant or distorted sense of taste. These manifestations are accompanied by ipsilateral loss of facial muscle tone. There is preservation of these functions associated with more distal lesions.

14. What is the manifestation of a lesion at the stylomastoid foramen?

A lesion at the styloid foramen or at that locale where the facial nerve superficially emerges from under the earlobe results in paralysis of the entire ipsilateral facial musculature. These are most obvious as a loss of the ability to wrinkle the forehead, whistle, or wink.

15. How does facial palsy of the upper motor neuron type differ from Bell's palsy, which is of the lower motor neuron type?

Supranuclear lesions by definition involve the upper motor neuron that traverses between the cerebral cortex, through the internal capsule, and terminates on the sensory or motor facial nuclei located in the brainstem. Clinically differentiating between a Bell's palsy and a facial palsy that occurred after a focal cerebrovascular accident is made easy by understanding the following neuroanatomy. The rostral portion of the motor nucleus is responsible for supplying nerve fibers to the superior facial muscles, that is, the area around the forehead and around the eyes. Unlike other portions of the nucleus, the rostral portion innervates its assigned area by both crossed and uncrossed corticobulbar tract collaterals. Because of this anomaly, facial paralysis after a stroke affects only the lower two thirds of the face while sparing the eyes and forehead. This bilateral innervation does not occur in the lower motor neuron, and therefore facial paralysis of the intranuclear kind, of which Bell's palsy is but one type, will involve the entire face and is only unilaterally innervated[27] (Fig. 23-5). A stroke above the level of the brainstem would also spare taste and hearing.

Additionally, with palsy resulting from an upper motor neuron lesion, the patient can partially often hide his palsy by smiling, since there is preservation of emotionally motivated movement. This fact implies that emotionally motivated output to the facial nucleus follows a pathway other than the corticospinal tract.

Finally, the degree of paralysis of facial musculature differs, depending on whether the lesion is of the upper or lower motor neuron type. An upper motor neuron lesion will result in contralateral *spastic* paralysis of the lower two thirds of the face, whereas a lower motor neuron lesion will result in ipsilateral *flaccid* paralysis to the entire face on one side.

16. What is the corneal blink test?

The *corneal blink reflex* is mediated by an afferent (sensory) component by cranial nerve V and an efferent

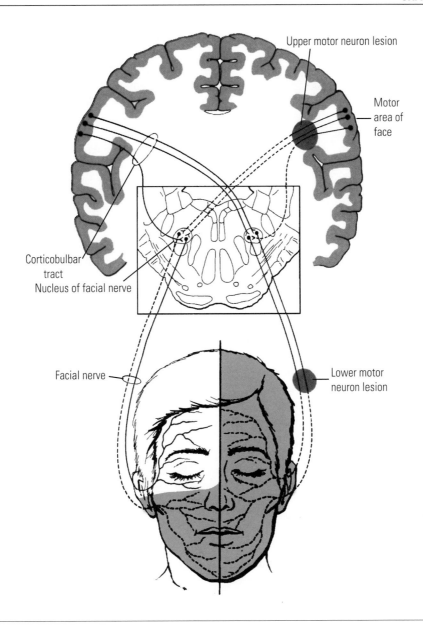

FIG. 23-5 Bell's palsy involves the lower motor neuron (infranuclear lesion) and manifests as a global facial asymmetry involving the ipsilateral upper and lower quadrants. Supranuclear lesions involving the primary (that is, upper) motor neuron result in facial asymmetry in the lower two thirds of the face. The shaded areas of the face show the distribution of paralyzed facial muscles. (From Gilman S, Winans S: *Essentials of clinical neuroanatomy and neurophysiology,* ed 6, Philadelphia, 1982, FA Davis.)

(motor) component controlled by cranial nerve VII. The correct way to elicit the corneal reflex is to touch a tiny swab of cotton to the *unilateral* colored cornea and not the white sclera (Fig. 23-6). The felt sensation is transmitted to the brain by the trigeminal nerve, whereas the efferent blinking response normally manifests in blinking of *both* eyelids. In true Bell's palsy, touching the cornea of the affected side will consensually cause the contralateral eye to close. This is not the case with upper motor neuron lesions.

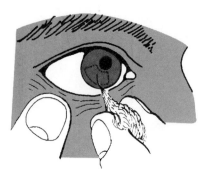

FIG. 23-6 The correct way to elicit the corneal blink test. (From Patten J: *Neurological differential diagnosis*, ed 2, London, 1996, Springer-Verlag.)

17. What is the differential diagnosis?

Bell's palsy has a diagnosis of exclusion. Diagnosis is reserved for patients in which an exhaustive search for a cause has proved fruitless. The following conditions also cause facial hemiparalysis.

- *Melkersson-Rosenthal syndrome,* perhaps a form of sarcoidosis, is distinguished from idiopathic facial palsy, since it also includes recurrent facial swelling (edema) particularly of the lip and eyelid that is nonpitting, painless, and short lived (that is, lasting several days). Cheilitis (chapping and swelling of edematous lips) as well as fissuring of the tongue,[24] though the latter is the least common component of this syndrome, present in approximately one third of all cases. Additionally, contralateral unilateral *facial palsy* characteristically accompanies this condition.[32]

- *Otitis media* is a bacterial or viral middle ear infection secondary to an upper respiratory infection that travels from the nasopharynx to the middle ear via the eustachian tube. Disease onset may occur at any age but is most common in young children. The very first complaint is severe earache with or without hearing loss. With time, the tympanic membrane may bulge and eventually rupture, releasing built-up exudate. Symptoms of impending complications include headache, sudden profound hearing loss, vertigo, chills, and fever. Among the complications of this unfortunate condition are *facial paralysis* and brain abscess.[9]

- *Ramsey-Hunt syndrome* (synonym: herpes zoster oticus or cephalicus, or geniculate herpes) is a condition that involves invasion of the eighth cranial nerve ganglion and the geniculate ganglion of the seventh cranial nerve by the same culprit responsible for shingles, chickenpox, and Bell's palsy. Clinical signs include ipsilateral hearing loss, vertigo or ataxia, and pain. The latter sign is almost always present and more severe when compared to Bell's palsy, and is accompanied by vesicle eruption developing over the four divisions of the facial nerve, that is, those sensory fibers supplying the posteromedial pinna and external auditory canal. Vesicles may be noticed before the onset of facial paralysis but may also appear up to 10 days later. *Facial paralysis* may be either transient or permanent. Because of involvement at the level of the geniculate ganglion, decreased taste, diminished salivary flow, and dry mouth will also manifest.[9]

- *Lyme disease* is a spirochete disorder spread by a deer tick and, in addition to facial palsy, is accompanied by a skin lesion characterized by a red macule or papule, usually on the proximal portion of the extremity or trunk, such as the thigh, buttock, or axilla. Malaise, fatigue, chills and fever, headache, stiff neck, myalgias, arthralgias, nausea and vomiting, as well as a sore throat also occur. The hallmark of this disease, however, is the skin lesion that is erythematous and macular with a pale center. *Facial palsy* is the commonest neurologic manifestation of mild meningitis that is characteristic of stage II of Lyme disease. The problem with definitive diagnosis is that there is no *good* test for Lyme disease. Unless treatment with broad-spectrum antibiotics or tetracycline is initiated early on, the disease may, in some instances, progress undetected to stage III, which is characterized by chronic fatigue syndrome and multiple sclerosis–like symptoms. One must be especially suspicious in cases of children diagnosed with juvenile rheumatoid arthritis who live in endemic areas.[9]

- *Botulism* caused facial palsy is bilateral and includes red (and parched) tongue, oropharynx, nasopharynx, and larynx. Botulism is a form of neuromuscular poisoning that decreases release of acetylcholine from presynaptic terminals. Neurologic symptoms are bilateral and symmetrical, and involvement begins with the cranial nerves and descends caudally. Neurologic symptoms are commonly preceded by nausea, vomiting, abdominal cramps, and diarrhea. Diagnosis is established by toxin isolation from stool specimen.[9]

- *Leprosy* (synonym: Hansen's disease) is a chronic infectious disease caused by a bacillus that has a predilection for cooler body areas, namely, skin, mucous membranes, and those peripheral nerves coursing closest to the surface of the body. Terminal cutaneous branches of the *facial nerve* typically become involved, including those branches to the orbicularis oculi, the orbicularis oris, and the medial parts of the corrugator supercilii muscles, manifesting in an inability to completely close one's eyes (lagophthalmos).[9]

- *Malignancies.* Neoplasms are suggested by a slowly progressing palsy that may spare some branches of the facial nerve but may culminate in complete involvement of that nerve (cerebellopontine angle tumor). Especially suspect are patients having a history of cancer, particularly of the breast, lung, thyroid, kidney, ovary, or prostate. Tumor is to be suspected when there is no recovery of *facial palsy* after 6 months. It is appropriate to palpate for masses in the parotid, submandibular gland, or neck. If the latter are found, referral is promptly made to a physician for skull imaging by radiographs or CT scan.[24]

- *Birth trauma.* Forceps injury can injure the nerve in the face or in the soft petrous bone, especially in light of the lack of a well-developed mastoid process that affords protection of the facial nerve. This is normally absent or poorly developed in the infant, although these children have a high incidence of recovery (approximately 90%). In the adult, injury to the facial nerve may occur after trauma either at the stylomastoid foramen, penetrating injury to the middle ear, facial injury, or fracture of the temporal bone. Such an injury will result in ecchymosis (Battle's sign) around the pinna and mastoid process. Barotrauma is caused by scuba diving and altitude paralysis.

- *Other manifestations.* Other manifestations of facial palsy that must also be ruled out include Guillain-Barré syndrome, poliomyelitis, multiple sclerosis, leukemia, osteomyelitis, Piaget's disease, meningococcal meningitis, infectious mononucleosis (Epstein-Barr virus), syphilis, malaria, cat-scratch disease, herpes zoster cephalicus, otitis media, myasthenia gravis, AIDS, alcoholic neuropathy, vitamin A deficiency, and polyneuritis. Toxic causes include arsenic, carbon monoxide, thalidomide, and ethylene glycol. Iatrogenic causes include mandibular block anesthesia; vaccine therapy for rabies, polio, or influenza; parotid surgery or mastoid surgery; or iontophoresis.[24]

18. What is the prognosis for recovery?

Prognosis very much depends on the extent of nerve damage. Generally the more proximal the lesion, the poorer is the prognosis. Complete resolution occurs in 75% to 80% of most patients who have succumbed to partial facial paralysis,[27] whereas the results after total

paralysis are variable. The likelihood of complete recovery is 90% if the nerve proximal in the face retains normal excitability to supramaximal stimulation but diminishes to 20% in the event that electrical excitability is absent.[9] Recovery, when it occurs, ordinarily begins within 1 to 4 weeks, may take longer than 8 months, but is always achieved by 12 months after onset.[24] Relapses are uncommon but occur in a minority of patients.

Ten to fifteen percent of all patients have incomplete or inappropriate reinnervation.[27] In the latter scenario, as the nerve regenerates, its sprouting branches may mistakenly innervate muscles not previously supplied by the facial nerve. This misdirected and aberrant growth may innervate lower facial muscles with periocular fibers or vice versa, resulting in contraction of unexpected facial movement on voluntary facial movement *(synkinesia).* For example, a patient may inadvertently smile when attempting a volitional blink. In contrast, the patient may cry *crocodile tears* instead of salivating when tasting or chewing (but not smelling) food.[9]

19. What is the medical management of Bell's palsy?

- Treatment with prednisone is not of proved benefit but seems to decrease acute pain and therefore ought to be administered soon (as within the first 72 hours) after onset.[2]

- Prevention of corneal ulceration caused by drying out of the exposed eye is mandatory. This is accomplished by use of methyl cellulose drops or use of an eye patch, especially at night.[9]

20. What is the traditional therapeutic management of Bell's palsy?

- Iontophoresis with hydrocortisone to decrease inflammation is appropriately applied before electrical stimulation. Treatment ought to be performed over the ipsilateral cheek, where that nerve runs subcutaneously, and not focally at the stylomastoid foramen. Phonophoresis may also be used.[21]

- Interrupted direct current and negative polarity, with the positive electrode on the ipsilateral forearm. Some 10 to 20 stimuli, repeated three times per session, are applied to the motor points of muscles of the facial nerve distribution.[21] The rationale behind electric stimulation is not that it will cause healing of the nerve; rather it simply maintains the involved muscles' tone until such time that reinnervation occurs. Thus electric stimulation prevents the muscles from becoming fibrotic or fatty after disuse.[9]

- Application of cold laser to the acupuncture points that relate to facial nerve distribution.[21]
- Massage to both involved and noninvolved facial musculature.
- Regimen of facial exercises.
- Of prime importance is psychologic support provided to the patient throughout the ordeal.

21. Why are nonspecific gross facial exercises inadequate to the management repertoire of Bell's palsy?

The efficacy of Craig's "face-saving exercises"[12] is questioned when we consider that gross exercises tend to reinforce abnormal movement patterns.[6] Asking a patient to open his or her mouth widely or move the lower lip from side to side does little but train compensatory movements by way of the masseter muscle or muscles. Asking the patient to move his or her eyes up, down, to the right, and to the left only trains eye movements. Requests such as close the eyes tightly, puff out the cheeks, or broadly laugh, may serve only to promote mass movement and synkinesis,[5] since the maximum effort needed to express these gross movements recruits excessive numbers of motor units.[14]

Because the ratio of muscle fibers to motor neurons is approximately 25 to 1, the facial muscles possess a high index for refinement of movement (compared to the 2000-to-1 ratio in the gastrocnemius).[23] As such, the intricacy and complexity of movement precludes the use of maximum-effort exercises, since motor units other than those targeted may be recruited because of overflow.[22]

22. What are the psychologic ramifications to the patient's being afflicted with facial palsy?

Our face is usually the first and often lasting impression and memory we have on others. How we look deeply affects our self-esteem. This sentiment was eloquently expressed by the Roman consul Cicero (106-43 B.C.) when he described how "The face is the image of the soul."[11] However, more than simply a cosmetic deformity, facial paralysis is very much a disability of communication. Minute changes in facial expression account primarily for human nonverbal communication. This is reflected in the proportionally large area of the motor homunculus that is associated with control of the facial muscles.

Depression, guilt, anger, hostility, anxiety, rejection, and paranoia have been noted after facial paralysis has occurred.[33] Patients may be considered mentally

deficient[19] and experience difficulties with interpersonal relationships, employability, making friends, and coping with looks of disgust or horror in others' faces.[16]

To the patient afflicted with facial paralysis, the psychosocial effect may be devastating. Feeling that they are freaks, patients will develop compensatory strategies that they believe will help hide their newfound deformity. Patients may maintain their faces relatively immobile and expressionless so as not to accentuate their paralysis. Patients may habitually sit with slouched postures, often with their head tilted with a hand covering and hiding the involved side from view.[7] Regrettably the sum total of these compensations may cause inhibition of the patient's natural affect and personality.[5] The therapist must gently work with the patient by providing emotional support by allowing the patient to vent his or her feelings. Suggested topics for discussion include discussing and identifying family and friends who, since the start of the patient's facial paralysis, are (1) no longer their friends, (2) are somewhat negative, (3) have always been supportive, and (4) are newly supportive (such as a facial paralysis support group).[5] With time and progress the patient is taught to reverse this denial and decreased facial awareness by encouraging self-esteem.[5]

23. What neuromuscular training (NMR) techniques are available to the patient after facial paralysis?

Facial neuromuscular retraining is a problem-solving approach to facial paralysis that utilizes specific reeducation techniques to promote symmetrical movement while inhibiting undesired movement patterns. The skilled therapist provides feedback training that is supplemented by mirror or electromyographic feedback tailored to the specific needs of the patient. An essential and key element to this approach is the successful implementation of a structured home program.

NMR emphasizes very small and slow, very symmetrical, and very isolated movements with an emphasis on quality of movement. This is in contrast to traditional gross motor strengthening exercises, which tend to reinforce mass movement and promote synkinesis. Normal facial movements are subtle and never harsh or performed with maximum effort.

Recapturing movement is an early goal of treatment. NMR often begins with an attempt to improve the critical function of eye closure. This is accomplished by having the patient focus on making controlled and small movements, aided by the therapist and a mirror. When the patient can execute a faint closure of the eye without other facial twitches occurring simultaneously, he or she may attempt a more definitive eye closure. For example, the patient learns to close his or her eyes very slowly while trying not to let the corner of the mouth move. With constant repetition, the patient learns to control eye closure with less and less conscious awareness. Over time the patient progresses to learn to perform the movement more quickly and forcefully and eventually automatically access that movement in a variety of different circumstances and settings. Accomplishing this milestone is followed by addressing the patient's own goals, such as having a normal smile, improving speech, and eating and drinking.

24. What is the premise of NMR, and for what population is it appropriate?

The premise behind a facial retraining program is the capacity of the central nervous system to modify its organization so as to engram new motor patterns within the existing motor repertoire. Facial retraining techniques may also be used in postacute patients suffering from facial paralysis caused by accidental injury, congenital reasons, carcinoma, postoperative nerve pain, postsurgical tumor resection, herpes zoster oticus, or Guillain-Barré syndrome.[14] NMR may be tailored to the many kinds of neurologic impairments ranging from spinal cord injury, peripheral neuropathy, and cerebrovascular accident.

25. What is the role of therapy in NMR?

The therapist's role is to formulate very specific goals, monitor progress, and serve as feedback to the patient. For example, the therapist may inform the patient, "The corner of your mouth is closing when you're chewing." Thus the therapist's role is to direct a recovery program rather than perform it.

26. What is the role of the home exercise program in NMR?

The patient with facial paralysis is typically involved in the NMR programs for 1 to 3 years during which time some 90% of treatment is performed by the patient at home.[13] Because no two patients have the same functional profile, no two treatment or home programs will be the same. The challenge to the therapist is that he or she must devise exercises to address very specific goals that the patient can perform a varying number of times throughout the day. A successful home program requires self-discipline on the part of the patient and tenacious persistence and adherence to performance of exercises. When the patient achieves success with a specific goal and replicates it with 75% accuracy, the therapist builds upon that success by slightly modifying the strategy.

Structuring therapy in this manner is cost effective in that it reduces the number of billed clinic hours while maximizing the number of patient participation hours. The demands of successful outcome often require a highly motivated patient who follows through with 30 to 60 minutes of consistent, concentrated practice every day. Patients periodically return to the clinic setting to refine movement patterns, learn new exercises, document progress, and establish new treatment goals.[13]

27. When is NMR management not appropriate?

Typically, two stages of recovery occur after the emergence of facial paralysis. During the first stage of nerve regeneration, healing occurs slowly and corresponds to a lack of any facial movement. Initiating intensive therapy at this early stage is inappropriate and may be detrimental to eventual recovery. Like a broken bone protected from stress by the cast,[13] the nerve must first recover before initiation of therapy. Active attempts at exercise before clinical evidence to reinnervation, that is, active facial movement serves only to exacerbate the condition[29] by causing overactivity in the musculature in the intact side.

Waiting for movement to occur can be frustrating for both patient and therapist, though most patients begin to demonstrate movement in 5 to 12 months.[15] The referral time for Bell's palsy is typically delayed until 3 months after onset because of the high probability of spontaneous recovery before that time. If paralysis persists after 3 months, recovery may be incomplete with the development of synkinesis,[4,25] at which point patients should be referred for NMR. Acoustic neuroma or the subsequent surgery is another common cause for facial paralysis. Since the auditory nerve (VIII) and the facial nerve (VII) course adjacent to each other, the facial nerve may incur damage by the tumor or operative procedure. Postoperative facial weakness, altered taste sensation, and excessively dry or wet eyes are attributable to the reaction of the nerve to the tumor itself or to separation during surgery. The optimal time for referral of these patients is when minimal facial movement becomes apparent, or as synkinesis begins to develop, or by 12 months after onset if no movement has occurred.

Recovery typically begins between 5 and 12 months after surgery.[30]

28. What is the optimal time for referral?

The second stage of recovery is characterized by the emergence of small facial movements. As recovery continues, the patient may notice movements beginning in areas of the face that they are not trying to move. This may manifest as eye closure during speech or pulling upward of the corner of the mouth when one is shutting the eye. The presence of this excess movement is known as *synkinesis* and is defined as abnormal synchronization of muscles that ordinarily do not contract together. These movements may occur with volitional or spontaneous movements. Synkinetic movement may pull antagonistically, like a tug-of-war, against the normal, primary movement. Synkinesis may vary in severity from subtle to severe and, in its worst form, mass action, may result in gross deformity of the affected side during any attempted expression. The involved side of the face may feel tight and even painful as the result of uncontrolled muscle contractions.

Thus patients should be referred to NMR when visible signs of return become apparent or once synkinesis is noted. There is no time limit for when facial retraining may begin. Improvements may even occur years after onset.[15]

29. What are the essential components to neuromuscular retraining?

Proper treatment environment. The proper learning environment is enhanced by a quiet, individual room where therapy may be conducted without distraction. This kind of privacy creates a "safe" setting for the patient embarrassed by his or her appearance. Here, they may work undistracted by social stigma and feelings of self-consciousness.

A thorough initial *evaluation* is imperative and determines the degree of available volitional movement, spontaneous movement, and presence of any synkinesis or mass action. The use of videotape is invaluable in capturing sequential facial movements as they occur. Photographic evaluation is valuable because it allows the patient to notice small changes occurring over time that may otherwise not be readily visible. Patients should view photographs reflected in a mirror to preserve the relative position of the paralyzed side.[14]

Patient *motivation* and *cognition* are necessary components to a successful outcome. Cognitive or attention deficits often associated with cerebrovascular accident or accidental brain injury may preclude participation in an NMR program. Similarly, it is imperative that the patient maintain consistency of practice with intense and disciplined concentration during his or her home program away from the clinic.

30. What is the method of NMR?

Patient education lays the foundation for learning selective movement patterns that lead to improved motor function. The therapist educates the patient in basic facial anatomy, kinesiology, angle of muscle pull (see Fig. 23-4), and physiology needed to understand the procedures and goals of treatment. Patients are made partners in their rehabilitation.

Exploration of facial movement. Most persons are not conscious of the specific movements involved in normal facial expression. The patient is instructed to perform small, specific movements on the contralateral side. The initial treatments are a time of discovery for the patient as he or she learns to identify specific areas of function and dysfunction and begin, with the therapist, to formulate strategies to improve facial movement.[14]

Biofeedback is used as an evaluative and a therapeutic tool. As an evaluative tool, surface electrode electromyography (seEMG) biofeedback is used to detect the presence of any functional return of hypoactive muscles before any visually observed facial movement. Weak electrical impulses may be demonstrated and made accessible to the patient in the form of a tone or visible oscilloscope trace in what appears to be an otherwise flaccid muscle. As a therapeutic tool seEMG may be used to increase activity in weak muscles, decrease activity in hyperactive muscles, and improve coordination of muscle groups.

The purpose of seEMG is to bring the normally unconscious control of specific muscles under conscious control. By correlating information from seEMG feedback with proprioceptive and mirror feedback, the patient slowly learns to reproduce new movement patterns outside the clinical setting in the context of a home exercise program.

31. What are the two categories of motor disturbance that facial paralysis is classified into?

Facial paralysis falls into one of two categories, each of which requires different treatment strategies:
- Flaccid paralysis or paresis in which *hypoactivity* dominates. The goal here is to increase muscle activity.

- Synkinesis or mass action. The goal here is to inhibit excess movement in *hyperactive* muscles so as to stave off abnormal and unsynchronous facial movement.
- Improve coordination of muscle groups.[14]

32. What NMR treatment strategy addresses the patient with flaccid paralysis or paresis?

Retraining strategies are an attempt to produce fine motor control of a single muscle or muscle group (such as the levator anguli oris–zygomaticus) are initially developed on the noninvolved side. This is accomplished by having the patient slowly contract these muscles (as in a broad smile) while observing the corresponding seEMG trace with the setting at a relatively low setting. The patient's task is to make appropriate contractions such that even a trace contraction appears as a ramp on the oscilloscope. This is repeated at even higher sensitivity levels until very small and slow facial contractions yield the same ramp function. The patient must focus on how the movement feels as it is being produced. Thus a base line is created for the normal function of that particular muscle. This is invaluable for the patient as the patient uses his or her newfound awareness of this isolated contraction to facilitate replication of this motor action on the involved side.[7]

Next, the patient is encouraged to "shift" his or her feeling of the fine motor control learned on the uninvolved side to the involved side. This painstaking process is aided by use of seEMG in which the patient sits in a darkened room and observes the EMG oscilloscope. The patient observes ramping produced by the uninvolved side and attempts to replicate that ramp by small facial movement on the involved side. This may be repeated thousands of times over as much as 25 1-hour sessions until a small isolated contraction is voluntarily and consistently performed. To prevent diminishment and extinguishment of this newfound contraction, amplification of this movement is necessary so that the patient may see small movements of the involved side in a mirror. Once visible movement is acquired EMG sensory biofeedback is immediately discontinued for that muscle and specific action exercises (SAE) are implemented with mirror feedback to obtain greater voluntary muscle control.[7] The patient is thus weaned from seEMG when he or she has successfully internalized a movement. The patient and a significant other, if possible, are trained in enhancing this motion by exercising exactly as instructed by the therapist. The therapist trains the patient to train himself or herself.

Self-esteem, improved physical function, and satisfaction improve as the patient learns to assume control of his or her recovery. Movements must be initiated slowly and gradually so that the patient may observe and modify the angle, strength, and speed of the excursion as it occurs. Otherwise, rapidly performed movements may revert to an abnormal motor pattern. Similarly, movements must be small in nature so as to limit motor-unit recruitment to those muscles targeted.[22] Large-scale movements serve only to recruit larger numbers of motor units resulting in overflow and diminished accuracy. Finally, movements must be equal on both sides to achieve symmetrical expression. Allowing the uninvolved side to dominate may possibly shunt excess tone to that side, resulting in diminishment of activity on the involved side.[7]

Approximately 90% of the patient's therapy program is carried out in the home setting. Treatment sessions may range from 2 hours per month (for local patients) to an intensive treatment session of 1 to 12 hours of space over 3 to 4 days every 6 months (for patients traveling a great distance). The entire course of therapy may last 18 months to 3 years.[34] During this time the frequency of clinic visits decreases as the patient becomes increasingly proficient in performing his or her home exercise program. Clinic visits involve identifying new problem areas and establishing new goals.

33. What NMR treatment strategy addresses the patient with synkinesis or mass action?

The first step in the treatment of synkinesis is to decrease hypertonus. Increased facial tone, tightness, or rigidity may be present on the affected side and is most likely caused by increased background muscle activity.[35] This activity may be observed as an increased nasolabial fold (musculus levator, m. zygomaticus), decreased palpebral fissure (m. orbicularis oculi), retraction of the corner of the mouth (m. zygomaticus, m. risorius), dimpling of the chin (m. mentalis or the depressors), drawing down of the corner of the mouth (depressors and platysma), and banding of the neck (platysma). Abnormal tone in the lips may manifest as thinning or "puffiness."[14]

Reduction of resting tone is imperative before the inhibition of synkinesis because normal movement cannot be superimposed on abnormal tone. The patient is taught to become aware that facial tightness or stiffness is caused by increased muscle activity at rest, followed by general relaxation training, and seEMG feedback.[5,10] Relaxation of all muscles of the face is necessary so as to prevent the muscles on the non-involved side from overacting during attempted voluntary movements. Massage of the affected side is helpful over those areas where thickening and immobility are observed.[8,31]

As an example of synkinesis, consider the patient who demonstrates zygomatic activity on attempted smiling but who also expresses synkinesis of the platysma and limited zygomatic excursion. Instead of the expected upward curl at the angle of the mouth (a smile), he or she demonstrates a drawing down at the angle of the mouth (a grimace). By focusing attention on the precisely correct movement pattern, the patient initiated the primary movement slowly while monitoring the areas of synkinesis vigilantly from the start. As synkinesis becomes visible, the primary movement is maintained while the synkinetic response is reduced. This difficult process requires complete concentration so as to "release" the synkinetic area. The exact timing of this sequence is essential for dissociation of synkinesis from primary movement. By inhibition of synkinesis of the platysma, the zygomaticus gains a more normal range of movement without the antagonistic effect of the platysma, resulting in a more natural smile. Once achieved, the patient may then relax the primary movement as inhibition of synkinesis requires less concentration, and excursion of the primary movement increases as control is learned. Initially this movement pattern may occur only volitionally, whereas over time these patterns are demonstrated spontaneously.[8,31]

34. What is the rationale behind electrical stimulation as a treatment modality?

Research during the 1960s has shown that electrical stimulation of a denervated muscle actually retards in growth of neurofibrils to the motor end plate.[7] The denervated neurofibril has no motivation to grow into the motor end plate if it's being electrically stimulated. In response to this, many insurance companies have since refused payment for a treatment that was deemed unjustified. This, in fact, was proved only during the initial 3 to 4 weeks during which fibrillation manifested. Rather, in deference to the aforementioned study, faradic (that is, direct-current) stimulation is appropriate but should rather begin some 28 to 30 days after onset, since that is the time when fibrillation has decreased.

The clinical use of electrotherapy remains controversial. Although nerve conduction and muscle contraction do occur, the reduction of circulatory stasis, increased muscle and nerve nutrition, and the reduction

of muscle atrophy have yet to be proved.[5] Furthermore, because of the small size and proximity of the facial muscles, it is difficult to produce an isolated contraction of a specific muscle using electric stimulation. Such large-scale contractions may cause mass action[14] and possibly contribute to synkinesis,[14] which serve only to reinforce abnormal motor patterns.

35. When is surgery appropriate?

In a small percentage of patients axonal regeneration is ineffective, and hypoglossal facial nerve anastomosis may partially restore facial function if none has returned in 6 to 12 months.[4]

REFERENCES

1. Adour KK: Medical management of idiopathic (Bell's) palsy, *Otolaryngol Clin North Am* 24(3):664, 1991.
2. Adour KK, Bell DN, Hilsinger RL Jr: Herpes simplex virus in idiopathic facial paralysis (Bell's palsy), *JAMA* 233:527-530, 1975.
3. Adour KK, Byl FM, Hilsinger RL Jr, et al: The true nature of Bell's palsy: analysis of 1000 consecutive patients, *Laryngoscope* 88:787-801, 1978.
4. Anderson RG: Facial nerve disorders, *Select Readings in Plastic Surgery* 6:1-34, 1991.
5. Balliet R: Facial paralysis and other neuromuscular dysfunction of the peripheral nervous system. In Payton OD, DiFabio RP, Paris SV, et al, editors: *Manual of physical therapy,* New York, 1989, Churchill Livingstone.
6. Balliet R, Lewis L: Hypothesis: Craig's "face saving exercises" may cause facial dysfunction, Edmonton, Alberta, April 1985, *Canadian Acoustic Neuroma Association.*
7. Balliet R, Shinn JB, Bach-y-Rita P: Facial paralysis rehabilitation: retraining selective muscle control, *Int Rehabil Med* 4:67-74, 1981.
8. Barat M: Principles of rehabilitation in facial paralysis. In Portmann M, editor: *Facial nerve,* New York, 1985, Masson.
9. Berkow R: *The Merck manual of diagnosis and therapy,* ed 15, Rahway, NJ, 1987, Merck Sharp & Dohme Research Laboratories.
10. Brundy J, Hammerschlag PE, Cohen NL, et al: Electromyographic rehabilitation of facial function and introduction of a facial paralysis grading scale for hypoglossal facial nerve anastomosis, *Laryngoscope* 98:405-410, 1988.
11. Cicero: In Stevenson B, editor: *Macmillan book of proverbs, maxims and famous phrases,* New York, 1948, Macmillan.
12. Craig M: *Face saving exercises,* New York, 1970, Random House.
13. Diels HJ: Neuromuscular retraining for facial paralysis, issue no 55, Sept 1995, *Acoustic Neuroma Association,* Carlisle, Penn.
14. Diels HJ: New concepts in nonsurgical facial nerve rehabilitation. In Myers EN, Bluestone CD, editors: *Advances in otolaryngology—head and neck surgery,* vol 9, St Louis, 1995, Mosby.
15. Diels HJ: Unpublished data. In endnotes of Ref. 14.

16. Elks MA: Another look at facial disfigurement, *J Rehabil* (Jan to Mar):36-40, 1990.

17. Hause SL, Levitt LP, Weiner HL: *Case studies in neurology for the house officer,* Baltimore, 1986, Williams & Wilkins.

18. Hause WA, Karnes WE, Annis J, et al: Incidence and prognosis of Bell's palsy in the population of Rochester, Minnesota, *Mayo Clin Proc* 46:258-264, 1971.

19. Hoos L, Devriese PP: The management of psychological problems of patients with facial paralysis. In Portmann M, editor: *Facial nerve,* New York, 1985, Masson.

20. Jansen JKS, Lomo T, Nicolaysen K, et al: Hyperinnervation of skeletal muscle fibers: dependence on muscle activity, *Science* 181:559-561, 1973.

21. Kahn J: *Principles and practice of electrotherapy,* ed 2, New York, 1991, Churchill Livingstone.

22. Kottke FJ: Therapeutic exercise to develop neuromuscular coordination. In Kottke FJ, Lehmann JF, editors: *Krusen's handbook of physical medicine and rehabilitation,* ed 4, Philadelphia, 1990, WB Saunders.

23. May J: Microanatomy and pathophysiology of the facial nerve. In May M, editor: *The facial nerve,* New York, 1986, Thieme.

24. May M, Klein SR: Differential diagnosis of facial nerve palsy, *Otolaryngol Clin North Am* 24(3):615-616, 1991.

25. May M, Podvinec M, Ulrich J, et al: Idiopathic (Bell's) palsy, herpes zoster cephalicus and other facial nerve disorders of viral origin. In May M, editor: *The facial nerve,* New York, 1986, Thieme.

26. Mendel GL, Douglas XX, Bennet JE: *Principles and practice of infectious diseases,* ed 3, New York, 1990, Churchill Livingstone.

27. Netter FH: *The CIBA collection of medical illustrations, vol 1: Nervous system,* part 2, Summit, NJ, 1986, CIBA-Geigy.

28. Peitersen E: The nature history of Bell's palsy, *Am J Otol* 4:107-111, 1982.

29. Ross B, Nedzelski JM, McLean JA: Efficacy of feedback training in long-standing facial nerve paresis, *Laryngoscope* 101:744-750, 1991.

30. Sataloff RT, Myers DL, Kremer FB: Management of cranial nerve injury following surgery of the skull base, *Otolaryngol Clin North Am* 17:577-589, 1984.

31. Schram G, Burres S: Nonsurgical rehabilitation after facial paralysis. In Portmann M, editor: *Facial nerve,* New York, 1985, Masson.

32. Stevens H: Melkersson's syndrome, *Neurology,* 15:263-266, 1965.

33. Twerski A, Twerski B: The emotional impact of facial paralysis. In May M, editor: *The facial nerve,* New York, 1986, Thieme.

34. Data compiled from the University of Wisconsin Neuromuscular Retraining Clinic fact sheet.

35. Valls-Sole J, Tolosa ES, Pujol M: Myokymic discharges and enhanced facial nerve reflex responses after recovery from idiopathic facial palsy, *Muscle Nerve* 15:37-42, 1992.

RECOMMENDED READING

Adour KK: Medical management of idiopathic (Bell's) palsy, *Otolaryngol Clin North Am* 24(3):663, 1991.

Balliet R: Facial paralysis and other neuromuscular dysfunctions of the peripheral nervous system. In Payton OD, DiFabio RP, Paris, SV, et al: *Manual of physical therapy,* New York, 1989, Churchill Livingstone.

Balliet R, Lewis L: Hypothesis: *Craig's "Face Saving Exercises" may cause facial dysfunction,* Edmonton, Alberta, April 1985, Acoustic Neuroma Association of Canada.

Balliet R, Shinn JB, Bach-Y-Rita P: Facial paralysis rehabilitation: retraining selective muscle control, *Int Rehabil Med* 4:67-74, 1991.

Diels HJ: Neuromuscular retraining for facial paralysis, issue no 55, Sept 1995, Acoustic Neuroma Association, Carlisle, Penn.

Diels HJ: New concepts in nonsurgical facial nerve rehabilitation. In Myers EN, Bluestone CD, editors: *Advances in otolaryngology–head and neck surgery,* vol 9, St Louis, 1995, Mosby.

Hauser SL, Levitt LP, Weiner HL: *Case studies in neurology for the house officer,* Baltimore, 1986, Williams & Wilkins.

Kahn J: *Principles and practice of electrotherapy,* ed 2, New York, 1990, Churchill Livingstone.

May M: Differential diagnosis of facial nerve palsy, *Otolaryngol Clin North Am* 24(3):613, 1991.

For more information regarding facial retraining, the reader is referred to: Neuromuscular retraining clinic. University of Wisconsin Hospital & Clinics, 2710 Marshall Court, Madison WI 53705.

24

Right Ape-Hand Deformity and Left Clawhand Deformity after Accident in Which Both Hands Were Thrust through a Glass Window

A 25-year-old man has visited from a third-world country and is referred to your hand clinic for evaluation of hand dysfunction. The hand surgeon, your associate, has not yet arrived but has left instructions asking you to begin the examination. The patient sustained a gunshot wound to the right upper trapezius muscle some 3 months ago while discovering a burglar in his home. He attempted to flee by punching out a glass window with both his hands and fell from a height of 6 feet only to dislocate his left shoulder. He was treated at the local emergency room. The significant results of your evaluation yielded the following data:

OBSERVATION   A right-shoulder droop is observed. The patient points to a scar site from the bullet at the superficial midcourse of the right upper trapezius muscle. The patient's hands appear as in Fig. 24-1.

PALPATION   When asking the patient to isometrically contract his left deltoid, a soft, noncontractile sensation is imparted to your hands, as compared to the contralateral deltoid.

RANGE OF MOTION   Within functional limits throughout the patient's extremities, except to the left shoulder, which demonstrates only 60° of shoulder elevation.

MUSCLE STRENGTH   Within normal limits throughout, except to left shoulder flexion, abduction, and extension, which score fair plus. Left external shoulder rotation scores good minus. When asked to shrug his right shoulder, he appears to do so at only half the height of the contralateral shoulder. His left-hand intrinsic muscles exhibit a poor plus grade, and his right hand exhibits an inability to oppose or flex his thumb. There is wasting of the right thenar eminence.

SENSATION   The patient is insensate only over a round area over the left middle deltoid muscle (Fig. 24-2).

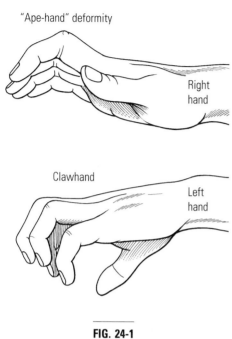

"Ape-hand" deformity

Right hand

Clawhand

Left hand

FIG. 24-1

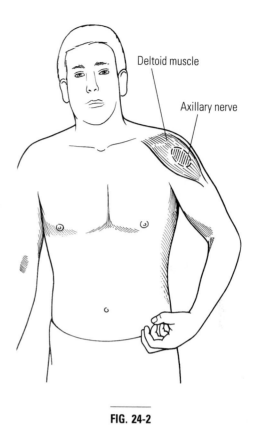

Deltoid muscle

Axillary nerve

FIG. 24-2

? Questions

1. What pattern of nerve injury has occurred to this man's hands?
2. What is the anatomy of the peripheral nerve?
3. What protective mechanism affords the peripheral nerve protection from compressive force?
4. What protective mechanism affords the peripheral nerve protection from tensile force?
5. What protective mechanisms are inherent in the vascular supply of the nerves?
6. What is the classification of peripheral nerve injury?
7. What is a first-degree injury to a peripheral nerve?
8. What is a second-degree nerve injury?
9. What is a third-degree peripheral nerve injury?
10. What are the mechanisms of nerve injury?
11. What are clinical examples of the acute compression mechanism of nerve injury?
12. What are clinical examples of the chronic compression mechanism of nerve injury?
13. What are clinical examples of the stretch injury mechanism of nerve injury?
14. What effect does an electrical injury have on the peripheral nerve?
15. How common are injection injuries to nerve tissue?
16. What happens to a nerve during a partial or complete transection from a knife stabbing?
17. What is the sequence of a progressive stretch of nerve resulting in rupture?
18. What is the difference between gunshot and shotgun wound injuries to the peripheral nerve?
19. What is long thoracic nerve palsy?
20. How does the spinal accessory nerve differ from other cranial nerves, and which muscles does it innervate?

21. What are the divisions and function of the trapezius muscle?
22. What is spinal accessory nerve palsy?
23. What is high median nerve entrapment?
24. What is the second most frequent upper extremity compressive neuropathy occurring after carpal tunnel syndrome?
25. What is the cause of tardy ulnar palsy?
26. What compressive neuropathy is associated with Guyon's tunnel?
27. What are the causes of injury to the ulnar nerve at Guyon's tunnel?
28. How is ulnar nerve compression at the wrist differentiated from a lesion at the elbow region?
29. What kind of injury results in radial nerve injury?
30. What are the clinical signs and symptoms of musculocutaneous nerve injury in the axilla?

31. What is the therapeutic management of nerve injury?
32. What is the efficacy of electrical stimulation to denervated musculature?
33. What is the faradic electrical stimulation technique to denervated musculature?
34. What is slow-pulse stimulation to denervated musculature?
35. What are four different operative procedures for nerves?
36. What are the goals of postoperative rehabilitation?
37. What is the role of motor reeducation after peripheral neurosurgery?
38. What is the role of sensory reeducation after microneurocoaptation?

1. What pattern of nerve injury has occurred to this man's hands?

- The patient's left-hand deformity is a combination of both median and ulnar nerve palsy with flexion of the proximal and distal interphalangeal joints and hyperextension of the metacarpophalangeal joints in what is known as *clawhand* or *clawfingers* (see Fig. 19-9). This deformity results from the loss of intrinsic muscle action and simultaneous overaction of the extrinsic extensor muscles. This deformity also occurs in syringomyelia.

- This is an *ape-hand deformity* of the right hand in which median nerve palsy causes thenar wasting such that the thumb falls into the plane of the fingers because of the overpull of the extensors. The patient is also unable to oppose or flex the thumb. This deformity may also accompany syringomyelia and amyotrophic lateral sclerosis.

  The patient's pattern of proximal muscle weakness implies damage to the axillary nerve, corresponding to paresis of the deltoid muscle as well as the teres minor muscle. Damage to this nerve may have been incurred from a shoulder dislocation as the humeral head pressed upon the posterior cord. This damage is confirmed by loss of sensation over the cutaneous distribution of that nerve. Additionally the droopy right shoulder, decreased ability to shrug the shoulder, and scar presence whose entry and exit sites correspond to the course of the spinal accessory nerve are suggestive of injury to that nerve.

2. What is the anatomy of the peripheral nerve?

Three kinds of nerve fibers are carried in the peripheral nerve—motor, sensory, and autonomic fibers. Several nerve axons running together form a densely packed bundle called a fascicle. There are three separate and distinct connective tissue elements serving as supportive tissue sheaths that are associated with nerve fascicles: *endoneurium, perineurium,* and *epineurium* (Fig. 24-3). These connective tissue sheaths facilitate a physiologic and a mechanical function of protecting the axons from excessive tensile force by virtue of their longitudinal collagen fiber orientation.[1]

The innermost viscous *endoneurium* resides between the fibers composing the individual fascicle. The next level of organization is the *perineurium* type of connective tissue that hugs each fascicle providing skeletal support, primarily tensile strength, to the enclosed neural tissue. The final supportive ensheathment is the outermost *epineurium* that surrounds, cushions, protects, and keeps the individual fascicles separate while collectively binding them together into a nerve trunk (Fig. 24-4). The outer epineurium facilitates gliding between fascicles, a necessary adaptation to accommodate extremity movement, especially when a peripheral nerve has to bend to an acute angle during limb movement. More epineural tissue is found where nerve trunks cross joints, or in tunnel areas such as the carpal tunnel.[1]

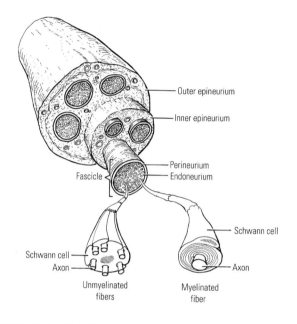

FIG. 24-3 Schema of peripheral nerve architecture. The connective tissue elements consist of the endoneurium, the perineurium, and the inner and outer epineuriums. Individual fascicles contain a heterogeneous mix of myelinated and unmyelinated fibers. (From Terzis JK, Smith KL: *The peripheral nerve: structure, function and reconstruction*, New York, 1990, Raven Press.)

3. What protective mechanism affords the peripheral nerve protection from compressive force?

Fascicles within the *epineurium* run a wavy course and constantly change position within the nerve trunk in what can be described as a fascicular mesh (Fig. 24-5). This arrangement affords both compressive and tensile protection. Furthermore, when a greater number of fascicles are present, a nerve is afforded better protection from compressive force. For example, at the knee crease the common peroneal nerve is composed of approximately eight fascicles, yet only a few centimeters distally at the head of the fibula there are approximately 16 fascicles, since the nerve is more likely to fall subject to external compressive force at that locale.[1]

4. What protective mechanism affords the peripheral nerve protection from tensile force?

The peripheral nerve attenuates applied tension by initially stretching out the undulations that compose the epineurium and the perineurium.[4] The *perineurium's* outer sheath is composed of collagen fibers that lie in three orientations: circumferential, longitudinal, and oblique.[27,28] As tension is applied, the perineurium lengthens because of the oblique perineurial fibers, much in the same way as a "Chinese finger trap."[26] Thus the epineurium lengthens but does so at the expense of creating a compressive force along the length of the nerve by way of increased intrafascicular pressures.[25,29]

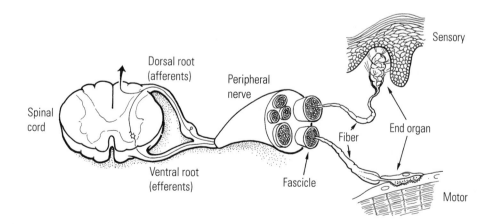

FIG. 24-4 The architecture of the peripheral nerve with central and peripheral connections. (From Terzis JK, Smith KL: *The peripheral nerve: structure, function and reconstruction*, New York, 1990, Raven Press.)

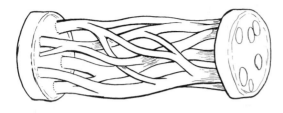

FIG. 24-5 Fascicular organization of the peripheral nerve. (From Terzis JK, Smith KL: *The peripheral nerve: structure, function and reconstruction*, New York, 1990, Raven Press.)

5. What protective mechanisms are inherent in the vascular supply of the nerves?

The peripheral nerve relies on continuous aerobic metabolism and is extremely susceptible to ischemia in the event of compression. In compensation of this vulnerability, the peripheral nerve is nourished by two integrated but functionally independent vascular systems referred to as the extrinsic and the intrinsic systems.[26] The arteries and veins composing the extrinsic system additionally possess the added advantage of being coiled in nature. This tortuous appearance in fact serves as a "reserve in length," which allows the nerve significant freedom of movement before the vessels become stretched and suffer traction injury.[17]

6. What is the classification of peripheral nerve injury?

Both Sedon and Sunderland developed classification schemes based on the direct relationship of prognosis for functional return as it correlates with the degree of intraneural disruption (Fig. 24-6). Sedon's triad classification includes neurapraxia, axonotmesis, and neurotmesis in increasing order of nerve injury.[26] Sunderland introduced a fourth- and a fifth-degree injury as part of the spectrum of nerve disorder. These latter types represent gradations of injury necessitating surgical intervention and are based upon integrity of the supporting elements of the nerve.

7. What is a first-degree injury to a peripheral nerve?

The first and most benign gradation of nerve injury is known as *neurapraxia* and describes the least type of injurious injury. Neurapraxia is defined as a *local conduction block* at a singular focal segment along a nerve because of compression or traction of the myelin sheath surrounding that nerve. However, because axonal continuity is maintained, axoplasmic transport is maintained, and the involved nerve remains capable of stimulation distal to the level of the lesion.[26] There is no evidence of wallerian degeneration, and electromyographic examination fails to demonstrate any electrical activity at rest. There will be no evidence of fibrillations or sharp positive waves seen if the patient is still paralyzed 3 weeks from onset.[26] Neurapraxia clinically manifests as motor loss that may be quite profound. Additionally, there is also a partial sensory loss and little or no sympathetic disturbance.[15] Classic neurapraxias include tardy ulnar palsy, Saturday night palsy, crutch palsy, or even one's foot falling asleep, with duration of paralysis from several moments to several weeks depending on how long the myelin sheath was compromised. Complete recovery usually occurs within 10 weeks and often less.[26]

8. What is a second-degree nerve injury?

Axonotmesis injury to the peripheral nerve exhibits all the characteristics of a first-degree injury, in addition to *disruption of the axon and myelin sheath with sparing of the Schwann sheath, endoneurium*, and successively larger subdivisions of the nerve.[15] Axonotmesis occurs from a more severe crush or traction injury or if the compression is severe or of such long-standing duration as to rupture the lamella of the myelin sheath and thus expose the unprotected axon to the direct brunt of compression. The resulting disability manifests as complete loss of motor and sensory function below the level of insult that is indistinguishable from a complete nerve transection. The segment of axon distal to the lesion suffers ischemia and begins to disintegrate some 3 to 5 days after the injury. The aforementioned was initially observed by Waller in the 1850s, hence the term *wallerian degeneration*. Corresponding electrical changes indicating denervation are observed after 3 weeks.[15] Fortunately, because the injury does not involve the endoneurial tube, attempted regrowth of the proximal part of the nerve may be guided back to reattach onto the distal portion of nerve at a growth rate of 1 mm per day, 1 cm per week, or approximately 1 inch per month.[4] The prognosis for recovery from second-degree nerve injury is excellent[15] because the return of function occurs within several months after the injury.

9. What is a third-degree peripheral nerve injury?

Neurotmesis involves complete severance of the axon and of the associated supporting connective tissue. This injury, like a second-degree injury, leads to wallerian

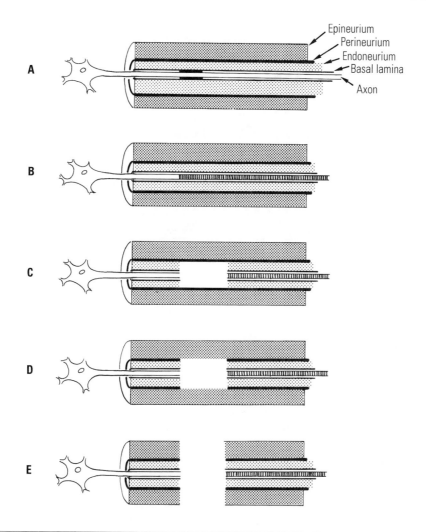

A

B

C

D

E

Epineurium
Perineurium
Endoneurium
Basal lamina
Axon

FIG. 24-6 Sunderland's classification of nerve injury. **A,** First-degree injury—local conduction blockade with minimal structural disruption. *Prognosis:* complete recovery within days to months. **B,** Second-degree injury—complete axonal disruption with wallerian degeneration. Basal lamina remains intact. *Prognosis:* complete recovery in months. **C,** Third-degree injury—axonal and endoneurial disruption with interruption of the basal lamina. *Prognosis:* intrafascicular axonal admixture with regeneration yields mild to moderate functional reduction. **D,** Fourth-degree injury—axonal, endoneurial, perineurial disruption. *Prognosis:* moderate to severe functional loss caused by interfascicular axonal admixture. Microsurgical manipulation can improve prognosis. **E,** Fifth-degree injury—complete structural disruption. *Prognosis:* no return without microsurgical manipulation. (From Terzis JK, Smith KL: *The peripheral nerve: structure, function, and reconstruction,* New York, 1990, Raven Press.)

degeneration of the axon but differs in that there is little chance for regrowth in the right direction. With a third-degree injury the loss of continuity of the supporting elements leaves the axon without directional guidance and results in misdirected axon growth. Without the benefit of an intact endoneurial tube the likelihood of blind axon sprouts reestablishing continuity with the appropriate end organ is remote.[26] This injury requires microsurgical intervention to reestablish continuity by means of fascicular realignment. Even then, the tips of the axons sprouting from the proximal stump often have little chance of being apposed with their correct endoneurial sheaths.[2] The result is often, at best, only an altered sensibility (Fig. 24-7). For example, heat or

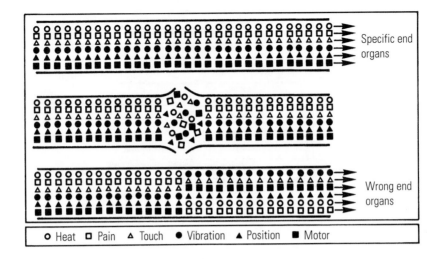

FIG. 24-7 Inappropriate reinnervation as a result of misdirected growth resulting in synkinesis. (From Dandy D: *Essential orthopaedics and trauma,* Churchill Livingstone, London, 1991.)

light touch may be experienced as pain because the incorrectly innervated patch of skin is hypersensitive.[3] Electromyographic findings after neurotmesis are the same as those observed after a second-degree injury, with additional or no action potentials on attempted voluntary contraction[15] of the denervated muscle.

10. What are the mechanisms of nerve injury?

The various mechanisms of nerve injury include acute and chronic compression, ischemia, traction, x radiation, inadvertent injection injury, or electrical injury. The common pathophysiologic denominator is mechanical deformation or ischemia-induced metabolic failure, or both.[26] An academic debate continues as to which factor contributes to nerve demise in certain mechanisms. Perhaps both factors are operative or even additive in their contribution toward nerve insult. Additionally, each category of injury carries with it a different prognosis. Thus, despite the fact that at the time of acute injury, there are clinical manifestations of numbness, pain, paralysis, or paresthesias, they by themselves shed very little light on the pathophysiologic course and ultimate prognosis. Because of this uncertainty, it is imperative that the examining clinician understand the nature and mechanism of injury.[26]

11. What are clinical examples of the *acute compression* mechanism of nerve injury?

Acute compression of the nerve is defined as any heavy force that compresses a nerve against an unyielding structure. Injury from this mechanism may take the

form of internal or external compression. Clinical examples of this class of nerve injury include high-velocity gunshot wounds or blast shrapnel wounds with severe fractures in which bone fragments compress the nerve, inadvertent crush by clamps or forceps during misguided attempts at hemostasis during surgery, and lengthy high-pressure tourniquet application.

12. What are clinical examples of the *chronic compression* mechanism of nerve injury?

Examples of *chronic internal compression* mechanisms of injury include tumors, ganglia, or callus. Carpal tunnel syndrome is another example of an internal chronic compression neuropathy. Whereas an example of a *chronic external compression* mechanism includes the comatose person whose nerve is compromised by pressure against a bed rail, a patient with chronic compression neuropathy rarely reports a history of trauma, and a great many present with complaints of pain, paresthesia, and weakness.

13. What are clinical examples of the *stretch injury* mechanism of nerve injury?

Nerve-stretch injuries are associated with fractures, fracture-dislocations, dislocations, obstetric trauma, and occasionally the state after inadvertent retraction during surgery. Stretch resulting in rupture or avulsion more commonly occurs with obstetrical brachial plexus injury than with peripheral stretch injury because spinal nerve roots lack perineurium. Spinal nerves thus represent a weak link in the peripheral nervous system by not having the protective cover of this middle nerve sheath.[25]

14. What effect does an electrical injury have on the peripheral nerve?

Electrical injury involves complicated and as-yet un-elucidated pathophysiologic features that clinically present from minor to life threatening. The most common site of electrical injury is the upper extremity by high-voltage linemen or by the home do-it-yourself handyman who contacts electrical lines with a metal ladder or while attempting to install an antenna.[7,21,22] Lightning strike injuries are exceedingly rare.[21]

Electrical current follows the path of least resistance, and resistance to flow increases in various tissues in the following order: nerve, blood vessels, muscle, skin, tendon, fat, and bone. Electrical current often follows the paths of existing neurovascular bundles and creates extensive deep (that is, subfascial) tissue destruction that is compounded by flash thermal burns at entrance and exit sites. The movement of current often enters peripherally at the neurovascular bundles and moves centrally. Subarachnoid bleeding is common. Patients are at risk for developing ischemic compartment syndrome. This horrible injury is further compounded by the often violent tetanic contractions accompanying electrocution that result in hemorrhage from muscle rupture or bone fracture, as muscles pull too hard on their bones. A major pathologic change is the conversion of electric energy to heat energy, resulting in coagulation necrosis. Electrical injuries are associated with a high percentage of extremity amputations.[7]

The resultant neurologic deficit occurring after electric injury is of immediate onset and typically involves the motor nerves, though the reason for this specificity is unclear. Although most injured nerves show some recovery with time, complete resolution is uncommon.

15. How common are injection injuries to nerve tissue?

Peripheral nerve injection injuries are all too common and are fraught with medicolegal overtones because of their frequent iatrogenic cause. Because of this, the tendency is not to publish such events, and the true incidence and outcome of nerve injection injury is probably unknown.[12] The cause of injury has been shown to be the result of injection of a neurotoxic substance and not the result of mechanical needle injury. This was confirmed in studies where repeated injection with normal saline failed to produce injury.[12,21]

The history of nerve injection injury is typical. The patient often complains of severe pain at the injection site, which radiates along the distribution of that nerve and is associated with neurologic deficit. For the first 3 months after the injury, observation is appropriate, and electrophysiologic studies are obtained approximately 6 weeks after the injury. Careful evaluation for clinical evidence of return is appropriate at 3-week intervals. Repeat electrodiagnostics are appropriate if no clinical evidence of return of function has occurred after 3 months.[12]

Early exploration with irrigation of the offending agent and external neurolysis is neither helpful nor indicated. Surgical exploration is indicated only after 4 months if no clinical recovery has occurred.

16. What happens to a nerve during a partial or complete transection from a knife stabbing?

A laceration of peripheral nerve results in a clearly defined area of motor sensory and autonomic deficit that results from an open wound caused by a low-velocity sharp instrument. Less often, these injuries may occur in a closed wound secondary to a fracture. A gap between the proximal and distal ends of the nerve occurs and is bridged by scar tissue. This situation will not improve without microsurgical intervention.[26]

17. What is the sequence of a progressive stretch of nerve resulting in rupture?

To sustain mechanical injury, the longitudinal stretch imposed upon a nerve must exceed the inherent limits of elasticity of that nerve. The sequence of compromise of the supporting elements of the peripheral nerve and finally of the nerve itself occurs along the following progression. Tension is first resisted by the outermost epineurium by way of stretching out redundant fascicular folds composing this outermost nerve cover. Tension is next withstood by the perineurium directly as a function of the number of fascicles within that middle protective nerve cover. The undulations composing this middle nerve cover similarly lengthen in an attempt to attenuate tensile force. Tensile force is also withstood by the orientation of collagen fibers making up the outer sheath of the perineurium. During the elongation of perineurium, axons begin to break and retract proximally and distally. Once perineurial rupture is complete, the proximal and distal nerve stumps are rapidly separated, since no strength is afforded by the endoneurium, myelin, or axons.[26]

18. What is the difference between gunshot and shotgun wound injuries to the peripheral nerve?

Gunshot wounds often involve "near-misses" of the nerves by *low-velocity* large bullets (200 msec) generating shock waves in soft tissue. These bullets drill a clean hole through soft tissue and occasionally cartwheel, in which case more damage is incurred. The cavitation that occurs here creates oscillation of wounded tissue that results in alternate stretching[15] and relaxation of the peripheral nerve as cavitation proceeds. The resultant nerve injury is of the first-degree type, in which focal conduction block without axon degeneration occurs after local stretching of the nerve.

On the other hand, *shotgun* wounds are a result of a high energy–*high velocity* (1000 msec) weapon, in which smaller projectiles can create massive injuries. When the muzzle velocity of a projectile reaches and exceeds the speed of sound, kinetic energy becomes proportional to the cube of velocity, and tissue damage, in turn, becomes largely dependent on velocity. What this translates into is that a small but high-velocity bullet causes severe intraneural disruption for a span of several centimeters proximal and distal to its path, rather than just focally, by means of *compressive force.* If cavitation follows, the subatmospheric pressures that follow the compressive way only compound the injury. With shotgun wounds, the nerve is frequently transected in close to 50% of cases and, if not, is often partially lacerated from adjacent shards of bone in associated bone fractures or is severely contused.[26]

19. What is long thoracic nerve palsy?

The *long thoracic nerve* exits from the pre-plexus locale, immediately after the exit of the C5, C6, and C7 nerve roots from the intervertebral foramina. Innervating the serratus anterior, this nerve falls heir to lesions from a variety of mechanisms resulting in paralysis of that muscle. Thus *isolated serratus palsy* may occur after viral illness, stab wounds, as a neuritis sequel to deltoid muscle serum immunization, recumbency for a prolonged period,[8] from infections such as diphtheria and infectious mononucleosis, or from prolonged wearing of a knapsack.

Isolated serratus palsy may occur after closed trauma to the upper limb or shoulder girdle by way of a traction lesion of the long thoracic nerve. Open injury of the long thoracic nerve is unusual, except when occurring as a complication of either breast surgery for cancer, or surgery done to relieve thoracic outlet compression.[15]

Some patients may become aware of a problem possibly because of significant shoulder pain coupled with difficulty in raising the arm, or they may suddenly realize that their scapula is winging (Fig. 24-8) because of an uncomfortable feeling when sitting in a high-backed chair. The loss of stabilization that the serratus conveys to the scapula alters the precise and interre-

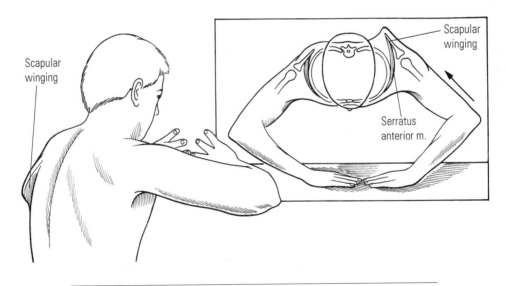

FIG. 24-8 Scapular winging caused by deinnervation of the serratus anterior muscle.

lated synchrony of balance in those muscles of the shoulder girdle. This altered biomechanical milieu results in less-than-ideal mechanical efficiency to those muscles originating on the scapula and will result in diminished shoulder elevation or even pain.[15]

The prognosis for recovery after closed injury or an atraumatic cause is usually favorable. If paralysis persists for a year, however, without any clinical or electromyographic evidence of recovery, the prognosis is poor. Complete paralysis after an open injury has a poor outlook for recovery. During the time waiting for recovery appropriate therapy includes joint mobilization to the scapulothoracic joint as well as all the major joints of the shoulder girdle to forestall the effects of stiffness, stretching, and strengthening of the muscles of the shoulder girdle so as to prevent their readjustment in length attributable to scapular winging, as well as electric stimulation to the motor point of the serratus anterior to maintain the contractility of the fibers of that muscle. Additionally, some patients experience relief from the dragging, painful feeling in the shoulder by the wearing of a pelvic-support orthosis.[5] There are good surgical options for the patient with poor prognosis that involve tendon transfers of the pectoralis minor or major muscles to the vertebral scapular border. Results of surgery are good in terms of pain relief, loss of winging, and return of function.[13]

20. How does the spinal accessory nerve differ from other cranial nerves, and which muscles does it innervate?

The *spinal accessory nerve* is only one of the cranial nerves that supplies muscles outside the head region but rather adjacent to the head in the neck and shoulder girdle. The name of this eleventh cranial nerve derives from the close structural continuity of this nerve root with the tenth cranial nerve. In fact, the eleventh cranial nerve has a dual origin from the spinal root contributions of cervical nerves C1 to C4 and a cranial nerve root contribution from the vagus nerve; hence our nerve is said to be an *accessory* to the vagus nerve.

The spinal accessory nerve is a motor nerve that innervates the sternocleidomastoid muscle and facilitates contraction that tilts the head ipsilaterally and rotates the head contralaterally. It also innervates the powerful trapezius muscle because of the following developmental reason. Embryologically the trapezius starts out as a high neck muscle and descends caudally on the neck and back during fetal elongation; as a result

the muscle drags down along its original source of innervation deriving from the head.

21. What are the divisions and function of the trapezius muscle?

The *trapezius* is a three-part back muscle that is the most superficial of muscles of the shoulder girdle. Although all three divisions of this muscle originate from essentially the same location, they are distinguished one from the other by their different distal attachment. Although the upper fibers of this muscle act to elevate the shoulder girdle by means of their distal attachment on the clavicle, the lower fibers act to depress the shoulder girdle by means of their distal attachment on the scapula. The paradox that emerges from these contradictory anatomic functions is clarified in the context of kinesiologically understanding the function of the trapezius as a *force couple* (Fig. 24-9). A force couple is defined as two forces working in opposite directions but acting on a single object so as to cause a rotational movement of that object. A familiar example is the turning of a steering wheel in an automobile with the driver's hands located at the 9 o'clock and 3 o'clock positions. If only one hand moved in one direction, the car would not turn, whereas the cooperative albeit diametrically opposed simultaneous movement does permit turning. Similarly, despite the seeming antagonism between the upper and lower fibers of this muscle, cocontraction manifests not as a tug of war but rather as rotation of the inferior angle of the scapula. This upward and outward mediolateral scapular rotation, known as *scapular protraction,* is facilitated by kinesiologic synergy between the upper and lower fibers of the trapezius. It is noteworthy to mention that the most important scapular protractor is the serratus anterior muscle.

The middle fibers of the trapezius do not retract the scapula despite their distal attachment on the root of the scapular spine; lateromedial scapular retraction is accomplished by the rhomboid muscles. The middle fibers instead elongate eccentrically to accommodate synergistic protraction.

22. What is spinal accessory nerve palsy?

Because the spinal accessory nerve is superficially located, it is quite vulnerable to injury,[15] as may occur from traction from a tight shoulder harness during a sudden stop from an automobile accident.[6] Because this nerve is so superficially located, it is also vulnerable to injury as a result of surgical operations to the neck. For

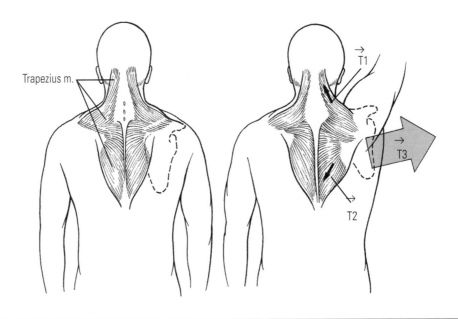

FIG. 24-9 Trapezius as a force couple. Graphical representation of vector subtraction of T_1 and T_2. T_3 represents the resultant displacement.

example, the nerve may be intentionally sacrificed during the course of a radical neck dissection for cancer. Inadvertent transection of this nerve may occur during the course of minor surgery to the neck area as from a lymph node biopsy.[30] Here the patient may not even realize that anything is wrong until several days after the biopsy when the pain of surgery should have receded, yet pain is still felt, especially when trying to elevate the shoulder. If complete paralysis of the trapezius persists both clinically and electromyographically for greater than 3 months, the nerve should be surgically explored. If the nerve is found to be caught up in scar tissue, neurolysis should be performed, whereas if a discontinuity is discovered, a suture or graft is appropriate if the gap cannot be closed without tension.[11]

The functional loss associated with spinal accessory nerve palsy includes torticollis with the head turned to the ipsilateral side and tilted contralaterally along with a drooping shoulder and an inability to shrug the shoulder ipsilaterally. Additionally the delicate balance of necessary length tension so important to normal shoulder kinesiology will have been altered because of injury of a significant scapular muscle. This will translate into a decreased ability of the scapula to glide synchronously and to provide the appropriate length ten-

sion to those muscles facilitating shoulder elevation. As a result there will be weakness of the shoulder abductors. Scapular winging may be accentuated by shoulder abduction and not by forward humeral flexion as seen in serratus anterior palsy.

23. What is high median nerve entrapment?

High median nerve entrapment includes proximal compression of that nerve in the region of the shoulder and proximal humerus as well as in the elbow region (pronator syndrome, see p. 27). The causes of injury at these sites are more often accidental in nature and may occur in the former following anterior shoulder dislocation. This mechanism, however, more often involves injury to the axillary nerve, which, unlike the median nerve, is unprotected by soft tissue. Another cause of high median nerve injury stems from the usage of improperly fitted axillary crutches by means of excessive external compression to that nerve; this mechanism may also injure the radial nerve. Finally, high median nerve compression may also occur alone or accompany radial and ulnar nerve palsies in inebriated individuals who happen to fall asleep while hanging their arms over a chair (Fig. 24-10) or park bench (Saturday night palsy).[28] Another mechanism contributing to high multiple nerve compression is *honeymoon palsy* in which a partner's

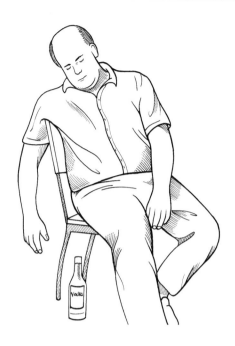

FIG. 24-10 Saturday night palsy: The radial and possibly median and ulnar nerves may be compressed by pressure from the backrest of a chair.

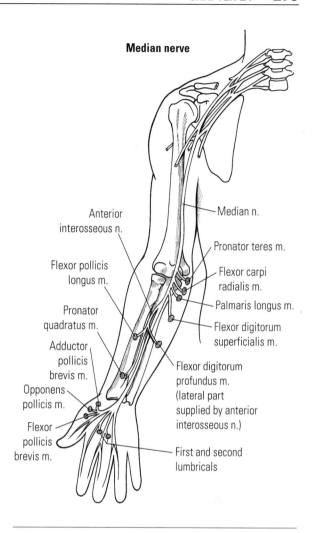

Median nerve

Anterior interosseous n.

Flexor pollicis longus m.

Pronator quadratus m.

Adductor pollicis brevis m.

Opponens pollicis m.

Flexor pollicis brevis m.

Median n.

Pronator teres m.

Flexor carpi radialis m.

Palmaris longus m.

Flexor digitorum superficialis m.

Flexor digitorum profundus m. (lateral part supplied by anterior interosseous n.)

First and second lumbricals

FIG. 24-11 Median nerve distribution and innervated musculature.

head presses on the brachial axillary angle or medial aspect of the arm.

The functional deficit associated with high median nerve lesions include significant compromise of forearm pronation as a result of paralysis of the pronator quadratus, though weak pronation can still be initiated by the brachioradialis and aided by gravity. Wrist flexion is weak, and there is weakness or absence of flexion of the interphalangeal joint of the thumb and of the proximal and distal interphalangeal joints of the index finger,[40] since the muscles producing these movements are supplied by the median nerve after it enters the forearm. Median nerve injuries spare flexion of the metacarpophalangeal joints, which are controlled by the ulnar innervated muscles. Proximal median nerve injury also results in a loss of sensation on the lateral portion of the palm, the palmar surface of the thumb, and the lateral two and one-half fingers.[18]

When a *Saturday night palsy* type of injury involves the median nerve alone, flexion of the distal interphalangeal joints of the ring and little fingers is unaffected, since the medial portion of the flexor digitorum profundus producing these movements is supplied by the ulnar nerve. However, the capacity to flex the metacarpopha-

langeal joints of the index and middle fingers will be compromised because the digital branches of the median nerve supply the first and second lumbrical muscles (Fig. 24-11).

A slightly different pattern of injury will manifest from median nerve injury occurring distally to the elbow in the forearm, as may occur from wounds to the forearm. When the median nerve is compromised in the cubital region, there will be loss of flexion of the proximal interphalangeal joints of all the digits as well as a loss of flexion of the distal interphalangeal joints of the index and middle fingers.[18]

The most common site of median nerve injury is distally just proximal to the flexor retinaculum, because of the frequency of wrist slashing from suicide attempts.[18]

24. What is the second most frequent upper extremity compressive neuropathy occurring after carpal tunnel syndrome?

Ulnar nerve entrapment at the elbow is the second most frequent upper extremity compression neuropathy. Whereas carpal tunnel syndrome is characterized by but not confined to sensory impairment, ulnar nerve entrapment results in motor loss that is characterized by considerably more significant disability. In the majority of cases of ulnar nerve lesion, initial symptoms are intermittent hypesthesia in the ulnar nerve distribution that is often associated with elbow flexion, whereas symptoms often abate when the patient extends his or her elbow. Use of the arm, especially in elbow flexion and extension, exacerbates symptoms. Patients are often awakened at night with elbow pain, shooting pain in the hand and fifth digit, and paresthesia and hypesthesia in the ulnar nerve distribution. Symptoms may vary from day to day and may even disappear for a period of time.[4] Signs of injury may include severe motor and sensory loss to the hand that include impaired power of ulnar deviation and impaired wrist flexion in the sense that the hand is drawn radially by the flexor carpi radialis when one is attempting to flex the wrist joint. In the hand there is difficulty in making a fist, since patients cannot flex their fourth and fifth digits at the distal interphalangeal joints. The resultant posture while attempting to make a fist is known as *main en griffe,* or *clawhand*[18] (see Fig. 24-12). The characteristic clinical sign of ulnar nerve damage is inability to adduct or abduct the medial four digits because of the loss of power of the interosseous muscles.[18]

The cause of ulnar nerve entrapment may be revealed by a history that includes elbow fracture or dislocation, acute blunt trauma at the medial epicondylar groove, or chronic occupational trauma in workers supporting themselves on their elbows; among such workers the neuropathy is more often seen on the nondominant side because the patient balances with one elbow while using the dominant arm for work.[4] Ulnar nerve trauma may also occur from chronic elbow arthritis in bedridden patients or after periods of unconsciousness as a result of intoxication, anesthesia, or coma caused by illness.[4] The most common site of ulnar nerve injury after insults to the forearm occurs where the nerve passes posteriorly to the medial humeral epicondyle. This most commonly occurs when the elbow hits a hard surface resulting in a medial epicondyle fracture.

More often than not, there is no history suggestive of a cause of compression, in which case the patient is diagnosed as having *cubital tunnel syndrome.* This syndrome is attributable to entrapment of the ulnar nerve between the fibrotic aponeurotic heads of the flexor carpi ulnaris. This aponeurotic band, arising from the medial humeral epicondyle and inserting on the medial border of the olecranon, represents a gateway through which the ulnar nerve enters the cubital tunnel to pass between the two heads of the flexor carpi ulnaris[4] (Fig. 24-13). The diameter of this tunnel is narrowly compromised upon elbow flexion for two separate reasons: (1) elbow flexion causes separation of the medial epicondyle and the olecranon; (2) during flexion, the medial collateral ligament bulges medially, causing further narrowing of the cubital tunnel diameter.[4]

Nonsurgical management entails avoidance of repetitive elbow flexion and extension, rest, or splinting

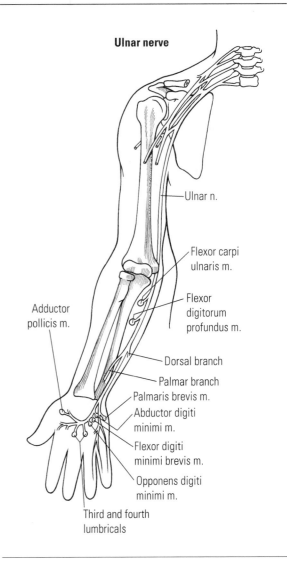

FIG. 24-12 Ulnar nerve distribution and innervated musculature.

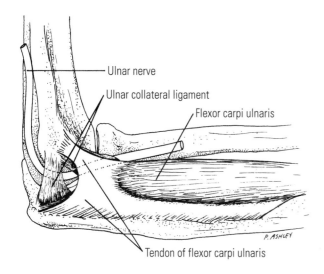

FIG. 24-13 Cubital tunnel. (From Magee DJ: *Orthopaedic physical assessment*, Philadelphia, 1987, Saunders.)

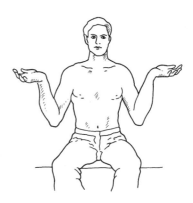

FIG. 24-14 The elbow flexion test for cubital tunnel syndrome. Symptoms may be reproduced or magnified by an upper extremity posture that places the ulner nerve on stretch. Superimposing additional components such as shoulder abduction, depression, and lateral rotation, as well as forearm supination, wrist extension, radial deviation, and contralateral neck flexion may further tense the nerve. (From Beuhler MJ, Thayer DT: The elbow flexion test: a clinical test for the cubital tunnel syndrome, *Clin Orthop* 233:213-216, 1988.)

the elbow in extension for a period of 2 to 3 months. The elbow flexion test for cubital tunnel syndrome provokes symptoms by placing the ulnar nerve on stretch (Fig. 24-14). Early diagnosis and treatment will result in complete cure.

25. What is the cause of tardy ulnar palsy?

Tardy ulnar palsy results from chronic stretch of that nerve secondary to a cubitus valgus deformity, often after a capitular fracture with arrest of the lateral humeral epiphysis and abnormal growth, or malalignment after supracondylar fracture.[4] A common cause of tardy ulnar palsy is chronic elbow arthritis in which the patient, in some cases, may have not noticed any elbow abnormality. When implicated, the patient typically lacks full elbow extension as compared with the contralateral side. Another mechanical cause of palsy is attributed to individuals with too shallow an olecranon fossa. This results in excessive movement of the nerve or even dislocation out of the groove during elbow flexion or extension.[24] Physical findings associated with ulnar nerve palsy include the following:

- Positive Froment's sign.[4] Loss of stability of the metacarpophalangeal joint as a result of ulnar paralysis causes metacarpophalangeal hyperextension with secondary interphalangeal joint flexion, which, together with weakness of the adductor pollicis, the flexor pollicis brevis, and the first dorsal interosseous muscle produces a thumb posture known as *Froment's sign* (Fig. 24-15).

- As the patient tries to pinch harder, the movement becomes less effective while the deformity accentuates.
- The ability to write deteriorates and becomes awkward as muscles weaken.
- Mild clawing and wasting of interosseous muscles.
- Weakness of flexor digitorum profundus of the fourth and fifth digits.
- An inability to adduct the index and pinky finger because of weakness of the volar interossei.
- Insidious onset of numbness and tingling in the little finger and ulnar half of the ring finger.[4]

Electrodiagnostic studies may show a nerve conduction block at the elbow. Nonsurgical management involves explicit instruction to the patient to keep his or her forearm in supination because this position will draw the ulnar nerve away from the site of pressure.[19]

26. What compressive neuropathy is associated with Guyon's tunnel?

Of the different ulnar nerve lesions near the wrist, the most common is compression of the *deep palmar branch* at the base of the palm where the ulnar nerve (and artery) enter the hand at the *ulnar tunnel* known as *canal de Guyon* (Fig. 24-16). Like the carpal tunnel, the

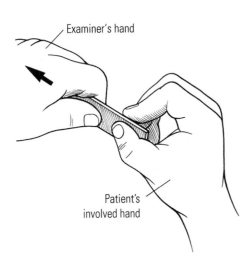

FIG. 24-15 Positive Froment's sign. *1,* Characteristic thumb posture on attempted pulp pinch between the thumb and adjacent digits. *2,* The patient is instructed to hold a sheet of paper between the thumb and index finger while the examiner attempts to pull it away. *3,* Weakness is attributable to diminished or absent innervation of the adductor pollicis, ulnar portion of flexor pollicis brevis, and the first dorsal interosseus. The former two muscles stabilize the metacarpophalangeal joint of the thumb. Weakness of the first dorsal interosseus results in impaired abduction of the index finger, which further impairs the pinch mechanism. The patient tries to retain the paper by flexing the thumb at the interphalangeal joint.

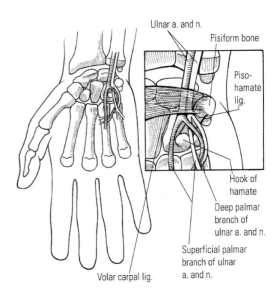

FIG. 24-16 Compression of the deep palmar branch of the ulnar nerve is shallow trough known as the ulnar tunnel. The walls of this tunnel are the pisiform and the hook of the hamate bone. The floor is bone covered by a carpetlike layer of ligament (pisohamate), and the roof of the trough is the volar carpal ligament and the palmaris brevis muscle.

ulnar tunnel is a closed space through which the ulnar nerve must pass. Located between the transverse carpal ligament and the volar carpal ligament, the bony parameters of this tunnel are defined by the pisiform medially and hook of the hamate laterally.[4] An ulnar lesion at this site may cause either motor or sensory symptoms, though the latter is less common. When present, sensory symptoms include wrist pain that radiates into the digits or forearm, is often worse at night, and is exacerbated by exercise or wrist motion.[4] Associated signs include Froment's sign, pronounced weakness of the first dorsal interosseous muscle, possible wasting between the thumb and the first finger, and weakened or absent flexion of the fourth and fifth digits. Ulnar nerve compression associated with Guyon's tunnel may occur at one of two sites. Proximal canal compression results in complete paralysis of all ulnar innervated intrinsic muscles. Long-term proximal compression results in

the typical *bishop's hand deformity* (Fig. 24-17) because of wasting of the hypothenar, interossei, and medial two lubricale muscles of the hand. Compression occurring distal to or at the level of the hook of the hamate results in the same pattern of muscle loss as before except for hypothenar function, which remains preserved.[4]

27. What are the causes of injury to the ulnar nerve at Guyon's tunnel?

Extrinsic causes of ulnar nerve compression at *Guyon's tunnel* may result from an acute blow over the hypothenar region, a laceration, or chronic occupational or avocational trauma resulting in a neuritis of that nerve. Injury commonly occurs to professional cyclists, pipe cutters, metal polishers, mechanics, from the repetitive use of pliers and screwdrivers or from using the palm as a hammer to put hubcaps back onto tires.[4] A characteristic callus at the base of the palm is often a good sign confirming such occupationally induced neuropathy. Injury may also occur after wrist fracture involving the pisiform, the body or hook of the hamate, or the metacarpals. Fracture injuries to the hamate are routinely ab-

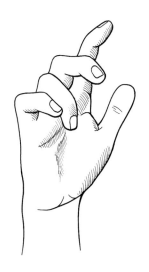

FIG. 24-17 Bishop's-hand deformity is named for its similarity to the ecclesiastical gesture of pronouncing benediction.

sent on radiographs and are discovered only by oblique views of the hand, lateral tomograms, bone scans, or computerized tomography.[4]

Intrinsic causes of injury include the presence of ganglions, ulnar artery diseases, scar tissue contracture, the presence of aberrant muscles, or pisiform bursitis.

Conservative management of the mild neuropathy includes the avoidance of inciting trauma with or without splinting. This generally results in complete return of function.[4]

28. How is ulnar nerve compression at the wrist differentiated from a lesion at the elbow region?

There are two ways in which elbow and wrist compression of the ulnar nerve are differentiated: (1) sparing of the flexor carpi ulnaris occurs when the nerve lesion originates at the wrist, and (2) there is normal dorsal ulnar sensation when the lesion originates at the wrist because the dorsal sensory branch bifurcates off the ulnar nerve some 6 to 8 cm proximal to the wrist.

29. What kind of injury results in radial nerve injury?

Injury to the *radial nerve* proximal to the origin of the triceps muscle results in paresis or paralysis of the triceps muscle, brachioradialis, supinator, and the extensors of the wrist, thumb, and fingers and is accompanied by sensory loss (Fig. 24-18). The characteristic clinical sign of radial nerve injury is *wristdrop,* defined as the inability to extend or straighten the wrist. This

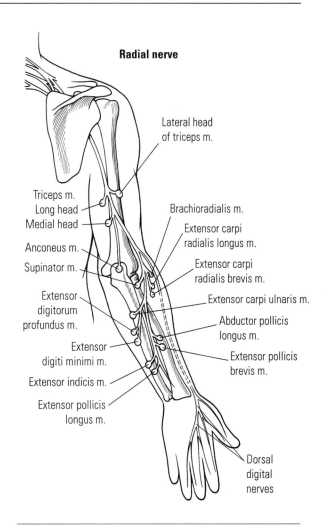

Radial nerve

Lateral head of triceps m.

Triceps m.
Long head
Medial head

Anconeus m.

Supinator m.

Extensor digitorum profundus m.

Extensor digiti minimi m.

Extensor indicis m.

Extensor pollicis longus m.

Brachioradialis m.

Extensor carpi radialis longus m.

Extensor carpi radialis brevis m.

Extensor carpi ulnaris m.

Abductor pollicis longus m.

Extensor pollicis brevis m.

Dorsal digital nerves

FIG. 24-18 Radial nerve distribution and innervated musculature.

may be confused with wristdrop after a stroke, especially when the onset is acute. Peripheral radial nerve palsy is differentiated from a focal central lesion in that fine movements of muscles innervated by the median and ulnar nerves are not affected with radial nerve lesions. Radial nerve palsy recovers in 8 to 12 weeks, provided that there is little or no axonal damage.

Radial nerve injury may also occur from deep wounds to the forearm, and severance of the deep branch of that nerve produces an inability to extend the thumb and the metacarpophalangeal joints of the fingers. There is no concomitant sensory loss, since the deep branch of this nerve is entirely muscular and articular in distribution. However, when the radial nerve proper or its superficial branch is cut, sensation will be lost on the posterior surface of the forearm, hand, and the proximal phalanges of the lateral three and one-half digits. However, just because there is no sensory loss experienced does not necessarily mean that the radial nerve is intact, because of the considerable overlap between the cutaneous nerves of the hand.[18]

When the radial nerve is injured at the radial groove, the triceps is not completely paralyzed, though other muscles supplied by that nerve distal to that groove suffer paralysis.

30. What are the clinical signs and symptoms of musculocutaneous nerve injury in the axilla?

Musculocutaneous nerve injury in the axilla from, say, a laceration, before its innervation of any musculature will result in paralysis of the coracobrachialis, biceps, and brachialis muscles. Functionally this manifests as significant weakening of elbow joint flexion and forearm supination. Both motions, however, will be somewhat preserved due to brachioradialis and supinator respectively. Additionally, there may also be sensory loss on the lateral surface of the forearm as a result of denervation of the lateral antebrachial cutaneous nerve.[20]

31. What is the therapeutic management of nerve injury?

Therapeutic management for nerve injury must attempt to maintain the appropriate range of the muscle or muscles innervated by the injured nerve, while helping prevent contracture in those muscles antagonistic to the denervated muscle by stretching. Joint mobilization is appropriate to the adjacent joints to stave off the development of joint stiffness. Muscle strengthening is appropriate to those uninjured agonistic and synergistic muscles.

32. What is the efficacy of electrical stimulation to denervated musculature?

There are no rigidly controlled human studies to prove the efficacy of electrotherapy. Animal studies have shown that direct electrical stimulation of denervated muscle was useful in retarding denervation atrophy for both type I and type II muscle fibers.[20] Electrical stimulation is appropriately applied to the motor points of the affected muscle to help maintain the state of contractility of that muscle. The intended strategy of electrical stimulation is artificially to allow the muscle to contract and, in this way, prevent muscle fibrosis until reinnervation permits normal muscle function.

33. What is the faradic electrical stimulation technique to denervated musculature?

One approach to electrical stimulation of denervated musculature is *interrupted direct current,* otherwise known as *galvanic current.* Before electrode placement, the skin site under the electrodes shoulder should be cleansed. The positive ground electrode is placed on the ipsilateral side of the body so as to minimize electrical resistance; however, the ground electrode is not to be placed too distant from the site of stimulation or on an antagonistic muscle group. With the stimulating electrode polarity set on negative the target muscle is stimulated at the motor point or slightly distally at 1-second intervals with about 20 repetitions. After a rest period the above procedure is repeated several times during each treatment session. Treatment is to be discontinued if and when the patient feels pain, skin irritation, or fatigue. After treatment, the skin areas under the electrodes should be massaged with an astringent (such as witch hazel) followed by a light dusting with talcum powder.[14]

Once regeneration has manifested clinically, electrical muscle stimulators may be utilized in lieu of faradic treatment. These units are mostly biphasic in nature (that is, of the alternating current type).

34. What is *slow-pulse stimulation* to denervated musculature?

Liberson developed a "slow-pulse stimulator" that delivers pulses at a rate of approximately 1 pulse every 10 seconds. This stimulator has a timer that limits applications to approximately 20 minutes, and this, unlike galvanic stimulation, has not been found harmful to the intervening skin or soft tissue. Treatment sessions are limited to 20 minutes each hour with an interval of at least an hour between sessions for a total stimulation time of 5 hours for adults and 3 hours for children per day.[16]

35. What are four different operative procedures for nerves? (See Fig. 24-19.)

- *Decompression* is the most commonly performed operation on nerves, such as median nerve decompression at the carpal tunnel.
- *Repair* of transected nerves by microsurgical suture of the perineurium.
- *Neurolysis.* Nerves can become enmeshed in dense scar tissue that tethers the nerve to bone or other tissue to such a degree that interference with function occurs. Neurolysis involves release of the nerve.

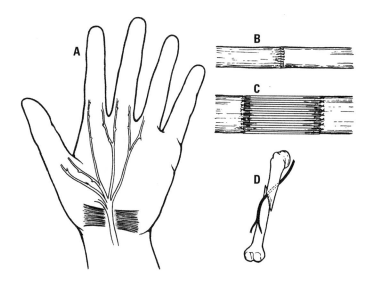

FIG. 24-19 Four different operative procedures for nerves. **A,** Decompression. **B,** Repair. **C,** Neurolysis. **D,** Grafting. (From Dandy DJ: *Essential orthopaedics and trauma,* Edinburgh, 1989, Churchill Livingstone.)

• *Grafting.* Large gaps in a nerve can be filled with a cable graft donated by a cutaneous nerve autograft such as the sural nerve. These operations are unreliable but are sometimes an attractive alternative to accepting serious disability.[3]

36. What are the goals of postoperative rehabilitation?

The whole purpose of immediate postoperative rehabilitation is the prevention of factors adverse to a satisfactory outcome.[26] This is accomplished by the maintenance of all involved structures in the best possible condition for reinnervation. The extent of therapy hinges on the magnitude of injury (Fig. 24-20). Obviously, a digital nerve laceration without any concomitant injury requires only little rehabilitation. On the other hand, a major proximal nerve injury will require a substantial amount of rehabilitation. A high degree of patient motivation is required for good therapeutic outcome.[26]

Joint range of motion and tendon excursion are maintained by passive joint motion, active assistive, active, and resistive exercise in that order. Insensate neurotrophic skin should be protected and kept supple by massage and appropriate moisturizers. Edema is appropriately addressed by edema-reducing strategies such as elevations, massage, and exercises.[26]

Substitution splinting in the form of passive or dynamic splints or a combination of both kinds of splints addresses the needs of remaining functional muscle groups and permits the gaining of stability so as to allow continued use of the extremity during the recovery period.[26]

37. What is the role of motor reeducation after peripheral neurosurgery?

Biofeedback is an especially important adjunct modality in the patient with a zero or grade 1 muscle function because it may help the patient to more quickly relearn control over those involved muscle groups. Biofeedback is essentially an external circuit that may actually help upgrade the function of denervated or partially denervated muscle function. Functional electrical stimulation is also helpful to the motor relearning process, in which the pattern of stimulation of weak, denervated muscle is included with a functional pattern of motion.[19,23]

38. What is the role of sensory reeducation after microneurocoaptation?

Regeneration of sensory nerve fibers are often imprecise, and the patient is faced with, at the very least, an unfamiliar volley of sensory input after repair. Without appropriate therapy, the patient may remain confused and unable to interpret these new patterns of sensory input leading to false localization and eventually absence of tactile gnosis. Sensory reeducation employs the use of higher cortical functions such as attention,

The most frequently encountered
causes of damage at the
various sites are indicated

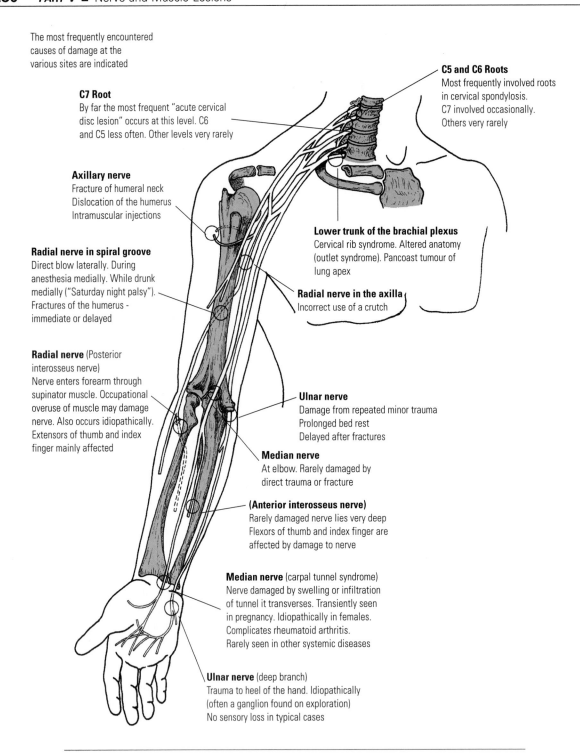

C5 and C6 Roots
Most frequently involved roots
in cervical spondylosis.
C7 involved occasionally.
Others very rarely

C7 Root
By far the most frequent "acute cervical
disc lesion" occurs at this level. C6
and C5 less often. Other levels very rarely

Axillary nerve
Fracture of humeral neck
Dislocation of the humerus
Intramuscular injections

Lower trunk of the brachial plexus
Cervical rib syndrome. Altered anatomy
(outlet syndrome). Pancoast tumour of
lung apex

Radial nerve in spiral groove
Direct blow laterally. During
anesthesia medially. While drunk
medially ("Saturday night palsy").
Fractures of the humerus -
immediate or delayed

Radial nerve in the axilla
Incorrect use of a crutch

Radial nerve (Posterior
interosseus nerve)
Nerve enters forearm through
supinator muscle. Occupational
overuse of muscle may damage
nerve. Also occurs idiopathically.
Extensors of thumb and index
finger mainly affected

Ulnar nerve
Damage from repeated minor trauma
Prolonged bed rest
Delayed after fractures

Median nerve
At elbow. Rarely damaged by
direct trauma or fracture

(Anterior interosseus nerve)
Rarely damaged nerve lies very deep
Flexors of thumb and index finger are
affected by damage to nerve

Median nerve (carpal tunnel syndrome)
Nerve damaged by swelling or infiltration
of tunnel it transverses. Transiently seen
in pregnancy. Idiopathically in females.
Complicates rheumatoid arthritis.
Rarely seen in other systemic diseases

Ulnar nerve (deep branch)
Trauma to heel of the hand. Idiopathically
(often a ganglion found on exploration)
No sensory loss in typical cases

FIG. 24-20 Common sites of nerve injury in the upper extremity. (From Patten J: *Neurologic differential diagnosis,* London, 1996, Springer-Verlag.)

learning, and memory to relearn the locale and identification of normal sensory input. For example, the patient's skin is stroked up and down with a firm, blunt object such as a pencil eraser. The patient sees what is happening and concentrates on the sensory input with his or her eyes closed so as to reconfirm the cause and localization of sensation. In such a fashion, each sensory submodality may be relearned.[26]

Once constant touch and moving submodalities are present in the previously numb area of the fingertips, late-phase sensory reeducation commences. The patient attempts to improve tactile gnosis by concentrating on the recognition of common objects of different shapes, textures, and sizes with his or her eyes open and closed. In such a fashion the patient memorizes the patterns of sensory input.[5]

REFERENCES

1. Butler DS: *Mobilisation of the nervous system,* Melbourne, 1991, Churchill Livingstone.
2. Cormack DH: *Introduction to histology,* Philadelphia, 1984, Lippincott.
3. Dandy DJ: *Essential orthopaedics and trauma,* Edinburgh, 1989, Churchill Livingstone.
4. Dawson DM, Hallet M, Millender LH: *Entrapment neuropathies,* ed 2, Boston, 1990, Little, Brown.
5. Dellon AL, Curtis RM, Edgerton MT: Reeducation of sensation in the hand after nerve injury and repair, *Plast Reconstr Surg* 53:297-304, 1974.
6. Diamond MC, Scheibel AB, Elson LM: *The human brain coloring book,* New York, 1985, Barnes & Noble.
7. Di Vinceti FC, Moncrief JA, Pruitt BA: Electrical injuries: a review of 65 cases, *J Trauma* 9:497-507, 1969.
8. Foo CL, Swann M: Isolated paralysis of the serratus anterior: a report of 20 cases, *J Bone Joint Surg* 65B:552-556, 1983.
9. Gentili F, Hudson AR, Hunter D, et al: Nerve injection injury with local anesthetic agents: a light and electron microscopic, fluorescent microscopic, and horseradish peroxidase study, *Neurosurgery* 6(3):263-272, 1980.
10. Gentili F, Hudson AR, Kline DG, et al: Peripheral nerve injection injury with steroid agents, *Plast Reconstr Surg* 69(3):482-489, 1982.
11. Harris HH, Dickey JR: Nerve grafting to restore function of the trapezius muscle after radial neck dissection, *Ann Otolaryngol* 74:880, 1965.
12. Hudson AR: Nerve injection injuries. In Terzis JK, editor: *Microreconstruction of nerve injuries,* Philadelphia, 1987, WB Saunders.
13. Jupiter J, Leffert RD: Non-union of the clavicle: associated complications and surgical management, *J Bone Joint Surg* 69A(5):753-760, 1987.
14. Kahn J: *Principles and practice of electrotherapy,* ed 2, New York, 1991, Churchill Livingstone.
15. Leffert RD: Neurological problems. In Hunter JM, Schneider LH, Mackin EJ, et al, editors: *Rehabilitation of the hand: surgery and therapy,* ed 3, St Louis, 1990, Mosby.
16. Liberson WT, Terzis JK: Contribution of neurophysiology and rehabilitation medicine to the management of brachial plexus palsy. In Terzis JK, editor: *Microreconstruction of nerve injuries,* Philadelphia, 1987, WB Saunders.
17. Lundborg G: The intrinsic vascularization of human peripheral nerves: structure and functional aspects, *J Hand Surg* 4(1):34, 1979.
18. Moore KL: *Clinically oriented anatomy,* ed 2, Baltimore, 1985, Williams & Wilkins.
19. Nelson AJ: Implications of electroneuromyographic examinations for hand therapy. In Hunter JM, Schneider LH, Mackin EJ, et al, editors: *Rehabilitation of the hand: surgery and therapy,* ed 3, St Louis, 1990, Mosby.
20. Pachter BR, Eberstein A, Goodgold J: Electrical stimulation effect on denervated muscle in rats: a light and electron microscope study, *Arch Phys Med Rehabil* 67:79-83, 1986.
21. Panse F: Electrical lesions of the nervous system. In Vinken PJ, Bruyn GW, editors: *Handbook of clinical neurology,* vol 7, New York, 1970, Elsevier.
22. Solem L, Fischer RP, Strate RG: The natural history of electrical injury, *J Trauma* 17(7):487-492, 1977.
23. Solomonow M: Restoration of movement by electrical stimulation: a contemporary view of the basic problems, *Orthopedics* 7(2):245-250, 1984.
24. Spillane JD, Spillane JA: *An atlas of clinical neurology,* ed 3, Oxford, 1982, Oxford University Press.
25. Sunderland S, Bradley KC: Stress-strain phenomenon in human peripheral trunks, *Brain* 84:102-119, 1961.
26. Terzis JK, Smith KL: The peripheral nerve: structure, function, and reconstruction, New York, 1990, Raven Press.
27. Thomas PK: The connective tissue of peripheral nerve: an electron microscopic study, *J Anat* 97:35, 1963.
28. Thomas PK, Olson Y: Microscopic anatomy and function of the connective tissue components of peripheral nerve. In Dyck PJ, Thomas PK, Lanber EH, editors: *Peripheral neuropathy,* Philadelphia, 1984, WB Saunders.
29. Wilgis EF, Murphy R: The significance of longitudinal excursion in peripheral nerves, *Hand Clin* 2(4):761-771, 1986.
30. Woodhall B: Trapezius paralysis following minor surgical procedures in the posterior cervical triangle, *Ann Surg* 136:375, 1952.

RECOMMENDED READING

Butler D: *Mobilisation of the nervous system,* Melbourne, 1991, Churchill Livingstone.
Dawson DM, Hallet M, Millender LH: *Entrapment neuropathies,* ed 2, Boston, 1990, Little, Brown & Co.
Kahn J: *Principles and practice of electrotherapy,* ed 2, New York, 1991, Churchill Livingstone.
Leffert RD: Neurological problems. In Hunter JM, Schneider LH, Mackin EJ, et al, editors: *Rehabilitation of the hand: surgery and therapy,* ed 3, St Louis, 1990, Mosby.
Liveson JA: *Peripheral neurology: case studies in electrodiagnosis,* ed 2, Philadelphia, 1991, FA Davis.
Patton J: *Neurological differential diagnosis,* ed 2, London, 1996, Springer-Verlag.
Spillane JD, Spillane JA: *An atlas of clinical neurology,* ed 3, Oxford, 1982, Oxford University Press.
Terzis JK, Smith KL: *The peripheral nerve: structure, function, and reconstruction,* New York, 1990, Raven Press.

25

Momentary Stabbing Pain in Groin and Ipsilateral Buttock and Loss of Ambulation after a Fall That Yanks the Ipsilateral Extended Leg into Excessive Abduction and Flexion

CASE 1: While skiing down an intermediate slope with a ski buddy in the Colorado Rockies, your friend loses control and falls in such a way as to position her left hip in exaggerated flexion and abduction with the knee straight out in extension. She cries out in anguish, and you run to help her as others seek emergency assistance. Before the arrival of the snowmobile that will deliver her to the medic at the first aid lodge, she tells you of a frightening and momentary stabbing pain in the left side of her groin and a pulling sensation near her left buttock at the moment of injury. As you help the ski patrol gently hoist her body out of its entangled posture, the sudden movement causes her to cry out and writhe in pain. Down at the lodge clinic the following clinical picture emerges during the examination.

OBSERVATION   The patient cannot walk because of pain and requires the use of crutches. There is slight ecchymosis and swelling over the proximal third of the upper inner and anterior thigh.

PALPATION   Moderate tenderness is present both at the left ischial tuberosity and over the upper third of the anterior left thigh within the muscular soft tissue.

PASSIVE RANGE OF MOTION   Passive left hip flexion and abduction are painful.

ACTIVE RANGE OF MOTION   Pain is elicited on active hip adduction while she is lying supine; active hip extension while in a side-lying or prone position. Antigravity hip extension is not possible.

MUSCLE STRENGTH   Judged to be fair plus, though adequate testing is hindered by the patient's pain.

RESISTED TESTS   Resisted adductor and knee extension are painful.

SPECIAL TESTS   Negative for knee stability. Radiographs taken show no evidence of fracture or avulsion and are otherwise normal appearing.

CASE 2: A 38-year-old male police officer takes his Great Dane out for a walk in the evening after work hours. While stopping at the corner to casually talk to a friend, he begins to feel a considerable tug on the leash held in his left hand. While talking and distracted, he pulls on the leash while widening his base of support by assuming a horse stance so as to counter the pull of his large dog. Eventually, his dog becomes frantic as another dog struts by only several feet past where dog and owner are standing, and the dog's barking culminates in a sideways lunge that forcefully yanks the owner sideways to his left and off balance. He feels an immediate excruciating pain and popping sensation in the left side of his groin and can barely stand. He returns home with great difficulty and only with the help of his friend. Clinical examination reveals the identical signs and symptoms as in case 1, minus pain and tenderness to the buttock area; additionally, active hip extension and passive hip flexion are painless and full in range.

? Questions

1. What is most likely to have occurred to these patients?
2. What are the two categories of injury to which muscle tissue is liable?
3. What accounts for distraction injuries often occurring in two joint muscles?
4. What are the degrees in the classification of muscle strain?
5. Why are distraction strains involving the upper extremity rare as compared to the incidence of these strains in the lower extremity?
6. What are eccentric contractions?
7. Why is the term "eccentric contraction" a misnomer?
8. What are the clinical findings in muscle injury?
9. What are differences of clinical presentation between a partial and a total rupture of muscle?
10. What is an intramuscular hematoma?
11. What is an intermuscular hematoma?
12. How are intramuscular and intermuscular hematomas differentiated?
13. What is the medical management of intramuscular hematoma?
14. What special problems are unique to the situation of lacerated muscle?
15. What common mechanism of injury results in pectoralis major rupture?
16. What common mechanism of injury results in a deltoid muscle rupture?
17. What common mechanism of injury results in a triceps muscle rupture?
18. What common mechanism of injury results in a biceps brachii rupture?
19. What common mechanism of injury results in a quadriceps contusion?
20. What common mechanism of injury results in a rectus femoris strain?
21. What common mechanism of injury results in a gluteus maximus strain?
22. What common mechanism of injury results in an adductor strain?
23. What is a pulled hamstrings injury?
24. What therapeutic management is appropriate for muscle strains?

1. What is most likely to have occurred to these patients?

The patients have most likely sustained a combined hamstring and adductor *strain* in case 1 and an adductor strain only in case 2. *Muscle injuries* are among the most common, misunderstood, and inadequately treated conditions in sports physical therapy.[12] The significance of these sorts of injuries is often understated because most patients, having sustained muscle injury, can continue on with their daily activities soon after injury. Chronic problems may develop either because of prolonged self-treatment or continued activity despite pain. The most commonly strained muscles of the lower extremities include the hamstrings, adductor longus, iliopsoas, rectus femoris, and the gastrocnemius muscles.[13]

2. What are the two categories of injury to which muscle tissue is liable?

Distraction ruptures are caused by (1) *overstretching* or (2) *contractile overload,* often occurring in the superficial aspect of muscle or at the origin and insertion. Overload occurs as a result of *intrinsic force,* whether concentric or eccentric, and generated by an individual's own muscle so that the demand made upon a muscle exceeds its innate strength. Examples of how this may occur include sudden deceleration (eccentric), rapid acceleration (concentric), or the potentially dangerous combination of deceleration and acceleration that accompanies sharp cutting movements. The common denominator to this sort of injury is that injury frequently occurs in activities requiring explosive muscular effort over a short period of time, and it occurs in sports such as sprinting, jumping, baseball, football, and soccer.[12] Overstretching of a specific muscle, however, occurs by way of excessive contraction of that muscle's *antagonist.*[3]

Compression ruptures result from direct trauma in which a forceful impact pushes muscle back against unyielding bone.[12] The subsequent contusion and tearing of muscle is generically termed a "charley horse" (possibly after the typical name of old lame horses) and results in the formation of a local mass of blood (hematoma) that escapes into the muscle from damaged vessels. The most common site of a charley horse involves the quadriceps muscle,[11] as may occur from a football tackle, or collision during a soccer game in which one player's knee rams into the anterior area of the thigh of another player.[12] Heavy bleeding may occur from compression injuries *deep* within the muscle,

since the momentum imparted from impact may be transmitted to the deep muscular compartment, which bears the brunt of injury by virtue of its being adjacent to bone. Or injury may cause bleeding to the *superficial* portion[12] of the muscle if the injurious force was delivered in a direction other than perpendicular to the surface of that muscle.

3. What accounts for distraction injuries often occurring in two joint muscles?

The hamstring muscle group and rectus femoris from the quadriceps muscle group, as well as the gastrocnemius and the biceps brachii, are all examples of two-joint muscles that are more prone to sustaining distraction injury by virtue of their extended span of length beyond more than one joint.[12] Muscle receptors have the unique task of maintaining an optimal milieu of muscle tone at both ends of the muscle (that is, across each joint) within the narrow confines of the Blix curve. Any deviation from optimum length and optimal tension will place muscle tissue at a greater potential risk for injury, since that muscle will then operate at less than optimum efficiency. Muscles normally operate within relatively narrow margins of length and tension before succumbing to decreased mechanical efficiency by even slightly excessive stretch or swelling of the muscle. Most muscles carry the burden of maintaining this milieu under constantly shifting conditions that move the muscle, lever like, across a single joint. Two-joint muscles are saddled with juggling this same task while moving two separate joints simultaneously! It is no wonder then that two-joint muscles are more likely candidates for injury. The actual site chosen for injury along the muscle's span is governed by the question: Where is the weakest link in the muscle-tendon-bone unit? The answer is that the location differs for each muscle.

4. What are the degrees in the classification of muscle strain?

A *strain* is a tear in the muscle-tendon complex. Mild to minimal strains are graded first degree, whereas second degree strains involve moderate disruption of the myotendinous unit. There are no clear criteria differentiating a first-degree from a second-degree strain. A designation may be made based on the amount of pain, swelling, and spasm present. Additionally, first-degree injuries tend to heal more readily and allow for an early return to athletic training than do second-degree injuries.[14a]

First-degree, or *mild,* strain represents an overstretching of the muscle or rupture of less than 5% of muscle fibers.[12] There is no significant loss of strength or restriction of movement, though active movement or passive stretching will cause some pain and discomfort. A first-degree strain will often resolve itself without treatment and without residual disability.[6]

Second-degree, or *moderate, strain* is more significant than a mild strain in that it involves greater than 5% of muscle fibers.[12] This kind of muscle injury is the one most frequently seen in the clinic, and must be treated cautiously, inasmuch as it may progress to a third-degree strain. Additionally, a second-degree strain, if untreated, may result in excessive scar formation with delayed healing.[14b]

Third-degree, or *severe, strain* involves total disruption of muscle.[12]

5. Why are distraction strains involving the upper extremity rare as compared to the incidence of these strains in the lower extremity?

Strains involving upper extremity musculature are, barring direct blows, relatively rare as compared to injuries occurring to the lower extremities. The lower extremities act as a transitional point for potentially disruptive forces entering the body by way of ground reaction forces incurred during locomotion. Because of this, the lower extremity evolved a larger bulk and breadth of muscle as well as the frequently recruited protective eccentric contraction as part of a repertoire of strategy that helps fend off disruptive forces. In contradistinction, although the upper extremity possesses the ability to contract eccentrically, it does so at times as a necessity of functioning within a gravitational environment and not additionally, as with the lower extremities, to absorb eccentrically the brunt of impact from normal forces. This, of course, excludes the professional trapeze artist or someone who locomotes by doing cartwheels all day.

For example, in bowling, the volar muscles of the dominant upper extremity eccentrically slow down the ball as it descends just before release across the floor toward the pins. From a functional point of view we can state that the upper extremity, like the lower extremity, contracts eccentrically but does so by choice rather than out of necessity. In other words, the lower extremity must eccentrically contract so that it may successfully cross terrain in a gravitational environment for the purpose of survival, that is, the foraging of food, if nothing else. On the other hand, most if not all tasks of daily living involving the upper extremity are simple open kinetic chain, ballistic movements.

6. What are eccentric contractions?

Whereas concentric contraction involves molecular cross-bridging that approximates the two Z lines composing the sarcomere unit (Fig. 25-1), an *eccentric contraction* works the muscle such that distraction of the Z lines actually occurs. Eccentric contraction represents the muscular system's coping strategy, recruited to absorb the energy of disruptive forces and deflect potential injury in those situations requiring high velocity or heavy resistive loads. This is not to say that the eccentric mode of muscle contraction is used only when excessive forces are imparted to the musculoskeletal system. Rather, eccentric muscle activity is part of the muscular repertoire of contraction used by the body and especially so for the lower extremities during locomotion. Interestingly, given the fact that humans, before the advent of modernity, have had to walk around quite

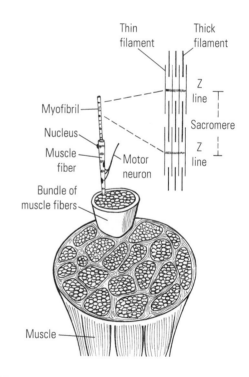

FIG. 25-1 Anatomic organization of skeletal muscle. *Sarcomeres* are arranged end to end, single file, forming a *myofibril.* Bundles of myofibrils make up a syncytial *muscle fiber.* Muscle fibers are grouped together to form *muscle bundles* together in dozens or hundreds to compose a *muscle.* (From Arms K, Camp PS: *Biology,* ed 2, Philadelphia, 1982, Saunders College Publishing.)

a bit, it is no wonder that eccentric work costs less energy than concentric work.[1,4]

Eccentric muscle activity involves the voluntary yielding of control in a graded fashion as a direct function of gravity or the opposition of internally generated forces. For example, if you suddenly wanted to squat down to eye level with a toddler, you could do so concentrically but would do so quite abruptly by whipping yourself down to 135° of knee flexion. This motion would be awkward and might cause you to lose balance, or even injure yourself. However, this abruptness and awkwardness is bypassed in the presence of gravity, and so we can easily drop down onto our haunches by means of a "lengthening" contraction of our hip extensor muscles. We become awkward without gravity. The paradox that emerges from this thought experiment

highlights the fact that what we normally refer to as flexor or extensor are actually semantically relative terms whose reference point is gravity. Thus, eccentric contractions would not occur to astronauts orbiting Earth who are in a state of weightlessness. What we come away with is that we rather have *agonist* and *antagonist* muscles.

7. Why is the term "eccentric contraction" a misnomer?

The term "contraction" is literally a semantic misnomer because what happens on a microanatomic level is actually a ***distraction*** (elongation) of the myofibril unit. Although the distracted state of the Z lines composing the sarcomere unit conjure up the state of a relaxed myofibril in the concentric framework, cross-bridging

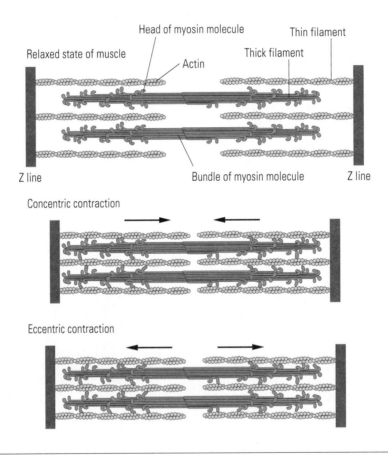

FIG. 25-2 Myosin and actin filaments are actively engaged during concentric and eccentric contraction. In the former, the Z lines approximate; in the latter, they distract. During muscular activity the filaments chemically interact when the heads of the myosin molecules (thick filaments) attach to the molecules (located along the length of the thin actin filaments). This cross-bridging of the filaments results in swiveling of the head of the myosin molecules.

of thick (myosin) and thin (actin) molecular filaments presumably still occurs in the eccentric framework. This is precisely the reason the heads of the myosin molecules do swivel, albeit in opposite direction, and thus permit the distraction of the Z lines and hence of the myofibril on a larger scale, in a graded controlled fashion (Fig. 25-2). Perhaps "muscle working," or "muscle activity," rather than "muscle contraction," is a more accurate term describing how energy is expended by muscle.

8. What are the clinical findings in muscle injury?

Pain is reported to emanate either from the muscle belly, its origin, or its insertion. Pain and stiffness may decrease during exercise, only to return after exercise with greater intensity. Active or resistive movement in the direction of action of the muscle will reproduce pain as will passive stretch in the opposite direction. Additionally the muscle may demonstrate a decrease in strength. It is not uncommon that there is a history of recurrence of disability in which a person reduces her or his activity level until pain has subsided, only to return to the same activity too soon and incur repeated injury.

9. What are differences of clinical presentation between a partial and a total rupture of muscle?

Although the pain after partial rupture can inhibit muscle contraction, the muscle that sustained a total rupture is unable to contract. In addition, with partial ruptures it is sometimes possible to feel a defect in part of the muscle during examination, whereas with total ruptures one can distinguish a palpable gap or defect across the entire muscle belly. In fact, the muscle may even "bunch up" to form a hump that resembles a local tumor.[12]

10. What is an intramuscular hematoma?

An *intramuscular hematoma* (Fig. 25-3) results from bleeding within the muscle sheath that further results in a rise of *intramuscular pressure*. This is actually a protective measure that counteracts a tendency to any further bleeding by way of compressing the vessels within that muscle. However, the pressure may rise so excessively high as to be counterproductive, leading to an *acute compartment syndrome.*[12]

This dangerous situation results in the occlusion of microcirculation secondary to ischemia or complete loss of blood supply, with potential loss of limb function. For example, after a supracondylar fracture the median nerve and radial artery can both be compressed by swelling within the anterior compartment of the forearm. In the event of paresthesia along the median nerve distribution accompanied by loss of finger extension on clinical examination, an emergency surgical fasciotomy is warranted, despite there being a radial pulse present, so as to avert disastrous loss of limb. Limb loss may occur as the swollen compartment clamps down on the blood vessel or vessels passing through it, thus starving itself of oxygen. The result is

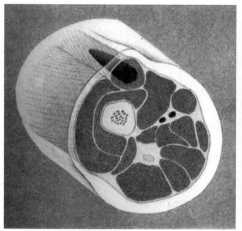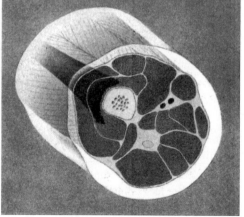

FIG. 25-3 Intramuscular hematoma. (From Peterson L, Renström P: *Sports injuries: their prevention and treatment,* London, 1986, Martin Dunitz, Ltd.)

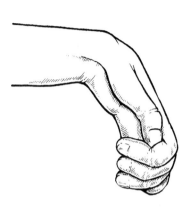

FIG. 25-4 Volkmann's ischemic contracture of the forearm. (From Dandy DJ: *Essential orthopaedics and trauma,* Edinburgh, 1989, Churchill Livingstone.)

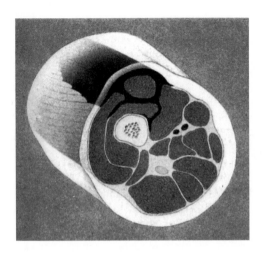

FIG. 25-5 Intermusculer hematoma. (From Peterson L, Renström P: *Sports injuries: their prevention and treatment,* London, 1986, Martin Dunitz, Ltd.)

muscle necrosis and eventual replacement of muscle tissue in the flexor compartment of the forearm with mats of fibrous tissue. This new tissue will subsequently undergo contracture and pull the limb and its joints into the disabling, permanent, and horrible posture of finger flexion, wrist flexion, and forearm pronation known as *Volkmann's ischemic contracture* (Fig. 25-4) of the forearm.[5]

11. What is an intermuscular hematoma?

An *intermuscular hematoma* (Fig. 25-5) is a relatively more benign situation that involves damage to the muscle sheath in addition to the muscle itself. This allows released blood to flow out of a given compartment and spread into that potential space between muscles, or out amongst the surrounding soft tissue. Thus pressure from the initial injury is not sustained, since there exists an avenue by which any damaging pressure is dissipated. Because of this, swelling is temporary, and muscle function will rapidly return to normal.[12]

12. How are *intra*muscular and *inter*muscular hematomas differentiated?

Rising intramuscular pressure can become dangerous if left unmonitored. Constant reexamination of the injured areas is necessary to distinguish between intermuscular and intramuscular bleeding. It is imperative that an accurate diagnosis be made because premature exercise of a muscle affected by extensive intramuscular hematoma or complete rupture can cause complications in the form

of further bleeding and sometimes increased scar formation. This in turn is likely to lead to a more protracted healing process and even permanent disability.

Decreased swelling and rapid recovery of function would be suggestive of *inter*muscular injury, whereas increased swelling with sustained poor function are suggestive of *intra*muscular injury. Additionally, if blood has spread and thereby causes bruising some distance from the site of injury, the hematoma is most probably intermuscular. Moreover, if the muscles' contractile ability does not show improvement and if swelling does not resolve itself, an intramuscular bleed is most likely present.[12]

13. What is the medical management of intramuscular hematoma?

If after 72 hours the symptoms caused by the injured muscle fail to improve, the possibility of intramuscular hematoma ought to be considered. The physician may take one or more of the following steps: measure intercompartmental pressure, puncture and aspirate the area with a wide-bore needle if pressure fluctuation is present, request soft-tissue radiographs with or without a contrast medium, administer an ultrasound examination, or undertake surgery. Surgery is especially appropriate if the muscle in question lacks compensatory agonists of equal size and power, as occurs with the pectoralis major. Surgery involves removal of any intervening blood clots, as well as repair of torn muscle by suturing the ends together such that the least possible scar formation will show. This is then followed by a period of immobilization in a plaster cast.[12]

14. What special problems are unique to the situation of lacerated muscle?

Muscle may be lacerated externally by a knife wound or internally from the sharp fragments of broken bone. In the event that muscle tissue is divided transversely, regardless of cause, the muscle will not hold sutures well enough to prevent normal muscle contraction from simply pulling apart the two sutured ends.[5] Another problem with invasive management is that operative insult may cause additional soft-tissue destruction[5] en route as the surgeon attempts to reach the injured area. Therefore, although the fascia surrounding muscle is amenable to repair, the risk of more soft-tissue destruction makes this unwise.[5] These kinds of injury and as well the nontransverse ruptures of a muscle belly cannot be repaired successfully. Healing takes at least 6 weeks, during which sound fibrous scar tissue is laid down to fill the gap.[5]

15. What common mechanism of injury results in pectoralis major rupture?

Pectoralis major rupture is a rare injury that, when occurring, has been reported to occur almost exclusively in males. This major and severe injury is accompanied by significant swelling and ecchymosis typically occurring from weight-lifting activities, particularly the bench press. An attempt to break a fall, resulting in severe force applied to a maximally contracted pectoralis major muscle, is yet another common mechanism of injury. Rupture may occur in that muscle's proximal or distal portion, resulting in immediate shoulder dysfunction, with visible or palpable defect. Partial ruptures are managed conservatively with initial icing and rest in the acute stage, followed by heat, ultrasound, and a program of passive and active assisted exercises of the shoulder subacutely. Although unresisted stretching exercises should be included early in the rehabilitation program, resistive exercises should follow a 6-week recovery period after good shoulder mobility is restored and the pain is resolved. A complete pectoralis rupture requires early surgical treatment in the active athlete.[3]

16. What common mechanism of injury results in a deltoid muscle rupture?

Deltoid muscle rupture is an extremely rare clinical entity, whereas minor strains of this muscle are common in athletic activity, especially in throwing sports. The anterior deltoid may suffer strain during the acceleration phase of throwing, when a forcible contraction and a forward body movement are simultaneously applied to an already stretched musculotendinous unit. The posterior deltoid acts to restrain the shoulder in the followthrough phase at the end of forward arm motion and is thus vulnerable to injury.

Clinical presentation varies with the site of rupture. In the event that the lesion is located near the deltoid's insertion, a defect may be palpable, as well as an associated mass that becomes firmer upon contraction of that muscle. If the deltoid has become avulsed from its origin, there would be a loss of normal contour of the muscle with weakness in flexion, abduction, or extension. If the rotator cuff was also involved, contraction of the spared deltoid will cause the humeral head to protrude in the direction of deltoid deficiency.

Minor strains and partial deltoid lesions are managed conservatively and usually restore the shoulder to full activity with a prescription of local cryotherapy in the acute stage, followed by heat, shoulder range of motion exercises and stretching, and gentle strengthening over a course of 6 weeks.[3]

17. What common mechanism of injury results in a triceps muscle rupture?

A *triceps rupture* is a rare injury that may result either from indirect injury or from a direct blow. Although the former is characterized by the application of excessive tension to the triceps muscle fibers from, say, a fall onto an outstretched hand, the latter mechanism may result from the elbow striking a fixed object. On examination, a palpable defect of the triceps tendon is usually present and accompanied by pain, swelling, bruising, and weakness of elbow extension. Complete rupture precludes antigravity elbow extension, whereas a false-negative clinical observation may be assessed if extension is allowed to be eccentrically performed by the biceps muscles. Radial head fracture is a common associated finding with tenderness and swelling over the fracture site.[8]

18. What common mechanism of injury results in a biceps brachii rupture?

A *biceps rupture* is ordinarily a rare injury[3] that does occur in greater frequency in military parachutists.[7,15] The mechanism of indirect injury involves the incorrect positioning of the static line in the front of the arm. When the paratrooper jumps, a severe force of 80 pounds per square inch is applied over the biceps, especially if the arm is simultaneously abducted after push-off. The patient will report a tearing or popping sensation at the time of injury, followed by severe pain, swelling, and loss of strength. A visible and palpable muscle defect may be detected if the patient is seen early before the onset of significant hematoma and swelling. Medical management of patients seen acutely after the rupture includes hematoma aspiration and immobilization of the elbow in acute flexion for 6 weeks, whereas subacute ruptures undergo open repair and immobilization in acute elbow flexion for 4 weeks. The angle is then decreased to 90° for an additional 2 weeks.[3]

19. What common mechanism of injury results in a quadriceps contusion?

Quadriceps contusion, otherwise known colloquially as a *charley horse,* is a term for a common injury in contact sports caused by a direct blow to the thigh that compresses the quadriceps muscle into the underlying femur. Examination reveals tenderness, swelling, often a large hematoma on the anterior part of the thigh, and a loss of knee range that may be severe enough to cause a total loss of knee flexion. Radiographic examination is appropriate to rule out the possibility of femoral fracture.[9]

Treatment begins acutely with the application of ice packs for 10 minutes every waking hour for 3 to 5 days after the injury. Knee flexion to the pain barrier is facilitated by the placement of pillows under the knee. The patient may ambulate using crutches, with weight bearing to pain tolerance. Although active range of motion exercise is to be performed within the pain-free range, the patient should avoid passive stretching, which can only increase muscle bleeding. Active hip flexion, though, ought to be encouraged. Once swelling has begun to decrease in the subacute stage, hot and cold compress applications may be initiated along with quadriceps-strengthening exercises. Active range of motion exercise ought to continue to be performed frequently. Only when regaining 90% of ipsilateral quadriceps length as compared with the uninjured contralateral side, measured in the prone position with both knees actively flexed, may the athlete return to his game.[9]

20. What common mechanism of injury results in a rectus femoris strain?

A *rectus femoris* strain (Fig. 25-6) refers to rupture of the origin, or upper third of this muscle, that is experienced as pain in the groin[12] and anterior area of the thigh.[9] These symptoms are preceded by a sudden stabbing pain or pulling sensation[9] during a vigorous hip-flexion motion that may accompany a sudden fast running start. Injury may also occur after a football tackle or during shooting practice in soccer. Additionally, injury may result from forced hip flexion against resistance or after excessive hip extension, especially when coupled with knee flexion, because this combination placed the two-joint rectus femoris on passive insufficiency and hence at greater risk for distraction strain.

Examination reveals tenderness to palpation that increases during resisted knee extension,[9] or resisted hip flexion as well as from a prone quadriceps stretch. Pain is more likely elicited on resistive knee extension than with resistive hip flexion, since the rectus femoris contributes to hip flexion in a rather minor capacity. Radiographs are indicated if an avulsion off the anterior superior iliac spine is suspected, especially in growing adolescents.[12] Treatment begins with ice massage and then progresses to contrast treatment of alternating ultrasound with cryotherapy. Range of motion and quadriceps setting exercises are appropriate immediately. Strengthening begins with concentric exercises and then progresses to eccentric activities. Backward walking and running is a good concentric workout of the quadriceps, whereas forward locomotion works that muscle eccentrically. The athlete may return to running when the motion shows 80% of range, as compared to the uninvolved side.[9]

Injury to iliopsoas (Fig. 25-7) may occur by way of the same mechanism as that of rectus femoris strain[6] and may occur from strength training with weights and simultaneous performing of deep knee bends, sit-ups, rowing, plowing through the snow for conditioning, running uphill, intensive shooting practice in soccer, badminton, long jump and high jump, hurdling, and steeple chasing. Unlike rectus femoris strain, here symptoms will be elicited from resistive hip flexion but not from resistive knee extension. In a similar vein, the same level of pain is perceived by the patient during the passive prone hip-extension test whether the examiner simultaneously bends the knee. Rupture of the iliopsoas muscle is rare, but when it occurs, it is usually located in the tendon, or tendon insertion on the greater trochanter.[12]

21. What common mechanism of injury results in a gluteus maximus strain?

An isolated *strain of gluteus maximus* is uncommon but can occur in sprinters. There is often associated sacroiliac joint involvement, and so the examiner must rule out any sacroiliac joint dysfunction, in addition to lumbar involvement or the piriformis syndrome. If the examiner finds tenderness in the muscle bulk of the glu-

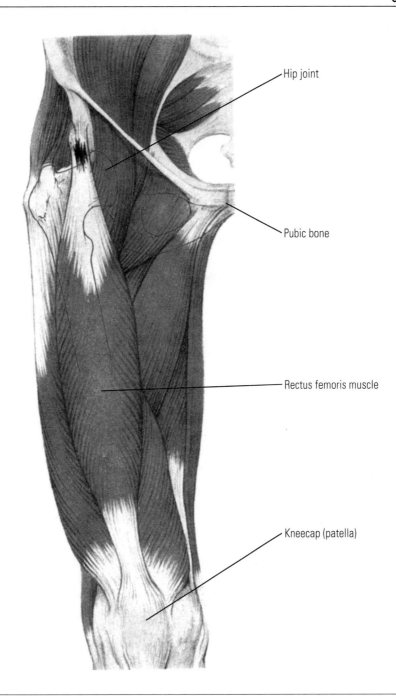

Hip joint

Pubic bone

Rectus femoris muscle

Kneecap (patella)

FIG. 25-6 Rectus femoris strain. (From Peterson L, Renström P: *Sports injuries: their prevention and treatment,* London, 1986, Martin Dunitz, Ltd.)

teus maximus but elicits no pain while palpating the sciatic notch, especially during resistive hip external rotation, then, having ruled out the piriformis syndrome, the clinician may suspect a gluteus maximus strain. This is confirmed when the patient reports a history of sudden sharp buttock pain during a burst of speed or sudden directional change.

Acute treatment involves ice massage to the sore area. Subacute treatment (after 72 hours) by deep heating of this thick muscle belly is achieved by means of

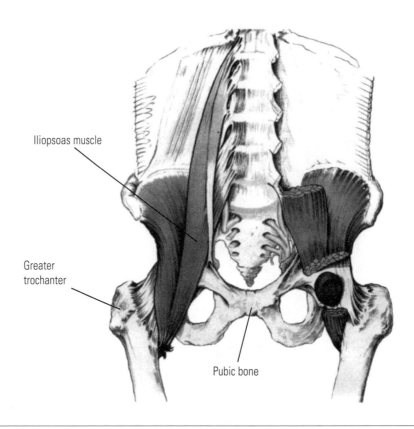

Iliopsoas muscle

Greater trochanter

Pubic bone

FIG. 25-7 Partial strain of the iliopsoas muscle. (From Peterson L, Renström P: *Sports injuries: their prevention and treatment,* London, 1986, Martin Dunitz, Ltd.)

ultrasound and followed by knee-to-chest exercises to stretch that muscle. As the pain subsides, one should commence a strengthening program that involves stair-climbing activities and the use of leg-press machines to strengthen that muscle.[9]

22. What common mechanism of injury results in an adductor strain?

Adductor strain, otherwise known as a *groin pull* (Fig. 25-8), is a debilitating injury caused by forced external rotation and abduction,[7] as may occur from a sudden directional change during sprinting, or repeated forceful adduction as may occur in soccer, when the ball and an opponent's foot are kicked together,[12] thus causing severe momentary stretching of a contracted adductor muscle. The patient feels a sudden momentary stabbing pain in the groin region that returns when he or she attempts to restart the activity.[12] Although local bleeding causes swelling and bruising, these do not often manifest until several days after the injury. Active or resis-

tive adduction, as well as passive or active abduction, should elicit pain. If the muscle cannot contract, there is reason to suspect total rupture.[12] Complete ruptures occur at that muscle's insertion onto the femur or, less likely, at its origin off the pubic bone. Partial ruptures usually occur in the muscle itself, or at its pubic origin. Radiographs are appropriate here, especially if there is bony tenderness present.[12] If the onset is insidious, the clinician should consider the possibility of proximomedial femoral-shaft stress fracture or periostitis.[9]

23. What is a pulled hamstrings injury?

A *pulled-hamstrings* injury (Fig. 25-9) involves strain rupture of one or more of the three hamstring muscles, usually as a result of excessive overload of those muscles. Sprinters show an especially high incidence of this injury.[10] The often violent muscular exertion[11] that occurs with sprinting or long-distance running[12] may tear or avulse part of the tendinous origin of one of these muscle from their common origin off the ischial tuberos-

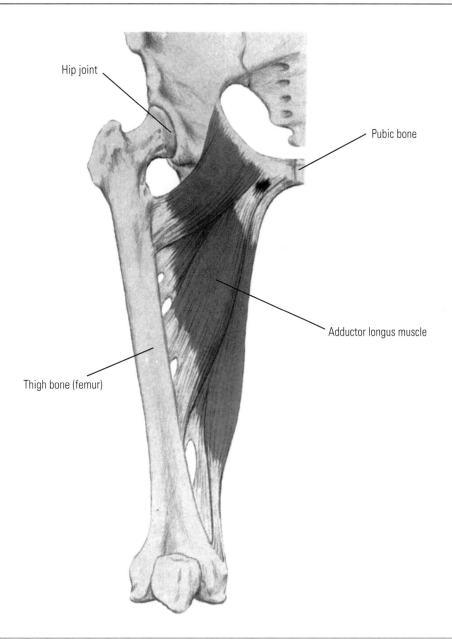

Hip joint

Pubic bone

Adductor longus muscle

Thigh bone (femur)

FIG. 25-8 Groin-pull injury. (From Peterson L, Renström P: *Sports injuries: their prevention and treatment,* London, 1986, Martin Dunitz, Ltd.)

ity[9]; injury may also occur in the midthigh region or more distally.[2] Injury will commonly occur during the last half of the swing phase, during which the hamstrings work eccentrically, or during early stance phase, when there is a large concentric boost of energy.[14]

Proposed causes of hamstring strain include an imbalance of strength between the hamstring muscles in each leg and tightness in these muscles. Hamstring strain injury may also occur after long or triple jumping and may occur during a badminton or tennis game,[12] or because of a very hard kick with the knee extended delivered to a football or soccer ball, which inadvertently creates a sudden forceful stretch or eccentric contraction to the hamstrings as the player attempts to decelerate his foot in an effort to control or aim the force delivered to the ball. The resultant injury usually extends

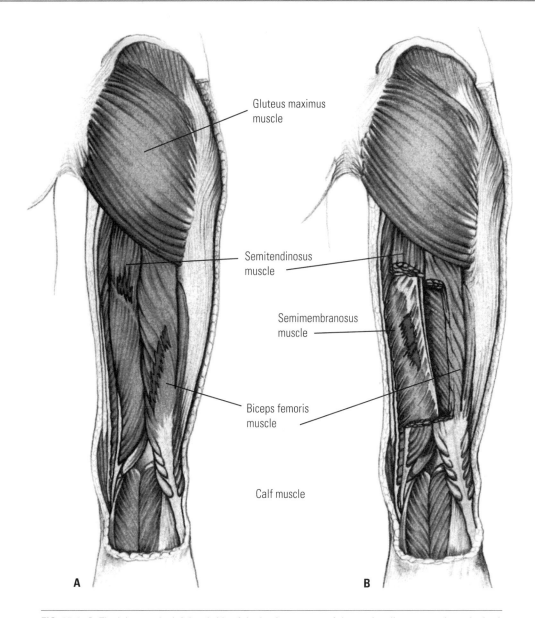

Gluteus maximus
muscle

Semitendinosus
muscle

Semimembranosus
muscle

Biceps femoris
muscle

Calf muscle

A

B

FIG. 25-9 A, The injury on the left-hand side of the leg is a rupture of the semitendinosus muscle at the back of the thigh. The injury on the right-hand side of the leg is a rupture of the biceps femoris muscle. **B,** Rupture of the semimembranosus muscle at the back of the thigh. The middle parts of the semitendinosus muscle and the biceps femoris have been removed to show the rupture. (From Peterson L, Renström P: *Sports injuries: their prevention and treatment,* London, 1986, Martin Dunitz, Ltd.)

longitudinally within the muscle strain, rather than transversely,[9] and the injury is so painful that the runner will often fall and writhe in pain.[11] The athlete may self-diagnose the problem at the time of injury and complain of a "pull" or "pop" sensation. Swelling occurs usually 2 hours[9] after the injury, since the hema-toma is initially contained by the dense fascia lata[11]; ecchymosis is observed within 48 hours.[9] Resisted knee flexion will increase symptoms, and the athlete is often unable to straighten the knee during the terminal swing phase of the gait. Avulsion fracture is suspected if the tibial tuberosity is exquisitely tender.[9]

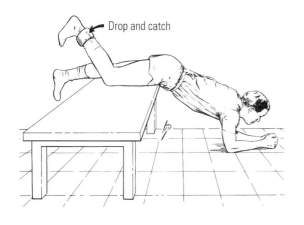

FIG. 25-10 Eccentric "catch" exercise for strengthening the hamstrings. The patient lies prone over the edge of the table so as to approximate the hip and knee angles during the late stance phase. (Modified from Stanton D. Purdham C: *J Orthop Sports Phys Ther* 10:347, 1989.)

The acute stage of management consists in the use of ice packs or ice massage to the site of injury, compression wraps, and possibly crutches. In the subacute phase (after 72 hours), when swelling begins to subside, a program of ice and heat contrasts is appropriate in conjunction with pulsed ultrasound (with or without the use of steroid cream)[2] and is followed by a 30-second passive hamstring stretch in the pain-free range.[9] Progression to active hip and knee hamstring range of motion may be incorporated once symptoms abate.[2] As healing progresses over time, contract-relax techniques to the hamstrings are followed by isometrics to those muscles at varying angles.[2] The final phase of treatment involves active strengthening by means of eccentric activity with gradual increase in both speed and weight. The eccentric-catch exercise is helpful and involves the patient who lowers an ankle weight at successively faster speeds so that he or she eventually progresses to the point of dropping the ankle and catching the weight before the knee reaches full extension[9] (Fig. 25-10).

Running should begin with a backward-running technique, which will help stretch the hamstrings. Forward running should begin with 60% of speed, with frequent hamstring stretch breaks interspersed throughout the workout.[9] Severe tears, more frequently seen in sprinters than in recreational or long-distance runners, may require immediate surgical repair. Chronic hamstring strain is a nonacute injury that develops slowly and is also implicated in inadequate stretching of these muscles before and after running.[2]

24. What therapeutic management is appropriate for muscle strains?

Studies have shown that healing is more rapid, with restoration of circulation and strength improvement, when rehabilitation is started early. The time required for healing of a third-degree muscle strain varies between 3 and 16 weeks, depending on location and extent of injury.

IN THE *ACUTE STATE*

- Ice treatment.
- Elevation.
- Pressure, from an elastic wrap applied from the knee to the groin.
- Rest, though protected weight bearing is generally permitted.
- No active range of motion exercise and no massage. Coagulation, the body's defense against excessive bleeding, springs to action as soon as injury occurs and continues to function for sometime thereafter. This repair mechanism, however, is unstable during the first 24 to 36 hours, and so further bleeding may occur from the impact of new force, vigorous muscle contraction, or unprotected weight bearing. Massage, which is, in effect, repeated minor trauma, should not be used during the first 48 to 72 hours after a muscle injury. After the acute stage, massage is actually beneficial because it can help decrease swelling and stiffness.
- Passive range of motion exercise to the joints of the involved extremity is begun distally and is moved proximally to decrease edema and maintain joint mobility.

IN THE *SUBACUTE STAGE*

Minor partial ruptures, intermuscular hematomas, and minor intramuscular hematomas are managed by the following progression:

- Heat treatment.
- Ultrasound.
- Deep transverse friction massage serves to prevent adherence of young unwanted fibrous tissue and separate existing adhesions between individual muscle fibers that are restricting movement.
- Pain-free passive stretching facilitates prevention of random alignment of new collagen fibers. Stretching does not, as some think, widen the distance between the muscle fibers; on the contrary, stretching permits

muscle fibers to lie more closely together. In a similar vein, pain-free contractile exercises performed early in the rehabilitation process also help structure scar tissue less randomly.

- Submaximal isometric exercises are appropriately begun once resistance to stretching is decreased to the point of achieving full painless range.
- Static (that is, isometric) exercises with light load.
- Pool therapy to encourage active movement.
- Limited dynamic muscle work in the form of short-arc active exercises. At this point, if movement during exercise becomes too painful, the exercises ought to be postponed until they can be performed with minimal pain.
- Dynamic exercises with increasing load.
- Gradually increasing the exercise level to include more aggressive training such as isotonics and isokinetics.
- Eccentric training as part of an injury-sparing strategy.
- Stretching exercises to improve flexibility to all the muscles of that region, including anatomic antagonists to the injured muscle. Stretching should be performed for at least 2 minutes per muscle for optimal results.

REFERENCES

1. Abbot BC, Bigland B, Ritchie JM: The physiological cost of negative work, *J Physiol* 117:380-390, 1952.
2. Brody DM: Running injuries: prevention and management, *Clin Symp* 39(3):1-36, 1987.
3. Caughey MB, Welsh PW: Muscle ruptures affecting the shoulder girdle. In Rockwood CA, Matsen FA, editors: *The shoulder,* vol 2, Philadelphia, 1990, WB Saunders.
4. Chauveau MA: La loi de l'équivalence dans les transformations de la force chez les animaux, *Acad* 122:113-126, 1896.
5. Dandy DJ: *Essential orthopaedics and trauma,* Edinburgh, 1989, Churchill Livingstone.
6. Gould JA: *Orthopaedic and sports physical therapy,* St Louis, 1990, Mosby.
7. Heckman JD, Levine MI: Traumatic closed transection of the biceps brachii in the military parachutist, *J Bone Joint Surg* 60A:369-372, 1978.
8. Levy M, Godberg I, Meir I: Fracture of the head of the radius with a tear or avulsion of the triceps tendon, *J Bone Joint Surg* 64B(1):70-72, 1982.
9. Lillegard WA, Rucker KS: *Handbook of sport medicine: a system-oriented approach,* Boston, 1993, Andover Medical Publishers.
10. Lysholm J, Wiklander J: Injuries in runners, *Am J Sports Med* 15:168-171, 1987.
11. Moore KL: *Clinically oriented anatomy,* ed 2, Baltimore, 1984, Williams & Wilkins.
12. Peterson L, Renström P: *Sports injuries: their prevention and treatment,* London, 1986, Martin Dunitz.
13. Renström P, Peterson L: Groin injuries in athletes, *Br J Sports Med* 14:30, 1980.
14. Stanton D, Purdam C: Hamstring injuries in sprinting—the role of eccentric exercise, *J Orthop Sports Phys Ther* 10:343-348, 1989.
14a. Subotnick SI: *Podiatric sports medicine,* Mount Kisco, NY, 1979, Futural Publishing.
14b. Subotnick SI, editor: *Athlete's feet,* Runner's World Publications.
15. Tobin WJ, Cohen LJ, Vandover JT: Parachute injuries, *JAMA* 117(16):1318-1321, 1941.

RECOMMENDED READING

Brody DM: Running injuries: prevention and management, *Clin Symp* 39(3):1-36, 1987.

Lillegard WA, Rucker KS: *Handbook of sport medicine: a system-oriented approach,* Boston, 1993, Andover Medical Publishers.

Peterson L, Renström P: *Sports injuries: their prevention and treatment,* London, 1986, Martin Dunitz.

PART VI

FOOT

26

Pain and Swelling of the Hallux, As Well As Difficulty Running Following Forceful and Excessive Forefoot Extension

A college football player enters your office with a mildly antalgic gait and complains of pain to his great toe following last week's preseason game. He explains how he got caught in a four-man pile-up with an opposing player falling backwards against his raised heel while his forefoot was raised. He initially thought nothing of it but found it hard to run. His toe has swelled as time has progressed, and he even has difficulty walking. The patient reports no history of hyperuricemia during puberty.

OBSERVATION   Moderate swelling and the presence of ecchymosis are observed.

PALPATION   Palpation reveals point tenderness and warmth at the metatarsophalangeal joint of hallux, particularly its plantar aspect.

ACTIVE RANGE OF MOTION   Active plantar flexion yields marked discomfort.

PASSIVE RANGE OF MOTION   Passive dorsiflexion of the great toe causes marked discomfort.

CLUE:

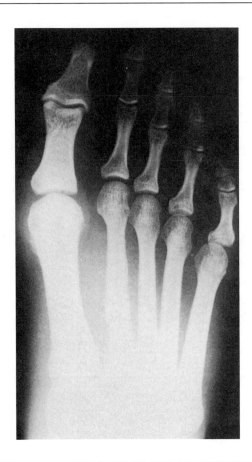

Dorsoplantar projection. (From Nicholas JA, Hershman EB: *The lower extremity and spine in sports medicine,* ed 2, St Louis, 1995, Mosby.)

? Questions

1. What is most likely wrong with this athlete's foot?
2. What anatomy is relative to understanding this disorder?
3. What are the three sources of stability to the first metatarsophalangeal (MTP) joint?
4. What are the kinetics of the first MTP joint?
5. What is the weight-distribution role of the sesamoids of hallux?
6. What dynamic role do the sesamoids of hallux offer the kinesiology of the first MTP joint?
7. What is the mechanism of injury?
8. What roles do playing surface and shoe wear have in hallux MTP sprain?
9. What is the classification of injury?
10. What therapeutic management is appropriate for first MTP joint sprain?

1. What is most likely wrong with this athlete's foot?

This athlete most likely has a *sprain* of the right plantar capsule and lateral collateral ligamentous complex of the metatarsophalangeal (MTP) joint of hallux, colloquially known as *turf toe.* Radiographic changes (see the Clue) associated with turf toe may be demonstrated on routine dorsoplantar projections and may consist only of soft tissue swelling about the first MTP joint, which reflects inflamed synovial tissue.[10] This significant athletic injury is common to sports such as American football (Fig. 26-1), soccer, and lacrosse. This injury may have significant short-term and potential long-term morbidity and disability that includes marked impairment of push-off, as well as compromise of forward drive and running.

2. What anatomy is relative to understanding this disorder?

The first MTP joint is composed of the first metatarsal head, the base of the proximal phalanx, and the superior surfaces of the medial and lateral sesamoids within a single synovial joint capsule. The convex condylar metatarsal head articulates with the concave condylar base of the proximal phalanx.

The MTP joints are *condyloid joints* between the rounded convex metatarsal heads and the concave, cuplike proximal segments of the proximal phalanges. Similar to the metacarpophalangeal joints of the fingers, each joint is enclosed by an articular capsule and reinforced by plantar and collateral ligaments. The *plantar plate ligament,* like its palmar counterpart, is a thick, fibrocartilaginous structure firmly anchored to

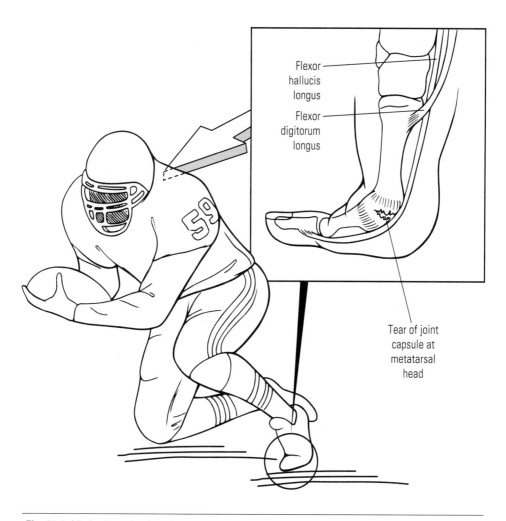

Flexor hallucis longus

Flexor digitorum longus

Tear of joint capsule at metatarsal head

Fig. 26-1 Mechanism of turf toe injury in American football resulting in hyperextension of the great toe.

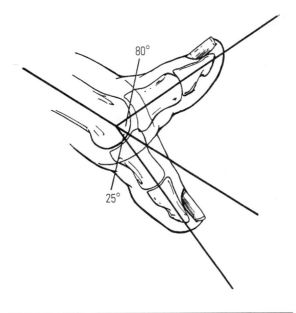

80°

25°

Fig. 26-2 Range of motion of the first metatarsophalangeal joint is 105° from extreme flexion to extension. (From Delee JC, Drez D Jr: *Orthopedic sports medicine: principles and practice*, Philadelphia, 1994, WB Saunders.)

the proximal plantar base of the phalanx and loosely attached to the neck of the metatarsal via the capsule. As such, the plantar ligament serves as part of the weight-bearing surface for the metatarsal head. At the great toe, the sesamoids and their interconnecting ligaments replace the plantar ligament.

The range of motion at the MTP of hallux is variable among the general population and averages 80°, although at least 60° of dorsiflexion is considered normal in barefoot walking on a level surface. Wearing still-soled shoewear reduces this range to 25° to 30° without significantly affecting gait.[3] Generally the range of dorsiflexion is greater than that of plantar flexion. Active plantar flexion averages 20° to 25°, although this excursion may decrease with advancing age[6] (Fig. 26-2).

3. What are the three sources of stability to the first MTP joint?

The static *capsuloligamentous complex* is the essential stabilizing component of the first MTP joint. Static stabilizers are composed of the strong *collateral ligaments* supporting the medial and lateral aspects of the joint. These strong collateral ligaments pass from the tubercles on each side of the metatarsal head to the sides

of the proximal end of the phalanx. The collateral ligaments along either side of the MTP of hallux are, in turn, composed of two components, namely a *metatarsophalangeal ligament* and a *metatarsosesamoid ligament*. The plantar ligaments are interconnected by the *deep transverse metatarsal ligament* connecting the heads and joint capsules of all the metatarsal heads (Fig. 26-3).

The osseous relationship of the elements of the first MTP joint affords minor static stability by virtue of the shallow socket of the proximal phalanx articulating with the biconvex surface of the metatarsal head. Musculotendinous insertions by way of short (intrinsic) muscles such as the abductor, adductor, and flexor hallucis brevis and possibly long (extrinsic) movers of the first MTP joint provide dynamic support between midstance and toe-off phases because of their blending into the joint capsule surrounding the joint.

4. What are the kinetics of the first MTP joint?

MTP joint motion occurs twice during the gait cycle. Active dorsiflexion occurs during late swing phase in preparation for heel strike, whereas passive dorsiflexion occurs during late stance phase of gait after heel lift.[1] Motion at the first MTP joint is initially hallux dorsiflexion, as well as a *rolling* motion for the first 20°, during which the joint behaves like a hinge.[16] Beyond 20° of dorsiflexion the head of the first metatarsal shafts *slides* in a plantar direction, which is described as plantarflexion of the first ray. This is followed by cam-like *compression* of the dorsal articular surfaces of the metatarsal head and the proximal phalanx as the end range of dorsiflexion is approached, in accordance with the rigid needs of the supinated foot during late stance[7] (Fig. 26-4). Open kinetic-chain dorsiflexion of the first ray during swing phase involves the sliding and compression, without the rolling, components of movement.

The kinetics of the first MTP joint thus involve four centers of motion[7] whose instant centers of velocity demonstrate an arc of movement in the closed kinetic chain. In the open kinetic chain, the lack of a rolling component and, consequently, the centers of rotation are more suggestive of a ring than an arc.[16]

5. What is the weight-distribution role of the sesamoids of hallux?

Any discussion of the sesamoids must be prefaced by mention of the flexor hallucis longus and brevis, as well as the abductor and adductor hallucis, because these

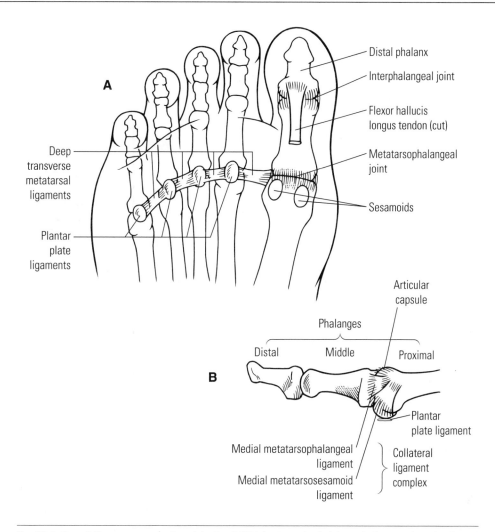

Fig. 26-3 Capsuloligamentous complex of the first MTP joint comprised of the articular capsule and collateral ligaments. The collateral ligament complex is comprised of the metatarsophalangeal ligament and metatarsosesamoid ligaments. No plantar plate ligament is present in the first ray. **A,** Palmar view. **B,** Lateral view.

muscles intimately relate to sesamoid function. The flexor hallucis brevis is an intrinsic two-bellied muscle that is interconnected by a tendinous raphe. Whereas the medial belly blends with the abductor hallucis to insert onto the medial side of the base of the proximal phalanx of hallux, the lateral belly combines with the tendon of the adductor hallucis muscle and inserts onto the lateral side of the base of the same phalanx. The common denominator of these three intrinsic muscles is the presence of two shared conjoint tendons consisting of a medial and lateral head. Embedded within the tendon heads are two sesamoid bones. The medial sesamoid is embedded within the medial head of the flexor hallucis brevis and abductor hallucis, whereas the lat-

eral sesamoid is embedded within the lateral head of the flexor hallucis brevis and the adductor hallucis[15] (Fig. 26-5). The extrinsic tendon of the flexor hallucis longus muscle passes through the groove between the intrinsic conjoint tendons to insert onto the base of the distal phalanx of hallux.

The *sesamoid* in each tendon of the short flexor muscle act as a *ball bearing* playing along the underside of the great metatarsal head. The sesamoids have both a *static* and *dynamic* function in locomotion. During quiet standing or foot-flat phase of stance, the foot functions as a supporting structure for the superincumbent body weight. Approximately half of the weight of each leg is transmitted to the heel, and the other half is

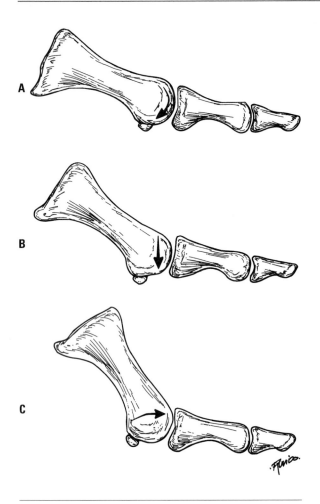

Fig. 26-4 Motion of the first metatarsophalangeal joint is comprised of both osteokinematic and arthrokinematic motion. **A,** *Rolling* motion of the metatarsal head during the first 20° of dorsiflexion. **B,** *Sliding* association with depression of the metatarsal head, known as first-ray plantarflexion. **C,** *Compression* at the end of range of motion. (From Valmassy RL: *Clinical biomechanics of the lower extremities*, St Louis, 1996, Mosby.)

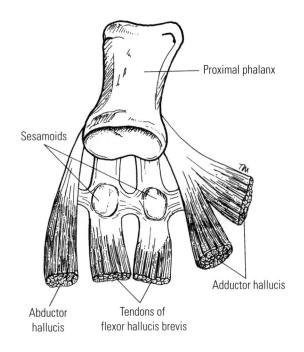

Fig. 26-5 A view of the sesamoids embedded within the conjoint tendon for flexor hallucis brevis, abductor hallucis, and adductor hallucis. (From Baxter D: *The foot and ankle in sport*, St Louis, 1995, Mosby.)

transmitted to the metatarsal heads. The virtue of having two sesamoids is that an additional surface area is provided on which to distribute body weight. It is as if there were now six metatarsal heads instead of five, so that each sesamoid bears one sixth of the forefoot weight. Thus the hallux, by virtue of its sesamoids, carries a full 30% of the forefoot share of superincumbent body weight. This amounts to more than twice the load carried by the lesser toes.[14] During walking, the forces acting across the first MTP joint are equal to 40% to 60% of body weight. During jogging and running, peak forces can increase by two or three times, whereas a running jump may increase forces active across the joint to almost eight times body weight.

6. What dynamic role do the sesamoids of hallux offer the kinesiology of the first MTP joint?

For effective heel rise during late stance, the first MTP joint muscle dorsiflexes between 65° to 70°. For this to occur the first metatarsal must depress in a plantarward direction. This is known as plantarflexion of the first ray, below the second ray and other metatarsals. This plantarflexion occurs during late stance because of activity of posterior compartment musculature, as well as the medial shifting of ground reaction force along the plantar surface of the foot.

In addition to providing additional surface area for weight distribution, the sesamoids offer a *biomechanical advantage* to the intrinsic muscles crossing the MTP articulation. Kinesiological analysis of the MTP joint is best understood by considering four muscle slips: the medial and lateral heads of the flexor hallucis brevis and the adductor hallucis brevis and abductor hallucis brevis. Two of these muscles provide a plantar flexion force to the head of the first MTP, and the other two oppose and effectively cancel each other. The abductor and adductor hallucis brevis function as a guy support and cancel the axis for abduction and adduction at the MTP joint during late stance. By functionally canceling the second degree of freedom, the MTP is reduced to a single-axis joint during late stance and effectively improves stability by preventing mediolateral wobbling and facilitating efficient thrust.

Dorsiflexion of the first MTP joint causes the sesamoids to move distally. Without the sesamoids, the effect of the contraction of the long and short great toe flexors would be to stabilize the hallux against the metatarsal head and not the ground. The sesamoids, located directly under the metatarsal, provide a mechanical advantage when they become positioned over the anterior aspect of the first metatarsal head. From this vantage point the sesamoids serve as a pulley to the long and short great toe flexors, increasing the lever arm for a plantar flexion moment, which stabilizes the hallux against the ground.[9]

The dynamic functions of the sesamoids are apparent during toe-off, when the foot propels the body forward. As the heel becomes elevated during the propulsion phase of stance, the sesamoids and first metatarsal head combine to form a pulley for the long and short great toe flexors. The sesamoids determine the angle of insertion of the tendons. Following heel-off and subsequent hallux dorsiflexion, the flexor hallucis brevis employs the sesamoids as a pulley so as to angle more obliquely up on its insertion on the base of the proximal phalanx and stabilize the first MTP joint against the ground during push-off.

7. What is the mechanism of injury?

The most common mechanism of injury involves excessive hyperextension of the great toe MTP joint. This may occur when one player falls toward the back of the leg and foot of another player whose heel is raised while his forefoot still contacts the ground. The force of the falling player drives the other player's foot into excessive hyperextension, causing a *plantar* tear of the joint complex at its weakest site, the metatarsal neck.

The turf toe injury may also occur from a *hyperflexion injury* of the great toe and results in a sprain of the *dorsal* capsule. This may occur in the case of a ball carrier who is tackled from behind, so that the knee is forced forward while the foot is plantar flexed. A *valgus stress* will sprain the *medial capsule* because of excessive and forceful push-off. In the normal foot a valgus stress to the great toe is created during late stance

phase as push-off is approached. Pronation of the foot causes an increased stress to the medial aspect of the foot. Thus a valgus stress of the MTP of hallux may be more likely in individuals with a functional flatfoot deformity.

8. What roles do playing surface and shoe wear have in hallux MTP sprain?

A common perception is that the incidence of sprain to the MTP joint of hallux is directly related to the introduction of artificial playing surfaces. Synthetic grass surfaces, unlike natural grass, lack the regenerative capacity to maintain resiliency and shock absorption capacity. Over time the fibers comprising Astroturf become worn and are less capable of providing a cushioning effect, which leads to an increase in surface friction.[11] This means that the forefoot of a player is more easily fixed on the turf, leaving the forefoot more vulnerable to injury.

When Astroturf was first introduced in the late 1960s, players complained of poor traction when using their grass shoes. The pursuit of improved performance led to a more flexible, soccer-type shoe. Unfortunately, these shoes have a relatively flexible forefoot, stressing the MTP joints of the foot and resulting in more sprains.

Other causative factors of great toe MTP sprain include player position, weight, age, years of participation, ankle range of motion, pes planus, a flattened first metatarsal head,[4] and the wearing of flexible shoes.[17] Soft-soled athletic shoes have a highly flexible insole that allows for hyperextension of the forefoot and little protection from a hyperextension injury.

9. What is the classification of injury?

The classification of injury is as follows[5]:

- *Grade I sprain* is a stretch injury or minor tearing of the capsuloligamentous complex of the first MTP joint. Clinical symptoms include localized medial or plantar tenderness, the absence of ecchymosis, minimal swelling, and minimal loss of joint range. Weight-bearing produces few symptoms, and the athlete may still continue to participate in sports despite mild pain, particularly during the push-off phase of running. This acute clinical profile is similar to that for the athlete with a chronic sprain of the MTP of hallux.

- *Grade II sprain* is a partial tear of the capsuloligamentous complex. Tenderness is more diffuse and intense than in a grade I sprain. There is usually mild to moderate range restriction, and moderate swelling and ecchymosis are present. During ambulation the athlete will experience moderate pain and display a slightly antalgic gait. Passive dorsiflexion of the joint causes marked discomfort.

- _Grade III sprain_ involves a complete tear of the capsuloligamentous complex and may also include tearing of the plantar plate from its origin on the metatarsal head-neck junction. The forces causing injury are of such magnitude as to cause injury to the articular joint surfaces by impacting the proximal phalanx into the metatarsal head dorsally. There may be an accompanying sesamoid fracture, separation of a bipartite sesamoid, or proximal sesamoid migration if sprain of the capsuloligamentous complex occurs distal to the sesamoid bones.

Clinical presentation includes severe pain and tenderness on both the plantar and dorsal aspects of the first MTP joint. Ecchymosis is obvious, swelling is marked, and the range of motion in the first MTP joint is severely restricted. The patient will be observed to negotiate stance phase of gait in discomfort, with a disproportionate amount of time spent bearing weight along the lateral border of the foot. This level of injury precludes athletic participation.

10. What therapeutic management is appropriate for first MTP joint sprain?

The majority of first MTP joint sprains, regardless of grade, will heal over a 3- to 4-week period if properly managed. Rest is the key component in management strategy, although it is often difficult to enforce. Difficulty in patient compliance stems from the misconception by both the player and coach that the injury may be relegated to the status of insignificance. Turf toe subsequently may be the precursor of hallux rigiditus,[12] characterized by progressive osteoarthritis. Unfortunately, an early return to competition almost always extends recovery time and may result in a prolonged disability. The long-term sequelae of a turf toe injury that is not appropriately managed include hallux rigidus, metatarsalgia, bunion, or ligament calcification.[2]

Cryotherapy is administered by placing the foot in a bucket of ice or a cold-water whirlpool for 10- to 20-minute intervals during the first 48 hours following injury. Progression to contrast whirlpool treatment may commence following the acute stage of the injury. Compression is provided by taping the toe or by wrapping the great toe with a compressive dressing. Elevation of the foot above the dependent position is appropriate. Early joint mobilization is crucial, because loss of motion is a common sequela of injury. Joint play simulating the normal arthrokinematic movement precedes osteokinematic movement. Once symptoms diminish, passive and active range-of-motion exercises may commence and progress from non–weight-bearing to weight-bearing exercises. Nonsteroidal antiinflammatory medications are helpful, whereas the use of cortisone or anesthetic injection is contraindicated because it may result in exacerbation of the original injury and lead to a more prolonged recovery.

Treatment may also include modifying equipment, such as reducing the flexibility of the shoewear. Increasing the stiffness of the shoe's sole reduces stress across the forefoot by reducing the amount of hyperextension and hyperflexion of the MTP joints. This may be facilitated by an insole modification that includes a stainless spring-steel plate in the forefoot region of the turf shoe. Alternatively, the use of plastic laminates placed inside the athletic shoes to inhibit flexion of the toe box have been gaining popularity. For chronic cases or for acute cases in which the patient does not tolerate a stiffened insole, a custom insole may afford better foot conformation. A Morton's extension should be incorporated into the design of this insole and should be stiff enough to limit first MTP joint movement. Because a hyperextension type of turf-toe injury is made worse with pronation,[13] maintenance of the foot in subtalar neutral is important to avoid exacerbating the sprain.

If the hindfoot is in valgus, management involves a 5° or 9° medial hindfoot wedge. A metatarsal pad is placed proximal to the greater MTP joint and is combined together with a stiff or rocker soled shoe and 1-mm heel height. If the hindfoot is in neutral, then management involves a neutral hindfoot wedge and 5° lateral forefoot wedge in conjunction with a metatarsal pad, a stiff soled shoe, and a 1-mm heel height.[12]

During the initial period of acute pain, the patient may be helped by spica taping of the hallux for short periods[12] to limit dorsiflexion. Taping, however, tends to lose efficacy after the first 10 to 15 minutes of athletic activity because of loosening. In patients with more severe involvement, a short-leg walking cast with the walker positioned to relieve stress on the plantar capsule of the hallux may be used for one week.

Following a grade I injury, an athlete may continue participation as symptoms allow. The toe is taped to neutral to stabilize the joint and prevent hyperdorsiflexion. Some authorities suggest taping the first toe to 45% of normal range and tethering that position with figure-eights using 1-inch tape. This position holds the toe up and out of the way when the athlete bends down, such as in a football stance. A stiffened insole may be used during practice and competition. There is usually no loss of playing time, whereas grade II sprains may result in a loss of playing time ranging from 3 to 14 days. A grade III sprain may necessitate a short-leg walking cast for 7 to 10 days with the walker positioned to relieve all stress on the plantar capsule of hallux. Alternatively, crutches may be used for ambulation. This is followed by taping of the first MTP joint to prevent hyperextension forces. The athlete should not begin running until he is asymptomatic. Thus loss of playing time may range from 2 to 6 weeks. After recovery a stiff-soled shoe with a steel spring plate or Orthoplast forefoot splint may be substituted for regular athletic footwear.[8]

REFERENCES

1. Bojsen-Moller F, Lamoreux L: Significance of free dorsiflexion of the toes in walking, *ACTA Orthop Scand* 50:411-479, 1979.
2. Brotzman SF: *Clinical orthopedic rehabilitation,* St Louis, 1996, Mosby.
3. Clanton TO, Butler JE, Eggert A: Injuries to the metatarsophalangeal joint in athletes, *Foot Ankle Int* 7:162, 1986.
4. Clanton TO, Eggert KE, Pivarnik JM, et al: First metatarsophalangeal joint of the great toe in athletes, *Am J Sports Med* 6:326-334, 1978.
5. Clanton TO, Ford JJ: Turf toe injury, *Clin Sports Med* 13(4):731-741, 1994.
6. Coker TP, Arnold JA, Weber DL: Traumatic lesions of the metatarsophalangeal joint of the great toe in athletes, *Am J Sports Med* 6(6):326-334, 1978.
7. Delee JC, Drez D Jr: *Orthopedic sports medicine: principles and practice,* Philadelphia, 1994, WB Saunders.
8. Heatherington VJ, Carnett J, Patterson B: Motion of the first metatarsophalangeal, *J Foot Surg* 28(1):13-19, 1989.
9. Jones DC, Singer KM: Soft-tissue conditions of the ankle and foot. In Nicholas JA, Hershman EB: *The lower extremity and spine in sports medicine,* ed 2, St Louis, 1995, Mosby.
10. Michaud T: *Foot orthoses and other forms of conservative foot care,* Baltimore, 1993, William & Wilkins.
11. Milbauer DL, Patel SA: Radiographic techniques. In Nicholas JA, Hershman EB: *The lower extremity and spine in sports medicine,* ed 2, St Louis, 1995, Mosby.
12. Nigg BM, Segesser B: The influence of playing surfaces on the load on the locomotor system and on football and tennis injuries, *Sports Med* 5(6):375-385, 1988.
13. Reiley MA: *Guidelines for prescribing foot orthotics,* Thorofare, NJ, 1995, Slack.
14. Rodeo SA, O'Brien S, Warren RF, et al: Turf toe: an analysis of metatarso-phalangeal joint sprains in professional football players, *Am J Sports Med* 18(3):280-285, 1990.
15. Sammarco GJ: Biomechanics of the foot. In Frankel VH, Nordin M, editors: *Biomechanics of the skeletal system,* Philadelphia, 1980, Lea & Febiger.
16. Stokes IAF, Hutton WC, Stott JRR: Forces under the hallux valgus foot before and after surgery, *Clin Orthop* 142:64-72, 1979.
17. Turco VJ: Injuries to the foot and ankle. In Nicholas JA, Hershman EB: *The lower extremity and spine in sports medicine,* ed 2, St Louis, 1995, Mosby.
18. Valmassy RL: *Clinical biomechanics of the lower extremities,* St Louis, 1996, Mosby.
19. Xethalis JL, Lorei MP: Soccer injuries. In Nicholas JA, Hershman EB: *The lower extremity and spine in sports medicine,* ed 2, St Louis, 1995, Mosby.

RECOMMENDED READING

Clanton TO, Ford JJ: Turf toe injury, *Clin Sports Med* 13(4): 1994.
Rodeo SA, O'Brien S, Warren RF, et al: Turf toe: an analysis of metatarsophalangeal joint sprains in professional football players, *Am J Sports Med* 18(3):280-285, 1990.

27

Painful Pebble Sensation Over Ball of Foot that Radiates Into Toes

Case 1 A 38-year-old woman works as a flight attendant on international flights for a major airline. The dress requirements of her job include wearing shoes with 2-inch heels. After 3 months of working five flights per week, she visits your office complaining of occasional sharp and throbbing pain over the ball of her right foot that radiates to the adjacent toes. She offers that the sensation is often akin to the feeling of getting a pebble in her shoe. Symptoms increase during the last hour or two of her work shift but are relieved by walking barefoot or removing her shoe and massaging her forefoot.

OBSERVATION A bunion is present with mild valgus of the first ray. Upon observation of the patient's gait, toe-off appears to reproduce pain.

PALPATION Palpation reveals the presence of a tender nodule between the third and fourth metatarsal heads. Pressure over the third and fourth metatarsal heads causes shooting pain into the fourth toe. Lateral compression of the forefoot reproduces the pain the patient describes.

RANGE OF MOTION Toe hyperextension increases pain, as does squatting or kneeling with the toes hyperextended. A hypermobile first ray is noted.

MUSCLE STRENGTH Muscle strength is normal.

SENSATION Sharp and burning intermittent pain and paresthesia along the adjacent sides of the third and fourth toes, with diminution of light touch and pinprick in the medial half of the fourth toe.

SPECIAL TESTS Positive compression test.

FOOT EVALUATION Foot evaluation indicates a 6° forefoot varus posture and a hypermobile first ray.

CLUE:

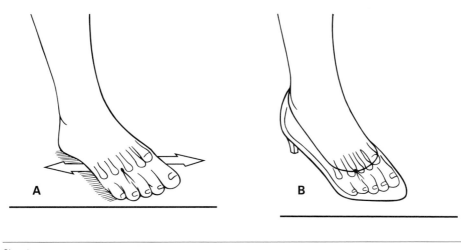

Clue 1

Case 2 A 40-year-old male electrician has spent the last 6 weeks working on base connections at a refurbished shopping mall complex. To do so he must spend at least 6 to 7 hours per day squatting on his right leg and dorsiflexing the ipsilateral metatarsophalangeal joint. Lately he complains of a dull and throbbing pain that comes on after several hours of work. The pain has been relieved somewhat by a change of shoes or by walking. There is no history of injury, nor does he experience any night pain. The patient reports being a noninsulin–dependent diabetic for several years. When asked, he admits to taking moderate doses of aspirin to relieve symptoms. Further probing reveals that he walks barefoot about the hardwood floors in his home.

OBSERVATION   Upon observation of the man's gait, it is noted that toe-off reproduces pain.

PALPATION   Palpation reveals the presence of a tender nodule between the third and fourth metatarsal heads. Pressure over the third and fourth metatarsal heads causes shooting pain into the fourth toe. Lateral compression of the forefoot reproduces the pain the patient describes.

RANGE OF MOTION   A rigid first ray shows increased rigidity and a decrease in great toe plantar flexion. Toe hyperextension increases pain, as does squatting or kneeling with the toes hyperextended.

MUSCLE STRENGTH   Muscle strength is normal.

SENSATION   The patient has dull and throbbing intermittent pain and paresthesia along the adjacent sides of the third and fourth toes, with diminution of light touch and pinprick in the medial half of the fourth toe.

SPECIAL TESTS   Positive compression test. A leg length discrepancy is detected, with the right lower extremity being ½ inch shorter than the other. There is no compensatory lift.

FOOT EVALUATION   Foot evaluation indicates a forefoot valgus posture and a hypomobile first ray.

CLUE:

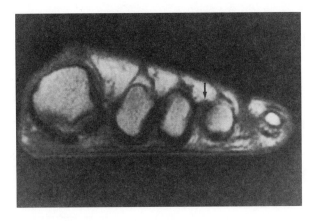

Clue 2 (From Nicholas JA, Hershman EB: *The lower extremity and spine in sports medicine,* ed 2, St Louis, 1995, Mosby.)

? Questions

1. **What soft-tissue injury is most likely causing pain in these patients?**
2. **What anatomy is essential to understanding this condition?**
3. **Interdigital neuritis may occur secondary to which other conditions or causes?**
4. **What type of foot malalignments may contribute to the development of interdigital neuroma?**
5. **What is the clinical presentation?**
6. **What is the differential diagnosis?**
7. **What is the association between interdigital neuroma and hallux valgus or the presence of a bunion?**
8. **What therapeutic management is appropriate to treating this condition?**
9. **What is the medical or surgical management for the patient with no relief from conservative treatment?**

1. What soft-tissue injury is most likely causing pain in these patients?

Morton's toe neuroma, or *interdigital neuritis* (Fig. 27-1), is the most common *entrapment neuropathy* in the foot. This condition was described by Thomas Morton in 1876.[8] The neuroma is a localized thickening of the plantar digital nerve. The condition is more often unilateral than bilateral and is more common in women than in men.[14] The exact cause of this condition is a matter of debate. The etiology is postulated to be traumatic and more likely to develop in people who walk, jog, or squat a great deal. High-heeled shoes are also a mechanical factor, which may account for the greater incidence in females.[6] Women's footwear often shifts weight to the forefoot, a situation compounded by high heels that force toe hyperextension while squeezing the forefoot into a narrow vamp. Foot posture has also been cited as contributory to the development of interdigital neuritis. Both an excessively pronated foot and a foot with an excessively high instep may cause anatomical and hence pathokinesiologic changes in the forefoot that may culminate in interdigital neuroma.

2. What anatomy is essential to understanding this condition?

The *metatarsal tunnels* lie between the superficial and deep transverse metatarsal ligaments. The tendons of the toe flexor and interosseus muscles contribute to forming these tunnels. The *posterior tibial nerve* gives rise to the *medial* and *lateral plantar nerves,* which are analogous to the medial and ulnar nerves of the upper extremity.[18] The plantar nerves, in turn, give rise to the *interdigital nerves.* As such, the interdigital nerves must come up from the sole of the foot to reach their dorsal destination. En route, the nerves course between

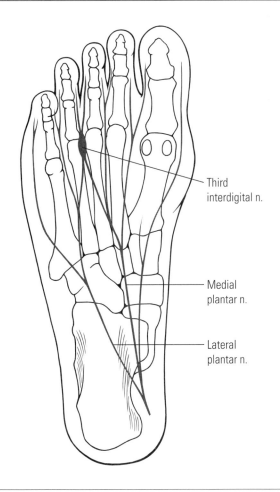

Fig. 27-1 Anatomical view of the interdigital nerve. The third web space receives branches from both the medial and lateral plantar nerves. Shaded area represents location of pain and numbness.

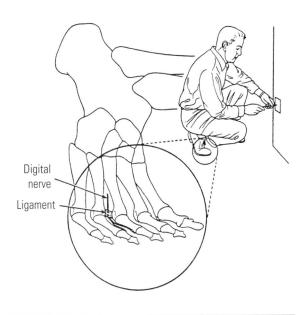

Fig. 27-2 The hyperdorsiflexed posture of the MTP joint will compromise this nerve by causing it to be stretched over the distal edge of the *intermetatarsal ligament*. (From Kopell HP, Thompson WAL: *Peripheral entrapment neuropathies*, Huntington, NY, 1976, Robert E Krieger.)

the metatarsal shafts and pass dorsally by coursing under and against the deep transverse metatarsal ligament known as the intermetatarsal ligament. This ligament binds the metatarsal heads together. The interdigital nerves are thus subject to both external compression from the ligament and to pinching between the metatarsal heads. The hyperdorsiflexed posture of the metatarsophalangeal (MTP) joint will especially compromise the bulbous nerve between the third and fourth metatarsals by causing it to be stretched over the distal edge of the *intermetatarsal ligament* (Fig. 27-2).

The interdigital nerve may be subject to both external compression and to pinching between the bulbous metatarsal heads during work or sport. Excessive angulation of the nerve over the intermetatarsal ligament is most marked when the toes are hyperextended at the

MTP joint. Certain work postures engender forced hyperextension of the MTP joints. For example, an electrician working on a base connection maintains a forced hyperextension of the MTP joint of one foot, whereas dance activities such as a relevé, grand plié, or whenever the foot assumes a demi-pointe position (Fig. 27-3). These postures exacerbate the stretching of the nerve because of repetitive and often extreme dorsiflexion of the MTP joints. Similarly, runners may sustain interdigital neuritis as a result of repetitive and often excessive dorsiflexion of the MTP joints during the toe-off phase of the running cycle.

Despite variation of distal lower extremity nerve patterns in humans, the medial and lateral plantar nerves most often anastomose as a nodular thickening between the third and fourth metatarsal heads before dividing and coursing distally over the ball of the foot to innervate the toes. The third interdigital nerve is therefore thicker and more readily traumatized than the other digital nerves. This *third plantar interdigital nerve* is the culprit implicated in this neuropathy, because the nerve is more vulnerable to ischemia as a result of its relatively large volume within the narrow tunnel formed by the metatarsal shafts. Chronic nipping of this nerve causes characteristic pathologic changes such

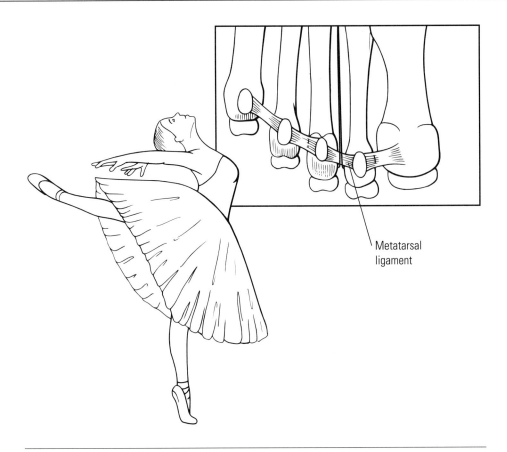

Metatarsal
ligament

Fig. 27-3 An interdigital neuroma may result from recurrent stretching of the interdigital nerve beneath the edge of the metatarsal ligament. This stretching is exacerbated by dorsiflexion of the toes as occurs in this ballerina performing a relevé.

as perineural fibrosis, fibrinoid degeneration, demyelination, and endoneural fibrosis[20] that manifests as scarring and eventual development of a local swelling known as a *neuroma.*

3. Interdigital neuritis may occur secondary to which other conditions or causes?

Interdigital neuritis may occur following an acute hyperdorsiflexion injury of the lateral digits with sprain of the ligamentous joint complex. This is similar in mechanism to a turf toe injury of hallux (see pp. 297-305). In this case repetitive dorsiflexion motions may stretch the interdigital nerve acutely over the distal edge of the intermetatarsal ligament. This may occur in sports during the toe-off phase of the running cycle, and in dance during a relevé, grand plié, or whenever the foot assumes a demi-pointe position (see Fig. 27-2). Idiopathic second MTP synovitis, a fairly common condition in runners, involves distention of the joint capsule,

causes local, bursal-like swelling between the second and third metatarsal heads,[4] and may lead to pressure of the interdigital nerve.

Interdigital nerve trauma may occur following a misstep on a descending step or pavement curb. This is the same mechanism implicated in the frequent tear of gastrocnemius. In this case the toe may be forced into passive hyperextension, stretching the nerve while the ligament is propelled by the forward force of body weight and leans against the nerve. If the foot moves into forced inversion, a peroneal neuropathy may also result. The interdigital nerve may also incur trauma when an individual runs barefoot on a hard surface while being unaccustomed to doing so.[9]

4. What type of foot malalignments may contribute to the development of interdigital neuroma?

Interdigital neuritis may also occur secondary to intrinsic foot malalignments. In the overpronated foot, such as may occur from a forefoot varus deformity (see p. 345), push-off is attempted on a loose, bony-articular complex. Because of this instability in the forefoot, abnormal shearing forces result between the metatarsal heads that may predispose for interdigital neuroma.* Thus this condition is often seen in basketball players or runners who have a hypermobile foot with excessive pronation.[17]

A compensated forefoot varus deformity translates into ineffective ligamentous and muscular stabilizers because of the pronated position of the subtalar joint, resulting in an unstable (hypermobile) first ray. Consequently, the lateral metatarsal heads, particularly the second head, undergo excessive loading, because the first ray cannot effectively contribute to propulsion. The increased shear forces between the lateral metatarsal heads may lead to irritation of the medial and lateral plantar nerves, which branch into an interdigital nerve in the third web space. Callus formation will be primarily under the second metatarsal head and is often extreme (pinch callus), because the foot remains abnormally pronated throughout the propulsion phase.

Overpronation also leads to excessive sagging of the transverse metatarsal arch, resulting in approximation of the metatarsal shafts and heads. Consequently, the interposed digital nerve located between the third and fourth shafts and heads will be compressed. In the excessively pronated foot, callous buildup will drift laterally and may be palpated under the medial great toe and second and third or even fourth metatarsal heads. This latter location coincides with the locale of Morton's toe neuroma. These calluses are often elongated because of lengthening of the foot with excessive pronation, whereas the medial hallux callus results from pinching against the shoe.

Excessive shear may also be implicated as a causative factor in the individual with a forefoot valgus (see pp. 346-347) deformity associated with a rigid (hypomobile) first ray. Normally the first MTP joint must have 60° to 75° of dorsiflexion as the heel rises off the ground during the propulsion phase of gait. For this amount of dorsiflexion to occur, the first ray must plantarflex more than the second ray during the propulsive sequence of locomotion. However, if the first ray is rigid, it will be incapable of moving into enough plantar flexion to provide the first MTP joint with the necessary dorsiflexion needed for normal propulsion. The burden of dorsiflexion, and hence propulsion, is shifted laterally to the other metatarsals, thereby altering the kinesiology of the forefoot. The first three metatarsals, which articulate with the cuneiforms, act as a single functional unit, whereas the fourth and fifth metatarsals, which articulate with the cuboid, act together as a separate functional unit. Excessive transverse plane movement between these two functional segments[25] may focus shear force at the confluence of the segments, which contain the interdigital nerve. Thus excessive movement between these two segments may contribute to the formation of a neuroma. The pes cavus foot may incur a lateral plantar numbness, because individuals with this foot posture spend a disproportionate amount of time along the lateral border of their feet. Callus patterns in the cavus foot rarely occur under the central metatarsal heads. They may be palpated under the medial great toe, between the second and third or third and fourth metatarsal heads, along the medial heel, and, uncommonly, along the lateral border of the foot.

5. What is the clinical presentation?

Morton's neuroma has a classic history of pain on the plantar aspect of the foot that is relieved by rest.[15] Initially the patient may complain only of transient mild ache, throbbing, or burning over the plantar aspect of the forefoot in the area of the third or fourth metatarsal head. The patient may report suddenly being seized with increasing severity by a burning or electric-like sensation along the lateral border of the forefoot. This pain may feel like a pebble or marble in the shoe. After a few minutes the pain abates and the patient may be able to walk comfortably. Because the digital nerves are purely sensory, symptoms is limited to pain and paresthesia, most commonly in the interspace between the third and fourth toes. Pain may radiate into the adjacent toes and occasionally may radiate proximally into the foot or calf. However, if multiple web spaces are involved, a more proximal nerve irritation may exist.

Symptoms of this condition are worsened by standing, walking, squatting, or kneeling with the toes extended and may be relieved by sitting, lying, or changing shoes. The examiner may reproduce pain by the application of pressure over the third or fourth metatarsal heads or by lateral compression of the forefoot. The compression sign[22] is elicited by squeezing the metatarsal heads together. This test is especially effective when combined with dorsiflexion of the toes and a pressing in on the plantar aspect of the affected web

---

*Other conditions that may also occur from this form of malalignment include metatarsalgias, metatarsal stress fracture, claw toes, hammer toes, hallux valgus, and plantar fasciitis.

space. Sensory testing may reveal decreased sensation in the adjacent sides of the affected toes. Diagnosis is made by clinical examination and the exclusion of any other foot disorder.

Electromyographic studies of the plantar nerves often are not performed, because they are unreliable. By age thirty the plantar surface of the foot has been so traumatized by walking that the foot muscles often register abnormal electromyographic signals.

6. What is the differential diagnosis?

• *Phalangeal* or *metatarsal stress* or *fatigue fractures* occur when normal bone is exposed to excessive deforming forces because of repeated unaccustomed impact loading. This may be precipitated by forefoot running or running uphill on hard surfaces or from unaccustomed walking, particularly in osteoporotic individuals. Fractures occur because of training errors that result in muscle fatigue with a diminished protective and energy absorbing role offered the bone by the intrinsic foot muscles. Stress fractures may also occur secondary to bony malalignment. Injury does not result from a single incident, but rather from cyclic trauma in which the ability to spontaneously heal is gradually lost with repetitive impact. Uncommonly, weak bones play a role in stress fractures in amenorrheic female athletes[12] and in rheumatoid patients.[2,7] Stress fractures are also called *march fractures,* because they commonly occur in military recruits unprepared for the rigors of boot camp. Stress fractures in the bones of the foot or ankle commonly occur in ballet dancers and include the metatarsal shafts, the sesamoids, the distal fibula, and tarsal navicular, but these fractures occur most commonly in the tibia.[1] Injury typically affects the beginning dancer, especially following a significant increase in rehearsal schedule. The experienced ballet dancer is less likely to sustain fatigue fractures, because of significant accumulated adaptive hypertrophy of bone in the foot and ankle. However, this injury may occur in the seasoned professional, especially when she or he performs on hard and unyielding floor surfaces. In ballet, metatarsal stress fractures usually occur in the proximal shaft, whereas in runners they most frequently occur in the metatarsal neck* following a sudden increase in mileage.

*Interestingly, stress fractures most commonly occur in humans, racehorses, and racing greyhounds. The common denominator to all three is training for maximum performance despite the presence of some pain.

Normally, living bone constantly remodels its internal structure by the concerted action of osteoblasts and osteoclasts. With repeated impact, bone reabsorption occurs faster than bone deposition, because osteoclastic activity is accelerated in the presence of deforming forces. Thus prior to new bone being formed (Wolff's law) to attenuate excessive stress, a linear fracture will have occurred. The process leading up to fracture begins as a gradual weakening of cortical bone that gradually enlarges as the bone is fatigued beyond its compressive, tensile, and shear limits. Eventually, a small crack may progress to involve the entire circumference of bone, and possibly bone displacement.

Etiologic factors contributing to the development of MTP stress fractures may be related to normal anatomy, as well as to biomechanical foot deviations. The most common sites of fracture are the second, third, and fourth metatarsals, in order of frequency.[17] The excessive forces focused at the medial foot during push-off are negotiated by the hallux by virtue of its having a metatarsal head that is twice the size of that of the second ray. As such, the hallux is capable of absorbing approximately 2 ½ times the force as that of the second metatarsal head. Thus while the first metatarsal is the most mobile, the second metatarsal is the most stable. The proximity of the most stable metatarsal with the hallux may place undue stress upon the metatarsal, especially during the toe-off phase of gait. The second and third rays are also less mobile than the fourth and fifth rays. This lack of mobility prevents the second and third metatarsal shafts from divesting themselves of potentially injurious forces associated with activity.

Biomechanical foot deviations contributing to the development of stress fractures are associated with either extreme of the foot posture spectrum. The ability of bones and joints in the rear and midfoot to absorb, disperse, and redirect excessive force away from the forefoot is compromised with a cavus foot. A cavus foot is inflexibly locked and rigid and has poor shock-absorbing capacity, and thus is a likely candidate for the development of stress fractures. Callosities or even plantar keratomas may be present under the metatarsal heads. In contrast, the forefoot varus-type malalignment may also develop a stress fracture. A forefoot varus is indicative of a mobile first ray, which rotates externally and superiorly during midstance. Displacement of the first ray requires the middle and lateral metatarsals to accommodate the force normally absorbed by hallux. Because the middle and lateral metatarsals are smaller in diameter, they require less force per gait cycle to acquire a fatigue fracture.

Clinical presentation of stress fracture includes the insidious onset of localized pain with weight bearing that is often relieved by rest. Over time, however, pain becomes localized to the area of the fracture. There is often local warmth, edema lying in a circular patch over the metatarsus that may extend to the dorsum of the forefoot, and tenderness of the metatarsal shaft and adjacent interosseous muscles. Palpation of the fracture site yields exquisite pinpoint pain, although there is a painless range of motion of the involved metatarsal joint. In runners the fracture is most often at the neck of the second through the fourth metatarsal. However, it may lie anywhere along the shaft; the fracture is often at the proximal neck in ballet dancers. Generally, there is no history of injury or of an audible crack. Children are also liable to develop marching fractures. Plain radiographs are initially negative for the first 3 to 4 weeks following injury; however, a technetium bone scan will demonstrate high blood flow and osteoblastic activity, confirming the clinical impression. After 2 or 3 weeks a callus may be palpated or viewed radiographically. Pinching of the interdigital nerve of the foot may occur because of callus formation. There is no fear of malunion and it is not necessary for the patient to stop walking during the period of union. The ability of the fractured bone to heal spontaneously is reduced following repeated traumatic loading of the foot. The forefoot should be firmly bound to enable the other metatarsal shafts to splint the broken bone, thus diminishing movement at the fracture site. The patient must decrease his or her level of activity. The use of a stiff-soled shoe or protective orthotic with metatarsal padding may be helpful. Weight bearing may continue to be painful, and the patient may be placed in a short-leg cast. After five weeks, support for the transverse metatarsal arch may be increased by inserting a medial or lateral longitudinal arch support and metatarsal pad proximal to the head of the involved metatarsal. Fractures of the second and third shafts require medial wedging, whereas fractures of the fourth and fifth shafts require lateral wedging.[19] With fractures of the second or third shafts, the use of a 5° to 9° medial hindfoot wedge is appropriate in the patient with hindfoot valgus. A medial forefoot wedge (5°) should be used if the hindfoot is in neutral. In contrast, with fractures of the fourth and fifth shafts, a lateral forefoot wedge (5°) is appropriate if the hindfoot is in neutral, and a lateral hindfoot wedge (5°) should be applied to the patient with hindfoot varus.[19] Casts are more effective for athletes who cannot be relied upon to decrease their activity. At four weeks an athlete may be allowed to gradually resume activity under supervision. A substantial shoe with an adequate arch support is vital for restoring normal biomechanics and preventing recurrence. Increases in activity should be guided by the presence or absence of pain. Cross-training consisting of bicycling or swimming is appropriate before running to maintain fitness during healing. When possible, the dancer is encouraged to perform barre exercises in the swimming pool. Full return to ballet is not permitted until there is radiographic evidence of healing.

• *Sesamoiditis* is inflammation and tenderness of either the tibial (medial) or fibular (lateral) sesamoid within the body of the two-headed flexor hallucis brevis tendon. During standing the extra surface area provided by the two sesamoids allows the hallux to bear a double portion of weight, compared with the adjacent metatarsal heads. During the toe-off phase weight is transferred from the lateral four metatarsals to hallux, which bears the brunt of body weight as it functions as the counterpoint for propelling the body into swing. The presence of the sesamoids helps distribute the considerable pressures focused at hallux during toe-off. The patient reports pain on toe-off that may be reproduced by pulling hallux into extension and palpating over the head of the first metatarsal.

The sesamoid bones offer a biomechanical advantage, similar to that offered by the patella in the knee, that increases mechanical advantage of the flexor hallucis brevis (FHB). The sesamoids deflect the tendons away so that the lever arm is increased, thus increasing mechanical advantage during toe-off. The sesamoids are pulled distally when the metatarsophalangeal joint is dorsiflexed. During late stance beyond heel rise, the sesamoids are placed directly under the first metatarsal and serve as a pulley for the FHB, thereby improving the lever arm for a plantar flexion force of hallux against the ground.[16] Thus the sesamoids are essential to effective propulsion. Chondromalacia and aseptic necrosis of the metatarsal sesamoids may also occur.[24]

Sesamoiditis is best treated with conservative management that includes an external modification, such as a rocker bottom, or an internal modification, such as orthoses with a C-pad or J-pad located proximal to the inflamed sesamoids. A sesamoid platform is a foot insert that has an elevation distal to the sesamoids. As such, it stabilizes the first metatarsal and reduces excess pressure on the first metatarsal head by shifting some of the load proximally to the first metatarsal shaft. An inner-sole excavation removes a portion of the inner sole corresponding to the head of hallux. The excavated area may then be filled with resilient material to reduce load and thereby cushion the sesamoids. A rocker bar is an external modification that has a firm convexity protruding 0.5 cm to 1.0 cm from the bottom of the sole of the shoes. The rocker bar serves several functions: 1) to shift superincumbent load from the phalangeal heads backward to the metatarsal shafts, thus reducing pressure to the heads; 2) to improve push-off; and 3) to reduce the distance the foot must travel during stance phase of gait. With a similar sole modification, the metatarsal bar, a firm piece of leather is placed across the widest portion of the sole. Other internal modifications include a domed metatarsal pad made of sponge rubber. Like the rocker bottom, the metatarsal pad reduces load on the metatarsal heads by shifting load to the shafts. Iontophoresis or the prudent injection of corticosteroids may help reduce inflammation. In recalcitrant cases avascular necrosis or stress fracture should be suspected.

- *Freiberg's disease* is a vascular osteochondrosis of a growth epiphysis similar to Perthes disease that follows the same cycle of rarefaction, collapse, and reformation. Repetitive stress from weight bearing may cause microfractures at the junction of the metaphysis and growth plate. The cumulative effect of these fractures deprives the epiphysis of adequate circulation, resulting in vascular insufficiency and avascular necrosis. Freiberg's differs from Perthes disease in that the osteochondral fragment may become loose, as in osteochondritis dissecans.

Freiberg's disease begins during the adolescent growth spurt in the teenage years between 13 and 18[21] and most commonly affects girls. Many of those affected have a congenital long second metatarsal or short first metatarsal, both of which may cause excessive pressure on the second metatarsal head. Freiberg's disease is associated with running-type activities, as well as with the hypermobile foot stemming from excessive pronation. Wearing high-heeled shoes may also be a predisposing factor, because these shoes deliver excessive forces to the forefoot. The third metatarsal is occasionally affected. The fourth and fifth MTP joints are rarely affected.[11] The adult form of this disorder is a different entity, most likely being an osteochondral stress fracture.[3]

Clinical manifestations of Freiberg's disease include insidious onset of forefoot pain and localized tenderness, usually at the MTP joint of the second toe. The pain usually is experienced on standing and walking and is relieved by rest. There appears to be localized arthritis of the MTP joint, including localized thickening, tenderness, warmth, and motion restriction in flexion and extension. Characteristic radiographic changes do not appear for approximately one month. This makes it difficult to differentiate from a march fracture, which does not become visible until approximately three weeks. Thereafter, x-ray examinations reveal changes typical of all osteochondroses. The first radiographic sign of Freiberg's disease is widening of the MTP joint space, which is seen relating to the effusion.[3] The metatarsal head will regenerate slowly as the blood supply becomes reestablished but will become widened, irregular, and flattened at its articular surface, presumably as a result of the continued stress of weight bearing on the soft, healing bone. Bony spurs, sclerosis, and irregular bone surfaces may be viewed. Diagnosis early in the course of the disease may be made based on increased uptake during a bone scan.

If the disease process is recognized early, cessation of sports activity and immobilization are indicated. However, it is not always possible to stabilize the joint and prevent the disorder from progressing to more advanced stages. Unfortunately, too often the condition is diagnosed only once the process has evolved to an advanced stage. If progression is halted and the disease process is quiescent, it is advisable to use an orthotic device with a metatarsal pad over the MTP joint. Recovery may occur spontaneously after one year with adequate, but not full, range of movement, although the metatarsal head may become permanently enlarged. This may be palpated as an increase in size compared with the contralateral side, as well as a prominent ridge on the bone at the dorsal aspect of its articular edge. Metatarsalgia may ensue, followed by the reappearance of symptoms that herald the onset of osteoarthritis. Eventually the joint may become fixed similar to hallux rigidus by age forty or fifty. Nonoperative management is accomplished by way of a rocker-bottom sole that renders limited toe extension symptomless. Additionally, a metatarsal bar or pad may be placed beneath the involved bone when the patient is wearing low-heeled shoes. Otherwise, orthoses for early stages of Frieberg's infarction are identical to management of sesamoiditis.[23] Activity should be limited to 4 to 6 weeks to permit molding of the metatarsal head into a shape that most closely resembles a normal head. Inflammation is addressed by rest and immobilization. If pain is severe or persistent, the foot may be immobilized in a short-leg walking cast for 3 to 4 weeks or until symptoms subside. If osteoarthritic symptoms persist beyond cessation of activity, surgery may be warranted to excise the metatarsal head or a portion of the shaft or to reshape the metatarsal head.

• *Metatarsalgia* is a commonly mentioned but loosely defined pathologic entity that refers to pain at the ball of the foot, particularly in the region of the metatarsal heads. The pain may be acute, intermittent, or chronic. This is in contrast to the tenderness between the metatarsal heads that corresponds to the course of the nerve in interdigital neuroma. Specific causes of metatarsalgia may include bunions, MTP joint arthritis, or other pathologic entities of the local osseous or soft tissue.[10] The etiology of metatarsalgia derives from numerous causes, many of which are related to the foot engaging in compensatory pronation. For example, first ray insufficiency syndrome is associated with a Grecian (atavistic or Morton's) foot profile in which the second toe is longer than the first. During stance phase excessive force is placed on the relatively less mobile second and third metatarsals, resulting in hypermobility at the first tarsometatarsal joint. This causes caudal migration of the first ray. Because a weight-bearing hallux is essential to locking of the midtarsal joint, the lack thereof during midstance leads to collapse of the midfoot into pronation. The foot is thus pronated when the needs of late stance require supination, resulting in overuse and abnormal stress at the second metatarsal. Management is accomplished by way of a sesamoid platform to support the first metatarsal so as to allow it to bear more weight.

Metatarsalgia may also occur secondary to a tight Achilles tendon, which causes increased stress on the forefoot. Gastrocnemius action progressively increases after its onset in early midstance, to peak action at toe-off. Gastrocnemius also assists in the stabilizing of the midfoot during this period by way of dynamic subtalar inversion, which then supinates the forefoot by way of the midtarsal joint. Thus gastrocnemius helps convert the foot from a "loose adaptor" to a "rigid lever." The foot and ankle require 10° of dorsiflexion for normal locomotion. A tight or congenital short gastrocnemius-soleus complex may prevent the ankle from reaching this position, and the subtalar joint will compensate by pronating during heel-off, when the foot should in fact be supinating. Stance phase will be completed with toe-off despite the foot not having converted into a rigid lever. The price is paid in potentially deranging forces delivered to the forefoot, particularly the MTP joints. Management is directed at stretching the Achilles tendon.

7. What is the association between interdigital neuroma and hallux valgus or the presence of a bunion?

With hallux valgus the flexor power of the toe is impaired by both the angular and rotation deformity occurring at the first MTP joint. Push-off is progressively compromised as the deformity evolves, so that the other MTP joints are passively forced into hyperextension because they are poorly suited to resist roll-over during push-off. Thus favorable conditions for interdigital nerve trauma are present in the presence of a bunion.

8. What therapeutic management is appropriate to treating this condition?

- Avoidance of offending activity.
- The use of an orthotic arch support to reestablish the medial longitudinal arch and transverse metatarsal arch.* If a foot-fault posture is detected, an appropriate orthosis is best prescribed to restore normal biomechanics and prevent stress to the forefoot. A metatarsal "cookie" (pad) may be placed on the superior surface of the orthosis proximal to the two involved adjacent metatarsal heads. This modification may help diminish excessive transverse plane metatarsal movement between the medial and lateral columns of the foot[25] by allowing the metatarsals to spread and facilitating toe flexion.
- Unloading of the metatarsal heads while loading the shafts via a metatarsal bar, rocker bottom, or the wearing of wider, flat shoes.
- Metatarsal pads that elevate the transverse in one of two ways, 1) by elevating the fourth metatarsal head or 2) by elevating the third and fifth metatarsal heads, will permit the fourth digit to sink down. Either method will keep the bones slightly enough out of line to prevent nerve pinching. The pad should be in place proximal to the pinched nerve.

---

*The theoretic basis for orthotic intervention is the hypothesis that by restoring the foot in a neutral position during support phase, and particularly by maintaining the posture of the foot within normal ranges for pronation and supination, abnormal compensations and concomitant stresses will be kept to a minimum or eliminated.

- Wearing of wider, flatter shoes with thicker soles and padding better suited to shock absorption. Wearing shoes with a wider, more spacious toe box and a lower heel is helpful in relieving pressure on the interdigital nerve. Wearing shoes with stiffer soles also may be of help, because these shoes lessen the range of digital dorsiflexion.[5]
- The use of oral nonsteroidal antiinflammatory medications.

9. What is the medical or surgical management for the patient with no relief from conservative treatment?

Relief may be provided by the occasional injection of a long-action corticosteroid with local anesthetic, at a 45° angle with the foot, into the interspace at the level of the dorsal aspect of the metatarsal phalangeal joint. If two or three repeated injections do not resolve this condition, surgical excision of this nerve and its neuroma often brings complete relief, although it leaves a sensory deficit.[9] Alternately, the surgeon may elect to release the intermetatarsal ligament or to partially release the ligament and resect the nerve. Common postsurgical complications are web space hematomas and stump neuromas, which may be avoided through careful hemostasis and the use of drains.[13]

REFERENCES

1. Bachner EJ, Friedman MJ: Injuries to the leg. In Nicholas JA, Hershman EB: *The lower extremity and spine in sports medicine,* St Louis, 1995, Mosby.
2. Baer GJ: Fractures with chronic arthritis, *Am Rheum Dis* 2:269-273, 1984.
3. Baxter D: *The foot and ankle in sport,* St Louis, 1995, Mosby.
4. Bossley CJ, Cairney PC: The intermetatarsphalangeal bursa: its significance in Morton's metatarsalgia, *J Bone Joint Surg* 62B:184, 1980.
5. Brotzman SB: *Clinical orthopedic rehabilitation,* St Louis, 1996, Mosby.
6. Dawson DM, Hallett M, Millender LH: *Entrapment neuropathies,* ed 2, Boston, 1990, Little, Brown.
7. Devas MB: Stress fractures, *Practitioner* 197:70-76, 1996.
8. Durlacher L: *Treatise on corns, bunions, the diseases of the nails and the general management of the feet,* London, 1845, Simption, Marshall.
9. Koppell HP, Thompson WAL: *Peripheral entrapment neuropathies,* Huntington, NY, 1976, Robert E Krieger.
10. Gould JS: Metatarsalgia, *Orthop Clin North Am* 20(4):553-562, 1989.
11. Gregg J, Das M: Foot and ankle problems in the preadolescent and adolescent athlete, *Clin Sports Med* 1(1):131-147, 1982.
12. Harrington T, Dracer KJC, Dip RACOG, et al: Overuse ballet injury of the base of the second metatarsal: a diagnostic problem, *Am J Sports Med* 21(4):591-598, 1993.
13. Jones DC, Singer KM: Soft-tissue conditions of the ankle and foot. In Nicholas JA, Hershman EB: *The lower extremity and spine in sports medicine,* St Louis, 1995, Mosby.
14. Magee DJ: *Orthopedic physical assessment,* Philadelphia, 1987, WB Saunders.
15. Mann RA, Reynolds JC: Interdigital neuroma: a critical analysis, *J Foot Ankle Surg* 3:238, 1983.
16. Michaud T: *Foot orthoses and other forms of conservative foot care,* Baltimore, 1993, Williams & Wilkins.
17. Milan KR: Injury in ballet: a review of relevant topics in the physical therapist, *J Sports Phys Ther* 19(2), 1994.
18. Patten J: *Neurological differential diagnosis,* ed 2, Berlin, 1995, Springer.
19. Reilley MA: *Guideline for prescribing foot orthotics,* Thorofare, NJ, 1995, Slack.
20. Schon LC: Nerve entrapment, neuropathy, and nerve dysfunction in athletes, *Orthop Clin North Am* 25(1):47-59, 1994.
21. Simillie IPS: Freiberg infarction, *J Bone Joint Surg* 147:553, 1957.
22. Spindler KP, Pappas J: Neurovascular problems. In Nicholas JA, Hershman EB: *The lower extremity and spine in sports medicine,* St Louis, 1995, Mosby.
23. Sproul J, Hobart K, Mannarino F: Surgical treatment of Freiberg's infarction in athletes, *Am J Sports Med* 21(3):381-384, 1993.
24. Turco VJ: Injuries to the foot and ankle. Leg. In Nicholas JA, Hershman EB: *The lower extremity and spine in sports medicine,* St Louis, 1995, Mosby.
25. Valmassy RL: *Clinical biomechanics of the lower extremities,* St Louis, 1996, Mosby.

28

Medial Calcaneal Heel Pain Upon Weight Bearing in an Intrinsic Foot Deformity

CASE 1: A 36-year-old female aerobics instructor complains of pain to the proximal plantar surface of her left foot and, to a lesser extent, to the area of her triceps surae tendon. She has taught low-impact aerobics part-time over the past 5 years and dates the origin of symptoms to a request by her supervisor some 5 weeks ago for her to include high-impact aerobics as part of her curriculum. This is a technique that she had not practiced previously. The instructor had occasionally severe pain at the end of the dance routines, and she experienced the pain again the next morning, after she got out of bed. Her family physician instructed her to ice the painful area and take naproxen (500 mg) orally twice daily for 2 weeks. The instructor returned to her physician to report no improvement in symptoms. Her physician twice injected the palmar surface of her right heel with cortisone at 1-week intervals, with no corresponding cessation of symptoms. Her physician then referred her for physical therapy. The patient rated her pain at "8" on an analogue pain scale (1 to 10).

OBSERVATION   Excessive pronation is observed at the heel during early stance phase of gait. Standing still, the patient demonstrates calcaneal valgus and tibial varus, left greater than right.

PALPATION   Palpation reveals exquisite point tenderness along the medial tubercle of the os calcis. Additionally, soft-tissue edema is palpated along the medial aspect of the calcaneus.

RANGE OF MOTION   Dorsiflexion of the first ray is limited to 45°. Ankle dorsiflexion is limited to two thirds of normal range and imparts an empty end-feel beyond that range.

MUSCLE STRENGTH   Muscle strength is normal.

MUSCLE FLEXIBILITY   Muscle flexibility testing reveals moderate tightness in calves and hamstrings, left greater than right. The patient's left medial hamstrings exhibit mild to moderate tightness.

SENSATION   The patient has intact sensation to light touch. No paresthesias are reported. The patient exhibits a negative Tinel's sign.

SPECIAL TESTS   Provocative, sudden, passive dorsiflexion of the left great toe causes searing pain at the medial calcaneus. The result of the hyperpronation test is negative.

RADIOGRAPHS   Radiographic examinations are unrevealing.

CLUE   Measurement of forefoot-to-rearfoot relationships indicates 12° of forefoot varus in the left foot and 10° in the right foot.

CASE 2:   A 48-year-old man received a pink slip from his white-collar desk job of 15 years and faced the prospect of maintaining support of his wife and family of five children. By day he began working for the postal service and delivered mail along his assigned route, and at night he began moonlighting until midnight as a walking guard at a local penitentiary. His duties include walking up and down the long corridors past the prison cells of the 2-acre complex. After 7 months at his newly found work, he visits your office with complaints of insidious pain along the center and inner aspect of his left sole after several hours of walking, but especially when he begins to walk after sleeping or sitting for long periods. The pain abates when he is sitting or standing. He denies any trauma to the foot. When asked, he offers that his mother had rheumatoid arthritis.

OBSERVATION   A slightly antalgic gait is observed, with no evidence of pronation during early stance phase of gait. Obesity is evident.

PALPATION   Palpation reveals exquisite point tenderness and a painful nodularity along the medial tubercle of the os calcis. Additionally, soft-tissue edema is felt at palpation along the medial aspect of the calcaneus.

RANGE OF MOTION   Dorsiflexion of the metatarsophalangeal joint of hallux is limited to 50°. An empty end-feel is felt when the therapist attempts to dorsiflex the left foot beyond 15° dorsiflexion.

MUSCLE STRENGTH   Muscle strength is normal.

MUSCLE FLEXIBILITY   The patient's left lateral hamstring and iliotibial band exhibit mild to moderate tightness.

SENSATION   The patient's sensation to light touch is intact. No paresthesia or anesthesia is reported.

SPECIAL TESTS   Sudden passive hyperextension of the left hallux reproduces symptoms. The patient exhibits a negative Tinel's sign. The result of a hyperpronation test is negative.

RADIOGRAPHS   Radiographic examination reveals a heel spur at the left medial calcaneal tuberosity.

CLUE   Measurement of the forefoot-to-rearfoot relationships indicates a rigid rear foot valgus deformity that is more pronounced in the left foot.

? Questions

1. What is the cause of pain in these patients?
2. What is plantar fasciitis?
3. What is the anatomy of the plantar aponeurosis?
4. How is the triceps surae complex in physical continuity with the plantar aponeurosis?
5. What are the arches of the foot, and what is their functional significance?

6. **What is significant about the foot having a more rigid arch laterally?**

7. **How does the *truss mechanism* maintain static arch support?**

8. **What is the windlass mechanism, and what primary function does it perform?**

9. **What osseous and dynamic factors contribute to resupination of the subtalar joint?**

10. **How many tight medial thigh structures result in the development of plantar fasciitis?**

11. **How may a cavus foot posture predispose to plantar fasciitis?**

12. **What is a calcaneal heel spur, and how is it related to inflammation of the plantar aponeurosis?**

13. **What is the clinical presentation of plantar fasciitis?**

14. **What is the differential diagnosis for plantar fasciitis?**

15. **What is lateral calcaneal neuritis?**

16. **What therapeutic management is appropriate in treatment of plantar fasciitis?**

1. What is the cause of pain in these patients?

Plantar fasciitis of the left foot is the cause of the pain in both case scenarios. In Case 1 the woman's abnormal foot alignment may have predisposed her to tissue breakdown and inflammation by way of excessive forces during repetitive, high-impact aerobics. *Low-impact aerobics* involve dancelike movements in which at least one foot is in contact with the floor at all times. Lower limb movements are typically low kicks and steps, and upper limb movements are typically large and sweeping. In contrast, *high-impact aerobics* involve movements in which both feet may be off the ground simultaneously. Additional resistance to movement, such as the use of held, weighted objects, may increase heart rate. In Case 2 plantar fasciitis has developed by an entirely different pathomechanical pathway.

2. What is plantar fasciitis?

Plantar fasciitis is a classic repetitive-stress injury that may occur in the posturally normal foot or may be precipitated in an abnormal foot. A majority of patients with plantar fasciitis demonstrate either a pronated or a cavus-type foot.[20] Excessive subtalar joint pronation, as from a forefoot varus-type deformity (pp. 345-346), leads to *excessive calcaneal eversion,* which results in stretching of the plantar fascia during the foot-flat subphase of gait. Moreover, if the foot fails to resupinate at toe-off, increased strain is placed along the plantar fascia. Conversely, a cavus foot occurs in the presence of *limited calcaneal eversion,* characteristic of diminished pronation, or supination of the foot, typical of a rigid forefoot valgus deformity (pp. 346-347). A cavus foot is intrinsically incapable of dissipating weight-bearing forces, particularly from heel strike to midstance. Thus

whereas a cavus-type foot stresses the plantar fascia during early stance, a hyperpronated foot stresses the plantar fascia from mid to late stance phase.[20]

Classic plantar fasciitis is an inflammatory condition that is commonly associated with prolonged standing, intense walking, stepping, or running. Repetitive traction stress[1] to the medial calcaneal tuberosity is incurred during gait as the plantar fascia pulls on its origin, causing microtears and painful inflammation. Whether caused by excessive activity in the normal foot or abnormal strain to the plantar fascia of the intrinsically deformed foot, plantar fasciitis will occur if the tensile distractive forces exceed the fascia's ability to withstand tension. If recognized and treated early, this condition may improve, whereas ignoring symptoms and continuing the precipitating activity despite pain may exacerbate inflammation, with disabling results.

Plantar fasciitis is common among dancers, tennis players, basketball players, and other athletes whose sport involves running. Ballet dancers who engage in demipointe and rolling in of the foot (Fig. 28-1) place excessive stress on the plantar fascia[23] and are prone to plantar fasciitis. This disorder is also common in nonathletes whose occupations require prolonged weight bearing on unyielding surfaces, particularly if those individuals are middle aged and overweight. Extrinsic factors that may precipitate a pathologic condition include a switch from activity on a resilient surface to one made of concrete or hardwood; the wearing of poorly cushioned or worn-out footwear, or shoes not designed for the activity; and a sudden increase in training intensity. The plantar fascia normally elongates with increased loads to act in a shock-absorbing capacity;

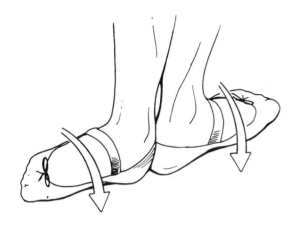

FIG. 28-1 Rolling-in is a maladaptive ballet technique that is characterized by extreme pronation, and places excessive stress upon the plantar fascia and other medial structures of the foot and ankle. (From Hardaker WT: Foot and ankle injuries in classical ballet dancers, *Orthop Clin of North Am* 20[4]:1275, 1989.)

however, with increasing age its elasticity is compromised.

Occasionally, plantar fasciitis occurs in the center of the medial longitudinal arch instead of at the calcaneal insertion of the plantar fascia. This occurrence is known as *midfoot plantar fasciitis.* Pain and tenderness are located in the non–weight-bearing portion of the plantar surface of the foot. Management is similar to that of the more classic form of this disorder.

3. What is the anatomy of the plantar aponeurosis?

The *plantar aponeurosis* (Fig. 28-2) is a broad, multi-layered, fibrous band of connective tissue lying atop the intrinsic foot musculature. The aponeurosis projects forward from the medial and lateral calcaneal tuberosities in the rearfoot distally, blending in with the flexor tendon sheaths and transverse metatarsal ligaments at the metatarsal head of each proximal phalanx. Before its distal insertion the aponeurosis divides to allow the extrinsic and intrinsic flexor tendons to pass through the aponeurosis en route to their plantar distal insertion; by inserting on the medial and lateral sides of the metatarsal heads, the plantar fascia stabilizes the flexor mechanism under the metatarsal heads. Thus by combining with the dynamic and static (joint capsule) structures at the metatarsal heads, the aponeurosis forms the plantar pads of the metatarsophalangeal (MTP) joints. Like the palmar aponeurosis in the hand, the plantar aponeurosis is composed of longitudinally arranged multilayered

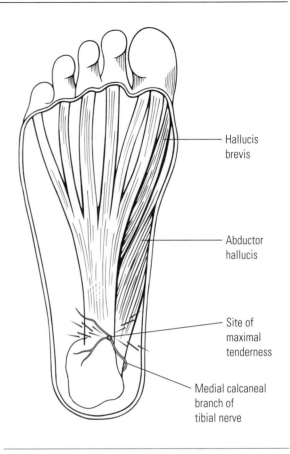

FIG. 28-2 Anatomy of the plantar aponeurosis and site of plantar fasciitis.

bands (medial, central, and lateral components) of fibrous connective tissue and spans the entire plantar aspect of the foot. The superficial central component is the major portion, extending from the plantar surface of the posterior *medial* calcaneal tuberosity to insert on the proximal phalanges of the five toes corresponding to the skin flexion creases between the skin and sole. It is the most superficial of four bowstring ligaments composing the static longitudinal arch supporters of the foot. The medial plantar fascia, known as the tibial component, originates distally and medially, covers the intrinsic muscles of the great toe, and is continuous with the abductor hallucis muscle.[28] The lateral plantar fascia, or peroneal component, is thick and well developed at the heel because it originates from the lateral margin of the medial calcaneal tubercle and is connected with the origin of the abductor digiti minimi muscle. The lateral plantar fascia grows thinner as it approaches the small toe; it is uncommonly implicated in plantar fasciitis.

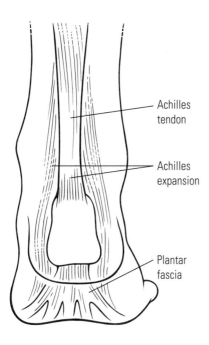

FIG. 28-3 The Achilles tendon has lateral and medial expansions that form broad sheets descending anteriorly and inferiorly to wrap around the sides of the calcaneus. These expansions thin out and wrap under the heel to blend with the plantar fascia. There is no break in continuity between the Achilles tendon and plantar fascia.

4. How is the triceps surae complex in physical continuity with the plantar aponeurosis?

It is significant that the plantar fascia actually originates at the calcaneal tuberosity as a direct continuation of the triceps surae tendon. The Achilles tendon has lateral and medial expansions that form broad sheets descending anteriorly and inferiorly to wrap around the sides of the calcaneus. These expansions wrap under the heel to blend with the plantar fascia (Fig. 28-3). Although the Achilles tendon mainly inserts on the inferior half of the calcaneus, it thins out and continues under the foot, running anteriorly and blending with the plantar fascia. There is no break in continuity between the plantar fascia and the Achilles tendon.[36] Because the plantar aponeurosis is in physical confluence with the Achilles tendon complex, the plantar fascia may be thought of as a quasisurrogate tendon to the triceps surae complex. The plantar fascia is similarly continuous with the dorsal fascia of the foot, as well as with the flexor retinaculum of the medial ankle. This is clinically significant because tightness of the triceps surae may relate to tightening of the plantar fascia

and, indeed, is often seen in patients who develop plantar fasciitis.[16]

5. What are the arches of the foot, and what is their functional significance?

The bones of the foot consist of 7 tarsals, 5 metatarsals, and 14 phalanges. The seven tarsals are the talus, calcaneus, navicular, three cuneiforms (medial, intermediate, and lateral), and cuboid. The arrangements of the 26 bones and 57 articulations composing the foot interlock to form an inherent bow, characteristic of an arch that spans between the hindfoot and forefoot.

The *arch* first came into use in Roman times and represented an innovative engineering principle that had a great advantage over *post-and-beam* architecture, which is limited by being subject to both compressive and tensile loads (Fig. 28-4). The uniqueness of the arch is that the principal stresses imposed upon it are entirely compressive.[5]

Bone is endowed with considerable resistance to compressive load. Since the foot represents the point of contact with the ground, it receives enormous compressive forces from ground reaction forces, as well as from superincumbent body weight. The foot can best adapt to negotiate these forces by assuming three different arches. The longitudinal arches of the foot run along the long axis of the foot and are subdivided into the medial and lateral aspects. The longitudinal arch is supported posteriorly on the calcaneal tuberosity; anteriorly, it rests on the heads of the five metatarsals. The transverse arch of the foot is located just posterior to the metatarsal heads.[8]

The *medial longitudinal arch* consists of the calcaneus, talus, navicular, three cuneiforms, and the medial three metatarsals. The talus is found at the summit of the arch, and the navicular serves as the keystone of the arch. Alternatively, the ligamentous supports of the long plantar arch may be thought of as a bowstring (Fig. 28-5). The bones that constitute the medial section of the longitudinal arch are interlocked by the bowstring action of the *bowstring ligaments,* which provide the highest relative contribution to medial arch stability in the following descending order: plantar aponeuroses, the long and short (calcaneocuboid) plantar ligaments, and the plantar calcaneonavicular (spring) ligament.[12] The elasticity of the *spring ligament,* which runs from the large medial extension of the calcaneus (sustentaculum tali) and supports (i.e., sustains) the talus, account for its name. A *bow* is created when a bowstring of a length shorter than the rod is affixed to the two ends of

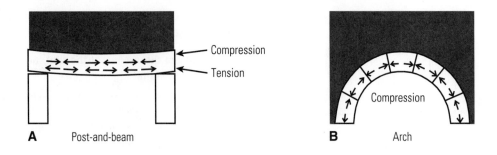

FIG. 28-4 A, While a post-and-beam structure undergoes both tension and compression; **B,** an arch must only bear compressive force. (Redrawn from Beiser A: *Physics,* ed 3, Menlo Park CA, 1982, Benjamin Cummings.)

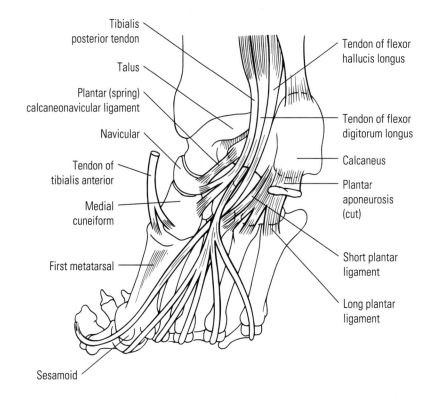

FIG. 28-5 The *medial longitudinal arch* is comprised of the calcaneus, talus, navicular, three cuneiforms, and the medial three metatarsals. The talus resides at the summit of the arch while the navicular serves as its keystone. The bones that constitute the medial section of the longitudinal arch are interlocked by the bowstring action of the *bowstring ligaments* which provide the highest relative contribution to medial arch stability in the following descending order: plantar aponeuroses, the long and short (calcaneo-cuboid) plantar ligaments, and the plantar calcaneonavicular (spring) ligament. The long extrinsic tendons may provide some arch support.

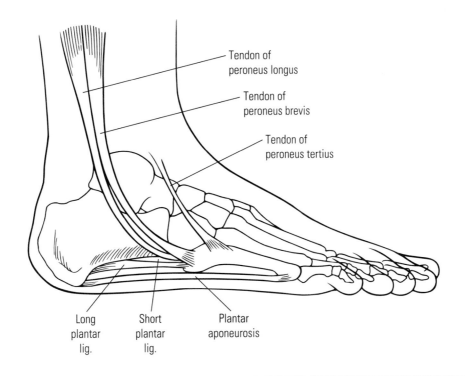

Tendon of
peroneus longus

Tendon of
peroneus brevis

Tendon of
peroneus tertius

Long
plantar
lig.

Short
plantar
lig.

Plantar
aponeurosis

FIG. 28-6 The *lateral longitudinal arch* consists of the calcaneus, cuboid and the lateral two metatarsal bones. While the lateral arch is primarily retained by its bony configuration, its secondary supports include three ligaments (i.e., the short and long plantar ligaments, and plantar aponeurosis) as well as three tendons (i.e., peroneus longus, brevis, and tertius).

the bow, thus creating the tension that pulls the rod into its bow or curved posture. Here, the osseous structures represent the rod that is pulled into a bow by the four bowstring ligaments running deep to the bow.

The plantar aponeurosis may be thought of as a "tie rod" for the medial longitudinal arch, resisting spread between its two ends. Weight bearing forces the forefoot and hindfoot apart, resulting in tension of the tie bar. The *forefoot* and *hindfoot* serve as the primary supports to the medial arch. Four tendons may serve a secondary, passive role by virtue of their orientation of span in relation to the long axis of the foot: the tibialis anterior, tibialis posterior, flexor hallucis longus, and flexor digitorum longus.[27] Thus the medial longitudinal arch relies primarily upon its soft tissue supports to maintain its elevation. Support for the compromised medial longitudinal arch may be provided with a medial forefoot or hindfoot wedge. If the uncorrected heel is in a neutral position, a medial forefoot wedge is helpful. If the uncorrected hindfoot is in valgus, a medial hindfoot wedge is indicated.[27]

The *lateral longitudinal arch* consists of the calcaneus, cuboid, and the lateral two metatarsal bones (Fig. 28-6). This arch, unlike the medial arch, which requires a tie rod to bowstring its configuration, is a true arch because its components are relatively wedge-shaped and interlock to configure a bow. The calcaneus forms the ascending flank, the talus and navicular are the keystones, and the fourth and fifth metatarsals form the descending flank. The lateral arch has a lower apex than the medial portion, rests on the ground during normal standing because of superincumbent body weight, and is the first to flatten during stance phase of gait. While the lateral arch is retained primarily by its bony configuration, its secondary supports include three ligaments (the short and long plantar ligaments and the plantar aponeurosis), as well as three tendons (the peroneus longus, brevis, and tertius.) Support for the lateral longitudinal arch is increased with either a lateral hindfoot or forefoot wedge. If the uncorrected foot of the patient has a varus hindfoot when viewed from behind, a lateral hindfoot wedge is prescribed. If the patient has

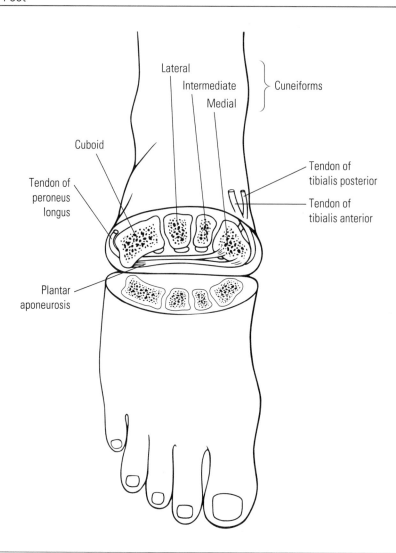

FIG. 28-7 The _transverse arch_ of the forefoot is located immediately behind the metatarsal heads and results from the shape of the distal tarsals and the bases of the metatarsals. The transverse arch runs from the medial aspect to the lateral aspect of the forefoot. It is formed by the cuboid bone, three cuneiform bones, and the bases of the metatarsal bones. The cuneiforms, being wedge shaped, act as keystones while the medial and lateral longitudinal arches act as forefoot pillars. The dynamic transverse arch supports include the peroneus longus tendon (a lateral arch support) the (plantar extension of the) posterior tibial tendon and the long toe flexor (medial arch support) the adductor hallucis muscle and the interosseous muscles. Static transverse arch supports include Lisfranc's ligament and the transverse metatarsal ligament.

a neutral hindfoot, a lateral forefoot wedge is prescribed.[27]

The _transverse arch_ of the forefoot is located immediately behind the metatarsal heads and results from the shape of the distal tarsals and the bases of the metatarsals (Fig. 28-7). These are generally broader dorsally so that, as they fit against one another, a domed con-

figuration results.[25] The transverse arch runs from the medial aspect to the lateral aspect of the forefoot. It is formed by the cuboid bone, three cuneiform bones, and the bases of the metatarsal bones. The wedge-shaped cuneiforms act as keystones, and the medial and lateral longitudinal arches act as pillars. The presence of this forefoot arch accounts for the greater prominence of the first and fifth metatarsal heads, also acting as pillars.[11] The osseous transverse arch, together with ligament and muscle, prevents splaying of the forefoot. The dynamic transverse arch supports include the peroneus longus tendon (a lateral arch support), the (plantar extension of the) posterior tibial tendon and the long toe flexor (medial arch support),[27] the adductor hallucis muscle, and the interosseous muscles. Static transverse arch supports include Lisfranc's ligament and the transverse metatarsal ligament.[35] Transverse arch problems result from forefoot splaying and are corrected by the use of a forefoot pad and a wedge insertion at one of the longitudinal foot arches.[27]

6. What is significant about the foot having a more rigid arch laterally?

The placement of a rigid longitudinal arch laterally and a relatively more flexible arch medially is not arbitrary. The placement of the longitudinal arches along the longitudinal axes of the foot is related to the lateral-to-medial pressure distribution along the foot, which indicates the location of ground reaction force beneath the foot during stance phase of gait. The requirements of early stance are characterized by a supinated foot that provides a rigid base during initial contact. Following initial contact the subtalar and transverse tarsal joints pronate, characterized by flattening of the medial longitudinal arch. Thus heel strike causes weight bearing along the lateral posterior border of the foot, producing pronation of the more rigid lateral longitudinal arch because the requirements of initial stance require a firm base. However, immediately following heel strike, the requirements of the foot include energy absorption of the forces incurred at heel strike and sole conformation to varied terrain. This is consistent with a medial drift of the path of center of pressure along the sole of the foot and corresponds to pronatory collapse of the medial longitudinal arch.

7. How does the *truss mechanism* maintain static arch support?

The longitudinal arches of the foot are not supported by muscle, since a fallen or flattened arch cannot be raised by exercise.[14] *Static* arch support is provided by the *truss mechanism* that converts compressive forces to tensile forces. The plantar aponeurosis is attached at the hindfoot and forefoot and thus traverses the sole of the foot. During static weight bearing, the function of the plantar aponeurosis may be compared to that of the tie rod tying together the two beams, namely the calca-

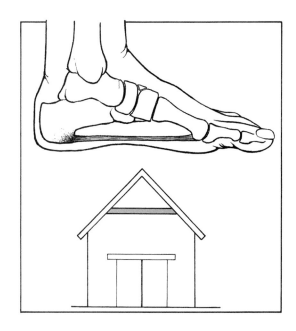

FIG. 28-8 The plantar aponeurosis may be thought of as a *tie rod* for the medial longitudinal arch, resisting spread between its two ends. Weightbearing forces the forefoot and hindfoot apart resulting in tension of the tie bar. (From Dandy DJ: *Essential orthopaedics and trauma,* Edinburgh, 1989, Churchill Livingstone.)

neus and the metatarsals. A *tie rod* is an engineering device in which a rod serves as a structural tie that keep the lower ends of a slanted roof truss or arch from spreading (Fig. 28-8). A *truss* is a triangular structure whose lower ends are connected by a tie rod or bar. The advantage of a truss is that it employs the design of a triangle, endowing it with a structural rigidity capable of withstanding significant *compressive* and tensile forces. The forefoot and hindfoot may be likened to the lower ends of a truss connected by the plantar aponeurosis as if by a tie rod. The vertical compressive forces on at the foot from superincumbent body weight are realized by the *truss mechanism* as *tensile forces* that distract the forefoot from the hindfoot. This increased tension of the plantar aponeurosis resists the tensile forces and becomes progressively stiffer because of the ability of dense collagen to attenuate tension. Increased tension along the tie rod is transmitted to both the lower ends of the truss and approximates the forefoot to the hindfoot. Thus arch support is maintained during standing, despite the vertical forces of superincumbent body weight.

8. What is the windlass mechanism, and what primary function does it perform?

The windlass mechanism* maintains *dynamic* arch support. The windlass action of the plantar aponeurosis is essential to resupination of the subtalar joint, reconstitution of the longitudinal arches, and reestablishment of the foot as a rigid lever during terminal stance phase of gait. Because of the strong distal attachment of the plantar fascia through the plantar pads of the MTP joints, ankle dorsiflexion and toe extension pull the aponeurosis around the metatarsal heads like a cable being wound onto a windlass. Tension is applied to the plantar aponeurosis as the MTP joints move into extension (dorsiflexion). This windlass action occurs passively during late stance as toe extension occurs with the forward momentum of the body.[10]

The kinesiology of the foot in relation to the plantar aponeurosis becomes apparent when the interim between midstance and late stance phase of gait is considered. During this interim the superincumbent body weight imposed on the talus causes inversion of the subtalar joint out of its everted posture, which, in turn, alters the relative alignment of the midtarsal joint (at the midfoot) and effectively locks that joint. As the sequence of superincumbent weight progresses from the hindfoot to the forefoot with heel rise, the ankle joint undergoes plantar flexion. As terminal stance is reached, the MTP joints (in the forefoot) passively dorsiflex during toe-off. During this motion the toes remain in contact with the floor, and the metatarsal shafts angle upward as the hind foot is lifted.

Because the distal insertion of the plantar aponeurosis occurs on the proximal phalanges of the toes, rolling over onto the ball of the foot during late stance of gait will cause winding of the distal aponeurotic fascia beneath the metatarsal heads. As the angle of 55° of toe dorsiflexion is approached at toe-off, the crank-and-winch–like assembly composed of the two osseous poles of the feet and the aponeurosis progressively tenses the aponeurosis, akin to a cable wound onto a windlass. The calcaneus is thus pulled closer to the forefoot, and the arch is elevated (supinated) (Fig. 28-9). This *windlass mechanism* is a passive mechanism and is entirely responsible for arch reconstitution,

known as *supination.* Because the primary origin of the plantar aponeurosis (central component) is the medial aspect of the calcaneus, tension of the aponeurosis promotes calcaneal inversion and thereby initiates subtalar joint supination.

The plantar fascia is composed of longitudinally arranged collagen fibers[22] capable of resisting considerable (e.g., 1.7 to 3 times body weight[10]) tensile forces. As increased loads are applied, the plantar fascia becomes progressively stiffer and more capable of resisting deformation.[37] Although weight bearing forces the metatarsals and calcaneus apart, increasing tension in the plantar aponeurosis negates distraction by binding the rearfoot to the forefoot. Tension at the anterior end of the tie rod (forefoot) is thereby transmitted to the posterior end (rearfoot) and pulls the two ends together. Thus the windlass mechanism is essential in converting a previously loose and adaptable foot to a rigid lever necessary to push-off phase of stance.

9. What osseous and dynamic factors contribute to resupination of the subtalar joint?

Although the passive windlass effect primarily accounts for resupination of the subtalar joint, other factors represent significant contributions to the same end. The integration of passive, osseous, and dynamic factors accounts for arch reconstitution and reversal of subtalar joint posture from pronation to supination.

During stance phase of gait the pressure distribution along the sole of the foot migrates from the proximal *lateral* border to the distal *medial* border. During early stance the lateral border of the heel strikes the ground. The ground reaction force acts lateral to the subtalar joint axis and thereby causes the calcaneal head to evert. Calcaneal eversion sets in motion a "domino effect" proximally as the head of the talus and the tibia internally rotate. In contrast, beyond midstance phase of gait the ground reaction shifts medial to the subtalar joint axis. This shift is demonstrated by medial migration of the path of center of gravity of the foot. This medial shift reaches a crescendo when the medial calcaneal condyle reaches the ground. Ground reaction force, now relocated medial to the subtalar joint axis, inverts the calcaneal head, causing the subtalar joint to reverse its direction and begin supinating. Calcaneal head inversion is accompanied by external rotation of the talus and tibia proximally.

The gastrocnemius-soleus complex may also play a dynamic role in resupinating the longitudinal plantar arch. During push-off phase of late stance, the triceps surae complex plantarflexes across the upper ankle joint

---

*A *windlass* or winch was a powerful machine used as far back as the twelfth century and utilized a rope or cable for hauling or hoisting. A small force applied at the outer edge of a winch handle is changed into a large force at the axle. Winches were used to raise a ship's heavy anchor, haul heavy buckets of water up from wells, or move other large objects. Based on the same principle as a lever which multiplies the force, a windlass basically pulls heavy objects with less effort.

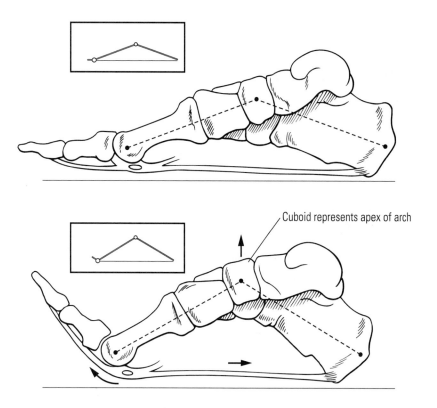

Cuboid represents apex of arch

FIG. 28-9 Windlass effect. The longitudinal arches of the foot and the plantar aponeurosis function as a windlass mechanism beyond heel rise phase of stance to passively resupinate the subtalar joint. The plantar aponeurosis reaches from the calcaneus to the proximal phalanges of the toes, and acts as a tie holding together the two portions of the arch during quiet standing. Beyond heel rise, the aponeurosis acts as a cable distally wound around the metatarsal heads with dorsiflexion. This dorsiflexion of the metatarsal phalangeal joints approximates the calcaneus closer to the forefoot, and results in increased height of the arch.

and falls to the medial side of the subtalar joint. As the line of pull lies medial to the subtalar joint axis, an inversion moment is generated across the subtalar joint. The calcaneous, rising from the ground, may be thought of as being essentially in an open chain condition with respect to the forefoot and is pulled into inversion—a component of arch (and subtalar joint) resupination. Moreover, because the plantar aponeurosis is in physical confluence with the Achilles tendon complex, the plantar fascia serves as a surrogate tendon to the triceps surae that pull the calcaneus into inversion. Concurrently, tension from the plantar aponeurosis, applied to the anteromedial heel, draws the calcaneous toward the forefoot as the arch lifts.

10. How many tight medial hamstring muscles result in the development of plantar fasciitis?

A tight medial hamstring muscle limits knee extension. At high velocities a limitation of knee extension mani-

fests as a lack of heel strike. Individuals with this condition demonstrate an inability to land on their heel and instead are characterized by a midfoot or forefoot strike. This lack of a normal heel-to-toe relationship may cause plantar fasciitis in long-distance runners. Unlike sprinters, who land on their forefoot for only a short period, long-distance runners land on their forefoot over an extended period of time. This causes the heel to sag and depress and in turn causes stretching of the aponeurosis.

11. How may a cavus foot posture predispose to plantar fasciitis?

A *pes cavus* foot may be loosely defined as one in which elevation of the arch of the foot is maintained by a limited (osseous) range of subtalar joint motion. The approximation of the hindfoot to the rearfoot results in shortening of the intervening plantar aponeurosis. The mild cavus foot is a dynamic deformity whose arch is

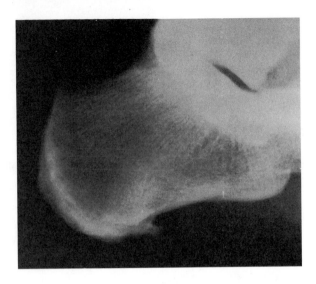

FIG. 28-10 Heel spur may accompany plantar fascitis, although many patients have asymptomatic spurs. (From Nicholas JA, Hershman EB: *The lower extremity and spine in sports medicine,* ed 2, St Louis, 1995, Mosby.)

still flexible enough to compress somewhat on weight bearing, although its shock-absorbing properties are compromised.[32] If this foot is then subjected to excessive, chronic, and repetitive loading, the plantar fascia may sustain strain at its (medial) calcaneal insertion, as relatively less soft-tissue length is available to absorb distractive stress. Furthermore, the patient with a cavus posture has a shortened plantar fascia that, over time, will lose extensibility because of the effects of age-related changes.

12. What is a calcaneal heel spur, and how is it related to inflammation of the plantar aponeurosis?

Regardless of the biomechanical source of plantar fasciitis, a secondary heel spur disorder may subsequently develop. Unrelenting pull of the plantar fascia on its proximal insertion will cause periosteal failure (periostitis), in which avulsion of the periosteum overlying the medial tubercle from the underlying cortical bone occurs. Referred to as a *tension reactive hyperostosis,* the void created by the lifting away of the periosteum is filled with calcium (exostosis), resulting in a *calcaneal plantar heel spur* (Fig. 28-10). Pain is associated with microtears in the plantar fascia and the resulting inflammatory response rather than with a sharp bony spur.

Although bone spurs may be associated with plantar fasciitis, they are not believed to be its cause. Statistically, 15% of normal feet have heel spurs and 50% of painful heels have no spurs.[33] Some patients with plantar fasciitis have an ipsilateral heel spur, and some have an identical spur on the contralateral asymptomatic foot. Similar to osteophytic spurring in the lumbar spine, the presence of a heel spur may be a normal variant; it is often present in the totally asymptomatic foot.

13. What is the clinical presentation of plantar fasciitis?

As with other overuse injuries, pain develops in the patient's foot at the beginning of a workout. The pain diminishes during the activity, only to recur at the finish or later that evening. The plantar fascia is a common site of heel pain in runners.[6] The patient may complain of pain along the instep (medial sole) when standing, walking, and especially running or carrying a heavy weight. This pain is quickly relieved by sitting. The hallmark of plantar fasciitis is severe pain in the heel when the patient first stands upright after a prolonged period of not bearing weight, probably because of the disruption of scar tissue that had begun to form during the period of rest. Slight to moderate to acute tenderness may be elicited on palpation over the midplantar region at the heel and radiating to the forefoot, or at the calcaneal insertion of the plantar fascia. A painful nodularity may be palpated over the proximomedial border of the plantar aponeurosis. When an associated heel spur is present, pinpoint pressing over the anterior medial heel while simultaneously dorsiflexing hallux (passively) tenses the aponeurosis and duplicates excruciating symptoms.

14. What is the differential diagnosis for plantar fasciitis?

The differential diagnosis for plantar fasciitis is extensive and includes systemic disorders such as Reiter's syndrome, psoriatic arthropathy, gouty arthropathy, ankylosing spondylitis, sarcoidosis, rheumatoid arthritis, hyperlipoproteinemia, and systemic lupus erythematosus.[18,19] A high index of suspicion for a systemic disorder is indicated in the young man (15 to 35 years of age) with a presentation of bilateral heel pain, recalcitrant symptoms, associated sacroiliac pain or multiple joint pain, and referral for rheumatologic workup is appropriate in this case. While an S1-level radiculopathy may cause a similar type of pain pattern, local tender-

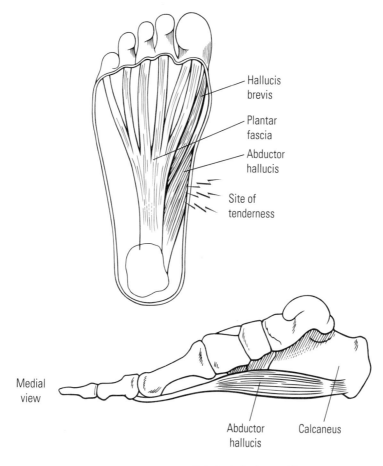

Hallucis brevis

Plantar fascia

Abductor hallucis

Site of tenderness

Medial view

Abductor hallucis

Calcaneus

Abductor hallucis myositis

FIG. 28-11 Abductor hallucis is prone to strain from overuse, overpronation, contusion, or shoe pressure.

ness is absent, and positive nerve stretch signs (e.g., straight leg raise or Lasegue's sign) are typical of a nerve root lesion. Nerve root lesions are often accompanied by a history of low back pain. Calcaneal tumors, stress fracture, or luminescent cysts indicating rheumatoid nodules may be ruled out with radiographic examinations.

- *Tarsal tunnel syndrome* (see Chapter 31) with entrapment of the tibial nerve causes burning or sharp shooting pain on the medial aspect of the heel and ankle. Paresthesias may radiate toward the toes or proximally, especially on percussion of the course of the nerve. The syndrome is frequently traced to *hyperpronation,* and symptoms may often be reproduced by stretching the course of the distal nerve via the *hyperpronation test*—maximal eversion of the

calcaneus of the involved foot for 30 to 60 seconds to reproduce symptoms.

- *Sever's disease* is a lesion similar to Osgood-Schlatter disease, occurring in the Achilles tendon at its insertion into the posterior apophysis of the os calcis (see Fig. 34-13). Common in 6- to 10-year-old children, this condition is characterized by pain, tenderness, and swelling along the calcaneal tendon. Relief is often obtained by elevation of the shoe heel (see Fig. 37-4C).
- *Abductor hallucis myositis,* or strain, is an overuse syndrome most common in men in the third decade of life (Fig. 28-11). The abductor hallucis brevis is an intrinsic foot muscle spanning from the rearfoot to the forefoot. It acts to abduct and assist in flexion of the great toe, as well as in adduction of the forefoot.[15]

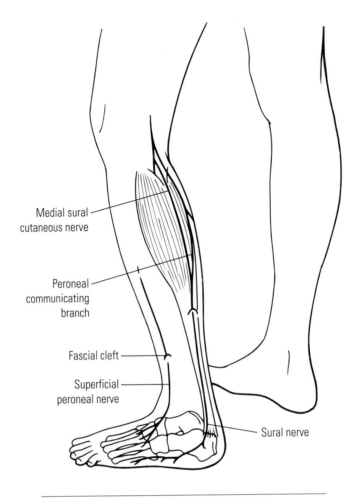

FIG. 28-12 Anatomic course of the sural nerve.

This muscle originates from the medial plantar surface of the os calcis and runs forward and medially to the plantar-medial base of the first phalanx of the great toe encapsulating the medial sesamoid. The posterior neurovascular bundle enters the sole of the foot beneath this muscle belly. During gait the abductor hallucis brevis (along with other foot intrinsic muscles, including the flexor hallucis brevis, flexor digitorum brevis, and abductor digiti minimi) acts to stabilize the transverse tarsal joint during stance phase of gait.[21] The abductor hallucis is singularly active during late stance phase, when it plantarflexes the first metatarsal during propulsion.[31] Once the sesamoids of hallux are firmly planted on the ground, the abductor hallucis is in a mechanically sound position to develop an effective lever arm to plantarflex the first ray.[34] Patients often complain of pain in the

foot with sprinting, aerobics, or dance-related activities. The common denominator of these activities is a lack of heel strike and excessive midfoot and especially forefoot landing. With myositis, pain may occur at the origin of the muscle on the medial aspect of the calcaneus or in the muscle belly along the medial aspect of the longitudinal arch, but not at the posterior tibial insertion on the navicular. Physical examination reveals tenderness in the soft tissue of the medial longitudinal arch,[34] which corresponds to the muscle belly of the abductor hallucis.[27] In contrast, *abductor hallucis brevis tendinitis* is characterized by pain at that tendon insertion at the medial aspect of the first metatarsophalangeal joint.[34] Whether myositis or tendinitis, inflammation of the abductor hallucis is often caused and exacerbated by overpronation of the foot.[34] Pain is elicited by having the patient pull the forefoot into adduction against pressure by the examiner. If the hindfoot is in valgus, a 5° or 9° medial hindfoot wedge and 1-mm heel height are appropriate, accompanied by daily calf stretching. If the hindfoot is in neutral, a 0° hindfoot wedge, 1-mm heel height, and 5° medial forefoot wedge are appropriate.[27]

- *Sural nerve entrapment* is another potential cause of calcaneal heel pain. The sural nerve at the ankle consists of the medial sural nerve and the peroneal communicating nerve. The medial sural nerve is a branch of the distal sciatic nerve that is formed by the union of several fascicles from both divisions of the sciatic in the popliteal fossa.[7] The medial sural nerve emerges from the fossa between the medial and lateral heads of the gastrocnemius muscle and travels down the posterior crural compartment to anastomose with the peroneal communicating nerve, becoming the sural nerve at the ankle. This nerve then emerges from the posterior crural fascia approximately 20 to 25 cm above the bottom of the heel,[7] descending along the border of the Achilles tendon. At the border of the Achilles tendon, just above the ankle joint, the nerve branches into a lateral branch that may anastomose with the superficial peroneal nerve and a posterior branch that runs just inferior to the peroneal sheaths subcutaneously. The nerve continues to branch by the region of the tuberosity of the fifth metatarsal (Fig. 28-12). The posterior branch provides sensation to the lateral part of the heel, lateral dorsal surface of the foot, and sole of the foot up to the base of the fifth toe.[30] The sural nerve at the ankle is most commonly entrapped or subject to laceration in the lateral ankle or foot,[30] primarily at the level of its exit through fascia. If this is the case, a positive Tinel's sign may be elicited at this point, with radiating paresthesias into the lateral foot. Sural nerve entrapment may develop in the feet of athletes who sustain a fracture of the base of the fifth metatarsal, fibula, calcaneus, or cuboid.[9,26] Recurrent lateral ankle sprains may cause fibrosis and nerve entrapment.[26] Ganglions and tumors of the peroneal sheath may also cause entrapment. A common cause of sural nerve pathologic conditions in athletes is an iatrogenic injury, in which the patient underwent a lateral ankle reconstruction using a peroneal tendon, during which time the sural nerve became entrapped in scar tissue or was transected during the surgical approach. Sural nerve compression may also stem from the nerve being adjacent to an inflamed and edematous Achilles' tendon.[13] Abnormality of the sural nerve

can be easily confirmed by studying its sensory action potential.[7] Conservative management is similar to that for other nerve problems in the foot and ankle.

15. What is lateral calcaneal neuritis?

A commonly overlooked cause of chronic heel pain *(calcodynia)* is entrapment of the *first branch of the lateral plantar nerve* (nerve to the abductor digiti minimi muscle). This branch commonly arises from the lateral plantar nerve, which originates in the posterior tibial nerve before passing behind the medial malleolus to enter the tarsal tunnel (Fig. 28-13).[17] This slip of nerve is composed of mixed motor and sensory fibers and changes direction from vertical to horizontal as it approaches the medial plantar aspect of the heel adjacent to the origin of the plantar fascia (see Fig. 31-4, *A*). Entrapment of the first branch occurs where the nerve passes just distal to the medial calcaneal tuberosity, which may precipitate nerve compression in the presence of a heel spur.[2] Alternatively, the nerve may sustain compression secondary to inflammation at the origin of the plantar fascia because of plantar fasciitis. The first branch may also undergo compromise as a result of overpronation, causing compression between the heavy, deep fascia of the abductor hallucis muscle (see Fig. 31-4, *B*), the medial caudal margin of the medial head of the quadratus plantae muscle,[30] and the most medial plantar fascia (Fig. 28-14).[2] Finally, the nerve may be compromised at the origin of the flexor brevis muscle which may cause sufficient swelling to result in compression of the nerve against the long plantar ligament and calcaneus. Nerve involvement may result from plantar fasciitis in approximately 10% to 15% of plantar fasciitis cases.[3,4] Etiology also includes excessive pronation, which, akin to compression of the *medial plantar nerve* (i.e., jogger's foot—see pp. 348-349) running beneath the spring ligament, traumatizes these nerves. Alternatively, these nerves may be compressed by an ill-fitting arch support. Clinical presentation includes tenderness over the course of the nerve maximally in the area of entrapment. Reproduction of neuritic pain with palpation of the *plantar medial aspect of the heel* along the proximal abductor of the plantar fascia is characteristic. Palpation should be performed along the tarsal tunnel and in the distal metatarsal interspaces over the interdigital nerve to determine the extent of involvement. Numbness may be found but is uncommon. Entrapment of the first branch of the lateral plantar nerve causes plantar medial heel pain that is often indistinguishable from plantar fasciitis. Motor

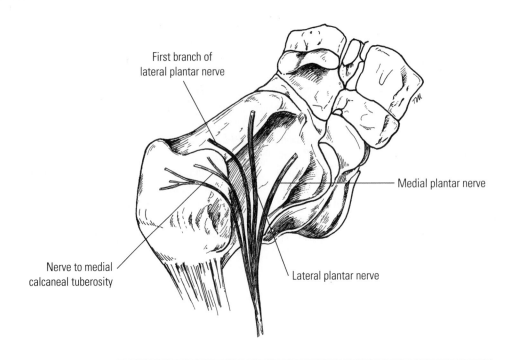

First branch of
lateral plantar nerve

Medial plantar nerve

Nerve to medial
calcaneal tuberosity

Lateral plantar nerve

FIG. 28-13 First branch of the lateral plantar nerve. (From Baxter D: *The foot and ankle in sport,* Mosby, St Louis, 1995, Mosby.)

weakness occurs in the *abductor digiti quinti muscle,* as well as paresthesia along the course of the nerve, without cutaneous sensory deficit. Occasionally a patient complains of a more neuritic pain, either in the medial aspect of the ankle or toward the lateral side of the foot. Symptoms of a neuroma involving three to four web spaces concurrent with the heel pain may be a clue to more proximal nerve involvement. This condition is managed by rest, nonsteroidal antiinflammatory agents, contrast baths, withholding of steroid injection, the use of a shock-absorbing heel insert, and medial longitudinal arch support to decrease tension on the nerve. The use of heel cups or pads with or without an accompanying heel lift in the shoes may be helpful. A stretching program focusing mostly on the Achilles tendon and plantar fascia should be instituted three times per day and after arising from bed. Surgical fasciectomy is reserved for recalcitrant cases.

16. What therapeutic management is appropriate in treatment of plantar fasciitis?

Patience is the virtue that is key to resolution of plantar fasciitis because the majority of cases resolve with therapeutic care. The *goals* of therapy include controlling the abnormal biomechanics of the foot, decreasing

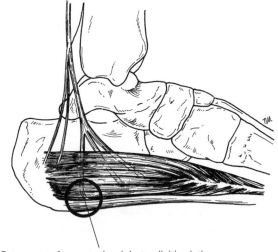

Entrapment of nerve to the abductor digiti quinti m.
between deep fascia of the abductor hallucis m.
and the medial caudal margin of the quadratus
plantae m.

FIG. 28-14 Entrapment of the first branch of the lateral plantar nerve to the abductor digiti minimi (quinti) muscle. (From Baxter D: *The foot and ankle in sport,* St Louis, 1995, Mosby.)

the inflammatory condition, and improving the flexibility of the triceps surae. The entire process may take 6 to 12 weeks. The patient must adhere to the conservative management program for as long as pain persists and avoid the temptation to return to vigorous activity prematurely; doing so may result in relapse and conversion of an acute condition into a chronic disability. An athlete may consider returning to the precipitating activity only when tenderness and morning symptoms (pain and stiffness) have consistently abated. Patients who remain symptomatic for 6 to 9 months after initiation of conservative care may be candidates for surgical intervention. Surgery is performed on an outpatient basis as a last resort and involves snipping away that portion of fascia undergoing excessive tension and inflammation.

• *Rest.* The key to effective management is early rest. The precipitating activity, such as high-impact aerobics, is temporarily stopped. The athlete may maintain cardiovascular conditioning through temporary substitution with non–weight-bearing activities such as swimming, cross-country skiing (e.g., using a Nordic Track), and stationary cycling. Recommended measures before getting out of bed in the morning include light stretching and warming of the calf muscles and plantar aponeurosis by pointing the toes toward the ceiling and making clockwise and counterclockwise foot circlets.

• *Night Splint.* Use of a *plantar fascia night splint* (Fig. 28-15) is effective in decreasing discomfort. Normal neuromuscular tone typically postures the foot in the equinus position during sleep, predisposing approximation of the forefoot to the rearfoot. This allows shortening of the plantar fascia during sleep, and hence a vicious circle of nocturnal contracture and early morning stretching of the aponeurosis with the first few morning steps is initiated. Using a splint to hold the involved foot in 90° dorsiflexion allows the aponeurosis to heal in the lengthened position and thereby circumvents reinjury on morning weight bearing. This position also addresses tightness of the calf muscle.

• *Iontophoresis.* This is performed by application of 10% hydrocortisone for 30 minutes to the inflamed area, with the drug electrode placed over the medial aspect of the calcaneus. This may be followed by ice massage over the same area. *Ice massage* may be applied for pain, up to three times per day, to the area of tenderness for 10 to 12 minutes at a time. One technique involves freezing water in an empty tennis ball and having the patient longitudinally roll the foot over the ball. The use of *whirlpool* treatment or *electrotherapy* by way of high-volt galvanic stimulation[24] or transcutane-

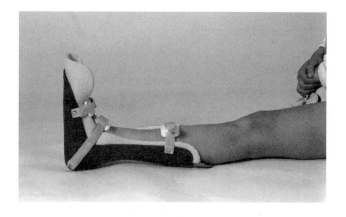

FIG. 28-15 Position of night splint during patient use. (From Brotzman SB: *Clinical orthopaedic rehabilitation,* St Louis, 1996, Mosby.)

ous electrical stimulation may also prove beneficial in reducing symptoms.

• *Stretching Exercises.* These include all the posterior lower extremity musculature, involving lengthening of the gastrocnemius-soleus muscle group and hamstring static stretching in combination with *ultrasound,* for 10 minutes. This may be followed by the application of *cold modality* for 20 minutes, with the patient in the same position as in the ultrasound treatment, to maintain gains in the plastic deformation accrued during stretching of the triceps surae. The clinician must address *imbalances in soft tissue* and attempt to redress them by appropriately identifying and applying stretching and strengthening modalities. If normal soft-tissue alignment is not reasserted in the lower extremity, the dysfunction may reassert itself and become chronic. Weakness found in either the lateral or medial hamstrings is managed by the strengthening of those muscles and stretching of the opposite side. The patient is instructed in a *home exercise program* of stretching.

• *Plantar Fascia Stretching.* This is accomplished by having the patient sit with the knees bent and feet flat on the floor (Fig. 28-16). The examiner holds the tips of the toes and gently bends them into dorsiflexion. The ankle is then gently dorsiflexed, and the metatarsophalangeal joints are gingerly hyperdorsiflexed. The patient should feel a stretch (not pain) along the plantar fascia. The examiner holds the stretch for 10 seconds and may superimpose gentle, simultaneous eversion of the calcaneus. This exercise may be performed up to 10 times a day. As pain recedes and recovery is initiated, stair stretching of the plantar fascia and calf complex may be initiated. Stair stretches are accomplished by

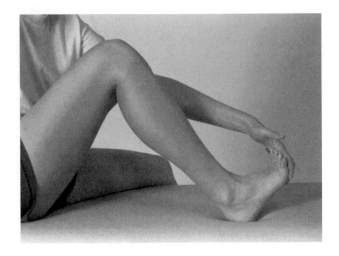

FIG. 28-16 The patient sits with her knees bent and feet flat on the floor. The patient or therapist holds the tips of the toes and gently bends them into dorsiflexion. The ankle is then gently dorsiflexed, and the metatarsophalangeal joints are carefully hyperdorsiflexed. A stretch (not pain) should be felt along the plantar fascia. The examiner holds the stretch for ten seconds and may superimpose gentle simultaneous eversion of the calcaneus. (From Brotzman SB: *Clinical orthopaedic rehabilitation,* St Louis, 1996, Mosby.)

having the involved heel hanging over the back of a step while supporting one's weight through the forefoot (Fig. 28-17). Steady downward pressure in the direction of the heel is gently applied.

• *Strengthening Exercises.* These include the muscles that cross the subtalar joint axes, particularly the tibialis posterior and anterior, because these muscles act eccentrically to decelerate pronation. Thus a patient with a foot-fault deformity in which excessive pronation is implicated as a causative factor in dysfunction would benefit from eccentrically working these muscles in an attempt to absorb excessive and potentially destructive forces resulting from quick collapse of the long plantar arch. The longitudinal arches are not supported by muscle, even though several musculotendinous structures pass under the midfoot en route to their distal attachment. A fallen or flattened arch cannot be raised by exercises. Because of this, exercises such as having the patient curl his or her toes around a towel and try to lift the towel with the toes are ineffectual vis-à-vis the long plantar arch. Eccentric strengthening of the triceps surae is also appropriate.

The use of oral nonsteroidal antiinflammatory *medications* may help relieve symptoms, although the patient and clinician must be on the lookout for such

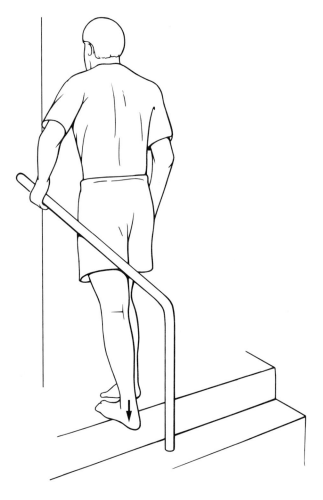

FIG. 28-17 Stair stretches are accomplished by having the involved heel hanging over the back of a step while supporting one's weight through the forefoot. Steady downward pressure in the direction of the heel is gently applied.

side effects as gastric irritation or black and bloody stools. *Shoe modification,* modification of the running surface (from concrete to a soft surface such as grass), or changing to good walking or running shoes are beneficial. Walking barefoot or wearing slippers and shoes without a heel is discouraged. A *weight reduction program* is essential to reduce tensile loading of the plantar aponeurosis. *Friction massage* at the origin of the plantar fascia is helpful in breaking down scar tissue. Taping may be employed to unload the plantar fascia.

• *Orthosis.* Correction of underlying intrinsic structural imbalance to correct biomechanics reduces the tensile forces acting to distract the plantar aponeurosis and thereby seeks to reverse the etiologic factors

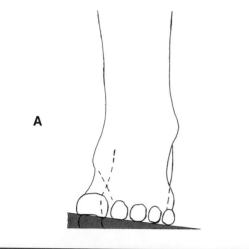

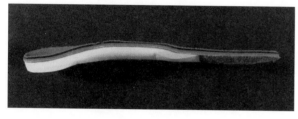

FIG. 28-18 A, Forefoot medial post for forefoot varus. **B,** Forefoot varus (medial post.) (From Brotzman SB: *Clinical orthopaedic rehabilitation,* St Louis, 1996, Mosby.)

predisposing to dysfunction. Before the therapist determines whether a patient would benefit from more expensive, custom-made orthoses, test pads consisting of wedges of high-density felt placed on the inside of the patient's shoes are appropriate to determine whether biomechanical alignment shows improvement. Alternatively, soft, spongy heel cups (e.g., Viscoheels) may be used. A mediolongitudinal arch support is often poorly tolerated because it pushes up on the plantar fascia and increases tension on its fibers.[2]

Orthotic management of a *forefoot varus deformity* involves supporting or balancing the forefoot by posting or building up an orthosis along the medial aspect of the foot (Fig. 28-18). This forefoot varus posting brings the surface or ground up to the suspended medial structures, under the weight-bearing aspects of the metatarsal heads. When this is done, the subtalar joint need not pronate as much to allow the medial aspect of the foot to contact the ground. A *rigid forefoot valgus* deformity is managed by lateral posting and heel lifts to take some tension off the Achilles tendon; additionally, rearfoot valgus posting is helpful to promote normal

pronation from heel strike to footflat. The correct height of the heel lifts is determined by having the patient stand with the hindfoot resting on wooden platforms of different heights until the ideal height that abolishes symptoms is found. Typically a ⅛-inch medial heel wedge is useful in taking tension off the plantar fascia. An elevated heel diminishes the angle between the hindfoot and forefoot, thereby relaxing the plantar fascia. The use of a doughnut placed under the painful anteriomedial calcaneus, or incorporation of a depression into the orthosis, may relieve painful weight bearing at the site of inflammation as load is disbursed peripherally.

If the patient's foot fits neither category of intrinsic deformity, orthotic treatment is keyed to the position of the hindfoot and mobility of the first ray for both classic and midfoot plantar fasciitis. Early orthotic management may require as much as an 8- to 9-mm heel height because of tight heel cords; this height is tapered down as symptoms improve. If the hindfoot is in valgus, a 5° to 9° medial hindfoot wedge and 1-mm heel height are appropriate. If the hindfoot is in neutral, a 0° hindfoot wedge with a 5° medial forefoot wedge and 1-mm heel height is appropriate.[27] If the foot has a neutral hindfoot and hypermobile first ray, a 0° hindfoot wedge, 5° lateral forefoot wedge, and 1-mm heel height are appropriate. If the hindfoot is in varus, the patient may require a 5° lateral hindfoot wedge and 1-mm heel height. Alternatively, the use of a University of California Biomechanics Laboratory (UCBL) orthosis may afford relief. This orthosis holds the heel in inversion and applies forces against the navicular and lateral aspect of the forefoot, without direct upward pressure on the soft tissue beneath the longitudinal arch.[1] This posture slackens the plantar fascia by approximating the proximal origin to the distal insertion (forefoot) of the aponeurosis.

Judicious use of *steroid injection* may be appropriate in recalcitrant cases. Although short-term steroid use may prove beneficial, long-term sequelae must also be considered. Possible long-term sequelae include plantar fascia rupture and subsequent loss of the medial longitudinal arch, fat pad atrophy, allergic reaction to corticosteroid, low infection risk, and a fairly painful injection.

• *Prevention.* Prevention includes warm-up before activity. Warm-up should include slow stretching of the calf muscles and the Achilles tendon. The intensity, frequency, and duration of workouts should be reduced. Runners must be reminded to avoid hills and speed work. Patients accustomed to one long workout should break the workout up into two shorter ones. Use of appropriate running shoes is essential.

REFERENCES

1. Baxter DE: *The foot and ankle in sport,* St Louis, 1995, Mosby.
2. Baxter DE, Pfeffer GB, Thigpen M: Chronic heel pain: treatment rationale, *Orthop Clin North Am* 20(4):563-569, 1989.
3. Baxter DE, Pfeffer GB: Treatment of chronic heel pain by surgical release of the first branch of the lateral plantar nerve, *Clin Orthop* 279:229-236, 1992.
4. Baxter DE, Thigpen CM: Heel pain: operative results, *Foot Ankle* 5(1):16-25, 1984.
5. Beiser A: *Physics,* ed 3, Menlo Park, Calif, 1982, Benjamin Cummings.
6. Bojsen-Moller F, Flagsted KE: Plantar aponeurosis and integral architecture of the ball of the foot, *J Anat* 121(3):599-611, 1976.
7. Dawson DM, Hallet M, Millendor LH: *Entrapment neuropathies,* ed 2, Boston, 1990, Little, Brown.
8. Goss CM, editor: *Gray's anatomy of the human body,* ed 29, Philadelphia, 1973, Lea & Febiger.
9. Gould N, Trevino S: Sural nerve entrapment by avulsion fracture at the base of the fifth metatarsal bone, *Foot Ankle* 2(4):213-219, 1987.
10. Hicks JH: The mechanics of the foot. II. The plantar aponeurosis and the arch, *J Anat* 88:25-30, 1954.
11. Hoppenfeld S: *Physical examination of the spine and extremities,* Norwalk, Conn, 1976, Appleton-Century-Crofts.
12. Huang CK et al: Biomechanical evaluation of the longitudinal arch stability, *Foot Ankle* 14(6):353-357, 1993.
13. Husson JL, Blouet JM, Masse A: Le syndrome du de file de l aponevrose superficielle posterieure surale (Entrapment syndrome of the superficial posterior sural aponeurosis), *Int Orthop* 11(3):245-248, 1987.
14. Jones RL: The human foot: an experimental study of its mechanics, and the role of its muscles and ligaments in the support of the arch, *Am J Anat* 68:1, 1941.
15. Kendall FP, McCreary EK: *Muscles: testing and function,* ed 3, Baltimore, 1983, Williams & Wilkins.
16. Kibler WB, Facsm CG, Chandler TJ: Functional biomechanical deficits in running athletes with plantar fasciitis, *Am J Sports Med* 19(1):66-71, 1991.
17. Kopell HP, Thompson WAL: *Peripheral entrapment neuropathies,* Huntington, NY, 1976, Robert E Krieger.
18. Kwong PK et al: Plantar fasciitis: mechanics and pathomechanics of treatment, *Clin Sports Med* 7(1):119-126, 1988.
19. Leach RE, Seavey MS, Salter DK: Results of surgery in athletes with plantar fasciitis, *Foot Ankle* 7(3):156-161, 1986.
20. Lutter LD: Running athletes in office practice, *Foot Ankle* 3(1):153-159, 1982.
21. Mann RA, Inman VT: Phasic activity of intrinsic muscles of the foot, *J Bone Joint Surg* 46A:469, 1964.
22. Mann RA: Surgical implications of biomechanics of the foot and ankle, *Clin Orthop* 146:111-118, 1980.
23. Milan KR: Injury in ballet: a review of relevant topics for the physical therapist, *J Orthop Sports Phys Ther* 19(2):121-129, 1994.
24. Moffat M: Course work materials for Therapeutic Exercise course offered in 1991.
25. Netter FH: *The CIBA collection of medical illustrations,* vol 8, part I, Summit, NJ, 1991, CIBA-GEIGY.
26. Pringle RM, Protheroe K, Mukherjee SK: Entrapment neuropathy of the sural nerve, *J Bone Joint Surg* 56B(3):465-468, 1974.
27. Reilly MA: *Guidelines for prescribing foot orthotics,* Thorofare, NJ, 1995, Slack.
28. Sarrafian SK: *Anatomy of the foot and ankle,* Philadelphia, 1983, JB Lippincott.
29. Schon LC, Baxter DE: Neuropathies of the foot and ankle in athletes, *Clin Sports Med* 9(2):489-508, 1990.
30. Schon LC: Nerve entrapment, neuropathy, and nerve dysfunction in athletes, *Orthop Clin North Am* 25(1):47-59, 1994.
31. Stormont DM et al: Stability of the loaded ankle: relation between articular restraint and primary and secondary static restraints, *Am J Sports Med* 13(5):295-300, 1985.
32. Subotnick SI: *Podiatric sports medicine,* New York, 1975, Futura.
33. Tanz SS: Heel pain, *Clin Orthop* 28:169-178, 1963.
34. Valmassy RL: *Clinical biomechanics of the lower extremities,* St Louis, 1996, Mosby.
35. Viladot A: The metatarsals. In Jahss MH, editor: *Disorders of the foot,* vol 1, Philadelphia, 1982, WB Saunders.
36. Waller JF Jr, Maddalo AV: Foot and ankle linkage system. In Nicholas JA, Hershman EB: *The lower extremity and spine,* ed 2, vol 1, St Louis, 1995, Mosby.
37. Wright DG, Rennels DC: A study of the elastic properties of plantar fascia, *J Bone Joint Surg* 46A:482, 1964.

RECOMMENDED READING

Hicks JH: The mechanics of the foot: the plantar aponeurosis and arch, *J Anat* 88:25, 1954.

Roy S: How I manage plantar fasciitis, *Phys Sports Med* 10:127-131, 1983.

29

Pain and Triggering Posterior to Medial Malleolus Just Lateral to Calcaneal Tendon That Is Exacerbated by Push-Off Phase of Gait and Reproduced by Flexing and Extending Hallux

CASE 1: A 19-year-old female ballet dancer complains of pain and tenderness posterior to the left medial malleolus, and an occasional snapping sensation when descending from the demipointe position. Symptoms are of 5 months duration and have become progressively worse. The patient reports practicing classical ballet 6 hours a day, with an emphasis on relevé pointe positions. She appears to have the classic "Balanchine" ballerina body silhouette, which includes a small head, slender neck, small waist, and slightly shortened torso with long slender legs. The patient reports that taking ibuprofen before and after dancing has afforded some relief. There is no history of recent ankle injury. When asked, she denies pain during downhill walking or wearing high heels.

OBSERVATION   A variance in cadence suggests a problem with the push-off phase of the left foot. No axial malalignment of the lower extremities is observed. Mild swelling is observed posterior to the medial malleolus. No peroneal muscle spasm is noted. A moderate left forefoot varus deformity is noted.

PALPATION   Slight crepitus is felt as the left great toe is alternately flexed and extended. Pinpoint tenderness is noted just medial to the left calcaneal tendon.

PASSIVE RANGE OF MOTION   Extremes of passive and active flexion and extension of the hallux reproduce pain. Passive extension of the left hallux is decreased by one third.

STRENGTH   Strength of left great toe flexion is decreased by one third of a grade.

SELECTIVE TENSION   Resistive left great toe flexion yields pain.

SENSATION   Sensation over the medial plantar area is normal.

REFLEXES   Reflexes are normal.

SPECIAL TESTS   Posturing the left foot in extreme plantarflexion or dorsiflexion is painless. A negative result is obtained on the hyperpronation test and tests for plantarflexion and Tinel's sign.

CASE 2: A 27-year-old prima ballerina complains of pain during the push-off phase of gait underneath her left great toe, particularly when toe dancing. Symptoms are of 6 months duration and are becoming worse. The patient reports definite triggering accompanied by pain while descending from the demipointe to foot flat or following the reassumption of demipointe. She occasionally is unable to assume the pointe posture because of triggering. No axial malalignment of the lower extremities is noted. The patient reports relief while taking aspirin before and after dancing. She reports no incident involving an ankle injury in recent memory.

OBSERVATION   Observation reveals mild swelling at the metatarsal head of the left first ray. A variance in cadence suggests a problem with the push-off phase of the left foot. No axial malalignment of the lower extremities is observed. No peroneal muscle spasm is noted. A moderate left forefoot valgus deformity is noted.

PALPATION   Palpation yields point tenderness deep in the posteromedial compartment of the ankle, just anterior to the Achilles tendon. A snap is imparted to the examiner's hand in this location as the hallux and ankle are flexed and extended.

PASSIVE RANGE OF MOTION   Extremes of passive and active flexion and extension of hallux reproduce pain. Passive extension range of the left hallux is decreased by one third.

STRENGTH   Strength appears decreased by one third in response to flexion of the left hallux.

SELECTIVE TENSION   Selective tension provokes reproduction of symptoms on resisted flexion of the left hallux.

SENSATION   Sensation is intact over the tibial nerve distribution.

REFLEXES   Reflexes are normal.

SPECIAL TESTS   Posturing the left foot in extreme plantarflexion or dorsiflexion is painless. A negative result is obtained on the hyperpronation test and the test for Tinel's sign.

? Questions

1. What is most likely causing these women's symptoms?
2. Why are dancers often at risk for injuries that are most commonly seen in the realm of competitive sports?
3. What is the classification of tendon pathophysiology?
4. What is the relevant anatomy of tendon disease?
5. How is the flexor hallucis longus (FHL) best palpated and assessed for muscular strength?
6. What areas along the distal tendon are predisposed to potential stenosis caused by overactivity?
7. What is the kinesiology of the flexor hallucis longus muscle?
8. What is the relationship between FHL function and the subtalar joint?
9. What two postural foot deformities are associated with the development of FHL tendinitis?
10. Which postural foot deformity is associated with FHL tendinitis caused by excessive *pronation?*
11. How may a compensated forefoot varus deformity compromise the structural integrity of the FHL tendon?

12. **Which postural foot deformity is associated with FHL tendinitis caused by excessive *supination*?**

13. **What external trauma mechanism may injure the FHL tendon?**

14. **What is the clinical presentation?**

15. **What is the differential diagnosis?**

16. **What therapeutic intervention is most appropriate to patient management?**

1. What is most likely causing these women's symptoms?

Flexor hallucis stenosing tenosynovitis occurs in the region of the fibroosseous canal posterior to the talus[25] and is suggested in case I. Tendinitis of the flexor hallucis longus (FHL) tendon, also called *dancer's tendinitis*,[40] is rarely seen with activities other than classical ballet. This is because dance frequently re-

quires the dancer to assume the relevé positions of demipointe (weight bearing on the metatarsal heads) and en pointe (the entire foot at 180° to the tibia), both of which are characterized by extreme plantarflexion of the ankle joint. With the ankle in plantarflexion, the FHL functions as a primary dynamic stabilizer of the medial foot, first ray, and ankle.[25] Both ballet positions place the foot in equinus and thereby stimulate late

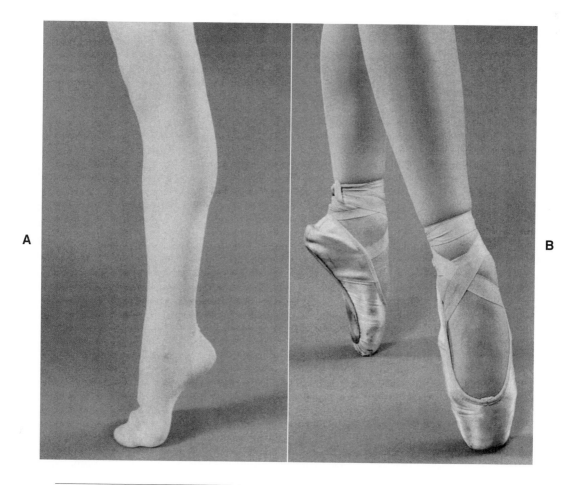

FIG. 29-1 A, Demipointe position, with the weight on the ball of the foot. This position is used by both male and female ballet dancers. **B,** A dancer "en pointe" wearing traditional pointe shoes. This technique is usually confined to female dancers. (From Baxter D: *The foot and ankle in sport,* St. Louis, 1995, Mosby.)

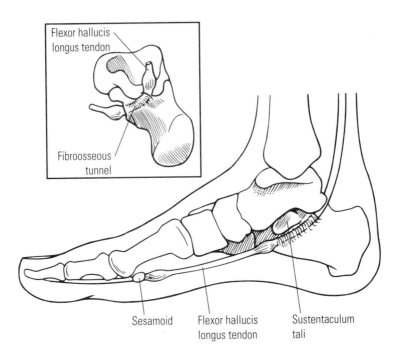

FIG. 29-2 Triggering occurs because of fusiform swelling of the flexor hallucis longus tendon at the fibroosseous pulley located between the medial and lateral tubercles on the posterior aspect of the talus, or beneath the sustentaculum tali.

stance of gait, during which the FHL contracts concentrically to help supinate the long arch of the foot. *Demipointe* corresponds to the heel rise phase of stance, and *pointe* may be compared with late toe-off (Fig. 29-1). Although aesthetically pleasing, repetitive *(sur le) pointe* dancing while maintaining an absolute "vertical line" of the foot with the proximal leg may stress, stretch, or produce partial tears in the FHL tendon.[10,11,34,35] Susceptibility to injury is increased in young, female dancers who are highly motivated and prematurely advanced beyond their ability. If ignored, FHL tendon disease may result in tendon rupture.[15]

Case II involves a *trigger toe of hallux* caused by partial rupture of the FHL tendon, with fusiform swelling of the tendon at the fibroosseous canal posterior and inferior to the medial malleolus. A rent in the FHL tendon and fusiform thickening of the distal tendon alter smooth gliding and may cause triggering of the great toe (Fig. 29-2). Triggering occurs because the swollen tendon is tethered at the flexor pulley as it passes through the fibroosseous canal or beneath the sustentaculum tali.

2. Why are dancers often at risk for injuries that are most commonly seen in the realm of competitive sports?

In the public eye, ballet dancers are considered artists and not athletes. Despite this perception the physical demands of dance choreography strain the limits of endurance such that the dancer is at risk for injuries frequently confined to the arena of competitive sports. Additionally, certain injuries are seen mostly in dancing and rarely in athletics.

The foot and ankle are common sites of injury in ballet dancers because of repetitive impact loading of the dancer's foot and ankle on a relatively hard, unyielding surface. Furthermore, unlike the athlete, who often wears footwear specifically designed to the needs of a given sport, the ballet dancer wears only a thin slipper or toe shoe. Because of this, the foot and ankle absorb the brunt of forceful impact and readily succumb to injury. Human willpower may readily push the body beyond the limits of endurance. Classical dance mandates rigid requirements of mastery of basic dance steps, concentration, balance, coordination, mental maturity, and physical strength

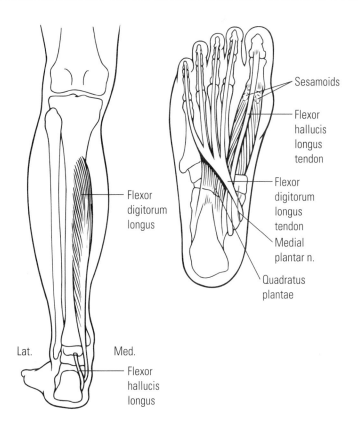

Sesamoids

Flexor hallucis longus tendon

Flexor digitorum longus

Flexor digitorum longus tendon

Medial plantar n.

Quadratus plantae

Lat.   Med.

Flexor hallucis longus

FIG. 29-3 Anatomic course of flexor hallucis longus. Note that the muscular portion of FHL shifts from the lateral to the medial crural compartment, while its tendon winds around the malleolus and travels posterior to anterior under the foot en route its distal insertion. This winding and transverse course may contribute toward increased friction within the substance of the tendon.

before a dancer advances to pointe dancing. Meeting these requirements is mandatory to advancement because advancing a dancer beyond her or his ability and training may lead to both acute and chronic injuries.[27]

3. What is the classification of tendon pathophysiology?

Tendons are composed of bundles of dense collagen fibers with a parallel orientation to the long axis of the tendon. Tendon strength is similar to that of bone and can often withstand 600 to 1000 kg of force. If excessive tensile force is applied to a tendon following violent (especially eccentric)[1] muscular effort, the tensile limit of the tendon will be exceeded, resulting in a strain. The blood supply nourishing tendons is generally tenuous and may be related to the tendon disease process.[4]

Tendon disease may be classified according to the various anatomic structures involved in the disease process. *Peritendinitis* is inclusive of *tenosynovitis* and *tenovaginitis*; the former refers to inflammation of the synovial nutrient sheath protectively covering the tendon, and the latter refers to scarring of that same sheath. *Tendinitis* refers to the condition in which the site of injury is the tendon itself and in which the injury is accompanied by an inflammatory response. Tendinosis refers to tendon degeneration without an inflammatory response.

Factors predisposing to tendon injury or disease include inadequate conditioning and warm-up, fatigue, prior muscle injury, scarring, overstretching, and prior steroid injection. Tendon failure occurs at the weakest point in the musculotendinous-skeletal system, and thus an individual's age is often determinant of the precise point of failure. An avulsion fracture at the

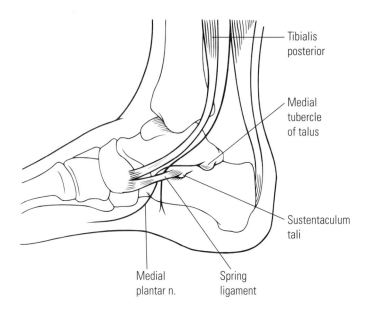

Tibialis posterior

Medial tubercle of talus

Sustentaculum tali

Medial plantar n.

Spring ligament

FIG. 29-4 Medial view of the ankle showing relationship between the sustentaculum tali, medial talar tubercle, and spring ligament. Note how the spring ligament and posterior tibial tendon respectively function to statically and dynamically maintain the medial longitudinal arch.

physeal plate is a more likely injury in children, because the growth plate is usually the weakest point. In middle age, increasing degeneration of collagen fibers within the tendon makes the tendon the weakest point.[1]

4. What is the relevant anatomy of tendon disease?

The FHL, located under the soleus, is the most robust of all posterior compartment leg muscles (Fig. 29-3). It arises from the distal two thirds of the posterior fibula, intermuscular septum, and interosseous membrane and distally courses lateromedial, passing medial to the Achilles tendon before entering the foot. Rather than wrapping posteriorly around the medial malleolus, as do the flexor digitorum longus (FDL) and the tibialis posterior tendons, the tendon of the FHL runs along the posteroinferior aspect of the ankle joint by way of a groove or *fibroosseous tunnel* between the medial and lateral tubercles on the posterior aspect of the talus. The tunnel is bordered anteriorly by the talar body, medially by the medial tubercle of the talus, laterally by the lateral tubercle of the talus (the os trigonum if separated), and posteriorly by the flexor retinaculum.[19] The fibrous tissue of the canal acts as a *simple pulley* for the FHL.[37]

The FHL tendon next passes under the sole of the foot by first traversing the undersurface of the *sustentaculum tali* (Fig. 29-4), the large medial calcaneal extension just inferior to the medial talar tubercle that is so essential to supporting the talus and a normal arch and that also functions as a *second simple pulley.*[41] The FHL tendon then passes forward in the sole, just medial to the overlying FDL tendon (where it offers a tendinous slip), beneath a fascial sling known as the *Master Knot of Henry* that is located under the base of the first metatarsal. After crossing the common toe flexor, the tendon crosses the metatarsophalangeal (MTP) joint and passes between the two sesamoid bones imbedded in the substance of the two heads of the flexor hallucis brevis. The tendon then crosses the interphalangeal joint and distally inserts into the plantar base of the distal phalanx of hallux.

5. How is the FHL best palpated and assessed for muscular strength?

Because the FHL is deeply located, it is often difficult to palpate. The tendon actually crosses the posterior aspect of the upper ankle joint rather than going around the medial malleolus. The FHL tendon runs along the posterior aspect of the tibia and grooves the posterior aspect of the talus between its medial and

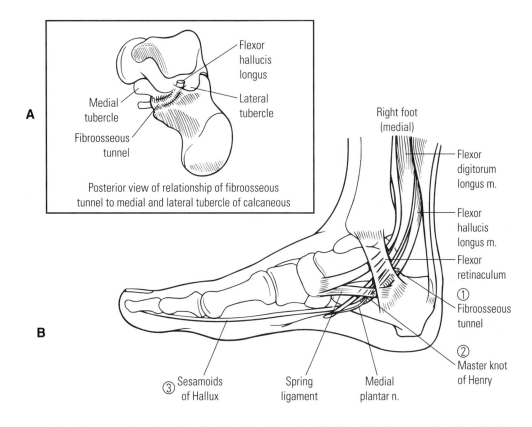

FIG. 29-5 Sites of potential tendon stenosis include the fibroosseous canals, Henry's knot corresponding to FHL crossing over flexor digitorum longus (FDL), and at the head of the first metatarsal where the tendon passes between the sesamoids of hallux. **A,** Posterolateral view. **B,** Medial view of the foot and ankle.

lateral tubercles.[16] Palpation is used for assessment most easily in the posteromedial compartment of the ankle, at the ankle joint line just anterior to the Achilles tendon.[33]

When manually assessing strength of the FHL, the examiner should ensure that the foot is not bearing weight. The examiner stabilizes the ankle joint midway between dorsiflexion and plantarflexion by fixing the calcaneus with one hand. Proximal stabilization is necessary because full dorsiflexion may yield passive flexion of the interphalangeal joint, whereas full plantarflexion would shorten the muscle, decreasing the muscle's mechanical advantage and thereby compromising its ability to generate maximum force.[20] The examiner uses the other hand to stabilize the MTP joint in neutral position while instructing the patient to curl his or her great toe against the examiner's opposition. The test should be performed on the uninvolved contralateral hallux first so as to determine a baseline.

6. What areas along the distal tendon are predisposed to potential stenosis caused by overactivity?

Because the distal route of the FHL tendon is fraught with areas of potential stress rise, the tendon may sustain tenosynovitis, partial ruptures, and nodules. Pathologic conditions may be manifested as pain, triggering, and problems with push-off.[41] Sites of potential tendon stenosis (Fig. 29-5) include the fibroosseous canals; *Henry's knot,* corresponding to the FHL tendon crossing over the FDL; and the head of the first metatarsal, where the tendon passes between the sesamoids of hallux.[40] Stenosis in the former location, the fibroosseous canal, predisposes the tendon to mechanical irritation and inflammation by virtue of an overactive tendon in a confined space, similar to extensor tendon tenosynovitis of the thumb in de Quervain's syndrome.[12] If inflammation is prolonged or the fibroosseous canal becomes stenotic, the disorder may evolve into a partial tendon strainwith snapping and triggering within the tunnel. The latter, more distal form of flexor hallucis stenosing tenosynovitis is rarer and more likely in runners. The sheath between the sesamoids undergoes chronic or intermittent inflammation and eventually heals in a constricted fashion, which impairs tendon passage.

7. What is the kinesiology of the flexor hallucis longus muscle?

Anatomically, the FHL primarily flexes the interphalangeal joint of the great toe and assists in flexion of the MTP joint, plantarflexion of the ankle joint, and inversion of the foot. The kinesiology of the FHL in relation to closed kinetic chain stance function is understood in relation to the subtalar joint, in which it performs an eccentric pronation function. Both pronation and supination are primarily passive occurrences. Whereas pronation is characterized by arch sag occurring as a direct function of superincumbent body load, supination is characterized by arch reconstitution and occurs as a direct function of the windlass mechanism of the plantar aponeurosis. Early stance is characterized by foot pronation to allow adaptation over varied terrain. The foot, serving as the point of confluence between superincumbent body weight and ground reaction force, may sustain injury in the absence of a force absorption strategy. Without the benefit of dynamic influence over the rate of pronation, the magnitude of forces at the foot following heel strike could easily result in injury. Energy absorption by the foot is afforded by controlled eccentric pronation. Controlled pronation that slows the rate of arch sag minimizes the jarring effect of impact; this may be accomplished by an eccentric contraction of the FHL and other extrinsic invertor muscles. These muscles demonstrate a peak of electromyographic output during early stance.

The FHL, like the tibialis posterior and the other posterior crural compartment musculature, concentrically contracts during late stance to provide the forward thrust necessary for push-off. Supination characterizes the foot during late stance, and the FHL and tibialis posterior may play a dynamic role in concentrically pulling the forefoot closer to the hindfoot (supination), thereby helping to reconstitute the long plantar arch. Hence a second peak of electrical activity for the FHL occurs between the heel-off and toe-off subphases of stance.

8. What is the relationship between FHL function and the subtalar joint?

FHL tendinitis stems from overuse, resulting in posterior and anterior shin splints. The pathokinesiology of the FHL[28] is best understood in relation to subtalar joint pronation and supination during the gait cycle.

Ten muscles, most of which have another primary function, are grouped according to their relationships to the subtalar joint axis (i.e., as the evertors, invertors, and plantar intrinsics). Muscles that cross the subtalar joint medially are listed in order of their inverting leverage; these include the tibialis posterior, tibialis anterior, FDL, and FHL. The common denominator of these muscles is their collective orientation of span; contraction approximates the forefoot to the hindfoot and thereby elevates the longitudinal plantar arch. An eccentric contraction of these muscles will allow flattening of the arch in a controlled fashion. This is important during the interval between early and midstance, when the foot must sequentially "crumple" as part of a strategy to absorb forces during heel strike.

The mechanism of injury in FHL tendinitis may be viewed against the backdrop of posterior shin splint syndrome. Like the latter, FHL tendinitis involves an extrinsic leg muscle that winds around the malleolus and may be overused because of an overpronated foot or a cavus foot posture. An additional complicating factor is present in the FHL tendon. The FHL shifts from lateral to medial, whereas its tendon winds around the malleolus and travels posterior to anterior under the foot en route to its distal insertion. This causes increased friction within the substance of the tendon.

9. What two postural foot deformities are associated with the development of FHL tendinitis?

Because of the intimate relationship the FHL has with subtalar joint function, any alteration in subtalar joint sequencing may compromise FHL function. After heel strike, the extrinsic invertor muscles (located along the medial side of the subtalar joint) eccentrically contract to pronate the arch, whereas during push-off, in conjunction with the triceps surae, these same muscles *concentrically* contract to propel the leg forward.[7] Abnormal sequencing of the subtalar joint may be expressed as one of two extremes: compensatory, and hence excessive, pronation, as in a forefoot varus deformity; or supination, as in a forefoot valgus deformity.[42] As a result, FHL function from either extreme will place the

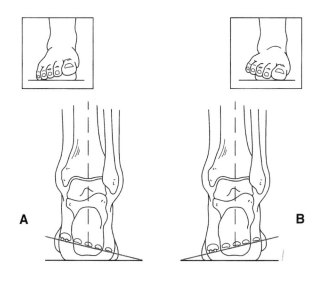

FIG. 29-6 A, In *forefoot varus* the forefoot is in structural inversion. **B,** In *forefoot valgus,* the forefoot is in structural eversion. (From Magee DJ: *Orthopedic physical assessment,* Philadelphia, 1997, WB Saunders.)

muscle at a mechanical disadvantage and result in muscle fatigue. If this condition is unresolved, tendinitis may develop at any one of three susceptible locations. The mechanism common to either foot deformity may contribute to FHL tendinitis through excessive tendon distraction by superincumbent body weight while the tendon concentrically contracts during supination or eccentrically contracts during pronation.

10. Which postural foot deformity is associated with FHL tendinitis caused by excessive *pronation?*

During quiet standing, a *forefoot varus deformity* is defined as a frontal plane malalignment characterized by an inversion of the forefoot on the rearfoot, with the subtalar joint held in neutral (Fig. 29-6).[7] Forefoot varus is one of the most common forefoot deformities, manifesting clinically as excessive weight borne along the lateral border of the foot and metatarsal heads, with calcaneal eversion. This increases the risk of inversion sprain. Forefoot varus usually appears in the compensated foot with a depressed arch and hindfoot valgus angulation. In the foot in which subtalar neutral has been restored, the medial forefoot is levered off the floor, creating a gap between the ball of the foot and the contact surface. From a management standpoint, the

gap would be filled with orthotic posting material so that normal forefoot and hindfoot alignment is restored. In the noncompensated condition the calcaneus everts and the longitudinal plantar arch depresses as the head of the talus bulges proximal to the tubercle of the navicular while the navicular adducts and plantarflexes on the talus and calcaneus. Excessive arch pronation tends to be prolonged beyond midstance and leads to late resupination at the end of stance phase of gait, thus delaying or preventing the foot from stiffening as a rigid lever during push-off. Push-off is inefficient, since the first ray cannot be recruited for effective propulsion. Hypermobility during late stance may lead to excessive soft tissue stress and injury. The functional results are poor forward propulsive thrust and inefficient transition from late stance to early swing. During stance phase, weight bearing will remain along the lateral plantar surface, placing excessive pressure under the fourth and fifth metatarsal heads. Palpation of a callus under the fifth metatarsal head is a clinical indicator of this uncompensated state.

To visualize compensatory forefoot changes, the examiner should view the foot from an anterior-to-posterior perspective. In the case of forefoot varus, in the non–weight-bearing condition (e.g., during swing phase of gait), the medial border of the foot rides higher than the lateral border. During early-to-mid stance phase of gait, as the plantar surfaces of the toes all make contact with the ground, there is a compensatory forcing of the subtalar joint into hindfoot valgus. In the case of a long-standing malalignment, correcting the hindfoot to subtalar neutral will have the effect of lifting the first ray (relative to the fifth). Thus while weight bearing in the corrected condition, and assuming that treatment involves orthotic control, the "gap" created between the great toe and the ground would be filled by a medial forefoot post.

11. How may a compensated forefoot varus deformity compromise the structural integrity of the FHL tendon?

By itself, forefoot varus is not destructive to the foot. However, the associated "unlocking" of the foot via subtalar joint pronation leads to loss of a rigid lever from midstance through push-off. This compensatory strategy involves pronation of the subtalar joint as midstance begins, continuing beyond midstance and into late stance at a time when the foot is resupinating.[14,17] When the subtalar joint compensates by pronating, the compensatory pronation occurs. When will this result in calcaneal eversion? Calcaneal eversion is a component of pronation and initiates a cascade of events proximally in what may be described as a "domino effect," in which the talus and tibia internally rotate.

Hypermobility of the foot during late stance (at push-off phase) causes severe stress on the tissues of the forefoot and can be destructive to the foot and the rest of the lower kinetic chain during propulsion.[31] Although this compensatory strategy improves the medial metatarsals in contact with the ground, it does so with the result that the foot loses its ability to become a rigid lever. The price the foot pays for pronatory compensation is the negation of the rigid lever function of supination that is so essential to adequate propulsion, since push-off is attempted on a loose bony-articular complex.*

The FHL produces concentric plantarflexion torque that peaks at late terminal stance, when the entire posterior compartment musculature generates propulsion. However, the tendon functioning out of temporal sequencing is being *distracted* along its length because of superincumbent body weight, while simultaneously attempting to concentrically *contract* during late stance. This may cause a tension rise within the tendon that may exceed the tendon's tensile limit and thereby compromise its structural integrity. Over time the FHL tendon may subsequently succumb to strain, degeneration, microtears, and inflammation because of chronic overload.

12. Which postural foot deformity is associated with FHL tendinitis caused by excessive *supination?*

When a patient's foot posture appears with the forefoot everted relative to the rearfoot, bringing the medial side below the lateral side, the patient is said to have a forefoot valgus deformity (see Fig. 29-6). When this foot posture cannot be eliminated in response to the standing posture, during which the ground reaction force pushes upward on the foot, the deformity is said to be a *rigid forefoot valgus deformity.* This deformity directly contrasts with the opposite-type forefoot varus posture, since the medial forefoot structures are in contact with the surface while the lateral aspect is suspended. An uncompensated forefoot valgus results in collapsing of the medial longitudinal arch because all of the body weight is borne on the medial side of the forefoot, thus effectively shortening the ipsilateral limb. A rigid forefoot valgus stems from an inherently insufficient range of motion in the longitudinal axis of the midtarsal joint.

Forefoot varus and valgus are the most common types of foot malalignments and may best be appreciated in the non–weight-bearing foot as a *twisting* of the forefoot relative to the hindfoot at the midtarsal joints when the ankle is maintained in *subtalar neutral.* In the case of forefoot valgus the fifth ray is elevated above the level of the great toe, theoretically subjecting it and the second digit to excessive loading, especially during the push-off phase of stance. Forefoot valgus may be thought of as the forefoot's twisting in the opposite direction such that the great toe and medial border of the foot are lifted above the fifth digit, subjecting the lateral forefoot to excessive loading. When the foot is in contact with the ground, during stance phase of gait, the clinical presentation of the forefoot changes and is best appreciated as a compensatory coupling with the hindfoot; forefoot deformities almost always manifest as hindfoot compensatory malalignments, thus distorting subtalar neutral alignment. Understanding the relationship of the hindfoot to the forefoot serves as the basis for treatment of the foot with posted in-shoe orthotics. Posting essentially fills the gap between the medial (forefoot varus) or lateral (forefoot valgus) border of the foot when the hindfoot is corrected to *subtalar neutral.* In many cases it is difficult to determine whether primary forefoot malalignments lead to hindfoot compensatory changes or vice versa, although the latter scenario may be more likely.

Bypassing the effects of this unstable foot posture as well as any ensuing biomechanical deviations, and continuing locomotion without interference are accomplished, once again, by the subtalar joint. Excessive pronation during contact phase is countered by subtalar joint supination as a compensation strategy during early stance, when the foot requires a loose adapter function characteristic of pronation. However, this requirement is bypassed to avoid gait-related instability caused by a functional, ipsilaterally shorter limb.

---

*Because of this instability in the forefoot, abnormal shearing forces between the metatarsal heads may predispose to interdigital neuroma, metatarsalgia, metatarsal stress fracture, claw toes, hammer toes, and hallux valgus, as well as plantar fasciitis. Because of instability in the rearfoot, pronation is expressed proximally along the tibial shaft as an internally rotated moment predisposing to Achilles tendinitis, shin splints, knee dysfunction, tethering of the sciatic nerve under the piriformis muscle, sacroiliac joint dysfunction, or low back pain. Thus, while pronatory compensation allows continued locomotion, it may alter the biomechanics of the distal and proximal extremity by generating a destructive imbalance to the biomechanics of the lower extremity.

Supinatory compensation for a rigid forefoot valgus occurs through the following sequence of events. Normally the subtalar joint begins to move from a locked, supinated position into a pronated posture at heel strike as the forefoot meets the ground in anticipation of foot flat during midstance phase of gait. With a rigid forefoot valgus, however, the medial side of the forefoot—particularly the first metatarsal—strikes the ground without the benefit of the lateral column loading. Locomotion in this fashion would eventually beat the foot into a pulp, were it not for the ability of the subtalar joint to allow for lateral metatarsal weight bearing along the supporting surface. The subtalar and midtarsal joints compensate by supinating, thus pulling the rearfoot into an inverted posture, which shifts weight bearing laterally. This early supination and resulting stability come at a high price, however, when the stance requires a pronated foot. The foot does not have a chance to return to pronation before midstance, resulting in the deleterious inability of the foot to absorb shock and adapt to changing terrain. Furthermore, vaulting over midphase of gait with weight now focused along the lateral border increases the likelihood of an inversion sprain of the ankle joint. Calluses form in the rigid forefoot valgus under the first and fifth metatarsal heads, corresponding to the initial and compensatory forefoot loading characteristic of this deformity.

Forefoot valgus manifests as essentially the opposite of forefoot varus. Given a raised fifth toe, during swing phase of gait, as the toes make contact with the ground during early approaching midstance, the hindfoot compensates and is forced into a varus angulation. In this case orthotic posting is applied to the lateral side of the forefoot after subtalar neutral is established.

Excessive stress may be delivered to the tendon of the FHL and to all of the invertor muscles that medially span the subtalar joint axis. A forefoot valgus deformity involves too little pronation during the interim between early stance and midstance as the subtalar joint is forced into supination immediately following heel strike. Aside from the jarring effects of this supinatory moment during early stance phase, the FHL and all of the invertor muscles that medially span the subtalar joint axis concentrically contract to approximate the forefoot to the hindfoot during that time when superincumbent body weight distracts the forefoot from the hindfoot. Thus the invertor muscles are mechanically disadvantaged, and sustain forces that *distract* them while they attempt to *contract*. Within the tendon, this may cause a tension rise that may exceed the tendon's tensile limit and thereby compromise its structural integrity. Over time the FHL tendon may subsequently succumb to degeneration and inflammation because of chronic overload.

13. What external trauma mechanism may injure the FHL tendon?

Laceration of the FHL commonly occurs in the region of the medial longitudinal plantar arch of the foot near the first MTP joint. Laceration injuries often occur secondarily to puncture wounds from stepping on sharp objects such as nails or broken glass.

14. What is the clinical presentation?

When the *proximal tendon* is inflamed, it is tender along its course posterior and lateral to the medial malleolus. The patient may complain of pain, tenderness, and mild swelling posterior to the medial malleolus, as well as problems with push-off. Posterior ankle pain extends just distal to the talus[15] but not as far as Henry's knot.[13] If the lesion has advanced to a stenosing tenosynovitis, the patient will additionally complain of a snapping sensation posteromedially. If a fibrotic nodule has developed, crepitus may be demonstrated on gentle palpation and the patient may report occasional difficulty in flexing the great toe. Triggering and pain may be reproduced by passively flexing and extending the great toe or by standing on the ball of the foot and descending to the floor. Triggering in these instances, as in trigger finger, is caused by a fibrotic nodule on the FHL tendon that yields a painful click because of tendon excursion through the fibroosseous stricture. The diagnosis is confirmed by palpating the tendon deep in the posteromedial compartment of the ankle at the ankle joint line anterior to the Achilles tendon and feeling the snap as the great toe and ankle are flexed and extended.

Tightness of the FHL may be observed in many individuals with chronic tenosynovitis of the FHL tendon. Tightness is assessed by noting the amount of passive extension of the first MTP joint with the foot and ankle in both neutral and plantarflexed postures. Contracture is demonstrated by an inability to passively or actively extend the MTP joint beyond neutral with the foot and ankle in neutral position, as compared with the passive extension possible with the ankle plantarflexed.[19] Contracture of the FHL tendon is one mechanism for the development of a *hammer toe deformity* of the great toe.[20]

Trigger toe may develop from proximal tenosynovitis, which can be caused by injury ranging from a minor strain to a partial rupture of the FHL tendon. The rent in the tendon, accompanied by a fusiform swelling at the entrance of the fibroosseous canal and occurring most commonly in female classical ballet dancers, is typically characterized by pain and triggering when an individual descends from the demipointe position to foot flat. However, symptoms may occur as the great toe and ankle joint are either flexed or extended and thus may be elicited during the pointe posture. Triggering of the hallux occurs because the thickened nodular portion of the FHL tendon is forced, by gravity and superincumbent body weight, through its sheath as the dancer descends to the floor after standing on the ball of her foot. This causes triggering of the great toe, similar to de Quervain's disease of the thumb. The tendon may occasionally lock distal to the tendon canal and prevent the dancer from standing en pointe efficiently. Despite the difficulty, the dancer may force herself to maintain this position despite the fact that she does so with mechanical disadvantage to the FHL. Thus locking not only prevents standing sur les pointes, but also predisposes the foot to additional strain to the tendon and other soft tissue structures of the foot. Diagnosis is made clinically by palpating for the tendon deep in the posteromedial compartment of the ankle just anterior to the Achilles tendon and feeling the snap as the great toe and ankle are flexed and extended.

Distal tendon inflammation is characterized by chronic or intermittent inflammation of the tendon sheath passing between the two sesamoid bones of hallux. The sheath eventually heals with a constrictor, which impairs tendon passage. Symptoms may often present as tenderness and swelling in the region of the sesamoids. A frequent finding is the patient's inability to flex the interphalangeal joint of hallux while the MTP joint is stabilized.[13] Tendinitis is evident on magnetic resonance imaging, as well as by computed tomography.[26]

15. What is the differential diagnosis?

Differential diagnosis includes the following:
- *Medial plantar nerve entrapment* is a rare condition occurring in the medial foot arch beneath the talus and naviculum, under cover of the master knot of Henry, and is colloquially known as *jogger's foot* (Fig. 29-7). After the medial plantar nerve courses underneath the flexor retinaculum, it runs beneath the spring ligament and accompanies the flexor digito-

rum longus muscle to the midfoot by passing through the master knot. The nerve may be compressed under the abductor hallucis muscle or may be bound by the master knot. However, because the medial plantar nerve runs in proximity to the flexor digitorum and hallucis longus muscles, it may be difficult to distinguish tendon problems from neuritis. There is often a history of a previous ankle injury, the use of a new orthosis, or excessive hyperpronation of the foot with heel valgus. In the latter case, the talar head displaces medially and plantarward and stretches the spring ligament. Subsequently, the medial plantar nerve, which passes beneath the spring ligament, may be compromised. Excessively built-up rigid arch supports may also compress the nerve. Pain may be of a burning, sharp, or shooting nature and radiates from the arch toward the plantar aspect of the second and great toes. Pain may radiate proximally into the ankle. Some patients report numbness beneath these medial digits as they increase activity. Although overpronation may increase susceptibility of this nerve to inflammation, symptoms will be worsened with high arch supports, particularly those of rigid materials. Examination reveals a point of maximal tenderness located anywhere from the superior edge of the abductor hallucis muscle to the distal aspect of the medial arch. Pain is worse with running on level ground, especially curves, but may also be induced by workouts on stairs.[2] Pain may be reproduced by everting the heel or by having the patient stand on the ball of the foot. The examiner may elicit tenderness while palpating anywhere from the superior edge of the abductor hallucis muscle to the distal aspect of the medial arch, with maximal tenderness at the medial plantar aspect of the arch in the region of the navicular tuberosity. Tinel's sign may be present on percussion. An area of numbness may be found on the plantar and medial aspects of the foot, but numbness usually occurs only after the patient has been running. Unlike flexion of the FHL tendon, flexion of the toes against resistance or passive hyperextension of the toes should not induce neuritic pain. Conservative management consists of elimination of high-arched orthoses, rest, antiinflammatory medication, a heel lift, or soft medial longitudinal arch support. The heel lift and arch support are used to limit foot pronation and thereby limit irritation of the medial plantar nerve at the area of the talonavicular joint. Occasionally a steroid injection into the area of maximum tenderness may be performed. Surgical fascial release is reserved

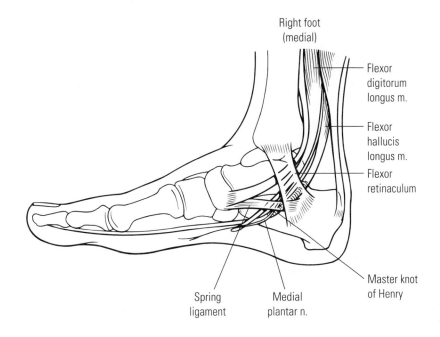

Right foot
(medial)

Flexor
digitorum
longus m.

Flexor
hallucis
longus m.

Flexor
retinaculum

Master knot
of Henry

Spring
ligament

Medial
plantar n.

FIG. 29-7 Medial plantar nerve entrapment also known as *jogger's foot* occurs beneath that fascial sling known as the Master Knot of Henry. After the medial plantar nerve courses underneath the flexor retinaculum, it runs beneath the spring ligament and accompanies the flexor digitorum longus muscle to the midfoot by passing through the master knot. (Because of its close proximity with FHL, neuritis of the medial plantar nerve may be confused with FHLT.)

for recalcitrant cases. Minimal postoperative immobilization is recommended, and early range-of-motion exercises should be performed.

• *Posterior tibial tendinitis,* also known as posterior shin splints (see Chapter 36), may be confused with FHL tendinitis because the location of symptomatic pain for both conditions is often the same. Posterior tibial tendinitis occurs more often in soccer players than in other athletes, probably because the tendon is subject to frequent microtrauma from repeated hyperpronation during the game.[44] This injury also occurs in other athletic competitions requiring quick directional changes, such as tennis, basketball, and ice hockey.[19] The key factor in understanding posterior tibial tendinitis is its relationship to the subtalar joint. Because of its orientation of span the tendon medially crosses the subtalar joint and spans the hindfoot to the forefoot by inserting via fibrous expansions on the navicular tuberosity, sustentaculum tali, spring ligament, and tarsal bones, including the cuboid, three plantar cuneiforms, and second, third, and fourth metatarsal bases. The tibialis posterior is thus similar to FHL in that it works during early stance to decel-

erate subtalar joint pronation. The tibialis posterior also decelerates forward tibial movement.[17] In contrast to the passive action of the windlass mechanism, which is primarily responsible for arch resupination, the tibialis posterior may contribute to supination of the foot by way of concentric activity[7] during late stance. Moreover, by reinforcing the spring ligament, this tendon helps dynamically support the talar head and helps prevent the talar sagging that is characteristic of pes planus. Before its insertion, the tendon intimately wraps around the medial malleolus, so that it functions much like a rope pulled through a pulley wheel. Attrition stresses may occur at the bone-tendon points of contact within this fibroosseous tunnel. During pronation the mechanical demands placed on the tibialis posterior are high and may exceed tendon capacity. The tendon may become inflamed (tendinitis), sustain inflammation of its synovial sheath (tenosynovitis), and eventually undergo degeneration or even rupture. Excessive friction may cause irregular osteophytes to develop in the region that further contributes to tendon disorders. The individual with a hyperpronated foot posture during stance phase is

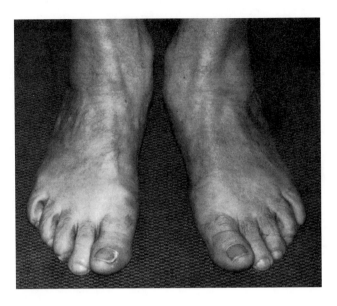

FIG. 29-8 This patient demonstrates elongation of the left tibialis posterior tendon with a pes planus deformity. (From Baxter D: *The foot and ankle in sport,* St. Louis, 1995, Mosby.)

more susceptible to this entity. Because the tendon is relatively superficial, it is subject to direct contusion with subsequent tendinitis and tenosynovitis as the result of a direct blow such as an opponent's kick. The tendon may also be injured by overstretching or by irritation caused by shoes. Pain is felt in the area of the navicular, with radiation to the posterior aspect of the medial malleolus and along the posteromedial tibial border. The player limps during athletic performance and is unable to accelerate or cut during running; running and jumping increase pain. Palpation of the tendon along its course from behind the medial malleolus to its insertion on the navicular elicits tenderness; frequently, there is associated crepitus. Resisting (concentric) supination or passive pronation the midfoot reproduces pain. Management includes rest, application of ice, use of antiinflammatory medication, transverse friction massage,[6] calf stretches, the wearing of firm soles, use of longitudinal arch supports, and the use of a medially posted heel wedge orthosis to decrease pronation during stance. Although steroid injection provides ready relief, it does so only temporarily and may increase the possibility of tendon attrition and rupture. In younger patients tendinitis is caused by overuse and is more amenable to conservative management. In older persons tendinitis is caused by degeneration and is less responsive to conservative intervention. Surgical decompression

of the flexor retinaculum at the fibroosseous tunnel with excision of the bony osteophyte is considered only in chronic cases that are recalcitrant to conservative management.

• *Posterior tibial tendon strain* involves stretching of the posterior tibial ligament and often occurs secondary to a pes planus deformity or chronic overpronation of the foot. Normally the plantar portion of the talar head is supported by the sustentaculum tali, whereas the anterior portion of the talus is supported by the posterior aspect of the navicular. A gap between these two supports exists and is compensated for by the tibialis posterior tendon and the spring ligament. In both pes planus and overpronation the talar head displaces medially and plantarward and stretches both soft tissue supports, resulting in loss of the medial longitudinal arch.[16] Initially, stretching of the tibialis posterior tendon will occur. Over time, however, attritional degeneration will give way to tendon rupture. The patient typically complains of pain over the medial aspect of the hindfoot. Progression from elongation (Fig. 29-8) to rupture may take months to years and is accompanied by a progressively increasing hindfoot valgus. Early diagnosis is essential if nonoperative management is to be effective.

• *Posterior tibial tendon rupture* is rare in young persons[19] and is most commonly seen in women over the age of 40 with no history of acute trauma.[18,23,24] The original injury involving tenosynovitis may evolve into a partial rupture of the central fiber tendons. The resulting inflammation results in a fusiform enlargement and loss of tendon strength, with eventual complete rupture. A grade II or III strain of the tibialis posterior tendon may also be caused by the same mechanism that causes peroneal nerve compromise: an acute inversion injury of the ankle joint. A rupture may also be iatrogenic in nature, stemming from multiple steroid injections.[39] Many cases of rupture have occurred in patients with flat feet, and excessive strain has been proposed as the mechanism.[3,5,21] Following rupture, decompensation of the spring ligament may promote progressive flat foot. The presence of unilateral flat foot in an adult is a primary indication of possible posterior tibial tendon compromise, particularly if rupture is long standing. This is because following rupture, there is a tendency for increased medial heel valgus and pronation as a consequence of the loss of medial restraint on the navicular; this eventually leads to lateral navicular subluxation. Observed from behind, the foot demonstrates increased heel valgus and forefoot pronation and abduction. The absence of heel varus is highlighted when the patient attempts to stand on tiptoes. With complete rupture, however, independent toe rise is impossible.[18,24] Stance phase of the involved foot is characterized by maintenance of the foot in an inverted posture as the longitudinal arch fails to reconstitute. This may result in osseous impingement of the anterior calcaneal process on the talus. The symptoms of a partial or complete tear of the tibialis posterior tendon include pain and swelling along the posteromedial ankle behind the malleolus, as well as pain at the tendon insertion onto the navicular.[40] Once the arch has collapsed, subjective complaints may include pain over the lateral aspect of the hindfoot, caused by calcaneal impingement against the lateral malleolus. Pathologic symptoms will eventually involve the sinus tarsi because of uneven loading of the subtalar joint with excessive forces laterally. This may result in osseous impingement of the anterior calcaneal process on the talus. The diagnosis is too often missed, and delay in early, aggressive treatment may lead to chronic, irreversible changes in the bones and soft tissues of the foot.[7] Early management includes tendon transfer using the flexor digitorum longus. If treatment is delayed, the secondary deformities of the heel valgus and forefoot supination will

occur and a triple arthrodesis may be necessary to achieve stabilization.[7]

- *Os trigonum pathology,* also known as *lateral trigonal impingement, posterior impingement syndrome of the ankle,* or *talar compression syndrome* is, like FHL tendinitis, also a source of posterior ankle pain and must be differentiated from FHL tendinitis. The posterior aspect of the body, or trochlea of the talus, has two bony tubercles—the medial and the lateral—that form a fibroosseous tunnel through which the FHL tendon courses en route to its distal insertion. Both tubercles are separated by a groove containing the FHL tendon. The smaller medial tubercle serves as the attachment for the posterior portion of the deep deltoid ligament, whereas the longer lateral tubercle projects more posteriorly and serves as the attachment for the posterior talofibular ligament. The lateral tubercle can be small or large. When it is large it is referred to as a *Stieda process,* or the *posterior talar process.* In approximately 10% of feet the lateral tubercle is a separate ossicle attached to the bone by a fibrous synostosis. This separate posterior talar process is a common assessory bone of the foot and is then called an *os trigonum.*[36] *The ossicle may be present unilaterally or bilaterally and is not truly a sesamoid bone within a tendon. Rather, it is a bony process, most likely a secondary center of ossification that has failed to unite with the talar body.*

The os trigonum also may result from repeated traumatic talar impingement against the posterior tibia or an acute fracture of the posterior talar tubercle during forced plantarflexion.[25] Here, the etiology of trigone injury is a *stress fracture,* which is frequently misdiagnosed as an ankle sprain or Achilles tendinitis.[9] The mechanism of injury involves sudden, forceful hyperplantarflexion of the ankle joint. This equinus posture compresses and may eventually crush the lateral tubercle between the posterior lip of the tibia and the underlying superior border of the posterior calcaneus.

Injury to the *os trigonum* or a *large Stieda process* (see Fig. 34-15) may also occur from repetitive overuse in ballet dancers performing the demipointe or full pointe position or from such jumping sports as soccer.[43] When the foot is positioned in hyperplantarflexion while enduring full weight bearing, the lower tibia and upper calcaneum come together, so that a large tubercle or os trigonum is caught like a nut in a nutcracker (see Fig. 34-17)[36] Posterior impingement syndrome of the ankle is common in ballet dancers and also occurs in athletes who jump or who play football. Clinical presentation includes posterior ankle pain and tenderness in the region of the Achilles tendon, particularly the lateral retrocalcaneal space, while walking on or pointing the toes. Point tenderness is noted behind the ankle joint, deep in the interval between the Achilles tendon and lateral malleolus. Forced maximal passive plantarflexion *(positive plantarflexion sign)* of the ankle also elicits pain, as does resisted plantarflexion of the great toe. Downhill walking or running or wearing high heels is painful. Wearing shoes that increase dorsiflexion relieves pain. A history of chronic ankle sprains is common. Swelling and signs of collateral ligament instability are absent. Tendinitis of the calcaneal, peroneal, and tibialis posterior tendons are ruled out as patients feel better in equinus and because palpation of those tendons is asymptomatic.[41] Whereas pathologic conditions of the os trigonum yield postero*lateral* pain, FHL tendinitis yields postero*medial* ankle pain. Posterior impingement syndrome is overdiagnosed by medical practitioners because of the dramatic appearance of the bone on lateral x-ray films. Diagnosis may be confirmed by the introduction of local anesthetic into the posterior soft tissues behind the peroneal tendons; the diagnosis is positive if the anesthetic provides pain relief. Treatment may vary from rest and a ½-inch heel lift[2] to casting for 6 weeks. Surgical excision of the trigone fragment is appropriate if conservative efforts have failed.

- *Anterior ankle impingement syndrome* may occur during extreme dorsiflexion where the anterior lip of the tibia contacts the talar neck. An exostosis may form where the tibia and talus meet, providing the basis for the anterior impingement syndrome (see Fig. 30-23). Factors influencing this condition include excessive posterior capsular and Achilles tendon extensibility, as well as lax lateral ankle ligaments that allow an increased amount of anterior tibial translation.[25]

- *Subtalar coalition* refers to cartilaginous bars of the tarsal bones that most commonly occur at the calcaneonavicular site and secondarily refers to the talocalcaneal coalition. The latter may occur in the region of the sustentaculum tali but may also be in the region of the posterior subtalar compartment. Simply stated, tarsal coalition causes restriction of motion at the subtalar joint. The subtalar joint acts as a torque converter and thereby permits dissipation of the enormous forces imparted to the foot during stance phase of gait. In the absence of normal motion as the result of restriction produced by the coalition, increased strain is placed on the foot, producing a cycle of strain, pain, and muscle spasm. Tarsal coalition means the union of two or more tarsal bones, which may be cartilaginous or osseous in nature. Tarsal coalitions begin as purely cartilaginous coalitions of bone that eventually ossify and cause restriction of motion, alteration of normal foot biomechanics, increased foot and ankle stress, and degenerative changes. Most patients with a tarsal coalition become symptomatic during adolescence. Formerly asymptomatic feet may become suddenly symptomatic following a simple ankle sprain or fracture. Conceivably, an ankle sprain may tax the foot's and ankle's ability to cope with an already disadvantaged biomechanical alignment. An ankle sprain by itself should not cause peroneal spasm, and coalition should be suspected when pain and peroneal muscle spasm persist beyond the usual disability time following fracture or sprain. Episodes of recurrent *peroneal spasm* occur as a protective reflexive response. The patient will complain of painful flat feet, and the examiner will notice decreased foot mobility on examination of range of motion. A common complaint is difficulty walking on uneven terrain. Special radiographic views, such as posterior subtalar views, and computed tomography delineate the coalition once diagnosis is confirmed. Conservative therapy may be attempted, consisting of rest in a short-leg cast, nonsteroidal antiinflammatory medication, and either an orthosis or a brace to decrease subtalar joint motion. The decision whether to resect the bar to perform triple arthrodesis is based on the presence or absence of degenerative changes.[41]

- *Achilles tendinitis* is characterized by pain above the insertion of that tendon on the os calcis. Pain is present on jumping activities, and patients often exhibit tight heel cords or pes planus foot postures. Pain is reproduced on forceful ankle dorsiflexion with the knee in extension (see Chapter 34).

- *Tarsal tunnel syndrome* refers to entrapment of the posterior tibial nerve as it passes through a fibroosseous tunnel along the medial ankle. Symptoms include burning or shooting pain from the medial side of the ankle and into the foot. Sensory loss may include the loss of two-point discrimination over the medial plantar area. Pain may be reproduced by positioning the foot in forced eversion, pronation, dorsiflexion, and toe abduction (see Chapter 31).

16. What therapeutic intervention is most appropriate to patient management?

Therapeutic intervention includes the following:

- *Cryotherapy* has positive effects when it is used in the treatment of tendon injury. The use of cold as an immediate care modality is useful in the acute stage because it causes circulatory vasoconstriction of the injured tendon. Musculoskeletal injury is accompanied by physiologic changes, including hemorrhage, inflammation, edema, muscle spasm, and pain.[30] Cold therapy affects all these factors and also affects local soft tissue metabolism by reducing enzymatic function.[30] The application of cold also facilitates reduction of pain by slowing the nerve conduction that bears pain messages centrally, as well as by affecting muscle spindles such that the stretch reflex is minimized or inhibited. However, it is important for the therapist to find the right balance of cooling so as not to provide undercooling or overcooling. Whereas the former does not provide the desired result, the latter risks tissue damage because significant reduction in circulation and inflammation during the initial 48 hours after injury may negatively affect healing. Decreased circulation contributes to secondary hypoxic injury, and the presence of some inflammation is a necessary prerequisite to resolution and subsequent wound healing.[22] Cryotherapy may be applied with ice, gel, vasocoolant spray, or whirlpool bath. The use of cold may also help during the rehabilitative phase following injury.

- *Thermotherapy.* The use of a heat modality causes physiologic, vasodilatory changes in tissue. Vasodilation causes an increase in the oxygen supply and therefore in the metabolic rate. Increased blood flow will also recruit more antibodies, leukocytes, nutrients, and enzymes that help anabolism of the injured tendon. This follows the acute period (after 48 hours), once the process of clearing away cellular debris has commenced. Heat is indicated during the rehabilitative phase because heating increases extensibility of the viscoelastic properties of the collagen that composes the tendon.[8] Heat modalities may include warm whirlpool, paraffin wax, hot packs, infrared heat, and therapeutic ultrasound.

  Management of FHL tendinitis also includes rest; nonsteroidal antiinflammatory medications; the use of a light, compressive dressing with an elastic bandage to strap the foot; the use of longitudinal arch supports; firm soles; and corrective orthoses. *Rest* is essential to proper healing and interruption of the in-flammatory cycle and includes withdrawal from both plié and pointe work. A *swimming program* is recommended until symptoms subside. Once symptoms subside, the dancer is encouraged to perform barre exercises while immersed in a swimming pool. Exercises are initially performed with the uninvolved leg as the support limb and the involved leg as the working leg. With further rehabilitation, the roles may be reversed.

- *Orthoses.* FHL tendinitis is aggravated by overpronation.[29] Thus if the hindfoot is in valgus, a 5° or 9° medial hindfoot wedge is appropriate, as is a 3-mm heel height. If the hindfoot is in neutral, a 5° medial forefoot wedge and 3-mm heel height are appropriate.[29] Dancers must stop all plié and pointe work to allow the tendon to heal.[40] Slow, gentle FHL strengthening, as well as calf stretching, is necessary for a complete rehabilitative management regimen.

The importance of early recognition and implementation of conservative management cannot be overemphasized because surgical intervention may add to the problem. If the original problem is ignored, the injury may evolve to partial rupture of the central fibers of the tendon. This results in a fusiform enlargement and loss of strength of the tendon itself. At this point the tendon may not recover, despite successful tendon decompressive release from the stenotic fibroosseous tunnel. Prognosis is guarded, since the now enlarged and partially ruptured tendon may eventually succumb to complete rupture.[32]

REFERENCES

1. Bachner EJ, Friedman MJ: Injuries to the leg. In Nicholas JA, Hershman EB, editors: *The lower extremity and spine,* ed 2, vol 1, St Louis, 1995, Mosby.
2. Baxter DE: *The foot and ankle in sports,* St Louis, 1995, Mosby.
3. Berndt AL, Harty M: Transchondral fractures (osteochondritis dissecans) of the talus, *J Bone Joint Surg* 41A:988, 1959.
4. Boland AL Jr, Hulstyn MJ: Soft-tissue injuries of the knee. In Nicholas JA, Hershman EB, editors: *The lower extremity and spine,* ed 2, vol 1, St Louis, 1995, Mosby.
5. Cozen L: Posterior tibial tenosynovitis secondary to foot strain, *Clin Orthop* 42:101-102, 1965.
6. Cyriax J, editor: *Textbook of orthopaedic medicine,* vol 2, Philadelphia, 1984, WB Saunders.
7. Donatelli RA: *The biomechanics of the foot and ankle,* ed 2, Philadelphia, 1996, FA Davis.
8. Drez D, editor: *Therapeutic modalities for sports injuries,* Chicago, 1989, Year Book Medical Publishers.
9. Glick JM, Sampson TG: Ankle and foot fractures in athletics. In Nicholas JA, Hershman EB, editors: *The lower extremity and spine,* ed 2, vol 1, St Louis, 1995, Mosby.

10. Hamilton WG: Stenosing tenosynovitis of the flexor hallucis longus tendon and posterior impingement upon the os-trigonum in ballet dancers, *Foot Ankle* 3(2):74-80, 1982.

11. Hardaker WT Jr, Margello S, Goldner JL: Foot and ankle injuries in theatrical dancers, *Foot Ankle* 6(2):59-69, 1985.

12. Hardaker WT Jr: Foot and ankle injuries in classical ballet dancers, *Orthop Clin North Am* 20(4)621-627, 1989.

13. Henry AK: *Extensile exposure,* ed 2, New York, Churchill Livingstone.

14. Hicks JH: The mechanics of the foot. 2. The plantar aponeurosis and arch, *J Anat* 88:25-30, 1954.

15. Holt KW, Cross MJ: Isolated rupture of the flexor hallucis longus tendon, *Am J Sports Med* 18(6):645-646, 1990.

16. Hoppenfeld S: *Physical examination of the spine and extremities,* Norwalk, Conn, 1976, Appleton-Century-Crofts.

17. Inman VT, Ralston HJ, Todd F: *Human walking,* Baltimore, 1981, Williams & Wilkins.

18. Johnson KA: Tibialis posterior tendon rupture, *Clin Orthop* 177:140-147, 1983.

19. Jones DC, Singer KM: Soft-tissue conditions of the ankle and foot. In Nicholas JA, Hershman EB, editors: *The lower extremity and spine,* ed 2, vol 1, St Louis, 1995, Mosby.

20. Kendall FP, McCreary EK: *Muscles: testing and function,* ed 3, Baltimore, 1983, Williams & Wilkins.

21. Kettlekamp DB, Alexander HH: Spontaneous rupture of the posterior tibial tendon, *J Bone Joint Surg* 51A:759, 1969.

22. Knight KL: *Cryotherapy: theory, technique, and physiology,* Chattanooga, TN, 1985, Chattanooga Corp.

23. Mann R, Specht L: Posterior tibial tendon ruptures: analysis of eight cases, *Foot Ankle* 2:350, 1981.

24. Mann R, Thompson F: Rupture of the posterior tibial tendon causing flat foot, *J Bone Joint Surg* 67(4):556-561, 1985.

25. Milan KR: Injury in ballet: a review of relevant topics for the physical therapist, *J Orthop Sports Phys Ther* 19(2):121-129, 1994.

26. Miller TT, Ghelman B, Potter HG: Imaging of the foot and ankle. In Nicholas JA, Hershman EB, editors: *The lower extremity and spine,* ed 2, vol 1, St Louis, 1995, Mosby.

27. Nixon JE: Injuries to the neck and upper extremities of dancers, *Clin Sports Med* 2(3):459-472, 1983.

28. Perry J: *Gait analysis: normal and pathological function,* Thorofare, NJ, 1992, Slack.

29. Reilly MA: *Guidelines for prescribing foot orthotics,* Thorofare, NJ, 1995, Slack.

30. Rivenburgh DW: Physical modalities in the treatment of tendon injuries, *Clin Sports Med* 11(3):645-659, 1992.

31. Root ML, Orien WP, Weed JN: *Clinical biomechanics,* vol 2. *Normal and abnormal function of the foot,* Los Angeles, 1977, Clinical Biomechanics.

32. Sammarco GJ, Miller EH: Partial rupture of the flexor hallucis longus tendon in classical ballet dancers: two case reports, *J Bone Joint Surg* 61(1):149-150, 1979.

33. Sammarco GJ: Dance injuries. In Nicholas JA, Hershman EB, editors: *The lower extremity and spine,* ed 2, vol 2, St Louis, 1995, Mosby.

34. Sammarco GJ: Diagnosis and treatment of dancers, *Clin Orthop* 187:176-187, 1984.

35. Sammarco GJ: The foot and ankle in classical ballet and modern dance. In Jahss MH, editor: *Disorders of the foot,* Philadelphia, 1982, WB Saunders.

36. Sarrafian SK: *Anatomy of the foot and ankle,* Philadelphia, 1983, JB Lippincott.

37. Scheller AD, Kasser JR, Quigley TB: Tendon injuries about the ankle, *Orthop Clin North Am* 11(4):801-811, 1980.

38. Schon LC: Nerve entrapment, neuropathy, and nerve dysfunction in athletes, *Orthop Clin North Am* 25(1):47-59, 1994.

39. Simpson RR, Gudas CJ: Posterior tibial tendon rupture in a world-class runner, *J Foot Surg* 22(1):74-77, 1983.

40. Trevino S, Baumhauer JF: Tendon injuries of the foot and ankle, *Clin Sports Med* 11(4):727-739, 1992.

41. Turco VJ: Injuries to the foot and ankle. In Nicholas JA, Hershman EB, editors: *The lower extremity and spine,* ed 2, vol 2, St Louis, 1995, Mosby.

42. Valmassy RL: *Clinical biomechanics of the lower extremities,* St Louis, 1996, Mosby.

43. Washington ZL: Musculoskeletal injuries in theatrical dancers: site, frequency, and severity, *Am J Sports Med* 6(2):75-98, 1978.

44. Xethalis JL, Lorei MP: Soccer injuries. In Nicholas JA, Hershman EB, editors: *The lower extremity and spine,* ed 2, vol 2, St Louis, 1995, Mosby.

RECOMMENDED READING

Hamilton WG: Stenosing tenosynovitis of the flexor hallucis longus tendon and posterior impingement upon the os-trigonum in ballet dancers, *Foot Ankle* 3(2):74-80, 1982.

Holt KW, Cross MJ: Isolated rupture of the flexor hallucis longus tendon, *Am J Sports Med* 18(6):645-646, 1990.

Sammarco GJ: The foot and ankle in classical ballet and modern dance. In Jahss MH, editor: *Disorders of the foot,* Philadelphia, 1982, WB Saunders.

PART VII

ANKLE

30

Painful and Unstable Upper Ankle After Jump Landing and Excessively Forceful Inversion Moment That Causes the Foot to Roll Inward

A student in his last senior-level clinical physical therapy affiliation participated in an interdepartmental rehabilitation basketball game between the physical and occupational therapy departments. He incurred an ankle injury following a leap upward toward the basket in an attempt to block a shot by the other team. The ankle was injured during this jump landing, and the student collapsed to the gym floor, grasping his right ankle, his eyes shut tight in pain. Watching the play, you notice that the student landed on an opposing player's foot, with a plantarflexed and internally rotated ankle. The student was helped off the court by two teammates while hopping toward the training room. During the evaluation, the patient reported no history of sprain, nor any audible "pop" during the injury. The following clinical data emerged during the examination:

OBSERVATION The patient hobbles with a characteristic foot flat–type gait, in which both heel strike and push-off are lacking in the injured extremity. A cavus-type foot is observed bilaterally and is secondary to a bilateral rigid forefoot valgus deformity. Ecchymosis is noted distal to the fibular malleolus.

PALPATION Palpation yields acute pain and tenderness over the anterolateral ankle at the tip of the fibula, lateral calcaneus, and sinus tarsi. Elevation of cutaneous skin temperature is noted.

ACTIVE RANGE OF MOTION Testing for active range of motion reveals difficulty in heel and toe walking.

PASSIVE RANGE OF MOTION Testing for passive range of motion reveals passive ankle movements limited in plantarflexion, inversion, and dorsiflexion, in that order.

STRENGTH Strength in the ipsilateral gluteus medius is graded good minus. Ipsilateral peroneals are good.

SELECTIVE TENSION Resisted movements, including isometric resistance to ankle eversion, are strong and painless.

SPECIAL TESTS The patient has a positive Achilles' bulge sign, positive anterior draw, negative talar tilt sign, and negative tibiofibular squeeze test.

SENSATION The patient has intact sensation to the peroneal cutaneous distribution.

REFLEXES Reflexes are normal.

RADIOGRAPHIC EXAMINATION   A lateral view of the ankle reveals a posterior hiatus when the talus is pulled away from the mortise.

CLUE:

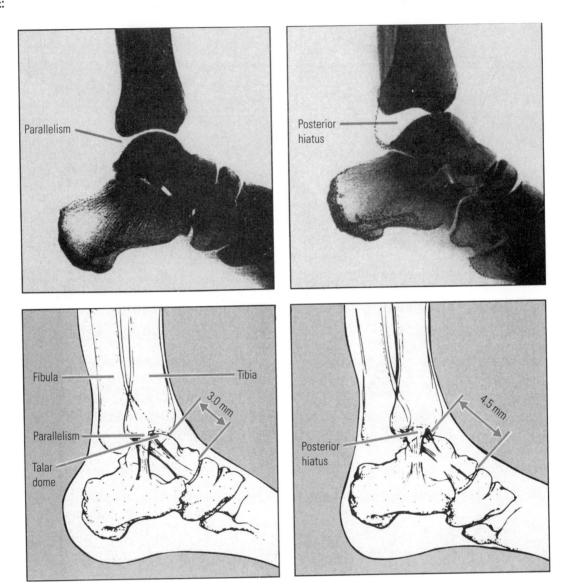

(From Lane SE: Severe ankle sprains, *The Physician and Sportsmedicine* 18[11]:46, 1990.)

The student was treated at your clinic over the subsequent weeks, and the conversation during these treatments inevitably drifted toward a discussion of the ankle joints and foot function. An appropriate appreciation of ankle joint kinesiology was accompanied by discussion of how the foot functions in relation to the ankle and preceded a discussion of the actual injury. Subsequently, you discussed the mechanisms and treatment of the injury. The talks were structured as a series of questions and answers sequenced as in the following material. Because of the complexity of the topic, repetition of key concepts inevitably crept into the discussion. This repetition was helpful in the student's assimilation of the information and is therefore preserved in the subsequent pages.

? **Questions**

1. What is most likely wrong with this man's ankle?
2. What is the osseous anatomy of the upper ankle joint?
3. What tarsal bone is common to the upper and lower ankle joints and the midtarsal joint, and how is this significant?
4. The upper and lower ankle joints and the transverse tarsal joint are in series, one with the other. How is the mutual interdependence of these joints demonstrated anatomically?
5. What is the significance of the wedge-shaped or domelike architectural configuration of the talus?
6. Why is describing the upper ankle joint as a modified hinge joint biomechanically more accurate than describing it as a pure hinge joint?
7. How does the asymmetric anteroposterior trochlear surface of the talus contribute to spin of the tibial shaft?
8. What is the sequence of talar motion within the ankle joint mortise during open chain plantarflexion and dorsiflexion?
9. Do the parameters of talar spin derived from the *upper ankle joint* depend on whether the lower extremity is bearing weight?
10. Do the parameters of talar spin derived from the *lower ankle joint* depend on whether the lower extremity is bearing weight?
11. Why does the lower limb, functioning in the weight-bearing capacity, engage the subtalar joint to yield more talar tibial rotation than might otherwise occur in the open kinetic chain?
12. Is the talus kinesiologically viewed as operating together with the proximal vertical crural column, or with the distal and horizontal heel-foot complex?
13. Why is a biomechanical understanding of foot-ankle biomechanics inadequate without the inclusion of the subtalar joint?
14. What is the anatomy of the subtalar joint?
15. What mechanical analogy lends itself to conceptualization of the subtalar joint?
16. Why is frontal plane motion the basis for measuring subtalar joint motion?
17. How is deviation from subtalar neutral determined?
18. What is the transverse tarsal joint?
19. What are the medial and lateral halves of the transverse tarsal joint?
20. How does motion at the transverse tarsal joint compensate for lack of motion in the upper and lower ankle joints?
21. What do pronation and supination mean in reference to the transverse tarsal joint?
22. How is the subtalar joint determinative of the transverse tarsal joint?
23. How does the talar-calcaneal interface serve as a transition point in the transfer of superincumbent body weight and ground reaction force?
24. What is meant by defining the triplanar motions of the subtalar joint as *pronation* and *supination?*
25. How are the components of pronation and supination altered and determined by whether the lower limb functions in the open or closed kinetic mode?
26. What is the relationship between energy dissipation of excessive force and subtalar joint pronation?
27. How does supination of the subtalar joint use the energy of ground reaction force to propel the body forward?
28. How do pronation and supination vary as a function of open and closed kinetic chain function during gait?
29. How is excessive torque conversion by the subtalar joint essential to understanding the origin of many proximal musculoskeletal dysfunctions?
30. Why is the cavus foot posture more likely to cause an inversion injury of the ankle joint?
31. Why is a rigid forefoot valgus deformity susceptible to inversion sprain at the ankle?
32. What is the mechanism of injury?
33. What are the ligamentous ankle joint stabilizers?
34. What are the components of the lateral collateral ligament complex, and what are the components' contributions to lateral ankle stability?
35. What is the anatomy of the anterior talofibular ligament, and what is its normal function?

36. What is the anatomy of the calcaneofibular ligament (CFL), and what is its normal function?
37. What is the anatomy of the posterior talofibular ligament (PTFL), and what is its normal function?
38. What is the sequence of lateral ligamentous defense against an inversion moment to the upper ankle joint?
39. How are lateral ligamentous ankle injuries classified according to anatomic and clinical criteria?
40. What deficits of proximal biomechanical linkage may contribute to lateral ankle sprain?
41. How is a suspected sprain of the lateral collateral ligament complex clinically confirmed?
42. What imaging techniques are appropriate?

43. What is the differential diagnosis?
44. What is the differential diagnosis for ankle sprain?
45. Why are fractures more likely than sprains to occur in children?
46. What therapeutic intervention is appropriate in management of lateral ankle sprain?
47. What management is appropriate for severe inversion sprain of the ankle joint?
48. What preventive measures decrease the likelihood of reinjury, sequelae, or chronic instability?
49. What is chronic lateral ankle instability?
50. What is a high ankle sprain?
51. What is sprain of the deltoid ligaments at the upper ankle?

1. What is most likely wrong with this man's ankle?

Ankle sprain of the lateral collateral ligamentous complex is most likely the problem. The provided clue demonstrates a forward talar shift, with applied stress of 25 lb, showing a total translation of 4 mm, as well as a posterior hiatus (a wedge-shaped space between the posterior tibial vault and the talar dome). Parallel lines are drawn along the anterior surface of the tibia and at the distal talus to quantify the exact amount of talar shift. This stress radiograph schematic shows clear evidence of severe joint instability and disruption of the anterior talofibular ligament (ATFL).

The ankle complex is the most frequently injured joint in athletics.[28] Every day approximately 23,000 people sustain an ankle sprain in the United States.[14] The national annual incidence of this injury has been estimated at 4.5 million, with restricted-activity days calculated at 20.7 million per year; bed-bound disability days at 5 million per year; and days lost from work or school at 5.8.[43] Up to 85% of these injuries involve sprain of the lateral collateral ligaments. Many studies cite basketball playing as being the most common cause of injury,[8,28,88] and ankle injury is considered *de rigeur* for basketball participation in North America.[63] Injury has also been reported in football,[25] soccer, skiing, cross-country running, volleyball, and falling from heights.[6,23] Ankle sprain is the most common acute injury affecting ballet dancers.[64]

Some authorities maintain that sprained ankles occur more frequently in women because of their greater ligamentous laxity.[45] However, statistics do not justify this assumption.[18,107] In fact, men sustain more ankle sprains than women overall, although there is no difference in incidence of injury when comparing sprains sustained from engaging in similar activities.[29]

Approximately one third of the population who sustain injury to the lateral ligaments of the ankle complain of residual dysfunction as long as 9 months after their injury. Previous ankle sprains appear to predispose an individual to future recurrent injury,[33,55] and chronic mechanical instability eventually develops in some 10% to 30% of persons with acute lateral ligament injuries. The significant emerging body of data suggests that clinicians should take this common yet potentially severe injury seriously, and not simply dismiss an ankle sprain with advice to use ice and an Ace bandage and instruction to let nature take its course. A simplistic dismissal of injury does not take into account such predisposing causes as proximal biomechanical linkage, intrinsic foot deformities, or the need for early mobilization to reorganize scar tissue. Rather, the need for a comprehensive and eclectic management strategy is imperative to minimize sequelae and the incidence of reinjury.*

---

*Caveat: The relationships and interrelationships of foot-ankle biomechanics are extremely complex and do not easily lend themselves to conceptualization. An appreciation of these concepts will not be achieved by a simple, quick read. The use of anatomic models may be of help. Emerging from a multitude of data regarding foot and ankle biomechanics is the relationship between the subtalar joint and talar rotation. Helical motions or moments in the entire lower extremity are referred to as *rotations* or *torsion* and occur in the transverse

2. What is the osseous anatomy of the upper ankle joint?

The *upper ankle joint,* also known as the *talocrural* or *talar joint,* includes the synovial articulation of the distal end of the tibia, fibula, and talus bones. Although intimately interrelated with the biomechanics of the foot, the ankle is the simpler of the two articulations that may be thought of as a point of linkage between the *vertical* shaft of the shin and the *horizontal* base of support (the foot). Superincumbent body weight is transferred to the talus via a malleolar "fork" (Fig. 30-1). The anatomic fit between the three osseous components of this joint is understood, by way of analogy, to be similar to a mortise and tenon joint. *Mortise* and *tenon* are carpentry terms meaning *square peg in square hole.* The *mortise* refers to the female receiver—the proximal two-pronged malleolar fork. The tenon is the head (trochlea) of the talus, or male counterpart, that projects and inserts upward into the concavity above. This analogy nicely describes a somewhat anteroposterior view of the ankle, in which the talus is not overlapped by either the tibia or fibula.[71] Some authorities classify this joint as a simple hinge joint. This is actually an oversimplification, since inherent variations in the malleoli and the talus lend this joint movement well beyond simple hinge function. Instead, the upper ankle joint is more accurately classified as a modified hinge joint.

3. What tarsal bone is common to the upper and lower ankle joints and the midtarsal joint, and how is this significant?

The key to understanding the biomechanics of the foot and ankle is the appreciation of the function of that largest tarsal bone known as the *talus* (also known as the *astragalus*). The quadrilateral-shaped talus articulates with many bones: the tibia and fibula above and on its sides, the calcaneus below, and the navicular in front. Because of its many articulations, the talus is an essential component of the *talo*crural joint, the sub*talar* joint, and the *talo*navicular (i.e., transverse tarsal) joints simultaneously. The talus is

plane. An understanding of the interrelationships among these key concepts serves as a guidepost in negotiating the maze of information regarding this topic. Moreover, the intricate set of relationships between the talus and the tibia and between the talus and calcaneus are more easily understood against the backdrop of a series of dualities such as open versus closed kinetic chain, internal versus external tibial torsion, medial versus lateral talar rotation, and superincumbent body weight versus ground reaction force.

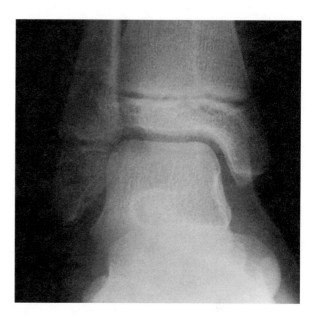

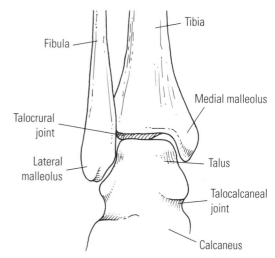

FIG. 30-1 *Upper ankle joint.* Superincumbent body weight is transferred to the talus via a malleolar "fork" comprised of the tibia and fibula fitting over and around the upwardly projecting talus. The anatomic fit between the three osseous components of this joint is understood, by way of analogy, to be similar to a mortise and tenon joint. Mortise and tenon are carpentry terms meaning square peg in a square hole. The mortise refers to the female receiver—the proximal two-pronged malleolar fork, while the head (trochlea) of the talus is the tenon, or male counterpart, that projects and inserts upward into the concavity above. (From Coughlin MJ, Mann RA: *Surgery of the foot and ankle,* ed 7, St. Louis, 1999, Mosby.)

the common denominator of all these bones simply because function of these joints cannot be viewed in solitary fashion. Rather, foot and ankle function is inextricably linked and understood in light of the mutual interrelationship and function of these joints as an integrative unit. Thus talar anatomy and function are focal points that help us appreciate the kinesiology of the foot-ankle complex.

4. The upper and lower ankle joints and the transverse tarsal joint are in series, one with the other. How is the mutual interdependence of these joints demonstrated anatomically?

The talocrural and subtalar joints share the same synovial and ligamentous capsule; moreover, the collateral ligament complex, particularly the calcaneofibular ligament (CFL),[53] spans both joints. Furthermore, the anterior and medial facets of the subtalar joint are in fact the medial half of the transverse tarsal joint; they are known as the talonavicular joint, and they have their own joint capsule. This joint capsule is an extension of the tissue surrounding the upper ankle joint. Thus the kinesiologic interdependence of these joints is ascribed to an intimately shared anatomy and to their adjacent relationship with each other.

5. What is the significance of the wedge-shaped or domelike architectural configuration of the talus?

The superior portion of the talus is known as the *trochlea,* a term that generically refers to any smooth, bony surface affording a smooth surface on which another glides. The trochlea, or dome, of the talus provides a convexity that articulates with the distal tibial plafond and presents an articular facet to articulate with each malleolus (Fig. 30-2). The majority of superincumbent body weight is thus borne through the tibia, whereas the fibula carries only approximately one-sixth the weight-bearing load. The saddle-shaped superior talar surface bears the weight of the body, transmitted via the tibia. The dome of the talus widens anteriorly because of its wedgelike shape and also appears wedge shaped as appreciated from a superior view. The clinical relevance of this is that ankle dorsiflexion snugly wedges the wider anterior dimension of the talus within the ankle mortise into a stable, closed-packed position. Most ankle injuries are more likely to occur when the ankle joint is in plantarflexion, since this posture places the narrower posterior aspect of the talus within the mortise, resulting in the open-packed position and subjecting the ankle to increased lateral instability.

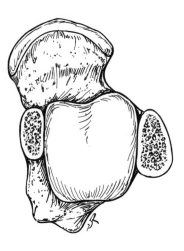

FIG. 30-2 Dorsal view of the right talus. The talar dome has a convex surface that articulates with the distal tibial plafond, and also presents an articular facet to articulate with each malleolus. The lateral malleolus is larger than the medial malleolus and extends more distally. (From Valmassy RL: *Clinical biomechanics of the lower extremities,* Mosby, St. Louis, 1996.)

6. Why is describing the upper ankle joint as a modified hinge joint biomechanically more accurate than describing it as a pure hinge joint?

The upper ankle joint is bounded medially and laterally by the malleolar processes of the distal tibia and fibula, respectively, and superiorly by the tibial plafond—the flat surface of the distal tibia. Clinical approximation of the ankle joint axis may easily be understood as the examiner creates an imaginary line running through the ankle by placing the ends of his or her index fingers at the distal bony tips of the malleoli (Fig. 30-3).[65] Anatomically, the fibular malleolus extends distally and posteriorly on the talus relative to the medial malleolus; biomechanically, this means that eversion is limited relative to inversion. The kinesiologic ramifications of this incongruity are important to fully appreciating the intricate biomechanical interplay of the foot-ankle complex. The most obvious consequence of this variation is that inversion is less limited than eversion. More subtly, however, the obliquity in the axis of the ankle joint dispels the idea of this joint as having a single plane of movement in the sagittal plane. Without this variation in malleolar length, motion at this joint would be confined to sagittal plane movement of dorsiflexion. However, because the transmalleolar axis is externally rotated ap-

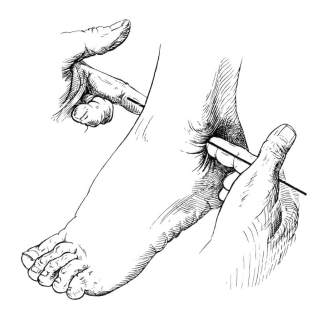

FIG. 30-3 Clinical approximation of *obliquity of the talocrural joint axis* may easily be appreciated by an imaginary line running through the ankle, created by placing the ends of the examiner's index fingers at the distal bony tips of the malleoli. Anatomically, the fibular malleolus extends more distally and posteriorly on the talus relative to the medial malleolus. The most obvious consequence of this difference in malleolar length is that inversion is less limited than eversion. (From Coughlin MJ, Mann RA: *Surgery of the foot and ankle,* ed 7, St. Louis, 1999, Mosby.)

proximately 15° to the coronal axis of the leg,[24] horizontal rotation is introduced in the foot or leg with movements of the ankle.

The deviation of motion of the upper ankle joint from the sagittal plane, as referenced to the midline of the shaft of the tibia, is known as *declination.* Declination of the ankle joint axis is such that it is directed laterally, posteriorly, and plantarly.[75] This inherent anatomic obliquity, further discussed in the following sections, imparts a *rotational component* to ankle joint function that differs during the open versus the closed kinetic chain.

7. How does the asymmetric anteroposterior trochlear surface of the talus contribute to spin of the tibial shaft?

In addition to upper ankle joint declination derived from the obliquity of the talocrural joint axis and the different malleolar lengths, rotational motion of the tibial shaft is also derived from another source. If we compare the anteroposterior dimension of the lateral and medial articular trochlear surface of the talus, we observe a different architectural configuration. The radii of the arches composing the talar trochlea are not uniform. Rather, the lateral articular trochlear talar surface is longer along its anteroposterior dimension, which means that it has greater excursion of movement than the shorter medial surface.[41] An analogy may be drawn to the knee joint, in which the longer and wider medial femoral condyle imparts a spin to the tibial or femoral shafts, depending on whether the lower extremity was functioning in the open or closed kinetic chain position, respectively.

8. What is the sequence of talar motion within the ankle joint mortise during open chain plantarflexion and dorsiflexion?

During ankle motion from plantarflexion to dorsiflexion, the talus rolls backward in the mortise and wedges up tightly between the two malleoli. However, because of the discrepancy in the anterior and posterior widths of the anterior aspect of the trochlea of the talus, talar movement is asymmetric. Because the lateral malleolus is larger, during dorsiflexion it engages the mortise before the medial side of the malleolus does, causing the talus to spin *dorsolaterally* until the smaller medial trochlear surface is in maximal congruence with the mortise (Fig. 30-4).

This dorsiflexion posture is the closed-packed position for the talocrural joint, in which both the larger lateral and narrower medial anterior aspects of the trochlear dome of the talus articulate tightly within the mortise. Conversely, during the reverse motion from dorsiflexion to plantarflexion, the talocrural joint may be said to unlock out of dorsiflexion. This disengagement of the talus out of a close-packed articulation with the malleolar mortise begins with the narrower medial aspect of the anterior aspect of the trochlear dome, followed by the larger lateral side as the talus rolls forward. In essence, the talus undergoes a reverse spin, or *medial-plantar rotation,* as movement progresses to plantarflexion. The relationship between the chain of motion and talar (and hence, tibial) rotation can be summarized as follows:

- Open-chain motion of plantarflexion to dorsiflexion: medioplantar talar and tibial rotation
- Open-chain motion of dorsiflexion to plantarflexion: dorsolateral talar and tibial rotation

While in the position of full plantarflexion, neither of the anterior arches of the trochlea articulates with the mortise. Only the narrow posterior aspect of the trochlea

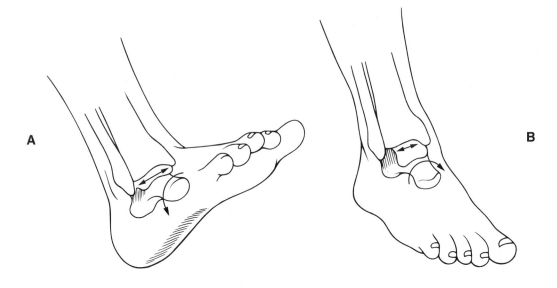

FIG. 30-4 A, During *dorsiflexion* the wider trochlear base wedges up tightly within the intermalleolar space corresponding to the closed packed position. Because of the larger lateral aspect of the trochlea of the talus, it engages the mortise asymmetrically, causing the body of the talus to undergo concomitant dorsolateral rotation. **B,** During *plantarflexion* the narrower trochlea of the talus rides up into the intermalleolar space corresponding to the open packed position for the joint. This disengagement of the talus out of a close packed articulation with the malleolar mortise begins with the narrower medial aspect of the anterior aspect of the trochlear dome, followed by the larger lateral side as the talus rolls forward. In essence, the talus undergoes a reverse spin or medioplantar rotation as movement progresses to plantarflexion.

engages the mortise, and stability is markedly decreased since small amounts of movement (side-to-side glide and rotation) are possible. It is with this anatomically less stable posture that sprains are most likely to occur.

9. Do the parameters of talar spin derived from the *upper ankle joint* depend on whether the lower extremity is bearing weight?

The motion of any body is a product of the *magnitude* of the force moving that body and the *direction* of that force. The answer to the question of talar spin and weight bearing is undoubtedly yes, because although the magnitude of angular momentum of the talus remains unaltered when the foot-ankle complex switches from open- to closed-chain mode, the direction of motion is not constant. Instead, the direction of talar spin changes and is *reversed*, or *opposite* in nature, to that of the open chain function.

Talar rotation is derived in part from the different architectural configuration of the anterior talar trochlear surface as the talus rolls backward with dorsiflexion or forward with plantarflexion. This medioplantar or dorsolateral rotation is obligatory in the sense that it must occur whether the foot functions in the open or closed

kinetic chain mode as a function of the anatomy of the upper ankle joint. In other words, the magnitude of the spin remains unaltered, whereas the direction of the spin is reversed according to whether the foot is bearing weight. Because of this directional change, the proximal and distal manifestations of this moment will differ. Most notably, the proximal changes refer directly to the direction of tibial rotation, whereas distal changes refer to rotational motion of the foot.

In the open kinetic chain, dorsiflexion is accompanied by lateral foot deviation (eversion), or toeing out, whereas plantarflexion is accompanied by medial deviation of the foot (inversion), or toeing in. In the closed kinetic chain, however, rotation of the distal foot complex is inhibited from expressing rotation because of the ground reaction and frictional forces. Motion is nevertheless preserved and instead expressed proximally as reverse rotation or spin of the tibia. Thus dorsiflexion, instead of rotationally expressing as toe-out, manifests as *medial tibial rotation*. Similarly, plantarflexion, instead of manifesting as toe-in during open chain function, manifests as *lateral tibial rotation* during closed chain function. Thus the component of lateral helical spin or rotation of the horizontal heel-foot complex is conserved and reexpressed during weight-bearing function as an opposite talar-tibial vertical column equal in magnitude but opposite in direction.

10. Do the parameters of talar spin derived from the *lower ankle joint* depend on whether the lower extremity is bearing weight?

As with the upper ankle joint, the magnitude and direction of subtalar joint-derived rotation are directly related to whether the lower limb is bearing weight. Interestingly, if we ascribe talar and other rotations only to the upper ankle joint, a discrepancy arises. In the closed kinetic function of gait, more tibial rotation occurs than can be accounted for simply by considering the upper ankle joint. The additional torsion is accounted for by considering the inferior aspect of the talus and its articulation with the superior aspect of the calcaneus to form the lower ankle, or *subtalar joint.* However, here our focus is specifically directed at the posterior facet, which articulates with the calcaneus (Fig. 30-5). The peculiar architecture of this articular interface endows the subtalar joint with the engineering capability of a mitered hinge, so that it may convert motion occurring at the foot complex into torque expressed as talar, and hence tibial, rotation.

11. Why does the lower limb, functioning in the weight-bearing capacity, engage the subtalar joint to yield more talar tibial rotation than might otherwise occur in the open kinetic chain?

The closed kinetic chain position during stance phase of gait is characterized by the movement of the (vertical) tibial-talar complex over a fixed (horizontal) calcaneal-foot complex. The ramifications of the closed kinetic function include the transmission of gravitational forces to and from the foot. These forces are routed through the subtalar joint. The forces include the equal but opposite forces of superincumbent body weight and ground reaction force. The passage of these forces through the subtalar joint activates the joint's inherent force-dissipating and torque-converting mechanisms such that locomotion may progress without injury to the foot. Relating these ideas to the foot means that biomechanically, motions described in the open kinetic chain at the foot yield an equal but opposite motion proximal to the foot in closed kinetic function. Those component motions of the foot in the sagittal and transverse planes manifesting as (dorso) *lateral calcaneal rotation* on the talar-tibial complex occurring during open chain function are preserved by way of reverse proximal reexpression as *medial* (plantar) *talar-tibial rotation* on the heel-

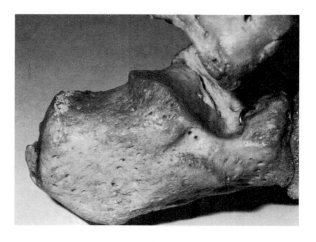

FIG. 30-5 The saddle-shaped posterior facet of the subtalar (talocalcaneal) joint is the broadest of all three facets comprising that articulation. (From Nicholas JA, Hershman EB: *The lower extremity and spine in sports medicine*, ed 2, St. Louis, 1995, Mosby.)

foot complex. Thus distal rotation of the calcaneus and foot is conserved as proximal but reverse rotation of the talus and tibial shaft.

12. Is the talus kinesiologically viewed as operating together with the proximal vertical crural column, or with the distal and horizontal heel-foot complex?

It is appropriate to momentarily detour and appreciate the stationary versus moving relationship the talus has with its proximal and distal segments in the open and closed kinetic chain positions. The talus, in direct line with the tibial shaft, may be thought of as part of the proximal crural column for the purpose of this discussion. In the open kinetic chain the foot and calcaneus complex move on the fixed talotibial complex; in other words, the distal segment moves on the proximal segment. In the closed kinetic chain the talotibial complex moves on the stationary calcaneal-foot complex because the foot is now fixed to the ground; here the proximal segment moves on the distal segment. Thus the talus may conceptually be considered as part of the vertical crural compartment that kinesiologically functions as a distal extension of the tibial shaft. This holds true regardless of whether the lower limb functions in the open or closed kinetic mode. It may be helpful to bear these ideas in mind when conceptualizing the various component alterations of motion of the talus and calcaneus as a function of the subtalar joint in open and closed chain function.

13. Why is a biomechanical understanding of foot-ankle biomechanics inadequate without the inclusion of the subtalar joint?

When rotational displacements of lower extremity function are calculated based on the rotational contribution of the upper ankle joint, they are found to match only when torsion is measured in the open kinetic chain. However, during closed chain locomotion (stance phase), much more rotation occurs than can be accounted for by simply considering the torsion contribution of the upper ankle joint. In other words, the degree of measured torsion during stance (i.e., the closed kinetic chain) is greater than what we would expect to find from the talocrural joint alone, suggesting another contributing source for rotation. It is only by examining the function of that articulation that is situated adjacent and immediately distal to the upper ankle joint that the examiner can reconcile the disparity. The *lower ankle joint* goes by a variety of names, including the *subtalar* or the *talocalcaneal joint.* It is the mutual cooperation of the upper and lower ankle joints that contributes to the total amount of tibial rotation incurred during the gait cycle.

14. What is the anatomy of the subtalar joint?

The subtalar joint is fascinatingly complex. It has three facets on the inferior talar surface that articulate with three facets on the superior calcaneal surface (Fig. 30-6). The talar-calcaneal interface consists of a biconvex *posterior calcaneal facet* articulating with a biconcave posterior talar facet located on the undersurface of the body of the talus. This facet is the broadest of all three and is *saddle shaped.* As such, this articulation allows for the frontal plane motions of eversion and inversion that, unlike other component motions of the subtalar joint, remain unaltered regardless of whether the lower limb functions in the open or closed kinetic chain position.

The subtalar joint also has an anteriorly placed calcaneal facet articulating with a talar facet on the neck of the talus, which together form a *horizontal surface.* In some persons an additional, more anteriorly placed concave calcaneal facet may articulate with a convex talar facet, forming an *inclined plane.*[16] These anterior and middle facets on the talus are convex, whereas the opposing facets on the calcaneus are concave.[41] If three facets exist, they are named *posterior, middle,* and *anterior* talar or calcaneal facets; if only two facets are present, they are simply called the posterior and anterior talar or calcaneal facets. The posterior facet is separated from the anterior and middle facets by a *tarsal*

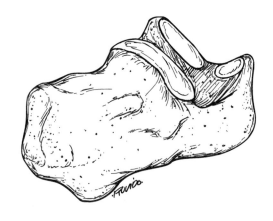

FIG. 30-6 The three inferior calcaneal facets of the subtalar joint correspond to *three superior talar facets.* (From Valmassy RL: *Clinical biomechanics of the lower extremities,* St. Louis, 1996, Mosby.)

canal that divides the subtalar joint into two joint cavities.[41] Transverse plane (abduction-adduction) motion and sagittal plane (dorsiflexion-plantarflexion) motions, unlike frontal plane motion and its relation to the posterior facet, cannot be identified as deriving from either the anterior or middle facet. The movements possible at these articulations are gliding and rotation. The movements occur in different planes and are thereby capable of motion in different directions. The joint axes of the subtalar joint cross all three body planes, and the joint is thus said to be *triplanar.* Sagittal plane motions include adduction and abduction; transverse plane motions include plantarflexion and dorsiflexion; and frontal plane motions include inversion and eversion. The latter two frontal plane motions are a function of the all-important posterior joint component of the subtalar joint. There is normally twice as much inversion available (40°) as eversion (20°). Thus a 2-to-1 ratio of supination to pronation exists as a function of the obliquity of the upper ankle joint axis, which itself is a direct function of the fibula's greater length.

15. What mechanical analogy lends itself to conceptualization of the subtalar joint?

The best mechanical analogy for understanding the subtalar joint in relation to the upper ankle joint is the *mitered hinge* (Fig. 30-7). Imagine a thought experiment in which a vertical piece of wood is attached to a horizontal board by an oblique hinge placed at 45°. If you twirl the vertical upper segment outwardly, the horizontal lower segment will of necessity rotate in the same magnitude and direction. Twirling the vertical segment inward will also turn the horizontal segment

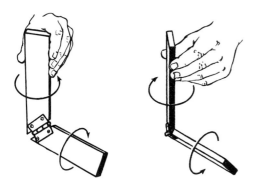

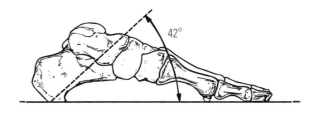

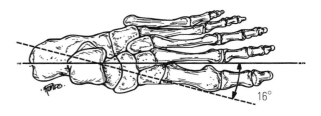

FIG. 30-7 The mechanism of a mitered hinge is analogous to function of the subtalar joint *(left)*. Action of a mitered hinge *(right)*. The vertical column corresponding to the tibia-talus complex, while the horizontal bar corresponds to the calcaneus and foot. (From Coughlin MJ, Mann RA: *Surgery of the foot and ankle,* ed 7, St. Louis, 1999, Mosby.)

FIG. 30-8 Axis of the subtalar joint. The angulation of axis has a 42° average inclination in a sagittal projection from the transverse plane as well as a 16° average medial deviation in a transverse projection from the sagittal plane. (From Valmassy RL: *Clinical biomechanics of the lower extremities,* St. Louis, 1996, Mosby.)

inward. This analogy shows the functional relationship between the vertical tibia and the horizontal foot platform. The subtalar joint acts as a hinge connecting the talus (and hence the tibia above it) and calcaneus (hence the foot distal to the calcaneus). This hinge, however, is "mitered" at a 45° incline, which has the mechanical effect of being a simple *torque converter* such that torque generated by either segment causes a torque of equal magnitude in the other segment. Thus every 1° of rotation of one segment must cause an equal rotation in the other segment. As such, the subtalar joint, aligned at a 42° angulation[68] of the horizontal axis and deviating from medial to lateral 16° in relation to the long axis of the foot (Fig. 30-8), is biomechanically defined as a torque converter or transmitter[46] that translates talocalcaneal movement into rotary motion of the tibial shaft. Tibial rotation is therefore a function of the subtalar joint, the talocrural joint, and rotation at the knee joint.

Any alteration in the angulation of our hinge will alter the one-to-one correspondence of the two segments in favor of either extreme. A more horizontally placed hinge results in greater rotation of the horizontal segment for each degree of rotation of the vertical segment; in this case the angle is less than 42°. Conversely, if the hinge is more vertically placed, a greater rotation of the vertical segment will occur for each degree of rotation of the horizontal segment; in this case the angle is greater than 42°. The former situation accounts for individuals with excessively pronated feet, whereas the latter characterizes individuals with excessive supination of the foot.[67]

16. Why is frontal plane motion the basis for measuring subtalar joint motion?

Frontal plane motion at the subtalar joint is a function of the unique posterior facet that is continuously perpendicular to the weight-bearing vector of the body. Because of this, frontal plane motions of inversion and eversion remain unaltered, regardless of whether the lower limb is functioning in the weight-bearing or non–weight-bearing positions. The clinical implication is that evaluative measurements taken in the non–weight-bearing position are applicable to weight-bearing conditions. Thus the therapist may make a determination of whether a given foot is excessively pronated or supinated during stance by evaluating the subtalar joint on the examining table.

Pronation and supination cannot be measured because they are triplane movements and also because two out of three of their components vary according to whether the foot operates in the open or closed kinetic chain. Despite this, movements in the frontal plane (calcaneal inversion and eversion) are identical for both open and closed kinetic chain function. Therefore calcaneal eversion and inversion are measured to reflect the subtalar joint motions of pronation and supination[44] and to determine whether a given foot is excessively pronated or supinated.

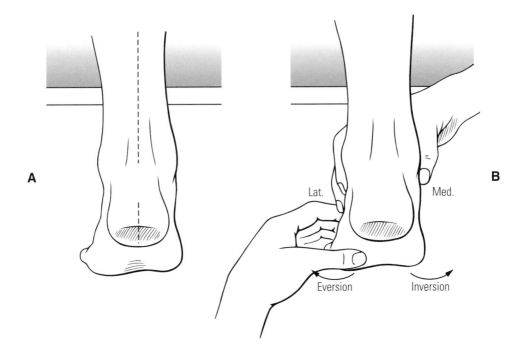

FIG. 30-9 Subtalar joint neutral is defined as the position in which the heel is aligned with the midline of the tibia. To determine subtalar joint neutral: **A,** First, lines are drawn over the midline of the calcaneus and lower ⅔ of the calf. **B,** The talus is then palpated both medially and laterally anterior to the malleoli as the foot is inverted and everted so as to gauge congruency between both sides. The examiner places his or her thumb and index finger on either side of the tibiotalar joint. For example, when examining the left ankle, the index finger is placed just in front of the anterior aspect of the fibula while the thumb is placed just anterior and inferior to the medial malleolus. By inverting and everting the hindfoot and ankle, one senses that the medial and lateral talar depressions are equal, implying a neutral position of the subtalar joint. This position of optimal foot function is necessary to determining the presence of intrinsic foot deformity and is used in making prescription orthotic devices.

17. How is deviation from subtalar neutral determined?

Determination of subtalar neutral is essential for detecting the presence of intrinsic foot deformity and for the satisfactory fabrication of an orthoses. *Subtalar joint neutral* is defined as the position in which the heel is aligned with the midline of the tibia (Fig. 30-9).[1] Alternatively, neutrality may be described as that joint position in which the foot is neither pronated nor supinated.[92] Another way of expressing this parameter is to say that subtalar neutral is the point of reference from which the foot may be maximally pronated or supinated.[50] This neutral position is likely present when the longitudinal axis of the lower one third of the tibia is perpendicular to the ground and its bisection is parallel to the posterior surface of the calcaneus and the vertical axis of the calcaneus. This is the biomechanically

sound posture of the lower extremity with the ground[101]; this posture may ideally be observed during quiet standing or midstance phase of gait as an imaginary or drawn vertical line bisecting both talus and calcaneus.[22] Overpronation increases the excursion of subtalar joint motion from 6° to 12°.

In the subtalar joint neutral position the talonavicular joint is maximally congruent, as can be observed by equal palpation of the margins of the talar head of the medial and lateral aspects of the ankle,[48] whereas the calcaneus is free to move in the frontal plane (as a function of the posterior talar-calcaneal facet) with twice as much inversion (20°) as eversion (10°). Palpation for subtalar joint neutral or either deviation from neutral involves palpation of either side of the talonavicular joint. This joint corresponds to both the anterior portion of the subtalar joint and the medial half of the transverse tarsal joint. The talonavicular joint thus provides the clinician a direct window of access for determining the osseous status of the other joints through palpation.

Clinical determination of subtalar joint neutral is an indispensable part of a lower extremity evaluation. For the examiner to best determine subtalar joint posture, the patient lies down prone and the knee of the examined foot is fully extended. Measurement may also be performed with the patient standing. Using a pen, the examiner bisects the Achilles' tendon and calcaneus of the ipsilateral extremity. The examiner asks the patient to try to relax completely, since inadvertent muscle contraction makes palpation of the neutral position difficult. The talus is palpated both medially and laterally, anterior to the malleoli, as the foot is inverted and everted to gauge congruency. The examiner places his or her thumb and index finger on either side of the talonavicular joint, while the other hand grasps the forefoot at the sulcus of the fourth and fifth digits, thereby locking the lateral column, and moves the forefoot into alternately pronated and supinated positions. At the extremes of pronation and supination the examiner will feel the talus pushing into the palpating thumb or index finger. For example, when the left ankle is examined, the index finger is placed just in front of the anterior aspect of the fibula and the thumb is placed just anterior and inferior to the medial malleolus. By inverting and everting the hindfoot and ankle, the examiner senses that the medial and lateral talar depressions are equal, implying a neutral position of the subtalar joint (see Fig. 30-9). Thus subtalar neutral may be defined as the middle position, in which neither palpating digit feels a bulge from the medial or lateral talar prominence.[93] When the examiner evaluates for subtalar neutral in the standing posture, the patient should actively invert and evert the foot until the talus feels equidistant between the examiner's palpating fingers. Deviations from this ideal position indicate the presence of an intrinsic foot deformity; conversely, deviations detected in subtalar joint neutral may be identified and measured.[14]

A pronated foot posture is observed and palpated as a valgus position of the calcaneus, and palpation of the talar head reveals a prominent medial bulge.[32] An excessively supinated foot is characterized by increased foot height because of excessive stacking of the talus atop the calcaneus, and observed as calcaneal varus and palpation of a laterally bulging talar head (Fig. 30-10).[68]

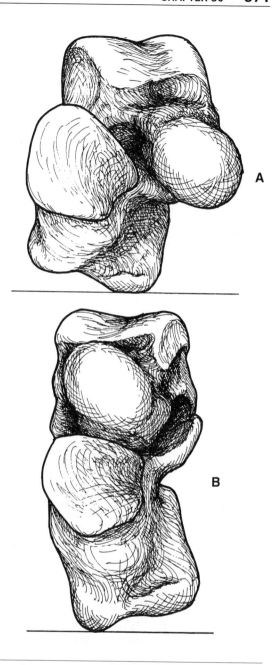

FIG. 30-10 Frontal view of talar calcaneal relationship during pronation and supination of the right foot. **A,** A pronated foot posture is observed and palpated as a valgus position of the calcaneus and palpation of the talar head as a prominent medial bulge. **B,** An excessively supinated foot is characterized by increased foot height due to excessive stacking of the talus atop the calcaneus and observed as calcaneal varus and palpation of a laterally bulging talar head. (From Root M, Weed J, Orien W: *Clinical biomechanics vol II: normal and abnormal biomechanics of the foot,* Los Angeles, 1977, Clinical Biomechanics Corp.)

Once the talonavicular position is deemed congruous, implying subtalar joint neutrality, the static positions of the forefoot and rearfoot may be assessed (Fig. 30-11). The forefoot and rearfoot relationships are evaluated, one relative to the other, to determine the presence of intrinsic deformity. This determination is made by using the metatarsal heads and the midline of the calcaneus (previously drawn) as reference landmarks. In the neutral subtalar posture the plane of the five metatarsals is said to be perpendicular to the midline of the calcaneus. Classification of deformity is based on observed or measured angular relationships among the calcaneus, Achilles tendon, and plantar surface of the forefoot. A *varus angle* created by an inverted-position calcaneus and Achilles tendon indicates a *rearfoot varus*; in this case the midline of the calcaneus is angled medially.[68] On the other hand, a *valgus angle* created by an everted position of the calcaneus and Achilles tendon indicates a *forefoot varus*; in this situation the forefoot takes on a valgus posture in relationship to the laterally angled calcaneus.[106] A third possibility involves the forefoot exhibiting a valgus posture relative to the calcaneus. This deformity is termed *forefoot valgus*.[103] These three basic foot types

all involve abnormal subtalar motion. Understanding the consequences of these deformities is pivotal to appreciating a host of distal and proximal biomechanical deviations resulting in dysfunction along the kinetic chain.

18. What is the transverse tarsal joint?

Consider again the previously described thought experiment describing motion of a vertical and horizontal segment connected by a mitered hinge. If the horizontal segment is divided into a short proximal and long distal segment with a pivot in between, the entire horizontal segment would be prevented from displacing in response to rotation of the vertical segment. This would allow the distal segment to remain stationary when vertical segment motion produces rotation of the proximal segment. This pivot on the horizontal segment corresponds to the *midtarsal* (*transverse tarsal* or *Chopart's*) *joint* and enables rotations of the leg and hindfoot to proceed without the forefoot leaving the ground.[105] Movement at this joint is understood in reference to the arches of the foot (pronation and supination). The subtalar joint appears to be a determinative joint of the foot.[1]

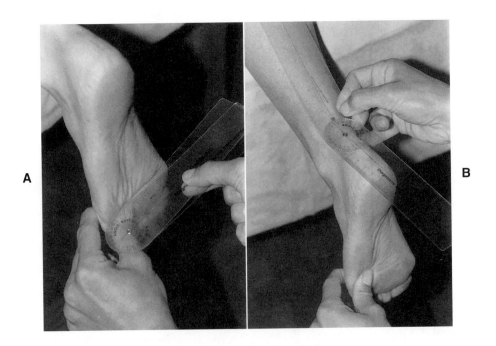

FIG. 30-11 A, Measurement of forefoot varus, and **B,** Rearfoot varus with the subtalar joint in the neutral position. (From Brotzman SB: *Clinical orthopaedic rehabilitation*, St. Louis, 1996, Mosby.)

19. What are the medial and lateral halves of the transverse tarsal joint?

The *transverse tarsal joint* (Fig. 30-12) is anatomically composed of both medial and lateral components. The medial side is composed of the *talonavicular articulation,* and is identical to the anterior and middle facets of the subtalar joint. The lateral aspect is composed of the *calcaneocuboid articulation;* thus the entire joint is aptly named the *talocalcaneonavicular joint.* The arrangement of these four tarsal bones has a transverse (cross), or S-shaped, side-to-side appearance when viewed from above, between the talus and calcaneus in the rearfoot and extending to the navicular and cuboid in the midfoot. Thus the transverse tarsal joint repre-

sents the functional articulation between the hindfoot and the midfoot.

20. How does motion at the transverse tarsal joint compensate for lack of motion in the upper and lower ankle joints?

The axes of the transverse tarsal joint are longitudinal and oblique and bear little correlation to the anatomic landmarks of this joint; rather, these axes are mechanical constructs useful to describing the behavior of the two separate anatomic articulations of the transverse tarsal joint as a single functional unit. The orientation of the longitudinal axis is similar to the longitudinal component of the oblique axis, permitting motion in the

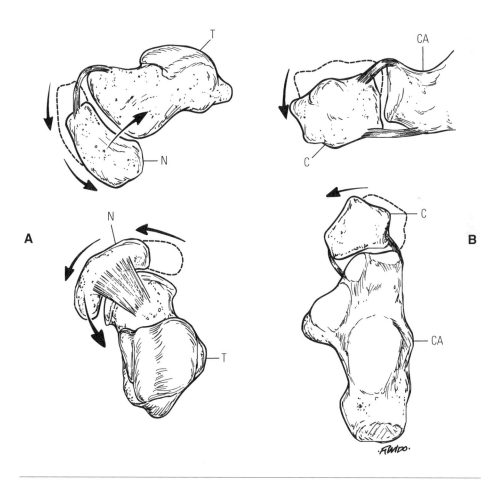

FIG. 30-12 Supination of the midtarsal joint involves **A,** plantar and medial movement of the navicular on the talus, and **B,** plantar and medial movement of the cuboid on the calcaneus. The reverse motions occur with pronation. *N,* navicular; *T,* talus; *C,* cuboid; *CA,* calcaneus. (From Valmassy RL: *Clinical biomechanics of the lower extremities,* St. Louis, 1996, Mosby.)

sagittal plane and allowing for significant amounts of dorsiflexion and plantarflexion. Thus the transverse tarsal joint amplifies the motion of both the talocrural and subtalar joints, which suggests that the loss of upper or lower ankle joint motion may be compensated for, at least partially, by motion of the transverse tarsal joint. For example, normal gait requires that there be at least 10° of dorsiflexion and 20° of plantarflexion when the knee is extended at midstance phase of gait. Many persons lack the necessary 10° of dorsiflexion, either congenitally or because of excessive tightness in the Achilles' tendon. The body must compensate to ensure that locomotion is preserved. One form of proximal compensation may involve genu recurvatum, whereas distal compensation may occur through early heel lift during the gait cycle. Alternatively, compensation may occur at the foot in the form of transverse tarsal joint motion in the sagittal plane; this motion has earned this articulation the appellation of "secondary ankle joint."

21. What do pronation and supination mean in reference to the transverse tarsal joint?

As in the subtalar joint, the component motions of the transverse tarsal joint are also defined as pronation and supination but are described in terms of the longitudinal arches of the foot. Conceptually, *pronation* of the transverse tarsal joint is understood as a *flattening* of the arches, whereas *supination* refers to *reconfiguration* of the long plantar arch. As one joint moves into pronation, it appears to pull the other joint toward pronation; conversely, supination at one joint appears to be accompanied by supination at the other.[78] The similar terminology describing the motions of both the subtalar joint and the transverse tarsal joint highlights their interdependent[68] relationship in function. Moreover, the axes of both joints pass through the center of the talar head.[42] Nevertheless, the subtalar joint appears to be the more significant player[1] orchestrating pronation and supination, and as such it is referred to as the more *dominant*[92] of the two joints.

22. How is the subtalar joint determinative of the transverse tarsal joint?

How the subtalar joint position relates to transverse tarsal joint function is most easily conceptualized by the following thought experiment. Consider a frontal plane view of the right rearfoot in the maximally pronated, neutral, and maximally supinated positions. When the subtalar joint is maximally pronated during early stance, the two axes of the transverse tarsal joint have a parallel relationship to each other, facilitating increased range of motion of the forefoot on the rearfoot as the midfoot unlocks on the hindfoot (Fig. 30-13). In other words, the hindfoot, midfoot, and forefoot are more flexible, and the long plantar arch sags. However, these axes converge after midstance, when the subtalar

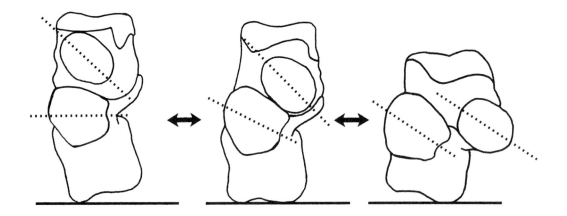

FIG. 30-13 Midtarsal joint reactions. When the subtalar joint is in its maximally pronated posture *(far right)*, the longitudinal axes of the talonavicular and calcaneal cuboid joints *(dotted lines)* are parallel with one another. In the subtalar joint neutral position *(middle)*, the angulation between the longitudinal axes has increased as the joint axes converge. Further divergence occurs on the *far left* with the subtalar joint in its maximally supinated posture. (From Seibel M: *Foot function: a programmed text*, Baltimore, 1988, Williams & Wilkins.)

joint supinates and thereby locks the forefoot on the midfoot and restricts movement of the midfoot on the hindfoot. The transverse tarsal joint is locked, and the foot is now rigid as the longitudinal arch is reconfigured in supination as a function of the nonparallel alignment of the joint axes.

The frontal plane subtalar joint component of calcaneal inversion and eversion is directly determinative of the parallel (arch pronation) or nonparallel (arch supination) alignment of the transverse tarsal joint.[66]

23. How does the talar-calcaneal interface serve as a transition point in the transfer of superincumbent body weight and ground reaction force?

By virtue of both shape and position in relation to the other tarsal bones, the talus receives superincumbent body weight at the ankle. Vertical load is received at the hindfoot by the talar dome and transmitted through the quadrilateral-shaped body of the talus to the calcaneus. Weight transmission is uniquely transmitted via two or three facets by the *subtalar joint*. This articulation is a transition point that allows dissipation of excessive forces through redistribution of load along the horizontal length of the foot and ultimately to the ground.

Motion may be divided into two components, *translation* and *rotation*.[58] Were motion confined to translation alone, the foot-ankle complex would not long endure the brunt of weight bearing. One mechanism that absorbs the force of impact is the group of fat cells, contained in the chambers formed by the fibrosepta in the heel pad, that act as shock absorbers.[2] Even more important, however, is the cascade of rotational motions constituting pronation of the subtalar joint. The introduction of rotation allows a dampening and redistribution of load over a larger number of bones and therefore over a larger surface area as an energy-dissipating strategy. In the foot and ankle the subtalar joint is engineered to orchestrate these rotations through the unique configuration bestowed on its architecture.

Between early and midstance phase of gait the superincumbent force of body weight is dampened (through arch pronation) and transferred to the ground. This transfer may be thought of as an incurred debt that is returned during the propulsive phase of stance between midstance and toe-off. During this latter interim, ground reaction force equal in magnitude but opposite in direction is received by the horizontal base, which is the foot. The foot is now configured in such a way (arch

supinated—rigid lever) so as to use that force for push-off as the path of the ground reaction force migrates past the subtalar joint and up the kinetic chain. The subtalar joint is the key player in these complex biomechanical actions, orchestrating both foot function and torque transfer between the body and ground, as well as between the horizontal foot component and the vertical leg component.

We may answer our original question by defining the subtalar joint as the point of transfer of superincumbent body weight and ground reaction force. The subtalar joint is analogous to a routing station that converts the angular components of the forces passing through so that locomotion may occur with respect to the ground. While accomplishing this, the subtalar joint simultaneously orchestrates force dissipation of superincumbent body weight and uses ground reaction forces as leverage for effective propulsion.

24. What is meant by defining the triplanar motions of the subtalar joint as *pronation* and *supination*?

The path of ground reaction force on the sole of the foot during stance phase courses from the hindfoot to the forefoot with each advancing step. The foot serves as the locus of collision of the forces of superincumbent body weight and ground reaction force. The foot negotiates these forces with the subtalar joint, which serves as a torque transmitter. By converting these potentially malevolent forces into rotations and transmitting them up the kinetic chain, the subtalar joint represents the machine behind the body's force-dissipating strategy that facilitates alternating bipedal locomotion. Subtalar joint pronation results in collapse of the medial longitudinal arch of the foot, whereas supination involves arch reconstitution. Pronation and supination are not static positions of the foot but are dynamic events that describe simultaneous component motions composed of triplanar component motions. Pronation and supination are passive occurrences. Pronation is primarily a function of superincumbent loading of the long plantar arch as body weight moves over the foot. Supination primarily occurs as a result of the windlass action of the long plantar fascia.

Pronation is a strategy that allows the foot to crumple into a loose adapter analogous to a "loose bag of bones" that dissipates the potentially injurious concussive forces of heel strike into the ground while allowing the foot to mold itself to the topography of varied terrain. Supination occurs briefly just before heel strike and provides a sturdy platform for stable ground contact. Beyond midstance phase, *supination* occurs again, converting the pliable foot into a rigid lever poised for effective propulsion during push-off, and accelerates the tibial shank forward as the leg moves into swing phase. Supination occurs beyond midstance. The extrinsic muscles of the foot cross the upper ankle and subtalar joints and may therefore play a secondary role in dynamically controlling pronation and supination. Eccentric contraction of the tibialis anterior and posterior may control both the rate and the magnitude of pronation.

The uniqueness of the subtalar joint stems from the fact that it lies in all three planes simultaneously. What this means is that the subtalar joint moves in an oblique direction through all three body planes, the sagittal, frontal, and transverse. The composite motions at the subtalar joint are called *triplanar motions* and are collectively understood as *pronation* and *supination*. A definition of these two triplanar motions does not simply involve a listing of their component motions, but also includes naming *a frame of reference* for these motions—namely, whether they occur in the open or closed kinetic chain.

Closed-chain pronation is different from open-chain pronation, and closed-chain supination is quite different from open-chain supination. Understanding both triplanar motions in both the weight-bearing and non–weight-bearing positions is essential to understanding foot-ankle biomechanics during locomotion. This is because swing phase involves supination in the open-chain mode, whereas stance phase involves pronation and supination in the closed kinetic mode of function. (Open-chain pronation does not occur in gait.) Thus, to appreciate the kinesiology and pathokinesiology of the lower extremity, the clinician must understand the minutiae of triplanar motion as it relates to open and closed kinetic chain function.

25. How are the components of pronation and supination altered and determined by whether the lower limb functions in the open or closed kinetic mode?

Open-chain function of the subtalar joint involves motion of the calcaneus and foot complex on the stationary talus. Closed-chain function of the subtalar joint involves motion of the talus (and tibia) on the stationary calcaneus-foot complex. These reverse relationships occur because whereas calcaneal-foot motion is unopposed in the non–weight-bearing posture, calcaneal-

foot motion is blocked during weight bearing by friction and ground reaction force. In other words, it is the opposing ground reaction force that reverses the direction of the sagittal and frontal plane components of pronation and supination while maintaining their magnitude. Thus *open-chain supination* of the subtalar joint is characterized by the calcaneus and foot inverting, plantarflexing, and adducting (*medioplantar rotation*) on the stationary talus; this is the posture of the foot during the entire swing cycle. In contrast, *closed-chain supination* involves talar abduction and dorsiflexion on a stationary calcaneus. Closed-chain supination begins after midstance phase of gait and peaks just before toe-off. The net sum of these component motions is dubbed *dorsolateral talar rotation*. Similarly, *open-chain pronation* of the subtalar joint involves calcaneal eversion, dorsiflexion, and abduction on a stationary talus (*dorsolateral rotation*). *Closed-chain pronation* involves talar adduction and plantarflexion on a stationary calcaneal-foot complex, whereas frontal plane movement is preserved and involves calcaneal eversion. The net sum of these component motions is dubbed *medioplantar rotation* of the talus.

The essential point of this question is that closed-chain pronation is accompanied by *medioplantar rotation of the talus* on a stationary heel-foot complex. Because the tibia articulates with the talus, it, too, undergoes a medial rotation. In contrast, closed-chain supination is accompanied by *dorsolateral rotation of the talus* on a stationary heel-foot complex. Because the tibia articulates with the talus, it, too, undergoes a lateral rotation (Fig. 30-14). Understanding these normal relationships is the key to understanding the critical pathways implicated in lower extremity dysfunction. Excessive medial (pronation) or lateral (supination) rotation of the vertical tibial-talar column disturbs the precisely orchestrated biomechanical milieu these joints require for optimal function. Consequently, many of the soft tissues are stressed beyond their limit or placed in mechanical disadvantage because of a disturbance of the precise balance of agonist-antagonist relationships.

26. What is the relationship between energy dissipation of excessive force and subtalar joint pronation?

The foot may be conceptualized as a medially incomplete hemisphere. The inherent value of this architectural design is that it endows the foot with the ability to undergo a radical flattening (pronation) during initial

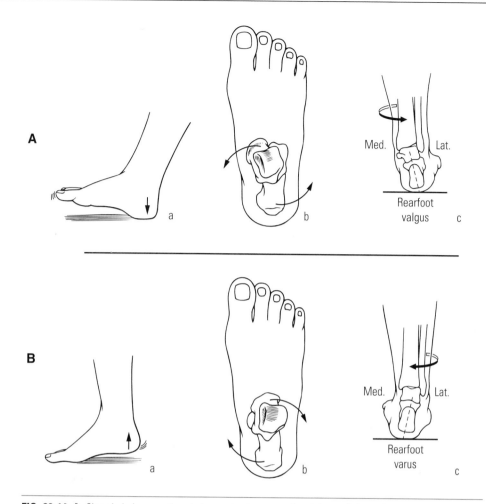

FIG. 30-14 A, Closed chain pronation during early stance causing right medial rotation of the vertical talar-tibial segment: *a,* heel strike; *b,* medioplantar rotation of the talus accompanying subtalar joint pronation indicated by arrows; and *c,* concomitant medial tibial rotation. **B,** Closed chain supination beyond midstance causing right external rotation of the vertical talar-tibial segment: *a,* heel rise; *b,* laterodorsal rotation of the talus accompanying subtalar joint supination indicated by arrows; and *c,* concomitant lateral tibial rotation.

weight bearing and to spring back (supination) during propulsion and swing phases of gait. An analogy may be drawn to the automotive industry, which developed the novel ability of body panels to spring back into shape after denting and side-impact collisions. The foot accomplishes this feat by a remarkable interplay among the many soft and osseous components of its 26 bones, 19 muscles, 107 ligaments,[89] and joints.[57] Without the presence of the subtalar joint, the foot would be doomed to early failure and arthrosis if it had to maintain its integrity as a dorsally convexed arch against the repetitive and unrelenting load of weight bearing during gait.

27. How does supination of the subtalar joint use the energy of ground reaction force to propel the body forward?

The foot has evolved a dynamic mechanism that dampens loading of the medial longitudinal arch, which would otherwise exceed the tolerance of the rigid medial arch and turn the foot to pulp. Because of its unparalleled articular ability to cross all planes, the foot has the ability to avoid injury by *medioplantar rotation* of the talus. Clinically, this is termed *pronation.* The primary locus of this motion occurs at the subtalar joint. Medioplantar talar rotation upon a stationary heel-foot complex is a helical movement whose component motions include *talar adduction* and *planatarflexion.* The sum of these movements allows redistribution of the forces of weight bearing by way of biomechanical linkage, both proximally and distally.

Supination is accomplished by two of three triplanar motions (*talar abduction* and *dorsiflexion*), whose collective movement causes a spin, or *dorsolateral rotation,* of the talus on the stationary calcaneal-foot complex. Early gait is characterized by an imparting of the force of superincumbent body weight to the ground. The purpose of supination is to convert the foot into a rigid structure that accepts the opposite ground reaction force and uses it to propel the body forward into yet another gait cycle (in accordance with Newton's third law). The foot-ankle complex has evolved a strategy that rapidly converts the loose and adaptable foot into a hard and rigid lever. Potential energy derived from ground reaction force is absorbed at the foot when its surface maximally contacts the ground during midstance. These forces, equal to superincumbent body weight although opposite in direction, are channeled through the subtalar joint and used to initiate yet another gait cycle.

28. How do pronation and supination vary as a function of open and closed kinetic chain function during gait?

The triplanar motions of the subtalar joint are complex and do not easily lend themselves to conceptualization. The essential concept here is that the components of subtalar joint pronation and supination differ in the closed and open chains. During swing phase of gait, characterized by the open kinetic chain, the calcaneus (and hence the entire foot) moves on the stationary tibial-talar column in the three composite motions of calcaneal-foot inversion, plantarflexion, and adduction. The motion of the foot and calcaneus is also described by the phrase *medioplantar rotation.* This is defined as open-chain supination. In contrast, closed-chain supination occurring during late stance phase of gait is characterized by a calcaneus that will still invert on the talus, although adduction and plantarflexion are thwarted by ground reaction force. Instead, the talus (and hence tibia above) rotates in the same magnitude, albeit in an opposite direction—namely, dorsiflexion and abduction. These latter two composite motions occur in the talus and may collectively be termed *dorsolateral rotation.* Thus the motion is not lost but rather conserved by being expressed proximally. This proximal expression occurs by way of the subtalar joint, which transmits calcaneal

motion or more aptly the medioplantar moment into an opposite talar dorsolateral moment. The preservation of *dorsolateral rotation* composed of plantarflexion and adduction of the foot and calcaneus is accomplished through transmission of motion as a counterrotation at the talar-calcaneus interface (subtalar joint).

The subtalar joint may best be conceptualized as an interface between the *vertical* superincumbent load derived through the tibial-talar complex and the *horizontal* base that is the foot, an interface that receives, dissipates, and transmits load to the ground so as to move forward. The joint also functions as a torque converter that converts the distal medioplantar torque of the horizontal foot into an opposite, dorsoplantar rotation of the vertical talotibial complex.

Pronation may be understood similarly to the action of the subtalar joint. Open-chain pronation does not occur during swing phase of gait but may be approximated when a patient is sitting on the edge of the table with the foot freely hanging in active dorsiflexion. In this situation the foot and heel are moving on a relatively stationary talar-tibia complex. What motions occur during open-chain pronation? The answer is the triplanar motions, consisting of simultaneous movement of the calcaneus and foot in the direction of calcaneal eversion, abduction, and dorsiflexion, which may be thought of as *dorsolateral rotation* of the heel and foot complex.

Closed-chain pronation occurs during the interim between heel strike and midstance. At heel strike the heel is lateral to the center of the ankle joint, where body weight is transmitted to the talus. This creates pronation at the subtalar joint that rotates the talus medially on the calcaneus. This movement of the talus on a fixed calcaneus occurs because of friction and ground reaction forces. As a result, the subtalar joint functions to maintain transverse and sagittal plane component of motion by way of proximal expression as an equal but opposite moment of the talus and tibia. Thus open-chain abduction and dorsiflexion of the distal horizontal segment are proximally reexpressed as closed-chain adduction and plantarflexion, or simply medioplantar rotation of the proximal vertical segment. The cumulative effect of these sequential relationships is to unlock the transverse tarsal joint and allow the longitudinal arch to pronate.

- Pronation—early stance—consistent with internal tibial rotation.
- Supination—late stance—consistent with external tibial rotation.

29. How is excessive torque conversion by the subtalar joint essential to understanding the origin of many proximal musculoskeletal dysfunctions?

Among the vast information available regarding structure and function of the foot-ankle complex, perhaps the most important emerging fact is that the subtalar joint is a *torque converter* or *transmitter* that translates the motions of the foot during early stance pronation into a medioplantar rolling of the talus into medial tibial torsion; conversely, laterodorsal talar rotation occurs in foot supination during late stance and is proximally expressed as external tibial torsion. It is essential to remember that many foot-fault dysfunctions are biomechanically derived from excessive tibial torsion that is caused by overpronation or excessive supination.

Of particular importance in understanding the subtalar joint is an appreciation of the relationship between two tarsal bones at the *posterior talar-calcaneal facet.* The posterior facet of the calcaneus is shaped as a one-quarter hemisphere, with its convex articular surface directed superiorly, medially, and anteriorly. This biconvex posterior calcaneal facet articulates with a biconcave posterior talar facet on the underside of the talus that is oriented inferiorly, laterally, and posteriorly. The posterior articulating component of subtalar joint alignment affords an articular surface that is *continuously perpendicular* to the weight-bearing vector of the body as the foot moves from supination-dorsiflexion at heel stroke to pronation-plantarflexion at the initiation of foot flat. Thus the articulating *interface* between these two tarsal bones at the inferior talar surface and superior calcaneal surface corresponds to a *transition point* of force between the vertical tibial-talus column and the horizontal calcaneal-foot complex. In the open kinetic chain, internally generated muscular forces are generated proximodistal and thus yield movement of the distal horizontal (foot) component on the proximal vertical (leg) component. In the closed kinetic chain the addition of externally generated, distal to proximal, ground reaction forces to the system reverses the direction of movement such that the proximal vertical (leg) segment moves on the horizontal (foot) component.

30. Why is the cavus foot posture more likely to cause an inversion injury of the ankle joint?

A cavus foot posture is characterized by a valgus or inverted heel in which the talus is excessively stacked over the calcaneus. The added height of the foot is colloquially referred to as a *high instep.* This posture locks the foot into a stiff and rigid structure that causes no problems when the individual comes up on the ball of the foot. In fact, this foot is capable of propelling the body forward beyond midstance. The shortcoming of this posture is that it fails to adequately dissipate forces during initial contact before midstance, because of a decreased ability to pronate. Instead of the normal lateral-to-medial route of plantar ground reaction force during locomotion, the varus posture of the heel diminishes the amount of medial weight along the plantar surface. In other words, individuals with cavus feet spend a disproportionately greater time during stance phase along the lateral border of their feet. In early stance this foot posture presents no problem as the foot progressively moves into relative dorsiflexion and hence into a safe, closed packed position. The foot is thus most stable just before heel-off because it is in maximal dorsiflexion. On the other hand, beyond heel rise the foot progressively plantarflexes and the upper ankle joint moves into an open packed position as toe-off is reached. Thus the foot is more vulnerable in the open packed posture. Because of this a jump landing often stresses the lateral collateral ligaments complex beyond its limit, resulting in sprain.

While in the position of full plantarflexion, neither of the anterior arches of the trochlea articulates with the mortise. Only the narrow posterior aspect of the trochlea engages the mortise, and stability is markedly decreased because small amounts of movement (side-to-side glide and rotation) are possible. It is in this anatomically less stable posture that sprains and other forms of traumatic foot injury are most likely to occur.

31. Why is a rigid forefoot valgus deformity susceptible to inversion sprain at the ankle?

A rigid forefoot valgus (see pp. 348-349) involves a forefoot that is everted relative to the rearfoot, bringing the medial side of the foot below the lateral side.[1] This results in an unstable base of support as body weight is borne on the medial side of the forefoot. Stability is achieved by countering and essentially negating forefoot eversion by way of inversion of the calcaneus at the subtalar joint. Thus compensation is achieved by subtalar joint supination.[1]

An adverse distal effect of an abnormally supinated foot is that the transverse tarsal joint is prevented from unlocking and negotiating uneven terrain. Thus the "loose adapter" capacity of the foot is diminished as more forces are absorbed by the foot rather than transferred to the ground. Moreover, this form of compensation brings the subtalar joint much closer to the end of its range of motion and negatively affects the reaction time of the peroneal muscles crossing the lateral aspect of the ankle. This deviation toward excessive supination places the peroneal tendons on stretch and thus reduces their efficiency. Thus, coupled with excessive lateral plantar weight bearing, compensatory supination in the rigid forefoot valgus is very susceptible to lateral inversion sprain[1,72] because the foot is more likely to roll inward and is less able to stave off inversion by way of reflexive distal contraction.

32. What is the mechanism of injury?

Whereas the upper ankle joint is stable in the dorsiflexed, closed-packed position, it is inherently unstable in the open-packed, plantarflexed posture. For example, during a jump landing following a rebound of a basketball, a player lands on the forefoot first, with the ankle plantarflexed and internally rotated.[25] The ankle mortise is least stable in this posture, and whatever stability is present is afforded by the surrounding ligamentous stabilizers rather than by an osseous locking mechanism. The inversion moment to the ankle is probably increased by the landing on the irregular surface of an opponent's foot, and the lateral ligament complex is strained beyond its ability to absorb stress. In football these same structures are placed at risk for excessive stress during running, cutting, and twisting and during tackling or collisions when the foot is trapped on the ground while the body is twisting above.[25] Lateral ankle sprain may also occur in persons wearing high-heeled shoes, who are more susceptible to an inversion moment of greater magnitude if their lateral sole enters a crack in the sidewalk. This may also occur after stepping off a curb and rolling onto the side of a plantarflexed foot.

33. What are the ligamentous ankle joint stabilizers?

The upper and lower ankle joints are supported by a common ligamentous capsule that includes a lateral ligament complex composed of 3 ligaments, the deltoid complex composed of 4 ligaments medially, and the tibiofibular ligaments of the distal tibiofibular joint (Fig. 30-15). The ligaments that make up the lateral ligament complex are known as collateral ligaments because they provide collateral (i.e., side-to-side) static stability. Collateral ligaments are thickenings of the articular capsule. Consequently, an intact collateral ligament complex stabilizes both the talocrural and subtalar joints. Individually named according to their origin

and insertion, collectively these ligaments serve as a guide to direct motion, aid in proprioception, and stabilize the ankle joint.[17] None of these ligaments are distinctly palpable. The deltoid ligament complex is a contiguous, thicker band of ligamentous tissue and is therefore relatively stronger than the separate thickenings that make up the lateral collateral ligaments.

34. What are the components of the lateral collateral ligament complex, and what are the components' contributions to lateral ankle stability?

The *lateral ligament complex* of the ankle consists of three structures, listed in order of increasing strength and decreasing susceptibility to injury: the *anterior talofibular* (ATFL); the posterior talofibular (PTFL); and the *calcaneofibular* ligaments (CFL). The ankle is most stable in dorsiflexion, whereas increasing plantarflexion allows more anterior talar translation (draw) of the talus and talar inversion (medial tilt) in the mortise.[34,39,69] Strain gauge measurement and selective cadaver sectioning of these ligaments elucidate the relative contributions of these ligaments to lateral ankle stability. The ATFL shows the highest strain in plantarflexion (Fig. 30-16) and decreasing strain in dorsiflexion. In direct opposition, the CFL shows the highest strain in dorsiflexion and decreasing strain in plantarflexion. The PTFL, like the CFL, exhibits the highest strain in full dorsiflexion, the position of greatest ankle stability; however, it is lax when the foot is in neutral.[52] As the ankle moves into a plantarflexed position, the CFL swings out of its "collateral" position. In this position the ligament is no longer able to effectively stabilize the lateral side of the ankle.

35. What is the anatomy of the anterior talofibular ligament, and what is its normal function?

The cylindrical ATFL consists of two portions, an upper and lower band, and is both intracapsular and intraarticular. This ligament courses from the anteroinferior border of the fibula to the neck of the talus. It runs parallel to the long axis of the fibula and talus and is therefore horizontal in orientation, and hence slack, when the ankle joint is in neutral or dorsiflexion and eversion. In contrast, the ATFL is more perpendicular to the long axis of the fibula and talus when the ankle joint is in equinus (plantarflexion and inversion),[25,62] and it takes a near vertical fiber orientation in this posture. This vertical slanting renders the ligament tense throughout plantarflexion.

As the ankle swings from dorsiflexion to plantar-

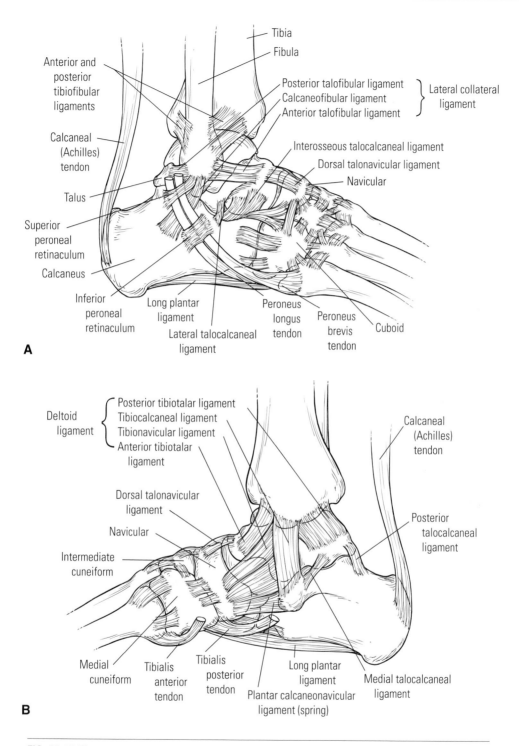

FIG. 30-15 The anatomical structures of the right ankle joint. **A,** Lateral view. **B,** Medial view. (From Greenstein GM: *Clinical assessment of neuromusculoskeletal disorders,* St. Louis, 1997, Mosby.)

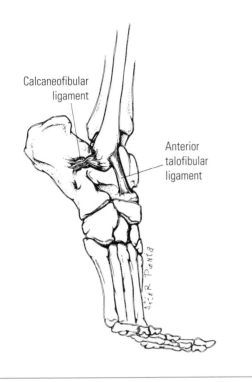

Calcaneofibular ligament

Anterior talofibular ligament

FIG. 30-16 The ATFL shows the highest strain in plantarflexion. (From Malone TR, Hardaker WT: Rehabilitation of foot and ankle injuries in ballet dancers, *JOSPT* 11:8, 1990)

flexion, the talus disengages from a closed-packed position with the malleolar mortise. The narrower medial aspect of the anterior aspect of the trochlear dome, followed by the larger lateral side of the talus, rolls forward by way of a *medial-plantar rotation.*

While in a position of full plantarflexion, neither of the anterior arches of the trochlea articulates with the mortise. Only the narrow posterior aspect of the trochlea engages the mortise, and stability is markedly decreased because small amounts of movement (e.g., side-to-side glide and rotation) are possible. It is in this anatomically less stable posture that sprains and other forms of traumatic foot injury are most likely to occur.

In the open packed posture the ATFL fulfills its primary function of preventing the talus from slipping forward from under the tibia. As such, the ATFL is considered a *primary talar stabilizer.* Normally the talus undergoes compressive forces near its base during plantarflexion, which tends to propel it toward the apex of the bony transverse arch of the foot. Forward slippage of the talus (which is the keystone of the osseous trans-

verse arch) is checked by the ATFL, which may be likened to a bridle restraining a running horse.

Biomechanical testing of ligament strength suggests that the ATFL has the lowest yield force and ultimate load of the entire lateral ligament complex.[98] Because of this, *the ATFL is the most frequently injured ligament during sprain* of the lateral collateral ligamentous complex.[13,25,30]

36. What is the anatomy of the CFL, and what is its normal function?

The CFL is a cordlike ligament that runs obliquely from the tip of the fibula to the calcaneal tubercle in a posterior-inferior direction,* under cover of the peroneal tendons. The fibers of the CFL run perpendicular, rather than parallel, under the peroneal tendons. Despite this, the peroneal tendons afford the CFL some dynamic protection by way of reflexive contraction in the event of sudden and violent ankle inversion. The CFL prevents the talus from slipping medially from under the tibia during normal function and is therefore considered a *secondary talar stabilizer.*[25] The CFL restrains excessive lateral calcaneal tilt in open-chain function, or medial talar tilt during closed kinetic function if forced ankle inversion occurs. During ankle eversion the ligament is slack, whereas it is taut during inversion and dorsiflexion. While the ankle is in neutral or dorsiflexion, the CFL lies perpendicular to the long axis of the talus.[88]

The CFL has the highest linear elastic modulus of the three ligaments and sustains higher yield forces and ultimate load (four times greater) than the ATFL.[20] Additionally, the CFL crosses both the upper and lower ankle joints.

37. What is the anatomy of the PTFL, and what is its normal function?

The PTFL is a stout, fanlike ligament originating from the posterior border of the distal fibula and inserting on a tubercle on the lateral talus. In addition to being strongest ligament of the lateral collateral complex (i.e., possessing the highest yield force and ultimate load),[25] the PTFL is rarely injured because its fibers are tensed only during hyperdorsiflexion, a movement that infrequently occurs to inversion. The significant function of the PTFL may be viewed as static dampening of excessive concussive force between the talus and the mortise as

---

*In other words, from front to back, and downward.

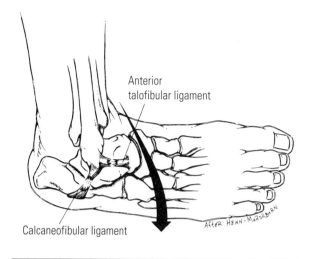

Anterior
talofibular ligament

Calcaneofibular ligament

After Henn-Morshorn

FIG. 30-17 Violent inversion and plantarflexion of the right ankle. The portion of the ATFL near its fibular origin is stretched taut over a ridge of bone created by the lateral articular facet of the talar body while the calcaneofibular ligament is tensed and torn as the fibular malleolus is distanced from the calcaneal tubercle. (From Malone TR, Hardaker WT: Rehabilitation of foot and ankle injuries in ballet dancers, *JOSPT* 11:8, 1990)

the upper ankle joint moves into osseous locking with dorsiflexion.

38. What is the sequence of lateral ligamentous defense against an inversion moment to the upper ankle joint?

When the ankle is violently plantarflexed (without inversion), the portion of the ATFL near its fibular origin is stretched taut over a ridge of bone created by the lateral articular facet of the talar body and the sunken neck of the talus, in much the same way that a length of adhesive tape is stretched until it tears when pulled on either side over the apex of granite rock (Fig. 30-17). The ATFL is the first line of static defense against excessive motion and is thus most susceptible to injury and the first ligament to be injured in an ankle sprain. Isolated sectioning of the ATFL shows increased laxity in draw and tilt parameters—more laxity in plantarflexion, but still a rather large increase in laxity in dorsiflexion.[25] However, if injurious forces are excessive, they are countered by the secondary restraint, the CFL. Thus as the foot continues to roll over into an inverted position, it is no longer in plantarflexion caused by ground reaction force, but rather in relative dorsiflexion. The CFL is taut in this position as it tries to check excessive motion. If the force is excessive, the tensile capacity of the

ligament is exceeded and the tropocollagen helical core composing the ligament unwinds as the ligament succumbs to tearing. This severe sprain of both ligaments renders the ankle joint *subluxated*[35,49,51,86] and unstable. If disruption of both ligaments is not enough to hinder progression of the injurious inversion moment, the PTFL is the final ligamentous line of defense. If this ligament is also sprained, the result is an inversion *dislocation* of the upper ankle joint.[25]

The majority of ankle sprains involve forced inversion and plantarflexion.[7,9,11] In approximately 65% of ankle sprains, injury involves the anterior talofibular ligament; with more violent inversion force (in 20% of cases), damage to the calcaneofibular ligament also occurs.[7,11,20] Isolated calcaneofibular ligament damage is rare, occurring in only 5% of grade III sprains. (Grading of sprains is discussed in the following sections.[7,11])

39. How are lateral ligamentous ankle injuries classified according to anatomic and clinical criteria?

The standard classification of ankle ligament injuries includes three grades. This is meaningful from both the anatomic and the clinical perspective. Such a grading system is based on ligamentous integrity and clinical assessment of function.

• *Grade I (mild sprain).* Grade I signifies stretching and some fiber tearing of the ATFL without significant ligamentous disruption. Quantitatively, this may be classified as having less than 25% of fibers torn.[10,20,26] Clinical presentation includes mild swelling and point tenderness, little or no hemorrhage of the lateral ankle, and mildly restricted range of motion. No instability is noted during examination, although the patient may have difficulty with full weight bearing. A zero to 1+ score on an anterior draw test is elicited on physical examination or radiographic examination.[85]

• *Grade II (moderate sprain).* Grade II signifies moderate injury to the lateral ligament complex, frequently with complete rupture of the ATFL and partial tear of the CFL. Quantitatively, this may be classified as having 25% to 75% of fibers torn.[19] The patient may report hearing an audible pop during the injury. Evaluation reveals restricted range of motion with localized swelling, ecchymosis, hemorrhage, and tenderness at the anterolateral ankle, although a defect of the ATFL is not palpable. Because the ATFL blends with the articular capsule, capsular tears usually accompany sprains of the ATFL. Subsequently there are palpable swelling and tenderness in the sinus tarsi because the ordinarily normal concavity is now filled with edematous fluid. Localized swelling and ecchymosis become more diffuse and within a few days extravasate (i.e., spread) beneath the deep fascia as far as the toes. Instability may be mild or absent, and the patient experiences additional functional loss in the form of an inability to toe rise or hop on the injured foot.[25,47] The patient may walk with a limp or may be unable to bear weight.[11] A grade II injury may be indistinguishable from a grade III injury in the acute phase.[25] The intermediate dorsal cutaneous nerve, a sensory branch of the superficial peroneal nerve, may also be injured because it crosses directly over the ATFL. The ligament will have a 2+ score on an anterior draw test and a negative result on the talar tilt test on a radiograph.[25]

• *Grade III (severe sprain).* Grade III signifies complete tear of the ATFL and capsule and rupture of the CFL. Quantitatively, this may be classified as having more than 75% of fibers torn.[11]* This state is referred to as *ankle subluxation,* whereas additional tear of the PTFL is classified as *ankle dislocation.* The PTFL is only infrequently the only ligament torn and is usually torn in conjunction with the other lateral collateral ligaments. A PTFL tear typically occurs secondary to application of force of a massive magnitude to the upper ankle joint. The PTFL has a rich blood supply by virtue of being intracapsular to the upper ankle joint. Because of this, swelling is rapid and, if observed within 2 hours after injury, is egg shaped and located over the lateral malleolus. Examination of a third-degree injury reveals a history of severe pain; diffuse swelling; ecchymosis on the lateral side of the ankle and heel; tenderness over the anterolateral capsule, ATFL, and CFL; and an inability to bear weight. A 3+ anterior draw sign is present, as well as a positive suction sign, and stress test. Radiographic examination reveals a positive anterior draw test and positive talar test result.[25] Bilateral malleolar ecchymosis occurs in approximately 60% of severe ankle sprains within 48 hours of the injury.[12,20]

40. What deficits of proximal biomechanical linkage may contribute to lateral ankle sprain?

It is erroneous to view an ankle sprain as merely an isolated, single-joint pathologic condition. The foot and ankle transmit ground reaction forces proximally up the

---

*Electromyographic studies show an 80% incidence of peroneal nerve damage after grade III sprains, supporting the notion that the lateral peroneal complex provides an additional inversion restraint. Whereas the peroneal nerve crosses the ATFL, the peroneal tendons cross the CFL.

kinetic chain. These forces are distributed, and hence dispersed, among the sagittal (front to back), transverse (rotational), and coronal (side-to-side) arcs of motion of those proximal joints, as well as among the muscles that move them. To engage in a thought experiment, we can extrapolate what happens proximally after an excessively violent inversion moment at the ankle joint. An ankle perturbation caused by an imbalance of force is detected in the form of excessive joint motion by proprioceptors in the lateral collateral ligament complex and the peroneal tendons. This volley of information is afferently transmitted to the spinal cord, where it synapses, or relays, information to an interneuron. The interneuron orders an efferent adjustment by way of activating an internally generated muscular counterforce. The body attempts to stave off potential injury by generating an equal but opposite torque offered by muscular forces. Which muscles of the lower limb are best able to generate an opposing everting force? The efferent reaction stimulates concentric contraction of the ankle evertors, namely the peroneals, as well as the hip abductors, specifically the gluteus medius (Fig. 30-18). In addition, the reaction reciprocally inhibits motor neurons of the antagonist muscles (i.e., ankle invertors and hip adductors).

To recapitulate, hip and ankle muscle recruitment is generated by a polysynaptic reflex that was initiated by ankle mechanoreceptors. This recruitment represents the body's protective strategy in the event of joint motion beyond the threshold of safety. Conversely, any weakness of the ipsilateral gluteus medius or peroneal musculature may conceivably predispose an individual to sustaining an inversion sprain of the ankle because of compromised muscle recruitment. This has direct bearing on the strategy for treating lateral ankle sprains.

41. How is a suspected sprain of the lateral collateral ligament complex clinically confirmed?

In the uninjured ankle the talus glides anteriorly and tilts medially within the mortise during plantarflexion and inversion, respectively. In treatment of lateral ankle sprain the foot is manipulated on the ankle to determine which motion elicits pain. If more pain is elicited during anterior draw, the ATFL integrity is suspect, whereas if the calcaneus or talus is tilted medially, CFL integrity is suspect. Both tests should be performed soon after injury, since muscle spasm and swelling may mask signs of talar instability.

The *anterior draw test* is a sagittal plane stress test that measures estimated millimeter shift of the talus on

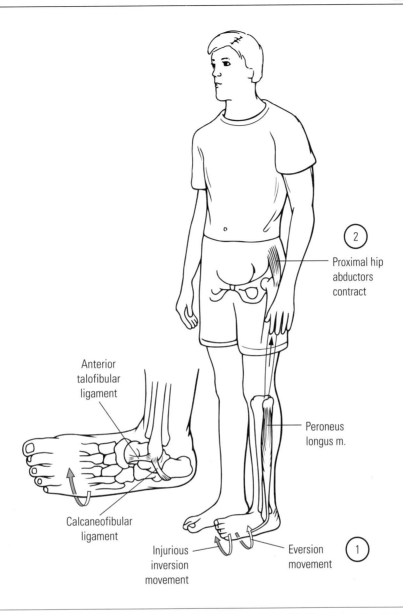

Anterior
talofibular
ligament

Peroneus
longus m.

Proximal hip
abductors
contract

Calcaneofibular
ligament

Injurious
inversion
movement

Eversion
movement

FIG. 30-18 Protective dynamic strategy to offset ankle perturbation beyond the ligamentous tensile threshold. Proprioceptors in the lateral ankle ligaments detect and relay excessive joint motion centrally where an efferent response *(1)* attempts to generate an equal but opposite muscular torque in the hip abductors *(2)* and peroneals, thus effectively cancelling the inversion moment and preventing further injury.

the tibia. The test is performed by simultaneously pulling forward on the heel while stabilizing the distal leg (Fig. 30-19). Before this the test is performed on the uninjured ankle to obtain a control value. When the normal ankle is viewed laterally, the heel cord can be seen to trace a posterior concavity. In the event of a complete sprain of the ATFL, this concavity will become flattened or even reversed as a convexity during a positive

anterior draw sign; this is known as a *positive Achilles bulge sign.*

The anterior draw test must be performed with the knee flexed and the ankle in slight plantarflexion. Ideally, the ipsilateral knee joint is placed in 90° flexion because this posture places the gastrocnemius muscle at mechanical disadvantage, thus dampening any reflex muscle tension derived from pain. Failing to place the

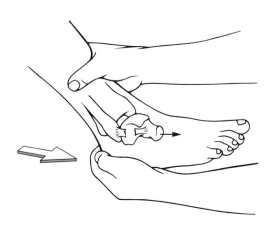

FIG. 30-19 The *anterior draw test* evaluates the integrity of the anterior talofibular ligament. In a positive test, the talus slides anteriorly *(arrow)* from under cover of the ankle mortise as the examiner draws the foot forward relative to a stationary tibia.

knee in 90° flexion may yield a *false negative* anterior draw sign. Similarly, the ankle joint is placed in as much plantarflexion as the patient will allow because a dorsiflexed ankle will mask evidence of sprain (false negative sign) as the result of bony locking within the mortise that prevents forward glide (draw) of the talus. Because of this, manual stress testing is best performed by having the patient sit on the end of the examining table with the knee in 90° flexion and the injured ankle in 10° plantarflexion.[3,19] Forward talar excursion of 3 mm more than the unaffected ankle is significant for positive instability caused by a torn ATFL.[3,11,19,26,54,95] A straight anterior draw bilaterally while the foot is in dorsiflexion implicates tear of both the medial and lateral collateral ligament complexes of the ankle joint.

A *talar tilt test* is an inversion stress test of the ankle performed by slightly plantarflexing the involved ankle during forced inversion. The examiner grasps the heel with one hand and purposefully inverts the heel on the stationary leg, while simultaneously palpating for lateral distraction of the talus on the tibia (Fig. 30-20). An excursion greater than 5 mm compared with the uninjured side is considered a positive sign for CFL impairment. Visible dimpling over the anterolateral aspect of the ankle, known as a positive suction sign, signifies incompetence of the ATFL. The presence of this sign indicates a grade III sprain.[2]

An isolated tear of the ATFL will not permit talar tilt because medial talar tilting in the ankle mortise is controlled by the calcaneofibular ligament. Despite this

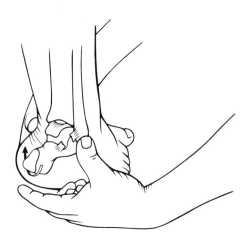

FIG. 30-20 A *talar tilt test* is an inversion stress test that primarily determines integrity of the calcaneofibular ligament performed by slightly plantarflexing the involved ankle during forced inversion. The examiner grasps the heel with one hand and purposefully inverts the heel on the stationary leg while simultaneously palpating for lateral distraction of the talus on the tibia.

talar tilting only occurs when both the anterior talofibular and calcaneofibular ligaments have been ruptured. If the CFL alone is ruptured and the ATFL remains intact, there will be neither talar tilt nor anterior draw. This rare injury manifests as subtalar tilt.[9]

42. What imaging techniques are appropriate?

Because of the difficulty of assessing the magnitude of injury during the acute stage, ancillary studies such as stress radiography and arthrography may be used to supplement the physical examination.

Because the anterior draw and talar tilt test involve small arthrokinematic movements, they may be quantitatively measured by *stress radiography,* which is performed with the patient under local anesthesia to eliminate pain and resultant muscle spasm. This is especially the case after swelling develops (within 24 hours of injury)[97] and makes it difficult for the examiner to estimate small amounts of motion. This type of testing requires examining the uninvolved extremity to determine the degree of normal joint laxity for that individual. For example, a ballet dancer who engages in toe dancing will probably have a much greater degree of joint laxity than will a nonathlete. Stress radiography is probably not accurate enough to distinguish between ATFL and combined ATFL and CFL tears.[25,51,77,91] Nevertheless, the presence of a posterior hiatus (a wedge-shaped space between the posterior tibial vault and the talar dome) is indicative of ATFL disruption (Fig. 30-21).[54] Radiographic examination of the anteroposterior, lateral, oblique, and mortise views may also be used to rule out avulsion fractures of the tip of the distal tibia, tuberosity of the fifth metatarsal, talar fractures,[3,19] and fractures of the medial malleolus.

Arthrography involves the injection of radiopaque isotope into the talocrural joint capsule. This test is most accurate during the first 24 hours after injury.[9] After this acute phase the result of arthrography is unreliable because of the formation of blood clots and fibrin that tend to seal off communication between the joint space and (torn) capsule. The premise of arthrography is based on the intimate relationship between the ATFL and the joint capsule, such that leakage of contrast material around the distal fibula indicates rupture of the ATFL (Fig. 30-22). Some authorities claim that arthrography cannot differentiate between a grade II and III injury.[25,74]

Peroneal tenography is, like arthrography, based on the intimate association between the peroneal tendons and the CFL; observation of contrast leakage indicates damage. Arthrography in combination with peroneal tenography offers the most precise assessment of lateral ankle ligament ruptures.[4] Magnetic resonance imaging is generally unreliable in visualizing ankle ligaments.[73]

43. What is the differential diagnosis?

Differential diagnosis includes acute rupture of the peroneal retinaculum with subluxation of the peroneal tendons, avulsion of the tuberosity of the fifth metatarsal, avulsion of the fibular malleolus, an epiphyseal fracture if the epiphyses are still open, osteochondral fracture of the talar dome, or fracture of the anterior process of the os calcis.[99] Dislocated peroneal tendons are observed to ride anteriorly over the lateral malleolus during dorsiflexion. Fracture is especially suspected following severe sprain, particularly when weight bearing is intolerable and severe tenderness or deformity is present over body prominences.[31] Talar dome fractures should be suspected in the ankle sprain that refuses to heal.

44. What is the differential diagnosis for ankle sprain?

- *Talotibial impingement syndrome.* Talotibial impingement syndrome goes by a variety of synonyms, including talotibial exostoses, athlete's ankle, footballer's ankle, or ankle impingement syn-

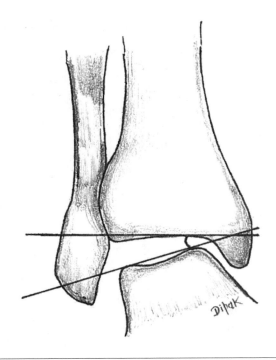

FIG. 30-21 Lateral instability is radiographically assessed by presence of a *posterior hiatus* (a wedge-shaped space between the posterior tibial vault and the talar dome) during talar tilt with maximal inversion stress exerted indicative of ATFL disruption. (From Patel DV, Warren RF: Ankle sprain: clinical evaluation and current treatment concepts. In Ranawat CS, Positano RG, editors: *Disorders of the heel, rearfoot, and ankle,* New York, 1999, Churchill Livingstone.)

drome.[36,57,70,76] This syndrome, common in such athletes as soccer players,[36] may occur either anteriorly or posteriorly. The syndrome involves compression of the talus against the tibia at the extremes of motion. *Anterior impingement syndrome* is the more common of the two.[57,84] It occurs in all competitive athletes,[79,83] including baseball catchers,[38] cross-country runners,[87] and dancers during the demi plié position, and results from hyperdorsiflexion of the upper ankle joint (Fig. 30-23). Posterior impingement syndrome occurs from hyperplantarflexion of the upper ankle joint (Fig. 30-24) and involves impingement of the posterior tubercle of the talus. Both forms of impingement can hinder athletic performance.

Normally a sulcus is present on the superior aspect of the talar neck. The sulcus accommodates the anterior tibial ridge. Excessive dorsiflexion, however, may cause direct contact between the tibia and the talus and cause minor fractures between the bone sur-

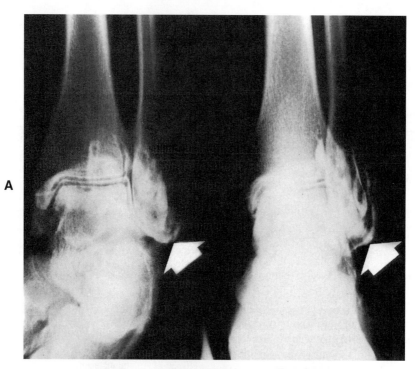

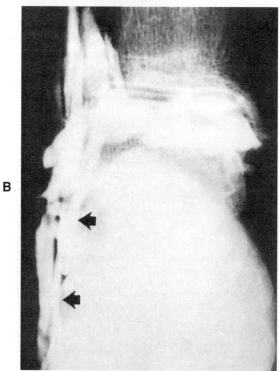

FIG. 30-22 A, Torn anterior talofibular ligament with extravasation of contrast medium from along the lateral aspect of the ankle around the tip of the lateral malleolus, best seen on a mortise view *(arrows)*. Normal articular cartilage of the ankle is well seen on a mortise view. **B,** Tear of the calcaneofibular ligament with profuse extravasation of contrast material and opacification of peroneal tendon sheath *(arrows)*. (From Nicholas JA, Hershman EB: *The lower extremity and spine in sports medicine,* ed 2, St. Louis, 1995, Mosby.)

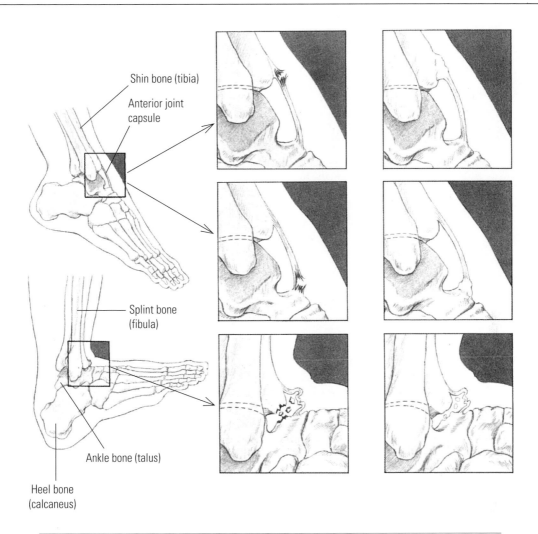

FIG. 30-23 Mechanism of injury in the most common form of *talotibial impingement syndrome* occurs by way of hyperdorsiflexion of the ankle joint which causes minor fractures between the bone surfaces. If the mechanism involves hyperplantarflexion, the soft tissue comprising the anterior joint capsule may undergo excessive traction resulting in sprain at the tibial or talar attachment. Here, the site of rupture is accompanied by palpable osteophytes as healing commences. (From Peterson L, Renstrom P: *Sports injuries: their prevention and treatment,* Chicago, 1983, Yearbook Medical Publishers.)

faces. Excessive plantarflexion imparts traction to the anterior joint capsule, which may entrap the synovium or sprain the capsule. Synovial entrapment typically occurs in the lateral gutter in the region of the talofibular articulation. Following repetitive impingement, marginal exostoses (bone spurs) form on the posterolateral aspect of the talus and tibia.[57] These bony deposits may cause inflammation of the joint capsule and tendon sheaths. Clinical presentation includes poorly localized ankle pain that becomes more localized to the anterior aspect of the ankle. Clinical presentation may also involve mild swelling.[37] Patients typically report a history of a blow or twisting injury to the ankle that has not resulted in ligamentous laxity and has been passed off as a mere sprain. Pain is heightened during push-off of the involved foot,[109] with point tenderness over the anterior aspect of the ankle between the anterior tibial tendon and the medial malleolus. Pain may be perceived as a band across the ankle joint, felt when performing such activities as kicking the ball forward in soccer.[57] Localized anterolateral swelling may be present. A palpable

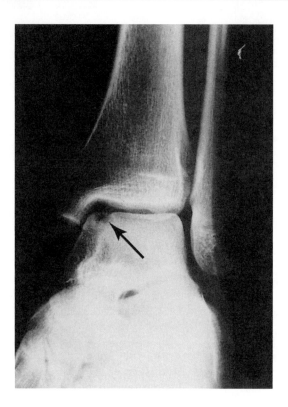

FIG. 30-24 A. Radiographic view of osteochondritis dissecans involving the superomedial aspect of the talus. (From Deltoff MN, Kogan PL: *The portable skeletal x-ray library,* St. Louis, 1998, Mosby.)

and tender osteophyte may be felt on the superior surface of the talar neck with the ankle in plantarflexion. Dorsiflexion is limited and painful and thus erroneously clues the unwary clinician to the mistaken diagnosis of Achilles tendinitis[57]; plantarflexion relieves symptoms. Lateral radiographs with the foot in dorsiflexion show hypertrophic sclerotic osteophytes along the anterior margins of the talus and tibia—the characteristic contact of the anterior lip on the talar neck. Initial treatment is nonsurgical and consists of Achilles' tendon stretching and strengthening of the anterior tibial and peroneal musculature.[2] Although talotibial impingement syndrome is irreversible, symptoms are relieved by wearing a half-inch heel, using antiinflammatory medication, and discontinuing excessive dorsiflexion activity. Exostectomy is a more definitive treatment[109] and is considered for patients who have not improved after a 3-month or longer regimen of physical therapy.

• *Osteochondritis dissecans.* Osteochondritis dissecans of the ankle joint refers to posttraumatic loose bone

fragments in the upper ankle joint following *transchondral talar dome fractures.* Similar to osteochondritis dissecans at the knee, in which a lesion develops on the bulbous aspect of the femoral condyle, this condition at the ankle has a traumatic etiology and causes a lesion on the bulbous projection of the talar dome. Moreover, transverse plane rotation, causing shear and torsional forces, is implicated in the mechanisms of both sites. The location of the lesion at the ankle is either the anterolateral or posteromedial portion of the superior margin of the talus. Anterolateral lesions are produced by a dorsiflexion and inversion mechanism. These motions compose pronation during weight bearing, which is accompanied by obligatory internal tibial and fibular rotation. In this case the fibular component of the malleolar fork impinges on the anterolateral talus. In contrast, posteromedial lesions are produced by a plantarflexion and eversion mechanism that compose the component motions of supination, which is accompanied by obligatory external tibial and fibular rotation. Here, the tibial component of the malleolar fork impinges on the posteromedial talus. Osteochondritis dissecans is more common in adolescent boys. Patients often have a history of trauma, although ankle injury may have occurred weeks or months before symptom presentation. Clinical presentation is similar to that of a ligament injury, with edema, ecchymosis, limited motion, pain on weight bearing, intermittent ankle swelling, and an increase in both anterior drawer and varus stress. Symptoms of osteochondritis dissecans may also be identical to those of chronic ligament instability, including activity-related stiffness that improves with rest. The absence of localized tenderness over the anterolateral fibular ligament may raise suspicion of osteochondritis dissecans. Because there are no pathognomonic signs and symptoms of osteochondritis dissecans of the ankle, diagnosis based only on clinical presentation is not certain. Radiographic examination from specific views is appropriate in the event of a suspected osteochondral lesion. A mortise view with the foot in full plantarflexion is best for viewing the medial posterior lesion, whereas bringing the foot to neutral or dorsiflexion will provide a better view of a lateral anterior lesion on the mortise view (Fig. 30-25).[109] Magnetic resonance imaging is the method of choice for confirming suspected osteochondritis dissecans because of its relatively low radiation exposure and its ability to grade the stages of pathology in a clinically relevant manner. The classification of transchondral fractures ranges from stage I, a small

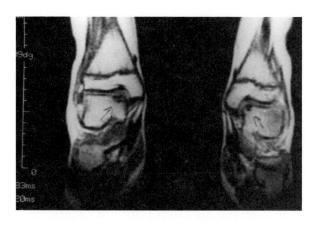

FIG. 30-25 Magnetic resonance imaging of bilateral osteochondritis dissecans of medial talus. (From Canale ST, editor: *Campbell's operative orthopedics,* St. Louis, 1998, Mosby.)

lesion, to stage IV, a displaced osteochondral fracture. Nonsurgical management is recommended for stage I and II lesions. Stage III and IV lesions may also initially be managed nonsurgically with protective splinting and with partial to full weight bearing, guided by the patient's symptoms. Exercises are directed at regaining a full range of motion and strength. Arthroscopic management is reserved for patients who do not respond to therapy, have unabated symptoms, and cannot participate in sports.

45. Why are fractures more likely than sprains to occur in children?

Sprains are relatively unusual before epiphyseal fusion. This is because the growth plates are inherently weaker than the ligaments spanning the joints.[57] Subsequently, injurious forces that would more likely cause a sprained ankle in an adolescent or adult will result in Salter-Harris fractures of the growth plate (i.e., the distal fibula, tibial physis)[100] or avulsion fracture of the distal tibia or fibula. In contrast to sprains, swelling from physeal fractures is less prominent and not as immediate, tenderness is noted over the epiphysis (rather than over the lateral ligament complex), and pain with motion is less marked.

46. What therapeutic intervention is appropriate in management of lateral ankle sprain?

An older management approach to treatment of lateral ankle sprain involves immediate immobilization of the ankle in neutral dorsiflexion and slight eversion[2] so as to allow maximal apposition of torn tissue ends, which will promote foreshortening of the healing ligaments. After approximately 3 weeks, presumably, enough scar tissue is laid down between the tattered ligament ends to regain some 65% of the original ligament strength, after which weight bearing may commence while this posture is maintained.

Ligaments are composed of dense connective tissue and demonstrate a histologic order of longitudinal alignment consistent with applied tension to the ligament. This alignment gives the ligament a unique tensile load–resisting capability, approaching that of steel. However, after a sprain injury, scar tissue composed of loose connective tissue and having the same random organization as superficial fascia is laid down between the torn ends of the ligament. Hence the new fibrils of connective tissue are randomly distributed in the connective tissue matrix that makes up the ligament. The problem with this approach is that the healed ligament is more likely to sustain reinjury because of weakness. Studies have borne out the belief that completely immobilizing joints for a prolonged period results in a poor capacity of the ligaments spanning that joint to functionally resist high stress loads.[94] Moreover, abnormal healing may occur, in which a ligament torn from one location reattaches at another.

Brostrom and Freeman, two of the most frequently quoted authorities regarding ankle sprain management, are major proponents of the more aggressive early-mobilization management strategy. Healing ligaments remodel in response to imposed stress demands by organizing collagen fibrils so that the fibrils lie parallel to the direction of greatest stress. The controlled application of external stress to the injured ligament stimulates reorganization of randomly deposited scar tissue in a functional manner consistent with the direction of applied stress so that the healing ligament is less likely to be reinjured. Both of these authorities concur that early mobilization yields results as good as those of cast immobilization, with a shorter period of disability.

The current trend in management of lateral ankle sprain leans to the more aggressive side of the nonoperative management controversy.[19,81] This strategy de-emphasizes *functional stability* as the major thrust of management while emphasizing *functional mobility,* or the application of *controlled stress* through rehabilitative exercise and protected function. Experimental evidence indicates that the latter approach enhances the strength of ligaments by making them heavier, wider, and thicker. In addition to promoting greater structural integrity, early mobilization encourages lymphatic drainage of fluid and necrotic debris, minimizes muscle atrophy, maintains joint proprioception, and inhibits development of adhesions and joint contractures.[19] Thus the current trend in lateral inversion sprain management emphasizes functional rehabilitation[19,108] involving the application of controlled stress that promotes organized functional remodeling of scar tissue. The following treatment protocol is an early course of ankle sprain management throughout which no heat whatsoever is applied. Heat is generally unnecessary until the second week, when pain is dull, if it is perceived at all.[90] This protocol was designed for the injured athlete and may be modified as necessary for the nonathlete. In the following program, treatment in the first 72 hours involves rest, ice, elevation, compression, and controlled motion by way of passive and active range of motion, gait training, and incline board usage.

Immediate Postinjury Regimen. During the first 24 hours treatment involves immediate *compression* of the sprained ankle with a compressive wrap or tape. Compression is most effective when used in conjunction with a felt or foam-rubber, horseshoe-shaped pad placed around the distal posterior and anterior aspects of the ipsilateral malleolus to fill the submalleolar depression. This allows even compression directly over the injury site,[5,56,93,108] despite the uneven topography of the lateral ankle, and prevents swelling in these areas that might otherwise occur from compression wrap alone. The importance of a horseshoe-shaped compression pad cannot be overemphasized. The two sides of the pad should cover the anterolateral aspect of the ankle joint over the anterior talofibular ligament and sinus tarsi.[19] Among the benefits of external compression is increased hydrostatic pressure that diffuses the gelled mass of subcutaneous fluid and necrotic debris. Increased hydrostatic pressure directly beneath the pad forces fluid toward areas in which hydrostatic pressure is lower (e.g., within the capillaries, the lymph vessels, or tissue spaces away from the injury site).[19] Thus the application of compression promotes an improved nutritive state of the injured tissue by causing more rapid absorption of excess proteins and fluid through the lymphatic system.[80,82] The compressed pad must be continually kept in position once it is applied because removal will result in rebound swelling for as long as the concentration of free proteins in the interstitial fluid is higher than normal.[19,82]

The materials chosen for constructing the compression pads should maximize patient comfort while maintaining adequate external compression. Felt is comfort-able against the skin and has an excellent absorptive quality. Other materials are less absorptive; using such materials may result in mild skin maceration occurring when moisture from perspiration is trapped against the skin by a nonabsorptive material. The problem with felt and other soft materials is that fluid tends to accumulate beneath them. Lightweight foam is an ideal compressive material. Preferably, foam that is used would have a teardrop shape, with the upper end of the drainage channel closed by the adjacent sides of the pad. This configuration allows the sides of the pad to spread when held against the ankle contour, facilitating maintenance of an open drainage channel. Hydrostatic pressure is lower in the open channel of the pad, and excess fluid is encouraged to drain up the side of the leg, where it is dispersed over a larger area, and where more lymphatic vessels would be recruited for its removal.[5] It is for this reason that the open area of the U is directed upward toward the heart; compression should be applied from the toes toward the heart to discourage fluid from flowing in a direction distal to the ankle joint.[19] Failure to maintain an open channel may cause pressure buildup around the ankle joint that would collapse blood and lymph vessels.

Patients may report discomfort that prevents restful sleep when wearing a compression pad beneath an elastic wrap. This perception of increased pressure may be caused by decreased competition from other sources of sensory stimuli while an individual is attempting to fall asleep.[19] As a result, patients often dismantle the compressive application (of pad and wrap) and do not reapply it, or reapply it improperly. Rebound swelling invariably results. For these reasons, compression boots have been designed such that the patient can easily adjust the degree of tightness and pressure with Velcro and elastic straps without disturbing placement of the compression pad. The Cyro/Cuff, developed by Aircast Corporation, is an ingenious device using chilled water and the principle of gravity to apply continuous cold compression.

A thin, less bulky, U-shaped pad should be kept in place around the lateral malleolus, beneath an Ace bandage or adhesive tape, when the patient begins weight-bearing exercises.[19] The compression pad may be removed for periods of time after blue or purple ecchymotic skin takes on a yellowish hue. This change in cutaneous coloration results from the hemoglobin breakdown of the pooled subcutaneous ecchymosis. Once this stage of healing has commenced, sudden rebound swelling will generally not occur, although the compression pad should immediately be reapplied after modality treatment and exercise. Use of the pad may be discontinued altogether when discoloration has disappeared and when delayed pooling of fluid around the ankle joint no longer occurs.[19]

A controversial issue in acute ankle strapping is the use of elastic wrap versus adhesive tape. Additionally, there is disagreement on the best method for application of taping, with proponents advocating both the *open* and *closed basket weave* approach. The three basic components for any taping technique are *anchor strips, checkreins,* and *figure-eights.* Anchor strips are snugly applied to the body and provide a firm point of attachment for other strips of tape. Checkreins may include any number of forms or shapes of strips of tape. Checkreins are placed between anchor strips to support a joint and prevent excessive motion while simultaneously accenting other motions necessary to perform the athletic task required. Figure-eights are applied in a circular fashion around the natural contours of the extremity so as to create a crisscross pattern that helps maintain joint integrity. Taping or wrapping should be applied in a distal-to-proximal fashion (as a function of edema control), beginning behind the toes and ending at the lower half of the leg. An alternative to ankle taping is the application of a lace-up or semirigid orthosis to limit ankle inversion and eversion.[19]

- *Cryotherapy.* Cryotherapy is best administered by placing the affected foot and ankle in a slush bucket of ice and water with the compression still intact. The level of water should reach the base of the calf, and the extremity should be immersed for 15 to 20 minutes. The patient should be supervised during the first 5 to 7 minutes of immersion, after which the foot becomes less sensitive and the ice bath tolerable. Wearing a sock or neoprene cover over the toes may be helpful in retaining toe warmth.
- *Modified weight bearing.* Modified weight bearing, such as partial weight bearing, is facilitated by the use of crutch walking with a three-point areciprocal gait.[68] Partial weight bearing, with a cane[19] held on the contralateral side and using either a three-point areciprocal or two-point reciprocal gait, is acceptable. Non–weight bearing is usually unnecessary and may be avoided except in severe ankle sprains because of its nonfunctional nature.
- *Edema and pain control.* Initially edema and pain control is accomplished by instructing the patient to elevate the ankle continuously. This may be facilitated by placing telephone books under the foot of the

bed or by inserting a dresser drawer at the foot of the bed between the mattress and box spring. The application of an edema- and pain-reducing electrical stimulation protocol is appropriate at this juncture of management. Transcutaneous electrical stimulation (TENS) may be applied to help relieve pain, with a nontetanic pulse rate setting (<40) and an intensity setting as high as tolerated. Additionally, massage therapy, beginning distally and moving proximally, is best performed with the foot elevated. A leg boot for intermittent compression may significantly reduce edema by increasing venous return from the injured limb. Whirlpool treatment is contraindicated while the ankle is still edematous because application of this modality places the ankle in a dependent position.

Day 1 Post Injury: Non–Weight-Bearing Phase. Active management of the ankle sprain begins the day after injury and consists of an alternation between cryotherapy and the application of intermittent air compression modalities. With a tape cast still applied, the patient immerses the injured ankle into a slush bucket of ice and water for 7 to 10 minutes. The tape is then removed, and the ankle is reimmersed for an additional 10 to 12 minutes. Immersion treatment is followed by the application of an intermittent air compression device for 20 minutes while the injured ankle is elevated above the heart. Tape cast or compression wrap is not necessary while the limb is undergoing intermittent compression. Once the foot is out of the slush bucket, no more than 1 to 2 minutes should elapse while the injured ankle is uncompressed with tape or bandage. After intermittent compression, the foot and ankle should undergo a brief and painless (1- to 2-minute) period of passive range of motion in a distal-to-proximal direction, with the foot elevated before reapplication of tape cast or bandage wrap. The motions emphasized include plantarflexion and dorsiflexion. This sequence should be performed for a minimum of three times during the first day.

Day 2 Post Injury. Day 2 begins with immersion in an ice bath for 12 to 15 minutes with the previous day's tape cast in place for the first 7 minutes, after which the patient is permitted to attempt beginning or increased weight bearing on the affected ankle. Immediate pain may preclude further weight bearing. The patient should not force weight bearing at any time, since bearing weight on a painful limb is premature. If weight bearing is accompanied by only minimal or no pain, active range of motion exercises and stationary bicycle riding may be initiated as long as motion does not extend into the painful range. Following stationary bicycle exercise, ice immersion is repeated, after which gait training may commence. With the ankle still numb from cold, the patient is asked to ambulate in a normal heel-toe manner until the ankle thaws out or pain returns. If an antalgic gait is present, or if the patient demonstrates an abnormal cadence or altered heel-toe relationship, it is too soon for the patient to be bearing this magnitude of weight. Thus if the patient cannot bear minimal weight without discomfort, the second-day program is identical to the first-day program. Otherwise, the entire sequence of cryotherapy, range of motion, cryotherapy, gait training, and pneumatic compression cast may be performed three times per treatment, with three treatments during this second day.

Day 3 Post Injury. By the third day, swelling may be considerably lessened and taping or wrap may be applied less tightly than previously. This is especially so if the patient demonstrated an ability to walk well on the second day. Treatment begins with ice bath immersion, followed by ambulation until pain reappears, followed by reimmersion in an ice bath. The patient then stands on an incline board to facilitate dorsiflexion and stretch the Achilles' tendon–hamstring linkage. A tightened heel cord complex is a predisposing factor in lateral ankle sprain because the upper ankle joint has less than adequate dorsiflexion. This may result in a relative increase in supination and an inversion moment across the subtalar joint, thereby shifting weight bearing along the plantar surface of the foot laterally and placing additional stress on the lateral ligaments.[15] This is followed by ice bath immersion and gait training, in which the patient attempts to ambulate with as normal a gait as possible. If necessary, the patient may walk with shortened stride lengths ("baby steps") to maintain the normal heel-toe sequence of gait. The sequence of day 3 management includes ice bath, gait training, ice bath, incline board, ice bath, gait training, ice bath, compression modality, and finally tape casting. The severity of injury is reevaluated between compression modality and tape casting. Compressive wrapping or taping is applied more lightly and in such a fashion as to allow for greater plantarflexion and dorsiflexion. Complete tape removal or cessation of compressive wrap may be considered at this time, depending on the patient's ability to ambulate forward without pain. The patient is encouraged to ride a stationary bicycle throughout the day, with the seat placed low so that ankle motions of

dorsiflexion (and plantarflexion) are encouraged, after which the ankle is iced.[19]

On the third day, proprioceptive training may be instituted via a sliding board or the *biomechanical ankle platform system (BAPS) board.* This system consists of an elliptical board on which one of five hemispheric attachments varying in diameter may be placed in an off-center position, allowing varying degrees of motion. Aside from proprioceptive training and nerve fiber stimulation, the BAPS board is also used to develop motion, strength, endurance, and balance.

Day 4 Post Injury and Beyond. When the patient can successfully ride a stationary bicycle (set at 10 inches or lower) without significant pain, prophylactic ankle taping is applied and the patient may commence running straight ahead. Although prophylactic ankle taping provides both physical and psychologic support for prevention of reinjury, it has no effect on such athletic performance as speed or agility. Moreover, as much as 40% of taping-support efficacy is lost after the first 10 minutes of athletic performance.[27] The preferred shoe type at this point in management is either a flat-bottomed turf shoe with the mountain climber (Vibram) or lug-type sole, or stiff (high-top) basketball sneakers.[19] If straight running is relatively painless, the patient may attempt *agility training* such as "lazy S" running or "sharp Z" running and progress to figure-eight sideways running. Each successive figure-eight should be smaller and faster. This is followed by backward running. These exercises may be accompanied by cariocas, side-to-side bilateral hopping (with progression to unilateral), front-to-back bilateral hopping (with progression to unilateral), diagonal patterns of hopping, minitrampoline jogging, and jumping rope.

- *Strength training* may be addressed with *progressive resistive strengthening exercises* in an isometric, concentric, and eccentric sequence. Isometric exercises are performed against an immobile object or manual resistance into eversion and dorsiflexion, respectively. Concentric strengthening into dorsiflexion and eversion emphasizes muscle shortening and may be performed with an elastic band for resistance. Eccentric contraction involves lengthening of muscle during the motions of eversion and dorsiflexion. This is accomplished by slow relaxation of muscle as the elastic band is allowed to overpower the deliberately slowly relaxing muscle. *Pliometric* step-ups and step-downs on the injured extremity are appropriate; the patient should begin these by negotiating the step from the side and progress to negotiating the step in a forward-backward manner. It must be emphasized that no single approach of therapeutic exercises best serves all lateral ankle sprains; rather, the treatment used depends on the needs of the individual patient and the severity of injury. For example, barre exercises may be performed in the pool setting, using the buoyancy of water to prevent excessive strain to the injured ligament while exercising the ankle in a more functional fashion.

- *Enhancing lateral lower limb muscle activation and recruitment as an injury-prevention strategy* is predicated on the concept of the biomechanical linkage chain. An invaluable component of management of lateral ankle sprain is the evaluative detection of weakness of the ipsilateral gluteus medius or peroneal musculature. An inversion torque to the ankle delivers an excessive tensile moment to the anterolateral ankle. The moment may be countered by the generation of a protective countertensile, or compressive, force by the ipsilateral hip abductors (gluteus medius) and the primary ankle evertors (peroneal muscles). A weak hip abductor may not be able to deliver enough compressive force quickly enough to realign the center of gravity and thereby shift the pelvis laterally and counter the steadily increasing injurious lever arm. Weakness of these muscles may thus predispose an individual to sustaining an inversion sprain of the ankle because of compromised muscle recruitment in the closed kinetic chain. Consequently, strengthening of the ipsilateral hip abductors and the ankle evertors may improve the rapidity and magnitude of force delivered by these muscles. Therapeutic techniques include closed kinetic chain exercises that require concurrent isometric hip and ankle activation, progressing to exercises that require active ankle stability, followed by contractile activation and recruitment of proximal and distal lateral lower limb stabilizers.
- Cyriax[21] advocates *transverse friction* massage for acute minor ligamentous sprain of the lateral ankle. Massage should not begin until 1 week after injury. Belief in the benefit of this modality is predicated on the assumption that application of a to-and-fro movement of the damaged ligament over bone therapeutically imitates the normal behavior of that ligament. This must be performed very gently and for short duration so as not to disturb the young and recently attached fibroblasts. In addition to providing stress consistent with normal function, deep transverse friction helps break down and stave off unwanted adhesions and maintain the normal mobility of the ligament. During the first 2 weeks, only 1 to 2 minutes of treatment is appropriate, followed by an increase of 5 to 15 minutes as tenderness and pain decrease.

47. What management is appropriate for severe inversion sprain of the ankle joint?

Severe inversion sprain of the ankle refers to unstable injuries than may be subcategorized as *minimal* and *moderate instability.* Although both degrees of instability share moderate to severe pain, marked swelling, diffuse tenderness, and an inability to bear weight, the former is characterized a talar tilt of 5° to 15° greater than the opposite ankle. Moderate instability is characterized by a talar tilt greater than 15° and a positive result from an anterior drawer test.[73] The anterior drawer test scores positive in both double- and triple-ligament injuries.[61] A talar tilt greater than 15° indicates a complete double tear of the CFL and ATFL along with the lateral capsule. If the posterior talofibular ligament is also torn, the talar tilt is greater than 30°.

The data are conflicting regarding the best approach to treat severe sprains resulting from instability. Suggested approaches range from conservative management to surgical intervention, especially when moderate instability is present. For the young, skilled, highly competitive athlete for whom a choice toward conservative management is made, a removable splint is applied and an intensive physical therapy program is instituted as outlined earlier. This requires a major commitment on the part of the patient; it may not be appropriate for the recreational athlete, who because of work or household responsibilities may simply not have the time, money, or inclination to pursue such a rigorous program. For such patients with severe sprains, the patient is immobilized in a short leg brace and may ambulate without bearing weight, with bilateral crutches.[73] Partial weight bearing may be allowed as soon as symptoms permit. During the entire time the ankle is casted, isometric exercises are performed within the cast.[59] The brace is removed after 3 to 6 weeks, and active range of motion is instituted, with continuous protection in an air cast. Most patients may continue to full activities in 2 to 4 months, but these patients should have additional protection for at least 4 months from the time of injury. The patient should be forewarned of the varying degrees of stiffness, atrophy, and functional disability that are possible sequelae of severe injury.[40]

48. What preventive measures decrease the likelihood of reinjury, sequelae, or chronic instability?

High-top shoes and prophylactic ankle taping that is used alone or in combination may decrease the severity and number of lateral ankle sprains.[30] The use of multiple-cleated molded sole shoes rather than shoes with fewer spikes also helps decrease the frequency of injuries.[28] Players may be taught to jump-land with a relatively wide-based gait. This should place the foot a bit more lateral to the falling center of gravity, thereby making an inversion stress to the ankle less likely.[14]

49. What is chronic lateral ankle instability?

Patients with *chronic lateral ankle instability* usually have a history of recurrent ankle sprain, ankle pain, swelling, giving way, and an inability to attain preinjury levels of function.* Diagnosis may be made by history, physical examination, routine radiographic examination,[25] or exclusion of other causes of symptoms such as occult osteochondritis dissecans,[17,60] posttraumatic or degenerative arthritis, synovitis, tarsal coalition, deltoid ligament injury, or peroneal tendon subluxation.[40] Stress radiographs may corroborate physical findings, but they are not essential.[25] Gait analysis reveals increased inversion at heel strike that was not correctable by peroneal strengthening or the use of a heel wedge in the ipsilateral foot.[39] Treatment includes restoration of full range of motion; strengthening of the peroneal, hip abductor, and other musculature; proprioceptive training; and bracing. Surgical reconstruction is indicated for patients who remain symptomatic after sufficient rehabilitation (6 months) and are unwilling to accept the necessary activity restrictions.[25]

50. What is a high ankle sprain?

A *high ankle sprain* (Fig. 30-26) is technically referred to as a *syndesmotic sprain* involving the *inferior tibiofibular syndesmosis,* also known as the *anterior* and *posterior inferior tibiofibular ligaments.* This type of injury results from a combination of hyperdorsiflexion and eversion, as, for example, in a running or jumping sport in which the athlete falls or is pushed forward after the foot is planted on the ground. Alternatively, a

hyperdorsiflexion mechanism may occur when an athlete abruptly stops while the foot is planted on the ground. In this case, forward momentum carries the foot dorsally so that as the athlete falls, the weight of the body stresses the mortise. Because the dorsiflexion posture tightly wedges the anterior body of the talus between the two malleoli, forceful hyperdorsiflexion and eversion act to push the fibula laterally, causing stretch or rupture of the anterior and posterior tibiofibular ligaments. Pain and swelling are present over this ligament and proximally over the interosseous membrane. Pain is reproduced by dorsiflexing the foot (wedging the syndesmosis), by externally rotating the leg, or with a combined plantarflexion-inversion movement.[6] Findings in acute tibiofibular syndesmosis injuries include point tenderness and swelling over the anterior and posterior tibiofibular ligaments; pain at the interosseous region of the lower leg, elicited by palpation and provoked by bimalleolar compression; a preference for toe walking; subjective complaints; and recovery out of proportion to the typical lateral ligament sprain. The area of injury may also extend to the region of the deltoid attachment on the medial malleolus as pain, swelling, and tenderness. Tenderness may occur if, concomitant to syndesmotic sprain, lateral displacement of the foot caused stretching of the deltoid ligament. Tenderness is typically present over the anterior aspect of the distal fibula at the level of the upper ankle joint, since the anterior tibiofibular ligament commonly pulls off the fibula rather than the tibia.[104] Squeezing the proximal tibia and fibula together (positive *squeeze test*) lessens pain.[19]

High ankle sprains occur in contact sports such as football. A high ankle sprain is more serious than an inversion sprain of the ankle joint because it involves a greater amount of playing time lost, practices missed, and treatments received. It is important to differentiate this sprain from a simple lateral ligament sprain. In general, tibiofibular involvement in ankle sprain prolongs the recovery period, and such a sprain is passed off as a lateral ankle sprain because the initial stress radiographs are negative except for a diastasis (widened space) between either malleolus and the talus. After several weeks, a repeat radiograph may indicate telltale evidence of hemorrhage in the interosseous are. The radiograph may also indicate partial deltoid avulsion, by a slight irregularity in the region of the medial malleolus or calcification in the interosseous space. Unlike simple lateral ankle sprains, syndesmotic sprains are characterized by maximal point tenderness and swell-

*Interestingly, pain on the first or second day after reinjury is often minimal.

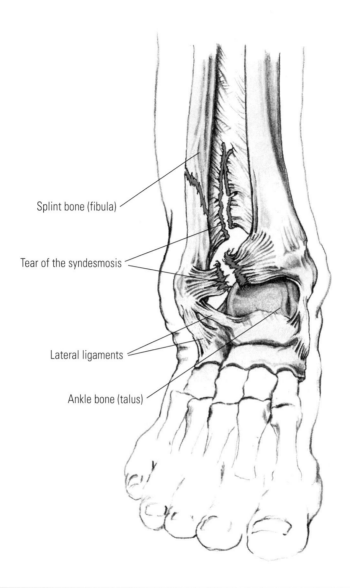

Splint bone (fibula)

Tear of the syndesmosis

Lateral ligaments

Ankle bone (talus)

FIG. 30-26 Sprain of the distal tibiofibular syndesmosis is often combined with a distal fibular fracture, injury to the deltoid or lateral ligaments of the ankle joint. (From Peterson L, Renstrom P: *Sports injuries: their prevention and treatment,* Chicago, 1983, Yearbook Medical Publishers.)

ing *above* the tip of the lateral malleolus. Although some swelling may extend below the fibular malleolus, gross swelling is confined above it. If this is missed early on, the athlete may experience weeks of frustration as he or she does not regain the ability to run on the injured foot within the time frame normally associated with healing of a simple lateral ankle sprain. Additional tearing of the posterior tibiofibular ligaments is indicated by pain and swelling that is localized posteriorly about the tip of the lateral malleolus, between the fibula and Achilles' tendon. A patient with this condition may complain of difficulty running uphill.[104] Treatment for severe high ankle sprain may involve control of swelling by immobilization in an ankle brace with slight heel elevation for 1 to several weeks after injury; this is followed by an aggressive protocol sequence of range of motion exercises, contrast baths, and ultrasound treatments. Gait training should progress from non–weight bearing to progressive weight bearing. Straight-ahead ambulation is permitted before agility training. This injury may linger or recur if the patient returns to full athletic involvement before becoming pain free. Thus gradual resumption of activities to the level of tolerance is essential to comprehensive rehabilitation of this injury. Heterotopic bone ossification of the syndesmosis is a common sequela of high ankle sprains.[102]

51. What is sprain of the deltoid ligaments at the upper ankle?

Less than 5% of ankle sprains involve the deltoid ligaments,[10] and the mechanism is usually eversion or eversion with external rotation.[73] Unlike inversion forces causing a lateral ankle sprain, eversion forces are more likely to result in an avulsion fracture of the tip of the medial malleolus than a sprain of the deltoid ligaments. This is because the deltoid ligaments composing the medial collateral ligament complex, unlike the discrete lateral collateral ligaments, fuse one with the other, lending the entire medial collateral ligament complex increased tensile strength. Additionally, unlike the lateral ankle sprain, which demonstrates equal gender distribution, eversion sprains are more common in females. This is most likely attributed to female hip alignment, with the weight line falling more medial in women than men.

REFERENCES

1. American Academy of Orthopaedic Surgeons: *Joint motion: method of measuring and recording,* Chicago, 1965, The Academy.
2. Baxter DE: *The foot and ankle in sport,* St Louis, 1995, Mosby.
3. Black HM, Brand RL, Eichelberger MR: An improved technique for the evaluation of ligamentous injury in severe ankle sprains, *Am J Sports Med* 6(5):276-282, 1978.
4. Bleichrodt RP, Kingma LM, Binnendijk D, et al: Injuries of the lateral ankle ligaments: classification with tenography and arthrography, *Radiology* 173(2):347-349, 1989.
5. Bonci CM: Adhesive strapping techniques, *Clin Sports Med* 1(1):99-116, 1982.
6. Bosien WR, Staples OS, Russell SW: Residual disability following acute ankle sprains, *J Bone Joint Surg Am* 37:1237-1243, 1955.
7. Brand RL, Black HM, Cox JS: The natural history of inadequately treated ankle sprain, *Am J Sports Med* 5(6):248-249, 1977.
8. Brand RL, Collins MD, Templeton T: Surgical repair of ruptured lateral ankle ligaments, *Am J Sports Med* 9(1):40-44, 1981.
9. Brody DM: *Clinical symposia: running injury—prevention and management,* vol 39, no 3, Summit, NJ, 1987, CIBA-GEIGY.
10. Brostrom L: Sprained ankles: anatomic lesions in recent sprains, *Acta Chir Scand* 128:483-495, 1964.
11. Brostrom L: Sprained ankles: clinical observations in recent ligament ruptures, *Acta Chir Scand* 130:560-569, 1965.
12. Brostrom L: Sprained ankles: treatment and prognosis in recent ligament ruptures, *Acta Chir Scand* 132(5):537-550, 1966.
13. Brostrom L: Sprained ankles: surgical treatment of "chronic" ligament ruptures, *Acta Chir Scand* 132:551-565, 1966.
14. Brotzman SB: *Clinical orthopedic rehabilitation,* St Louis, 1996, Mosby.
15. Cahill BR: Chronic orthopedic problems in the young athlete, *J Sports Med* 1(3):36-39, 1973.
16. Cailliet R: *Foot and ankle pain,* ed 3, Philadelphia, 1997, FA Davis.
17. Chapman MW: *Sprains of the ankle,* American Academy of Orthopaedic Surgeons instructional course lectures, 24:294-308, Rosemont, Ill, 1975, The Academy.
18. Clarke KS, Buckley WE: Women's injuries in collegiate sports, *Am J Sports Med* 8(3):187-191, 1980.
19. Cox JS, Brand RL: Evaluation and treatment of lateral ankle sprains, *Phys Sports Med* 5(6):51-55, 1977.
20. Cox JS: Surgical and nonsurgical treatment of acute ankle sprains, *Clin Orthop* 198:118-126, 1985.
21. Cyriax J: Treatment by manipulation, massage, and injection. In Cyriax J: *Textbook of orthopedic medicine,* ed 11, vol 2, London, 1984, Bailliere Tindall.
22. Donatelli R: *The biomechanics of the foot and ankle,* Philadelphia, 1990, FA Davis.
23. Evans GA, Hardcastle P, Frenyo AD: Acute rupture of the lateral ligament of the ankle: to suture or not to suture? *J Bone Joint Surg Br* 66(2):209-212, 1984.
24. Fetto JF: Anatomy and physical examination of the foot and ankle. In Nicholas JA, Hershman EB, editors: *The lower extremity and spine,* ed 2, vol 1, St Louis, 1995, Mosby.
25. Fochios D, Nicholas JA: Football injuries. In Nicholas JA, Hershman EB, editors: *The lower extremity and spine,* ed 2, vol 2, St Louis, 1995, Mosby.
26. Freeman MA: Treatment of ruptures of the lateral ligament of the ankle, *J Bone Joint Surg Br* 47(4):661-668, 1965.
27. Fumich RM, Ellison AE, Guerin GJ, et al: The measured effect of taping on combined foot and ankle motion before or after exercise, *Am J Sports Med* 9(3):165-170, 1981.
28. Garrick JG: Epidemiologic perspective, *Clin Sports Med* 1(1):13-18, 1982.
29. Garrick JG, Requa RK: Role of external support in the prevention of ankle sprains, *Med Sci Sports* 5(3):200-203, 1973.
30. Garrick JG: The frequency of injury, mechanism of injury, and epidemiology of ankle sprains, *Am J Sports Med* 5(6):241-242, 1977.
31. Garrick JG: When can I? A practical approach to rehabilitation illustrated by treatment of an ankle injury, *Am J Sports Med* 9(1):67-68, 1981.
32. Giallonardo LM: *Clinical evaluation of foot and ankle dysfunction,* Boston, Boston-Bouve College of Human Development Professions.
33. Glick JM, Gordon RB, Nishimoto D: The prevention and treatment of ankle injuries, *Am J Sports Med* 4(4):136-141, 1976.
34. Gould N, Seligson D, Gassman J: Early and late repair of lateral ligament of the ankle, *Foot Ankle* 1(2):84-89, 1980.

35. Gronmark T, Johnsen O, Kogstad O: Rupture of the lateral ligaments of the ankle: a controlled clinical trial, *Injury* 11(3):215-218, 1980.

36. Hamilton WG: Stenosing tenosynovitis of the flexor hallucis longus tendon and posterior impingement upon the os trigonum in ballet dancers, *Foot Ankle* 3(2):74-80, 1982.

37. Hardaker WT Jr: Foot and ankle injuries in classical ballet dancers, *Orthop Clin North Am* 20(4):621-627, 1989.

38. Hardaker WT Jr, Moorman CT : Foot and ankle injuries in dance and athletics: similarities and differences. In Shell CG, editor: *The dancer as an athlete,* Proceedings of the Olympics Scientific Congress, 1984.

39. Harper MC: Talar shift: the stabilizing role of the medial, lateral, and posterior ankle structures, *Clin Orthop* 257:177-183, 1990.

40. Harrington KD: Degenerative arthritis of the ankle secondary to long-standing lateral ligament instability, *J Bone Joint Surg Am* 61(3):354-361, 1979.

41. Hertling D, Kessler RM: *Management of common musculoskeletal disorders: physical therapy principles and methods,* ed 2, Philadelphia, 1990, JB Lippincott.

42. Hicks JH: The mechanics of the foot, the joints, *J Anat* 88:345-357, 1954.

43. Holbrook TL: *The frequency of occurrence, impact and cost of selected musculoskeletal conditions in the United States,* report of the American Academy of Orthopaedic surgeons, Chicago, 1984, The Academy.

44. Hunt GC: Examination of lower-extremity dysfunction. In Gould JA, editor: *Orthopedic and sports physical therapy,* ed 2, St Louis, 1990, Mosby.

45. Hunter L et al: Common orthopedic problems of the female athlete. In *American Academy of Orthopaedic Surgeons instructional course lectures,* vol 31, St Louis, 1982, Mosby.

46. Inman VT: *The joints of the ankle,* Baltimore, 1976, Williams & Wilkins.

47. Jackson DW, Ashley RL, Powell JW: Ankle sprains in young athletes *Clin Orthop* 101(01):201-215, 1974.

48. James SL: Chondromalacia of the patella in the adolescent. In Kennedy JC, editor: *The injured adolescent knee,* Baltimore, 1979, Williams & Wilkins.

49. Jaskulka R, Fischer G, Schedl R: Injuries of the lateral ligaments of the ankle joint: operative treatment and long-term results, *Arch Orthop Trauma Surg* 107(4):217-221, 1988.

50. Jepson KK: Biomechanical evaluation of the running athlete, *Phys Ther Forum* Northeast edition, 3, 1987.

51. Johannsen A: Radiological diagnosis of lateral ligament lesion of the ankle, *Acta Orthop Scand* 49(3):295-301, 1978.

52. Johnson EE, Markoid KL: The contribution of the anterior talofibular ligament to ankle laxity, *J Bone Joint Surg* 65(1):81-88, 1983.

53. Kaumeyer G, Malone TR: Ankle injuries: anatomical and biomechanical considerations necessary for the development of an injury prevention program, *J Orthop Sports Phys Ther* 173, 1980.

54. Kelikian H, Kelikian AS: *Disorders of the ankle,* Philadelphia, 1985, WB Saunders.

55. Kjaersgaard-Andersen P, Sojbjerg JO, Wethelund JO, et al: Watson-Jones tenodesis for ankle instability, *Acta Orthop Scand* 60(4):477-480, 1989.

56. Klafs CE, Arnheim DD: *Modern principles of athletic training,* ed 5, St Louis, 1981, Mosby.

57. Kleiger B: Anterior talotibial impingement syndromes in dancers, *Foot Ankle* 3(2):69-73, 1982.

58. Kotwick JE: Biomechanics of the foot and ankle, *Clin Sports Med* 1(1):19-34, 1982.

59. Lane SE: Severe ankle sprains: treatment with an ankle-foot orthosis, *Physician Sports Med* 18(11), 1990.

60. Lassiter TE, Malone TR, Garrett WE: Injury to the lateral ligaments of the ankle, *Orthop Clin North Am* 20(4):629-640, 1989.

61. Lauren C, Mathieu J: Sagittal mobility of the normal ankle, *Clin Orthop* 108:99-104, 1975.

62. Leonard MH: Injuries of the lateral ligaments of the ankle, *J Bone Joint Surg* 31:373-377, 1949.

63. Liu SH, Jason WJ: Lateral ankle sprains and instability problems, *Clin Sports Med* 13(4):793-809, 1994.

64. Malone TR, Hardaker WT: Rehabilitation of foot and ankle injuries in ballet dancers, *J Orthop Sports Phys Ther* 11(8):355, 1990.

65. Mann R: Biomechanics of the foot and ankle. In Mann R, editor: *Surgery of the foot,* ed 5, St Louis, 1986, Mosby.

66. Mann RA: Biomechanics of running. In Nicholas JA, Hershman EB, editors: *The lower extremity and spine,* ed 2, vol 1, St Louis, 1995, Mosby.

67. Mann RA: Surgical implications of the biomechanics of the foot and ankle, *Clin Orthop* 146:111-118, 1980.

68. Manter JT: Movements of the subtalar and traverse tarsal joint, *Anat Red* 80:397-409, 1941.

69. McCullough CJ, Burge PD: Rotatory stability of the load-bearing ankle, *J Bone Joint Surg* 62(4):460-464, 1980.

70. McMurray TP: Footballer's ankle, *J Bone Joint Surg Br* 32:68, 1950.

71. Meals RA: *One hundred orthopedic conditions every doctor should understand,* St Louis, 1992, Quality Medical Publishing.

72. *Merck manual,* ed 15, Rahway, NJ, Merck, Sharp, & Dohme Research Laboratories.

73. Milbauer DL: Principles of radiographic evaluation and imaging techniques. In Nicholas JA, Hershman EB, editors: *The lower extremity and spine,* ed 2, vol 1, St Louis, 1995, Mosby.

74. Moller-Larsen F, Wethelund JO, Jurik AG, et al: Comparison of three different treatments for ruptured lateral ankle ligaments, *Acta Orthop Scand* 59(5):564-566, 1988.

75. Morris JM: Biomechanics of the foot and ankle, *Clin Orthop* 122:10-17, 1977.

76. Morris LH: Athlete's ankle, *J Bone Joint Surg Am* 25:220, 1943.

77. Nyska M, Amir H, Porath A, et al: Radiological assessment of a modified anterior drawer test of the ankle, *Foot Ankle* 13(7):400-403, 1992.

78. Oatis CA: *Biomechanics of the foot and ankle under static conditions,* Philadelphia, Philadelphia Institute for Physical Therapy.

79. O'Donoghue DH: Impingement exostosis of the talus and tibia, *J Bone Joint Surg Am* 39:835, 1957.

80. O'Donoghue DH: *Treatment of injuries to athletes,* ed 3, Philadelphia, 1976, WB Saunders.

81. Ouillen WS: An alternative management protocol for lateral ankle sprains, *J Orthop Sports Phys Ther* 2(4):187-190, 1981.

82. Ouillen WS, Rouillier LH: Initial management of acute ankle sprains with rapid pulsed pneumatic compression and cold, *J Orthop Sports Phys Ther* 4(1):39-43, 1982.

83. Parkes JC, Hamilton WG, Patterson AH, et al: The anterior impingement syndrome of the ankle, *J Trauma* 20(10):895-898, 1980.

84. Patterson JD: Ankle injuries. In Lillegard WA, Rucker KS, editors: *Handbook of sports medicine,* Boston, 1993, Andover Medical Publishers.

85. Pennal GR: Subluxation of the ankle, *Can Med Assoc J* 49:92-95, 1943.

86. Peterson L, Renstrom P: *Sport injuries: their prevention and injury,* Chicago, 1986, Year Book Medical Publishers.

87. Prins JG: Diagnosis and treatment of injury to the lateral ligament of the ankle: a comparative study, *Acta Chir Scand* 486:143-149, 1978.

88. Ratcliff JD: *I am Joe's body,* New York, 1975, Berkeley Books.

89. Reese RC Jr, Burruss TP, Patten J: Athletic training techniques and protective equipment. In Nicholas JA, Hershman EB, editors: *The lower extremity and spine,* ed 2, vol 1, St Louis, 1995, Mosby.

90. Rijke AM, Jones B, Vierhout PA: Stress examination of traumatized lateral ligaments of the ankle, *Clin Orthop* 210:143-151, 1986.

91. Root ML, Orien WP, Weed JH: *Biomechanical examination of the foot,* vol 1, Los Angeles, 1971, Clinical Biomechanics.

92. Roy S, Irvin R: *Sports medicine: prevention, evaluation, management, and rehabilitation,* Englewood Cliffs, NJ, 1983, Prentice-Hall.

93. Roy S, Irvin R: *Sports medicine,* Englewood Cliffs, NJ, 1983, Prentice-Hall.

94. Rubin G, Witten M: The talar-tilt angle and the fibular collateral ligaments: a method for the determination of talar tilt, *J Bone Joint Surg Am* 42:311-326, 1960.

95. Ruth CJ: The surgical treatment of injuries of the fibular collateral ligaments of the ankle, *J Bone Joint Surg Am* 43:229-239, 1961.

96. Sauser DD et al: Acute injuries of the lateral ligaments of the ankle: comparison of stress radiography and arthrography, *Radiology* 148(3):653-657, 1983.

97. Siegler S, Block J, Schneck CD: The mechanical characteristics of the collateral ligaments of the human ankle joint, *Foot Ankle* 8(5):234-242, 1988.

98. Singer KM, Jones DC, Taillon MR: Ligament injuries of the ankle and foot. In Nicholas JA, Hershman EB, editors: *The lower extremity and spine,* ed 2, vol 1, St Louis, 1995, Mosby.

99. Spiegel PG, Cooperman DR, Laros GS: Epiphyseal fractures of the distal ends of the tibia and fibula, *Bone Joint Surg Am* 60(8):1046-1050, 1978.

100. Subotnick SI: *Podiatric sports medicine,* New York, 1975, Futura Publishing.

101. Taylor DC, Englehardt DL, Bassett FH: Syndesmosis sprains of the ankle: the influence of heterotopic ossification, *Am J Sports Med* 20(2):146-150, 1992.

102. Tiberio D: *Pathomechanics of structural foot deformities,* Storrs, Conn, On-Site Biomechanical Education and Training.

103. Turco VJ, Gallant GG: Occult trauma and unusual injuries in the foot and ankle. In Nicholas JA, Hershman EB, editors: *The lower extremity and spine in sports medicine,* ed 2, vol 2, St Louis, 1995, Mosby.

104. Valmassy RL: *Clinical biomechanics of the lower extremities,* St Louis, 1996, Mosby.

105. Vetter WL, Helfet DL, Spear K, et al: Aerobic dance injuries, *Phys Sports Med* 13, 1935.

106. Whiteside PA: Men's and women's injuries in comparable sports, *Phys Sports Med* 8(3):130, 1980.

107. Weiker GG: Ankle injuries in the athlete, *Primary Care* 11:101-108, 1984.

108. Xethalis JL, Lorei MP: Soccer injuries. In Nicholas JA, Hershman EB, editors: *The lower extremity and spine,* ed 2, vol 2, St Louis, 1995, Mosby.

RECOMMENDED READING

Hicks JH: The mechanics of the foot: the joints, *J Anat* 87:345, 1953

Hicks JH: The foot as a support, *Acta Anat* 25:34, 1955.

Inman VT: The influence of the foot-ankle complex on the proximal skeletal structures, *Artif Limbs* 13(1):59-65, 1969.

Liu SH, Jason WJ: Lateral ankle sprains and instability problems, *Clin Sports Med* 13(4):793-807, 1994.

Malone TR, Hardaker WT: Rehabilitation of foot and ankle injuries in ballet dancers, *J Orthop Sports Phys Ther* 11:8, 1990.

Mann RA: Surgical implications of the biomechanics of the foot and ankle, *Clin Orthop* 146:111-118, 1980.

Subotnick SI: Biomechanics of the subtalar and midtarsal joints, *J Am Podiatry Assoc* 65(8):756-764, 1975.

Wilkerson GB: Treatment of ankle sprains with external compression and early mobilization, *Phys Sports Med* 13(6), 1985.

31

Burning Pain and Paresthesia over Medial Side of Ankle
That Radiates to Foot and Sole After Excessive Walking That Is
Relieved by Sitting

A 47-year-old overweight female complains of pain and paresthesia over the medial left foot during prolonged standing and walking of 2 months duration. Symptoms are reported to be focused at the ball of the left foot just proximal to the first ray. Paresthesia include the medial aspect of the foot and sole. The patient reports a history of carpal tunnel syndrome, insulin-dependent diabetes, and she sustained a fracture dislocation of the ankle 16 months ago. There is no other history of lower extremity disorders.

OBSERVATION   Both feet are observed to pronate excessively during ambulation. A pes planus foot posture is observed in both feet when non–weight bearing. There is no redness observed anywhere on the left foot or ankle.

PALPATION   There is slight warmth in the area of the left medial malleolus, as well as palpable tenderness between the tendons of the flexor digitorum and flexor hallucis longus.

PASSIVE RANGE OF MOTION   Moving the calcaneus into valgus while everting the foot reproduces pain.

ACTIVE RANGE OF MOTION   Active range of motion is full and painless in the spine and all joints of bilateral lower extremities.

MUSCLE STRENGTH   Muscle strength is decreased in the left foot interossei when compared with the contralateral lower extremity. Strength is otherwise normal.

SENSATION   Testing for sensation indicates loss of two-point discrimination over the medial plantar surface of the left foot.

SPECIAL TESTS   The patient has positive Tinel sign in the vicinity of the left medial malleolus, positive hyperpronation test, and negative straight leg raise (SLR).

? Questions

1. What is most likely causing symptoms in this woman's foot?
2. What is tarsal tunnel syndrome?
3. Why is the tibial nerve unlikely to sustain injury along its proximal route?
4. What is the anatomy of the tarsal tunnel?
5. What are the contents of the tarsal tunnel?
6. Where are the potential sites of nerve damage at the tarsal tunnel?

7. What is the etiology of tarsal tunnel syndrome?
8. Does overpronation contribute to incidence of tarsal tunnel syndrome?
9. What is the clinical presentation?
10. What is Tinel's sign?
11. What is the differential diagnosis?
12. What is anterior tarsal tunnel syndrome?
13. What therapeutic management is appropriate?

1. What is most likely causing symptoms in this woman's foot?

Tarsal tunnel syndrome of the left foot is the most likely cause of this woman's symptoms. This compressive neuropathy is analogous to the carpal tunnel of the wrist, resulting in similar clinical presentation characteristic of posterior tibial nerve entrapment.

2. What is tarsal tunnel syndrome?

Tarsal tunnel syndrome refers to entrapment of the neurovascular bundle comprised of the posterior tibial nerve and tibial artery at the medial ankle. Entrapment occurs at the level of the medial malleolus, the point from which the nerve supplies motor innervation to the intrinsic foot muscles and sensation to the sole. This syndrome often has a traumatic basis[7] such as a fracture or dislocation at the ankle, although symptoms may not develop until some time after the injury. Etiology may be idiopathic or may derive from intrinsic or extrinsic factors. Similar to carpal tunnel syndrome at the wrist, any process that compromises the caliber of the tarsal tunnel, either intrinsic or extrinsic, may causes pressure neuropathy of the tibial nerve. Thought to be underdiagnosed by many physicians,[15] this uncommon condition is usually unilateral, but may occur bilaterally.

3. Why is the tibial nerve unlikely to sustain injury along its proximal route?

Tibial nerve (L4-S3) lesions are uncommon since it runs a course in the lower extremity that protects it from injury. In the region of the hip joint and throughout the thigh it lies in a deeply protected position. Behind the knee the tibial nerve is deeply located and well protected from knee trauma, although it may sustain damage by a fracture dislocation of the knee. Proximal entrapment of the tibial nerve may occur from tethering of the nerve due hypertrophy of the soleus and plantaris muscles[22] or compressed by tumor, aberrant muscles, or head of the gastrocnemius muscle.[22] In the calf region, the nerve lies deep to triceps surae and becomes superficial only where it trifurcates at the region of the flexor retinaculum into the medial plantar, lateral plantar, and calcaneal branches. The former two nerves are analogous to the median and ulnar nerves in the upper extremity.[17] These branches supply the skin of the sole, plantar and apposing surfaces of the toes, as well as the plantar intrinsic musculature.

4. What is the anatomy of the tarsal tunnel?

The *tarsal tunnel* (Fig. 31-1) is composed of the bones of the ankle and the laciniate ligament (flexor retinaculum). The unyielding osseous floor of the tunnel is a groove behind and underneath the medial malleolus. The lateral wall of this tunnel is comprised of a bony sulcus along the medial wall of the calcaneus, the posteromedial aspect of the talus, and the posteromedial distal tibia. The medial wall is formed by the tendinous arch of the abductor hallucis muscle and the *ligamentum laciniatum,* both of which are comprised of two layers extending from the medial malleolus to the medial surface of the calcaneus, forming the soft roof of the tarsal tunnel. The length of the tunnel spans from the medial aspect of the calcaneal tuberosity to the sustentaculum tali.[6]

In addition to the (posterior) tibial nerve and its branchings, the tunnel houses the artery, veins, and

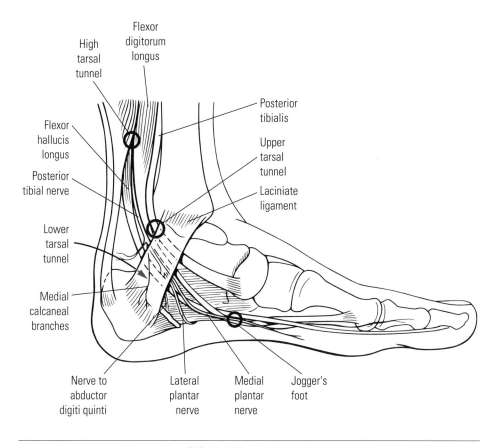

FIG. 31-1 The tarsal tunnel.

three tendons including the tibialis posterior, the flexor digitorum longus, and the flexor hallucis longus. The nerve sulcus along the medial calcaneus many vary from shallow (8-10 mm, 23%), or medium (11-13 mm, 64%), to deep (14-16 mm, 13%). Conceivably, nerves running in a shallow sulcus are possibly more susceptible to compression.

The tarsal tunnel may be divided into a proximal and distal tarsal tunnel. *Proximal tarsal tunnel* syndrome consists of entrapment of the tibial nerve in the retromalleolar region, whereas *distal tarsal tunnel* syndrome involves the divisions of the tibial nerve. The classic form of tarsal tunnel syndrome involves pathology at both the proximal and distal zones comprising the tarsal tunnel. However, localized entrapment of only one of the divisions of the tibial nerve may occur.[22]

Prior to entering the proximal tarsal tunnel, the tibial nerve branches off to send a calcaneal branch[22] to supply the medial aspect of the skin of the heel. This nerve may be compressed by the edge of the laciniate ligament resulting in heel pain known as *calcaneal nerve entrapment.* Thus the tarsal tunnel may be thought of as the hilum of the plantar surface as virtually all of its neurovascular supply enters through it making the nerves passing this juncture relatively more vulnerable to injury.[2]

At the entrance to the proximal tarsal tunnel the tibial artery and nerve arborize into medial plantar and lateral plantar arteries and nerves as well as the first branch of the lateral plantar and medial calcaneal nerves. Once beyond the proximal tarsal tunnel, the tibial nerve trifurcates into the medial and lateral[12,20,26] plantar nerves. A branching off the lateral plantar nerve known as the *nerve to the abductor digiti quinti muscle* (see Fig. 28-14) may be compressed by a calcaneal heel spur and result in chronic heel pain. The *medial plantar nerve* supplies sensory innervation of the medial aspect of the plantar surface of the foot and to the medial three and one half toes as well as motor innervation to the abductor hallucis, flexor digitorum brevis and first lumbrical. The *lateral plantar nerve* provides sensory innervation to the lateral one and one half toes and the sole of the foot as well as motor innervation to the remaining plantar intrinsics.

5. What are the contents of the tarsal tunnel?

In addition to the posterior tibial nerve, artery, and vein, the tunnel contains the flexor tendons along the posteromedial aspect of the ankle, each of which has its own separate synovial sheath. This group includes from anteromedial to posterolateral, the tibialis posterior, the flexor digitorum longus, and the flexor hallucis longus. The neurovascular bundle lies between the latter two tendons.[25] The spatial relationship among these posterior compartment tendons just above the medial malleolus, like their anterior analog along the dorsal surface, are expressed by the *Tom, Dick, and Harry* pneumonic: "Tom" for tibialis posterior, "Dick" for flexor digitorum longus, and "Harry" for flexor hallucis longus; Harry is the deepest while Tom is the most superficial.

6. Where are the potential sites of nerve damage at the tarsal tunnel?

Although the tarsal tunnel may be anatomically divided into proximal and distal portions, it is clinically subdivided into proximal, middle, and distal thirds. At the tarsal tunnel, nerve compression may occur at one of three different sites. *Proximal* (or *high*) *tunnel syndrome* results from compression of the posterior tibial nerve above the lancinate ligament. In classic tarsal tunnel syndrome, nerve compression occurs in the retromalleolar region under the laciniate ligament. *Distal tarsal tunnel syndrome* results from compression of the medial plantar nerve by the abductor muscle and fascia.[9] Damage to the tibial nerve can occur via two mechanisms. Vascular embarrassment via pressure on the vasa nervosum results in initial symptoms of sensory loss without motor loss, whereas direct pressure neuropathy upon the nerve will present with both sensory and motor loss.[14,16]

7. What is the etiology of tarsal tunnel syndrome?

The etiologies for tarsal tunnel syndrome are quite diverse. Connective tissue diseases that may alter spatial relationships within the tunnel include rheumatoid arthritis, gout, scleroderma, sarcoidosis, amyloid, or dermatomyositis. Metabolic/hormonal causes result in soft tissue effects and include diabetes, pregnancy, myxedema, hyperlipidemia, and acromegaly osteoporosis. Tumors and other space occupying lesions include the presence of a ganglion, lipoma, neurilemoma, cysts, and neurofibroma. Congenital causes that affect the initial tunnel configuration include malformation of the posterior process of the talus and hypertrophy of the abductor hallucis muscle. Vascular causes that compromise tunnel space include varicose veins, early collagen vascular disease, peripheral occlusive disease, and stasis secondary to activities requiring long periods of standing. Traumatic changes in anatomical tunnel configuration include exostosis, medial malleolar fracture, fracture of the posterior process of the talus, ankle dislocation, and post traumatic arthritis.[23] The common denominator in these pathologies is a regional space alteration resulting in mechanical pressure from changes in either the osseous or the soft tissue relationships within the tunnel and resulting in neuropathy of the posterior tibial nerve. Trauma, congenital, or acquired anomalies predispose these individuals to a higher risk of nerve compression due to *bony changes* in the tunnel's configuration that reduce tunnel volume. Autoimmune and inflammatory diseases decrease tunnel volume by way of *soft tissue changes,* particularly tendon swelling, that causes cramping of the tunnel contents. Regardless of etiology, the histologic changes seen in pressure neuropathy of the posterior tibial nerve at the tarsal tunnel are classified into three stages that include local edema, moderate axonal degeneration, and Wallerian degeneration, respectively.[4]

8. Does overpronation contribute to incidence of tarsal tunnel syndrome?

Compensatory *overpronation* of the subtalar joint during stance phase of gait, especially in runners,[15] is most definitely a possible mechanical mechanism for the development of tarsal tunnel syndrome[12,20,26] (Fig. 31-2). The pronated foot is characterized by increased valgus of the hindfoot. This posture serves to place the posterior tibial nerve and its branchings on stretch while simultaneously tensing the neurovascular bundle against the edge of the laciniate ligament.[13] In other words, in an individual with a hypermobile (pronated) foot the talar head becomes extremely prominent during foot flat phase of stance resulting in compression of the posterior tibial nerve as it is stretched around the talus. For a track runner with normal feet, it is typically the inside foot that hyperpronates and more likely to develop tarsal tunnel syndrome. Similarly, in runners who run along banked roads, the foot on the high side of the road crown will overpronated and more likely sustain pathology.[22]

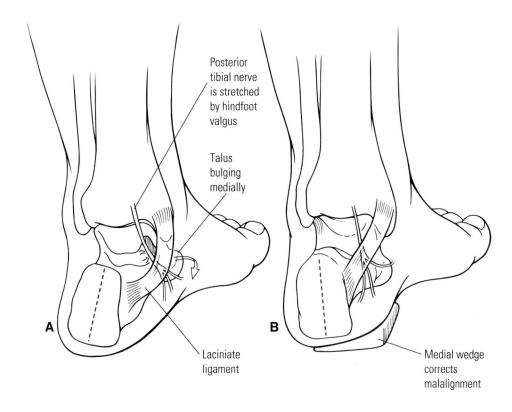

Posterior
tibial nerve
is stretched
by hindfoot
valgus

Talus
bulging
medially

A

B

Laciniate
ligament

Medial wedge
corrects
malalignment

FIG. 31-2 Stretching of the posterior tibial nerve due to a valgus deformity of the hindfoot. **A,** In an individual with a hypermobile (pronated) foot, the talar head becomes extremely prominent during flat foot phase of stance resulting in compression of the posterior tibial nerve as it is stretched around the talus and causes tensing of the neurovascular bundle against the edge of the laciniate ligament. **B,** A medial wedge corrects the misalignment.

Controversy exists regarding whether a hindfoot valgus or varus is implicated as a causative intrinsic foot deformity causing tarsal tunnel syndrome. Tarsal tunnel syndrome presents in the pronated foot with either a valgus[5] or varus heel[18] Hindfoot valgus is the rearfoot component of a pes planus deformity, whereas rear foot varus posture is compensated for by excessive pronation of the subtalar joint.[27] Some authorities attribute stretching of the posterior tibial nerve to a valgus deformity of the hindfoot.[19] However, treatment of tarsal tunnel with a medial hindfoot wedge afforded no benefit to some patients. Other authorities ascribe this pathologic syndrome to a varus hindfoot which causes kinking of the posterior tibial nerve (Fig. 31-3) and is relieved by treatment with lateral hindfoot wedge[19] that attempts to place the hindfoot into valgus. Thus, tarsal tunnel syndrome is the only medial hindfoot problem that is treated with a lateral hindfoot wedge.[19]

9. What is the clinical presentation?

Symptoms vary and are not typical. Sharp shooting pain from the medial side of the ankle may radiate into the medial or plantar aspect of the foot and sole and often centers around the first metatarsophalangeal joint. Pain may have a burning quality (dysthesia), and may occur nocturnally[15] similar to that described in carpal tunnel syndrome.[17] Paresthesias may mediate toward the toes, or proximally.[22] Radiation of pain from the site of stenosis proximally is often seen and known as a *Valleix phenomenon.* This occurs because of proximal excitation of autonomic nerve fibers.[5,11,28] Similarly, pain is often nocturnal, but may also occur after long periods of standing of walking. However, whereas the effects of carpal tunnel syndrome may be quite noticeable, the effects of distal tibial nerve compression may go unnoticed since the foot is not typically used for precise movements. Sensory symptoms predomi-

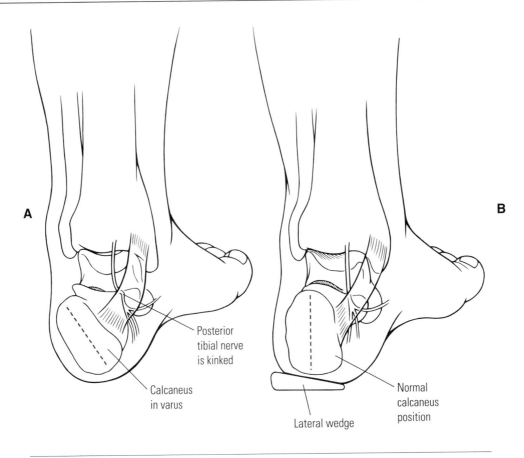

FIG. 31-3 Tarsal tunnel syndrome may also be attributable to a varus hindfoot that causes kinking of the posterior tibial nerve **(A)** and is relieved by treatment with the lateral hindfoot wedge **(B).**

nantly affect the toes, particularly the metatarsophalangeal joint of hallux,[15] and may be accompanied by paresthesia such as burning, numbness, pressure, or feelings of pins and needles. Sweating may occasionally be observed. Motor weakness and wasting the of intrinsic foot musculature is not seen until later disease progression.

Objective signs include hypesthesia and loss of two-point discrimination as early signs of nerve compression. Sensory loss is most easily tested where the skin is thinnest over the medial plantar area rather than over the tips of the toes. Swelling of the involved foot may occur, despite the lack of hand swelling in carpal tunnel syndrome.[17] There is palpable tenderness and/or tingling over the posterior tibial nerve located between the flexor digitorum and flexor hallucis longus tendons.[27]

Muscle weakness may occur in the intrinsic foot muscles including the flexor digitorum brevis, the flexor hallucis brevis (medial plantar nerve), the quadratus plantae, the interossei, and the lumbricals (lateral plantar nerve). Early on, muscle weakness may be difficult to detect since the long foot and toe flexors are preserved, and patients will exhibit no difficulty in standing or walking. Over time, muscle dysfunction may lead to changes in foot conformation that ultimately posture the foot in pes cavus with toe clawing. This muscle weakness is observed by loss of flexion at the metatarsophalangeal joints and extension at the interphalangeal joints,[12,20,26] which impairs push-off during stance.

The most consistent finding during electrodiagnostic testing is a decreased amplitude and an increased duration of evoked potentials in the abductor hallucis or the abductor digiti minimi when compared with the normal foot. One usually also sees an increased latency to these same muscles.[10]

Provocative maneuvers include forced eversion,

pronation, and dorsiflexion, as these movements may reproduce pain and paresthesia in the nerve's distribution. Forcing the heel into varus (toward midline) may provide sufficient slack in the laciniate ligament to decrease symptoms.[12,20,26] Abduction of the toes may also cause pain. The *hyperpronation* test involves positioning the ipsilateral foot and ankle into the extremes of the triad postures comprising the triplanar motion known as pronation: dorsiflexion, eversion, and abduction. This may be easily performed by taking the calcaneus of the involved foot and maximally everting it and maintaining that posture for 30 to 60 seconds.[1]

10. What is Tinel's sign?

Named after Jules Tinel (1879-1952), *Tinel's sign* is an exaggeration of the tingling sensation that occurs when a normal nerve is percussed (for example, the "funny bone" at the elbow). In an injured nerve this phenomenon may be evoked more readily and may persist longer. Tinel's sign is not a guide to the condition of the nerve as the test may score positive even when there is an anatomic gap at the site of nerve injury. Tinel's sign simply indicates the presence of regenerating fibers and, as such may be used to localize the site of injury.[24] In tarsal tunnel syndrome, Tinel's sign is produced by gentle percussion over the tarsal tunnel just below and behind the medial malleolus.[3]

11. What is the differential diagnosis?

The differential diagnosis includes, among others, lumbosacral root disorders with radicular symptoms, metatarsalgia, heel spur, stress fracture, bursitis at the insertion of the anterior tibial muscle, interdigital neuroma, peripheral vascular disease, sciatica, peripheral neuritis, and plantar fasciitis.[8] Tarsal tunnel syndrome yields more medial heel and arch pain (at the abductor hallucis muscle) than at the origin of the plantar fascia.[16] The clinician must also rule out arthritic tarsal joints, interdigital neuroma, and systemic peripheral neuropathy.

- *Diabetic neuropathy* causing painful burning feet may be very difficult to distinguish form bilateral tarsal tunnel syndrome, but is differentiated by the use of electrophysiologic testing.[1] In early, confusing cases, electrodiagnostic studies may be of considerable value in evaluation, progression of compression, and nerve recovery. Electromyography (EMG) must evaluate both the medial and lateral plantar nerves (motor and sensory) as well as the muscles of the foot and leg.[3,21] However, negative electromyographic and normal conduction velocity studies do not

exclude the possibility of tarsal tunnel syndrome. Radiographs are usually normal.

- *High tarsal tunnel syndrome* refers to a more proximal posterior tibial nerve compression at the lower edge of the gastrocnemius muscle in the middle aspect of the posteromedial tibia. Compression of various branches of the posterior tibial nerve may occur distal to the laciniate ligament but are not relieved following laciniate release as the cause of compression differs from classical tarsal tunnel syndrome. The *medial calcaneal branch* of the posterior tibial nerve may be compressed under the fibrous border of the abductor hallucis muscle. This may occur in runners secondary to swelling or hypertrophy of this muscle, and is symptomatic during vigorous running or immediately after. A positive Tinel sign over the muscle or at its superior border is helpful in confirming diagnosis. Similarly, the first branch of the *lateral plantar nerve* may be compressed (Fig 31-4) and result in heel pain, as it changes direction from vertical to horizontal at the medial plantar aspect of the heel adjacent to the origin of the plantar fascia, secondary to plantar fasciitis. Electrodiagnostic studies, including prolonged terminal latency of the lateral plantar nerve to the abductor digiti minimi and decreased amplitude in this muscle of the evoked potential, aid in the diagnosis. Surgical release of the laciniate ligament for either of these neuropathy would not be expected to relieve symptoms. Release of the abductor hallucis and of the plantar fascia, respectively, provide relieve of symptoms.

12. What is anterior tarsal tunnel syndrome?

The term "tarsal tunnel syndrome" is colloquially reserved for the posterior syndrome and refers to compressive entrapment or kinking of the posterior tibial nerve. There is yet another potential tunnel of nerve constriction in close relation to the anterior tarsus. *Anterior tarsal tunnel syndrome* (See Chapter 32) refers to compression of the deep peroneal nerve along the dorsum of the foot as it passes under the inferior extensor retinaculum. A high index of suspicion for anterior syndrome is suggested in the patient with exertional anterior compartment pain, weakness of toe hyperextension, and transient numbness of the first web space.

13. What therapeutic management is appropriate?

Conservative therapy includes correcting faulty foot posture by way of an accommodative medial *arch support* or molded in-shoe *orthosis* to decrease the exces-

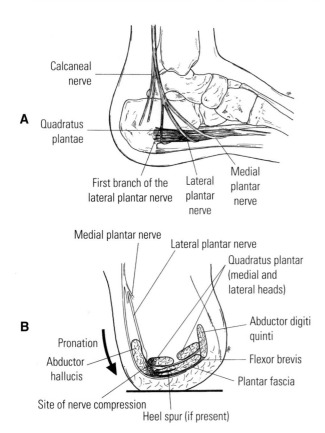

A

Calcaneal nerve

Quadratus plantae

First branch of the lateral plantar nerve

Lateral plantar nerve

Medial plantar nerve

B

Medial plantar nerve

Lateral plantar nerve

Quadratus plantar (medial and lateral heads)

Abductor digiti quinti

Flexor brevis

Plantar fascia

Pronation

Abductor hallucis

Site of nerve compression

Heel spur (if present)

FIG. 31-4 A, Entrapment of the first branch of the lateral plantar nerve occurs as the nerve changes direction from vertical to horizontal adjacent to the origin of the plantar fascia at the medial plantar aspect of the heel. Compression may occur from inflammatory swelling at the origin of the plantar fascia secondary to plantar fascitis. **B,** Site of compression of the first branch of the lateral plantar nerve to the abductor digiti minimi (quinti) muscle. The exact site of compression is between the abductor hallucis muscle and the medial caudal margin of the medial head of the quadratus plantae muscle. Compression is accentuated in the presence of overpronation. (From Baxter D: *The foot and ankle in sport,* St Louis, 1995, Mosby.)

nonsteroidal antiinflammatory medication, as well as well as prudent injection of corticosteroids into the tunnel may be indicated.[15] The physician may recommend a trial of a tricyclic compounds.[22] Physical therapy strengthening of the flexors and tibialis posterior is appropriate.[22] When these measures do not afford relief after 2 months of conservative management, surgical retinacular release of the tarsal tunnel to free the entrapped the plantar nerves. Operative results boast a high success rate.

Postoperative management involves crutch walking for 1 to 2 weeks. Early range of motion is encouraged and may become increasingly aggressive as wound healing commences. Recovery may range anywhere between 2 weeks and 6 months, depending on the individual.

REFERENCES

1. Bordelon RL: Subcalcaneal pain: A method of evaluation and plan for treatment, *Clin Orthop* 177:49, 1983.
2. Butler DS: *Mobilisation of the nervous system,.* Melbourne, 1991, Churchill Livingstone.
3. Dawson DM, Hallett M, Millender LH: *Entrapment neuropathies,* ed 2, Boston, 1990, Little, Brown & Co.
4. Denny-Brown, Brenner C: Paralysis of nerve induced by direct pressure and by tourniquet, *Arch Neurol Psychiat,* 1944; 51:1-26.
5. Edwards WG, Lincoln CR, Bassett FH, et al: The tarsal tunnel syndrome: diagnosis and treatment, *JAMA* 207:716, 1969.
6. Fetto JF: Anatomy and physical examination of the foot and ankle. In Nicholas JA, Hershman EB, editors: *The lower extremity and spine,* ed 2, vol. 1, St. Louis, 1995, Mosby.
7. Goodgold J, Kopell HP, Speilholz NI: The tarsal tunnel syndrome, *N Engl J Med* 273:742, 1965.
8. Jackson DL, Haglund B: Tarsal tunnel syndrome in athletes: case reports and literature review, *Am J Sports Med* 19:61, 1991.
9. Jones DC, Singer KM: Soft-tissue conditions of the ankle and foot. In Nicholas JA, Hershman EB, editors: *The lower extremity and spine,* ed 2, vol. 1, St. Louis, 1995, Mosby.
10. Kaplan PE, Kernahan WT: Tarsal tunnel syndrome: an electrodiagnostic and surgical correlation, *J Bone Joint Surg* 63A:96-99, 1981.
11. Keck C: The tarsal-tunnel syndrome, *J Bone Joint Surg* 1962; 44A:180.
12. Kopell HP, Thompson AL: Peripheral entrapment neuropathies of the lower extremity, *N Engl J Med* 262:56-60, 1960.
13. Kopell HP, Thompson WAL: *Peripheral entrapment neuropathies,* New York, 1976, Robert E. Krieger Publishing Co.
14. Lam SJS: Tarsal tunnel syndrome, *J Bone Joint Surg,* 49B:87, 1967.
15. Lillegard WA, Rucker KS: *Handbook of sports medicine,* Boston,1993, Andover Medical Publishers.

sive hindfoot valgus. The therapist may also attempt to check for excessive hypermobility due to excessive pronation by the use of a supplemental medial heel and sole wedge in the shoe[22] to correct valgus of the hindfoot. If the hindfoot is in varus the application or a 5° or 9° lateral hindfoot wedge with a 3-mm heel height is helpful. If the hindfoot is in neutral then orthotic management includes a 5° lateral forefoot wedge, a 1-mm heel height, and a 0° hindfoot wedge.[27] An ankle support stocking, ankle stirrup brace or walking brace may be beneficial.[22] Rest, ice, heat,[25] flexibility training,

16. O'Malley GM, Lambdin CS, McCleary GS: Tarsal tunnel syndrome: a case report and review of the literature, *Orthopedics,* 8 (6), 1985.

17. Patten J: *Neurological differential diagnosis,* ed 2, London, 1995, Springer.

18. Radin EL: Tarsal tunnel syndrome, *Clin Orthop* 181:167-170, 1983.

19. Reilly MA: *Guidelines for prescribing foot orthotics,* Thorofare, NJ, 1987, SLACK Inc.

20. Roegholt MN: Een nervus calcaneus inferior als overbrenger: van de pijn bij cananeodynie of calcaneusspoor en de daavuit volgend therapie, *Ned Tijdschr Geneeskd* 84: 1898-1902, 1940.

21. Rzonca EC, Baylis WJ: Common sports injuries to the foot and leg, *Clin Podiatr Med Surg* 5:591, 1988.

22. Schon LC: Nerve entrapment, neuropathy, and nerve dysfunction in athletes, *Orthop Clin North Am* 25(1):50, 1994.

23. Schumacher HR, Bomalaski JS: *Case studies in rheumatology for the house officer,* Baltimore, 1993, Williams & Wilkins.

24. Spillane JD, Spillane JA: *An atlas of clinical neurology,* Oxford, 1982, Oxford University Press.

25. Subotnick SI: *Podiatric sports medicine,* New York, 1975, Futura Publishing Co.

26. Tanz SS: Heel pain. *Clin Orthop* 28: 169-177, 1963.

27. Tiberio D: Pathomechanics of structural foot deformities. *Phys Ther* 68(12):1840-1849, 1988.

28. Wileman WK: Tarsal tunnel syndrome: a fifty year survey of the world literature and a report of two new cases, *Orthop Rev* 8:111-117, November 1979.

RECOMMENDED READING

Schon LC: Nerve entrapment, neuropathy, and nerve dysfunction in athletes, *Orthop Clin North Am* 25(1):50, 1994.

Jackson DL, Haglund B: Tarsal tunnel syndrome in athletes: case reports and literature review, *Am J Sports Med* 19:61, 1991.

O'Malley GM, Lambdin CS, McCleary GS: Tarsal tunnel syndrome: a case report and review of the literature, *Orthopedics,* 8(6), 1985.

Pecina MM, Krmotic-Nemanic J, Markiewitz AD: *Tunnel syndromes,* Boca Raton, FL, 1991, CRC Press.

32

Pain, Crepitus, and Snapping Over the Lateral Malleolus After Ankle Injury

CASE 1: A 22-year-old college football player caught a ball and proceeded to run toward the end zone for a touchdown. To avoid being tackled, the player suddenly cut sharply to the right with his right stance leg. He felt an immediate pain in the lateral ankle that was accompanied by a snapping sensation. The following clinical picture has emerged from on-field and later examinations of the player.

OBSERVATION Swelling and ecchymosis are noted at the retromalleolar area and just superior to that locale. The patient shows a mild cavus foot posture bilaterally.

PALPATION Tenderness is noted immediately posterior to the right fibular malleolus. A "click" is imparted to the examiner's hand as resistive ankle dorsiflexion and foot eversion were attempted. No tenderness was noted at the right tuberosity of the fifth metatarsal.

PASSIVE RANGE OF MOTION Yields mild discomfort during plantarflexion and inversion of the ankle-foot complex.

STRENGTH Eversion scores are one entire grade weaker in the right foot, compared with the left.

SELECTIVE TENSION Resisted dorsiflexion with ankle eversion reproduces symptoms and manifested as a visible, subcutaneous, thin, and cord-like movement over the lateral malleolus.

SPECIAL TESTS Negative anterior draw and talar tilt tests of the right ankle.

RADIOGRAPHIC EXAMINATION An avulsion fracture of the lateral ridge of the distal fibula is observed with radiographic examination.

CASE 2: A 26-year-old male professional soccer player complains of pain over the lateral ankle after each of his last 7 games. The patient has a history of multiple inversion sprains to the left ankle, the last of which occurred at the end of last year's playing season, for which he underwent and completed an extensive rehabilitation program. The patient walks with a slight limp and reports that taking oral antiinflammatory medication affords slight relief. After watching him play at one of the games, you notice his method of kicking the ball to be more often than not confined to kicking with the outer aspect of the left leg. On two occasions, an opponent accidentally kicked the patient along the left ankle while attempting to steal the ball.

OBSERVATION   Shows swelling inferior to the lateral malleolus. The patient walks with an antalgic gait with increased stance time on the right lower extremity and decreased swing time on the left. A rearfoot varus deformity is present in both feet, left greater than right.

PALPATION   Pain and tenderness are present over the lateral ankle, particularly behind the left fibular malleolus, with maximal tenderness at the left peroneal tubercle. Crepitus is noted during active ankle joint eversion.

PASSIVE RANGE OF MOTION   Forced passive inversion with plantarflexion yields pain.

ACTIVE RANGE OF MOTION   Range of motion of the subtalar joint is decreased.

STRENGTH   Eversion is decreased by one grade during a manual muscle test. The patient complains of discomfort and symptom reproduction when asked to walk along the medial borders of his foot for 30 feet.

SELECTIVE TENSION   Resistive eversion and dorsiflexion of the left foot are acutely uncomfortable.

CLUE   For both cases:

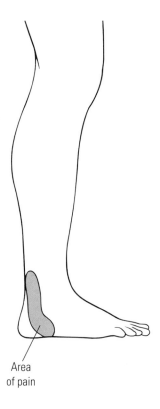

Area
of pain

? Questions

1. What is most likely wrong with these patients?
2. What is the relevant anatomy of this disorder?
3. What is the etiology of peroneal tenosynovitis?
4. What is the kinesiology of the peroneal muscles during early stance?
5. What role in stabilization of the plantarflexed foot do the peronei perform in synergy with dynamic extrinsics spanning the subtalar joint medially during late stance?
6. What is the mechanism of peroneal subluxation?
7. What anatomic anomaly may predispose some persons to peroneal tendon instability?
8. What is the mechanism of injury resulting in strain of the peroneal tendons?
9. What is the clinical presentation of pathologic condition of the peroneal tendon?
10. How are the peronei best palpated and assessed for muscular strength?
11. What is peroneal spastic flatfoot?
12. What therapeutic management best addresses peroneal tendon disease?

1. What is most likely wrong with these patients?

Case I involves a patient whom has sustained *subluxation of the left peroneal tendons,* whereas Case II involves a patient with *tenosynovitis of the right peroneal tendons.* Subluxation was precipitated by sudden, sharp eversion while the right foot was in relative dorsiflexion, just after midstance phase of gait. Tenosynovitis involves the confluence of the peroneus brevis and longus, which share a common tendon sheath, and extends from the level of the fibular malleolus to the peroneal tubercle distally. Inversion sprains of the ankle joint are frequently associated with peroneal tendon pathologic conditions. Case II involves an inflammation of the tendon or the synovial sheath enveloping the peroneal tendons.

2. What is the relevant anatomy of this disorder?

The *peroneal muscles,* innervated by the superficial branch of the common peroneal nerve, comprise the lateral crural compartment of the leg. The *peroneus longus muscle,* bipennate in form and more superficial than the brevis,[30] arises higher in the leg, from the proximal half of the lateral fibula and intramuscular septa. The smaller and shorter *peroneus brevis* originates from the distal half of the lateral fibula and intramuscular septum. At the level of the fibular malleolus, the peroneal tendons usually unite within a common synovial tendon sheath to distally course across the ankle joint through two fibroosseous tunnels before their distal insertion. The peroneus brevis is closest to the lateral malleolus, whereas the longus is posterior and more superficial. A fascial band known as the *superior peroneal retinaculum* tethers both tendons to the *peroneal groove,* or *sulcus,* posterior to the lateral malleolus, and represents a simple pulley.[12] A pulley is a simple machine that is merely a modification of simple lever. A single rope-and-pulley system multiplies neither force nor distance; it merely changes the direction of the applied force.* This sulcus may cause a sudden indentation along the course of the peroneal tendons with certain motions of the ankle, and thus represents a site of heightened friction and potential irritation.

Together, beyond the lateral malleolus, the tendons distally course toward the sole of the foot by passing across the lateral calcaneus, where they are separated by an approximately 1-cm osseous lateral projection[19] of the calcaneus, known as the *peroneal tubercle.* The tendons are tethered on either side of this *peroneal trochlea* by an *inferior peroneal retinacula* that acts as a second pulley system. At this level the longus tendon passes forward and inferior to the brevis tendon and angles medially into the foot through a plantar groove along the anterior slope of the cuboid. A sesamoid within the tendon protects it from excessive pressure

---

*A *pulley* is a rounded structure that relates to a rope passing over its edge. Trochlea means *resembling a pulley,* and the peroneal tubercle acts as a trochlea with regard to the peroneal tendons crossing over it. Although a simple pulley provides the advantage of merely changing the direction of force, it does so at the cost of increased friction as the rope, in this case the peroneal tendons, moves across its protruded surface.

from the *cuboid tuberosity*.[30] The longus tendon then proceeds distally by crossing the sole of the foot lateromedially to insert on the plantar base of the first metatarsal. Because of its oblique line of pull across the breadth and length of the sole, the peroneus longus, like the tibialis posterior, has a bowstring effect upon the long plantar arch of the foot. The peroneal brevis tendon however, unlike its companion tendon, remains on the lateral side of the foot for its entire course and distally inserts on the tuberosity on the base of the fifth metatarsal.

3. What is the etiology of peroneal tenosynovitis?

The peroneal tendon is an uncommon site for tendinitis.[2] The cause of peroneal tenosynovitis derives from stenosis of the tendon sheath at any one of three sites of potentially increased friction. The pulley sites and the angulation under the cuboid bone represent potential stress risers to the tendons (Fig. 32-1). Stenosis of the peroneal tendons with subsequent tendinitis may also occur at one of three anatomic sites corresponding to tendon passage through fibroosseous tunnels or passage at an acute angulation. These potential sites of stress rise include: the first simple pulley, located posterior to the lateral malleolus at the peroneal sulcus; the second simple pulley, at the peroneal trochlea; and the angulation of the peroneus longus tendon as it winds under the cuboid bone.[4,13] The effect of the tendons running through the fixed pulley system along the lateral ankle is to cause oblique stress to the tendon(s). This results

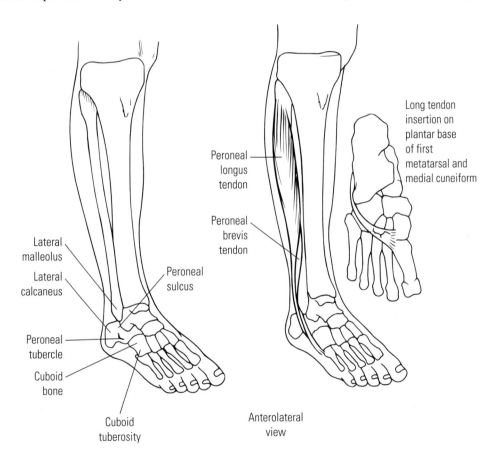

Peroneal longus tendon

Peroneal brevis tendon

Long tendon insertion on plantar base of first metatarsal and medial cuneiform

Lateral malleolus

Lateral calcaneus

Peroneal tubercle

Cuboid bone

Peroneal sulcus

Cuboid tuberosity

Anterolateral view

FIG. 32-1 Anterolateral view of the right leg and ankle showing the *peroneal muscles* origins and insertions. Prior to their insertion the peroneal tendons course along the osseous surface topography of the lateral ankle and foot. In doing so, the tendons cross three sites of potential friction. Should friction occur, the accompanying inflammation may cause nodular swelling and stenosis of the tendon sheath at those sites: *1,* posterior to the lateral malleolus at the peroneal sulcus; *2,* at the peroneal trochlea; and *3,* the peroneus longus tendon passing under the cuboid tuberosity.

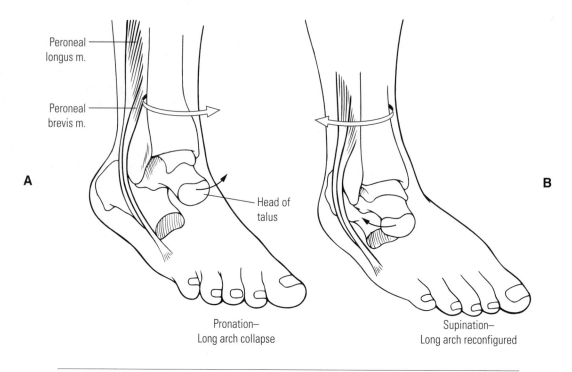

A

Peroneal longus m.

Peroneal brevis m.

Head of talus

Pronation— Long arch collapse

B

Supination— Long arch reconfigured

FIG. 32-2 Tendon stress may be increased by torsion of the tendon, secondary to excessive tibial torsion, derived from either extreme of the spectrum of foot deformity ranging from (**A**) excessive pronation or from (**B**) diminished pronation in the rigid forefoot valgus posture.

in compromised tendon vascularity and consequently predisposes the tendon to such pathologic conditions as irritation, tenosynovitis, and, eventually, tendinitis.[36] Tendon stress at those junctions may be increased by torsion of the tendon secondary to excessive tibial torsion, derived from either extreme of the spectrum of foot deformity, ranging from excessive pronation in the forefoot or rearfoot varus posture to too little pronation in the rigid forefoot valgus posture (Fig. 32-2).[43] Tendinitis may also be precipitated by traumatic etiology derived from inversion ankle injuries, lateral malleolar stress fractures,[19] and calcaneal fractures.[41] Soccer players may sustain peroneal tendinitis after a direct kick to the tendons.[45]

Tenosynovitis refers to roughening of the synovial surfaces of a long tendon that possesses a protective synovial sheath. Excessive gliding of the tendon within its synovial sheath may result in excessive longitudinal friction that causes roughening of the inner aspect of the synovial sheath by crepitus imparted to the examiner's hand. Movement is not limited because no adhesions are present. Continued movement between the close-fitting sheath and the tendon heightens symptoms, which if unabated, evolve into a vicious cycle of inflammation. As this pathologic condition of the tendon evolves, the tendon surface is also roughened,[7] and inflammation spreads to involve the tendon itself (tendinitis).

4. What is the kinesiology of the peroneal muscles during early stance?

Collectively, the peronei evert the foot and plantarflex the ankle. These peronei are the primary ankle evertors and secondary plantar flexors. The peronei may pull anterior to the axis of the upper ankle joint such that they also have a tertiary function of dorsiflexion. The peroneus longus has the additional function of depressing the head of the first metatarsal by virtue of its distal insertion. Because the line of pull of the longus tendon extends obliquely across the length and breadth of the foot, it functions to bowstring the long plantar arch. A primary role of the peronei is determined by their function during the closed kinetic mode, particularly during early stance phase of gait.

The two peroneal muscles begin their action early in the gait cycle with the onset of forefoot loading.[5,40,43a] The kinesiology of peronei function during gait is understood in relation to the subtalar joint, in which the peronei perform an eccentric pronation function during early stance. Early stance is characterized by foot pronation to absorb the jarring effects of heel impact. Eccentric contraction of the peronei during the interim between early to midstance phase of gait allows flattening of the longitudinal arch in a controlled manner and not all at once, so that the disruptive energy of impact is absorbed without causing injury. The peronei also exhibit a second peak of electrical activity during late stance, corresponding to a lateral, dynamic, concentric, and stabilizing role.

To appreciate peroneal function in relation to gait, we must focus on the ankle and subtalar joints and their relationship to ground reaction forces during early stance. In the interim between heel strike to foot flat, the ground reaction force is located behind the ankle axis for dorsiflexion and plantarflexion. This causes a passive plantarflexion moment at the ankle joint at the foot-flat subphase of gait. The forefoot, if unrestricted, will slap down. The extrinsic muscles of the foot, such as the peronei and tibialis anterior and posterior work eccentrically to lower the forefoot to the floor (Fig. 32-3). By absorbing the passively generated plantarflexion moment they prevent a jarring transition from early to middle stance. Simultaneously, their eccentric contraction along either side of the subtalar joint allows controlled motion at that joint.

Energy absorption of the ground reaction force by the foot is best accomplished by deliberately controlled pronation. This is accomplished through eccentric contraction of those extrinsic muscles crossing the subtalar joint medially and laterally. The peronei and other extrinsic evertor muscles laterally cross the subtalar joint. The peronei may be considered anatomic antagonists when they are compared with those extrinsic muscles passing along the medial side of the subtalar joint during the open kinetic mode of function. The peroneus longus also functions with the extrinsic invertors before midstance, in relation to subtalar joint pronation. This closed-chain synergic relationship among open-chain anatomic antagonists occurs because their common denominator is a collective orientation of span that crosses the hindfoot to insert in the midfoot and forefoot (Fig. 32-4).

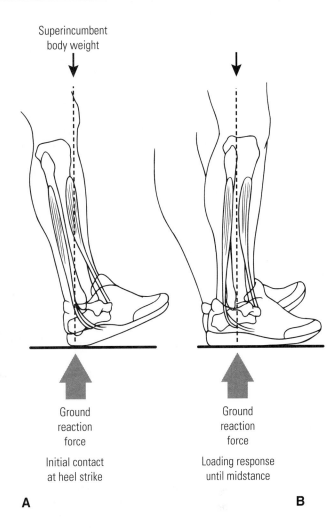

Superincumbent body weight

Ground reaction force

Initial contact at heel strike

A

Ground reaction force

Loading response until midstance

B

FIG. 32-3 Dynamic extrinsic eccentric control during early stance preventing foot slap. The kinesiology of peronei function during gait is understood in relation to the subtalar joint in which it performs an eccentric pronotary function during early to middle stance. **A,** At heel strike the ground reaction force vector lies behind the ankle joint axis for flexion and extension, and generates a passive plantarflexion moment. **B,** The dynamic response of the extrinsics act as shock absorbers to restrain the rate and magnitude of pronation either directly as with tibialis posterior and the peronei, or indirectly via tibialis anterior, which decelerates the anteriorly moving tibial shank. These muscles collectively prevent a jarring transition from early to middle stance that accompanies foot slap. Arrow indicates direction of motion.

During midstance the tibia moves directly over the foot and the ground reaction force shifts from behind the ankle to forward of the ankle. The resulting strong passive dorsiflexion moment inclines the tibia forward through the range of available dorsiflexion. Once the

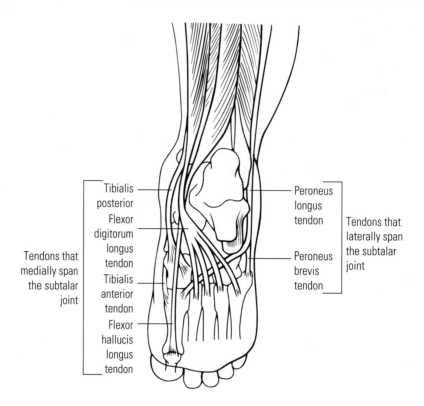

Tibialis posterior

Flexor digitorum longus tendon

Tibialis anterior tendon

Flexor hallucis longus tendon

Tendons that medially span the subtalar joint

Peroneus longus tendon

Peroneus brevis tendon

Tendons that laterally span the subtalar joint

FIG. 32-4 Kinesiologic synergy of foot extrinsics. The extrinsic muscles of the foot passing medial (long invertors) and lateral (long evertors) to the subtalar joint axis are viewed as anatomic antagonists performing inversion and eversion functions. Kinesiologically, however, the tendons of these muscles work in eccentric synergy prior to midstance phase of gait to control the rate and magnitude of pronation as an energy absorption strategy. The pretibial muscles (tibialis anterior and the long toe extensors) reach peak contractile intensity during early loading to restrain the rate of passive ankle plantar flexion. In such fashion, tibialis anterior restrains the downward motion of the forefoot and prevents foot slap. Tibialis posterior action demonstrates an early peak of electrical activity. Both tibialis anterior and posterior are invertor muscles. The peronei demonstrate activity early in the gait cycle. The common denominator among many of the cruel extrinsics is that their eccentric contraction prior to midstance phase of gait has a diminishing effect on both the rate and magnitude of pronation.

limits of that range are reached, the forward inclination of the tibia continues as a function of forward body momentum. Forward tibial inclination levers the heel off the floor during heel rise and initiates the passive windlass mechanism that resupinates the foot. Once this occurs, all the posterior compartment muscles start to increase their contractile output to the level necessary to thrust the body forward into the next stance cycle. Thus late stance is characterized by passive reversal of the ankle joint from dorsiflexion to one of decided plantarflexion as a function of ground reaction force.

5. What role in stabilization of the plantarflexed foot do the peronei perform in synergy with dynamic extrinsics spanning the subtalar joint medially during late stance?

During late stance phase of gait, between heel rise and push-off, the foot is postured in decided plantarflexion. The relationship of the parts of the ankle mortise during plantarflexion is unstable because the narrow posterior trochlea of the talus lies between the two malleoli. A decrease of bone-on-bone contact within the mortise results in greater intramalleolar distance and represents potential instability of the ankle joint. As the foot postures into plantarflexion, the thruster muscles such as the triceps surae and other posterior compartment musculature exhibit peak electrical activity as they collectively contract. Both the tibialis posterior and the flexor hallucis longus concentrically contract. However, the tendons of these muscles wind around the medial malleolus and pass medial to the subtalar joint axes and thereby create an inversion moment. In the absence of osseous stability within the mortise, contraction of these two muscles results in inversion. The tendency toward inversion is increased by the osseous architectural obliquity of the axis of the upper ankle joint, in which the fibula projects more distal than the tibia. Unrestrained inversion causes weight bearing to be concentrated along the lateral border of the sole and predisposes the ankle toward an inversion sprain. An excessive inversion moment is normally countered by the static restraint of the anterior talofibular lateral collateral ligament.

During late stance, the peronei, whose alignment is consistent with the anterior talofibular ligament, are active as dynamic stabilizers to provide lateral ankle stability during push-off. The peronei work as dynamic ligaments and provide a counter-inversion moment, thereby restoring rotary balance to the foot (Fig. 32-5). Thus in the closed kinetic chain during gait the peronei do not evert, but rather concentrically contract to counterbalance the inversion moment generated by the middle and deep layers of the posterior compartment of the leg (the flexor hallucis, flexor digitorum, and posterior tibialis, respectively). This *synergic guy support mechanism* between the evertors and the inverters has a net effect of maintaining the ankle in neutral so that a maximal plantarflexion moment successfully propels the body forward without injury to the ankle.*

6. What is the mechanism of peroneal subluxation?

The peroneal tendons are considerably more prone to subluxation than to tearing.[41] Peroneal instability is more common in younger athletes, particularly those participating in sports such as soccer, basketball, football, ice skating, and skiing.[21] Traumatic etiology of subluxation and dislocation is ascribed to sudden forceful dorsiflexion of the inverted foot, along with reflex contraction of the peroneal tendons, causing a tear of the superior peroneal retinaculum (Fig. 32-6). This may occur during a skiing injury in which passive ankle dorsiflexion and inversion moments occur when a ski tip digs into the snow and the skier falls forward.[1,44] In football, tendon instability may be precipitated by the high magnitude of torque generated over the lateral ankle during cutting movements; this may result in tearing of the peroneal retinaculum.[16] Injury may also occur from forceful and repetitive equinus positions characteristic of classical ballet.[42] An alternative mechanism causing subluxation involves inversion of the slightly plantarflexed foot, as would occur with a lateral ankle ligament sprain.[7] Finally, tendon dislocation may occur 25% to 40% of the time in conjunction with intraarticular fractures of the calcaneus.[9,34]

7. What anatomic anomaly may predispose some persons to peroneal tendon instability?

Most individuals have a definite sulcus behind the fibula for the passage of the peronei across the ankle joint. However, anatomic variations in malleolar groove size and shape may be related to the incidence of tendon instability, in much the same way that the long biceps tendon relates to the bicipital groove at the anterior proximal humerus. It is speculated that some individuals possess a groove that is relatively flat or even convex suggesting an anatomic predisposition to subluxation. Generally, some 11% of the population have flat grooves, whereas approximately 7% have convex grooves. The range of sulcus width ranges between 5 mm and 10 mm.[7]

Another anatomic variation predisposing an individual to peroneal tendon instability may be related to an absent posterior crest.[26] The superior peroneal retinaculum attaches to the periosteum of the posterior fibular malleolus. Incompetence or absence of this crest may occur from repetitive stress that causes the retinaculum to strip the periosteum away from the lateral malleolus, leaving the retinaculum lax.[10] This degenerative process may be related to a common radiologic finding of tendon instability including spurs on the distal fibula. Thus the restraining retinaculum may be compromised as a result of acute injury, stretching by repetitive trauma, or overuse.[41] Finally, a cavus or val-

---

*Interestingly, the tendons of the flexor hallucis longus, tibialis posterior, and the peronei span the subtalar joint inferiorly as they insert upon the medial, central, and lateral borders of the forefoot. Their collective concentric contraction acts to approximate the hindfoot to the forefoot. Thus these extrinsics may offer a dynamic role in assisting the primary resupinating passive windlass effect.

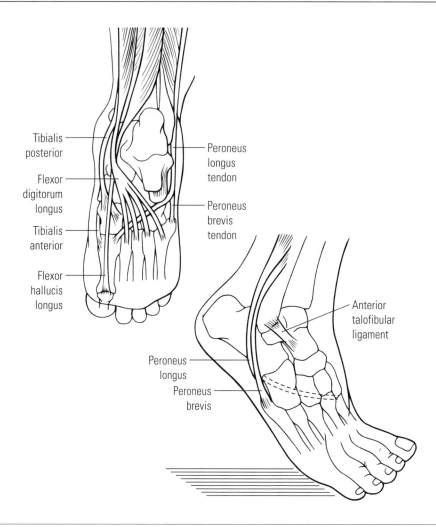

Tibialis posterior

Flexor digitorum longus

Tibialis anterior

Flexor hallucis longus

Peroneus longus tendon

Peroneus brevis tendon

Anterior talofibular ligament

Peroneus longus

Peroneus brevis

FIG. 32-5 Guy support mechanism represents synergistic cooperation between the evertors and invertors during late stance. The decided plantarflexion posture of the foot during late stance results in diminished osseous contact within the mortise at the upper ankle joint. Consequently, a condition of potential instability exists. Simultaneously, the posterior compartment musculature collectively fire and exert a thruster force to the inversion side of the ankle and subtalar joints. Subsequently, the foot and ankle complex may sustain an inversion sprain of the ankle during late stance phase of gait. Normally, this is prevented statically by the anterior talofibular ligament and dynamically by the peronei which share a similar orientation to the anterior talofibular ligament. The peronei provide a counter-inversion moment by generating an eversion moment during late stance phase, thus restoring rotary balance to the foot and ankle complex. Total forefoot contact with the surface is thus assured by the eversion force generated by the peronei.

gus hindfoot posture may also be a contributory factor by biomechanically altering tendon pull.[42]

8. What is the mechanism of injury resulting in strain of the peroneal tendons?

Partial tear or *strain* of the peroneal tendons may occur with inversion ankle sprain or dislocation. This tear is usually an incomplete longitudinal splitting[35] of the peroneus brevis, which is in close contact with the fibula. Strain may also occur as an isolated injury in soccer as, for example, when the tendons are subjected to sudden forceful stretch during an attempted outside kick.[43] This is accomplished by sudden inversion and plantar flexion that is immediately followed by forceful peroneal contraction into dorsiflexion and eversion. Patients clinically exhibit soft tissue swelling

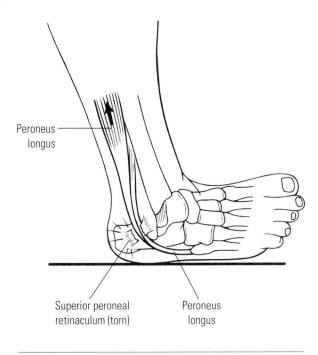

Peroneus longus

Superior peroneal retinaculum (torn)

Peroneus longus

FIG. 32-6 Traumatic etiology of peroneal subluxation/dislocation is ascribed to sudden forceful dorsiflexion of the inverted foot with reflex contraction of the peroneal tendons causing a tear of the superior peroneal retinaculum.

over the peroneal tendon just proximal to the lateral malleolus.

9. What is the clinical presentation of a pathologic condition of the peroneal tendon?

The clinical presentation of *peroneal tendon disease* includes pain and tenderness along the course of the peroneal sheath. Symptoms are accentuated by forced passive inversion with plantar flexion or resistive eversion of the inverted foot. Swelling may be present inferior to the lateral malleolus. The patient may exhibit an antalgic gait, limitation of subtalar joint motion, and point tenderness at the inferior peroneal retinaculum. There may be a history of trauma or a biomechanical foot deviation at either extreme of subtalar joint neutral. If peroneal tendon pathology is ignored, it may progress to a lateral shin splint syndrome (see p. 504).

Peroneal tendon *subluxation* and *dislocation* are characterized by swelling and ecchymosis superior to[36] the retromalleolar area and tenderness over the peroneal tendons.[7] The patient usually reports a snapping sensation and pain in the posterior lateral ankle. Subluxation

may be observed by having the patient attempt to actively evert and dorsiflex the foot. Although this may not be possible acutely, it is frequently demonstrated in the subacute stage. Both the peroneal retinaculum may be stressed and subluxation may be reproduced through resisted dorsiflexion with ankle eversion. Instability may be observed as a palpable clicking or visible snapping of the tendons out of their groove, both behind the lateral malleolus and distal to it.[6,8,17] Diagnosis is radiographically confirmed by the presence of an avulsion fracture of the lateral ridge of the distal fibula.

10. How are the peronei best palpated and assessed for muscular strength?

The peroneal longus and brevis cross the tarsus distal to the lateral malleolus and course obliquely forward of the calcaneus by crossing the peroneal tubercle. In the event of inflammation at either of these pulleys, the site behind the fibular malleolus and in the area of the peroneal tubercle feels thick and is tender to palpation. The insertion of the peroneus brevis tendon may be palpated at its insertion into the styloid process, particularly as the patient actively everts and plantar flexes the foot. Tenderness here may be secondary to reflexive contraction of the peronei, in association with a lateral ankle sprain that involves the tendon avulsing off the tip of the styloid process. In the absence of trauma, tenderness at this site may derive from an inflamed bursa over the process.[14]

The peronei are tested simultaneously for muscular strength. Functional testing involves asking the patient to walk on the medial borders of the feet. A patient demonstrating a decreased ability or inability to do so indicates probable weakness of the peronei. By watching the exposed lateral ankle, the examiner may observe prominence of the tendons as they wind around the lateral malleolus.

To perform manual muscle testing of the peronei, the examiner stabilizes the leg just above the ankle joint and postures the patient's foot in maximal inversion and eversion. The examiner then requests the patient to evert against resistance. Counterpressure is delivered against the lateral border and sole of the foot, in the direction of foot inversion and ankle dorsiflexion. Weakness indicates that the patient has decreased ability to rise the toes and an increased likelihood for inversion ankle sprain secondary to decreased lateral stability of the ankle joint.[23] It is important to avoid applying pressure to the toes, since they may move and skew the results of the test.[3,14,22,25,28,31,38]

11. What is peroneal spastic flatfoot?

Peroneal spastic flatfoot is not a neurologic condition, but rather a pathologic condition of the tarsal joints of the foot. This condition most commonly occurs at the calcaneonavicular site and secondarily at the talocalcaneal coalition. The diagnostic term "tarsal coalition" has essentially replaced the term "peroneal spastic flatfoot" because the former term describes the cause of the condition.[22] A tarsal coalition is the union of two or more tarsal bones, which may be fibrous (syndesmosis), cartilaginous (synchondrosis), or osseous (synostosis) in nature.[28] Simply stated, a tarsal coalition occurs when movement between two or more tarsal bones is restricted or absent and motion is restricted at the subtalar joint. The most common sites of tarsal coalitions are the calcaneonavicular and talocalcaneal joints.[38] Talocalcaneal joint coalitions most commonly occur over the middle and posterior facets of the subtalar joint.[25] A subtalar coalition is a form of tarsal coalition in which a fibrous or cartilaginous bar calcifies to become completely ossified or remains osteocartilaginous; the presence of this bar hinders normal arthrokinematic and osteokinematic motion among the tarsal bones. The subtalar joint acts as a torque converter and thereby permits dissipation of the enormous forces imparted to the foot during stance phase of gait. In the absence of normal talocalcaneonavicular motion because of restriction produced by the coalition, increased stress is placed upon the foot and ankle, producing a cycle of strain, pain, and muscle spasm,[3] with eventual degenerative changes in the subtalar synostosis.

Coalitions are often asymptomatic at first, only to become symptomatic after injury; alternatively, they may present as recurrent episodes of peroneal muscle spasticity. The peroneal tendons, running closely along the lateral aspect of the subtalar joint, protectively react by reflex muscle spasm. The magnitude of spasm of the evertors is so exaggerated that it merits the descriptions *spasticity* and *clonus,* terms normally reserved for pathologic conditions caused by upper motor neuron disorders. *Clonus,* meaning turmoil in Greek, refers to an abnormal state in which spasticity means involuntary alternate muscular contraction and relaxation of the evertors in rapid succession. Clonus is induced by sudden passive stretch into inversion of the ankle joint. This results in excessive eversion muscle tone dominating the mid and hindfoot. Calcaneal eversion is a component of pronation of the foot, and hence the foot is postured into pronation. Over time, the peronei and other soft-tissue and osseous-tissue components of the

foot adapt to this posture, resulting in a *rigid flatfoot* or *pes planus* deformity caused by depression of the medial longitudinal arch and posturing into abduction and eversion. The peronei pass posterior to the ankle axis, whereas the longus inserts at the base of the first metatarsal. Consequently, the ankle may be postured into plantarflexion while the longus acts to depress the head of the first metatarsal.[11,12,15,20,24] On occasion, pain may be so disabling as to require a period of plaster immobilization. The clinician is alerted to this condition by recurrent episodes of peroneal spasm and decreased mobility of the talocalcaneonavicular complex in the flatfooted patient. Patients with other forms of tarsal coalition may have a foot posture other than a rigidly pronated foot, such as an adducted and inverted foot.[3]

Not all individuals with tarsal coalition develop symptoms.[11] If symptoms do occur, they usually occur during adolescence, although they occasionally manifest in adulthood.[20] Most patients with a tarsal coalition become symptomatic during adolescence. In most cases symptoms are provoked by mild traumatic episodes, usually inversion sprains of the ankle that may cause disruption of the fusing or already fused articulation.[12] Formerly asymptomatic feet may become suddenly symptomatic following a simple ankle sprain or fracture. An ankle sprain per se should not cause peroneal spasm, and coalition should be suspected when pain and peroneal muscle spasm persist beyond the usual disability time after fracture or sprain. The clinician is alerted to this condition by recurrent episodes of peroneal spasm and by decreased mobility of the calocalcaneonavicular complex in the flatfooted patient.[32,41,42]

Subtalar joint coalition is characterized by muscle spasm of the evertors coalition that results in reduced subtalar joint mobility and a pes planus posture of the foot. The patient will complain of painful flatfeet only during weight bearing, and decreased foot mobility is noted upon examination of range of motion. A common complaint is difficulty walking on uneven terrain. Common observations of radiographs in persons with tarsal coalition include a talar beak, narrowing of the talocalcaneal space, rounding of the lateral process of the talus, failure to visualize the middle facet of the subtalar joint on a lateral view, inability to visualize the tarsal sinus, and a positive halo sign. The halo sign is an increase in trabecular bone density, having a ring-like appearance, seen in the calcaneus below the lateral process of the talus. The halo sign is thought to be caused by altered compressive forces from the talus, secondary to loss of subtalar joint motion.[32] Computerized tomography is the diagnostic test of choice in determination of suspected tarsal coalition. Once talocalcaneal coalition is identified, the therapist should determine whether the calcaneus is in a neutral, inverted, or everted position. The position of the rearfoot while the patient is at rest appears to predict the effectiveness of nonoperative treatment. Conservative therapy consists of rest in a short-leg cast applied in the subtalar neutral position, nonsteroidal antiinflammatory medication, and an orthosis such as a medial heel wedge and medial longitudinal arch support to decrease subtalar joint motion (Fig. 32-7). Conservative treatment is less likely to be successful if the rearfoot is everted, and more likely to be successful if the rearfoot is capable of being positioned at or near subtalar joint neutral.[22] Pain may, on occasion, be so disabling as to require a period of plaster immobilization. The decision of whether to resect the bar to perform triple arthrodesis is based on the presence or absence of degenerative changes.[42] Alternatively, surgery may include calcaneal osteotomy.

12. What therapeutic management best addresses peroneal tendon disease?

Management of peroneal tendinitis includes rest, iontophoresis, cold and heat modalities, oral antiinflammatories, eccentric strengthening of the peronei, and a management regimen similar to other forms of foot tendinitis. Crutches may occasionally be employed to rest the overworked tendons from weight bearing.[36] Steroid injections are not indicated, and may contribute to tendon degeneration.

Whereas the causative factor in peroneal tendinitis is overuse by way of excessive longitudinal friction (as discussed earlier), the curative factor is transverse *friction massage*. When the tendon sheath on the tendon is rubbed transversely with a to-and-fro motion instead of and up-and-down motion, the roughened surfaces are made smooth again. During the massage it is best to stretch the tendon so as to provide an immobile base against which to move the tendon sheath circumferentially. The patient may require 2 to 4 weeks of treatment, with 20-minute treatment sessions given 3 times per week.[19] Pretreatment and posttreatment ice massage may be effective at minimizing inflammation.

Management of peroneal tendon strains is identical to that of inversion ankle sprains (see pp. 391-395). Ice bath treatment is often helpful in reducing early symptoms. An L-shaped or horseshoe-shaped pad is placed around the fibular malleolus to help maintain pressure over the peroneal sheath.[33] The pad may be held in place

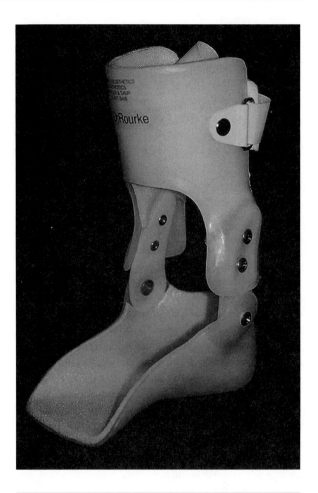

FIG. 32-7 Short articulated ankle foot orthosis used to decrease the pain of a tarsal tunnel coalition by restricting subtalar joint motion. (From Coughlin MJ, Mann RA: *Surgery of the foot and ankle,* ed 7, St. Louis, 1999, Mosby.)

by tape. Application of tape with a technique identical to that used for inversion ankle sprain promotes eversion and minimizes inversion. A lateral heel wedge or heel lift is placed in the shoe to further limit inversion and thereby minimize tension on the peroneal tendons.

Recognizing and implementing treatment for tendon dislocation is essential. Failure to implement early treatment may lead to chronic lateral instability.[27] Axial imaging is helpful in confirming a suspected diagnosis of tendon instability because clinical observation of soft tissue swelling may hinder palpation of the displaced tendons and be mistakenly attributed to a sprained ankle.[1]

Management of acute dislocation is controversial. Some authorities hold that conservative treatment is beneficial[39]; however, others maintain that it always fails, and recommend early surgical intervention.[10,29] In the more active, competitive athlete, conservative management is not likely to prove successful in preventing recurrence, and surgery may be appropriate early in management.[7] Nevertheless, it is recommended that an initial trial of nonsurgical management be attempted in the occasional athlete. Gentle pressure may be applied over the peroneal tendons with a compression dressing with a felt pad cut in the shape of a keyhole; the dressing should be strapped over the lateral malleolus and reinforced with a plaster splint. After the acute symptoms have abated, a well-molded cast is applied and worn for a total of 5 to 6 weeks. Aggressive ankle rehabilitation similar to management of lateral ankle sprains (see pp. 391-396) is begun after the cast is removed.

In cases of chronic instability or in the acute condition in the professional athlete, surgical management includes excision of the torn portion of tendon,[41] deepening of the groove,[37] and retinacular repair. If the lateral ligament was also injured, it may be repaired at the same time. Immobilization is continued for 1 week, with the patient instructed not to bear weight, after which a walking cast is used for 5 weeks. The subsequent rehabilitation program includes taping to provide support, as well as an emphasis on strengthening the lateral compartment muscles (see p. 395). Athletes require 4 to 6 months of management before they can return to sports participation.

REFERENCES

1. Arrowsmith SR, Fleming LL, Allman F: Traumatic dislocations of the peroneal tendons, *Am J Sports Med* 11(3):142-146, 1983.
2. Bachner EJ, Friedman MJ: Injuries to the leg. In Nicholas JA, Hershman EB, editors: *The lower extremity and spine,* ed 2, vol 1, St Louis, 1995, Mosby.
3. Baxter DE: *The foot and ankle in sports,* St Louis, 1995, Mosby.
4. Burman M: Stenosing tenosynovitis of the foot and ankle, *Arch Surg* 67:686, 1953.
5. Close JR, Todd FN: The phasic activity of the muscles of the lower extremity and the effect of tendon transfer, *J Bone Joint Surg Am* 41(2):189-208, 1959.
6. Cohen I, Lane S, Koning W: Peroneal tendon dislocations: a review of the literature, *J Foot Surg* 22(1):15-20, 1983.
7. Cyriax: *Textbook of orthopedic medicine, vol 2, Treatment by manipulation, massage and injection,* ed 11, London, 1984, Bailliere Tindall.
8. Duddy RK et al: Tendon sheath injuries of the foot and ankle, *J Foot Surg* 30(2):179-186, 1991.
9. Ebraheim NA et al: Radiologic evaluation of peroneal tendon pathology associated with calcaneal fractures, *J Orthop Trauma* 5(3):365-369, 1991.
10. Eckert WR, Davis EA: Acute rupture of the peroneal retinaculum, *J Bone Joint Surg Am* 58(5):670-672, 1976.
11. Ehrlich MG, Elmer EB: Tarsal coalition. In Jahss MH, editor: *Disorders of the foot and ankle: medical and surgical management,* ed 2, vol 1, Philadelphia, 1991, WB Saunders.
12. Elkus RA: Tarsal coalition in the young athlete, *Am J Sports Med* 14(6):477-480, 1986.
13. Evans JD: Subcutaneous rupture of the tendon of peroneus longus, *J Bone Joint Surg Br* 48(3):507-509, 1966.
14. *Compton's interactive encyclopedia,* 1995, Compton's NewMedia.
15. Fetto JF: Anatomy and physical examination of the foot and ankle. In Nicholas JA, Hershman EB, editors: *The lower extremity and spine,* ed 2, vol 1, St Louis, 1995, Mosby.
16. Fochios D, Nicholas JA: Football injuries. In Nicholas JA, Hershman EB, editors: *The lower extremity and spine,* ed 2, vol 2, St Louis, 1995, Mosby.
17. Frey CC, Shereff MJ: Tendon injuries about the ankle in athletes, *Clin Sports Med* 7(1):103-118, 1988.
18. Reference moved to no. 43a.
19. Gray EG, Basmajian JV: Electromyography and cinematography of leg and foot ("normal" and flat) during walking, *Anat Rec* 161(1):1-16, 1968.
20. Hoppenfeld S: *Physical examination of the spine and extremities,* Norwalk, Conn, 1976, Appleton-Century Crofts.
21. Jack EA: Bone anomalies of the tarsus in relation to "personal spastic flatfeet," *J Bone Joint Surg Br* 36:530-542, 1954.
22. Jones DC, Singer KM: Soft-tissue conditions of the ankle and foot. In Nicholas JA, Hershman EB, editors: *The lower extremity and spine,* ed 2, vol 1, St Louis, 1995, Mosby.
23. Kelo MJ, Riddle DL: Examination and management of a patient with tarsal coalition, *Phys Ther* 78(5):518-525, 1998.
24. Kendall FP, McCreary EK: *Muscles: testing and function,* ed 3, Baltimore, 1983, Williams & Wilkins.
25. Kendrick JI: Tarsal coalitions, *Clin Orthop* 85:62-63, 1972.
26. Lapidus PW: Spastic flatfoot, *J Bone Joint Surg* 28:126-136, 1946.
27. Miller JW: Dislocation of the peroneal tendon: a new operative procedure, *Am J Orthop* 9(7):136-137, 1967.
28. Miller TT, Ghelman B, Potter HG: Imaging of the foot and ankle. In Nicholas JA, Hershman EB, editors: *The lower extremity and spine,* ed 2, vol 1, St Louis, 1995, Mosby.
29. Mosier KM, Asher M: Tarsal coalitions and peroneal spastic flatfoot: a review, *J Bone Joint Surg Am* 66(7):976-984, 1984.
30. Murr S: Dislocation of the peroneal tendon with marginal fracture of the lateral malleolus, *J Bone Joint Surg Br* 43:563, 1961.
31. Netter FH: *The Ciba collection of medical illustrations,* vol 8, part 1, Summit, NJ, 1991.
32. Percy EC, Mann DL: Tarsal coalition: a review of the literature and presentation of 13 cases, *Foot Ankle* 9(1):40-44, 1988.
33. Perlman MD, Wertheimer SJ: Tarsal coalitions, *J Foot Surg* 25(1):58-67, 1986.

34. Reese RC Jr, Burruss TP, Patten J: Athletic techniques and protective equipment. In Nicholas JA, Hershman EB, editors: *The lower extremity and spine,* ed 2, vol 1, St Louis, 1995, Mosby.

35. Rosenberg ZS et al: Peroneal tendon injury associated with calcaneal fractures: CT findings, *AJR* 149(1):125-129, 1987.

36. Sammarco GJ, DiRaimondo CV: Chronic peroneus brevis tendon lesions, *Foot Ankle* 9(4):163-170, 1989.

37. Scheller AD, Kasser JR, Quigley TB: Tendon injuries about the ankle, *Orthop Clin North Am* 11(4):801-811, 1980.

38. Steadman JR, Scheinberg RR: Skiing injuries. In Nicholas JA, Hershman EB, editors: *The lower extremity and spine,* ed 2, vol 2, St Louis, 1995, Mosby.

39. Stormont DM, Peterson HA: The relative incidence of tarsal coalition, *Clin Orthop* 181:28-36, 1983.

40. Stover CN, Bryan DR: Traumatic dislocation of the peroneal tendons, *Am J Surg* 103:180, 1962.

41. Sutherland D: An electromyographic study of the plantar flexors of the ankle in normal walking on the level, *J Bone Joint Surg Am* 48(1):66-71, 1966.

42. Trevino S, Baumhauer JF: Tendon injuries of the foot and ankle, *Clin Sports Med* 11(4):727-739, 1992.

43. Turco VJ: Injuries to the foot and ankle. In Nicholas JA, Hershman EB, editors: *The lower extremity and spine,* ed 2, vol 2, St Louis, 1995, Mosby.

43a. Valmassy RL: *Clinical biomechanics of the lower extremities,* St Louis, 1996, Mosby.

44. Yulish BS, Mulopulos GP, Goodfellow DB, et al: MR Imaging of osteochondral lesions of talus, *J Comput Assist Tomogr* 11(2):296-301, 1987.

45. Xethalis JL, Lorei MP: Soccer injuries. In Nicholas JA, Hershman EB, editors: *The lower extremity and spine,* ed 2, vol 1, St Louis, 1995, Mosby.

RECOMMENDED READING

Trevino S, Baumhauer JF: Tendon injuries of the foot and ankle, *Clin Sports Med* 11(4):727-739, 1992.

Frey CC, Shereff MJ: Tendon injuries about the ankle in athletes, *Clin Sports Med* 7(1):103-118, 1988.

Gudas CJ: Sports-related tendon injuries of the foot and ankle, *Clin Podiatr Med Surg* 3(2):303-313, 1986.

Arrowsmith SR, Fleming LL, Allman F: Traumatic dislocations of the peroneal tendons, *Am J Sports Med* 11(3):142-146, 1983.

33

Slim Young Woman With Painless, Sudden Foot Drop After Cross-Legged Posture

CASE 1: A 19-year-old woman had just lost 32 pounds by following a weight reduction program, which she began following the birth of her child. She presents the following history relating to a wedding she attended on the night before she visits you. Before meeting friends and relatives, she drank a whole bar-glass full of scotch whiskey to help her relax. She reported sitting down after the ceremony for at least 2 hours in the crossed-leg posture and chatting with friends and family. After dessert she decided that it was time to go home, but discovered that she could not stand up. When she attempted to stand, her right foot gave way, causing her to topple to the floor. She felt no pain. During her pregnancy she demonstrated gestational diabetes. The patient reports a brief history of childhood anorexia from which she completely recovered. When asked, she admits to having a history of recurrent right lateral ankle sprain and having worn high-heeled shoes that night for the first time since she gave birth. She now weighs 98 pounds.

OBSERVATION   A steppage gait is observed.

PALPATION   Palpation yields tenderness at the right fibular head.

RANGE OF MOTION   Range of motion is normal.

STRENGTH   A poor grade for both right dorsiflexion and eversion are noted, whereas right inversion is fair. The right hip adductors are normal, whereas the hip abductors are good.

SENSATION   Partial sensory loss is demonstrated over the anterolateral leg and dorsum of the foot, but the loss does not follow a dermatomal or specific cutaneous nerve distribution.

DEEP TENDON REFLEXES   Normal right lateral hamstring reflex.

SPECIAL TESTS   Positive Tinel's sign at the right fibular neck.

CASE 2: A 26-year-old prima ballerina with a history of recurrent lateral sprain to her left ankle celebrated a successful season opening at the ballet by celebrating with friends and family at a posh restaurant, followed by dancing in high-heeled shoes. That night she was startled awake by pain and paresthesia in the left ankle and foot. The pain and paresthesia were relieved by wagging her ankle back and forth. She reports using a commercially purchased knit ankle sleeve that, like a tight glove, affords increased stability to her ankle during performances. When asked about the location of shoe straps, she admits that her shoe has a proximal and distal dorsal strap. She offers that a similar aching sensation at the ankle and dorsum of her left foot occurs during prolonged practice, while in the pointe posture, particularly when she wears an elastic ankle sleeve. After practice, holding the ankle in a posture of extension and eversion afford relief from pain. There is no history of back pain or injury.

OBSERVATION   There is no erythema or swelling of the foot or ankle.

PALPATION   A positive Tinel's sign is present adjacent to the dorsalis pedis artery. No tenderness is noted over the fibular neck. Palpation over the left extensor digitorum brevis yields a firm muscular mound with no evidence of atrophy.

RANGE OF MOTION   Range of motion is within functional limits. Extreme plantarflexion of the left ankle reproduces foot pain.

STRENGTH   Resisted extension of the left great toe, performed with the foot in maximal dorsiflexion, is identical to the unaffected contralateral extremity. Right biceps femoris strength is normal.

SENSATION   Sensation is diminished to the web space of the left foot.

DEEP TENDON REFLEXES   The patient has 2+ left ankle jerk reflex.

SPECIAL TESTS   Electromyographic studies show chronic denervation of the extensor digitorum brevis.

? Questions

1. What is most likely wrong in these patients?
2. What is the anatomic course of the peroneal nerve?
3. What is the peroneal tunnel at the knee?
4. What are the mechanisms of injury that result in compression of the common peroneal nerve?
5. What mechanism of injury involves traction of the common peroneal nerve at the fibular neck?
6. How would compromise of the common peroneal nerve at the fibular neck give rise to recurrent ankle sprain?
7. What is superficial peroneal nerve entrapment?
8. How can exertional compartment syndrome compromise peroneal nerve function?
9. What are the extensor retinacula at the ankle?
10. What is anterior tarsal tunnel syndrome, and at which other sites may the deep peroneal nerve sustain injury?
11. How would contusion occur to the dorsal cutaneous nerves of the foot?
12. What is the clinical presentation of peroneal neuropathy?
13. What is the differential diagnosis?
14. What is peroneal muscle atrophy?
15. What therapeutic intervention would best manage these patients?

1. What is most likely wrong in these patients?

Acute peroneal palsy, implicated in Case 1, is a focal, peripheral, compressive mononeuropathy of the common peroneal nerve. For a slender person, sitting with the left leg crossed over the right lateral knee causes compression of the right common peroneal nerve by the weight of the left lower leg. The patient may not have been aware of any developing paresthesia because she had ingested a substantial amount of alcoholic beverage, which may have had an anesthetic effect on her sensory capacity. The neural supply to the lateral hamstrings conveys the lateral hamstring reflex through the S1 root. This enables clinical differentiation of a lesion to the common peroneal nerve above or at the level of the knee. Alcoholics, diabetics, and patients with Guillain-Barré syndrome are particularly vulnerable to acute common peroneal palsy. *Anterior tarsal tunnel syndrome* is implicated in Case 2, in which the deep peroneal nerve was trapped within the anterior tarsal tunnel or just distal to the tunnel, secondary to osteophytes at the dorsal midtarsus. The nerve may have been predisposed to prolonged ischemia that is secondary to the high-heeled shoes that stretch the nerve and to the placement of the dorsal straps that represent an external source of compression.

2. What is the anatomic course of the peroneal nerve?

The common peroneal and tibial nerves compose the terminal branches of the sciatic nerve. Both nerves are considered the sciatic nerve when they are bound together in a common sheath. The nerves divide just proximal to the knee in most persons,[33] at the superior border of the popliteal fossa. The *common peroneal nerve* contains fibers from the posterior divisions of the ventral rami of L4 through S2, and is considered the smaller and lateral terminal branch.* Of the 2 branches of the sciatic nerve, the peroneal branch is 6 times more likely to sustain pressure injury than the posterior tibial. This increased susceptibility relates to the variation in intraneural topography of the fiber bundles of the 2 components of the sciatic nerve.[44,45] Also, the common peroneal nerve is more vulnerable to the effects of ischemia because it has a poorer blood supply than the adjacent tibial nerve.

Before division, the common peroneal gives off only one branch in the entire thigh to the short head of the biceps femoris (the lateral hamstring muscle), which conveys the lateral hamstring reflex through the S1 root. This is clinically relevant in establishing the level of a peroneal nerve root lesion, in which reflex preservation will only occur if the offending lesion is at or below the knee.[31] After entering the popliteal fossa, the common peroneal nerve courses down the lateral aspect of the popliteal fossa, beneath the head of the biceps femoris tendon and superficial to the lateral head of the gastrocnemius en route to the posterior aspect of the fibular head.† It is of clinical significance that compression of the nerve may occur at this site from an enlarged *fabella*[22] that most often forms within the smaller lateral head of the gastrocnemius.[30] The nerve then winds lateral and forward around the neck of the fibula piercing the peroneus longus muscle, where it lies exposed subcutaneously. At this site the nerve, vulnerable to external compression, bifurcates into two terminal branches, known as the *superficial* and *deep peroneal nerves.*

Whereas the deep division of the nerve supplies a larger number of muscles and covers a smaller sensory area, the superficial branch supplies a smaller number of muscles and relatively large cutaneous area. The deep branch provides dorsiflexor motor function to the anterior crural compartment that consists of the tibialis anterior, extensor digitorum longus, and extensor hallucis longus. The deep branch terminates in the first metatarsal space by providing cutaneous innervation to the first dorsal web space via a twig of the deep peroneal nerve known as the *dorsal digital nerve.* The superficial peroneal nerve enters the lateral compartment and supplies the peroneal longus and brevis muscles that compose the lateral crural compartment. The superficial peroneal nerve also supplies sensation to a triangular area on the anterolateral dorsum of the foot and toes via the *dorsal cutaneous pedal nerves,* with exception to the first web space and the dorsum of the fourth and fifth toes. (Fig. 33-1).‡

3. What is the peroneal tunnel at the knee?

As the common peroneal nerve winds around the fibular neck, it does so in the gap between the origin of the peroneus longus and the bone. This gap consists of a fibroosseous *fibular* or *peroneal tunnel,*[2,25] in which the

---

*The medial, larger branch of the tibial nerve is rarely damaged because it lies in a deeply protected position within the thigh and leg. It only becomes vulnerable where it divides at the ankle into the medial and lateral plantar nerves.

†Proximal to the fibular head, the lateral sural cutaneous nerve branches from the common peroneal nerve.

‡The dorsum of the lateral fourth and fifth toes are innervated by the sural nerve via the lateral dorsal cutaneous pedal nerve. The sural nerve can trapped at three locations. The first is an exit point in the fascia just above he ankle, the second is behind the lateral malleolus, and the third is at the fifth metatarsal following a displaced fracture.

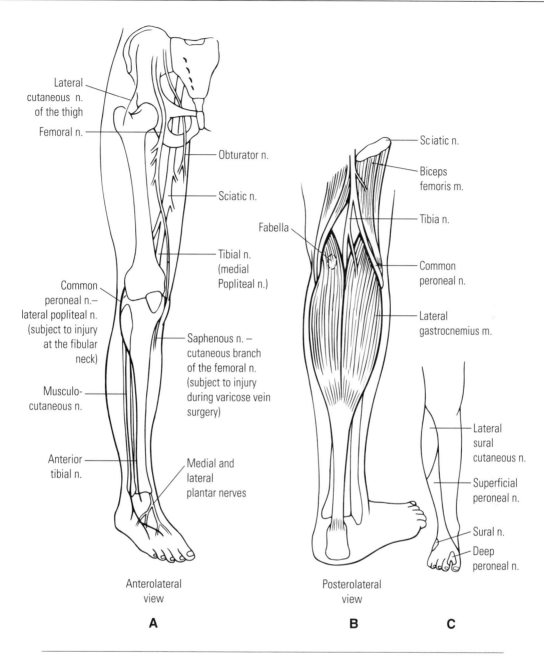

Lateral cutaneous n. of the thigh

Femoral n.

Obturator n.

Sciatic n.

Tibial n. (medial Popliteal n.)

Common peroneal n.– lateral popliteal n. (subject to injury at the fibular neck)

Saphenous n. – cutaneous branch of the femoral n. (subject to injury during varicose vein surgery)

Musculo-cutaneous n.

Anterior tibial n.

Medial and lateral plantar nerves

Anterolateral view

A

Sciatic n.

Biceps femoris m.

Fabella

Tibia n.

Common peroneal n.

Lateral gastrocnemius m.

Lateral sural cutaneous n.

Superficial peroneal n.

Sural n.

Deep peroneal n.

Posterolateral view

B

C

FIG. 33-1 Anatomy of the peroneal nerve. **A,** Anterolateral view. **B,** Posterolateral view. **C,** Anterolateral view of cutaneous innervation deriving from the peroneal nerves.

common peroneal nerve and its initial branches are drawn tightly by fascia over the periosteum of the fibular neck and under cover of the tendinous origin of the peroneus longus muscle. The floor of the tunnel is the fibula, and the root is composed of the tendinous edge of the origin of peroneus longus.[45] This tendinous edge manifests as a hook or "J" on the left leg or a reversed J on the right leg (Fig. 33-2).[15] The bifurcated branches

of the common peroneal nerve are bent over the fibrous edge over the bottom of the J.[16] The clinical significance here is that this site represents a site of potential tension and entrapment of the nerve, especially when plantar flexion and inversion of the ankle occur simultaneously.[32] Farm workers who spend considerable time in the squatting position may be at increased risk for peroneal nerve damage because this posture draws

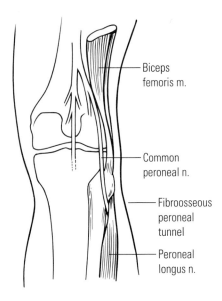

- Biceps femoris m.
- Common peroneal n.
- Fibroosseous peroneal tunnel
- Peroneal longus n.

FIG. 33-2 The peroneal tunnel is a fibroosseous tunnel comprised of the fibular neck and the tendinous hooked origin of the peroneus longus.

the arched fibrous border of the head of the peroneus longus against the common peroneal nerve.[36] This activity or using a squat-type toilet[19] may provoke a sudden yet painless footdrop.[14]

4. What are the mechanisms of injury that result in compression of the common peroneal nerve?

The most common mechanism of injury to the common peroneal nerve is acute compression at the fibular neck, where the subcutaneous nerve lies protected only by skin and fascia. It is significant that although the common peroneal nerve consists of approximately only eight fascicles at the level of the popliteal fossa it consists of approximately 16 fascicles just several centimeters farther distally, at the fibular head.[44] The increased number of fascicles may be a protective strategy for shielding the subcutaneous position of the nerve at the level of the fibular head. Acute trauma to the common peroneal nerve is the most common nerve injury seen in soccer,[48] and may occur from receiving a kick to the lateral knee. Even modest direct compression at this superficial location may result in a local conduction blockage (neuropraxia) after sitting for long periods with the legs crossed (crossed peroneal palsy), and certainly following a sharp blow to that site. Pressure against the nerve may also occur from lying in the lithotomy position during surgery, in which the feet and

legs are placed in stirrups. A spiral fracture of the upper end of the fibula may directly injure the nerve, and subsequent callus formation during the healing process may indicate a space-occupying lesion that compresses the nerve. This represents a chronic form of entrapment that results in nerve ischemia. Hematoma, as a space-occupying lesion, has also been implicated in hemophiliacs.[20] Among vascular causes of ischemia to the common peroneal nerve is acute thrombus or embolus of the femoral or popliteal arteries. Correction of valgus knees during knee arthroplasty may also injure the nerve.[35] A space-occupying lesion, such as a ganglion cyst[46] or fabella, in the lateral aspect of the popliteal fossa may also impinge on the nerve.

The *fabella* (Latin for *bean*) is an oval nodule of bone that, like all sesamoids, is found where tendons of two jointed muscles cross the ends of long bones in limbs, particularly the lower extremities. These bones are typically embedded within the substance of the muscle or tendon adjacent to the proximal or distal attachment. Sesamoids function to alter the angle of the tendon as it passes to its insertion, and thereby improve mechanical advantage to the adjacent joint while protecting the tendon or muscle from excessive wear.[27] The fabella, visible on a lateral view of radiographic examination, lies at the site of high intersecting tensile stresses along the posterolateral corner of the knee joint, and acts as a pulley to redirect tensile forces and equalize stress along the posterolateral knee joint capsule. The fabella is present only in approximately 20% of the population.[28] The presence of the fabella may cause compression to the common peroneal nerve.

Injury to the common peroneal nerve or its proximal branches may be caused by tight ski boots or roller blades[10]; tight, high stockings; garters; or from a below-knee cast. Similarly, patients who have recently lost a lot of weight through diet reduction[40] or because of cancer or acquired immune deficiency syndrome are more vulnerable to compression because the protective effect of body fat is lessened. This is especially so in the bedridden patient whose lateral knee makes contact against the bed rail. Neuropathy may result from falling asleep with the lateral aspect of the calf resting against a sharp or protruding object, and is more likely in the person who is unconscious from drug ingestion or anesthesia. Various disease states may result in peroneal nerve lesion as the result of impaired nutrition of the nerve; this includes diabetes as the most common cause, followed by polyarteritis nodosa, other collagen vascular diseases, and endemic leprosy.[31]

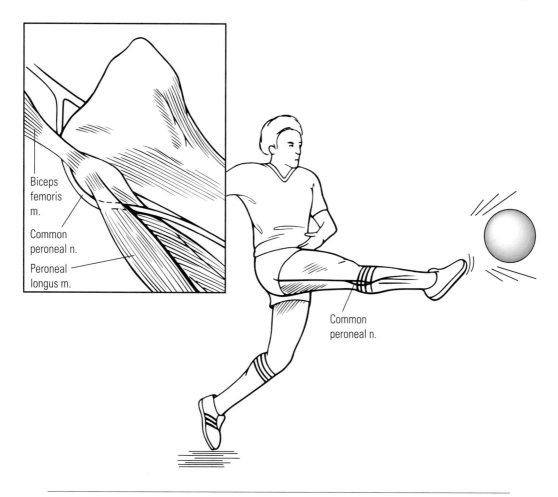

Biceps
femoris
m.

Common
peroneal n.

Peroneal
longus m.

Common
peroneal n.

FIG. 33-3 The sudden violent soccer outside kick has the effect of tensing the common peroneal nerve, both proximal as well as distal to the knee, causing tethering and compression of the nerve as it winds about the fibular neck.

5. What mechanism of injury involves traction of the common peroneal nerve at the fibular neck?

Because the nerve is tethered around the fibular neck, it is vulnerable to acute traction from excessive stretch on the length of the nerve, and thereby results in a neuropraxic lesion. A sudden plantar-inversion moment applied distally at the foot and ankle tenses the peroneus longus muscle and tautens the fibrous edge of its origin over the common peroneal nerve at the fibular neck.[8] Moreover, because of the course of the common peroneal nerve distal to the knee, this same motion stretches the nerve along its length and further tenses it proximally over the lower hook on the tendinous arch,[16,32,33] resulting in hemorrhage within the nerve.[26] Injury to the common peroneal nerve may also occur by a violent twisting[42] of the lower extremity during athletic activity that involves the combined postures of straight leg raising, hip adduction, medial rotation, and ankle plantar flexion and inversion. The superimposition of these lower limb postures has the simultaneous effect of tensing the entire length of the common peroneal nerve, thus causing focal compression at the fibular neck (Fig. 33-3). A severe varus injury to the knee may also cause traction of the nerve.

6. How would compromise of the common peroneal nerve at the fibular neck give rise to recurrent ankle sprain?

The relationship between the common peroneal nerve and ankle sprain injury is understood against the backdrop of peroneal muscle function at the foot and ankle. During late stance phase of gait between heel rise and push-off, the foot is postured in decided plantarflexion. The relationship of the mortise to components of the ankle during plantarflexion is unstable because the narrow posterior trochlea of the talus lies between the two malleoli. The reduction of bone-on-bone contact within the mortise results in greater intramalleolar distance and causes potential instability of the ankle joint. As the foot postures into plantar flexion, the thruster muscles such as the triceps surae and other posterior compartment musculature exhibit peak electrical activity as they collectively contract. Both the tibialis posterior and flexor hallucis longus concentrically contract. However, the tendons of these muscles wind around the medial malleolus and pass medial to the subtalar joint axes, which endows the muscles with an inversion role. In the absence of osseous stability within the mortise, contraction of these two muscles results in inversion. The tendency toward inversion is additionally biased by the osseous architectural obliquity of the axis of the upper ankle joint, in which the fibula projects more distally than the tibia. Unrestrained inversion causes weight bearing to be concentrated along the lateral border of the sole and predisposes the ankle toward an inversion sprain. An excessive inversion moment is normally countered by the static restraint of the anterior talofibular ligament.

During late stance, the peroneals—whose alignment is consistent with the anterior talofibular ligament—act as *dynamic stabilizers* to provide lateral ankle stability in marked plantar flexion associated with push-off. The peroneals work as dynamic ligaments and provide a counter-inversion moment, thereby restoring rotary balance to the foot (see Fig. 32-5). Thus in the closed kinetic chain during gait, the peroneals do not evert but, rather, concentrically contract to counterbalance the inversion moment generated by the middle and deep layers of the posterior compartment of the leg (the flexor hallucis, flexor digitorum, and posterior tibialis, respectively). This synergic *guy support mechanism* between the evertors and the inverters has the net effect of maintaining the ankle in neutral so that a maximal plantarflexion moment successfully propels the body forward without injury to the ankle. Palpation of the common peroneal nerve as it winds subcutaneously around the neck of the fibula is critical because entrapment at the fibular tunnel may give rise to recurrent lateral ankle sprain caused by loss of the lateral peroneal component of the guy support mechanism at the foot.

7. What is superficial peroneal nerve entrapment?

The superficial peroneal nerve descends between the extensor digitorum longus and peroneal muscles and innervates both peroneals proximally as it courses through the anterolateral compartment of the leg. After providing motor innervation to the peroneals, the nerve descends under cover of the peroneus brevis to the deep crural fascia at the level of the middle and distal third of the leg. It pierces the fascia approximately 10 to 12 cm above the tip of the lateral malleolus to become subcutaneous. In the majority of persons,[17] bifurcation of the nerve occurs beyond the crural fascia and approximately 6.5 cm[13] above the lateral malleolus, where the nerve divides into the intermediate and medial dorsal cutaneous nerves. The medial dorsal cutaneous nerves divide into the dorsal digital nerves at the lower border of the inferior extensor retinaculum.

Entrapment of the superficial peroneal nerve has been described in both young dancers and athletes,[39] with the lesion site located where the nerve pierces the deep crural fascia of the anterior or lateral compartment of the leg to become superficial. The site of entrapment is located distal to the point of innervation of the peroneus muscles, and thus the symptoms are purely sensory, manifesting as pain and altered sensation in its cutaneous distribution. The loss of cutaneous innervation associated with a lesion of the superficial branch is extensive, covering the distal lateral calf, the lateral malleolus, the dorsum of the foot, and the medial three or four toes up to the interphalangeal joint. Nerve trauma may occur as a result of compression from ski boots and tight-fitting shoes as the nerve is compressed between the tongue of the footwear and the underlying bone on the dorsum of the foot. Postulated etiologies for compression include a sprain of the anterior talofibular ligament[12] and peroneal muscle herniation caused by an anterolateral fascia defect.

In contrast to situations involving compression, the superficial peroneal nerve may also undergo stretching at the site where it becomes superficial, similar to stretching of the common peroneal nerve within the fibular tunnel. The crural fascia forms a narrow *fascial tunnel* for the superficial peroneal nerve that ranges between 1 and 11 cm in length.[43] Because the nerve is fixed by the length of the tunnel, that site represents a potential stress riser. Forced inversion of the ankle, as may occur during a lateral ankle sprain (Fig. 33-4), may irritate or stretch the superficial peroneal nerve[2] over the fascial border of the tunnel. This may result in scar-

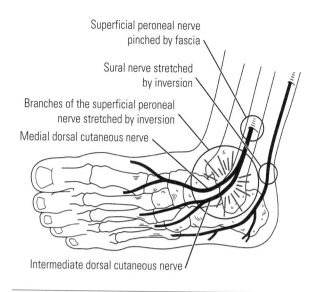

Superficial peroneal nerve
pinched by fascia

Sural nerve stretched
by inversion

Branches of the superficial peroneal
nerve stretched by inversion

Medial dorsal cutaneous nerve

Intermediate dorsal cutaneous nerve

FIG. 33-4 Both the superficial peroneal and sural nerve may be stretched during an ankle sprain. (From Magee DJ: *Orthopedic physical assessment,* Philadelphia, 1997, WB Saunders.)

ring of the tunnel opening, which leads to stenosis and further irritation.

8. How can exertional compartment syndrome compromise peroneal nerve function?

Exertional compartment syndromes are often exercise induced, and typically occur either chronically in well-trained athletes[24] or acutely in individuals performing unaccustomed exercises, such as marching or prolonged running (see pp. 505-507). A compartment syndrome occurs when increased pressure within a limited space compromises the circulation to the contents of that space, resulting in reduction of muscle and nerve perfusion. In both traumatic and exercise-induced compartment syndromes, the muscles within the compartment enlarge with lactate[34] and cause a reduction in blood flow to the relatively small anterior and lateral crural compartments. Muscle bulk increases by 20% after exercise.[47] This is not to be confused with anterior shin splint syndrome, which shows no pressure elevation within the anterolateral compartment of the leg.[7] Individual variation in the relationship of muscle bulk to compartment volume may account for the susceptibility of certain persons to exercise-induced compartment syndrome.[1] Although the pathophysiology of both forms of compartment syndrome are essentially the same, the end result of the acute form differs from that of the chronic. In both conditions, ischemia resulting from abnormal pressure causes pain. In the acute syndrome, however, continued, mounting pressure causes pain out of proportion, pulselessness, and dramatic pain on passive stretching of the muscles in the involved compartment; this causes irreversible tissue necrosis. With the chronic form, the changes are reversible and the involved muscles may be completely normal between episodes. The patient's initial complaint includes a deep ache or pain over the anterior or lateral compartments of the leg during or after a relatively long period of exercise; the pain disappears with cessation of activity. Symptoms often interfere enough to cause the athlete to either rest or reduce the intensity of the activity, and the symptoms may be reproduced by either dorsiflexion or plantar flexion of the foot. This patient may have decreased sensation in the first web space. Patients with recurrent exertion compartment syndrome are at risk for developing peroneal muscle herniation at the fascial tunnel in the anterolateral distal leg. This tunnel serves as a hiatus and source of intracompartment relief of pressure buildup. The herniated muscle may suffer ischemia projecting beyond the hiatus, whereas the superficial peroneal nerve is compressed. In contrast, because the deep peroneal nerve descends through the leg in the anterior compartment between the peroneus longus (lateral compartment) and the extensor digitorum longus (anterior compartment) adjacent to the anterior intermuscular septum, it may also be compressed, accounting for sensory loss at the first web space. Management involves fasciotomy of the lateral compartment.

9. What are the extensor retinacula at the ankle?

The *retinacula* function to hold down the tendons deriving from muscles of the anterior crural compartment, thus preventing anterior bowstringing during dorsiflexion of the ankle joint.[27] The superior extensor retinaculum is a strong, broad band of deep crural fascia passing from the fibula to the tibia, proximal to the malleoli. The inferior extensor retinaculum is a Y-shaped band of deep fascia, consisting of a stem and two rami, overlying the dorsum of the foot and front of the ankle joint. The stem of the Y originates on the upper border of the lateral calcaneus and courses medially over the front of the ankle, where the limbs of the Y diverge. The upper limb, known as the *oblique superomedial band,* attaches on the medial malleolus, whereas the lower limb, known as the *oblique inferomedial band*, attaches to the plantar aponeurosis.*

10. What is anterior tarsal tunnel syndrome, and at which other sites may the deep peroneal nerve sustain injury?

The *deep peroneal nerve* courses down the anterior compartment of the leg and sends branches to the muscular contents of that compartment that includes the tibialis anterior extensor digitorum longus, extensor hallucis longus, and peroneus tertius. Several centimeters (3 to 5 cm) above the ankle joint, the nerve exits from beneath the muscle belly of the extensor hallucis longus and passes beneath the superior and inferior extensor retinacula in an area known as the *anterior tarsal tunnel.*[23] In the region underneath the oblique superomedial band of the inferior extensor retinaculum, the nerve gives off a lateral branch that innervates the extensor digitorum muscle. The medial branch of the deep peroneal nerve continues forward alongside the dorsalis pedis artery, underneath the oblique inferomedial band, and over the talonavicular joint. The medial (sensory) branch then passes underneath the tendon of the extensor hallucis brevis at the junction of the first and second cuneiforms with the metatarsals, and pierces the dorsal aponeurosis of the foot to supply sensation the first web space.[37]

Compression of the deep peroneal nerve (Fig. 33-5) may occur at a number of sites because of intrinsic factors such as tendon constriction or osteophytic irritation. The most commonly described area of entrapment is known as the *anterior tarsal tunnel,* whose roof is defined by a tight inferior extensor retinaculum in proximity to the floor of the tunnel defined by the talus. The tunnel contains the tendons and tendon sheaths of the tibialis anterior and extensor hallucis longus muscles, as well as the dorsalis pedis artery and vein. Consequently, the volume of the tunnel will be altered by space-occupying lesions such as osteophytes or ganglion cysts, by callus formation, or by vascular disorders.[18] It is within the tarsal tunnel that the deep peroneal nerve bifurcates and provides motor innervation to the extensor digitorum brevis. Consequently, compression within the tunnel results in motor weakness of this muscle, and not of the anterior compartment extrinsic muscles that were innervated prior to the nerve's entrance into the anterior tarsal tunnel.

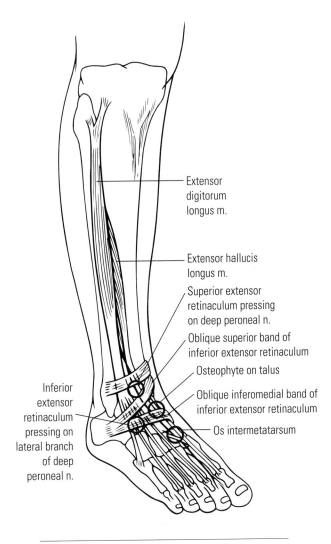

FIG. 33-5 Compression sites of the deep peroneal nerve.

If only the lateral division of the deep peroneal nerve is compromised, the primary symptom is pain in the foot. Weakness of the extensor digitorum brevis confirms that compression occurred before the bifurcation of the deep peroneal nerve.† However, if there is weakness of the long extensors of the foot, a more proximal lesion is suspected. Although lesions stemming from compression of the common peroneal nerve

---

*Two additional retinacula exist, including the flexor retinaculum, as well as the peroneal (superior and inferior) retinacula.

†To assess the strength of extensor digitorum muscle strength the foot is maximally dorsiflexed, thus eliminating the action of the extensor digitorum longus. The patient is then asked to further extend his or her great toe. This muscle is palpated as a small mound of tissue on the lateral side of the foot. The deep peroneal nerve also supplies the first dorsal interosseous muscle, but atrophy or loss of function is not practically assessable.

are typically mixed and involve both superficial and deep divisions of the nerve that include motor and sensory loss, this is not always the case. Patients with lesions at the fibular level may demonstrate affectations of only the deep branch.[9]

The deep peroneal nerve may also become entrapped at other locations in the foot and ankle. The nerve may be compressed under the superior edge of the inferior retinaculum, where the extensor hallucis longer tendon crosses over the nerve.[5] Alternatively, the nerve may be trapped under the tendon of the extensor hallucis brevis.[15,16] Similarly, bony osteophytes from the medial midtarsus, including the talonavicular joints, naviculocuneiform joints, cuneiform metatarsal joints, or between the bases of the first and second metatarsals (os intermetatarseum) have also been implicated.[29,38] Some ballet dancers have prominent dorsal ridges of the tarsal joints that compress the nerve when assuming the pointe position (Fig. 33-6).

External factors may also cause compression of the deep peroneal nerve. Among these factors are tight-fitting ski boots and blows to the dorsum of the foot, as occurs in soccer players (described in the next section). Patients may have a history of recurrent lateral ankle sprain in which the ankle and foot is plantar flexed and inverted. This posture places the deep peroneal nerve under maximal stretch over the dorsal capsule covering the tarsal joints. The equinus posture of the foot associated with wearing high heeled shoes also places increased tension on the deep peroneal nerve.[6] A common design of women's shoes places the dorsal straps over two anatomically vulnerable sites for the deep peroneal nerve, and thus represents a form of external double crush. The proximal strap is placed over the anterior tarsal tunnel, and the distal strap compresses the tendon of the extensor hallucis brevis.[21]

11. How would contusion occur to the dorsal cutaneous nerves of the foot?

Traumatic neuropathy caused by forceful impact to the dorsum of the foot may contuse the medial or intermediate dorsal cutaneous branches of the deep peroneal nerve.[11] These nerves are especially susceptible at the tarsal-metatarsal area, where they lie superficial over a bony prominence.[48] In soccer this neuropathy is most commonly caused by tight-fitting shoes. Injury may also involve the lateral dorsal cutaneous nerve that is a continuation of the sural nerve distal to the lateral malleolus. A positive Tinel's sign may be elicited, with varying degrees of paresthesias and numbness in the

cutaneous distribution of these nerves. Management includes restriction of activities until symptoms subside, appropriate shoe wear, and appropriate padding over the areas of compression.

12. What is the clinical presentation of peroneal neuropathy?

- *Common Peroneal Palsy.* The clinical presentation of common peroneal palsy varies according to whether the lesion is acute or slowly progressive. The most common form of neuropathy is the acute compressive variety, in which external trauma compresses the nerve against the underlying bone. The patient initially feels local pain from the impact and pain (likened to an electric shock) radiating down the anterior leg and into the dorsum of the foot. Evidence of abrasion or ecchymosis over the site of impact may be present. Presentation consists of painless loss of motor power manifesting as *foot drop.* The foot drop is caused by transient neuropraxia following contusion to the nerve that lasts 1 to 2 days.[48] A positive Tinel's sign at the site of injury is a common finding. Prolonged sensory symptoms are few; if present, they manifest as a partial sensory loss in either the superficial or deep peroneal cutaneous territories.[9]

  In contrast with the acute form, patients with entrapment or chronic progressive lesions have radiating pain and slowly progressive motor and sensory disturbance. Pain is initially focused at the lateral knee and spreads distally to the lateral aspect of the leg and foot in the cutaneous distribution of both the deep and superficial peroneal nerves. In severe cases pain may radiate in retrograde fashion into the thigh. Motor weakness involves the distribution of both the superficial and deep peroneals, causing weakness of eversion and dorsiflexion.* Weakness of eversion is usually unnoticed by the patient because of the drop foot. Peroneal muscle weakness becomes evident when the patient cannot walk along the medial borders of his or her foot. Forced inversion and plantar flexion of the foot will increase pain. The pretibials also provide a significant contribution to inversion as a function of their relation to the ankle joint axis, despite the fact that the tibial nerve via the posterior compartment muscles supply the primary inversion moment at the ankle. The patient may be so preoccu-

---

*Although the muscles of the anterior compartment contribute to inversion, it is the posterior compartment muscles, innervated by the posterior tibial nerve that invert the foot and ankle.

pied with other symptoms that he or she does not notice weakness of ankle inversion.

- *Superficial Peroneal Nerve Entrapment.* The clinical presentation of superficial peroneal nerve entrapment includes the symptoms of burning, superficial pain; numbness; and paresthesia along the nerve distribution that are worse with activity and improve with rest. Retrograde pain may also occur.[15,16] There is no motor loss. Point tenderness is found exactly over the area at which the nerve pierces the fascia. Nerve enlargement or nodular fibrosis may be palpated in persons with sparse subcutaneous fatty investiture, and may exacerbate radiating pain. Positive results of three provocative tests provide clinical evidence of superficial peroneal entrapment. In the first test, the therapist palpates the nerve at the impingement site while the patient dorsiflexes and everts the ankle against resistance. In the second test the clinician passively plantar flexes and inverts the foot without palpating the nerve, and thereby imparts a stretch to the nerve. In the third test the examiner stretches the nerve as in the second test, all the while percussing the nerve as it emerges from the fascial tunnel.[43] A positive result for these provocative tests is the reproduction of pain and paresthesia over the nerve's cutaneous distribution. Electromyographic studies of the peroneal and anterior tibial muscles help identify this syndrome.

- *Deep Peroneal Nerve Entrapment.* Features of neuropathy depend on whether the sensory or motor fibers of the deep peroneal nerve are affected. Weakness of the extensor digitorum brevis will occur only if compression occurred proximal to the anterior tarsal tunnel. Sensory symptoms include numbness and paresthesias in the first dorsal web space. The patient may feel an aching at the ankle and dorsum of the foot. Nocturnal pain and paresthesias may awaken the patient; the pain and paresthesias are relieved by moving the foot about. The patient may report that certain postures provide pain relief, such as extension and ankle eversion, which relieve tension on the nerve from investing fascia forming the roof of the tunnel.[9] A positive Tinel's sign may be present over the nerve. When the entrapment is long standing, atrophy of the extensor digitorum brevis[12] and trophic changes[32,33] of the metatarsal bones (e.g., osteoporosis) may occur. Electromyographic studies demonstrate an increased distal latency of the deep peroneal nerve, along with active and chronic denervation of the extensor digitorum brevis.[12]

13. What is the differential diagnosis?

The key to diagnosis of entrapment neuropathy is a thorough knowledge of the peripheral neuroanatomy of the lower extremity. The examination for and location of pain, as well as the presence of Tinel's sign and the distribution of the altered sensation or radiation, is specific for each type of entrapment.

- *Ganglion cysts* can be very difficult to distinguish clinically from an entrapment disorder. Ganglia may arise from the peroneus longus muscle or superior tibiofibular joint, whereas tumors of the nerve itself may develop. Ganglia are easily detected by computed tomography or magnetic resonance imaging.

- *Sciatic nerve lesions* may occur in the pelvis as a result of neoplasms spreading from the colon or rectum; these lesions may cause sciatic nerve compression. In the buttock, penetrating trauma from a knife or gunshot wound or from a misplaced deep intramuscular injection may injure the sciatic nerve. Alternatively, injury to the sciatic nerve may be caused by a hip fracture or dislocation or by a hip arthroplasty. These represent more proximal causes of foot drop that must be differentiated from foot drop that is caused by common peroneal palsy (as, for example, in the case of a patient who suffered a posterior dislocation of the hip with subsequent fracture as a result of trauma, followed by open joint surgery, and who demonstrated a foot drop postoperatively). The question arises as to whether the patient's foot drop was caused by traumatic injury or surgical insult to the sciatic nerve, or whether it was simply a result of pressure on the common peroneal nerve caused by limb positioning during surgery. Answering this question is extremely important in determination of prognosis for full recovery and the time required to recover and for medicolegal issues. Weakness or wasting of the biceps femoris suggests a proximal lesion, whereas normal lateral hamstring strength suggests that palsy derives from pressure at the fibular neck and head during surgery.[31] Another way to differentiate a sciatic nerve lesion from a common peroneal nerve injury is to test the ankle invertors by having the patient walk on the lateral borders of the feet. The muscles that invert the foot are innervated by the posterior tibial nerve, not by the common peroneal nerve. The patient who cannot ambulate along the lateral border of the foot, in addition to having a foot drop, also has a sustained injury proximal to the division of the sciatic nerve (i.e., above the knee). Electrophysiologic data from a sciatic nerve lesion show no focal slowing at the fibular head, and possibly an abnormal sural nerve. Electromyographic data may be abnormal outside the territory of the peroneal nerve, *excluding* the paraspinal muscles.[9]

- *Lumbosacral nerve root lesions* are typically characterized by a history of low back pain that migrated distally as sciatica. An L5 radiculopathy may resemble peroneal palsy. The motor and sensory loss present as myotomal and dermatomal loss, and do not present according to peripheral nerve distribution. Furthermore, an L5 radiculopathy manifests as a depressed tibial posterior reflex,* whereas peroneal neuropathy does not. Electromyographic data deriving from a root lesion demonstrate denervation of muscles outside the peroneal nerve territory, such as the tibialis posterior, the short head of the biceps femoris, the popliteus, the tensor fasciae latae, *and* the paraspinal musculature. The peroneal sensory action is normal and shows no focal slowing at the fibular head.[9]

- *Mononeuritis multiplex* is a syndrome involving major nerve trunks such as the radial, peroneal, and sciatic nerves in an asymmetric or symmetric profile. The syndrome is caused by systemic illness such as diabetes, leprosy, polyarteritis nodosa, rheumatoid arthritis, or systemic lupus erythematosus. Mononeuritis multiplex commonly affects the peroneal nerve, causing clinical neurologic signs that are indistinguishable from those of a pressure palsy. The electrophysiologic findings may be identical, except that mononeuritis multiplex does not show focal slowing or decrement of the muscle action potential across the fibular head since the lesion is not demyelinating.[9]

14. What is peroneal muscle atrophy?

Peroneal muscle atrophy (otherwise known as Charcot-Marie-Tooth disease or Dejerine-Sottas disease) is a relatively common, hereditary, axonopathy-type disorder of the peripheral nervous system that is characterized by an autosomal dominant pattern of inheritance. The disorder manifests as weakness and atrophy, primarily in the peroneal and distal muscles of the leg. This manifestation is a result of a slow but progressive muscle paresis in the distribution of the peroneal and posterior tibial nerves. Family members who carry the trait exhibit high pedal arches, clubfoot, and absent ankle jerks.[41] Attention is first drawn to the case of the child who has difficulty in fitting shoes secondary to a high instep, hammer toes, and wasting of the small muscles of the feet. The legs become progressively thinner, and eventually the lower limbs take on a "stork-" or spindle-like appearance similar to an inverted champagne bottle. Patients typically demonstrate foot drop and associated steppage gait. Instead of shrinking and wasting as in motor neuron disease, the atrophy slowly creeps up the limb and is accompanied by a stocking-glove decrease in vibration, pain, and temperature.[4] Deep tendon reflexes are absent. Intrinsic muscle wasting of the hands develops later, at approximately age 20, with eventual wasting of both the thenar and hypothenar musculature; the fingers tend to curl up. The muscles of the face and limb girdles are unaffected, and sphincter function remains intact. Despite the deformities, the degree of disability is so slight as to become hidden when the patient wears trousers. The disease becomes arrested in midlife and is compatible with a normal life span. Treatment is nonspecific and includes bracing to correct for foot drop.

15. What therapeutic intervention would best manage these patients?

When the compressive lesion derives proximally at the fibular head, the motor disturbance should consist of bracing to offset the foot drop and thereby allow normal ambulation. Normal function should return once neuropraxia resolves. As active motion of the involved ankle dorsiflexors and foot evertors returns, gravity-assisted active contraction is encouraged and progressed through neutral-gravity and, finally, to an antigravity mode. Once active motion reasserts itself, walking may begin in a mode that is protective of the healing nerve. Toward this end, a lateral sole wedge and flare are appropriate to maintain an eversion posture of the foot and thereby relax tension on the common peroneal nerve.[15,16]

Entrapment of the superficial peroneal nerve is managed by removal of the offending compression, rest, and the use of a lateral sole wedge and shoe flare to increase eversion of the foot and relax the fascia of the lateral aspect of the leg. Entrapment of the deep peroneal nerve involves identification and removal of any external source of compression. Occasionally, a short-leg walking case or cast-brace is used to rest the affected lower limb by posturing the foot and ankle in

---

*A tibialis posterior reflex is assessed in the following manner: hold the forefoot in slight dorsiflexion and eversion and tap the tibial posterior tendon with a reflex hammer on the medial side of the foot just before its tendon's insertion into the navicular tuberosity; a 2+ grade generates a slight plantar inversion.

slight dorsiflexion and eversion. This position eliminates tension to the irritated nerve and allows the nerve
to recover.[3] Padding around the nerve is appropriate.

Gently introducing tension to the peroneal tract
and progressively increasing the tension with patient
tolerance frees the nerve from binding as it courses
throughout the distal lower extremity. Nerve mobilization of the peroneal axis begins with plantar flexion at
the foot and flexion of the knee and hip joints. Eventually, tension on the peroneal tract is maximized by superimposing plantar flexion and inversion of the foot,
on knee extension, and by medial hip rotation and adduction.[6] There is evidence that the "B" family of vita-
mins provides nutritional maintenance and has healing
properties for peripheral nerves.

REFERENCES

1. Bachner EJ, Friedman MJ: Injuries to the leg. In Nicholas JA, Hershman EB, editors: *The lower extremity and spine in sports medicine,* ed 2, St Louis, 1995, Mosby.
2. Banerjee T, Koons DD: Superficial peroneal nerve entrapment, *J Neurosurg* 55(6):991-992, 1981.
3. Baxter D: *The foot and ankle in sports,* St Louis, 1995, Mosby.
4. Berkow R, Fletcher AJ, editors: *The Merck manual of diagnosis and therapy,* ed 15, Rahway, NJ, 1987, Merck Sharp & Dohme Research Laboratories.
5. Borges LF, Halle HM, Selkoe DJ, et al: The anterior tarsal tunnel syndrome: report of two cases, *J Neurosurg* 54(1):89-92, 1981.
6. Butler DS: *Mobilization of the nervous system,* Melbourne, Australia, 1991, Churchill Livingstone.
7. D'Ambrosia RD, Zelis RF, Chuinard RG et al: Interstitial pressure measurements in the anterior and posterior compartments in athletes with shin splints, *Am J Sports Med* 5(3):127-131, 1977.
8. Davies JA: Peroneal compartment syndrome secondary to rupture of the peroneus longus, *J Bone Joint Surg Am* 61(5):783-784, 1979.
9. Dawson DM, Hallett M, Millender LH, editors: *Entrapment neuropathies,* ed 2, Boston, 1990, Little, Brown.
10. Dewitt LD, Greenberg HS: Roller disco neuropathy, *JAMA,* 246(1):836, 1981.
11. Hoadley AF: Six cases of metatarsalgia, *Chicago Med Rec* 5:32, 1893.
12. Jones DC, Singer KM: Soft-tissue conditions of the ankle and foot. In Nicholas JA, Hershman EB, editors: *The lower extremity and spine in sports medicine,* ed 2, St Louis, 1995, Mosby.
13. Kernohan J, Levack B, Wilson JN: Entrapment of the superficial peroneal nerve, *J Bone Joint Surg Br* 67(1):60-61, 1985.
14. Koller RL, Bland NK: Strawberry pickers' palsy *Arch Neurol* 37(5):320, 1980.
15. Kopell HP, Thompson WAL: *New Engl J Med* 262:56, 1960.
16. Kopell HP, Thompson WAL: *Peripheral entrapment neu-*

17. *ropathies,* Huntington, New York, 1976, Robert E Krieger Publishing.
18. Kosinski C: The course: mutual relations and distribution of the cutaneous nerve in the metazonal region of the leg and foot, *J Anat* 60:274, 1926.
18. Kravatte MA: *J Am Podiatr Assoc* 61:457, 1971.
19. Kumaki D: The facts of Kathmandu: squatter's palsy, *JAMA* 257(1):28, 1987.
20. Large DF, Ludlam CA, MacNicol MF: Common peroneal nerve entrapment in a hemophiliac, *Clin Orthop* 181:165-166, 1983.
21. Macinnon SE, Dellon AL: *Surgery of the peripheral nerve,* New York, 1988, Thieme.
22. Mangieri JV: Peroneal-nerve injury from an enlarged fabella: a case report, *J Bone Joint Surg Am* 55(2):395-397, 1973.
23. Marinacci AA: Neurological syndromes of the tarsal tunnels, *Bulletin of the Los Angeles Neurological Society* 33:90-100, 1968.
24. Martens MA et al: Chronic leg pain in athletes due to a recurrent compartment syndrome, *Am J Sports Med* 12(2):148-151, 1984.
25. Maudsley RH: Fibular tunnel syndrome, *J Bone Joint Surg Br* 49:384, 1967.
26. Meals RA: Peroneal nerve palsy complicating ankle sprain, *J Bone Joint Surg Am,* 59(7):966-968, 1977.
27. Moore KL: *Clinically oriented anatomy,* ed 2, Baltimore, 1985, Williams and Wilkins.
28. Muller W: *The knee: form, function, and ligament reconstruction,* New York, 1983, Springer-Verlag.
29. Murphy PC, Baxter DE: Nerve entrapment of the foot and ankle in runners, *Clin Sports Med* 4(4):753-763, 1985.
30. Pagnani MJ, Warren RF, Arnoczky SP, et al: Anatomy of the knee. In Nicholas JA, Hershman EB, editors: *The lower extremity and spine in sports medicine,* ed 2, St Louis, 1995, Mosby.
31. Patten J: *Neurological differential diagnosis,* ed 2, London, 1995, Springer.
32. Pecina MM, Krmpotic-Nemanic J, Markiewitz AD: *Tunnel syndromes,* Boca Raton, Fla, 1991, CRC Press.
33. Pecina M: Ostecenja zivcanog stabla (ogranaka ishijadikus uvjetovana posebnim topograskoantosskim odonosima, disertacija), *Medicinsi Fafultet,* 1969.
34. Qvarfordt P et al: Intramuscular pressure, muscle blood flow, and skeletal muscle metabolism in chronic anterior tibial compartment syndrome, Clin Orthop 179:284-290, 1983.
35. Rose HA, Hood RW, Otis JC, et al: Peroneal-nerve palsy following total knee arthroplasty: a review of The Hospital for Special Surgery experience, *J Bone Joint Surg Am* 64(3):347-351, 1982.
36. Sadhu HS, Sandberg BS: Occupational compression of the common peroneal nerve at the neck of the fibula, *Aust NZ J Surg* 46:160, 1976.
37. Sarrafican AK: *Anatomy of the foot and ankle: descriptive, topographic, functional,* Philadelphia, 1983, JB Lippincott.
38. Schon LC, Baxter DE: Neuropathies of the foot and ankle in athletes, *Clin Sports Med* 9(2):489-508, 1990.
39. Schon LC: Nerve entrapment, neuropathy, and nerve dysfunction in athletes, *Orthop Clin North Am* 25(1):47-59, 1994.

40. Sherman DG, Easton JD: Dieting and peroneal nerve palsy, *JAMA* 238(3):230-231, 1977.

41. Spillane JD, Spillane JA: *An atlas of clinical neurology,* ed 3, Oxford, 1982, Oxford University Press.

42. Spindler KP, Pappas J: Neurovascular problems. In Nicholas JA, Hershman EB, editors: *The lower extremity and spine in sports medicine,* ed 2, St Louis, 1995, Mosby.

43. Styf J: Entrapment of the superficial peroneal nerve: diagnosis and results of decompression, *J Bone Joint Surg Br* 71(1):131-135, 1989.

44. Sunderland S, Bradley KC: The cross-sectional area of peripheral nerve trunks devoted to nerve fibers, *Brain* 72:428-439, 1949.

45. Sunderland S: *Nerves and nerve injuries,* ed 2, London, 1978, Churchill-Livingstone.

46. Tupmann GS: *Br J Surg* 45:23, 1957.

47. Wright S: *Applied physiology,* ed 10, London, 1961, Oxford University Press.

48. Xethalis JL, Lorei MP: Soccer injuries. In Nicholas JA, Hershman EB, editors: *The lower extremity and spine in sports medicine,* ed 2, St Louis, 1995, Mosby.

RECOMMENDED READING

Dawson DM, Hallett M, Millender LH, editors: *Entrapment neuropathies,* ed 2, Boston, 1990, Little, Brown.

Pecina MM, Krmpotic-Nemanic J, Markiewitz AD: *Tunnel syndromes,* Boca Raton, Fla, 1991, CRC Press.

34

Pain over Posterior Aspect of the Ankle after Brisk Walking and When Rising on Tiptoe, with a Lower Extremity Profile of Tightness in Right Posterior Lower Extremity Musculature and Calcaneal Deviation from Subtalar Joint Neutral

CASE 1: A 38-year-old seasoned jogger was accustomed to jogging in the city for 30 minutes every day before moving to a rural area following a company incentive offer to relocate. Enjoying the fresh air, he now spent 45 minutes each day jogging over a long stretch of grass-covered hilly terrain. As the meadow was wet from dew during his morning jog, he put away his running shoes and invested in spiked running shoes with a rigid heel counter. Over the last few weeks he complains of a diffuse painful swelling along the posterior aspect of his distal leg just above his heel bone. In response, he has initiated warm-up exercises and stretching activities, which seem to offer some measure of relief. He enters your office for a consultation, which reveals the following clinical presentation:

OBSERVATION   A cavus foot posture is noted bilaterally, left greater than right.

PALPATION   Palpation yields diffuse painful swelling and crepitus over the left Achilles tendon. The fat pad is neither painful nor tender. Callous formation is noted under the first and fifth metatarsal heads.

MALALIGNMENT   A bilateral forefoot valgus is noted, left greater than right.

PASSIVE RANGE OF MOTION   Passive range of motion of left ankle joint demonstrates a painful arc of movement at the neutral position during excursion from dorsiflexion to plantarflexion and vice versa.

ACTIVE RANGE OF MOTION   Active range of motion is full but mildly uncomfortable. Plantarflexion is more uncomfortable than dorsiflexion.

MUSCLE STRENGTH   Normal for dorsiflexion of the left ankle. The patient cannot sustain standing left tiptoe for long secondary to discomfort.

FLEXIBILITY   Demonstrates tightness in several bilateral lower extremity structures including the right hamstring muscle group and gastrocnemius-soleus complex.

SPECIAL TESTS   Negative Thomas sign, negative leg length discrepancy, and a normal Q angle.

CASE 2: An obese 42-year-old house wife followed her physician's advice to incorporate an exercise regimen as part of a weight reduction strategy. She began by walking briskly every morning precisely at 6 AM for 3 miles along with two other friends despite the cold winter weather. She wore her old, but comfortable, soft, worn tennis shoes that she normally used for gardening in the warmer months. Four weeks later and 8 pounds lighter she began to feel an uncomfortable burning pain over the posterior aspect of her right ankle in her daily walk. The pain became less severe as she continued to walk, only to worsen about 1 hour after she finished. She reports that negotiating steep inclines, stairs, as well as rising up on to her tiptoes provokes similar pain. The patient reports no significant medical history, but admits to walking along the banked shoulder of a well-paved concrete road. Symptoms intensified as she attempted to ignore them and she began to take aspirin twice per day that provided some relief. Two weeks later, she complains of early morning pain and stiffness when getting out of bed during her first few steps that gradually subsides during the day. Symptoms are reproduced during running.

OBSERVATION   Slight erythema over her right Achilles tendon as compared to the uninvolved side. During weight bearing you notice bilateral valgus position of both heels and pronation of both feet. In the non–weight-bearing posture, both feet demonstrate a forefoot varus foot posture.

PALPATION   There is slight crepitus, warmth, and swelling over the right calcaneal tendon 4 cm above its insertion into the os calcis. Extreme tenderness is provoked during gentle palpation. Tenderness does not extend to the plantar aspect of the rearfoot.

ACTIVE RANGE OF MOTION   Within functional limits to all motions of the foot and ankle as compared with the contralateral extremity. A painful arc is noted as the right ankle is sagittally moved from extreme plantarflexion to dorsiflexion and vice versa that is not confined to a particular juncture in the range, but rather moves with tendon excursion.

PASSIVE RANGE OF MOTION   Passive range of motion of right ankle in the sagittal plane is pain free, although uncomfortable upon dorsiflexion.

MUSCLE STRENGTH   Resistive dorsiflexion is mildly uncomfortable. Resistive plantarflexion is moderately painful. Right pretibial muscles are graded G only.

FLEXIBILITY TESTING   Demonstrates tightness is several bilateral lower extremity structures including the right hamstring muscle group and gastrocnemius-soleus complex.

ALIGNMENT   A pattern of miserable malalignment of femoral anteversion and genu varum emerges.

SPECIAL TESTS   Negative squeeze test and Homan's sign. There is no leg length discrepancy. Q angle is measured at 20° bilaterally.

CLUE:

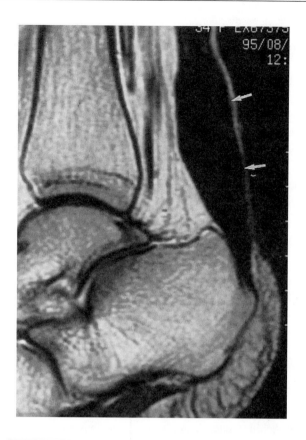

(From Taylor JAM, Resnick D: *Skeletal imaging: atlas of the spine and extremities,* Philadelphia, 2000, WB Saunders.)

? Questions

1. What is most likely the cause of pain in the patients in Cases 1 and 2?
2. What is the relative anatomy of the triceps surae muscle-tendon complex?
3. In what three ways is the gastrocnemius-soleus muscle unique?
4. What is the physiologic difference between the type of muscle fibers comprising the gastrocnemius and soleus muscles?
5. What is the biomechanical significance of deviation of the Achilles tendon insertion from the midline of the os calcis?
6. How is a shortened gastrocnemius differentiated from a shortened soleus muscle?
7. What is the etiology of gastrocnemius-soleus muscle shortness or weakness, and how does this contribute to suboptimal triceps surae contraction?
8. How do gastrocnemius and soleus act synergistically in relation to the ankle joint and antagonistically in relation to knee joint function?
9. What portion of the Achilles tendon is most vulnerable to compromise of vascular perfusion as related to tendon inflammation and degeneration?
10. What is the significance of the lateromedial spiral alignment of the distal tendon insertion?
11. How does excursion of the Achilles tendon contribute to pathologic dysfunction?

12. What is the evolution of Achilles tendon disease?
13. What are the progressive stages of Achilles tendon disease?
14. What training errors predispose this condition?
15. How would running on inclines predispose tendinitis?
16. What biomechanical problems of the foot may contribute to the development of calcaneal tendinitis?
17. What is a forefoot equinus deformity?
18. What extrinsic and intrinsic variables serve as predisposing factors in the development of Achilles tendon overuse injuries?
19. How are dancing or cycling activities related to the onset of Achilles tendinitis?
20. What is the clinical presentation?
21. What is the differential diagnosis for Achilles tendinitis?
22. What is tennis leg?
23. What is the therapeutic management of Achilles tendinitis?

---

1. What is most likely the cause of pain in the patients in Cases 1 and 2?

Paratendinitis of the calcaneal tendon in Case 1 and *Achilles tendinitis* in Case 2. The Clue in Case 2 demonstrates a magnetic resonance image of the Achilles tendon in which the bulbous enlargement of the tendon's diameter is in excess of 9 mm measured 2 cm above the bursal projection. Achilles tendinitis is the most common form of tendinitis in runners and track athletes. In basketball players, Achilles tendinitis ranks second after patellar tendinitis as the most frequent overuse injury. Considered the thickest and strongest tendon in the body, the calcaneal tendon is about 15 cm long, begins at the midleg, and receives muscular fibers almost to its termination.[61] The Achilles tendon does not have a true synovial sheath but is rather enveloped by a paratenon—an avascular synovium that surrounds and nourishes the tendon via diffusion from the epitenon. The evolution of Achilles tendon disease often begins with paratenonitis and involves a degenerative thickening of the paratenon in the absence of inflammation, which impairs tendon gliding. The Achilles tendon has a relatively poor blood supply, particularly at that junction most liable to degeneration—the insertion of the tendon midsubstance into the calcaneus.[52] Paratenonitis typically progresses to tendinosis involving degenerative changes in the tendon itself, particularly in the poorly perfused midsubstance. The suffix *-osis* in the latter infers a lack of the acute inflammatory process because the tissue at hand is avascular in nature. Rather, tendinosis is characterized by degenerative changes in the tendon only. In contrast, the suffix *-itis* (as in tendinitis) refers to an inflammatory response of white blood cells that occurs in vascularized tissue. Eventually, the entire tendon undergoes degeneration as well as inflammation in which case the condition has progressed to a full-blown tendinitis.

Authorities have alternately implicated both a hyperpronated and cavus foot as having a greater risk of Achilles tendon disorders during physical activity owing to the diminished shock absorption capacity correlated with theses malalignments.[6,39,73] Although a forefoot varus (see p. 347) or equinus deformities are often implicated with Achilles tendinitis due to compensatory subtalar joint pronation, forefoot valgus (see pp. 348-349) is cited as causative of Achilles tendinitis secondary to compensatory subtalar joint supination.[76,78]

2. What is the relative anatomy of the triceps surae muscle-tendon complex?

Triceps surae (three-headed calf muscle) is comprised of the 2 heads of gastrocnemius and the soleus muscle and share a distal conjoint tendon. These two muscles share both structural and functional roles. Running behind the axis for plantarflexion/dorsiflexion of the ankle joint, these posterior compartment muscles powerfully lift the weight of the body onto the metatarsal heads (plantarflexion). Together with flexor hallucis longus, these 3 muscles perform the propulsive function during late stance phase of gait

The *gastrocnemius* (Greek; gaster, *belly,* and kneme, *knee*) muscle is a (predominantly phasic) two-joint muscle that proximally originates from the medial and lateral femoral condyles by way of 2 separate tendon heads (Fig. 34-1). It is here that the 2 tendons form the inferior border of diamond shaped popliteal fossa. Deep to each head lies a bursa with the medial one frequently communicating with the knee joint. Within the lateral head a cartilaginous or osseous sesa-

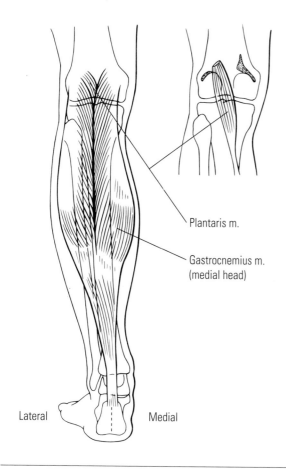

FIG. 34-1 Gastrocnemius is a two-jointed and predominantly tonic-type muscle. Plantaris also spans two joints and assists gastrocnemius in knee flexion and ankle plantarflexion.

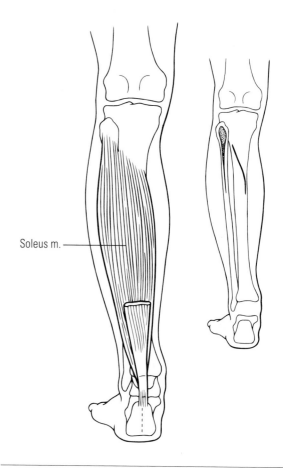

FIG. 34-2 Soleus is predominantly a phasic single jointed muscle.

moid known as the *fabella* may form.[62],* The medial head is the larger of the two and its muscular portion descends further distally behind the shaft of the tibia than that of the lateral head; this may be observed from behind when an individual rises on tiptoes. The muscle fibers of the two heads converge to distally attach to a broad tendon-aponeurosis, which fuses with the aponeurosis over the soleus muscle to distally narrow and form the Achilles tendon some 5 to 6

---

*The *fabella,* which is present in approximately one-fifth of the population as an osseous structure or as a cartilaginous analogue. Similar to the patella, the fabella is a sesamoid bone that lies at the site of high intersecting tensile stresses along the posterolateral corner of the knee joint. The fabella, connected to the fibula via the fabellofibular ligament, acts like a pulley to redirect tensile forces and equalize stress along the posterolateral knee joint capsule. (From Muller, W: *The knee: form, function, and ligament reconstruction,* New York, 1983, Springer-Verlag.)

cm above the os calcis. From their point of confluence into one homogeneous tendon, the tendon fibers take a slightly spiral course en route to their destination on the calcaneus.

The *soleus* (Fig. 34-2) is a (predominantly tonic) single-joint muscle that proximally originates from two heads of the posteromedial and lateral sides of the proximal tibia and proximal fibula, respectively. The soleus forms a broad aponeurosis that parallels the gastrocnemius before uniting with it and distally inserting on the posterior calcaneal tubercle. Manual muscle testing of soleus alone involves isolating soleus muscle function distinct from gastrocnemius activity. This may be done by placing gastrocnemius at mechanical disadvantage (active insufficiency) by flexing the knee to 90°[40] while the patient lies in the prone position[51] or while short sitting. Testing for plantarflexion in this fashion may isolate soleus while diminishing gastrocnemius contribution to plantarflexion as a function of approximating that muscles' attachments.

The 2 heads of the gastrocnemius and the soleus are collectively known as the triceps surae. The gastrocnemius muscle is the more superficial of the two. Together, both muscle share a conjoint tendon—the Achilles tendon that is the thickest, strongest, and perhaps longest (6 cm) tendon in the body.[2] Named for the only vulnerable portion of the legendary Greek warrior who fought in the war against ancient Troy, Achilles was felled by Paris who shot an arrow at his heel. The tendon inserts just medial and inferior to the posterior calcaneal tubercle (i.e., tuberosity). Instead of being surrounded by a synovial sheath, the Achilles tendon is instead covered by a pseudosheath or peritenon, as well as two small bursae: the retrocalcaneal bursa (or anterior calcaneal bursa) located anteriorly and the tendo Achillis bursa (or posterior calcaneal bursa) located posteriorly and thus subcutaneously to the distal end of the tendon as it inserts on the calcaneus[59] (Fig. 34-3). The purpose of these bursae is to minimize frictional stress to the tendon owing to the projection of the calcaneal tuberosity.[24] Prominence of the posterior tubercle may be causative in bursal inflammation.[81] The posterior calcaneal bursa is more commonly enlarged, a condition often due to wearing high heels, or tight and oversized shoes.

The *plantaris* muscle, like gastrocnemius, originates from the lateral aspect of the lateral femoral condyle posteriorly is also a two joint muscle located in the posterior compartment leg. The *muscle* belly of this muscle ranges between 7.5 to 10 cm in length and rapidly tapes to a long, thin tendon that courses between the gastrocnemius and soleus muscle. Distally, plantaris attaches on the posterior calcaneal tubercle, although medial to Achilles tendon attachment. The musculotendinous junction of plantaris is in the lateral popliteal area beneath the lateral head of gastrocnemius. Because its access tendon begins high in the leg, plantaris is therefore insignificant in function despite its holding title to the muscle with the longest tendon in the body. Plantaris is a rudimentary muscle that is analogous to the palmaris longus of the forearm. Some 30 inches long, this tendon is often harvested by surgeons as an autograft for tendon-transfer procedures. No weakness or diminished function occurs following surgical removal of plantaris. Running between gastrocnemius and soleus, plantaris may become inflamed from excessive activity of the two former muscles. This may occur in tennis players.

It is significant to note that the plantar fascia actually originates at the calcaneal tuberosity as a direct continuation of the triceps surae tendon. The Achilles tendon has lateral and medial expansions that form broad sheets descending anteriorly and inferiorly to wrap around the sides of the calcaneus; these expansions wrap under the heel to blend with the plantar fascia. Although the Achilles tendon mainly inserts on the inferior half of the calcaneus, it thins out and continues under the foot, running anteriorly and blending it with the plantar fascia. There is no break in continuity between the plantar fascia and the Achilles tendon.[79] The

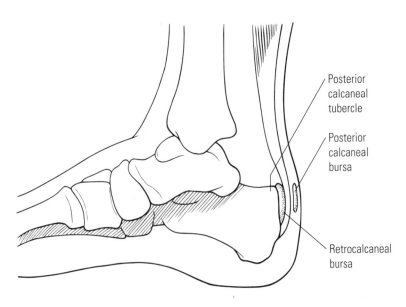

FIG. 34-3 Calcaneal bursae include the posterior calcaneal bursa and retrocalcaneal bursa.

plantar fascia is similarly continuous with the dorsal fascia of the foot as well as the flexor retinaculum of the medial ankle. The pathokinesiologic significance of this continuity means that a similar mechanism is causal for both plantar fasciitis as well as Achilles tendinitis.

3. In what three ways is the gastrocnemius-soleus muscle unique?

- *Balance maintenance during quiet standing.* The standing posture of humans is extremely energy efficient when compared with the stance of quadrupeds, who must stand on flexed extremities. In the human, the line of gravity falls very close or through the joint axes so that only one muscle group in the lower extremities need be active to maintain balance. In the relaxed standing posture, the vertical projection of the center of mass falls behind the hip joint, in front of the knee joint, and in front of the ankle joint. As a result, the center of gravity falls slightly forward of the body and may cause toppling forward in the sagittal plane. This tendency is countered by active tonic contraction of the soleus muscle, which generates a constant low-grade internally generated counter force (Fig. 34-4). Soleus, like other postural muscles, is comprised of the red, oxidative metabolic type muscle fiber that can generate continuous contractile output without succumbing to significant fatigue.*
- *Vascular return function.* Because the triceps surae comprises the major portion of the muscles of the calf they, by way of continuous contractile tension during ambulation, largely contribute to the vascular function of venous return. However, despite gastrocnemius's antigravity function, prolonged standing (especially in a hot environment) causes excessive pooling of venous blood known as hypostasis.†
- *Active insufficient function.* Purposeful (useful) movement rarely demands a muscle spanning two joints to simultaneously contract over both ends.

---

*Minimal contraction of several other muscles include the temporalis (jaw closure), trapezius, and erector spinae. Some people may also have slight contraction of the hamstrings and iliopsoas due postural alignment deviations such as the sway-back, or flat-back postures in the former and kyphosis-lordosis, or the "military-type" postures in the latter.

†*Venous hypostasis* is commonly reported in military recruits who must stand at attention for prolonged periods in the hot sun. This decline in venous return reaches a critical point in which cardiac output is insufficient to maintain blood pressure in the arteries of the brain. This mild anoxia to brain cells provokes reflexive fainting as part of the body's very efficient early warning system. As soon as the head comes down to the level of the heart the flow of blood is restored to the brain.

Such a contraction is physiologically disadvantageous as the muscle loses length very rapidly and the graphic profile on the Blix curve (see Fig. 39-6) shifts to the left in what is known as active insufficiency. Compensation for this physiologic shortcoming of

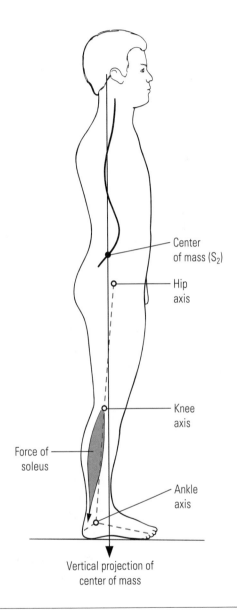

FIG. 34-4 Tonic contraction of soleus maintaining balance during quiet standing. In the relaxed standing posture, the vertical projection of the center of mass falls behind the hip joint, in front of the knee joint and in front of the ankle joint. As a result, the center of gravity falls slightly forward of the body and may cause toppling forward in the sagittal plane. This tendency is countered by active tonic contraction of the soleus muscle, which generates a constant low-grade internally generated counter force.

muscle occurs such that while one end of a muscle is contracting and therefore being shortened over a joint, the other end of the muscle is elongated over the other joint. Thus, the net change in total muscle length is kept at zero. This strategy preserves the optimum tension (and hence power) generating ability of that two-jointed muscle.

- Gastrocnemius function is the exception to the human body's intentional avoidance of active insufficiency in two jointed muscles. Gastrocnemius is actively insufficient during late stance phase of gait. During push-off, the knee flexes to approximately 40° while the ankle moves into significant plantarflexion to thrust the body forward into toe-off.

4. What is the physiologic difference between the type of muscle fibers comprising the gastrocnemius and soleus muscles?

Most striated muscle fibers occur as a heterogeneous mosaic comprised of all three histologically distinct types of muscle types. Histological and histochemical studies differentiate three muscle types, each differing in the type of neuromuscular junctions they contain, the activities of their glycolytic and oxidative enzymes, and their contractile characteristics.

Type I, or *slow intermediate fibers* are red in color due to having a large reservoir of myoglobin (muscle hemoglobin that stores oxygen.) Their energy production is a slow twitch oxidative enzyme system (pyruvic acid). They have many mitochondria, are surrounded by many capillaries, and possess a preponderance of oxidative enzymes (associated with aerobic metabolism.) These small, thin fibers show little or no fatigue and are well adapted for sustained tonic activity. Tetany is defined as a maximal sustained level of contraction output over an extended time. This is accomplished by asynchronous contraction meaning that individual fibers will contract briefly and then briefly relax as others take over; in this fashion, contractile output is continuous such as in the postural muscles of the back that must keep working throughout the day. The soleus muscle is another example of a postural muscle as 80% of its muscle fiber is type I. Because of their poorly developed glycolytic system, if circulation is occluded, as for example from peripheral vascular disease, the patient will experience pain and soreness from fatigue as well as shaking tremors. Slow intermediate fibers do not grow in bulk with exercise, or decrease in size with bed rest.

Type II, or *fast white fibers,* have diminished myoglobin as well as mitochondria and therefore a low ca-

pability for oxidative metabolism. These large, wider diameter fibers are best suited for powerful bursts of energy, characteristic of running, metabolize via a fast twitch glycolytic activity and thus fatigue more quickly. Pale fibers have a preponderance of glycolytic enzymes (associated with anaerobic metabolism.) These muscle fibers are recruited during short periods of intense work such as lifting a heavy object or running a 40-yard dash. As lactic acid debt accumulates, fatigue rapidly sets in as these muscles are incapable of the same power output after approximately 3 minutes. The gastrocnemius muscle is comprised of type II muscle fibers and will rapidly hypertrophy with exercise and quickly atrophy during bed rest.

Type III, or *fast red fibers,* have both oxidative and glycolytic capabilities, have an intermediate fiber size, many mitochondria, a short contraction time, and are relatively resistant to fatigue. These characteristics make fast twitch fibers ideal for prolonged phasic contractions, typical of the diaphragm.[71]

The juxtaposition of the soleus muscle together with the gastrocnemius muscle before their confluence as a conjoint tendon may be related to the development of Achilles tendon disorders. It has been postulated[17] that excessive shear develops between these two muscles. How shear develops may be related to a contractile differential in the power output of these two muscles, particularly during a state of fatigue. Shear forces, are not confined to deriving from opposing forces only, but also include those derived from a relatively varying rate or magnitude of contraction. As such, gastrocnemius and soleus may experience the buildup of shear stress owing to the differing twitch tensions of the muscle fibers comprising these respective muscles.

5. What is the biomechanical significance of deviation of the Achilles tendon insertion from the midline of the os calcis?

The Achilles tendon inserts slightly medial to the midline of the calcaneus. Although this is not immediately obvious while viewing the heel posteriorly, it becomes more apparent as proportionately more skin wrinkle medial to the distal insertion when patients stand on their toes. The biomechanical significance of the distal medial tendon insertion is that it causes tension to be delivered across the medial side of the upper and lower ankle joints. Contraction of the triceps surae therefore results in plantarflexion of the upper ankle joint and an inversion moment across the subtalar joint.

Moreover, because the Achilles insertion deviates

medially from midline, tightness of the triceps surae complex invariably pulls the heel into a rearfoot varus posture. Compensation at the foot occurs by way of overpronation of the subtalar joint. However, excessive pronation increases the degree of twisting that the tendon undergoes, resulting in increased rotational and shear forces within the tendon[20,39,60] that "wrings out" the least perfused central portion of the tendon.

6. How is a shortened gastrocnemius differentiated from a shortened soleus muscle?

Differentiating between a shortened gastrocnemius and soleus muscle is accomplished by flexing the knee and passively dorsiflexing the ankle joint. Whereas a shortened soleus muscle prevents 10° of ankle joint dorsiflexion with the knee joint flexed, a shortened gastrocnemius, by virtue of it spanning two joints, limits dorsiflexion with the knee joint extended.

7. What is the etiology of gastrocnemius-soleus muscle shortness or weakness, and how does this contribute to suboptimal triceps surae contraction?

Excessive strength of the ankle plantarflexors occurs secondary to muscle imbalance derived from shortness or even contracture of the gastrocnemius-soleus complex. This may occur for a variety of intrinsic or extrinsic reasons ranging from excessive tightness of the hamstrings group[5] in the former, to constant wearing of high-heeled shoes[40] in the latter. Plantarflexion shortness tends to manifest as an equinus posture of the foot both in the non–weight-bearing as well as weight-bearing foot posture.

Sudden trauma to the triceps surae may occur following landing from a jump in a position of ankle dorsiflexion and knee flexion. Gradual trauma to the soleus muscle may occur from repeated deep knee bending while the ankle is fully dorsiflexed. Either mechanism may result in muscle weakness.

Weakness of the triceps surae complex causes a heel drop posture of the foot. During standing, the patient demonstrates an inability to marshal enough plantarflexion power to rise on their toes. Over time, this pulls the foot into a cavus posture owning to excessive dorsiflexion tone. During gait, compensation for an inability to plantarflex is most obvious during late stance as the patient attempts to clear the heel from floor by tensing the plantarflexors and simultaneously flexing the knee. This deviation occurs at a time when maximal thrust is normally facilitated by knee extension. Evi-

dence of plantarflexion weakness is thus observable as a gastrocnemius limp[40] that manifests as an inability to normally transfer weight to the involved limb.

Stretching of the Achilles tendon, which occurs beyond midstance phase of normal gait primes the triceps surae complex for optimal concentric propulsion contraction during toe off phase of late stance. This occurs because of forward tibial inclination beyond mid-stanced positions the upper ankle in dorsiflexion and thereby stretches the triceps surae. Prestretch (overload) of the triceps surae complex immediately prior to concentric contraction utilizes the viscoelastic properties of the whole muscle to produce greater forces than by sarcomere shortening alone. This magnitude of force generation is necessary for push-off phase of gait. However, in the presence of a tightened posterior leg musculature, triceps surae contracts suboptimally, and the Achilles tendon undergoes excessive stress.

8. How do gastrocnemius and soleus act synergistically in relation to the ankle joint and antagonistically in relation to knee joint function?

Gastrocnemius, by virtue of its proximal origin, acts as a knee flexor in synergy with the hamstring muscles and antagonistically to the quadriceps muscle. Under normal circumstances, it acts to prevent knee hyperextension. Thus weakness of the gastrocnemius manifests as a tendency toward knee joint hyperextension. Paresis of the soleus manifests as knee joint flexion or forward compensatory inclination of the body above the ankle. In contrast, soleus shortness manifests as knee hyperextension whereas gastrocnemius shortness manifests as knee joint flexion. Thus, although the action of the gastrocnemius is the same as the soleus on the ankle joint, the two muscles act antagonistically in relation to the knee joint both during muscle shortness and weakness.[40]

9. What portion of the Achilles tendon is most vulnerable to compromise of vascular perfusion as related to tendon inflammation and degeneration?

The Achilles tendon is unusual in that it is not surrounded by a true synovial sheath. Instead there is a pseudosheath—a *peritenon,* which is comprised of an inner epitenon and superficial paratenon that surround the Achilles tendon.[70] Most of the tendon vascular supply derives from the *epitenon*—a thick, vascular connective tissue layer that invests the tendon surface and nurtures its substance.[46,74] The *paratenon* is actually a series of thin membranes that enhance tendon gliding by minimizing friction between the tendon and the surrounding tissue,[46,47,74] and demonstrate excursions of up to 1.5 cm.[46] The triceps surae has a relatively good blood supply and heals predictably well following injury.[53] Unfortunately, an exception to this is the Achilles tendon where there is a *critical zone* of relative avascularity (Fig. 34-5). The vascular supply of the Achilles tendon consists of longitudinal arterioles that course the length of the tendon that are supplemented by vessels from the paratenon. This vascular watershed exists at 4.5 cm[49] above the tendon insertion and is vulnerable to ischemic insult. This central portion of the tendon is the least well perfused and consequently the most vulnerable to ischemic insult. In addition, the tendinous vessels decrease in size and number with increasing age.[29] The combination of these factors accounts for increased

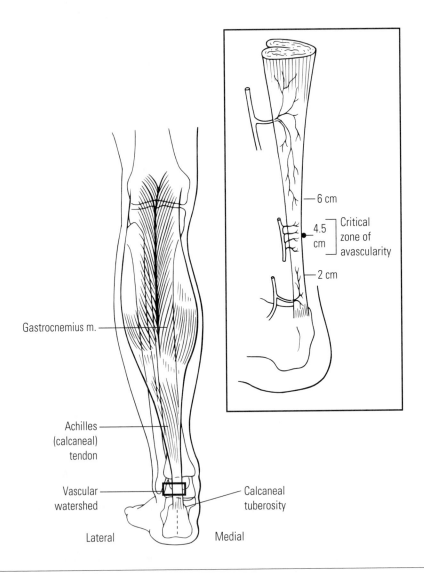

FIG. 34-5 The Achilles tendon has a relatively poor blood supply. Although the longitudinal vessels supply the tendon proximally and distally, the central portion of the tendon is supplied at its surface by transverse vessels. Incomplete vascular anastomosis occurs at the central portion of the tendon. The vascular watershed region refers to a poorly perfused area located 2 to 6 cm above the tendon insertion. The *critical zone* of minimal vascularity is located at 4.5 cm above the distal tendon insertion.

susceptibility to chronic inflammation and degeneration at the central aspect of the tendon located at 2 to 6 cm proximal to the calcaneal insertion.[36,55]

10. What is the significance of the lateromedial spiral alignment of the distal tendon insertion?

The insertion of the triceps surae is a *conjoint tendon* alternately referred to as the Achilles tendon, tendo calcaneus, tendo Achillis, and tendon of the triceps surae. The tendon inserts on a rectangular area at the posteromedial aspect of the calcaneal tuberosity. However, because the calcaneal tuberosity is medial to the midline of the os calcis, the distal tendon travels along a gentle spiral from its point of confluence in what may be characterized as a slight internal rotation. During gait this generates tensile stress along the lateral convex aspect on the tendon. Similarly, the individual with an overpronated foot may, even during ordinary walking, incur magnified tension along this site and thereby incur increased susceptibility to overuse.

11. How does excursion of the Achilles tendon contribute to pathologic dysfunction?

Understanding the rotation of the distal Achilles tendon is clarified by considering calcaneal excursion during gait. During the latter part of swing phase of gait the foot is locked into supination and dorsiflexion in preparation for heel strike. This foot posture necessitates obligatory external tibial rotation with the heel inverted. Once heel strike occurs, the foot everts as a function of subtalar joint, and thereby allowing the foot to become a mobile adapter at contact.

Thus, early stance phase is characterized by a sudden alteration from calcaneal inversion to eversion during heel strike as the foot pronates. This process is reversed beyond midstance when the foot supinates and the calcaneus is said to undergo relative *inversion* as the body moves medially over the heel. The cumulative effect of repetitive calcaneal excursion has a whipping effect on the calcaneal tendon, which pulls it *medial to lateral*[20] during pronation at heel strike, (see Fig. 35-3) and conversely, whipping the tendon lateral to medial at maximal supination during toe-off phase of gait. This "sawlike" action of the tendon may be heightened due to the rotation of the distal Achilles tendon fibers.[17]

12. What is the evolution of Achilles tendon disease?

Achilles tendon disease may be viewed as a spectrum of related disorders that are characterized by the site of involvement. Because sports-induced inflammation is a localized tissue response initiated by injury or destruction of vascularized tissue exposed to excessive mechanical load,[50] there is an evolution from the most benign type of Achilles disorder to complete rupture.

- *Peritendinitis.* Overuse injuries to the Achilles tendon initially manifest as inflammation of the surrounding paratenon known as peritendinitis. This most benign form of pathology clinically presents as diffuse painful swelling that is sometimes associated with crepitus.[2] Crepitus may result from thickening of the paratenon that impairs the gliding function of this tissue, thereby intensifying the inflammatory stimulus.[74] Pain is perceived along the Achilles tendon and disability with plantarflexion activities.[48] If the inciting stimulus is removed, peritendinitis is often self-limited and may heal without consequence.

- *Tendinosis.* Refers to focal degenerative changes of the tendon midsubstance without peritenon involvement causing a local, pain-free, swelling. This less benign stage leads to paratenon scarring and structural tendon disruption begins.[33] Normal tendon is composed of tightly arranged bundles of collagen capable of withstanding enormous tensile loads.[74] Tendinosis represents a form of tendon failure and causes microtearing[18,39,60] at its weakest point. Tendinosis may also occur to normal tendon that has not sustained peritendinitis when loads in excess of physiologic magnitude are applied.[33] Histologic changes associated with tendinosis shown collagen degradation owing to release of proteolytic enzymes by inflammatory cells,[60] followed by focal proliferation of poorly organized scar tissue that only weakens the tensile strength of the tendon.

- *Tendinitis.* Refers to diffuse tendon inflammation and degeneration within the substance of the Achilles tendon. Tendinitis is a more form of Achilles tendon pathology that represents a magnification of the histological failure occurring with tendinosis. The stage is thus set in which the most poorly vascularized portion of the tendon midsubstance is degraded by microtearing, collagen fraying, or even calcification in advanced states. These factors coupled with the spiraling architecture of the Achilles tendon causing a cyclic wringing out of the avascular portion and vascular insult, as well as a variety of extrinsic (shoe wear, running surface) and intrinsic (biomechanical malalignment) factors priming the tendon for eventual partial or complete rupture.

- *Tendon rupture.* Represents the most serious Achilles tendon injury and typically occurs 3 to 6 cm proximal to the calcaneal insertion site. Although there is some evidence that tendinitis is present in surgical patients, many patients deny any symptoms before injury.[64] This suggests that there are two separate groups of patient who sustain Achilles tendon ruptures: acute injury in younger, more active male individuals without any previous symptoms, and middle aged adults, particularly to males in their third to fifth decades, following chronic Achilles pain and weakness. Pathogenesis has thus been attributed to either chronic degeneration of the tendon or excessive mechanical failure.

13. What are the progressive stages of Achilles tendon disease?

The *acute stage* (symptoms of less than 2 weeks duration) involves the paratenon and not the tendon, and is characterized by dull aching pain after the precipitating activity. Tenderness is limited to a 4-cm area, 3 to 6 cm above the proximal tip of the os calcis. Symptoms become more intense about an hour after activity. Initially, these symptoms are only bothersome and the athlete may ignore them as he or she continue to train and compete. However, as the tendon is subjected to continued undue stress, injury progresses to the next stage. The subacute stage (3 to 6 weeks duration) occurs when the athlete continues running without treatment with pain in the tendon during the activity that increases with sprinting. Symptoms increase from one day to the next and the athlete becomes worried about them. In addition, crepitus may be noted during active plantarflexion and dorsiflexion. The *chronic stage* (over 6 weeks duration) is characterized by several changes occurring within the tendon, such as longitudinal fissures, microtears with mucoid degeneration, as well as the presence of scar tissue. Pain is present over an ever-increasing area possibly before activity, when walking, and the patient is unable to run effectively. Athletic participation and training becomes impossible at this point. On palpation, the tendon is found to be markedly thickened and often nodular and may be observed as reddened. The end result may cause partial (first to second degree strain) to full-thickness tear of the calcaneal tendon (third degree strain).[72]

14. What training errors predispose this condition?

Changes in running surfaces (grass to concrete), training in cold weather, and running on very soft surfaces predispose an increased likelihood of sustaining Achilles tendinitis. In addition, tendinitis may be caused by sudden changing from flats to spikes, or a change from endurance to speed running.[72] Running against an inflexible outer sole, or wearing shoes with an inadequately padded heel wedge or soft heel counter that does not stabilize the heel may also contribute to injury. During autumn when the ground becomes soft, football quarterbacks and defensive backs are particularly susceptible to increased tension due to stretching of the heel cord complex.[65]

15. How would running on inclines predispose tendinitis?

Increased forceful heel strike while running downhill, as well as toe off during uphill running contribute to increased strain of the calcaneal tendon.[61] During uphill running (Fig. 34-6), the Achilles tendon of the stance leg undergoes excessive prestretch before and during toe off. This places the triceps surae at physiologic disadvantage as it concentrically contracts to propel the leg forward. During downhill running, the gastrocsoleus complex is recruited to halt excessive speed and disorganized foot-slapping corresponding to a shortened interval between heel strike and foot flat phase of gait. This is accomplished by an eccentric contraction

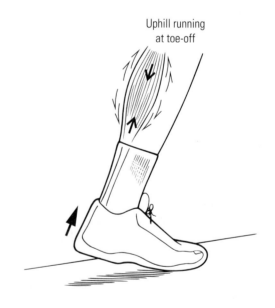

Uphill running
at toe-off

FIG. 34-6 Running uphill places excessive strain on the Achilles tendon. During uphill running, the Achilles tendon of the stance leg undergoes excessive prestretch before, and during toe off. This places the triceps surae at physiologic disadvantage as it *concentrically* contracts to propel the leg forward under less than favorable conditions of stretch.

of triceps surae that attempts to dampen uncontrolled forward motion that begins with heel strike. These high-speed forces are focused at the Achilles tendon insertion and place it at increased risk for injury (Fig. 34-7).

16. What biomechanical problems of the foot may contribute to the development of calcaneal tendinitis?

Biomechanical foot alterations that contribute to development of Achilles tendinitis include both the pronated and supinated foot in the closed kinetic chain. The former refers to as a pes planus deformity, while the latter is known as a pes cavus deformity. A valgus position of the calcaneus on the talus is associated with pronation at the subtalar joint, whereas a varus hindfoot is associated with supination at the subtalar joint.

In the normal foot, stretching of the Achilles tendon occurs uniformly along its course. With either excessive pronation or supination, excessive torsion is im-

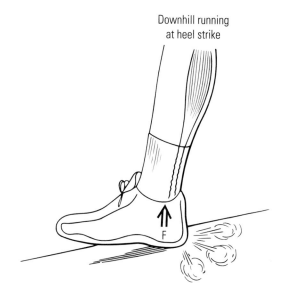

Downhill running
at heel strike

FIG. 34-7 Running downhill places excessive strain on the Achilles tendon owing to transmission of forceful *(arrow)* impact to the tendon. Also, during downhill running, the gastroc-soleus complex is recruited to halt excessive speed and disorganized foot-slapping corresponding to a shortened interval between heel strike and foot flat phase of gait. This is accomplished by an *eccentric contraction* of triceps surae that attempts to dampen uncontrolled forward motion that begins with heel strike. These high-speed forces are focused at the Achilles tendon insertion and place it at increased risk fatigue, failure, and injury.

parted to the lateral convex side of the tendon resulting in excessive stress to those fibers. The over-pronated foot will result in a rear foot valgus deformity causing excessive contractile focus and distraction along the medial convex border of the tendon. In contrast, the patient with an observed heel varus (supination) will focus distractive and contractile forces along the lateral convex aspect of the Achilles tendon. The difference between a flat foot with a tight calcaneal tendon and a high-arched foot with a tight calcaneal tendon is that although the flat foot has the ability to compensate for tightness by excessive pronating the foot, the cavus foot does not.[58]

A cavus foot is poorly designed to absorb the forces incurred during the gait cycle. A pes cavus foot demonstrates a high arch and limited range of motion of the subtalar joint causing locking of the bones comprising the arch. This results in approximation of the hindfoot and forefoot, which, over time results in the contracture of the plantar fascia. A cavus foot is neither flexible nor pliant, and the foot, as a whole, has diminished capacity to absorb impact incurred during heel strike. Normally, the forces incurred during weight bearing are absorbed by bone, ligament, and muscle-tendon units. An individual with a cavus type foot is biomechanically disadvantaged as their locked bony foot is characterized by a paucity of movement of its osseous components which deprives the foot of a mechanism for energy dissipation. Consequently, the responsibility for dissipating potentially injurious forces is shifted to the adjacent muscle-tendon and ligaments. However, because the intrinsic muscles of the cavus foot as well as the ligaments connecting its osseous components undergo contracture secondary to lack of arthrokinematic and osteokinematic motion within the foot, the next level of tissue to absorb the force of impact are the extrinsic muscle-tendon units. The concussive forces incurred during heel strike will be delivered proximally, as the foot is incapable of dissipating the impact of ground reaction force. These concussive force incurred during early stance migrate proximally and are absorbed by the muscles spanning the crural compartment. The posterior tibial tendon is thus forced to work harder to take up the excess force. Because its distal tendon is tethered around the medial malleolus, tibialis posterior is subject to the development of overuse more distally (than tibialis anterior) in the form of tendon inflammation.

Supination associated with a cavus foot posture causes excessive calcaneal inversion during stance phase that causes obligatory lateral to medial whipping of the Achilles tendon. This excessively early supination delivers and external rotary torque to the distal tibia when it should be internally rotating. The conflicting torsions are absorbed by the Achilles tendon and may have a wring-out effect of the vessels in the zone of relative avascularity.

Abnormal deviation from subtalar neutral during stance may present as either excessive or inadequate pronation of the subtalar joint. Two forms of intrinsic foot deformities that represent diametrically different deviations from subtalar joint neutral are forefoot varus (see p. 347) and rigid forefoot valgus (see pp. 348-349). Although the former represents an over mobile foot due to excessive pronation and a planus type foot posture, the latter represents a rigid foot owing to inadequate pronation and a cavus type foot posture. Both represent extremes of biomechanical function in relation to subtalar joint neutral. Consequently, the length-tension relationships of the extrinsic muscles moving the foot will deviate from ideal and cause these muscles to overwork. Relentless overuse of muscle results in muscle fatigue that predispose the calcaneal tendon, as well as other structures, to a spectrum of proximal and distal disorders.

17. What is a forefoot equinus deformity?

Some persons may have shortening of the gastroc-soleus muscle complex either because of overdevelopment of these muscles[12] or because of congenital shortening of the gastrocnemius or hamstring muscle. Regardless of the exact etiology, the outcome of this muscle imbalance results in a plantarflexed or equinus posture of the forefoot when compared with the rear foot.[30] This form of intrinsic sagittal plane deformity of the ankle is called forefoot equinus and may overstress and thereby predispose the Achilles tendon to pathology.

18. What extrinsic and intrinsic variables serve as predisposing factors in the development of Achilles tendon overuse injuries?

Intrinsic malalignment may be osseous (deformities) or soft tissue (imbalance) in nature. Pronation causes internal tibial rotation and causes increased midfoot flexibility. Increased femoral anteversion increases the duration of subtalar pronation by forcing the limb into internal rotation. A varus deformity of the knee, tibia, heel, or forefoot (supination) results in the heel striking the ground in a varus position and promotes a compensatory pronation to maintain the foot in a more planti-

grade position.[39] A tight triceps surae with simultaneous weakness of the dorsiflexors and invertors creates a functional heel varus that is accompanied by increased pronation.

It is important to realize that although the Achilles tendon may suffer increased stress from a distal malalignment, such as an over-pronated foot derived from an intrinsic foot deformity, it may also fall prey to inflammation and degeneration owing to a proximal osseous or soft tissue deformity. Proximal deformities such as increased femoral anteversion, varus deformity of the knee or tibia, or a pattern of tightness in the triceps surae with weakness of the pretibials share a common denominator of subtalar joint pronation. Thus, whether the malalignment is proximal or distal, injurious force is delivered to the Achilles tendon by way of the subtalar joint. This point underscores the significance of this joint in lower extremity biomechanics. Excessive pronation is often the final pathway resulting in increased shear and rotational forces of the Achilles tendon leading to inflammation and tendon degeneration.

19. How are dancing or cycling activities related to the onset of Achilles tendinitis?

Although the foot acts a flexible lever during running, particularly during early stance, it acts as a rigid lever in cycling.[66] Achilles tendinitis may occur in cyclists as a result of excessive "ankling" while pedaling from an overflexible foot and soft shoe, or a foot that is placed too far behind the pedal spindle.[31] Achilles tendon injuries are more common in dancers who perform on surfaces with poor shock-absorbing properties.[25,28] In addition, the classic ballet positions of en pointe and relevé focus force on the Achilles tendon by virtue of their demanding extreme ankle plantarflexion. The grande plié and demi plié positions required marked ankle dorsiflexion with eccentric contraction of the triceps surae complex that may also contribute to tendon overuse.[33]

20. What is the clinical presentation?

The patient may present a history of varying extrinsic factors contributing to the onset of Achilles tendinitis including increases in mileage, hill running, interval training, changes in footwear, too rapid return from a layoff from running, insufficient warm-up, and running surface. Intrinsic factors may include anatomic malalignment that result in abnormal foot strike secondary to abnormal hindfoot mobility. Other intrinsic factors include tight hamstring and gastroc-soleus muscles. Because the entire lower extremity functions as a linked

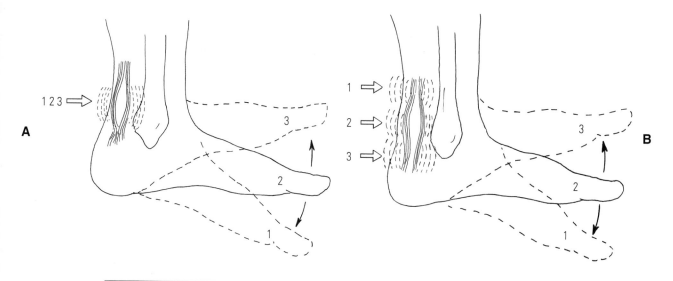

FIG. 34-8 *Painful arc sign.* **A,** In peritendinitis, where pathologic involvement is confined to the synovial paratenon surrounding the Achilles tendon, tenderness remains in one position despite moving the foot from dorsiflexion to plantarflexion. **B,** When pathology involves the tendon itself, as in tendinitis or partial rupture, the point of tenderness moves throughout the arc of sagittal plane motion. (Redrawn from Williams JGP: Achilles tendinitis, *Sports Med* 3:114, 1986.)

unit, a tightened hamstrings complex will place an inordinate amount of tension on the triceps surae complex;[5] the converse is true as well.

In the early phase of Achilles tendon disease, patients may complain of pain primarily following strenuous activities such as running or jumping. This results in overuse that inflicts small cumulative tears in the paratenon causing an inflammatory response. If ignored, damage will progressively increase as inflammation invades the tendon and producing pain during athletic activities that may eventually limit participation. The patient may complain of early morning pain and stiffness as they get out of bed and take a few steps, that gradually subsides during the day. If ignored, the patient may eventually report pain during sprinting or acceleration that almost always correlates with surgical findings of tendinosis or partial rupture.[60] A palpable defect (hatchet sign) indicates significant or complete rupture.

Physical findings vary with the degree of tendon involvement and typically include, marked restriction of passive ankle dorsiflexion with the knee extended due to pain,[81] hamstring tightness, static tenderness to palpation present approximately 3 to 6 cm above the tendon insertion, tender nodular swelling or crepitus in more severe cases,[33] and strong but slightly painful resisted plantarflexion.[23] Patients often complain of pain

when climbing stairs, although normal walking does not produce discomfort.[5] If the tendon is tender on gentle palpation, the tendinitis is considered serious.[65]

The *painful arc* sign (Fig. 34-8) is helpful in differentiating peritendinitis from tendon involvement ranging from tendinitis to partial rupture. When pathology is confined to the peritenon only, pain and tenderness remain fixed during ankle excursion from plantarflexion to dorsiflexion. When pathology involves the tendon however, pain is not stationary during sagittal ankle excursion but rather moves with the tendon.[15]

21. What is the differential diagnosis for Achilles tendinitis?

Focal causes of plantar heel pain are numerous. Peripheral neuropathy should be ruled out when heel pain is diffuse and bilateral. Chronic pain at rest is an unusual presentation for plantar heel pain and may suggest a calcaneal tumor. Radiculopathy in the L5-S1 distribution should be considered in the patient with low back pain. Prior to arriving at a diagnosis of Achilles tendinitis, the following pathological conditions must additionally be ruled out:

- *Achilles tendon rupture.* In the same way that disease of the peritenon is differentiated from tendinitis or partial rupture by a moving painful arc, several signs help the clinician differentiate between partial and full rupture of the Achilles tendon. An acute total rupture is characterized by an inability to resistively plantarflex, considerable decrease in the ability to actively plantarflex, and slightly excessive dorsiflexion of the involved foot. Moreover, their is often a "snap" or "pop" associated with total rupture, a positive Thomas test, and palpable gap felt in the substance of the Achilles tendon particularly if examined early on before swelling and ecchymosis sets in. Finally, the patient cannot walk tiptoe, and heel drop (loss of active dorsiflexion) is a pathognomonic sign in the absence of neuromuscular or spinal disease. The normal state of balance between the antagonistic pre- and posttibial musculature places the foot in neutral or in slight equinus (as during sleep). Following total rupture, a loss of tonal output to the posterior musculature is expressed as an imbalance in a muscular tug of war, resulting in the pretibial muscle pulling up the forefoot slightly as the heel drops downward. Partial rupture is differentiated from complete rupture by active dorsiflexion, resistive although painful dorsiflexion, and an ability to rise on toes; a slight notch may be felt at the midportion of the tendon. In contradistinction to total rupture, partial rupture does not preclude the ability to ambulate following injury.

- *Haglund's disease,* also known posterior calcaneal tendon bursitis, is an inflammation of the superficial (posterior) bursa lying between the skin and the calcaneal tendon. Because the insertion of the Achilles tendon is distal to the peak of the calcaneal tuberosity, a tendo calcaneal bursa is necessary between these two structures to reduce frictional stress. This disorder may occur as a function of bursal irritation between the peaklike prominence of the calcaneal tuberosity owing to an intrinsic deformity such as a rearfoot varum posture associated with the supinated foot. Alternately, it may be extrinsically caused by a hard heel counter rubbing against the posterior aspect of the calcaneus. Pathology may also occur in individuals with an abnormal prominence of the posterosuperior surface of the calcaneal surface known as the bursal projection. Regardless of the etiology, inflammation of this region at the site of the calcaneal tuberosity and subsequent excessive frictional stress on the bursa will result in swelling, erythema, and painful thickening of the surrounding soft tissues known as Haglund's disease. Pain is present 2 to 3 cm proximal to the tendon insertion. Palpation at this region yields pain. Swelling or erythema is usually absent.

The heel counter of a shoe is ideally designed to fit a convex surface. When it is rigid (new) or poorly manufactured, it can irritate the subcutaneous tissues. When the cause of irritation is external as from excessive shoe pressure on the posterior aspect of the calcaneus, it may cause a thickening of the subcutaneous calcaneal bursa known as a "pump bump." This is located immediately lateral to the attachment of the Achilles tendon onto the posterosuperior aspect of the os calcis along the convex aspect of that insertion. A red "bump" is attributed to a reactive thickening of the subcutaneous calcaneal bursa at the tendo Achilles insertion as well as a bony enlargement (exostosis) of the calcaneus at that level, corresponding to where a low-cut, high-heeled shoe (pump) rubs. This reddened area may yield tenderness and pain upon palpation. A pump bump (Fig. 34-9) initially begins as an irritation of the skin when the calcaneus everts within the shoe that results in a blister. This is followed by a bursa reactively forming owing to excessive irritation which, if uninterrupted, is compli-

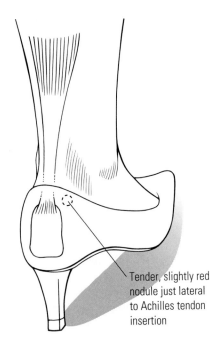

Tender, slightly red nodule just lateral to Achilles tendon insertion

FIG. 34-9 A *pump-bump* is a nodular thickening of the subcutaneous calcaneal bursa. Reactive bursal enlargement occurs from wearing low-cut, high-heeled shoes. Similar to the bunion mechanism at the forefoot, a pump-bump begins as a blister and progresses into a bursitis. If the offending friction continues, this condition will evolve into a retrocalcaneal exostosis as a function of calcaneal overgrowth.

cated by osseous overgrowth of the adjacent calcaneus. This may lead to inflammation of the Achilles tendon. This retrocalcaneal exostosis appears at the upper outer aspect of the heel bone and causes increased rubbing of the calcaneal tendon over the outgrowth. Haglund's disease may have radiographically observable characteristics known as Haglund's deformity. (Fig. 34-10) Pump bumps are common in adolescent females, and both male and female ice skaters. It may also occur in persons who have rheumatoid arthritis.

In addition to a cavus foot posture, another cause of Haglund's deformity may be attributed to footwear with a stiff shoe counter particularly if the upper posterior edge projects inward. Management involves elevating the heel to eliminate shoe counter pressure, placing padding around the bursa to relieve irritation, the use of ice to decrease inflammation, correction of rearfoot varus posture by an orthosis that will appropriately align the position of the heel, wearing shoes with a high heel counter, nonsteroidal antiinflammatory oral medication, or infiltration of soluble corticosteroid with local anesthetic via iontophoresis to reduce inflammation. Because a bursa is inert rather than contractile, differentiating a subcutaneous posterior calcaneal bursa from a tendon-related lesion is

accomplished by asking the patient to rise on tiptoe. If this maneuver is painless, then the bursa is implicated.[21]

- *Albert's disease,* also known as Achilles tendon bursitis, anterior calcaneal tendon bursitis, or precalcaneal bursitis, is inflammation of the deeply located bursa known as the retrocalcaneal bursa. The calcaneal tuberosity is located along the posteroinferior portion of the calcaneus. It is rough and striated for the attachment of the calcaneal tendon, in contrast to its superior-most surface, which is smooth for the subtendinous bursa of the calcaneal tendon. The Achilles tendon attaches to the lower part of the posterior calcaneus. This distal, rather than proximal, attachment affords the tendon maximal leverage when rising on the ball of the foot or when running. However, the price paid for this mechanical advantage is that the inner portion of the distal tendon intermittently contacts a small area of calcaneal bone but is not attached to it. As pressure is defined as force-per-unit area, the friction accrued from the tendon rubbing across this small area of bone may be considerable. Toward this end a retrocalcaneal bursa is present to facilitate smooth gliding between the tendon and bone. In some persons, the superior posterior calcaneal tuberosity is prominent or angles sharply. In

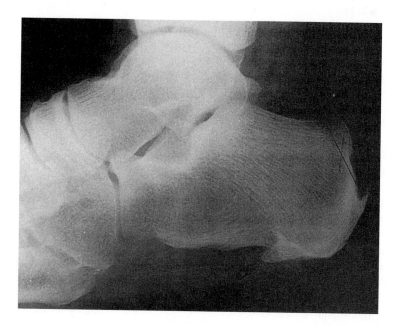

FIG. 34-10 Radiographic appearance of Haglund's deformity. (From Guten GN: *Running injuries,* WB Saunders, 1997, Philadelphia.)

these persons, or in persons such as dancers who may engage in repetitive equinus posturing of the foot, the bursa may become inflamed, distended, and painful. This disorder is more common to young females,[9] and may occur if performance continues unabated through the pain. Dancers may admit to overuse of the ankle in preparation for an audition, examination, or performance. Retrocalcaneal bursitis also occurs in athletes with boot-type shoes, such as skiers, skaters, and basketball players.[32] Abnormal pronation occurring during heel strike phase of stance predisposes for anterior calcaneal tendon bursitis. Here, excessive pronation occurs in association with a tibial varum deformity and a valgus posture of the calcaneus during heel strike. Palpating with the thumb and index finger elicits tenderness anterior to the tendon attachment onto the calcaneus and not posteriorly over the paratenon or substance of the tendon.

Pain, swelling, and heat are felt in the retrocalcaneal space, and complaints of difficulty when walking even while wearing a worn-in pair of shoes. In less severe cases, palpating with the thumb and index finger in front of the Achilles tendon yields a spongy resistance in contrast to the firm texture of the unaffected heel. When more involved, the bursa may be easily palpated where it bulges on either side of the Achilles tendon. Swelling is initially localized anterior to the Achilles tendon but over time will extend medially and laterally. Pain localized primarily within soft tissue differentiates this condition from a fractured posterior lateral tubercle, although x-rays should be ordered. Similarly, bursitis is distinguished from a tendinous lesion as rising on tiptoe is relatively painless. Bursography (an x-ray with contrast medium) is sometimes used to confirm the diagnosis of bursitis, although this procedure is invasive and may be painful. Ultrasound will show the size of the bursa, whether or not it contains fluid and is the imaging procedure of choice.[7] Conservative treatment includes the wearing of shoes without a back (such as sandals or clogs), correcting any postural biomechanical foot deviation by way of an orthosis, wearing shoes with a softer and lower shoe counter, the use of a heel lift, ice, the use of ultrasound, moist heat, phonophoresis or iontophoresis, and nonsteroidal antiinflammatory medications. Local steroid injections must be avoided. When conservative treat fails, excision of the bursa provides relief.

- *Rheumatic conditions.* Rheumatoid arthritis, gout, or pseudogout, demonstrate sharp contrasts between signs and symptoms. The Achilles tendon is very warm to touch, is often swollen and very tender, although crepitus is not present. Complaints of pain are mainly restricted to when the patient's heel cord catches against an object when they walk barefoot, while standing on one's toes is not uncomfortable. The latter is not the case in true Achilles tendinitis. In pseudogout, a localized swelling occasionally forms and lasts for one month without causing interference with function. Bone erosion at the calcaneal insertion of Achilles tendon is described in rheumatoid disease. Symptomatic onset is gradual when tendinitis is attributed to a systemic disease such as rheumatoid arthritis.

Entrapment of the first branch of the lateral plantar nerve to the abductor digiti quinti muscle is one of the most commonly over looked causes of chronic heel pain.[8,68] Entrapment of this nerve occurs as the nerve changes from a vertical to horizontal orientation around the medial plantar aspect of the heel (See Fig. 31-5 A). This is accentuated by overpronation of the foot. The site of compression is located between the heavy deep fascia of the abductor hallucis and the medial caudal margin of the medial head of the quadratus plantae (Fig. 34-11). The patient presents with tenderness over the course of the nerve maximally in the area of entrapment. Compression of that area may elicit paresthesias. Although motor weakness in the abductor digiti quinti may be detected, no cutaneous sensory deficit occurs. Electromyography is of little help in diagnosing this condition. Treatment includes the application of a medial longitudinal arch support as well as a shock absorbing heel insert.

- *Fat pad injury (bruised heel).* The fat pad at the heel absorbs the concussive forces of impact during early stance. The adipose tissue comprising the heel pad is organized as U-shaped or comma-shaped fat filled septa that are vertically oriented to resist compressive loads.[75] The fat cells within these fibrosepta act to cushion the foot with each heel strike. The fascia comprising these fibrosepta are attached to the skin of the heel and hindfoot. Unlike the skin on the dorsum of the foot, the skin on the sole of the foot cannot slide backward and forward over the tissues beneath. Repetitive jumps from landing on the heels that occurs with hurdling, long and triple jumping can rupture these septa. Alternately, these fibrosepta are pressed outwards from the area of the heel, which contacts the running surface, causing the cushioning effect of the fat pad to be reduced. If the activity con-

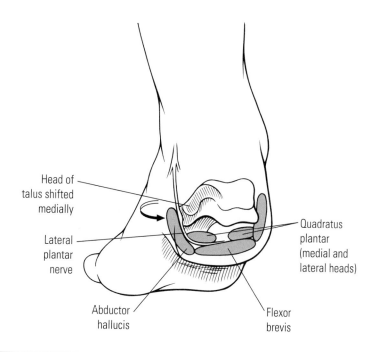

FIG. 34-11 Overpronation of the subtalar joint causes medial prominence of the talar head, which compresses the quadratus plantae muscle against the abductor hallucis muscle. The interposed lateral plantar nerve undergoes subsequent compression.

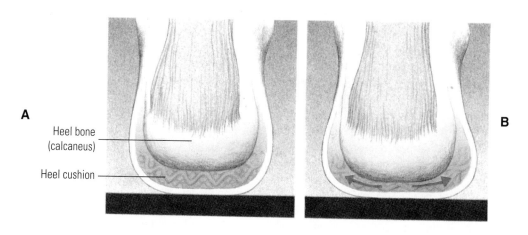

FIG. 34-12 A, Normal heel cushion. The calcaneus is protected by fatty tissue. **B,** A painful heel cushion. Here the adipose tissue comprising the fat pad is pressed outward toward the sides of the heel and causes apposition of the calcaneus to the skin. This represents impaired protection to the heel bone. (From Peterson L, Renstrom P: *Sports injuries: their prevention and treatment,* Chicago, 1983, Yearbook Medical Publishers.)

tinues unabated, the skin will come to appose the bone, and subsequently, the rearfoot becomes more sensitive to pain with loading (Fig. 34-12). Deterioration of this adipose tissue occurs insidiously after age forty. Calcaneal fat pad trauma or shear presents as plantar heel paid that is exacerbated with weight bearing and especially with heel impact. Diffuse tenderness is limited to the fat pad, with pain provoked as the pad is grasped and mobilized. If trauma to the fat pad is prolonged, the underlying bone may be felt be-

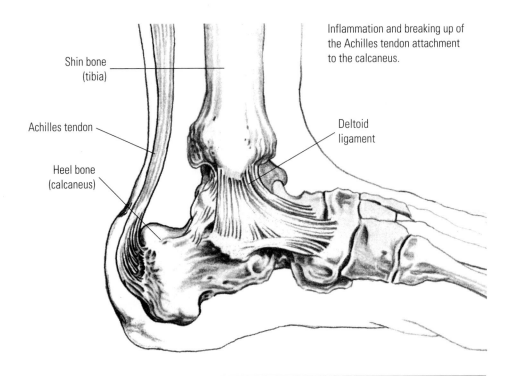

Shin bone
(tibia)

Inflammation and breaking up of
the Achilles tendon attachment
to the calcaneus.

Achilles tendon

Deltoid
ligament

Heel bone
(calcaneus)

FIG. 34-13 Apophysitis calcanei was described by J.W. Sever and involves inflammation and breaking up of the Achilles tendon attachment on the calcaneus. (From Peterson L, Renstrom P: *Sports injuries: their prevention and treatment,* Chicago, 1983, Yearbook Medical Publishers.)

neath the skin.[63] Fat pad shear is associated with a high arched and supinated foot. Early detection and prevention is essential, as the condition becomes difficult to treat once the calcaneus is felt beneath the skin[7]. The clinician must also rule out the possibility of calcaneal stress fracture, which has a similar presentation to calcaneal fat pad trauma. A bone scan is the only definitive test that rules out calcaneal stress fracture. Intervention for both fat pad trauma and calcaneal stress fracture includes decreased activity, heel cushioning, and running on low-impact surfaces. A shoe with a loose-fitting heel counter allows the calcaneal fat pad to spread at heel strike, increasing transmission of impact to the heel. In contrast, a firm, well-fitting heel counter maintains compactness of the fat pad, which buffers the force of impact.

• *Sever's disease (calcaneal apophysitis).* This is a painful condition of the heel before epiphyseal closure that affects children between 8 to 16 years of age who are involved in running sports, (Fig. 34-13). Boys are affected twice as frequently as girls. Soccer, basketball, gymnastics, and track are the sports most frequently associated with this syndrome.[57] Ossifica-

tion of the cartilage connecting the calcaneus' two centers of ossification begins after the eighth year and may extend beyond age 16. These years, characterized by a rapid growth spurt, may focus excessive strain upon the epiphysis due to jumping or other athletic activities may break the cartilaginous union between the two parts of the calcaneus or disrupt Sharpey's fibers of the tendinous insertion at the apophysis.[3,38] Localized tenderness due to compression on the medial and lateral side of the heel without erythema, edema, or skin tenderness. Ankle dorsiflexion may be limited due to pain of activity and decreased Achilles tendon mobility. There is no correlation between symptoms and radiographic appearance. Both parents and child should be reassured that healing will occur by way of fibrocartilage replacement over a period of several months duration. Treatment is similar to that of Achilles tendinitis and include gastroc-soleus stretching and anterior tibial strengthening. Heel pads may be placed in the shoe to alleviate the pull of the Achilles tendon on the heel, or immobilization of the foot in a plaster or fiberglass cast.[10] if the condition is markedly painful. Recovery may take months to one year and supplemented by a maintenance program of stretching, strengthening, and endurance exercises. Changing from running or jumping sports to bicycling or swimming may be helpful. Students may require an elevator pass to avoid negotiating stairs while in school. Sever's disease is a self-limiting process if allowed to become quiescent through rest.

- *Xanthomatosis.* This is a genetic disorder of lipid metabolism characterized by elevated serum cholesterol, accelerated atherosclerosis, and early death (age 40) from myocardial infarction. The hallmark of this disorder are xanthomas (lipid-laden tumors) over joints, blood vessels, and tendons such as the Achilles, patellar,[21] and digital extensor tendons of the upper and lower extremities. When the Achilles tendon is involved the patient may complain of pain in both heels during walking. Both tendons may be thickened and palpation reveals enlargement and diffuse nodularity.[21] Morbidity can be forestalled by effective cholesterol lowering.[10]

- *Posterior impingement syndrome* or *os trigonum pathology*, or dancer's heel, involves compression of soft tissues from structures present from birth. Fractures of the posterior process of the talus are uncommon but often-missed athletic injuries. The posterior aspect of the body or trochlea of the talus has two bony tubercles separated by a groove containing the FHL tendon (Fig. 34-14). The smaller medial tubercle serves as the attachment for the posterior portion of the deep deltoid ligament whereas the longer lateral tubercle projects more posterior and serves as attachment for the posterior talofibular ligament. In approximately 10% of feet the lateral tubercle is a separate ossicle attached to the bone by a fibrous tissue known as the os trigonum (Fig. 34-15).[67] The flexor hallucis longus tendon runs just medial to the lateral tubercle as that tendon crosses the posterior surface of the talus. At times the ossicle may appear fused to the talus or calcaneus or both, and may be unilateral or bilateral.[43,44] It appears in children between the ages of 8 and 10 years and usually unites with the talus within a year of appearance. The ossicle, located at the posterior aspect of the talus behind the posterior tubercle, may be unilateral or bilateral and is not truly a sesamoid bone within a tendon. Rather, it is a bony process, most likely a secondary center of ossification that has failed to unite with the talar body (Fig. 34-16). A posterior talar process compression injury may occur in which the more promi-

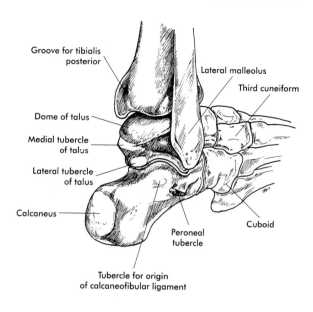

FIG. 34-14 Posterior process of the talus is comprised of the posterolateral and posteromedial tubercles separated by the groove for the flexor hallucis tendon. (From Harper MC: Stress radiographs in the diagnosis of lateral instability of the ankle and hindfoot, *Foot Ankle* 13:435, 1992.)

nent lateral tubercle (known as *Stieda's process*) is compressed resulting in *trigone injury*. This stress fracture is frequently misdiagnosed as an ankle sprain or Achilles tendinitis.[35] The mechanism of injury involves sudden, forceful, hyperplantarflexion of the ankle joint. This equinus posture compresses and may eventually crush the lateral tubercle between the posterior lip of the tibia and the underlying posterior calcaneus (Fig. 34-17). Injury may also occur from repetitive over use in ballet dancers en pointe or from jumping sports such as soccer.[80] Clinical presentation includes posterior ankle pain and tenderness located in the region of the Achilles tendon, particularly the lateral retrocalcaneal space while walking on one's toes. Point tenderness is noted deep in the interval between the Achilles tendon and lateral malleolus. Forced maximal plantarflexion of the ankle also elicits pain, as does resisted plantarflexion of the great toe. Downhill walking or running, or wearing high heels are painful. Wearing shoes that increase dorsiflexion relieves pain. A history of chronic ankle sprains is common. Swelling and signs of collateral ligament instability are absent. Tendinitis of the calcaneal, peroneal, and tibialis posterior tendon is ruled out as patient feel better in equinus and because pal-

Posterior view of talus   Superior view of talus

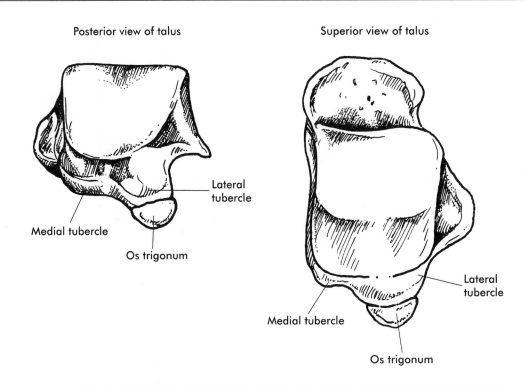

FIG. 34-15 Os trigonum from a posterior and superior view of the talus. (From Baxter D: *The foot and ankle in sport,* St. Louis, 1995, Mosby.)

pation of those tendons in asymptomatic.[77] Treatment may vary from rest and a one-half inch heel lift to ankle taping to resist excessive plantarflexion to casting for 6 weeks. Surgical excision of the trigone fragment is appropriate if conservative efforts have failed.

22. What is tennis leg?

Tennis leg refers to acute strain of the gastrocnemius muscle (Fig. 34-18) and does not refer to rupture of the plantaris tendon or injury to the Achilles tendon. Tennis leg is a common injury in athletes who participate in racket sports, running, basketball, or skiing. Tear of this muscle typically occurs at the proximal confluence of the medial muscle belly and Achilles tendon, and may relate to its unique ability, as a two-jointed muscle, to contract across the knee and upper ankle joints simultaneously. Gastrocnemius undergoes a rapid active insufficiency during push-off that flexes the knee to approximately 40° while the ankle moves into significant plantarflexion to thrust the body forward. Strain of the gastrocnemius may also occur while making a sharp cutting movement or during stair descent during a mis-

step. The foot that has missed the step beneath it protectively postures into ankle plantarflexion and knee flexion so as to absorb the brunt of unexpected landing. *Active insufficiency* of gastrocnemius results in concentric activity across both the knee and upper ankle joints simultaneously and subjects the juncture of the medial gastrocnemius and Achilles tendon to rupture. The mechanism implicated in tennis leg is when the athlete extends the knee while in the crouched position with the ankles dorsiflexed (Fig. 34-19). This position simultaneously pulls on both the origin and insertion of gastrocnemius, placing the muscle on excessive stretch with passive insufficiency. Tear occurs in the push-off leg in the athlete lunges forward to meet the ball or anticipate the movement of an opponent player.[7] Tear typically occurs at the juncture of the distal medial gastrocnemius belly with the calcaneal tendon in the push-off leg as the athlete lunges forward to meet the ball or anticipate the movement of an opponent player. Often, the patient will report sudden intense calf pain in the upper third of the posterior medial calf that is felt as a tearing sensation or blow, and may be followed by swelling, cramping, and discoloration (bruising) sec-

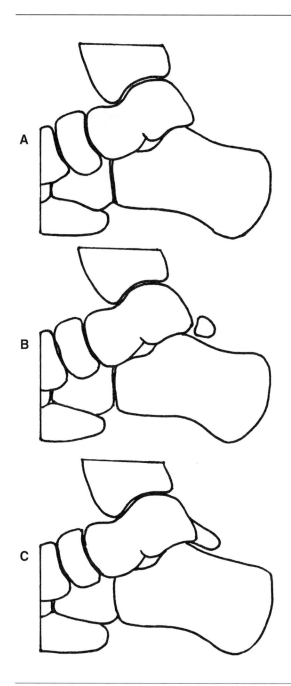

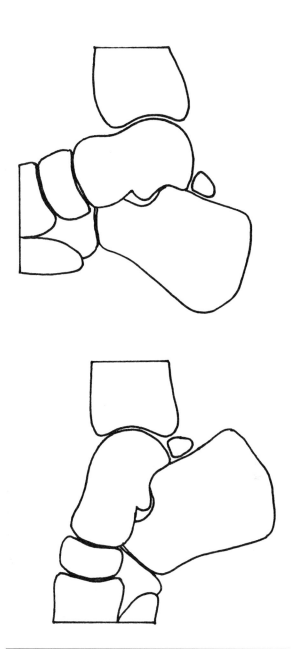

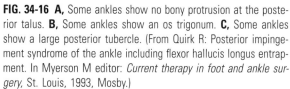

FIG. 34-16 A, Some ankles show no bony protrusion at the posterior talus. **B,** Some ankles show an os trigonum. **C,** Some ankles show a large posterior tubercle. (From Quirk R: Posterior impingement syndrome of the ankle including flexor hallucis longus entrapment. In Myerson M editor: *Current therapy in foot and ankle surgery,* St. Louis, 1993, Mosby.)

FIG. 34-17 When the ankle is plantarflexed the os trigonum becomes entrapped between the lower tibia and upper calcaneus. (From Quirk R: Posterior impingement syndrome of the ankle including flexor hallucis longus entrapment. In Myerson M editor: *Current therapy in foot and ankle surgery,* St. Louis, 1993, Mosby.)

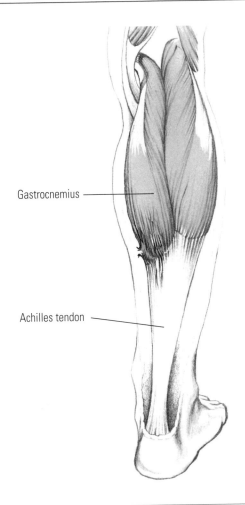

FIG. 34-18 Tennis leg involves rupture of the inner gastrocnemius at the merger of muscle and tendon. (From Peterson L, Renstrom P: *Sports injuries: their prevention and treatment*, Chicago, 1983, Yearbook Medical Publishers.)

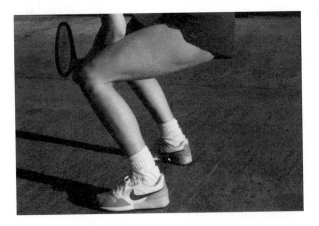

FIG. 34-19 Gastrocnemius tear occurs when the athlete extends the knee from the crouched position with the ankles dorsiflexed. This causes stretching of gastrocnemius at both its proximal and distal ends simultaneously (passive insufficiency). (From Baxter D: *The foot and ankle in sport*, St. Louis, 1995, Mosby.)

ondary to hemorrhage. The injury often causes the patient to stop activity and seek medical attention. The classic findings include swelling and tenderness at the medial calf may present as late as 24 hours later. Bruising may be dramatic and is caused by bleeding from the torn ends of the ruptured muscle. A gap may be palpated over the site of injury. Passive ankle dorsiflexion is painful, and weakness and pain occur with resisted ankle plantarflexion. Rising up on one's toes and the toe off portion of gait are often uncomfortable for the patient. Tennis leg is often missed or misdiagnosed. In middle aged and elderly patients a calf rupture may be misinterpreted as deep vein thrombosis. This can be ruled out by a negative Homan's sign, venography or duplex ultrasound. Treatment is critically important to good healing because the untreated strain leads to scarring which carries with it the risk of a repeated rupture if the muscle is overexerted. Immediate treatment involves cooling the site of injury, applying gentle compression, elevation, and avoidance of contracting the torn muscle. Partial or complete nonweight bearing is essential to minimize swelling. After several days, a one-half inch heel lift is used to relax stress on the tendon during the initial 2 weeks of weight bearing.[26] After 6 weeks of healing active range of motion may be initiated gently. Gentle stretching may be performed during contrast baths, depending on the magnitude of symptoms. Gentle gradual stretching facilitates aligning the healing of scar tissue within the torn muscle. No ballistic activity is permitted until motion, strength, and power are restored to premorbid levels. Tears require at least 6 weeks to heal and this cannot be accelerated[22] and may take up to 3 months for complete recovery. Ultrasound is helpful as it reduces localized swelling, while passive knee and upper ankle motion maintains joint mobility. The patient must perform a preexercise stretching routine of the hamstrings and triceps surae complex. Tennis leg has an excellent prognosis provided rehabilitation is initiated appropriately and in a timely manner. An athlete may expect a full return to athletic competition, as permanent disability does not occur.

23. What is the therapeutic management of Achilles tendinitis?

A conservative program instituted early and carefully adhered to allows the patient with acute tendinitis to experience improvement over a period of 2 to 3 weeks. Return to most activities may be extended within 3 to 4 months of beginning nonoperative management, although resumption of running may require a wait-period of up to 6 months. The following rehabilitative program is appropriate for the spectrum of Achilles tendon disease ranging from peritendinitis to tendinitis to (small) partial tendon rupture. It is recommended that patients undergo at least 6 months of physical rehabilitation before surgical rehabilitation.[18] Therapeutic management of calcaneal tendinitis includes:

- *Rest.* Because mature tendons have no active fibroblast of their own they require migration of healing elements from outside the tendon. This, however, results in an inflammatory process of the tendon sheath and narrows the orifice in which the tendon glides. Without sufficient resting of tendon excursion, a vicious cycle may be set into motion whereby the continued tendon excursion within the inflamed sheath contributes to increased tendinitis.[72]
- *Therapeutic exercise.* Gentle passive, active, resistive stretching as well as strengthening exercises in conjunction with cryotherapy may be implemented after the swelling has subsided when the condition is no longer acute. Ice provides an anesthetic effect helpful in alleviating patient's symptoms after exercises. Once tenderness has subsided, more vigorous strengthening and stretching may begin, with an emphasis on eccentric muscle activity.

Passive gentle **stretching** represents the most important treatment component in management of the patient with an Achilles tendon overuse injury.[33] Stretching leads to lengthening of the muscle-tendon unit and consequently minimizes the deleterious effects of harmful tension build-up in the Achilles tendon during exercise.[27] Stretching may be accomplished by way of a wall lean stretch with the knee in both full extension and 45° extension to isolate both the gastrocnemius and soleus component of the muscle complex. Patients must be cautioned to preface stretching with a brief period of warm-up, and to perform the stretch gently, slowly, with a 10-second hold, and without bounce. Stretching may also be performed with a "foot-on-chair" method or by employing stairs. The use of an incline board is indispensable in proper stretching of the triceps surae complex, and

feet should be gradually worked to the base of the incline board. An incline board should measure 12 inches wide, 18 inches deep at the base, 6 inches high, and thus create an incline of approximately 15° to 18°. The patient begins by standing near the top of the board with the knees in full extension, making sure that the heels are flat and touching the board at all times. A stretch sensation should be felt in the proximal gastrocnemius area[65] or musculotendinous junction[65] and not in the tendinous portion of the heel cord. Recommended treatment time is 3 to 5 minutes six to eight times per day. Small doses of treatment many times a day are more effective than one large dose; whereas prolonged stretching for an extended period may exacerbate symptoms of tendinitis. As stretching and flexibility are achieved, the patient may move down toward the base of the board while leaning his or her back against a wall. Beyond this, added elevation may be placed under the board to create more tilt and hence more stretch once the patient feels that they are not gaining any more flexibility on the incline board.[65] Aggressive hamstring stretching are an indispensable part of the flexibility program as tight hamstrings may contribute toward triceps surae tightness.

Gentle passive, active, resistive **strengthening** as well as stretching exercises in conjunction with cryotherapy may be implemented after the swelling has subsided when the condition is no longer acute. Ice provides an anesthetic effect helpful to alleviating patient's symptoms after exercises. Once tenderness has subsided, more vigorous strengthening and stretching may begin, with an emphasis on eccentric muscle activity.

Maximal tensile load on the Achilles tendon occurs during eccentric contraction.[27] Because the eccentric mode of contraction is thought of as contributory to the development of Achilles tendon disorders, it is appropriate to specifically strengthen the triceps surae in this mode. This is accomplished by performing plantarflexion activities with elastic bands. If tolerated, toe-ups are performed using a stair with special attention paid to the descent (eccentric) phase of the exercise (Fig. 34-20). Although ascent involves a concentric contraction of the triceps surae, the eccentric descent component is performed slowly; hand weights maybe added to increase resistance as tolerated. The value of performing closed kinetic chain exercises is that they better simulate functional activities that require specific recruitment patterns of

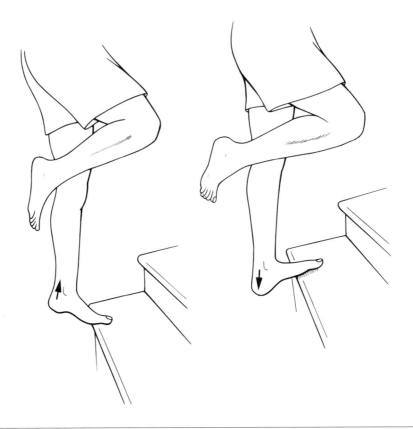

FIG. 34-20 Stairs may be used for both stretching and strengthening. Before stretching a maximal contraction of the triceps surae may be performed *(left)* by way of a toe raise, and followed by stretching *(right)*. Alternately, an eccentric strengthening exercise may be performed by posturing the involved foot in equinus *(left)* and slowly descending into ankle dorsiflexion *(right)*.

different muscles as well as proprioceptive responses than do open kinetic chain strengthening exercises.[37] Thus, exercises such as calf raises, squats, and step-ups are appropriate toward the final stages of triceps surae rehabilitation.

• *Plyometric exercise.* This uses the viscoelastic properties of the whole muscle and thereby produces greater forces than by sarcomere shortening alone. Studies have shown that an eccentric muscle contraction immediately preceding a concentric muscle contraction significantly increases the force generated concentrically.[4,11,13,16] This mechanism is known as a stretch-shortening contraction and occurs during plyometric training, which consists of a quick powerful movement involving pre-stretching or countermovement. The additional force generated during the stretch-shortening contraction is due to two mechanisms:

1. Prestretching of the elastic or noncontractile portions of the muscle, resulting in stored energy that is then quickly released.
2. Elicitation of the myotatic stretch reflex, which is a proprioceptive reflex.

Plyometric exercise involves rapid overload (prestretch) placed on the muscle immediately before concentric contraction. This both stretches the connective tissue and places an eccentric load on the muscle, which facilitates maximal fiber recruitment of the entire muscle and thereby peak concentric-generated force from that muscle.[45,56,69] The incorporation of plyometric exercises into an Achilles tendon rehabilitation program is helpful and utilizes an incline board to simulate the closed-chain functional mode. The patient postures the ankle in passive dorsiflexion to stretch the triceps surae complex, followed by active concentric contraction into equinus.

- *Modality use.* The use of iontophoresis with 10% hydrocortisone is effective in reducing inflammation. The use of oral antiinflammatory medications is appropriate. Electric stimulation (i.e., high or low volt galvanic stimulation[14] may be followed by contrast baths.

  Cryotherapy is a time-honored method of modifying the acute inflammatory response. This may be accomplished by way of ice massage applies 4 to 5 times a day for approximately 25 minutes for the first 24 to 48 hours. In addition to decreasing blood-flow, cooling also reduces the metabolic demands of tissue and thereby minimizes the zone of injury.[42] Elevation, together with rest and cold will help decrease swelling. The use of oral nonsteroidal antiinflammatory medication is helpful, although it has not conclusively shown to shorten recovery time.[1]

  Once the acute state has subsided (i.e., after 10 to 12 days), the application of moist heat should be employed often.[65] The use of ultrasound, although not helpful in modifying the acute inflammatory response, may have a role in the later stages of inflammation. When employed in the proliferative phase of wound healing, ultrasound has been shown to increase collagen production and possibly improve both the orientation and strength or the collagen comprising new scar tissue.[34] This effect may be highlighted by concomitant passive stretching.[33]

  Lower extremity alignment must be carefully assessed in patient presenting with Achilles tendon pathology, particularly for the presence of femoral anteversion, genu varum, tibia varus or either extreme of subtalar joint posture. These malalignments may result in excessive Achilles tendon excursion and subsequent degeneration.[20] Compensation for malalignment is accomplished by an appropriate orthosis that minimizes Achilles tendon excursion by way of subtalar joint realignment.

- *Patient education.* This is paramount as the athlete who fails to warm up with appropriate flexibility exercises invites recurrence. Modification of athletic program includes termination of hill running, decreased running mileage, stop interval training, change from a hard to a soft running surface, and increases cross-training in low impact sports such as swimming.

- *Orthotic management.* The use of an orthosis to maintain subtalar neutral, as well as a heel lift (ranging between 5/16 of an inch and 2 inches) to decrease

tendon excursion is part of the repertoire of management. Heel lifts should be placed in both shoes so as to prevent an abnormal gait. For players running in cleats, a disk or bar heel may be applied to keep the athlete from sinking into the soft turf.[65] For the cyclist, treatment is directed at correction of foot placement by moving it forward on the bike pedal, or the wearing of a more rigid shoe.[31] Heel pads have not shown to be beneficial in management of Achilles tendon overuse injuries.[54] For the patient with the cavus foot posture, the use of a padded heel cup absorbs the energy incurred by the foot during early stance.

Choosing the appropriate footwear is very important and differs for the patient with a flatfoot to a high-arched type foot. As a general rule, however, choosing a shoes with a flexible sole, a well-molded Achilles pad, a heel wedge at least 15 mm high, and a rigid heel counter will stave off stress to the Achilles tendon.[14] It is essential for the athlete to return to premorbid level of activity in a graduated manner.

- *Transverse friction massage.* This must address the entire portion of the inflamed tendon, and may include the medial, lateral, and anterior portions of the Achilles tendon. The duration of massage is fifteen minutes every other day for 1 to 2 weeks.

- *Taping.* This is generally not recommended for Achilles tendon disorders as it may intensify the problem more than alleviating it. Taping is generally done to prevent rupture and preferably done at the end of the season when the disorder will have a chance to properly heel or near the end of the season when there is only a limited period of participation. The clinician may tape using a short Achilles strap or a long Achilles strap. Taping is discouraged at the beginning of the season because of the potential of turning an acute problem into a chronic one.[65]

Intratendinous steroid injection is contraindicated as it may result in tendon rupture.[41] If any injection is attempted it must be carefully directed into the paratenon sheath or the space between the tendon and paratenon in the case of refractory peritenonitis, but not into the tendon itself.[22] This should be followed by a week's rest from vigorous activity. It is difficult to reliably confine injection to the region of the paratendon.[33] A more conservative approach would emphasize an initial trial or ultrasound, or phonophoresis with steroid cream.

The patient should not participate in any activity until the Achilles tendon has minimal tenderness on palpation. Chronic Achilles tendinitis require a 4 to 8 week mandatory rest period.[65] Severe cases may require immobilization in a short-leg walking cast for 1 to 2 weeks in the event that the above measures are unsuccessful.

The adage that prevention is easier than treatment certainly holds true for Achilles tendinitis. Once a patient is cured of Achilles tendinitis, they must always engage in proper warm-ups, range of motion activities, and stretching of the triceps surae complex.

Severe or chronic Achilles tendinitis that progresses to the point where the player can no longer participate mandates that all aggressive treatment should temporarily stop with the exception of moist heat or ultrasound application. Instead, the athlete is treated with cast immobilization or instructed to wear high heeled shoes or cowboy boots at all times; even getting out of bed in the middle of the night requires clogs with a minimum of a 2-inch heel.[65]

When tendinitis is unresponsive to some 6 to 8 weeks of conservative treatment the patient is considered for surgical excision of the thickened sheath. Pathology has evolved into tenovagitinis[21] in which the tendon and paratenon are adhered one to the other and can no longer glide relative to each other. In such refractory cases, tenolysis is performed and consists of surgically freeing the tendon from the paratenon and the removal or any nodules or scar tissue.

REFERENCES

1. Abramson SB: Nonsteroidal anti-inflammatory drugs: mechanisms of action and therapeutic considerations, In Leadbetter WB, Buckwalter JA, Gordon SL editors: *Sports-induced inflammation: clinical and basic science concepts.* Park Ridge, IL, 1990, American Academy of Orthopaedic Surgeons.
2. Allenmark C: Partial Achilles tendon tear, *Clin Sports Med* 11(4):759, 1992.
3. Andrish JT: *Overuse syndrome of the lower extremity in youth sports,* Champaign, Ill, 1984, Human Kinetics.
4. Asmussen E, Bonde-Peterson F: Storage of elastic energy in skeletal muscle in man, *Acta Physiol Scand* 91:335, 1974
5. Bachner EJ, Friedman MJ: Injuries to the leg, In Nicholas JA, Hershman EB editors: *The lower extremity and spine in sports medicine,* St. Louis, 1995, Mosby.
6. Bates BT et al: Foot orthotic devices to modify selected aspects of lower extremity mechanics, *Am J Sports Med* 7:338-342, 1979.
7. Baxter D: *The foot and ankle in sport,* St. Louis, 1995, Mosby.
8. Baxter DE: Chronic heel pain-treatment rationale. *Orthop Clin North Am* 20(4), 1989.
9. Bergfield J: The ankle and foot, instructional course, American Academy of Orthopaedic Surgeons Annual Meeting, St. Louis, January, 1982.
10. Berkow R, Fletcher AJ: *The Merck manual of diagnosis and therapy,* ed 15, Rahway, NJ, 1987, Merck & Co.
11. Bobbert MF: Drop jumping as a training method for jumping ability, *Sports Med* 9:7, 1990.
12. Bodgan RJ, Jenkins D, Hyland T: The runner's knee syndrome. In Rinaldi RR, Sabia M, editors: *Sports medicine,* Mount Kisco NY, 1978, Futura Publishing.
13. Bosco C, Komi PV: Potentiation of the mechanical behavior of the human skeletal muscle through prestretching, *Acta Physiol Scan* 106:467, 1979.
14. Brody DM: Running injuries. In Nicholas JA, Hershman EB editors: *The lower extremity and spine in sports medicine,* St. Louis, 1995, Mosby.
15. Brotzman SB: *Clinical orthopaedic rehabilitation,* St. Louis, 1996, Mosby.
16. Cavanga G, Saibene F, Magaria R: Effect of negative work on the amount of positive work performed by an isolated muscle, *J Appl Physiol* 20:157, 1965.
17. Christensen IB: Rupture of the Achilles tendon: analysis of 57 cases, *Acta Chir Scand* 106:50, 1953.
18. Clancy WG: Runner's injuries, *Am J Sports Med.* 8:287-289, 1980.
19. Clancy WG, Neidhart D, Brand RL: Achilles tendinitis in runners: a report of five cases, *Am J Sports Med* 4:46-57, 1976.
20. Clement DB, Taunton JE, Smart GW: Achilles tendinitis and peritendinitis: etiology and treatment, *Am J Sports Med* 12:179-184,1984.
21. Cyriax J: *Textbook of orthopaedic medicine, Diagnosis of soft tissue lesions,* ed 8, vol 1, London, 1982, Bailliere Tindall.
22. Dandy DJ: *Essential orthopaedics and trauma,* Edinburgh, 1989, Churchill Livingstone.
23. Donatelli RA: *The biomechanics of the foot and ankle,* ed 2, Philadelphia, 1996, FA Davis.
24. Fetto JF: *Anatomy and physical examination of the foot and ankle,* In Nicholas JA, Hershman EB editors: *The lower extremity and spine in sports medicine,* St. Louis, 1995, Mosby.
25. Fernandez-Palazzi F, Rivers S, Jujica P: Achilles tendinitis in ballet dancers, *Clin Orthop* 257-261, 1990.
26. Froimson AI: Tennis leg, *JAMA* 209:415, 1969.
27. Fyfe I, Stanish WD: The use of eccentric training and stretching in the treatment and prevention of tendon injuries, *Clin Sports Med* 11(3):601, 1992.
28. Hardaker WT: Foot and ankle injuries in classical ballet dancers, *Orthop Clin North Am* 20:621-627, 1989.
29. Hastad K, Larsson LC, Lindholm A: Clearance of radiosodium after local deposit in the Achilles tendon, *Acta Chir Scand* 116:251-256, 1976.
30. Hlavac HF: Compensated forefoot varus, *J Am Podiatr Assoc* 60:229-233, 1970.
31. Holmes JC, Pruitt AL, Whalen NJ: Cycling injuries. In Nicholas JA, Hershman EB editors: *The lower extremity and spine in sports medicine* St. Louis, 1995, Mosby.
32. Hunter-Friffin LY: Aspect of injuries to the lower extremity unique to the female athlete. In Nicholas JA, Hershman EB editors: *The lower extremity and spine in sports medicine,* St. Louis, 1995, Mosby.

33. Galloway MT, Jokl P, Dayton OW: Achilles tendon overuse injuries, *Clin Sports Med* 11(4), 1992.

34. Gieck JH, Saliba E: Therapeutic ultrasound: influence on inflammation and healing, In Leadbetter WB, Buckwalter JA, Gordon SL editors: *Sports-induced inflammation: clinical and basic science concepts,* Park Ridge, IL, 1990, American Academy of Orthopaedic Surgeons.

35. Glick JM, Sampson TG: Ankle and foot fractures in athletics, In Nicholas JA and Hershman EB editors: *The lower extremity and spine in sports medicine,* St. Louis, 1995, Mosby.

36. Gould N, Karson R: Stenosing tenosynovitis of the pseudosheath of the tendo-Achilles, *J Foot Ankle Surg* 1:3, 1980.

37. Greenfield BH, Tovin BJ: The application of open and closed kinematic chain exercises in rehabilitation of the lower extremity, *J Back Musculoskel Rehabil* 2:38, 1992.

38. Gregg J, Das M: Foot and ankle problems in the preadolescent and adolescent athlete. *Clin Sports Med* 1:131, 1982.

39. James SL, Bates BT, Osternig LR: Injuries to runners, *Am J Sports Med* 6:40-50, 1978.

40. Kendall FP, McCreary EK: *Muscles: testing and function,* ed 3, Baltimore, 1983, Williams and Wilkins.

41. Kleinman M, Gross AE: Achilles tendon rupture following steroid injection, *J Bone Joint Surg* 65A:1345-1347, 1983.

42. Knight KL: Cold as a modifier of sports-induced inflammation, In Leadbetter WB, Buckwalter JA, Gordon SL editors: *Sports-induced inflammation: clinical and basic science concepts,* Park Ridge, IL, 1990, American Academy of Orthopaedic Surgeons

43. Kohler A: *Roentgenology,* ed 2, London, 1935, Balliare, Tindall & Cox.

44. Kohler A, Zimmer EA: *Borderlands of the normal and early pathologic in skeletal roentgenology,* ed 3, New York, 1968, Grune & Stratton.

45. Komi PV, editor: *Strength and power in sport,* London, 1992, Blackwell Scientific Publications.

46. Kvist M et al: Chronic Achilles paratenonitis in athletes: a histologic and histochemical study, *Pathology* 19:1-11, 1987.

47. Kvist MH et al: Chronic Achilles paratenonitis: an immunohistologic study of fibronectin and fibrinogen, *Am J Sports Med* 16:616-623, 1988.

48. Landvater SJ, Renstrom PAFH: Complete Achilles tendon ruptures, *Clin Sports Med* 11(4), 1992.

49. Largergren C, Lindholm A: Vascular distribution in the Achilles tendon, *Acta Chir Scand* 116:491, 1958.

50. Leadbetter W, Buckwalter J, Gordon S editors: *Sports-induced inflammation,* Chicago, 1990, Am Acad Orthop Surg.

51. Lehmkuhl LD, Smith LK: *Brunnstrom's clinical kinesiology,* ed 4, Philadelphia, 1989, FA Davis.

52. Lillegard WA, Rucker KS: *Handbook of sports medicine: a symptoms-oriented approach,* Boston, 1993, Andover Medical Publishers.

53. Ljungqvist R, Eriksson E: Partial tears of the patellar tendon and the Achilles tendon, In *American Academy of Orthopedic Surgeons Symposium on the foot and leg in running sports,* St Louis, 1982, Mosby.

54. Lowdon A, Bader DL, Mowat AG: The effect of heel pads on the treatment of Achilles tendinitis: a double blind trial, *Am J Sports Med* 12:431-435, 1984.

55. Lundqvist R: Partial subcutaneous of the patellar tendon. Proceeding of the First Scandinavian Sportsmedicine Conference, *Syntex Ter* 2:89 1977.

56. McArdle WE, Katch FI, Katch VL: *Exercise physiology: energy, nutrition and human performance,* ed 3, Philadelphia, 1991, Lea & Febiger.

57. Micheli LJ: Overuse injuries in children's sports, the growth factor, *Orthop Clin North Am* 14:337, 1980.

58. Micheli LJ et al: Athletic footwear and modifications, In Nicholas JA, Hershman EB editors: *The lower extremity and spine in sports medicine,* St. Louis, 1995, Mosby.

59. Miller TT, Ghelman B, Potter HG: Imaging of the foot and ankle. In Nicholas JA, Hershman EB editors: *The lower extremity and spine in sports medicine,* St. Louis, 1995, Mosby.

60. Nelan G, Martens M, Burssens A: Surgical treatment of chronic Achilles tendinitis, *Am J Sports Med* 17:754-759, 1989.

61. Netter FH: The Ciba Collection of Medical Illustrations, vol 8, *Musculoskeletal System, Part I, Anatomy, Physiology, and Metabolic Disorders,* Summit, New Jersey, 1991, CIBA-GEIGY.

62. Pagnani MJ et al: Anatomy of the knee. In Nicholas JA, Hershman EB editors: *The lower extremity and spine in sports medicine,* St. Louis, 1995, Mosby.

63. Peterson L, Renstrom P: *Sports injuries— their prevention and treatment,* Chicago, 1986, Year Book Medical Publishers.,

64. Puddu G, Ippolito E, Postacchini F: A classification of Achilles tendon disease. *Am J Sports Med* 4:145-150, 1976.

65. Reese RC Jr, Burruss TP, Patten J: Athletic training techniques and protective equipment. In Nicholas JA, Hershman EB editors: *The lower extremity and spine in sports medicine,* St. Louis, 1995, Mosby.

66. Sanderson DJ: The biomechanics of cycling shoes, *Cycling Sci* 2(3):27, 1990.

67. Sarrafian SK: *Anatomy of the foot and ankle,* Philadelphia, 1983, JB Lippincott.

68. Schon LC, Baxter DE: Neuropathies of the foot and ankle in athletes, *Clin Sports Med* 9:489-508, 1990.

69. Sharkey BJ: Training for sport. In Catu RC, Michelli LJ, editors: *ACSM's Guidelines for the team physician,* Philadelphia, 1991, Lea & Febiger.

70. Simpson RR, Gudas CJ: Posterior tibial tendon rupture in a world-class runner, *J Foot Surg* 22:74, 1983.

71. Strand FL: *Physiology: a regulatory systems approach,* ed 2, New York, 1983, Macmillan Publishing.

72. Subotnick S: *Podiatric sports medicine,* Mt. Kisco, NY, 1975, Futura Publishing.

73. Subotnick S, Sisney P: Treatment of Achilles tendinopathy in the athlete, *J Am Podiatr Med Assoc* 76:552-557, 1986.

74. Teitz CC: Overuse injuries. In Teitz CC editor: *Scientific foundation of sports medicine,* Toronto, 1989, BC Decker.

75. Titze A: Ueber den architektonischen aubau des biodegenebes in der neuschilchen fuss-sohle, *Beitr A Klin Chir* 123:493, 1921.

76. Tiberio D: Pathomechanics of structural foot deformities, *Phys Ther* 68(12), 1988.

77. Turco VJ: Injuries to the foot and ankle, In Nicholas JA, Hershman EB editors: *The lower extremity and spine in sports medicine,* St. Louis, 1995, Mosby.

78. Valmassy RL: *Clinical biomechanics of the lower extremities,* St. Louis, 1996, Mosby.

79. Waller JF, Maddalo AV: *Foot and ankle linkage system,* In Nicholas JA, Hershman EB editors: *The lower extremity and spine in sports medicine,* St. Louis, 1995, Mosby.

80. Washington ZL: Musculoskeletal injuries in theatrical dancers: site, frequency, and severity, *Am J Sports Med* 6:75, 1978.

81. Xethalis JL, Lorei MP: Soccer injuries, In Nicholas JA, Hershman EB editors: *The lower extremity and spine in sports medicine,* St. Louis, 1995, Mosby.

RECOMMENDED READING

Galloway MT, Jokl P, Dayton OW: Achilles tendon overuse injuries, *Clin Sports Med* 11(4), 1992.

Soma CA, Mandelbaum BR: Achilles tendon disorders, *Clin Sports Med* 13(4), 1994.

35

Popping Sensation Above Heel Followed by Intense, Immediate Pain, Loss of Ambulation, and Slight Bulge Over Left Calf

CASE 1: A 53-year-old male executive plays a vigorous game of basketball with his teenage children one Sunday afternoon, and experiences sudden, sharp, and severe pain after lunging forward while dribbling the ball. This occurs after a perceptibly audible snap that he felt at the right heel. Bystanders remember him immediately swinging around looking behind himself to see if someone had accidentally kicked or bumped him from behind; no one had done so. Immediately overcome with pain, he sat down. After several minutes, he could no longer walk normally. The patient later admits to no history of any leg or foot tendinitis, nor any history of syphilis or gout.

OBSERVATION   Swelling and ecchymosis are present above the right heel, with a loss of normal outline of the Achilles tendon. An increase in right calf prominence is observed as a lump at the midcalf region. The patient walks with an antalgic gait that lacks push-off, and demonstrates a forefoot varus foot posture.

PALPATION   Palpation yields a palpable defect 5 cm above the right os calcis, especially when the non–weight-bearing right foot is passively dorsiflexed with the patient prone on the examination table. Palpation of the sole of the right foot indicates predominant weight borne along the lateral border of the foot, with a callus under the fifth metatarsal.

PASSIVE RANGE OF MOTION   Dorsiflexion of the right ankle appears slightly increased, compared with the contralateral ankle.

ACTIVE RANGE OF MOTION   Good plantarflexion of the right ankle. Complete loss of active dorsiflexion is present, and heel drop is noted.

STRENGTH   Fair to Fair+ manual muscle test grade to right resistive ankle plantarflexion, although this becomes minimally possible several days later. The patient cannot rise on his right tiptoe.

FLEXIBILITY   Tightness is present in the ipsilateral hamstring muscle and contralateral triceps surae and hamstring.

SPECIAL TESTS   Positive squeeze sign, sulcus sign, and heel drop test; negative Homan's test.

CLUE:

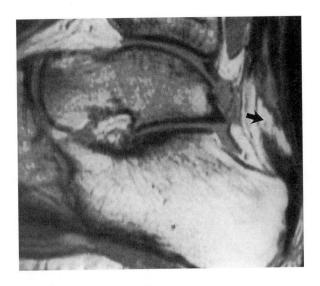

(From Nicholas JA, Hershman EB: *The lower extremity and spine in sports medicine,* ed 2, St Louis, 1995, Mosby.)

CASE 2: A 28-year-old competitive track runner with a history of unresolved Achilles tendinitis took part in a charity race. Although she won the race, she did so at the expense of an explosive take-off at the beginning of the race. The pain she felt after the "runner's high" after the race was temporarily relieved when she placed her left foot in an ice bucket for 20 minutes. Since the race she complains of pain at the beginning of activity. The pain gradually subsides and returns following cessation of activity. The pain is most acute as she accelerates. She also reports stiffness after rest and sleep. When asked, she admits to having received several injections to her Achilles tendon over the past several years. The results of an x-ray examination are negative. Anterior and posterior draw signs for both the ankle and knee are negative.

OBSERVATION   A forefoot valgus deformity of both feet is noted.

PALPATION   A tender fusiform swelling at the midportion of the left Achilles tendon is noted, as is as a slight notch in that tendon. Callus buildup is noted under the first and fifth metatarsal heads of both feet.

PASSIVE RANGE OF MOTION   Passive range of motion is normal and full for both left ankle plantarflexion and dorsiflexion.

ACTIVE RANGE OF MOTION   A slight loss of left ankle dorsiflexion is noted when compared with the contralateral ankle.

STRENGTH   Left ankle plantarflexion is G−, whereas dorsiflexion is good. The patient can heel walk and toe walk.

FLEXIBILITY   Tightness of bilateral heel cords, triceps surae, and hamstring muscles are noted.

SPECIAL TESTS   Negative squeeze test and negative Homan's sign. Electromyographic tests reveal less than maximal plantarflexion muscle recruitment of the left triceps surae muscle group. Positive heel drop test.

CLUE:

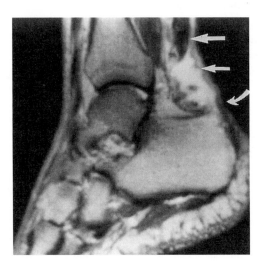

(From Nicholas JA, Hershman EB: *The lower extremity and spine in sports medicine,* ed 2, St Louis, 1995, Mosby.)

? | Questions

1. What injury did these people sustain?
2. What is the incidence of Achilles tendon rupture?
3. What is the pathogenesis of Achilles tendon rupture?
4. What is the mechanism of Achilles tendon rupture in the younger, athletic population?
5. What is the degenerative etiology of Achilles tendon rupture?
6. What is the histopathology of the Achilles tendon prior to rupture?
7. How is the vascularity of the Achilles tendon complex essential to an understanding of the location of pathologic tendon degeneration and rupture?
8. What are the spiral and rotational courses of the insertional fibers of the Achilles tendon?
9. What are the parameters of calcaneal excursion during gait?
10. How does rapid alternation between calcaneal eversion and inversion result in Achilles stress caused by excessive tendon excursion?
11. How would a forefoot varus and forefoot valgus deformity predispose for Achilles tendinitis?
12. How may the rapid alternation between the eccentric and concentric functions of a tight triceps surae result in pathologic conditions of the Achilles tendon?
13. How may the disparity in the rate and magnitude of contraction between the gastrocnemius and soleus contribute to Achilles tendon degeneration as a function of shear-force buildup within the conjoint tendon?
14. How does tightness of the triceps surae complex affect stress on the Achilles tendon?
15. What is partial rupture of the Achilles tendon?

16. What is the clinical presentation of total rupture?
17. What provocative tests confirm suspicion of a torn Achilles tendon complex?
18. Why does the ability to plantarflex against resistance return several days after injury?
19. What imaging techniques help clinical diagnosis in the delayed examination of a suspected rupture?
20. Which criteria determine whether a torn tendon is conservatively or surgically managed?
21. What are the problems and benefits with surgical and nonsurgical management of rupture?

22. What is percutaneous repair of the Achilles tendon?
23. What therapeutic intervention is appropriate after Achilles tendon rupture?
24. What is the surgical approach to treatment?
25. What is the postoperative therapeutic regimen?
26. What accounts for a greater rerupture rate with the nonsurgically managed patient?
27. How is a partial rupture of the Achilles tendon managed?

1. What injury did these people sustain?

Complete rupture of the *Achilles tendon* in case I is demonstrated by tendinous discontinuity seen by magnetic resonance imaging (MRI). Moreover, the proximal end of the tendon is retracted, the distal end is seen *(curved arrow)*, and fluid is present between the two torn ends *(small arrow.)* The clue in Case II indicated a *large partial rupture* of the Achilles tendon with herniation of pre-Achilles fat *(arrow)* into the site of the defect. The Achilles tendon is the strongest and largest tendon in the body, and yet is also commonly ruptured. This patient has incurred a third-degree strain of the myotendinous junction of the tendo Achilles. Authorities have alternately implicated both a hyperpronated and cavus foot deformity in the etiology of Achilles tendon disorders, ranging from the more benign tendon inflammation to a full-blown full-thickness rupture. Patients with these intrinsic foot deformities are at greater risk for injury or rupture during physical activity because of the diminished shock-absorption capacity correlated with these malalignments.[4] The physical therapist applies a spectrum of diagnostic and rehabilitation techniques to identify etiologic extrinsic or intrinsic factors contributing to disorders of the Achilles tendon ranging from tendinitis to rupture (Fig. 35-1). Correction of pathomechanic factors, modality application, and aggressive postoperative rehabilitation are among the strategies that allow early return to function or sport without significant loss of strength or mobility.

2. What is the incidence of Achilles tendon rupture?

The incidence of Achilles tendon rupture has dramatically increased over the last few decades,[27,36] and may be related to the increased participation of individuals older than 30 years of age in recreational and physical fitness activities.[43] Classically, the patient is a middle-aged, male, former college athlete who has a sedentary or white-collar type of occupation but enjoys an occasional weekend volleyball game with his colleagues or children. Recreational sports such as skiing, basketball, and tennis or other racquet sports often involve sudden acceleration or jumping that may unduly stress the tendon and result in rupture. Ruptures are more common in mesomorphic[60] men, with the male-to-female ratio ranging anywhere from 2:1 to 12:1.[7,58] A statistical correlation between the incidence of Achilles tendon rupture and ABO blood groups exists, in which patients with tendon ruptures demonstrate a significantly higher incidence of the O blood group.[36] The significance of this finding is unknown.

3. What is the pathogenesis of Achilles tendon rupture?

The exact pathogenesis of Achilles tendon rupture remains obscure, and may be multifactorial in origin. An academic query as to why an otherwise typically healthy 30- to 40-year-old individual should suddenly sustain spontaneous midsubstance strain of the Achilles tendon remains unanswered. Theories attempting to identify the mechanism of pathogenesis include degeneration, mechanical failure caused by cyclic loading and disruption of collagen bundles, hypoxia caused by compromised vascularity, stress concentration at the lateral convex aspect of a spiraling tendon insertion, excessive shear stress between the gastrocnemius and soleus tendons before their confluence,[35] excessive mediolateral tendon excursion, or perhaps a complex interplay of these factors. Rupture may also occur as the result of a direct blow to the Achilles tendon while

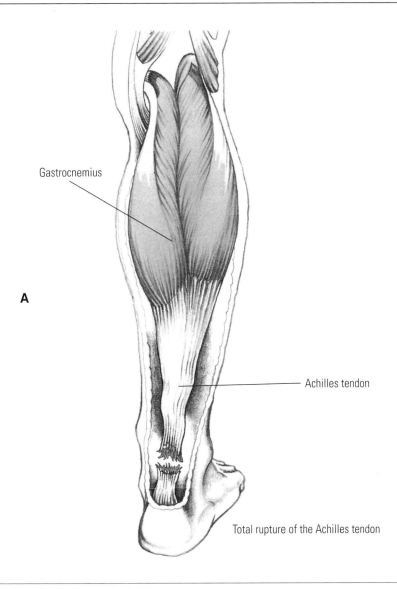

Gastrocnemius

Achilles tendon

A

Total rupture of the Achilles tendon

FIG. 35-1 A, Total rupture of the Achilles tendon. (From Peterson L, Renstrom P: *Sports injuries: their prevention and treatment,* Chicago, 1983, Yearbook Medical Publishers, Inc.)

(Continued)

the muscle is strongly contracted,[16,30] or iatrogenically from steroid injection.[45,50]

There is mounting evidence that Achilles tendon ruptures are sustained by two separate groups of patients: acute injury in younger, more active male individuals without any prior symptoms; and middle-aged adults, particularly males in their third to fifth decades, after chronic Achilles pain and weakness. Pathogenesis has thus been attributed to either chronic degeneration of the tendon or excessive mechanical failure. Rupture

occurs approximately 3 cm proximal to the tendon's insertion on the calcaneus.

4. What is the mechanism of Achilles tendon rupture in the younger, athletic population?

Tendon rupture may occur in healthy, active, athletic individuals who have rarely experienced pain in the calf or heel before their injury. In these cases, the Achilles tendon may be torn by the same mechanism that tears the medial head of the gastrocnemius muscle, such as a

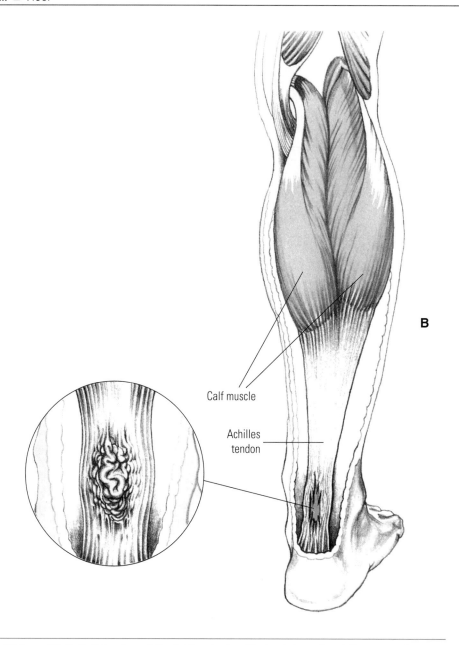

Calf muscle

Achilles
tendon

B

FIG. 35-1, cont'd B, Partial rupture of the Achilles tendon. The inset shows how inflammatory tissue can form in the injured site following partial rupture.

sudden jump or lunge on the sports field. Injury is predisposed by sudden, explosive effort, such as the run-ups and take-offs at the start of a 100-meter race. The resulting sudden recruitment of the entire triceps surae imposes tension to the Achilles tendon that exceeds its inherent tensile limit. The Achilles tendon is practically avulsed through its midsubstance; occasionally, avulsion of the calcaneal insertion may occur instead.

5. What is the degenerative etiology of Achilles tendon rupture?

The Achilles tendon begins to demonstrate degenerative histologic changes at the early age of 25 to 30 years, which over time results in ischemia secondary to compromised blood supply. Soft tissue changes associated with maturation and senescence include alteration of tendon collagen with increased cross-linking of tropocollagen, increased tendon stiffness, decreased tensile strength, and fiber shrinkage.[53] Consequently the tendon becomes more injury prone. Progressive degeneration continues into middle age and acts to lower the tensile yield point of tendon strength. Subsequently a trivial misstep, stumble, or startle (as may occur when crossing the street) may cause a middle-aged mesomorphic male to break into a sudden run in the attempt to catch himself. The resultant sudden and forceful distractive tension imparted to the tendon may exceed the tendon's tensile tolerance and result in heel cord rupture. Alternatively, injury may follow intermittent, aggressive athletic activities in which the individual demonstrates effort out of proportion to his age and activity level by attempting to perform as he did during those idyllic years of young adulthood. Injury frequently occurs in entertainers (such as tap dancers) who carry on beyond the prime of their life. Injury may also occur after unusual activity that follows a sedentary period. There may be a history of previous intermittent pain suggestive of long-standing mild chronic Achilles disease, or no history whatsoever.

6. What is the histopathology of the Achilles tendon prior to rupture?

A *musculotendinous unit* is composed of contractile (muscle) and passive (tendon) components. The tensile strength of a tendon is more than twice the strength of its associated muscle.[3] Tendons are composed of closely packed, parallel, cross-linked collagen fiber bundles interposed with elastin fibers. Whereas *collagen* is characterized by tensile strength and poor ability to recoil, *elastin* is characterized by a capacity to recoil and a relatively weak tensile strength. Together, these two substances lend the tendon its unique ability to tolerate large magnitudes of tension and yet recoil following tension release. When the tendon is loaded under tension, the parallel, wavy fibers of collagen straighten along the direction of load. Once the load is released, the elastin fibers facilitate reorientation of the collagen into its resting wavy configuration. However, once the physiologic limit (yield point) of these fibers has been surpassed by excessive tensile stress (8% strain), the tendon fails because of breakage of the collagen cross-links,[60] and sudden rupture may occur.[3] The tensile strength of the Achilles tendon has been measured at 4000 to 5000 N, and an elongation at rupture of 1 to 2 cm.[1]

7. How is the vascularity of the Achilles tendon complex essential to an understanding of the location of pathologic tendon degeneration and rupture?

The Achilles tendon is unusual in that it is not surrounded by a true synovial sheath (tenosynovium). Instead there is a pseudosheath—a *peritenon,* which is composed of an inner epitenon and superficial paratenon that surround the Achilles tendon.[65] The majority of the tendon vascular supply derives from the *epitenon*—a thick, vascular connective tissue layer that invests the tendon surface and nurtures its substance.[41,62] The *paratenon* is actually a series of thin membranes that enhance tendon gliding by minimizing friction between the tendon and the surrounding tissue[39,41,62] and demonstrate excursions of up to 1.5 cm.[41] The triceps surae complex has a relatively good blood supply and heals predictably well after injury.[7,58] Unfortunately, an exception to this good vascular supply exists in the Achilles tendon where there is a *critical zone* of relative avascularity[1] akin to the critical zone in the rotator cuff at the shoulder. The vascular supply of the Achilles tendon consists of longitudinal arterioles that course the length of the tendon and are supplemented by vessels from the paratenon. This vascular watershed exists at 4.5 cm[42] above the tendon insertion, and is vulnerable to ischemic insult. This central portion of the tendon is the least well perfused and consequently the most vulnerable to ischemic insult. Additionally, studies have shown that the tendinous vessels decrease in size and number with increasing age.[26] The combination of these factors accounts for increased susceptibility to chronic inflammation and eventual rupture[23,47] at the central aspect of the tendon, located 2 to 6 cm proximal to the calcaneal insertion.[50]

8. What are the spiral and rotational courses of the insertional fibers of the Achilles tendon?

The tendon of insertion of the triceps surae muscle group is a conjoint tendon known by a variety of synonyms, including Achilles tendon, tendocalcaneus, tendo Achillis, and tendon of the triceps surae. Regardless of nomenclature, a key point in understanding the pathokinesiology of the Achilles tendon is its rotational component prior to its distal insertion. The tendon inserts on a rectangular area at the postero*medial* aspect of the calcaneal tuberosity. Hence since the calcaneal tuberosity is medial to the midline of the os calcis, the distal tendon travels along a gentle spiral from its point of confluence in what may be characterized not as a vertical, but rather a slightly curved tendon. When the posterior right foot is viewed, the Achilles insertion is thus described as being slightly convex laterally and concave medially (Fig. 35-2). Consequently, the tendon may have a higher tensile load along its convex aspect. Additionally, from the point of confluence of the gastrocnemius and soleus 5 to 6 cm proximal to the insertion of the Achilles tendon, the tendon fibers assume a slightly spiral course. The posterior fibers obliquely course from medial to lateral, whereas the anterior fibers pass from lateral to medial.[14,25]

9. What are the parameters of calcaneal excursion during gait?

Any understanding of how rotation of the distal Achilles tendon relates to pathokinesiology must be prefaced by a discussion of calcaneal excursion during gait. During the latter part of swing the foot is locked into supination and dorsiflexion in preparation for imminent heel strike; this foot posture necessitates obligatory external tibial rotation. What is the calcaneal posture? Since supination is a triplanar motion consisting of a combination of forefoot plantarflexion and adduction and rearfoot inversion, the calcaneus is said to be *inverted.*

Once heel strike occurs, the foot unlocks out of supination into the extreme opposite triplanar directions characteristic of pronation—forefoot dorsiflexion and abduction and rearfoot eversion. This is consistent with obligatory internal tibial rotation. What is the calcaneal posture? *Eversion.* This eversion of the heel allows the foot to become a mobile adapter at contact.

10. How does rapid alternation between calcaneal eversion and inversion result in Achilles stress caused by excessive tendon excursion?

Early stance phase is characterized by a sudden alternation from calcaneal inversion to eversion during heel strike as the supinated foot becomes pronated. This process is reversed beyond midstance when the pronated foot becomes resupinated. The repetitive calcaneal excursion has a whipping effect on the calcaneal tendon that pulls the tendon *mediolaterally*[20] during pronation at heel strike and, conversely, whips the tendon *lateromedially* at maximal supination during toe-off phase of gait (Fig. 35-3). Conceivably, excessive tendon hypermobility may follow excessive running or other sports that may concentrate stress at the central avascular portion of the tendon and cause mechanical wear and tear. This saw-like action of the tendon may be heightened

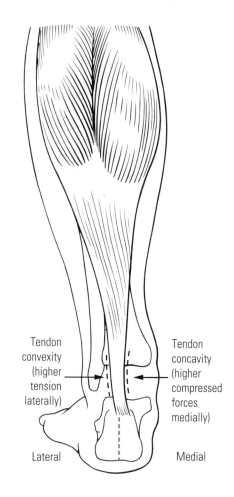

Tendon convexity (higher tension laterally)

Tendon concavity (higher compressed forces medially)

Lateral

Medial

FIG. 35-2 When viewing the posterior right foot, the Achilles insertion is thus described as being slightly convex laterally and concave medially.

as a result of the rotation of the distal Achilles tendon fibers.[8] Additionally, because of the rotational insertion of the distal Achilles tendon medially to the calcaneal midline, stress may be nonuniformly delivered to the tendon, which may serve to accentuate stress and compound the problem. The tension within the tendon may be increased because of the spiraling architecture of the anterior and posterior fibers composing the tendon, which would produce a "wring-out" effect of the least perfused central portion.[10,11] If unabated, stress will be focused at the tenoperiosteal junction at the heel, causing periosteal avulsion away from the underlying cortical bone. The resulting void may be filled by a spur thatoffers mechanical obstruction to tendon function and initiates a vicious cycle of pathologic conditions.

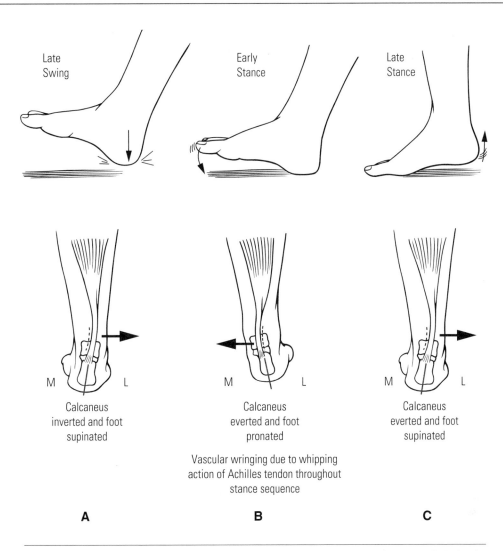

FIG. 35-3 *Achilles tendon excursion* as a function of alternating hindfoot posture during stance. **A,** During the transition from late swing to early stance, the subtalar joint alternates from a supinated posture to a pronated one. At the rearfoot, this manifests as an alteration from inversion to eversion of the calcaneus. **B,** This rapid alteration causes a *mediolateral* whipping of the Achilles tendon, subjecting its distal fibers to vascular wringing at its relatively avascular central aspect. With overpronation, avascularity of the tendon is magnified due to excessive and prolonged tendon excursion, concentrating stress and causing mechanical wear and tear on the tendon. **C,** In contrast to early stance, whipping of the tendon *lateromedially* at maximal supination during toe off phase of gait occurs.

11. How would a forefoot varus and forefoot valgus deformity predispose for Achilles tendinitis?

Whereas as a forefoot varus deformity (see p. 347) compensates by way of excessive *pronation,* a rigid forefoot valgus deformity (see pp. 348-349) compensates by minimizing pronation or *supination.*[63] Thus both extremes of the spectrum of foot deformities have been implicated as being causative of Achilles tendinitis,[66] albeit via two diametrically differing mechanisms.

A *forefoot varus deformity* (see p. 347) is characterized by subtalar joint *compensatory pronation* during midstance and propulsion phases of gait. Excessive pronation causes excessive calcaneal eversion during stance phase, which causes excessive obligatory mediolateral whipping of the Achilles tendon. The abnormal temporal sequencing characteristic of a forefoot varus means that pronation persists beyond midstance, during that time when the foot should be supinating. The net result is counter rotary forces along the tibia during midstance; simultaneously, external rotation occurs in the proximal tibia (as a function of the screw-home mechanism of the knee) while the pronating foot imparts an internal rotation along the distal tibia.[6] These conflicting torsions magnify the bowstringing effect on the tendon, and potentially wreak havoc on the Achilles tendon, increasing rotational and shear forces[10,34,51] that "wring out" those vessels in the zone of relative avascularity. This establishes the appropriate setting for inflammation and degenerative changes within the tendon.[7,58]

Stress concentration of the Achilles tendon is amplified in the excessively pronated foot by an additional factor. Because the tendon inserts medial to the calcaneal tuberosity, lateral calcaneal excursion that accompanies pronation subjects the Achilles tendon to a slight lateral twisting. This imparts a higher tensile load along the lateral convex aspect of the tendon, further concentrating deleterious stress at the vulnerable central portion.

A *forefoot valgus deformity* (see pp. 348-349) is characterized by a reduction in pronation because of *compensatory supination* that precludes enough pronation during contact phase of gait. Excessive supination causes excessive calcaneal inversion during stance phase, which causes obligatory lateromedial whipping of the Achilles tendon. This excessively early supination delivers an external rotary torque to the distal tibia during a time when the proximal tibia is medially rotating the knee out of its locked extended position and into flexion. The conflicting torsions are absorbed by the Achilles tendon and other soft tissue running longitudinally along the tibia bone; these tissues may sustain inflammatory and degenerative changes.

12. How may the rapid alternation between the eccentric and concentric functions of a tight triceps surae result in pathologic conditions of the Achilles tendon?

Tendon rupture is the most serious, and often the end stage, of a long history of Achilles tendon disorders. The role of eccentric versus concentric loading in the etiology of Achilles tendonopathy and rupture remains a source of debate.[12] Many authorities consider a large and unmanageable eccentric loading of the tendon as the final insult that precedes full thickness rupture[9,34,51,62] as the foot and ankle are in dorsiflexion and the knee is extended.[60] A similar mechanism results in tear of the medial head of the gastrocne-

mius. Others maintain that rupture follows a sudden, concentric contraction of the triceps surae that had been previously undergoing an eccentric contraction.[67] Perhaps an imbalance in the concentric and eccentric interplay of these two modes of contraction may be culpable as a contributing mechanism of injury. How this occurs during stance phase must be understood in relation to contraction of the two-jointed gastrocnemius muscle.

The gastrocnemius is a kinesiologically complex muscle that plays a key role in lower extremity biomechanics by virtue of heavily influencing the knee, ankle, and subtalar joint.[55] At midstance phase of gait the knee is in relative extension, the ankle is neutral, and the gastrocnemius is placed on stretch from its proximal origin. Just beyond midstance the vertical projection of the center of gravity (at the pelvis) moves behind the knee joint and generates a flexor moment. Excessive knee flexion is dampened by eccentric contraction of the quadriceps muscle proximally and the gastrocnemius muscle distally. Proximal distraction, which was initially facilitated by knee extension, is consistent with midstance phase of gait just prior to heel rise. The gastrocnemius undergoes an eccentric contraction along its length to slow down knee flexion that accompanies heel-off. As this occurs the foot is dorsiflexed, resulting in stretching of the gastrocnemius muscle distally because of dorsiflexion at the upper ankle joint. Thus although the source of gastrocnemius stretch is minimized and lost proximally, it is simultaneously being generated distally by dorsiflexion, so that the muscle retains a state of constant stretch. This point is essential because for the gastrocnemius to undergo an efficient eccentric contraction, it must be first stretched as tension is developing. Stretching of the tendon is consistent with distraction of one or both of the muscle attachments.

As knee flexion increases, the stance leg must catch up with the forward displacement of the center of gravity by initiating toe-off. The gastrocnemius accomplishes this by rapidly switching to a concentric contraction during the impending toe-off phase of late stance. What has occurred during the short interim between midstance and late stance is a two-fold reversal, involving the rapid alternation from an eccentric to concentric contractile mode of the gastrocnemius muscle, as well as a rapid change in sagittal ankle motion (and hence, Achilles excursion) from maximal dorsiflexion to maximal plantarflexion. It is this dual rapid alternation that may, in the presence of a shortened gastroc-soleus complex, focus a locus of stress on the Achilles tendon.

13. How may the disparity in the rate and magnitude of contraction between the gastrocnemius and soleus contribute to Achilles tendon degeneration as a function of shear-force buildup within the conjoint tendon?

The Achilles tendon is a true conjoint tendon bound by collagen fibers known as Sharpey's fibers. Although collagen loads well under tension, it frays under shear. The anatomic juxtaposition between the gastrocnemius (consisting primarily of type II, fast-twitch fibers) and soleus (consisting primarily of type I, slow-twitch intermediate fibers) during cocontraction may result in shear* buildup between the two components of the conjoint distal tendon because of a differential in the rate of contraction. This disparity in the rate of contraction may loosen the junction between the two portions of tendon because of increased friction.

14. How does tightness of the triceps surae complex affect stress on the Achilles tendon?

Stretching of the Achilles-gastrocnemius unit, which occurs beyond midstance phase of normal gait, primes the triceps surae complex for optimal concentric propulsive contraction during toe-off phase of late stance. This occurs because forward tibial inclination beyond midstance postures the upper ankle in dorsiflexion and thereby stretches the triceps surae. This prestretch (overload) of the triceps surae complex immediately before concentric contraction uses the viscoelastic properties of the whole muscle to produce greater forces than are produced by sarcomere shortening alone. This magnitude of force generation is necessary for push-off phase of gait. However, in the presence of a tightened posterior leg musculature, the triceps surae contracts suboptimally, and the Achilles tendon undergoes excessive stress.

In the presence of a tight gastroc-soleus muscle group, the gastroc-soleus lacks the ability to appropriately stretch before eccentric contraction. Thus an ineffective eccentric contraction precedes the concentric contraction, possibly resulting in a violent concentric contraction that sends a sudden jerk through the gastroc-soleus–Achilles tendon–plantar facial system that

---

*Shear, by definition, is not confined to opposing forces only, but may also include forces that derive from a varying rate or magnitude in contraction.

may exceed the strength of one of these structures, damaging the weakest link in the system. The calf may tear, the Achilles tendon may rupture, the plantar fascia may be strained, or a combination of these injuries may occur.[67]

15. What is partial rupture of the Achilles tendon?

Unlike total Achilles tendon ruptures that tend to occur in middle-aged, deconditioned individuals, partial ruptures occur in well-trained athletes and are usually secondary to multiple microtrauma caused by overuse.[1] Athletes susceptible to partial tears include runners, jumpers, throwers, and participants in racquet sports.[57] Partial ruptures are usually along that aspect of the Achilles tendon subject to the greatest concentration of stress—the lateral convex aspect of the tendon.[65] Partial ruptures may occur in the central tendon fibers without breaking tendon continuity.[15] The type of tear, whether longitudinal, transverse, or a combination thereof, is variable. Additionally, the magnitude of fiber involvement may vary from only a few to just short of a complete rupture.

Partial Achilles tendon tears are frequently misdiagnosed as chronic Achilles tendinosis because of the absence of many of the signs associated with classic full-thickness rupture.[57] Because of this, a diagnosis of chronic Achilles tendinosis is not a certain conclusion, and remains suspect until confirmed by appropriate imaging. Diagnosis of partial tears is thus difficult, but enhanced by diagnostic imaging, including ultrasound, sub-Achilles bursography, computed tomography, magnetic resonance imaging, or electromyography. Electromyography allows electrophysiologic evaluation of muscle function in a dynamic way that reveals maximum fiber recruitment with effort and increased resistance; extrapolation of possible partial rupture is made based on a minimal magnitude of fiber recruitment for that muscle. A soft tissue roentgenogram using a mammography machine demonstrates local swelling of the tendon and a local edema in the fat pad just anterior to the tendon.[46,61]

Clinically, the patient with a partial Achilles tendon rupture demonstrates a negative result on the squeeze (i.e., Thompson) test, and the test also yields a tender, fusiform swelling in the tendon's midportion.[64] The patient shares many of the same signs and symptoms as patients with less benign Achilles tendon disease (see pp. 454-455). However, in contradistinction to total rupture, partial rupture does not preclude the ability to ambulate following injury. The onset of symptoms may be acute or insidious.[52] A common complaint is the so-called pain cycle, characterized by pain at the beginning of activity that gradually subsides and returns after cessation of activity. Pain is most acute during sprinting or acceleration and almost always correlates with surgical findings of either tendinitis or partial rupture.[1] Stiffness after rest and sleep is a common complaint.[44] In the case of large partial ruptures, the examiner may feel a notch in the tendon (Fig. 35-4). The patient may exhibit both a slight loss of ankle dorsiflexion and calf muscle hypotrophy in the case of long-standing pain.[46]

Although it might be assumed that a partial rupture is a less benign injury than a full-thickness rupture, this is not necessarily the case from the point of view of tendon healing. Whereas complete rupture is followed by a sufficient recruitment of fibroblasts and other tendon-healing variables, partial tendon rupture with sparse vascularity is compromised by a hypoxic state in the peritendinous tissues, and leads to an immature scar, chronic inflammation, and persistent pain with delayed or absent healing.[1]

16. What is the clinical presentation of total rupture?

Many patients who have sustained Achilles tendon rupture have no symptoms before rupture. If symptoms are present, they manifest as tenderness, stiffness, or discomfort in the area of subsequent tendon rupture.[37] The historical presentation of Achilles tendon rupture may often be accompanied by a sudden, sharp, and severe pain, and occasionally patients report hearing an audible snap. Patient may report feeling as if they had received a blow to the Achilles tendon from behind, as though they had been kicked. There have been reports of patients turning around and punching the person standing behind them in retribution for a supposed kick. Occasionally, the pain associated with rupture may be slight or even absent.[43] Diagnosis of heel cord rupture is based on sudden loss of plantarflexor strength, palpation of a gap in the tendon, a positive result from the calf-squeeze test, and instantaneous weakness in push-off, accompanied by pain and swelling. Clinical presentation often includes the following:

- Immediate decreased ability or inability to walk or tiptoe while standing
- *Heel drop* is pathognomic for complete rupture, when accompanied by appropriate history in the absence of neuromuscular or spinal disease (Fig. 35-5)[57]
- Swelling caused by bleeding, and eventual ecchymosis

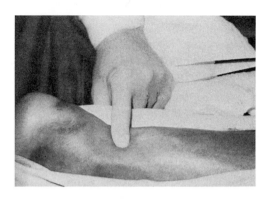

FIG. 35-4 Defect in Achilles tendon clinically apparent with rupture. Palpable sulcus (*hatchet* or *sulcus sign*) at the site of rupture (i.e., 3 to 6 cm proximal to the calcaneus) is felt as a distinct gap or defect when the foot is gently passively dorsiflexed in the acute state. This is more easily assessed with the patient in the prone (i.e., non–weight-bearing) position and the foot over the end of the examining table. However, the longer the time elapsed since the time of injury, the greater the subsequent formation of edema and hematoma, and the more difficult it is to positively palpate for a defect at the site of rupture. (From Nicholas JA, Hershman EB: *The lower extremity and spine in sports medicine,* ed 2, St. Louis, 1995, Mosby.)

- Loss of the normal outline of the Achilles tendon
- Palpable sulcus (*hatchet* or *sulcus sign*) at the site of rupture (i.e., 3 to 6 cm proximal to the calcaneus) felt as a distinct gap or defect when the foot is gently, passively dorsiflexed in the acute state; more easily assessed with the patient in the prone (i.e., non–weight-bearing) position and the foot over the end of the examining table; however, the longer the time elapsed from the time of injury, the greater the subsequent formation of edema and hematoma, and the more difficult it is to positively palpate for a defect at the site of rupture
- Increase in calf prominence observed as a calf lump, caused by shortening of the triceps surae
- Impaired ability to plantarflex the non–weight-bearing ankle
- Positive result on Thompson test (i.e., *squeeze test*)

17. What provocative tests confirm suspicion of a torn Achilles tendon complex?

The *Thompson* or *squeeze test* (Fig. 35-6) involves squeezing the calf. A positive test result is failure to achieve plantarflexion secondary to discontinuity of the muscle-tendon complex. Squeezing the gastrocnemius produces plantarflexion of the foot only if the Achilles

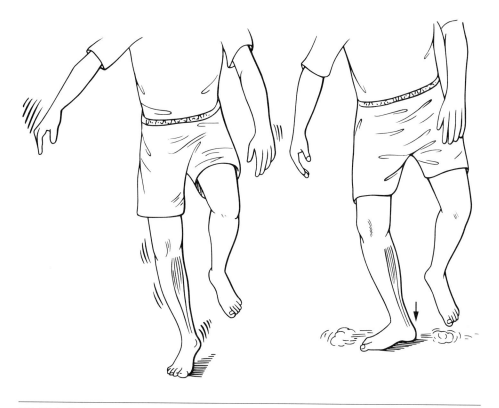

FIG. 35-5 *Heel drop* is pathognomic from complete rupture when accompanied by appropriate history in the absence of neuromuscular or spinal disease.

tendon is intact. When the muscle belly of a normal gastroc-soleus complex is squeezed, the stretch reflex is initiated and, in turn, shortens the motor unit and pulls the ankle into plantarflexion when the heel cord is intact. This passive contraction eliminates any influence that the secondary ankle flexors may have while the patient attempts to actively move the ankle. As such, in the acute setting in which pain precludes asking the patient to actively or resistively plantarflex to determine tendon integrity, the clinician confirms tendon patency by passively facilitating contraction of the muscle-tendon unit.

A commonly misleading feature during physical examination is the ability of the involved foot to actively (but not resistively) plantarflex because of the action of the intact tibialis posterior, peroneals, and long toe flexors. Thus although resistive plantarflexion may be painful in the acute stage, an inability to plantarflex is a positive score for rupture of the gastrocnemius-soleus–Achilles tendon complex. A positive result from the *resistive plantarflexion test* selectively isolates for strain of the resistive ankle plantarflexors, either manu-

ally or during an inability to perform a single toe rise.[43]

Copeland described a new diagnostic clinical test to detect Achilles tendon rupture. With the knee flexed 90°, a sphygmomanometer cuff is inflated to approximately 100 mm Hg with the ankle plantarflexed. The examiner then passively dorsiflexes the ipsilateral ankle by pressing upward on the sole of the foot. If the tendon is intact, the mercury column will rise to approximately 140 mm Hg, or whatever value was obtained earlier in the contralateral uninjured lower extremity. However, the presence of a total rupture is reflected in only a flicker of movement in the mercury column, since pressure can no longer be effected in the absence of an effective resistive contraction of the triceps surae complex.

18. Why does the ability to plantarflex against resistance return several days after injury?

Once pain abates several days after injury, the patient may plantarflex against minimal resistance by contracting the secondary ankle flexors (tibialis posterior and peroneus longus and brevis). However, these muscles

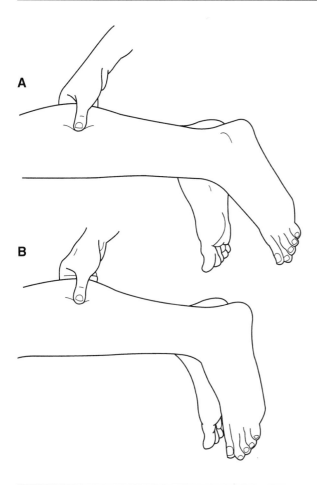

FIG. 35-6 *Thompson test* for rupture of the Achilles tendon. **A,** No pressure on the gastrocnemius. **B,** Squeezing the gastrocnemius and associated plantarflexion. If the Achilles tendon is ruptured, plantarflexion will not accompany pressure, and is indicative of a discontinuous muscle-tendon unit. (From Mercier LR: *Practical orthopedics,* ed 5, St. Louis, 2000, Mosby.)

are too weak to permit standing on tiptoes. This maneuver is too painful to attempt in the acute state.

19. What imaging techniques help clinical diagnosis in the delayed examination of a suspected rupture?

Complete ruptures are diagnosed clinically, but clinical evaluation may be hampered once excessive time has elapsed between the trauma and examination. Although magnetic resonance imaging (MRI) is expensive, it provides unparalleled soft tissue discrimination.[17,59] In sagittal and coronal images, MRI is able to detect *flap-folded tears,* which occur in 10% to 20% of all ruptures and are not amenable to conservative management.[43]

Sonographic examination may detect rupture of the Achilles tendon, but it has the shortcoming of having a limited field of view and limited soft tissue discrimination, as well as being operator dependent. Lateral radiographs may also show disruption of soft tissue.

20. Which criteria determine whether a torn tendon is conservatively or surgically managed?

Management of Achilles tendon rupture remains controversial in orthopedic and sports physical therapy circles. Advocates of the divergent approaches to management have a common, identical goal: to restore normal length and tension to the Achilles tendon. Neither method is ideal for every case of rupture; each management approach has virtues and deficits that must be weighed against the unique needs of the patient. Variables include patient age, the presence of systemic disease, a history of steroid injection, and whether the tear is chronic or acute. Generally, surgical management is superior in the younger, more athletic patient in whom re-rupture and residual lengthening has resulted in significant functional disability; it is precluded in patients with an underlying systemic disease such as diabetes or in patients who are taking steroids for any reason. On the other hand, low-demand, recreational athletic and nonathletic patients, especially those more than 50 years of age, show good results when conservative management is implemented soon after rupture.[24,38,54]

21. What are the problems and benefits with surgical and nonsurgical management of rupture?

Over the years, the pendulum has swung to either extreme with regard to enthusiasm for operative versus nonoperative management of severe strain of the heel cord. The Achilles tendon does not usually rupture in a clear fashion, but rather as a shredded, multiply torn tendon analogous to two "mop ends," that is technically difficulty to repair.[43] Proponents of conservative management point out that the torn ends are frayed, not cut evenly across (heelstrung); as such, an operation would sloppily appose the two torn ends, causing the ends to assume the appearance of "two untidy shaving brushes." These two ends of the tendon are brought into adjacent contiguity by simple plantarflexion, and if held in this posture long enough would allow gradual elimination of the defect through healing. Additionally, because the tendon ends are avascular, surgical exposure further robs the tendon of its blood supply. Surgery also carries the risk of wound infection, skin sloughs, and sural nerve injury. On the other hand, surgically repaired tendons demonstrate significantly more muscle power during isokinetic testing when compared with conservatively managed ruptures. Complications of conservative treatment of Achilles tendon rupture include a higher rate of rerupture and residual tendon lengthening that both result in significant functional disability.[32,33,56] Failure of conservative management is thought to stem from an undetected folded flap tear, which precludes the possibility of good apposition during healing despite early initiation of treatment.

22. What is percutaneous repair of the Achilles tendon?

Percutaneous repair of the Achilles tendon may be thought of as bridging the gap between open repair and nonoperative management of Achilles tendon rupture. This technique, having the benefit of being performed under local anesthesia and with a tourniquet, involves suturing together and drawing tight the torn tendon ends while the ends are approximated during ankle plantarflexion.[7,58] That portion of the tendon is then protectively wrapped (augmented) with a fascia lata autograft that is sutured into the body of the tendon. Percutaneous repair is associated with such problems as sural nerve entrapment, and although it produces better cosmetic results, the method has a higher rerupture rate than open repair.[5,29]

23. What therapeutic intervention is appropriate after Achilles tendon rupture?

Achilles tendon ruptures may be conservatively managed low-end, recreational athletic or nonathletic patients, particularly those older than 50. Physical therapy should ideally be instituted within a week of initial injury to return the patient to the preinjury activity level. If a delay in management exceeds one week, surgical repair may be indicated. For a more complete discussion of physical therapy management of Achilles tendon pathology, refer to pp. 465-468)

Conservative treatment for closed, complete rupture of the Achilles tendon involves application of a below-knee plaster cast with immobilization in equinus angulation for 4 weeks. This is followed by the application of a short leg cast, with the ankle set in reduced plantarflexion for an additional 4 to 8 weeks. The benefit of the equinus posture is that it facilitates maximal approximation of the torn tendon ends. When the second cast is removed the patient may walk while wearing shoes with a heel lift under the involved foot, for

1 month or until the patient can dorsiflex his or her ankle to approximately 10°. Moist heat, stretching, and massage are invaluable modalities for regaining normal Achilles tendon length. Strengthening and stretching of the triceps surae complex and the entire extremity are appropriate for regaining normal muscle bulk and soft tissue extensibility as compared with the uninvolved lower extremity. Strengthening follows a sequence of active, resistive, eccentric, and pliometric exercises. It is essential to be cautious and not overaggressive in the implementation of the therapeutic exercise program, so as to allow remodeling of the tendon consistent with lines of stress.

24. What is the surgical approach to treatment?

If the decision is made to operate, the operation should be performed at the earliest possible time. After the use of spinal or general anesthesia, the site of rupture is exposed by a longitudinal incision, with care taken to avoid the sural nerve. Alternatively, a straight medial incision may be employed. The retracted ends of the tendon are gently apposed and undergo anastomosis. The plantaris may be used as a living suture to reconstruct the tendo Achilles.

Although equinus immobilization is recommended following surgical repair, it should not exceed the 7- to 10-day period typically required for wound healing. Because tendon tension improves orientation of collagen fibers and improves strength, it is important to place the foot in neutral with no more than 0° to 20° of plantarflexion range once wound healing is complete.[43] In addition to its positive effect on collagen fiber orientation, early motion is also beneficial in promotion of nutrient transport and the reduction of adhesions.[60]

25. What is the postoperative therapeutic regimen?

It is largely believed that rehabilitative care after repair is important in the final outcome of tendon repair. Research has borne out that immobilization of healing wounds compromises overall outcome. Conversely, early controlled mobilization of the healing tendon leads to reduction of adhesion formation,[21,31,49] promotion of nutrient transport, improved collagen orientation, and hence stronger tendons upon final healing.[28,31,49] Three different approaches exist to postoperative management of Achilles tendon rupture. Program 3 advocates the early but controlled movement management strategy, and is perhaps the cutting edge of postsurgical management. The advantage of such a carefully planned rehabilitation program is that it emphasizes early functional activities[18,19,48] that promote tendon healing by accelerating parallel alignment and polymerization of fibrils into collagen, thereby augmenting the tensile strength in the healing tendon.

PROGRAM 1

Postoperatively, the limb is encased in a long leg cast with the foot postured in as much dorsiflexion as possible. This position will increase tension along the length of the newly repaired tendon to the limit of endurance, so as to prevent calf muscle contracture. After 4 weeks, a short walking cast with a ½-inch heel lift is applied, with slightly more tension on the tendon, for an additional 4 weeks. It is usually necessary to allow a 6- to 8-month break in competition following surgery and a break of at least 9 to 12 months after nonsurgical plaster cast treatment.

PROGRAM 2

Postoperatively the limb is placed in a long leg cast for 1 month with the foot postured in equinus. This is followed by a short walking cast with the foot still postured in equinus for an additional month. The following 6 months are characterized by the wearing of a ½-inch heel lift, accompanied by rehabilitation similar to that for Achilles tendinitis (see pp. 465-468); however, the Achilles tendon may be stretched no earlier than 3 months after surgery. When these guidelines are followed, normal strength may be achieved 1 year after surgery.

PROGRAM 3

During the *first week* after surgery, the foot is splinted in neutral with a removable splint. The splint is removed for gentle, passive range of dorsiflexion and plantarflexion motion several times a day, and the patient is not bearing weight. During the *second week,* inversion and eversion may be added, as may clockwise and counterclockwise circumduction ankle exercises. Strength exercises may commence with isometric inversion and eversion, as well as toe curls with a towel and weight, while the foot is in neutral. For the next 3 to 6 weeks the foot is placed in a removable walking cast, which is removed several times per day for passive and active range of motion.

During *week 3,* progressive partial weight bearing may begin in a walking splint. All of the aforemen-

tioned active and isometric exercises continue, in addition to isometric plantarflexion and gentle passive stretching into dorsiflexion with a strap or towel. Cryotherapy may be of benefit. Conditioning exercises may begin at week 3; these include stationary cycling for approximately 7 to 12 minutes with minimal resistance. Water exercises may begin with the use of a flotation device. At approximately *3 to 4 weeks,* cowboy boots may be worn as the patient begins to ambulate with a cane.

From *weeks 5 to 6,* weight bearing may progress to full load, and strengthening may progress from a level-I to a level-III resistance factor rubberband. Passive dorsiflexion is continued with the knee at full extension and approximately 35° of flexion. Gentle cross-fiber massage is applied to the Achilles tendon to dislodge adhesions binding the peritenon from the tendon. Ultrasound, phonophoresis, and electrical stimulation may be administered to decrease excessive scar formation or for chronic swelling.

Beyond *week 6* the patient may ambulate in full weight bearing, without a cast, provided he or she wears a 1-inch heel lift or cowboy shoes with a 1-inch heel. Passive and isometric activities should be discontinued, and level-III resistance rubberband strengthening exercise should be continued in all directions. Double-legged toe rises should be initiated with body weight, as tolerated. Balance board exercises are begun for proprioceptive training. Conditioning exercises include stationary cycling, treadmill walking, stair-climbing activities, water exercises in chest-deep water, and modality application as needed.

Beyond *12 weeks,* toe raising should progress to include the use of additional weight at least as great as body weight or up to 1.5 times body weight for the injured athlete; single-leg toe raises are begun as tolerated. Conditioning activities include jogging on a trampoline and then running on a treadmill, together in a walk-run program. This is followed by steady-state outdoor running for up to 20 minutes before performing figure-eight and cutting drills. Water exercises such as hopping, bounding, and jumping drills may be performed in waist-deep water. The completely rehabilitated Achilles tendon repair allows between 15° to 20° of ankle dorsiflexion. Rehabilitative management attempts to develop strength, endurance, and flexibility to preinjury levels.[60]

It is imperative to inculcate the athlete with the importance of warming up and cooling down. Prophylactic warm-ups allow creep, stress relaxation, and the temperature rise in the tendon and peritendinous tissues. It is essential to minimize all extrinsic contributors toward Achilles tendon compromise by selecting shoes with good shock absorption, avoiding high-mileage training, running on hard surfaces, and running hills. The athlete should understand that the maintenance of a constant level of activity may counteract the structural changes within the muscle and tendon that is caused by normal aging or inactivity.[1]

26. What accounts for a greater rerupture rate with the nonsurgically managed patient?

Conservative management of Achilles tendon rupture consists of casting the lower leg and foot, with the latter positioned in plantarflexion. The intention of this strategy is that scar tissue is laid down to it bind together the torn tendon ends as closely as possible. With surgical repair, very little scar tissue is involved in the repair because living tendon (plantaris) is used in the repair.

Both scar tissue and tendinous tissue are composed of connective tissue. Scar tissue is generally *loose connective tissue,* and tendinous tissue is generally *dense connective tissue.* The loose connective tissue that composes scar tissue is characterized by sparse and randomly oriented collagen fibers. Tendons consist of regular, well-organized, and tightly packed parallel bundles of collagen fibers.[13] It is no wonder, then, that nonsurgical management carries the risk of approximately a 10% rerupture rate, nearly twice that of operative management.

27. How is a partial rupture of the Achilles tendon managed?

When a relatively small tendon defect is acutely detected, a decision to manage conservatively may be made in which a plaster cast is applied for 2 to 3 weeks, with the ankle in slight plantarflexion.[1] Excessive immobilization may have deleterious effects on tissue, including joint stiffness, muscle atrophy, and damage to joint cartilage.[13] On the other hand, immediate immobilization during the early phases of tendon healing may lead to increased separation of tendon fibers and enlargement of the rupture site.[18] It is therefore advisable to wait approximately 2 or 3 weeks before initiating controlled tendon mobility. Mobilization at this relatively early time may benefit the healing tendon by accelerating healing and the increase of tendon strength.[40,48] Alternatively, one may apply a combination of heel lifts, cryotherapy, and rest.[7,58]

If either the patient or caregivers delay in dealing

with a negligible or small tear, scar formation and inflammation may set in and preclude conservative management, in which case management is similar to that of an involved partial tear.[1] In such a case, a small chronic tear or a larger, acute partial tear is surgically managed by removal of scar tissue or any cyst found in the center of the tendon, corresponding to the site of rupture of the original central fibers.[64] Surgery restores approximately 75% of high-performance athletes to competitive activities and approximately 90% of recreational athletes to full activity.[22] Convalescence is twice as long as the time for which the below-knee plaster cast is worn, and the athlete should not resume competition for at least 4 to 6 months.[1] The average rehabilitation period from surgery to the previous level and intensity of activity may last up to 8 months.[2]

REFERENCES

1. Allenmark C: Partial Achilles tendon tears, *Clin Sports Med* 11(4):759-769, 1992.
2. Allenmark C, Peterson L, Renstrom P, et al: Persistent pain in the distal part of the Achilles tendon: surgical treatment. Submitted for publication.
3. Bachner EJ, Friedman MJ: Injuries to the leg. In Nicholas JA, Hershman EB, editors: *The lower extremity & spine,* ed 2, vol 1, St Louis, 1995, Mosby.
4. Bates BT, Osternig LR, Mason B, et al: Foot orthotic devices to modify selected aspects of lower extremity mechanics, *Am J Sports Med* 7(6):338-342, 1979.
5. Bradley JP, Tibone JE: Percutaneous and open surgical repairs of Achilles tendon ruptures, *Am J Sports Med* 18(2):188-195, 1990.
6. Brotzman SB: *Clinical orthopaedic rehabilitation,* St Louis, 1996, Mosby.
7. Carden DG, Noble J, Chalmers J, et al: Rupture of the calcaneal tendon, *J Bone Joint Surg Br* 69(3):416-420, 1987.
8. Christensen IB: Rupture of the Achilles tendon: analysis of 57 cases, *Acta Chir Scand* 106:50-60, 1953.
9. Clancy WG, Neidhart D, Brand RL: Achilles tendinitis in runners: a report of five cases, *Am J Sports Med* 4(5):46-57, 1976.
10. Clement DB, Taunton JE, Smart GW: Achilles tendinitis and peritendinitis: etiology and treatment, *Am J Sports Med* 12(3):179-184, 1984.
11. Clement DB, Taunton JE, Smart GW, et al: A survey of overuse running injuries, *Physician Sports Med* 9:47-58, 1981.
12. Connell MD, Jokl P: The aging athlete. In Nicholas JA, Hershman EB, editors: *The lower extremity & spine,* ed 2, vol 1, St Louis, 1995, Mosby.
13. Cormack DH: *Introduction to histology,* Philadelphia, 1984, JB Lippincott.
14. Cummins EJ, Anson BJ, Carr BW, et al: The structure of the calcaneal tendon in relation to orthopaedic surgery with additional observations on the plantaris muscle, *Surg Gynecol Obstet* 83:107-116, 1946.

15. Dandy DJ: *Essential orthopaedics and trauma,* Edinburgh, 1989, Churchill Livingstone.

16. DeStefano V: Pathogenesis and diagnosis of ruptured Achilles tendon, *Orthop Rev* 4:17, 1975.

17. Ehman RL, Berquist TH: Magnetic resonance imaging of musculoskeletal trauma, *Radiol Clin North Am* 24(2):291-319, 1986.

18. Enwemeka C, Spielholz N, Nelson A: The effect of early functional ambulatory activities on experimentally tenotomized Achilles tendons in rats, *Am J Phys Med Rehabil* 67(6):264-269, 1988.

19. Enwemeka C: The effects of early function on tendon healing [abstract]. *Med Sci Sports Exerc* 20(suppl):33, 1988.

20. Galloway MT, Jokl P, Dayton OW: Achilles tendon overuse injuries, *Clin Sports Med* 11(4):771-782, 1992.

21. Gelberman RH, Manske PR, Van de Berg JS, et al: Flexor tendon repair in vitro: a comparative histologic study of the rabbit, chicken, dog, and monkey, *J Orthop Res* 2(1):39-48, 1984.

22. Gillstrom P, Ljungqvist R: Long-term results after operation for subcutaneous partial rupture of the Achilles tendon, *Acta Chir Scand* 482(suppl):78, 1978.

23. Gould N, Karson R: Stenosing tenosynovitis of the pseudosheath of the tendo-Achilles, *J Foot Ankle Surg* 1:3, 1980.

24. Haggmark T, Liedberg H, Eriksson E, et al: Calf muscle atrophy and muscle function after non-operative versus operative treatment of Achilles tendon ruptures, *Orthopedics* 9(2):160-164, 1987.

25. Hart T, Napoli R, Wolf J: Diagnosis and treatment of the ruptured Achilles tendon, *J Foot Surg* 27(1):30-39, 1988.

26. Hastad K, Larsson LC, Lindholm A: Clearance of radiosodium after local deposit in the Achilles tendon, *Acta Chir Scand* 116:251-256, 1976.

27. Hattrup SJ, Johnson KA: A review of ruptures of the Achilles tendon, *Foot Ankle* 6(1):34-38, 1985.

28. Hitchock TF, Light TR, et al: The effect of immediate controlled mobilization on the strength of flexor tendon repairs, *Trans Orthop Res Soc* 11:216, 1986.

29. Hockenbury RT, Johns JJ: A biomechanical in-vitro comparison of open versus percutaneous repair of tendon Achilles, *Foot Ankle* 11(2):67-72, 1990.

30. Hooker C: Rupture of the tendocalcaneus, *J Bone Joint Surg Am* 58A:990, 1976.

31. Hu HP, Ferris B: Tendons. In Bucknell TE, Ellis H, editors: *Wound healing for surgeons,* London, 1984, Bulliere-Tindall.

32. Inglis AE, Scott WN, Sculco TP, et al: Ruptures of the tendo Achillis: an objective assessment of surgical and nonsurgical treatment, *J Bone Joint Surg Am,* 58(7):990-993, 1976.

33. Jacobs D, Martens M, Van Audekercke RV, et al: Comparison of conservative and operative treatment of Achilles tendon rupture, *Am J Sports Med* 6(3):107-111, 1978.

34. James SL, Bates BT, Osternig LR: Injuries in runners, *Am J Sports Med* 6(2):40-50, 1978.

35. Jones DC, Singer KM: Soft-tissue conditions of the ankle and foot. In Nicholas JA, Hershman EB, editors: *The lower extremity & spine,* ed 2, vol 1, St Louis, 1995, Mosby.

36. Jozsa L, Kvist M, Balint BJ, et al: The role of recreational sport activity in Achilles tendon rupture, *Am J Sports Med* 17(3):338-343, 1989.

37. Kannus P, Jozsa L: Histopathological changes preceding spontaneous rupture of a tendon, *J Bone Joint Surg Am* 73(10):1507-1525, 1991.

38. Kellam JF, Hunter GA, McElwain JP: Review of operative treatment of Achilles tendon rupture, *Clin Orthop Rel Res* 201:80-83, 1985.

39. Kvist MH, Lehto MUK, Jozsa L, et al: Chronic Achilles paratenonitis, *Am J Sports Med* 16(6):616-623, 1988.

40. Kvist M, Jarvinen M: Clinical, histochemical and biomechanical features in repair of muscle and tendon injuries, *Int J Sports Med* 3(suppl 1):12-14, 1982.

41. Kvist M, Jozsa L, Jarvinen MJ, et al: Chronic Achilles paratenonitis in athletes: A histologic and histochemical study, *Pathology* 19(1):1-11, 1987.

42. Largergren C, Lindholm A: Vascular distribution in the Achilles tendon, *Acta Chir Scand* 116:491, 1958.

43. Landvater SJ, Renstrom PAFH: Complete Achilles tendon ruptures, *Clin Sports Med* 11(4):741-758, 1992.

44. Leach RE, James S, Wasilewski S: Achilles tendinitis, *Am J Sports Med* 9(2):93-98, 1981.

45. Lee HB: Avulsion and rupture of the tendo calcaneus after injection of hydrocortisone, *Br Med J* 2:395, 1957.

46. Lungqvist R: Subcutaneous partial rupture of the Achilles tendon, *Acta Orthop Scand Suppl* 113, 1968.

47. Lundqvist R: Partial subcutaneous ruptures of the patellar tendon. Proceedings of the First Scandinavian Sportsmedicine Conference, *Syntex Ter* 2:89, 1977.

48. Mabit C, Bellaubre JM, Charissoux JL, et al: Study of the experimental biomechanics of tendon repair with immediate active mobilization, *Surg Radiol Anat* 8(1):29-35, 1986.

49. Marske PR, Lester PA: Histological evidence of intrinsic flexor tendon repair in various experimental animals: an in vitro study, *Clin Orthop* 192:297-304, 1984.

50. Melmed EP: Spontaneous bilateral rupture of the calcaneal tendon during steroid therapy, *J Bone Joint Surg Br* 47:104, 1965.

51. Nelen G, Martens M, Burssens A: Surgical treatment of chronic Achilles tendinitis, *Am J Sports Med* 17(6):754-759, 1989.

52. Nichols A: Achilles tendinitis in running athletes, *J Am Board Fam Pract* 2(3):196-203, 1989.

53. O'Brien M: Functional anatomy and physiology of tendons, *Clin Sports Med* 11(3):505-520, 1992.

54. Percy EC, Conochie LB: The surgical treatment of ruptured tendo Achillis, *Am J Sports Med* 6(3):132-136, 1978.

55. Perry J: *Gait analysis: normal and pathological function,* Thorofare, NJ, 1992, Slack.

56. Persson A, Wredmard T: The treatment of total ruptures of the Achilles tendon by plaster immobilization, *Int Orthop* 3(2):149-152, 1979.

57. Peterson L, Renstrom P: *Sport injuries: their prevention & treatment,* Chicago, 1986, Year Book Medical Publishers.

58. Puddu G, Ippolito E, Postacchini F: A classification of Achilles tendon disease, *Am J Sports Med* 4(4):145-150, 1976.

59. Quinn SF, Murray WT, Clark RA, et al: Achilles tendon: MR imaging at 1.5 T', *Radiology* 164(3):767-770, 1987.

60. Soma CA, Mandelbaum BR: Achilles tendon disorders, *Clin Sports Med* 13(4):811-823, 1994.

61. Smart GW, Taunton JE, Clement DB: Achilles tendon disorders in runners: a review, *Med Sci Sports Exerc* 12(1):231-243, 1980.

62. Teitz CC: Overuse injuries. In Teitz CC, editor: *Scientific foundation of sports medicine,* Toronto, 1989, BC Decker.

63. Tiberio D: Pathomechanics of structural foot deformities. On-Site Biomechanical Education and Training, Connecticut.

64. Turco VJ, Gallant GG: Occult trauma and unusual injuries in the foot and ankle. In Nicholas JA, Hershman EB, editors: *The lower extremity & spine,* ed 2, vol 1, St Louis, 1995, Mosby.

65. Turco VJ: Injuries to the foot and ankle. In Nicholas JA, Hershman EB, editors: *The lower extremity & spine,* ed 2, vol 2, St Louis, 1995, Mosby.

66. Valmassy RL: *Clinical biomechanics of the lower extremities,* St Louis, 1996, Mosby.

67. Waller JF Jr, Maddalo AV: Foot and ankle linkage system. In Nicholas JA, Hershman EB, editors: *The lower extremity & spine,* ed 2, vol 1, St Louis, 1995, Mosby.

RECOMMENDED READING

Carden DG, Noble J, Chalmers J, et al: Rupture of the calcaneal tendon, *J Bone Joint Surg Br* 69(3):416-420, 1987.

Hattrup SJ, Johnson KA: A review of ruptures of the Achilles tendon, *Foot Ankle* 6(1):34-38, 1985.

36

Lateral or Medial Exertional Shin Pain in Hyperpronated Feet During Running Activity

CASE 1: A 27-year-old professional soccer player began intensive preseason training 3 weeks ago after not playing the entire previous season because of a dislocated shoulder. He now complains of pain in his lateral shin while running, especially when slowing down. When asked, he admits to not adhering to his off-season regimen of strengthening, stretching, and endurance training because of his recent marriage and honeymoon. He complains of pain and tenderness along the area of his leg corresponding to the right anterior area of his shin bones.

OBSERVATION A forefoot varus deformity is noted. Callus formation occurs under the second metatarsal head. A right pinch callus is noted. The heel counter of the patient's right shoe demonstrates a valgus tilt.

PALPATION Yields pain and tenderness to the touch over the right anterolateral border of the proximal tibia. The skin over the pretibial muscles feels warm to the touch.

PASSIVE RANGE OF MOTION Eversion of the foot yields pain on right plantarflexion of the ankle joint. All trunk movements are full and pain free.

ACTIVE RANGE OF MOTION Repetitive dorsiflexion of the ankle joint and foot inversion yields mild reproduction of symptoms. All trunk movements are full and pain free.

MUSCLE STRENGTH The patient exhibits normal ability to stand on his right heel, but reports pretibial soreness when asked to heel-walk. Collective testing of pretibial ability to dorsiflex against resistance yields a G/G+ grade when compared with the opposite side. Selective muscle testing of the right extensor hallucis longus yields a good grade; similarly, left foot inversion also yields a good grade. Isolated muscle testing of the tibialis anterior yields a G− grade and is painful.

SELECTIVE TENSION Reproduces symptoms to the right anterolateral shin during resisted dorsiflexion of the ankle and foot eversion.

FLEXIBILITY Moderate tightness is noted in the hamstrings, quadriceps, and Achilles tendon bilaterally.

SPECIAL TESTS Negative Homan's sign and hyperpronation test. A normal Q angle is measured. Negative leg-length discrepancy and Lasègue's sign.

CLUE:

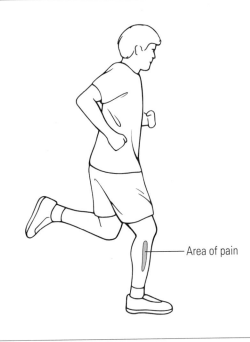

Area of pain

CASE 2: A 41-year-old, hard-driving attorney had just made partner in a prestigious law firm and decided that she would run every day to get into shape. She began by jogging 3 miles every morning before work along the hilly foothills of her suburban neighborhood, while wearing her old, worn-out tennis sneakers. Four months later and 14 pounds lighter, she enters your office with a complaint of right medial leg pain of 3 weeks' duration. Symptoms are localized to her right medial area of the shin and to her inner ankle area. When questioned, she admits to running along the banked surface of the beach close to the surf, and despite the onset of symptoms, she continued running through her pain in the hope that it would abate. Although initially she felt the pain only just after her run, she now reports feeling symptoms toward the end of her run that linger on after activity. She complains that symptoms begin to manifest when she climbs stairs. There is no history of peripheral vascular disease, or any recent penetrating skin wound. There is a positive history of juvenile rheumatoid arthritis, which was managed by gold therapy and later resolved.

OBSERVATION Deviation from right subtalar neutral is very obvious when both feet are observed to be weight bearing. The talar head appears displaced medially and plantarward, whereas the os calcis and Achilles tendon complex deviate in bilateral valgus. A right rearfoot varus deformity is noted. Gait appears normal. A thick callus is palpated under the right second metatarsal, and to a lesser degree under the third and fourth metatarsal heads; a right pinch callus is noted. The heel counter of the patient's right running sneaker demonstrates a varus tilt.

PALPATION   Point tenderness is localized behind the right medial malleolus. Tenderness is also localized more proximally, over the substance of the tibialis posterior tendon in the sulcus between the Achilles tendon and the tibia, and extending up to the distal two thirds of the medial tibia.

PASSIVE RANGE OF MOTION   Passive dorsiflexion and eversion reproduce left leg pain. All trunk movements are full and pain free.

ACTIVE RANGE OF MOTION   Active inversion of the right ankle reproduces mild discomfort. All trunk movements are full and pain free.

MUSCLE STRENGTH   Inversion of the foot with plantarflexion of the ankle joint yields a G— grade. The patient cannot rise on her right toes as well as she can on her left toes.

SELECTIVE TENSION   Resisted foot inversion and plantarflexion of the ankle joint reproduce pain.

FLEXIBILITY   Moderate tightness is noted in the hamstrings, quadriceps, and Achilles tendon bilaterally.

SPECIAL TESTS   Negative Homan's sign and hyperpronation test. A normal Q angle is measured. Negative leg-length discrepancy and Lasègue's sign.

CLUE:

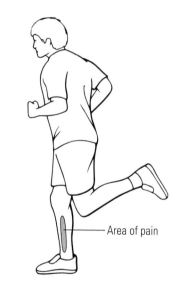

Area of pain

? Questions

1. What are the causes of these patients' leg pain?
2. What are shin splints?
3. What factors contribute to the development of shin splint syndrome?
4. What is the relationship of the tibialis anterior to the longitudinal arch of the foot?
5. What is the anatomy of the tibialis posterior and what is its relationship to the longitudinal arch of the foot?
6. What are the kinesiologic roles of the anterior and posterior tibialis during the gait cycle?
7. What are subtalar joint pronation and supination?

8. **What is the role of the extrinsic muscles of the foot in relation to subtalar joint pronation and supination?**

9. **What synergic relationship do the anterior and posterior tibial tendons have with regard to the subtalar joint during early stance phase of gait?**

10. **What two postural foot deformities are associated with the development of shin splints?**

11. **Why does posterior shin splint syndrome clinically manifest more distally than anterior shin splints?**

12. **How is the tibialis posterior stressed twice during each stance cycle as compared with function of the tibialis anterior?**

13. **What is a rearfoot varus deformity?**

14. **What athletic training errors may contribute to anterior shin splint syndrome?**

15. **How would jogging or long-distance running compromise pretibial muscle function and predispose for anterior shin splint syndrome?**

16. **How may muscle imbalance between the anterior and posterior tibial muscle groups predispose for anterior shin splints during level and hill running?**

17. **What is *snowshoe leg?***

18. **What are lateral shin splints?**

19. **What is the clinical presentation?**

20. **Unattended shin splint syndrome may progress to which osseous tissue pathology?**

21. **What is compartment syndrome?**

22. **What is the differential diagnosis for shin splint syndrome?**

23. **What therapeutic management is appropriate?**

24. **What is chronic shin splint syndrome?**

---

1. What are the causes of these patients' leg pain?

Anterior shin splints in Case 1 and *posterior shin splints* in Case 2 are the causes of the pain. Anterior shin splints may occur during preseason training in soccer players, because this sport involves large, active dorsiflexion and plantarflexion forces across the ankle when the athlete is kicking the ball. This repetitive action causes stretching and tearing of the origins of the anterior compartment musculature on the anterior surface of the tibia, and players who run excessively on unconditioned legs are predisposed to the condition.[19] In Case 2, note that a positive history of rheumatoid arthritis suggests a possible rupture of the posterior tibial tendon. This may account for medial talar prominence and accompanying heel valgus that are associated with the pronated foot posture; however, this is ruled out by a normal strength grade for ankle inversion.

2. What are shin splints?

Shin splint syndrome of the lower extremity encompasses several disorders that were previously considered unrelated but today are viewed as belonging to the same spectrum of disorders. Once used to describe any pain between the knee and ankle, "shin splints" now refers to pain only along the distal two thirds of the tibial shaft.[3] This syndrome is characterized by a sequential progression of pathology that progresses from *tendinitis* to *myositis* to *periostitis,* which may then progress to either *compartment syndrome* or *stress fracture.*[24] Shin splints are an overuse-type syndrome that may occur in the anterior, posterior, or lateral muscle groups of the lower leg, and are unified by a similar mechanism of injury.

Shin splint syndrome, whether anteriorly or posteriorly derived, results from excessive activities such as distance running that involve cyclic pronation loading. Anterior shin splints are caused by repetitive trauma to the origins of the *tibialis anterior* primarily, and the extensor hallucis longus and extensor digitorum longus muscles secondarily. Posterior shin splints involve the origins of the muscles of the deep posterior compartment, including the *tibialis posterior* primarily and the flexor hallucis longus and flexor digitorum longus muscles secondarily. Whereas anterior shin splits are characterized by a myositis and eventual periosteal avulsion, posterior shin splits are, in fact, a posterior tibial tendinitis.

3. What factors contribute to the development of shin splint syndrome?

Shin splints represent a classic *overuse syndrome* resulting in tissue overload. This syndrome may be influenced by a variety of intrinsic and extrinsic factors. Extrinsic factors include training errors such as poor conditioning, running on hard surfaces with poor shoes, excessive mileage, and running on a banked track or the shoulder of the road. Intrinsic factors include soft tissue imbalances and limb alignment abnormalities such as excessive femoral anteversion, external tibial torsion, hyperpronation, or increased heel eversion characterized by excessive valgus angulation greater than 5°.[8]

4. What is the relationship of the tibialis anterior to the longitudinal arch of the foot?

The *anterior tibialis* (Fig. 36-1) is named for its location and point of origin, and gives a rounded contour to the shinbone anteriorly. This muscle attaches at the proximal half of the anterior tibia. The muscle is unique among the leg muscles in that it does not wind around either malleolus en route to its distal insertion on the dorsomedial aspect of first cuneiform and base of the first metatarsal. Innervated by the deep peroneal nerve (L4), the tibialis anterior is primarily a dorsiflexor and secondarily an invertor as it courses medially to the subtalar joint. The tendon of the tibialis anterior arises well above the ankle joint in the distal two thirds of the leg and is prevented from bowstringing dorsally during

contraction by the superior and inferior extensor retinacula, (otherwise known as the transverse crural and cruciate crural ligaments) which act as a simple pulley. Thus despite the fact that its tendon does not wind around either malleolus, this unique muscle-tendon complex travels from a dorsolateral position proximally to a dorsal medial position distally. The kinesiologic ramification of this insertional reversal is that the anterior tibialis muscle affects and helps control the longitudinal arch of the foot. This has direct bearing upon the kinesiology of the foot during stance and swing phases of gait. The anterior muscle group is normally active during the swing, heel contact, and after toe-off phase of stance.

The distal insertion of the tibialis anterior is Y-shaped, with two slips of tendon that attach to the dorsomedial aspect of the base of the first metatarsal and the dorsomedial base of the first cuneiform, respectively. The significance of both insertions at the level of the midfoot is that together, they work as a sling to raise the apex of the long plantar arch. Correspondingly, if only one slip was present, instead of two, the arch would sag. Thus the tibialis anterior has an additional function as a dynamic arch support.

5. What is the anatomy of the tibialis posterior, and what is its relationship to the longitudinal arch of the foot?

The deep and intermediate layers of the posterior compartment of the leg includes the posterior tibialis, flexor digitorum longus, and flexor hallucis longus muscles. During contraction the tendon of the tibialis posterior (Fig. 36-2) is drawn against the calcaneus and talus as it courses down the medial ankle to wind around the medial malleolus en route to its distal insertion, among others, on the navicular, the keystone of the longitudinal plantar arch. As a primary inverter of the ankle joint, the tibialis posterior is especially subject to irritation as it wraps around the narrow groove behind the medial malleolus. Tension along the length of the tendon will be compounded in the hyperpronated foot. Patients will complain of pain along the medial distal two-thirds of the tibial shaft, or more vaguely of calf pain[3] deep to the triceps surae.

The *tibialis posterior,* innervated by the tibial nerve, is the deepest of the calf muscles and is the primary invertor of the ankle. The muscle originates from the proximal half of the posterior tibia, runs down the posterior calf, and deviates medially toward the medial malleolus. Its tendon enters the foot under cover of the

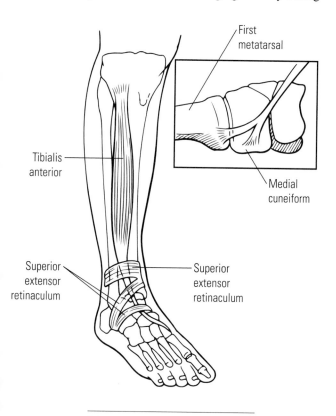

FIG. 36-1 Anatomy of tibialis anterior.

First metatarsal

Tibialis anterior

Medial cuneiform

Superior extensor retinaculum

Superior extensor retinaculum

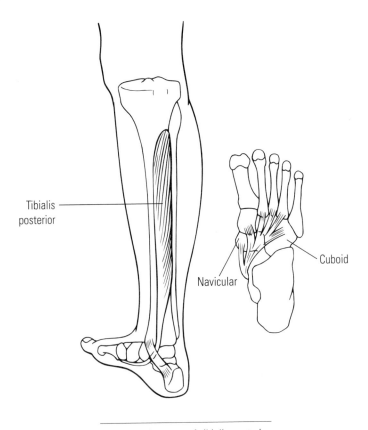

FIG. 36-2 Anatomy of tibialis posterior.

flexor retinaculum, winds around the tibial malleolus, and distally inserts primarily onto the navicular tuberosity. The tendon also inserts as several assessory slips onto the bases of the second, third, and fourth metatarsals. The distal attachments suggest that, like tibialis anterior, the orientation of span and distal insertion of the tibialis posterior muscle have a dynamic sling-like effect on the longitudinal plantar arch, in addition to a bowstring action akin to the bowstring ligaments. Thus during early stance the tibialis posterior may act as both a bowstring *and* a sling.

Because the tibialis posterior muscle, unlike the anterior tibialis, winds around a malleolus, it serves as a simple pulley en route to its insertion onto the midfoot. This is clinically significant because it accounts for why posterior shin splints, in contrast to anterior shin splints, typically involve the distal tendon and symptomatically present more distally. Posterior shin splint syndrome stems from a similar mechanism to that of flexor hallucis longus tendinitis (see Chapter 29). The tethering of the posterior tibial tendon around the medial malleolus acts as a stress riser, concentrating force distally in the tendon if overuse of the muscle-tendon occurs.

6. What are the kinesiologic roles of the anterior and posterior tibialis during the gait cycle?

The kinesiology of the anterior tibialis is best understood in relation to the ankle and subtalar joints during the gait cycle. During the interim between heel strike and foot flat subphases of stance, the ground reaction force is located behind the ankle axis. This results in an obligatory plantarflexion moment at foot flat subphase of stance. If unrestricted (as in the individual with a common or deep peroneal nerve palsy), the rapidly plantarflexing foot will slap down the forefoot, as occurs in a drop-foot condition. The pretibial muscles demonstrate a peak level of electromyographic activity to eccentrically lower the foot to the floor. In this manner the pretibials play an energy-absorbing role that minimizes the jarring transition from early stance to midstance. In addition to dampening unrestrained foot slap at the ankle joint eccentric activity smooths pronation at the subtalar joint.

The tibialis posterior exhibits a peak of electromyographic activity during stance phase of gait, from just after heel strike to the period just after heel-off. During early stance the tibialis posterior works in synergy with the anterior tibialis to eccentrically dampen the concussive forces of heel strike by pronating the foot at the subtalar joint. The tibialis posterior also demonstrates a burst of electrical activity during late stance just beyond heel rise, and together with other plantarflexors, concentrically thrusts the leg forward.

7. What are subtalar joint pronation and supination?

The sequence of muscle control within the foot during stance progresses from the hindfoot to the forefoot with each advancing step. The foot serves as the locus of the colliding forces of superincumbent body weight and ground reaction force. The foot negotiates these forces with the subtalar joint, which serves as a torque transmitter. Subtalar joint pronation results in the collapse of the medial longitudinal arch of the foot, whereas supination involves arch reconstitution. Both are passive actions. Pronation is primarily a function of superincumbent loading of the long plantar arch as body weight moves over the foot. Supination primarily occurs as a result of the windlass action of the long plantar fascia.

Pronation dissipates the potentially injurious, concussive forces of heel strike allowing the foot to mold itself to the topography of varied terrain. Supination converts the pliable foot into a rigid lever* that allows for effective propulsion during push-off and accelerates the tibial shank forward as the leg moves into swing phase. Eccentric contraction of the tibialis anterior and posterior may control both the rate and magnitude of pronation.

8. What is the role of the extrinsic muscles of the foot in relation to subtalar joint pronation and supination?

Ten muscles, most of which have another primary function, are grouped according to their relationship to the subtalar joint axis (i.e., as the long evertors, long invertors, and plantar intrinsics.) Muscles that cross the subtalar joint medially are listed in increasing order of their inverting leverage: the tibialis posterior, tibialis anterior, flexor digitorum longus, and flexor hallucis longus.[20]

*The windlass effect is a passive occurrence allowing resupination of the arch. It occurs by the plantar fascia tensing during late stance as the metatarsophalangeal joints move into hyperextension.

Eccentric contraction represents a dynamic bone and soft-tissue sparing strategy that diminishes potentially injurious forces.

9. What synergic relationship do the anterior and posterior tibial tendons have with regard to the subtalar joint during early stance phase of gait?

The function of the tibialis anterior muscle prevents foot slap immediately after heel strike. Where the tibialis anterior passes superior to the subtalar joint the tibialis posterior spans the underside of the subtalar joint. Tibialis posterior slows the rate and diminishes the magnitude of pronation by controlling anterior inclination of the tibia just after heel strike. Thus both the anterior and posterior tibialis provide a dynamic control of pronation flattening the arch in a controlled fashion, minimizing the injurious effects of concussive forces incurred during initial contact.

10. What two postural foot deformities are associated with the development of shin splints?

Alteration in subtalar joint temporal sequencing may result in macrophysiologic compromise of function to the muscles and tendons of the tibialis anterior and tibialis posterior. Forefoot varus and rearfoot varus deformities represent abnormal deviation from subtalar neutral during stance that may present as either excessive magnitude or rate of pronation, or prolonged pronation of the subtalar joint. Consequently the length-tension relationships of the extrinsic muscles moving the foot will deviate from the optimum and cause these muscles to overwork. Relentless overuse of muscles result in fatigue that may predispose anterior and posterior shin splints.

Pronation is a triplanar motion including talocrural joint dorsiflexion and subtalar joint calcaneal abduction and eversion. Excessive pronation elongates the distal anterior (Fig. 36-3) and posterior tibial tendons (Fig. 36-4) by distracting them along their longitudinal axis at their distal insertion. If relieved, tension will mount, elongating the tendons, and eventually exceeding their tensile capacity leading to injury.

11. Why does posterior shin splint syndrome clinically manifest more distally than anterior shin splints?

Because the tibialis posterior curves around the medial malleolus and the calcaneous en route its distal insertion, these bony prominences serve as frictional stress-raisers; this may account for why posterior shin splints clinically manifest as posteromedial distal crural pain

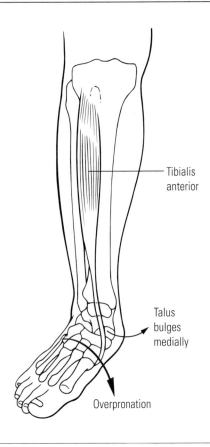

FIG. 36-3 Excessive pronation of the subtalar joint results in distractive tension of tibialis anterior.

consistent with tendinitis. This may result in posterior tibial tendon attrition, tendinitis, and eventual rupture. In contrast, the tibialis anterior passes into the foot under cover of the extensor retinaculum. Although the extensor retinaculum also serves as a simple pulley, it lacks the stress-raising capability inherent in the osseous pulley that is present with the tibialis posterior. Subsequently, muscle-tendon overuse caused by overpronation migrates proximally to stress the muscle (myositis), ultimately evolving into *periostitis*.

12. How is the tibialis posterior stressed twice during each stance cycle as compared with function of the tibialis anterior?

The tibialis posterior demonstrates two periods of electrical activity during stance. During early stance, the tibialis posterior contracts eccentrically in conjunction with the tibialis anterior to facilitate pronation of the subtalar joint. During late stance the tibialis posterior,

in conjunction with the other muscles of the posterior compartment, concentrically contracts to thrust the leg forward. In contrast, the tibialis anterior demonstrates a single peak of electrical activity during early stance. This peak of electrical activity eccentrically prevents foot slap (plantarflexion) across the talocrural joint and absorbs the jarring, concussive impact of ground reaction force through eccentric subtalar joint and transverse tarsal joint pronation. Thus the tibialis posterior undergoes a rapid alternation between two different modes of contraction, which subjects the tendon to twice the strain per stance cycle as compared with the anterior tibialis.

13. What is a rearfoot varus deformity?

A rearfoot varus deformity (Fig. 36-5) is the most common structural foot deformity[26] that is dominated by compensatory pronation. To understand a *rearfoot varus deformity* and its compensatory subtalar joint deviation it is essential to understand normal calcaneal inversion during heel-strike phase of stance. During late swing just before heel strike, the lower limb is adducted and the subtalar joint is slightly supinated as a function of a dorsiflexed foot posture in preparation for heel strike. This results in a strike pattern that begins along the lateral border of the rearfoot and proceeds medially as stance phase ends at toe-off (Fig. 36-6). To cushion the ankle-foot complex from traumatic concussive forces incurred at heel strike subtalar joint pronation causes increased weight distribution medially along the foot. Unlocking of the subtalar joint allows calcaneal eversion and flattening of the longitudinal plantar arch so that superincumbent body weight is distributed over its medial plantar surface.

Some individuals have a type of intrinsic foot deformity that involves excessive inversion of the calcaneus, which results from a failure of the posterior calcaneus to completely derotate from its original infantile posture.[27] *Rearfoot varus deformity* manifests as a varus angle created by the calcaneus and the Achilles tendon. During heel strike, because of the excessively inverted calcaneus, the medial condyle of the calcaneus and hence the entire medial side of the arch of the foot is farther from the ground. If an individual walks in this manner for very long, the foot, lacking shock-absorbing ability associated with pronation, would soon be severely contused; thus this uncompensated state is rare. Instead, the subtalar joint allows calcaneal eversion to neutralize the effects of excessive inversion. This permits the medial side of the foot to contact the

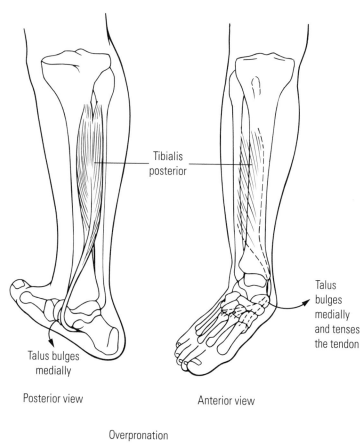

Tibialis
posterior

Talus
bulges
medially
and tenses
the tendon

Talus bulges
medially

Posterior view

Anterior view

Overpronation

FIG. 36-4 Excessive pronation of the subtalar joint causes excessive traction on the tendon of tibialis posterior.

ground increasing foot–surface-to-ground contact, thereby transmitting potentially injurious force to the ground.

Suspected rearfoot varus may be confirmed by palpation of callus formation under the second metatarsal head, and to a lesser degree under the third and fourth metatarsal heads.[9] Biomechanically, the lack of foot stabilization during forward propulsion causes the metatarsal heads to move across the skin, resulting callus buildup. Because a pronated foot decreases the physiologic advantage of the peroneus longus muscle, the stability of the first metatarsal head is compromised, and a callus does not occur at that location. Rather, the first metatarsal is hypermobile (unstable), and the second metatarsal suffers the brunt of callus formation.

The pathokinesiologic price paid for compensation

of rearfoot varus is that the subtalar joint undergoes excessively rapid pronation. Whereas the distal (forefoot) effects of abnormal subtalar joint pronation secondary to rearfoot varus are frequently insignificant, the proximal effects are substantial. The acceleration and increased magnitude of pronation during contact places excessive stress on the muscles that decelerate subtalar joint pronation, particularly the tibialis posterior muscle. Tensile forces along the tendon during the eccentric contraction (in early stance) are increased by the speed of motion.[23,28] Symptoms of overuse result from high tensile forces that may exceed the limit of the muscle-tendon unit to eccentrically attenuate forces.[27] Symptoms may occur at the distal tendon attachment to the navicular and first cuneiform, in the tendon sheath as it glides around the medial malleolus, and at the proximal muscle *(myositis)* or its attachment to the

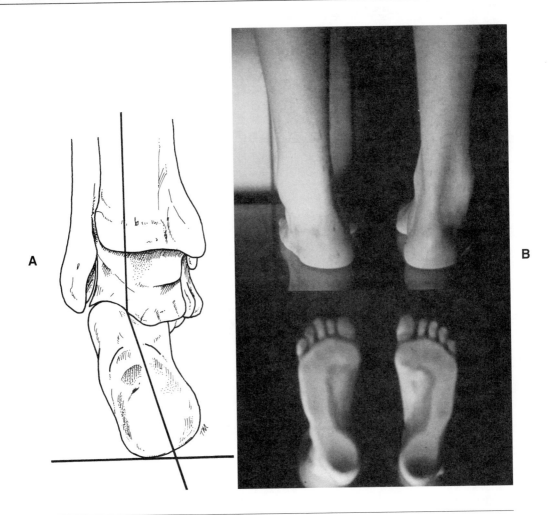

FIG. 36-5 Rearfoot varus deformity. **A,** Although the subtalar joint is in the neutral position, there is an inversion deformity of the calcaneus. **B,** Patient with rearfoot varus. (From Baxter D: *The foot and ankle in sport,* St. Louis, 1995, Mosby.)

proximal posterior tibia (*periostitis*—a tearing away of muscle fibers from bone).[27]

Excessive medial tibial rotation associated with overpronation cause more proximal stress along the kinetic chain. An attempt to dissipate excessive rotation may pathologically manifest as dysfunction at the knee, hip, sacroiliac joint, or intervertebral segments. For example, excessive medial tibial torsion translates into excessive valgus force at the knee. Over time, this force exceeds the threshold of the medial stabilizing knee structures and may additionally manifest as lateral patellar subluxation, excessive wear of the medial patellar facet, or a mild (grade 1) sprain of the medial collateral ligament.

14. What athletic training errors may contribute to anterior shin splint syndrome?

The anterior muscle groups include the tibialis anterior, extensor digitorum longus, and the extensor hallucis longus. These dorsiflexors of the ankle joint are particularly prone to shin splint syndrome, and may occur when a runner suddenly changes running styles, such as from a flat-footed running style to a forefoot running style characteristic of sprinters; changes shoes—for example, to an overly flexible sole; changes running surfaces, as from a soft to a hard running surface; or subjects the foot to overuse to compensate for biomechanical foot imbalance. A combination of any or all of these factors increases the likelihood of injury.

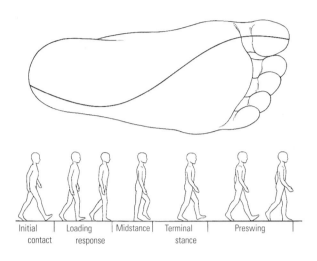

Initial | Loading | Midstance | Terminal | Preswing
contact | response | | stance |

FIG. 36-6 Center of pressure distribution during stance phase of gait in the balanced foot begins proximolaterally with heel strike in early stance and migrates medially and distally during late stance toward the sesamoids under the metatarsal head of hallux during propulsion phase. (From Greenstein GM: *Clinical assessment of neuromusculoskeletal disorders,* St. Louis, 1997, Mosby.)

15. How would jogging or long-distance running compromise pretibial muscle function and predispose for anterior shin splint syndrome?

The muscles of the anterior compartment are active during the first 80% of stance phase, and maintain activity throughout swing phase. During early stance phase, the pretibial muscles assist in the deceleration of the tibia over a fixed foot in an eccentric manner. This cushions the impact of the body against the ground and allows excessive energy to be dissipated as the foot assumes pronation immediately after heel strike. In long-distance runners and joggers, the ground-to-shoe contact is made with the foot in a flatfoot or slightly flat-heel to flatfoot position. The consequences of locomotion in the absence of heel strike rob the foot of its primary energy-absorption strategy, in which the excessive forces of gait are minimized by controlled pronation during the interim between heel strike and foot-flat phase of gait. To prevent foot slap, in which the foot is passively rotated plantarward over the fulcrum at the heel, the pretibials are forced to work harder and more rapidly. In the absence of the heel strike component, excessively large forces are borne by the pretibials, which may result in muscle overload and eventual pathologic conditions.

16. How may muscle imbalance between the anterior and posterior tibial muscle groups predispose for anterior shin splints during level and hill running?

A muscle imbalance between the posterior (triceps surae) and anterior (pretibial) muscle groups may contribute to the development of shin splints, especially during hill running.[25] During uphill running the pretibial muscles forcefully contract to clear the surface of the ground by acutely dorsiflexing the foot. If the posterior compartment muscles are tight, the pretibials will not begin contracting from a position of slight stretch. Denied their full excursion, the pretibials will decrease tension production because the length-tension relationship is compromised from overuse. Additionally, the anterior muscles may suffer overstrain during *overstriding* when an individual is running on level surfaces. Forceful contact on hard surfaces begins with a forceful heel strike that may result in foot-slap. This will recruit the anterior muscle group to *eccentrically* contract, to increase the time interval between heel strike and foot-flat phase of stance. This same mechanism may be implicated during downhill running, during heel strike in which the pretibial muscles eccentrically contract to control ankle plantarflexion and prevent foot-slap. Overactivation of these muscles may occur in the presence of a tight triceps surae, resulting in microtrauma and inflammation of the pretibial muscles, tendons, and bony attachments.

The end result of the muscle imbalance is an overload of the anterior compartment muscles that produces pain in the anterior leg or along the extensor tendons of the ankle and foot. Repeated tension on the tendon will cause tendinitis. If unrelieved as the patient continues to run through the initial injury, the tendinitis will migrate distally to inflame the muscle (myositis). Alternatively, continued training, unrelieved by treatment, may cause distal periosteal avulsion (periostitis) of the tendon(s) off their insertion on the bone. The sequelae of untreated shin splint syndrome in the presence of continued training is either stress fracture of the tibia or fibula, or a full-blown compartment syndrome.

17. What is *snowshoe leg?*

Snowshoe leg refers to anterior shin splint syndrome that is specific to people living in high temperate zones such as Alaska and northern Canada. Following the first snowfall of the winter season, snowshoes are donned and the pretibial muscles are suddenly subjected to severe contractile demands. During swing phase of gait the pretibial muscles contract concentrically just before heel strike, but do so in midair against no resistance. The pretibial muscles are not accustomed to concentric contractions against resistance; therefore, the repetitive concentric raising of the toe end of these snowshoes in the effort to keep them straight during gait amounts to an excessive strain upon the pretibial muscles because of the weight of the shoes.

18. What are lateral shin splints?

The *peroneus longus* and *brevis* occupy the lateral compartment of the leg. Both muscles, as they descend, pass behind the fibular malleolus and evert the ankle; they are also secondary plantarflexors as a function of their relation to the posterior ankle joint axis. A peroneal retinaculum on the dorsum of the foot tethers the peroneal tendons against the dorsum of the ankle, preventing bowstringing during contraction. The deep peroneal nerve also passes under this retinaculum. Thus this retinaculum is responsible for both anterior tarsal tunnel syndrome, and acts as a friction raiser in the development of tendinitis at this locale. If ignored, tendinitis may develop into a full-blown lateral shin splint syndrome. Pain is felt along the lateral ankle area, and peroneal muscle weakness may be assessed.

19. What is the clinical presentation?

The clinical presentation of anterior shin splints includes pain and tenderness over the pretibial muscles and warmth over the anterolateral aspect of the tibia bone. Stretching of the involved foot into extremes of ankle plantarflexion and foot eversion, as well as resisted ankle dorsiflexion and foot eversion, may reproduce pain. Additionally, the patient may complain of soreness upon heel walking, callus buildup under the second metatarsal head, and a valgus tilt wear pattern of the shoe worn by the involved foot. There is often tightness of the triceps surae muscle complex.

Signs and symptoms of posterior shin splints include pain and tenderness over the distal third or distal two thirds of the posteromedial shin bone. Alternatively, tenderness may present at the navicular insertion or just behind the medial malleolus, along the tendon.[22] Passive stretching into ankle dorsiflexion or plantarflexion and foot eversion reproduces pain, as does resistive foot inversion and ankle plantarflexion. Pain may duplicate when the involved foot is passively plantarflexed with eversion and with active inversion. Associated tight calf musculature may be found.

The patient with shin splints may complain of soreness while toe walking. The patient may also show callus patterns, predominantly under the second metatarsal head, and a varus tilt wear pattern in the shoe. Tightness of the proximal posterior soft tissue of the ipsilateral extremity may be present. Pain derived from posterior tibial tendinitis gradually increases after running. In severe cases, pain may be present both during and after the run. Tenderness often presents along the distal third or distal two thirds of the medial aspect of the tibia bone.[4]

Inspection of the feet and footwear provides biomechanical clues about the origin of dysfunction. Callus patterns along the plantar surface of the feet indicate primary weight-bearing areas, and may provide clinical information regarding clearly identifiable patterns characteristic of pathokinesiology. A callus is a dermatologic strategy to protect the skin from excessive shearing forces between the underlying bones and the insole of the shoe. Callus buildup typically occurs under the second metatarsal head for both forefoot and rearfoot varus.[23,28] Additionally, a *pinch callus* may also form on the medial side of the distal phalanx of hallux as it rubs against the inside of the shoe; this happens predominantly in the forefoot varus-type deformity, although it may also manifest in the rearfoot varus deformity.[27] A rearfoot varus may additionally exhibit a thickened callus posterolaterally.[12] Wear patterns along the sole and heel of the patient's footwear often mimic callus patterns. Whereas a forefoot deformity is characterized by a valgus tilted heel counter, a rearfoot deformity exhibits a varus tilted heel counter.

20. Unattended shin splint syndrome may progress to which osseous tissue pathology?

Stress fractures of the lower extremities account for 95% of all lower extremity fractures in athletes. Fracture may be sustained when a poorly conditioned athlete attempts to suddenly increase mileage or speed too rapidly, or as a sequela to running "through" an injury instead of resting and allowing soft tissue to recuperate. In the latter scenario, bone represents the body's last defense when soft tissue has been stressed beyond its capacity to attenuate stress. Stress fractures may occur close to the source of the disruptive ground reaction force at the sesamoids of the great toe, metatarsals, navicular, calcaneus, tibia, and fibula, and may migrate up along the closed kinetic chain to occur at the femoral neck or shaft, symphysis pubis, sacroiliac joint, iliac crest, pars interarticularis, or even the lumbar vertebral bodies.

Shin splint syndrome may culminate as a fatigue fracture anywhere along the proximal tibia and junction of the middle and distal two thirds of the tibial shaft. Stress fractures of the proximal medial tibia commonly occur in bowlegged runners.[3] In runners the most common site of stress fracture is 3 cm to 7 cm above the level of the fibular malleolus. Approximately one half of all lower extremity stress fractures occur in the tibia or fibula. However, a simultaneous tibial and fibular stress fracture is rare.

Osseous tissue normally remodels its internal structure by the concerted action of osteoblasts (deposition) and osteoclasts (resorption). According to Wolff's law, bone adapts to change by first resorbing trabeculae and then forming new trabeculae along lines of applied stress. A vulnerable interim period or window exists after the old trabeculae have been resorbed but before the new trabeculae have been laid down. If stress continues during this period of transient weakness, focal microfractures may occur. This stage of injury is referred to as a stress reaction of bone, and is not radiopaque.

Stress injury is often precipitated by participation in new forms of activity, overtraining, or a change in the way a sport is performed. This change may be as trivial as the wearing of a new pair of jogging sneakers or changing the direction of a regular jogging route. Stress injury is also common after foot surgery; for example, stress reaction and subsequent fracture may follow bunionectomy as weight-bearing forces are transferred to the second metatarsal.

A stress reaction is painful, and the only clinical findings are localized swelling and point tenderness. If the patient discontinues the activity at this time, the stress reaction of bone usually resolves. But if the stress-specific activity is resumed through the pain, the microfractures coalesce to form a complete fracture line known as a stress fracture. An analogy may be drawn to the repeated bending of a paper clip; although no single bend is sufficient to break the wire, repeated bending results in metal fatigue and an eventual break. What begins as a small crack may progress to involve the entire circumference of bone, and possibly bone displacement. Bone displacement is particularly problematic in stress fractures of the femoral neck, which may be incurred by both young and healthy military recruits and older persons with osteoporosis. Continued weight bearing causes tension that acts to distract and displace the two fracture fragments.

The initial diagnosis of stress fracture is difficult because plain x-ray films taken within the first 3 to 4 weeks after symptom onset are negative. This is because the fracture line is not visible before the microfractures have coalesced as subperiosteal new bone formation (callus), indicating a healing reaction. Hence diagnosis is based on clinical findings, including point tenderness and pain that occurs with activity but subsides during rest. Swelling may also be present. Technetium 99m bone scan shows increased radioisotope uptake into the region of new bone formation as early as 3 days after injury. This is considered the gold standard in diagnosis of stress fracture and even stress reaction. False-positive scan results are infrequent.[14]

An important distinction in the bone-scan pattern readily differentiates stress fracture from the tibial stress characteristic of shin splint syndrome. Tibial stress fractures are round and fusiform on the bone scan; the patterns seen in tibial periostitis are markedly different. In tibial periostitis, posterior cortical activity at the tibial midshaft[11] is typically linear ("streaking") and diffuse in nature and corresponds to tibial periostitis of the tibia in the region of the soleus insertion.[17,18] Similar findings at other locations such as the anterolateral cortex and the distal tibia suggest that more than one form of periostitis may cause shin splint syndrome.[15,29] On the other hand, a focal zone of increased activity on the medial portion of the tibia represents a stress fracture.[6]

If the injury is identified in the stress-reaction phase, healing will occur if the stress load is simply eliminated for a period of 10 days to 2 weeks. If a stress fracture has already occurred, repair may take some 6 to 12 weeks or longer. However, because persistently painful nonunion may result from stress fractures of the navicular, the sesamoid bones of hallux, and the proximal shaft of the fifth metatarsal, cast immobilization and complete elimination of weight bearing may be required for 6 to 8 weeks. Immobilization in a fiberglass cast may be necessary for lower extremity fatigue fractures if pain is severe. The sine qua non treatment for stress fracture of the tibia is rest from weight bearing; however, running in water while wearing a waterskiing vest is an excellent conditioning exercise during fracture healing.[3] Water provides a medium for low-impact kinetic exercise that minimizes body weight through buoyancy and significantly reduces concussive forces.

21. What is compartment syndrome?

Following the evolutional sequence of tendinitis-myositis-periostitis is yet another disorder that may occur in the lower extremity; unlike mere stress fracture, this disorder is potentially devastating. This disorder, known as *effort-related* or *exercise-induced compartment syndrome,* involves a loss of microcirculation of the muscles because of osteofascial compartments of unyielding size. This loss may occur after strenuous muscle activity that increases soft tissue pressures through fluid accumulations, resulting in lower leg claudication. The end result of restricted volume expansion is reversible ischemia. If ignored, ischemia may easily reach a critical point of no return, resulting in partial muscle necrosis and thereby necessitating immediate surgical intervention. Exercise-induced anterior compartment syndrome may be viewed as the end result of a pathologic process that begins with anterior shin splint and which, if not adequately addressed, may progress to a full-blown compartment syndrome.

This condition most commonly affects the anterior compartment of the leg, and occurs in athletes in the absence of significant atherosclerotic disease. The disorder most frequently occurs in men with a mean age of 23 years. The right leg is affected twice as commonly as the left leg. Ischemic involvement of the pretibial muscles first occurs in the extensor hallucis longus muscle, followed by the anterior tibial muscle, and lastly by the extensor digitorum longus muscle. This sequence may be related to the fact that the former two muscles are more active during athletic involvement than is the third muscle. Several factors may predispose certain individuals to this condition, including muscle hypertrophy, a congenitally small or inelastic fascial compartment, or venous hypertension.

The *fascia lata* of the thigh extends distally into the leg, where it is designated as the *crural fascia* (Fig. 36-7).Deep extensions of the crural fascia define the intramuscular septa, or boundaries of the leg, so as to form separate compartments defining the *anterior, lateral, deep posterior, and superficial posterior compartments* of the leg. The former three fascial compartments are relatively unyielding and are each supplied by one major vessel and nerve. The superficial posterior compartment houses the gastrocnemius muscle, which is sensitive to any interruption in its blood supply because it lacks intramuscular anastomosis. However, compartment syndrome of the superficial posterior compartment is unlikely since expanding muscle tissue may swell unhindered against the posterior skin of the leg.

Normally, the pressure of tissue fluid is less than 30 mm Hg, permitting blood to flow freely through large arteries, smaller arterioles, and capillaries to nourish

and oxygenate tissues. During athletic activity compartment pressures may increase to 3 to 4 times baseline values after vigorous activity; the pressures rapidly return to normal within several minutes. However, if vigorous activity persists, the oxygen debt incurred results in the accumulation of high concentrations of lactic acid. As mounting intrafascial pressure rises to or above 40 mm Hg, a critical impasse is rapidly reached in which small nutrient arterioles and capillaries feeding the muscles are compressed (decreased arteriole perfusion). Larger vessels such as arteries will remain patent because their contiguous pressure is normally 100 mm Hg. Thus blood flow in these larger and more resistant vessels will persist, accounting for palpable dorsalis pedis or posterior tibial pulses and giving a false impression of adequate circulation. Continuing intractable swelling may result in compartment tamponade and ischemic damage to muscles and nerves. The resulting ischemia produces further edema in a self-perpetuating cycle that may climax into a full-blown acute compartment syndrome. If this continues for several hours, the natural course of this emergency situation is muscle necrosis and nerve damage known as Volkmann's ischemic contracture. The only effective treatment is surgical compartment release (fasciotomy). Loss of pulses is a late finding, and surgery should not be delayed until this sign is present. Delay beyond 4 to 6 hours after onset may result in significant, irreversible damage.

The earliest clinical finding of acute compartment syndrome is a swollen, palpably tense compartment that is subjectively tight. The appearance of the limb is reddened and glossy. On palpation, the skin over the anterior compartment feels warm and firm. Pain on stretch or active movement of the involved ischemic muscles may be elicited, but this depends on the patient's pain threshold. Also, differentiating pain caused by ischemic muscle from pain caused by a fracture is sometimes difficult. Muscle paresis of the foot dorsiflexors may be caused by nerve involvement, muscle ischemia, or guarding secondary to pain; as the condition progresses, a foot drop may occur. The most reliable physical finding in a conscious and cooperative patient is sensory deficit. Sensory deficit may manifest as paresthesia initially but may progress to hypesthesia and anesthesia if treatment is delayed. Thus pain that was originally present may become diminished or absent. An anterior compartment syndrome may involve exhibited sensory loss on the dorsum of the foot in the first interdigital cleft, caused by compression of the

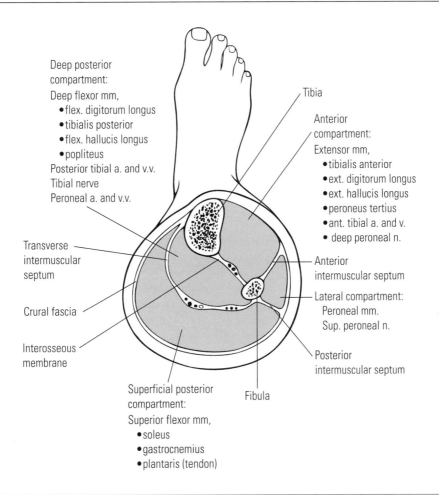

Deep posterior
compartment:
Deep flexor mm,
- flex. digitorum longus
- tibialis posterior
- flex. hallucis longus
- popliteus
Posterior tibial a. and v.v.
Tibial nerve
Peroneal a. and v.v.

Transverse
intermuscular
septum

Crural fascia

Interosseous
membrane

Superficial posterior
compartment:
Superior flexor mm,
- soleus
- gastrocnemius
- plantaris (tendon)

Tibia

Anterior
compartment:
Extensor mm,
- tibialis anterior
- ext. digitorum longus
- ext. hallucis longus
- peroneus tertius
- ant. tibial a. and v.
- deep peroneal n.

Anterior
intermuscular septum

Lateral compartment:
Peroneal mm.
Sup. peroneal n.

Posterior
intermuscular septum

Fibula

FIG. 36-7 Compartments of the lower leg. Deep extensions of the crural fascia define the intramuscular septa or boundaries of the leg so as to form separate compartments defining the *anterior, lateral, deep posterior,* and *superficial posterior compartments* of the leg.

deep peroneal nerve. Pulses are intact in approximately 90% of all patients suffering from compartment syndrome. Additionally, capillary refill is often present, and the limb remains pink in color.

Educating athletes about the danger of compression syndrome is important. Initially there is a cramplike feeling that may be accompanied by weakness or numbness. The patient should stop exercise, rest, have his or her limb packed in ice, and be carefully observed.[24] Ischemia can be reversed with resolution of symptoms by exercise. Symptoms will ordinarily resolve within a few minutes if the activity is immediately stopped, but may persist much longer if the athlete continues to perform through pain.[13] Full recovery may take up to several months if the warning signs are ignored. Occasionally there may be

some residual muscular fibrosis and concomitant slight residual disability.[1]

22. What is the differential diagnosis of shin splint syndrome?

The differential diagnosis includes thrombophlebitis, osteomyelitis, cellulitis, bone tumors, and intermittent claudication. Although rare in runners, these conditions must be ruled out. Early acquired syphilis may stimulate shin splints in a jogger.[16]

23. What therapeutic management is appropriate?

- *Rest* from causative activity is the first line of treatment. Because shin splints are often brought on by overuse, it is recommended that athletes with serious cases eliminate practice sessions and active work for a period as short as 1 to 2 days, or many weeks in severe cases. Players returning from a rest period should be allowed to practice when they are asymptomatic but should be excused from all agility drills.[21] Immediate modality treatment includes ice baths and ice massage. A brief course of antiinflammatory medications may be helpful. Local steroid injections are not advisable.[23,28]

The biomechanical alignment of the foot must be analyzed so as to detect as contributory hyperpronation. Orthosis management to regain subtalar joint neutral *(arch support)* will realign the foot while simultaneously unloading the posterior tibial tendon by allowing it to slightly slacken. The use of a lateral heel wedge or a rigid heel counter, as well as soft arch supports or a rigid orthotic device, may be helpful in reducing compensatory pronation and tibial rotation in the individual with posterior shin splints. Since the tibialis anterior and posterior help support the medial longitudinal arch, support of the arch may be accomplished by the application of a medial longitudinal arch support in conjunction with medial posting. If the uncorrected hindfoot is in valgus, a medial hindfoot wedge is prescribed; if the uncorrected heel is in neutral position, then a medial forefoot wedge is appropriate.[4] The use of a heel lift or neutral orthosis is prescribed for anterior shin splints. The heel lift prevents pretibial muscle overuse by allowing a quicker plantarflexion and thus decreasing the time required for the foot to move from midstance to late stance phase of gait. Immobilization is not recommended because it may lead to further muscle atrophy and prolong the treatment period.[2]

The patient should *rest* for up to 1 week, especially if pain persists,[24] then *slowly resume activity* when asymptomatic. Ice massage is appropriate for the first 3 to 5 days. The ice massage should be followed by alternating heat and cold modalities. The use of oral nonsteroidal antiinflammatory medication is helpful. Phonophoresis with steroid cream may relieve inflammation. Iontophoresis (10% hydrocortisone)[7] may be applied over the posteromedial aspect of the tibia bone or where the posterior tibial tendon runs superficially behind the medial malleolus. The athlete should run on a level, soft surface and wear good running shoes such as an air sneaker and a Sorbothane insert. Taping is occasionally effective and attempts to pull the anterior muscles toward the tibial to relieve tension.[23,28] The patient must be educated about the importance of stretching before and after exercise, and instructed in the recognition of symptoms and the avoidance of compartment syndrome. The patient must be inculcated with the vigilant attitude that prevention is the best management against future recurrence.

When a muscle is subject to myositis, inflammation results in fibrotic adhesions binding the muscle fibers together. As a muscle contracts, it broadens. When the ability to broaden is diminished by restricting adhesions, the muscle's ability to recruit its full complement of muscle fibers is compromised. Hence the muscle's power is diminished, and it is more likely to sustain injury as it fails to meet the demands placed upon it. This may be remedied by *deep transverse friction massage* to help forcibly broaden out the muscle. This does not mean widening the distance between the muscle fibers, but rather rupturing and separating the adhesive-like scar between the individual fibers that serves to restrict full muscle broadening.[5]

- *Strengthening* of the tibialis anterior, extensor hallucis longus, and extensor digitorum communis muscles. The anterior muscle group is often weaker than a relatively stronger posterior muscle group by virtue of the greater bulk of the latter. A dynamic imbalance may occur between these two antagonistic muscle groups that may accentuate anterior muscle group susceptibility to overuse. This may account for the higher incidence of anterior versus posterior shin splint syndrome. It is therefore essential to increase strength of the pretibial muscle group in an *eccentric* fashion, so that the anterior group is trained consistent with the demands of its function. Moreover, eccentric contractions are an injury-sparing strategy as they, by virtue of distraction during contraction, tend to absorb disruptive force. Strengthening may be accomplished using cuff weights or elasticized material.
- *Stretching* of the antagonist muscles group, predominately the triceps surae in the patient with anterior shin splints, is essential to alleviating muscle imbalance and restoring a balanced soft-tissue milieu. Gentle stretching of the inflamed muscles (e.g., the pretibials in anterior shin splints) also helps gain soft-tissue extensibility. A gain in extensibility may help alleviate tension build-up during intense muscle contraction, since an increase in the viscoelastic slack of the muscle-tendon unit(s) may unload tension deliv-

ered to the periosteal tendon junction. Stretching of the anterior compartment musculature may be accomplished by having the patient sit on his or her heels, or by having the patient stretch the dorsum of one foot while standing normally on the contralateral foot with a bent knee.

In the presence of tight heel cords, it is imperative to provide an adequate heel cord stretching program so as to unload stress to the pretibial muscles during intense activity. Stretching of the gastrocnemius-soleus-calcaneal tendon complex may be accomplished by using an incline board. This may be performed 10 to 12 times per day, 5 minutes per session, for a total of 1 hour. Heel cord stretching is also helpful to the individual with posterior shin splints who is following a strengthening program of the muscles that compose the deep layer of the posterior compartment.

The athlete must cross-train—that is, participate in sports that do not stress the affected musculature—during the entire length of the treatment program. Bicycling (while using the heel to push off), swimming without kicking or using a kickboard, stair climbing, rowing, cross-country skiing, or circuit weight training is mandatory for maintenance of muscle tone, cardiovascular fitness, and aerobic capacity.

Correction of training errors includes wearing athletic shoes having a firm, but not hard, well-cushioned heel. Additionally, shoes may have a padded or cutout area over the calcaneal tendon. Runners should be instructed to initially limit their speed and mileage and progress cautiously and incrementally. They should not run daily at first and should run along a soft, level surface.[24]

24. What is chronic shin splint syndrome?

When the shin splint syndrome does not respond to therapeutic management, the patient should be referred for a series of x-ray examinations at 2-week intervals to detect a possible stress fracture.[24] Multiple views may be necessary, since only a single cortex of bone is often involved.[1] *Chronic* or *recurrent shin splint syndrome* may show irregularity and new bone formation at the tendon attachments. A bone scan may reveal increased uptake in longitudinal (streaking) patterns in periostitis, and shows localized transverse uptake in the presence of a stress fracture.[3] Chronic shin splint syndrome may require an injection of corticosteroid to increase strength and flexibility.[24]

REFERENCES

1. Zitelli BJ, Davis HW, editors: *An atlas of pediatric physical diagnoses,* ed 3, St Louis, 1997, Mosby.
2. Bachner EJ, Friedman MJ: Injuries to the leg. In Nicholas JA, Hershman EB, editors: *The lower extremity and spine,* ed 2, vol 1, St Louis, 1995, Mosby.
3. Brody DM: *Clinical symposia: running injury—prevention and management,* vol 39, no 3, Summit, NJ, 1987, CIBA-GEIGY.
4. Brody DM: Running injuries. In Nicholas JA, Hershman EB, editors: *The lower extremity and spine,* ed 2, vol 2, St. Louis, 1995, Mosby.
5. Cyriax J: *Textbook of orthopaedic medicine. Vol. 1. Diagnosis of soft tissue lesions,* ed 8, London, 1982, Bailliere Tindall.
6. D'Ambrosia RD, Zelis RF, Chuinard RG et al: Interstitial pressure measurements in the anterior and posterior compartments in athletes with shin splints, *Am J Sports Med* 5(3):127-131, 1977.
7. Donatelli RA: *The biomechanics of the foot and ankle,* ed 2, Philadelphia, 1990, FA Davis.
8. Fetto JF: Anatomy and physical examination of the foot and ankle. In Nicholas JA, Hershman EB, editors: *The lower extremity and spine,* ed 2, vol 1, St Louis, 1995, Mosby.
9. Gray GW: *When the feet hit the ground everything changes. Program outline and prepared notes—basic manual,* Toledo, Ohio, 1984, American Physical Rehabilitation Network.
10. Hamilton JJ, Ziemer LK: Functional anatomy of the human ankle and foot, *American Association of Orthopedic Surgeons, symposium on the foot and ankle,* St Louis, 1983, Mosby.
11. Holder LE, Matthews LS: The nuclear physician and sports medicine. In Freeman LM, Weissmann HS, editors: *Nuclear medicine annual,* New York, 1984, Raven Press.
12. Jepson KK: Biomechanical evaluation of the running athlete, *Phys Ther Forum* 6(43), 1987.
13. Lillegard WA, Rucker KS: *Handbook of sports medicine—a symptom-oriented approach,* Boston, 1993, Andover Medical Publishers.
14. Markey KL: Stress fractures, *Clin Sports Med* 6(2):405-425, 1987.
15. Matin P: Basic principles of nuclear medicine techniques for detection and evaluation of trauma and sports medicine injuries, *Semin Nucl Med* 18(2):90-112, 1988.
16. Meier J, Mollet E: Acute periostitis in early acquired syphilis simulating shin splints in a jogger, *Am J Sports Med* 14(4):327-328, 1986.
17. Michael RH, Holder LW: The soleus syndrome: a cause of medial tibial stress (shin splints), *Am J Sports Med* 13(2):87-94, 1985.
18. Mubarak SJ, Gould RN, Lee YF, et al: The medial tibial stress syndrome: a cause of shin splints, *Am J Sports Med* 10(4):201-210, 1983.
19. Orava S, Puranen J: Exertion injuries in adolescent athletes, *Br J Sports Med* 12(1):4-10, 1978.
20. Perry J: *Gait analysis: normal and pathological function,* Thorofare, NJ, 1992, Slack.

21. Reese RC Jr, Burruss TP, Patten J: Athletic training techniques and protective equipment. In Nicholas JA, Hershman EB, editors: *The lower extremity and spine,* ed 2, vol 1, St Louis, 1995, Mosby.

22. Reiley MA: Guidelines for prescribing foot orthotics, Thorofare, NJ, 1995, Slack.

23. Stanish WD, Curwin S: Tendinitis: its etiology and treatment, Lexington, Mass, 1984, DC Health & Co.

24. Subotnick SI: *Podiatric sports medicine,* New York, 1975, Futura.

25. Subotnick SI: The shin splints syndrome of the lower extremity, *Podiatr Sports Med* 66:43, 1976.

26. Tiberio D: Pathomechanics of structural foot deformities, *Phys Ther* 68(12):1840-1849, 1988.

27. Werneck J, Langer S: *A practical manual for a basic approach to biomechanics,* Deer Park, NY, 1973, Langer Laboratories.

28. Winter DA: *Biomechanics of human movement,* New York, 1979, John Wiley & Sons.

29. Zwas ST, Elkanovitch R, Frank G: Interpretation and classification of bone scintigraphic findings in stress fractures, *J Nucl Med* 28(4):452-457, 1987.

RECOMMENDED READING

Brody DM: Running injuries. In Nicholas JA, Hershman EB, editors: *The lower extremity and spine,* ed 2, vol 2, St Louis, 1995, Mosby.

Jones DC, James SL: Overuse injuries of the lower extremity, *Clin Sports Med* 6(2):273-290, 1987.

Subotnick SI: The shin splints syndrome of the lower extremity, *J Am Podiatry Assoc* 66(1):43-45, 1976.

37

Tall Adolescent Male with Anterior Knee Pain After Basketball Activities

A 14-year-old athletic male is brought to your office by his father with complaints of a history of gradually increasing pain and swelling in the right anterior knee. The boy reports playing team basketball several hours a day since school classes were finished 2 weeks ago. Pain is particularly acute, he reports, when he crouches down in a low defense posture. In addition, he spends 4 afternoons per week in the crouched catcher position for the baseball team sponsored by the local Police Athletic League. Although his knee bothers him when he rides his bicycle, kneeling is sheer agony. Discomfort is relieved by rest, with full knee extension. His father points out a palpable lump below his right patella. When asked, he admits to occasionally limping slightly following athletic activity. There is no significant medical history, or history of knee injury. Upon questioning, the patient reports negatively to queries about the presence of giving way, locking, sudden swelling, or any popping sound.

OBSERVATION   Shows prominence over the right tibial tubercle. Both quadriceps femoris muscles seem strong and slightly hypertrophied. Bilateral pronation posture of both feet is observed.

PALPATION   Pinpoint tenderness is noted over the tibial tuberosity. There is mild swelling over the area of the right tibial tuberosity and distal patellar tendon insertion.

PASSIVE RANGE OF MOTION   Reveals limitation of acute knee flexion secondary to painful reproduction of symptoms.

ACTIVE RANGE OF MOTION   Range of motion is grossly in functional limits for the entire right lower extremity, although pain is reproduced when the right knee is flexed beyond 120°. A 5°-extensor lag is noted in the right knee.

MUSCLE STRENGTH   Muscle strength is grossly in normal limits for the right lower extremity. Resistive right knee extension reproduces pain.

FLEXIBILITY TESTING   Right lower extremity soft tissue demonstrates normal length with exception of bilateral hamstring, quadriceps, and calf tightness.

SELECTIVE TENSION   Reproduces symptoms of resisted right knee extension.

GIRTH TESTING   No quadriceps femoris atrophy noted.

SENSATION   Intact to light touch and pressure throughout the right lower extremity.

SPECIAL TESTS   The right Q angle measures 13°; the right hip is neither anteverted nor retroverted. Positive Ely test. Negative camel sign.

CLUE:

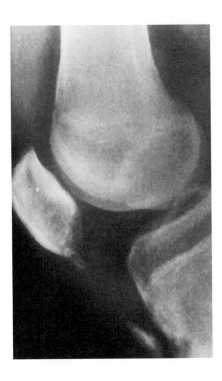

(From Scuderi GR, McCann PD, Bruno PJ: *Sports medicine: principles of primary care,* St Louis, 1997, Mosby.)

? **Q**uestions

1. What is most probable the cause of this boy's condition?
2. What is the difference between epiphysis and apophysis, and how is this important to the classification of this form of osteochondrosis?
3. What is the cause of this disorder and how does it relate to early adolescence?
4. What is the pathophysiology of this disorder?
5. What distal biomechanical deviation would cause excessive traction on the patellar tendon?
6. What is Sinding-Larsen-Johansson disease and how is it differentiated from sleeve fractures of the inferior patellar pole?
7. What distal site of osteochondrosis secondary to traction apophysis occurs in the lower extremity?
8. What is the clinical presentation of this disorder?
9. What do radiographs reveal?
10. What is the therapeutic management of this condition?
11. When is surgery considered?

1. What is the most likely the cause of this boy's condition?

Osgood-Schlatter disease is a form of traction periostitis of the tibial apophysitis type that manifests as a partial avulsion of the tibial tuberosity with subsequent avascular necrosis of the fragmented bone. This overuse syndrome seems to be precipitated by athletic activities in late childhood or early adolescence by basketball in particular. Although this condition was once confined to pubescent males,[28] it is now typical of females involved in athletic activity, particularly soccer and gymnastics.[33] Thus the development of this disorder seems to be dependent on the degree of skeletal maturity and activity level rather than gender. There may also be a genetic predisposition to Osgood-Schlatter disease because siblings of affected persons are more likely to develop this disorder.[14] This condition, simultaneously described in 1903 by Osgood in the United States and Schlatter in Germany, is usually unilateral but may occur bilaterally. There is no accompanying systemic disturbance. This disease is self-limiting and spontaneously remitting over a period of 6 to 24 months as the tibial tubercle ossifies.[37]

2. What is the difference between epiphysis and apophysis, and how is this important to the classification of this form of osteochondrosis?

Osgood-Schlatter disease is classified as a *juvenile osteochondrosis* and, as such, is a disorder of the physis. Growth cartilage is present at 3 sites in the developing child: the epiphyseal plate, the joint surface, and the apophysis or tendon insertion (Fig. 37-1).[16] The former and latter are types of physis (epiphysis and apophysis) that represent the weakest structure in growing bone, being much weaker than ligaments or tendons.[7] *Epiphyses,* located at either head of long bones, are growth plates by which longitudinal growth (by way of cartilaginous proliferation) occurs away from the middle of long bones. The epiphyses are entirely cartilaginous during growth and ossify only when growth is complete, which usually coincides with puberty. Before closure of the physis, the growth plate is weaker than adjacent ligaments or tendons. Subsequently, the growth plate represents an inherently weak link, so that injuries that occur near joints are more likely to result in physeal disruption. As such, the physis may be subjected to excessive pressure by the joints on either end of their articulations and are vulnerable to epiphyseal or apophyseal injury or failure; for example as in Legg-Calve-Perthes disease of the proximal hip or Osgood-

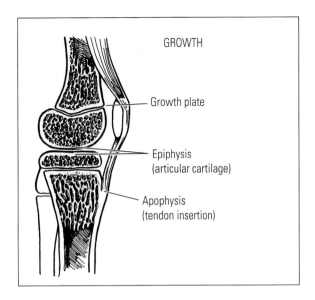

FIG. 37-1 Growth cartilage is present at three sites—the growth plate, the articular surface, and the apophysis—and is susceptible to overuse injury at each of these sites. (Adapted from Micheli LJ: Overuse injuries in children's sports: the growth factor. *Orthop Clin North Am* 14: 337-360, 1983.)

Schlatter disease at the proximal tibia, respectively. The *epiphyseal growth plate* has been reported to be particularly vulnerable to linear and torsional tears.[29]

Apophyses are also cartilaginous growth plates, but differ from epiphyses in that they occur alongside certain bones to form bony prominences for tendon attachment. The tibial tuberosity is an example of an apophysis defined as protuberant projections that are a bony outgrowth that are separated from the main body of bone by a layer of cartilage and eventually unite with the bone through further ossification. Consequently, apophysis such as the tibial tuberosity may be subject to *traction* (tension) rather than *pressure* (compression). Osgood-Schlatter disease is therefore most accurately described as *tibial apophysitis,* and represents an avulsion fracture of the developing ossification center of the proximal tibia[5,7,8,19] secondary to traction at the proximal tibial physis.

During fetal development the tibial tuberosity develops independently of the proximal tibia as 3 merging areas of a tongue-shaped downward extension of the tibial plateau. After birth the apophysis migrates distally and forms its own growth plate with an associated center of ossification by 7 to 9 years of age. If not interfered with, the ossification center will fuse with that of the tibial epiphysis. Osgood-Schlatter disease will occur when excessive *tensile* force upsets this vulnerable stage of endochondral ossification, resulting in avulsion of the superficial portion of the tuberosity. Unlike the proximal tibia, which is composed of hyaline cartilage that better attenuate stress, the tibial tuberosity is composed of fibrocartilage and thus less likely to stave off tensile-related stress.

3. What is the cause of this disorder and how does it relate to early adolescence?

Somatic muscle growth is stimulated by skeletal growth because of the increasing distance imposed on the muscle attachments as bone growth. Thus skeletal muscles may increase their parallel length in response to osseous growth.[18] Osgood-Schlatter disease is unique to ages 10 to 15 years due to the *rapid growth differential* between osseous and soft tissue structures corresponding to the adolescent growth spurt. This spurt results in an imbalance in the rate of maturity of the quadriceps mechanism and the tibial tuberosity. The quadriceps muscle group is stimulated to grow by an increase in femoral length and width. Although the quadriceps muscles have enlarged to near maturity, an osseous maturation lag exists at the proximal tibia in which the tibia apophysis has not yet fused with the tibial epiphysis.

In adolescents the strength of the tendons, ligaments, and muscles is greater than that of the bones, whereas the reverse is true for adults. The bony attachment of the tendon or ligament is commonly torn away from its attachment instead of the tendon or ligament themselves tearing.[22] Hence, vigorous physical activity common to this age group may cause excessive traction to the patellar ligament on its immature apophyseal insertion as result in traction apophysitis (Fig. 37-2). Repeated running and jumping activities involve rapid and forceful quadriceps contraction and are implicated as causative in fragmentation and separation of the secondary ossification center of the tibial tubercle. This is known as the *physeal fracture theory* of Osgood-Schlatter disease. Initially, the fragment is cartilaginous, but with stimulation of callus formation as well as childhood growth and development the tuberosity enlarges, ossifies, and may separate from the tibia.

4. What is the pathophysiology of this disorder?

In the physeal fracture theory of Osgood-Schlatter disease, a traumatic etiology is postulated. Presumably, excessive traction of the quadriceps tendon due to re-

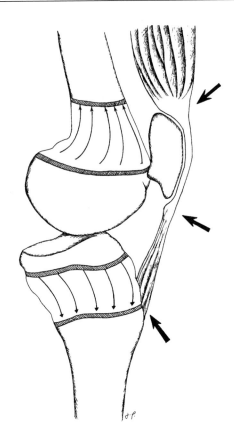

FIG. 37-2 Rapid longitudinal skeletal growth may lead to tightness of soft-tissue structures at the knee. Problems may arise at a number of places *(arrows)* corresponding to suprapatellar tendinitis, Sinding-Larsen-Johansson disease or infrapatellar tendinitis, and Osgood-Schlatter disease in proximodistal order. (From Nicholas JA, Hershman EB: *The lower extremity and spine in sports medicine,* ed 2, St Louis, 1995, Mosby.)

peated, forceful contraction on the less mature tibial tuberosity might culminate in an avulsion fracture of the developing ossification center of the proximal tibia[3] known as *traction apophysitis.* This may occur in the pubescent child involved in organized sporting events that involve repeated jumping or running. This may result in separation or fragmentation of the secondary ossification center of the tibial tubercle. This fragment is initially cartilaginous but, with growth, development, and stimulation of callus formation, the tuberosity will enlarge and the fragments ossify. Although partially avulsed fragments will continue to grow by virtue of their attachment, entirely avulsed fragments will undergo avascular necrosis. The intervening site undergoes reactive inflammation and the body reacts by fill-

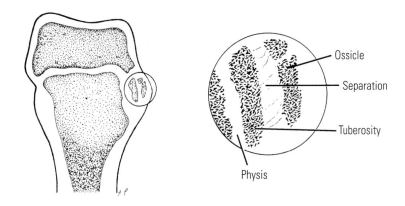

FIG. 37-3 Possible mechanisms of formation of an Osgood-Schlatter lesion. The primary lesion involves avulsion of small areas (ossicles of anterior portions of the developing ossification center of the tibial tuberosity with callus formation in the intervening area, and thereby building up the anterior portion of the tuberosity). The growth plate of the tuberosity remains intact. (From Nicholas JA, Hershman EB: *The lower extremity and spine in sports medicine,* ed 2, St Louis, 1995, Mosby.)

ing the gap with newly generated bone that is viewed and palpated as a pronounced bump (Fig. 37-3). Subcutaneous swelling is due to a combination of bone traction as well as inflammation by adjacent soft tissue. Some 5% of patients[4] have persistent pain from an ununited spicule of bone in the tubercle. Spicule excision should be considered only after conservative treatment has failed.

5. What distal biomechanical deviation would cause excessive traction on the patellar tendon?

Excessive pronation during stance phase of gait results in corresponding proximal biomechanical deviations along the kinetic chain. An alteration in the degree of tibial rotation, specifically medial tibial torsion, will occur in proportion to the magnitude of hyperpronation. This excessive torsion will, in turn, cause excessive medial torsion along the length of the patellar tendon with respect to that tendon's insertion. This may contribute to traction at the distal insertion of that tendon. Thus excessive pronation may be causative in the development of Osgood-Schlatter disease.[31]

6. What is Sinding-Larsen-Johansson disease and how is it differentiated from sleeve fractures of the inferior patellar pole?

Sinding-Larsen-Johansson disease (SLJD—also known as *jumper's knee, patella baja, high-riding patella*) is another form of osteochondrosis secondary to traction apophyses, affecting the lower extremity. This condi-

tion was independently described in the early 1900s by Sinding, Larsen,[26] and Johansson[12] as pain at the inferior patellar pole accompanied by radiographic findings of fragmentation of the pole. This condition, caused by traction of the patellar tendon, occurs 1 to 2 years earlier than does Osgood-Schlatter disease. This condition is an apophysitis of the inferior patellar pole, or less commonly the superior patellar pole, and may be thought of as the counterpart of Osgood-Schlatter disease at the patellar poles. Although Osgood-Schlatter disease is confined to the tibial tuberosity, it is a disorder involving both osseous and soft tissues at the bone–tendon junction. It is not unusual to see tibial tubercle apophysitis develop synchronously to Sinding-Larsen-Johansson syndrome,[35] although the latter condition typically occurs 1 to 2 years (age 8 to 13) before the former. This condition is most common in normal males at puberty, but may also occur in spastic children. SLJD is an extraarticular lesion resulting from a chronic traction phenomenon with avulsion of the patellar ligament fibers that undergo necrosis and calcification. The recurrent pull of the quadriceps mechanism may avulse a small piece of bone and periosteum from the anterior-inferior surface of the patella. The avulsed fragment consisting of bone, periosteum, and patellar ligament undergoes calcification and new bone formation.[9]

The presentation of SLJD normally occurs in the healthy, vigorous patient between the ages of 10 and 14 years.[2,15,17] The etiology of Sinding-Larsen-Johansson syndrome is ascribed to excessive traction on the patellar tendon secondary to chronic extensor mechanism overloading. Apophysitis is exceeded by a history of chronic anterior knee pain that has an initially gradual onset related to activity such as jumping, running, ascending stairs, and prolonged sitting. The duration of symptoms ranges from 1 or 2 days to several months. Although most patients typically present with a pattern of chronic pain, some patients may present with acute onset of symptoms, although all patients do not have a history of direct knee trauma. Repetitive loaded knee activity leads to a progression of extensor tendinitis, partial ligament avulsion, or stress fracture of the inferior patellar pole. Pain and swelling at either patellar pole as well as a relatively weak quadriceps mechanism are universally present. Tenderness is localized to the inferior patellar pole. Presentation to the primary care provider is often preceded by an acute trauma (such as a sporting event) that amplifies ongoing symptoms to an intolerable level. Occasionally, a prominence is present and is best viewed with the patient supine and the knee hyperflexed.

Lateral radiographic evaluation may show irregularity or fragmentation at the distal patellar pole, superior patellar ossification, patellar elongation, or even bony avulsion. Pain and swelling at either the inferior or superior patellar pole in the absence of radiographic findings are suggestive of attritional partial ligament rupture. The diagnosis of SLJD is usually clinical and is suggested by mild pain and point tenderness at the inferior patellar pole. Radiographic confirmation is not always possible, as the lesion may not be initially detectable, and only then as calcification progresses.

Sleeve fractures as well as SLJD occur at the inferior pole of the patella in adolescents between the ages of 10 and 14 years. Because sleeve fractures occur infrequently, they may be overlooked on initial evaluation.[10,24] Sleeve fractures occur as an acute injury in the adolescent patient following forceful contraction of the quadriceps mechanism against a partially flexed knee. This may occur during high jumping or hurdling, or while propelling oneself on a skateboard. The quadriceps mechanism undergoes a forceful, often violent contraction against firm resistance. This sudden eccentric loading causes avulsion of articular cartilage as well as a small fleck of patellar bone. It is imperative to recognize the differences in clinical presentation between SLJD and cartilage fractures as the latter represents an acute, intraarticular injury that requires open reduction and internal fixation of the avulsed articular cartilage. There is no history of direct trauma to the knee.[23] Patients classically describe a sudden, painful giving way of the knee and inability to bear weight. Palpation reveals a swollen, tender knee, with point tenderness and a palpable gap felt in the patellar ligament at the inferior patellar pole. Similar to SLJD, sleeve fractures may also present with a small bone fragment and patella alta that are radiographically detectable. However, with SLJD, a patella alta may or may not be present, whereas it is always radiographically detected following sleeve fracture. Moreover, the physical finding of a palpable gap is exclusive to cartilage fractures. Radiographs following a suspected cartilage fractures may only show a knee effusion and patella alta; the small avulsed fragment of bone may not be detectible.[9] It is essential not to minimize the severity of this fracture simply because of its benign radiographic appearance. Postoperatively, the knee is immobilized in a cylinder cast with 5° of knee flexion for 4 to 6 weeks. A program of range of motion and 4 to 6 weeks of strengthening and stretching is appropriate following cast removal.

SLJD typically runs its course in 2 to 14 months. Treatment is conservative and consists of rest by way of activity restriction, followed by stretching of the hamstring musculature, and strengthening, particularly eccentric working, of the quadriceps musculature, especially as the patient often presents with tight hamstring and weak hip flexors.[17] In the patient with acute and severe pain, a knee immobilizer or cylinder cast may be applied for 3 to 4 weeks. When chronic symptoms are exacerbated, cylinder casting is used for 4 to 6 weeks before instituting an exercises program. Healing is often rapid, with symptom abatement after 3 to 4 weeks and complete radiologic healing in 6 to 8 weeks following onset of treatment. Normal activity may be resumed when the patient is pain free and fully rehabilitated. Incorporation of the calcific lesion is not a prerequisite for activity resumption.[9] Typically, no residual disability occurs as the child returns to preinjury status. There is no evidence to suggest that children with this problem are more susceptible to the development of jumper's knee in early adulthood (Fig. 37-4).

7. What distal site of osteochondrosis secondary to traction apophyses occurs in the lower extremity?

Sever's disease is a partial avulsion of the calcaneal apophysis at the Achilles tendon insertion onto the posterior apophysis on the os calcis. The calcaneus is the only tarsal bone that derives from two centers of ossification: one from the calcaneal body and the other

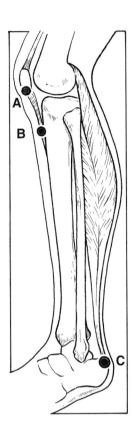

FIG. 37-4 Sites of osteochondritis involving apophysis: **A**, Sinding Larsen-Johansson disease; **B**, Osgood-Schlatter disease; **C**, Sever's disease. (From Dandy DJ: *Essential orthopaedics and trauma,* ed 2, Edinburgh, 1993, Churchill Livingstone.)

from its apophysis, which later forms the posterior portion of this bone. Ossification of the calcaneal body begins at birth whereas apophyseal ossification lags behind and does not begin until age 8, although complete ossification and union of both centers certainly occurs by age 16. However, if excessive jumping or athletic activity occurs between ages 8 and 16, a fracture of the cartilaginous union of these two bones may occur. The child may experience pain behind the heel and walk with a little spring in his or her step *(calcaneus gait)* in an unconscious attempt to reduce the powerful pull of the Achilles tendon on the apophysis. Local tenderness and slight swelling may present over the posterior aspect of the heel. This self-limiting disorder spontaneously improves in less than a year, with healing occurring by fibrocartilaginous replacement. Differential diagnosis for heel pain in children includes rheumatoid arthritis. Management emphasizes symptomatic relief

as well as elevating heel height by 1 cm to minimize Achilles tendon pull.

8. What is the clinical presentation of this disorder?

Osgood-Schlatter disease is diagnosed as a painful swelling at the tibial tubercle[21] that is accentuated by vigorous physical activity, kneeling, or crawling activity, and is relieved by rest. When the affected knee is examined, a prominence of the proximal tibia may be palpated and elicit tenderness (Fig. 37-5). Swelling may be apparent in the distal portion of the patellar tendon, over the tibial tubercle, and occasionally in the local subcutaneous tissue;[28,34] intraarticular effusion is absent. Active flexion and extension may be limited by pain or swelling, and resistive knee extension may also yield pain. Occasionally, an extensor lag may present in the ipsilateral knee.[33] Some patients have findings of limitation of knee flexion with reproduction of pain.[37] This may occur because patellofemoral forces increase with flexion; subsequently, acute flexion will transmit extreme tension throughout the extensor mechanism and focus tension at the tibial tubercle. Tightness or contracture may be present in several muscle groups including the hamstrings, gastrocnemii,[33] but especially the quadriceps, demonstrated by a positive *Ely test* (Fig. 37-6). Quadriceps atrophy is common.[33]

9. What do radiographs reveal?

The radiographic features of Osgood-Schlatter disease are observed at the lower attachment of the patellar tendon. Films of the contralateral knee should be obtained for comparison. Lateral radiographs of the knee are also useful to exclude other pathologic entities such as tumor and infection. Early on in the disease process, lateral knee radiographs will show widening of the space between the tibial apophysis and metaphysis. As the condition evolves into a chronic one, fragmentation occurs due to prominent irregular ossification of the tibial tubercle. This is followed by fragment coalition, separation, and displacement of a separate superficial and proximal ossicle away from the tibial tuberosity.[6,21] The tibial tubercle normally develops irregularly from 1 or 2 ossification centers. Thus despite positive radiographs, diagnosis relies heavily upon clinical correlation as ossification patterns of the tubercle are variable.[33] Ossification of the patellar tendon does not represent Osgood-Schlatter disease and is more common in skeletally mature individuals. Magnetic resonance imaging of the knee may also be useful.

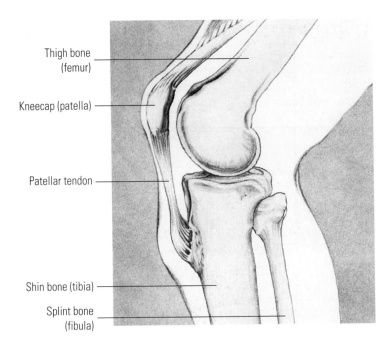

Thigh bone
(femur)

Kneecap (patella)

Patellar tendon

Shin bone (tibia)

Splint bone
(fibula)

FIG. 37-5 Diagnosis of Osgood-Schlatter disease is made by confirmation of painful swelling at the tibial tubercle, as well as an accompanying history of physical activity. Clinical diagnosis is confirmed by positive lateral radiographs. (From Peterson L, Renstrom P: *Sports injuries: their prevention and treatment,* Chicago, 1983, Yearbook Medical Publishers.)

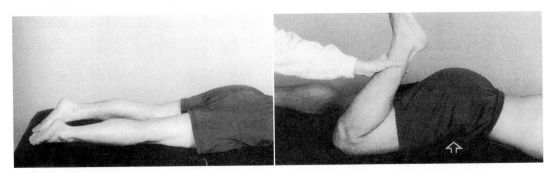

FIG. 37-6 Ely test for rectus femoris tightness. The patient lies prone *(left)* and receives passive knee flexion *(right)*. This posture places the two jointed rectus femoris on *passive insufficiency* as it is pulled at its origin as well as insertion. A positive test is indicated if the ipsilateral hip spontaneously flexes and viewed as an ipsilateral buttock rise secondary to tightness of the rectus femoris muscle on that side *(arrow)*. Both sides should be tested and compared. (From Magee DJ: *Orthopedic physical assessment,* Philadelphia, 1997, WB Saunders.)

10. What is the therapeutic management of this condition?

Treatment of Osgood-Schlatter disease is conservative[1,28] and similar to management of adult patellar tendinitis[3] (see pp. 533-536). In the acute state *ice, compressive wrap,* and *oral analgesics* provide symptomatic benefit. Corticosteroid medication is contraindicated as a form of treatment because of the potential for deleterious skin complications[25] to the relatively thin dermis covering the tubercle.

It is important to reassure parents that, despite the serious sounding name of this condition, their child will be fine. It must be emphasized than Osgood-Schlatter disease is a benign entity. If this condition is only occasionally bothersome and does not limit activities, then treatment is unnecessary. However, when symptoms are bothersome during sporting activities, the goal of treatment is the prevention of further irritation during the healing phase. This is accomplished by imposing mandatory *rest* in the form of minimizing or avoidance of activities such as jumping, kneeling, deep knee bending, and the avoidance of strenuous or excessive exercise to the involved lower extremity. This is accompanied by an exercise program of short-arc hamstring exercises for approximately 6 weeks until symptoms subside to avoid the risk of separation of the tibial tubercle. However, if the patient complains of pain toward the end of one day but is asymptomatic the following day, then only activity modification is recommended. Encouraging the adolescent to take frequent rest periods while maintaining involvement with sports may be arranged by having the parents and coaches discuss the situation.[27] Should pain persist for longer periods of time and cause limping, it may be necessary for the child to sit out the remainder of the sporting season. Cycling or swimming is often good substitutes for exercise,[20] but the patient should avoid extremes of flexion. Weight bearing is permitted, and it is not necessary to immobilize the knee or restrain the child from running.

Bracing or the use of a sleeve cast are appropriate only if the child experiences severe pain and a limp is observed during nonsporting activities and the child demonstrates difficulties with activities of daily living or walking over level ground. The brace is then worn for at least 5 weeks. Generally, immobilization is rarely used although this may be necessary for the unreliable patient who will not or who cannot comply with a program of relative rest.[33] The use of *ice massage* may relieve acute symptoms. The use of oral aspirin, or locally applied *iontophoresis* may be prescribed by the physician. Steroid injection is contraindicated as this may cause patellar tendon deterioration, and provides little in the way of long-term relief.

The key to conservative management of Osgood-Schlatter disease lies in regaining adequate flexibility of the extensor mechanism at the knee. A muscle imbalance between the anterior and posterior musculature in favor of quadriceps hypertrophy may contribute to the onset on Osgood-Schlatter disease. This may occur due to excessive pull of the strong quadriceps on the tibial tubercle. Any difference in strength among muscle antagonists should be noted, and a combination of appropriate *stretching* and *strengthening* exercises should be prescribed and instituted to negate and reverse any soft tissue imbalance. A strengthening exercise program

emphasizing working the weaker hamstring muscle group should be emphasized to restore muscle balance, and relieve excessive tensile force on the tubercle exerted by the quadriceps. *Eccentric* quadriceps strengthening is appropriate as it involves distraction of muscle fibers. Conversely, eccentric contractions will develop greater muscle force, compared with concentric contractions and accordingly should be prescribed with caution. Stretching of tight musculature, particularly the quadriceps muscle group in the nonpainful range may be helpful by way of increasing soft tissue extensibility; stretching of the hamstring muscle group may also prove helpful. These strategies may help minimize excessive stress delivered to the tibial tuberosity during quadriceps femoris contraction.

Exercise should begin with *stretching* activities of the quadriceps and hamstrings on a 3-times-daily basis, followed by a 20-minute application of ice to the area of the tibial tubercle. When the patient can easily touch the heel of the affected leg to the buttock while in the prone posture, quadriceps strengthening may be added.[30] Progressive resistive straight leg raising exercises are indicated as a useful way to isometrically strengthen quadriceps while controlling excessive tension being applied to the tibial tuberosity compared with isotonic exercises where the knee would be flexed. The addition of weight is guided by avoiding any extensor lag or knee pain.[33] Slow resumption of activity is allowed once flexibility and strength have improved. The use of neuromuscular *electrical stimulation* to the quadriceps muscle as well as *biofeedback,* particularly to the vastus medialis oblique portion of quadriceps, may be helpful in diminishing any extensor lag. Young athletes are gently informed during treatment that a residual deformity may persist in the tuberosity.[33]

The use of knee orthoses such as the Marshall or Palumbo braces may be used to dampen the pull of the extensor mechanism upon the vulnerable tibial apophysis. *Protective kneepads* may be used to reduce by applying direct pressure over the tubercle. "Off the shelf" cushioned *foot orthoses* may be helpful in diminishing the impact of heel strike upon the extensor mechanism,[33] although a custom-fabricated *foot orthoses* is appropriate for those feet exhibiting excessive or deficient pronation. The musculoskeletal system is malleable until fusion of all primary and secondary epiphysis. Because of this, correction via therapeutic reversal of deformity, especially in the foot-ankle complex, exists until late puberty when the growth centers fuse.[32] Early diagnosis of foot deformity accompanied by intervention before mid-adolescence is important as the period of rapid growth and relative plasticity offer the best opportunities for effective orthotic intervention.[11] Moreover, early access to a foot, which is in deviation from subtalar joint neutral, may prevent the development of secondary problems.

11. When is surgery considered?

A small percentage of adolescents do not improve with conservative therapy because of inadequate compliance with a stretching program.[33] For adolescent patients close to physis closure, patience is indicated[36] because completion of tuberosity growth is often associated with amelioration of symptoms. In the skeletally mature symptomatic patient, or in the younger athlete with a wide, open physis and 2 to 3 years of athletic participation lost during the turbulent years of adolescence, surgery is considered after 6 months of uneventful conservative management. Surgery involves excision of loose ossicles under the patellar tendon[13] and any underlying bony tubercle prominence.[33] Athletic resumption following surgical epiphysiodesis may begin once bony union has occurred.[33]

REFERENCES

1. Beddow FH: Treatment of 103 patients with Osgood-Schlatter's disease. *J Bone Joint Surg* 48A:384, 1960.
2. Blazina ME, Kerland RJ, Jobe FW et al: Jumper's knee. *Orthop Clin North Am* 4:665-667, 1973.
3. Boland AL Jr, Hulstyn MJ: Soft-tissue injuries of the knee. In Nicholas JA, Hershman EB, editors: *The lower extremity and spine,* ed 2, vol 1, St Louis, 1995, Mosby.
4. Dandy DJ: *Essential orthopedics and trauma,* ed 2, Edinburgh, 1993, Churchill Livingstone.
5. Dunkerly GE: Osgood-Schlatter and Sinding-Larsen-Johansson disease, *J Bone Joint Surg* 49B:591, 1967.
6. Edeiken J: *Roentgen diagnosis of diseases of bone,* ed 3, Baltimore, 1981, Williams & Wilkins.
7. Ehrlich M, Hulstyn M, D'Amoto C: Sports injuries in children and the clumsy child, *Pediatr Clin North Am* 39:433, 1992.
8. Ferretti A et al: Jumper's knee, *Am J Sports Med* 11:58, 1983.
9. Gardiner JS, McInerney VK, Avella DG, et al: Injuries to the inferior pole of the patella in children, *Orthopedic Review* 19(7):643-9, 1990.
10. Houghton GR, Ackroyd CE: Sleeve fractures of the patella in children: a report of three cases, *J Bone Joint Surg* 61B:165-168, 1979.
11. Jahss M, editor: *Disorders of the foot,* vol 1, Philadelphia, 1982, Saunders.
12. Johansson S: En forut ecke beskriven sjukdom I patella, *Hygiea* 84:161-166, 1922.
13. King AG, Bludell-Jones G: A surgical procedure for the Osgood-Schlatter lesion, *Am J Sports Med* 9:250, 1981.
14. Kujala UM, Kvist M, Heinonen O: Osgood-Schlatter's disease in adolescent athletes: retrospective study of incidence and duration, *Am J Sports Med* 13:236, 1985.
15. Medlar RC, Lynne ED: Sinding-Larsen-Johansson disease, its etiology and natural history. *J Bone Jt Surg* 60A:1113-1116, 1978.
16. Micheli LJ: Overuse injuries in children's sports: the growth factor. *Orthop Clin North Am* 14:337-360, 1983.
17. Nicholas J, Herschman E: *The lower extremity and spine in sports medicine,* New York, 1986, CV Mosby.
18. O'Dwyer NJ, Neilson PD, Nash J: Mechanisms of muscle growth related to muscle contracture in cerebral palsy, *Dev Med Child Neurol* 31:543-552, 1989.
19. Ogden JA, Southwick WD: Osgood-Schlatter's disease and tibial tubercle development, *Clin Orthop* 116:180, 1976.
20. O'Neill DB, Micheli LJ: Overuse injuries in the young athlete, *Clin Sports Med* 7:591, 1988.
21. Osgood RB: Lesions of the tibial tubercle occurring during adolescence, *Boston Med Surg J* 148:114, 1903.
22. Peterson L, Renstrom P: *Sport injuries: their prevention and injury,* Chicago, 1986, Year Book Medical Publishers.
23. Rang MC: *Children's fractures,* Toronto, 1982, JB Lippincott.
24. Rockwood CA, Wilkens KA, King RE: *Fractures in children,* San Antonio and Atlanta, 1984, JB Lippincott.
25. Rostron PKM, Calver RF: Subcutaneous atrophy following methylprednisolone injection in Osgood-Schlatter epiphysitis, *J Bone Joint Surg* 61(A):627, 1979.
26. Sinding-Larsen MF: A hitherto unknown affection of the patellain children, *Acta Radiol* 1:171-173, 1921.
27. Singer KM, Henry J: Knee problems in children and adolescents, *Clin Sports Med* 4(2):385-97, 1985.
28. Soren A, Fetto JF: Pathology, clinical findings, and treatment of Osgood-Schlatter's disease. *Orthopedics* 7:230, 1984.
29. Speer DP, Braun JK: The biomechanical basis of growth plate injuries, *The physician and sports medicine* 13:72-78, 1985.
30. Strizak AM: Knee injuries. In Nicholas JA, Hershman EB, editors: *The lower extremity & spine,* ed 2, vol 2, St Louis, 1995, Mosby-Year Book.
31. Subotnick SI: *Podiatric sports medicine,* New York, 1975, Futura Publishing.
32. Tachdjian M: *The child's foot,* Philadelphia, 1985, WB Saunders.
33. Thabit G III, Micheli LJ: Patellofemoral pain in the pediatric patient, *Orthop Clin North Am,* 23(4):578, 1992.
34. Wiley JJ, Baxter MP: Tibial spine fractures in children, *Clin Orthop,* 225:54, 1990.
35. Wolf J: Larsen-Johansson disease of the patella. Seven new case reports. Its relationship to other forms of osteochondritis. Use of male sex hormones as a new form of treatment, *Br J Radiol* 23:335-347, 1950.
36. Woolfrey BE, Chandler EF: Manifestations of Osgood-Schlatter's disease in late teenage and early adulthood, *J Bone Joint Surg* 42A:327, 1969.
37. Zitelli BJ, Davis HW: *Atlas of pediatric physical diagnosis,* St Louis, 1987, Mosby-Wolfe.

RECOMMENDED READING

Singer KM, Henry J: Knee problems in children and adolescents, *Clin Sports Med* 4(2), 1985.
Thabit G, Micheli LJ: Patellofemoral pain in the pediatric patient, *Orthop Clin North Am* 23(4), 1992.

38

Pain and Tenderness at Inferior Patellar Pole and Ligament After Descent From Repetitive Jumping Activities

A 26-year-old female plays varsity basketball at the local town college. She complains of a 2-week-old right anterior knee pain during basketball that subsides about 10 minutes after the game has begun. However, pain is most acutely felt when she lands on her feet following jumping up at the basket. After practice she feels an aching anterior knee pain and stiffness. In the evening following practice, walking upstairs, stooping, and kneeling are painful. She denies any history of trauma to the knee. She also denies any locking or catching sensation, or buckling of the right knee joint.

OBSERVATION   Her right stance foot posture seems moderately pronated and slight genu valgum. A double hump characteristic of the positive camel sign is present at her right knee.

PALPATION   Point tenderness is noted at the right inferior patellar pole with no evidence of knee joint effusion.

PASSIVE RANGE OF MOTION   Yields painful passive right terminal knee flexion.

ACTIVE RANGE OF MOTION   Normal, although at full knee flexion the patella seems to occupy a high position in the proximal femoral trochlear groove.

MUSCLE STRENGTH   Relative right concentric quadriceps strength is graded at G−.

SELECTIVE TENSION   Shows uncomfortable resistive right knee extension.

FLEXIBILITY TESTING   Shows bilateral hamstring tightness. There seems to be excessive ligamentous laxity of the terminal extensor mechanism as well as the medial and lateral patellar retinacula due to excessive patellar mobility. Tightness is present in the triceps surae muscle group.

SPECIAL TESTS   Positive patella grinding, negative limb-length discrepancy, Thomas, Lachman, McMurray, and Apley tests. Right Q angle is measured to be in excess of 18° in the open kinetic chain as patient lies on the examination table. A leg length discrepancy of 8 mm, longer on the left side, is noted.

RADIOGRAPHS   Show the distal patellar pole elongated, and are otherwise negative. The patella seems to rest slightly higher when compared with the contralateral lower extremity.

CLUE   A lateral view of the right knee at 30° of flexion which indicates a patellar length vs. patellar tendon length, shows an increase greater than 20% of patellar tendon length (see illustration on next page):

521

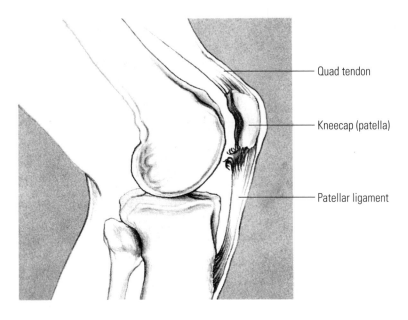

Quad tendon

Kneecap (patella)

Patellar ligament

(From Peterson L, Renstrom P: *Sports injuries: their prevention and treatment,* Chicago, 1983, Yearbook Medical Publishers.)

? | Questions

1. What knee disorder is most likely implicated?
2. What is jumper's knee?
3. What are patella alta and baja, and how do they relate to jumper's knee?
4. What anatomy is relevant to understanding the spectrum of these disorders?
5. What are the histologic changes associated with jumper's knee?
6. What is the mechanism of injury?
7. What is the Q angle, how does it normally bias patellar ligament excursion laterally, and how does this bias minimize the length-tension of the extensor mechanism?
8. How may an excessive Q angle or over-pronated foot result in jumper's knee owing to excessive frontal plane excursion of the extensor tendon?
9. How may asynchronous rotations occur along the tibial shaft?
10. How may a patella alta disorder predispose to other forms of knee dysfunction?
11. What sporting activities are most often implicated in patellar alta syndrome?
12. What are the clinical stages of tendinitis?
13. What is the clinical presentation?
14. What is patella baja?
15. How may inflammation of the infrapatellar fat pad result in patella baja?
16. What is Sinding-Larsen-Johansson disease?
17. What therapeutic management is appropriate for patellar tendinitis?

1. What knee disorder is most likely implicated?

Jumper's knee or *patellar tendinitis* of the right knee localized to the *right infrapatellar tendon*. Her injury is classified as a stage II type because pain begins with athletic practice but decreases as the activity continues. Although predisposing factors such as tightness of posterior leg musculature and subtalar joint over-pronation were present, the patient's right lower extremity demonstrates a leg length discrepancy that serves to magnify the shortening of that limb already present because of right subtalar joint pronation. Consequently, the magnitude of internal rotatory torsion imparted proximally to the right knee will be of greater magnitude than at the left knee. Subsequently, the right infrapatellar tendon (patellar ligament) will be subject to excessive lateral excursion as well as torsion.

2. What is jumper's knee?

Jumper's knee is categorized as traction overuse injury secondary to both extrinsic and intrinsic overload on the extensor mechanism of the knee. This *insertional tendinopathy* of the extensor tendon most commonly involves the patellar ligament insertion at inferior patellar pole. This disease entity demonstrates a high incidence in athletes preoccupied with jumping, kicking,[11,12,14,20,21,23,26,27,29,31,37,47,48] climbing, and running.[18] There is no particular age predilection for the development of *extensor tendon injury,* although this disorder is most common in skeletally mature individuals. Jumper's knee is the most benign form of *extensor tendon disease,* a progressive condition that may culminate as full thickness tear of the patellar tendon or ligament.

Extensor tendon injury is a degenerative process secondary to chronic overuse resulting in repetitive microtrauma. This disorder is not a benign, self-limiting process that resolves with time. Rather, patellar tendon injury may be viewed as a continuum of disorders that begin with tendinitis and may progress to tendon rupture as the end-stage of this pathologic process. Unfortunately, there is no "pre-rupture" prodrome that suggests impending tendon strain.

3. What are patella alta and baja, and how do they relate to jumper's knee?

Patella alta represents a disruption of the knee extensor mechanism because of an abnormally *high-riding patella* in relation to the femur both during standing and sitting postures. Patella alta may also result from stretching or tearing of the patellar retinaculum. This disorder results from *patellar tendon disease* that may include tendinitis, partial, or even complete rupture of the *infrapatellar tendon* (patellar ligament) at the patellar bone–patellar tendon junction, that is, the proximal posterior portion of its origin. Indeed, the sequence of pathology of the distal stretch of the extensor mechanism at the knee (the quadriceps tendon and patellar ligament) often begins as tendon disease that progresses to full thickness rupture. Eventually, cephalic migration of the patella may occur so that the patella will lie between the femoral condyles. The articular underside of the patella will then rest upon cortical bone which, over time, will lead to breakdown of articular cartilage. Thus patella alta is but a sign of chronic overloading characteristic of injury to the knee extensor mechanism.

Patellar tendinitis of the *suprapatellar tendon* (quadriceps tendon) is another form of jumper's knee whose site of occurrence is confined to the superior patellar pole, and may be associated with *patella baja* (Fig. 38-1). Either site of patellar tendinitis, as well as the adolescent form of infrapatellar tendinitis, known

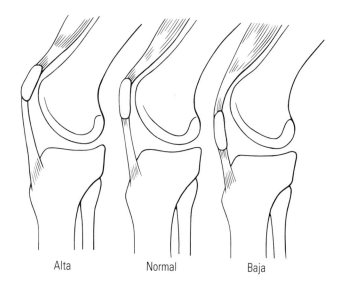

Alta   Normal   Baja

FIG. 38-1 *Patella alta* and *baja* are associated signs accompanying jumper's knee. If the site of involvement is the junction of the patellar ligament (infrapatellar tendon) junction with the inferior patellar pole, then stretching or tearing at that site will result in cephalic patellar migration characteristic of patella alta. If the site of pathologic involvement occurs at the junction of the quadriceps tendon (suprapatellar tendon) with the superior patellar pole, then stretching or rupture at that site may result in the patella sliding caudally. Patella posture is most easily viewed from the lateral view with the knee in 45° flexion.

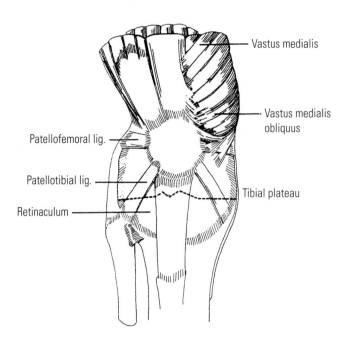

FIG. 38-2 The patellofemoral and patellotibial ligaments. (From Jacobson KE, Flandry FC: Diagnosis of anterior knee pain, *Clin Sports Med* 8[2]:191, 1989.)

as Sinding-Larsen-Johansson disease, are referred to as *jumper's knee*. The latter condition represents stress concentration at the accessory ossification center at the inferior patellar pole that leads to traction epiphysitis and eventual fragmentation at the tendon-bone junction.[39]

4. What anatomy is relevant to understanding the spectrum of these disorders?

The *extensor mechanism* at the knee includes the quadriceps femoris muscle group, the quadriceps femoris tendon, the patellofemoral joint, and the patellar ligament. The medial and lateral retinacula are static patellar restraints composed of the medial and lateral patellofemoral ligaments, respectively. Together, they serve as static patella stabilizers that act as check ligaments to restrict excessive mediolateral movement. In addition, they restrain the patella from excessive cephalic glide on the femur (Fig. 38-2).

The *patellar ligament* (also known as the *infrapatellar tendon*) is the physical continuation of the quadriceps femoris suprapatellar tendon (Fig. 38-3). A relatively flat and extremely strong band, it attaches above the patella and continues over its front with fibers distally attaching on the tibial tuberosity. Its function is to

unilaterally provide stabilization to the patellofemoral joint by restraining excessive cephalic patellar glide. The patellar ligament is cushioned by a large subcutaneous infrapatellar bursa as well as a deep infrapatellar bursa between the ligament and bone. The nomenclature describing that portion of the quadriceps tendon distal to the patella as a (patella) ligament is based upon the fact that it spans from (the patellar) bone to bone (tibial tubercle). In actuality, the collagenous tissue comprising the patellar ligament is identical to its precursor, the quadriceps ligament. The patellar ligament is, in fact, a continuation of the quadriceps tendon distally beyond the patella as the latter envelops the patella before giving rise to the former. Thus the patellar ligament is actually a dynamic ligament in the indirect service of the quadriceps muscle group.

5. What are the histologic changes associated with jumper's knee?

The histologic changes associated with jumper's knee involve sequential pathologic changes in the tendon matrix and bone–tendon junction as a direct result of persistent microtrauma. The quadriceps tendon or patellar ligament undergo microtears in their substance that serve as the site of focal mucoid collagen degen-

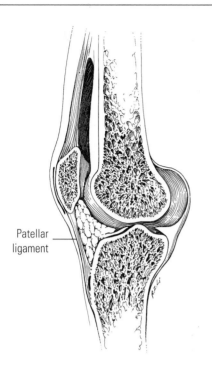

Patellar
ligament

FIG. 38-3 The *patellar ligament* is the continuation of the quadriceps tendon, and represents the distal aspect of the extensor mechanism. Note how the patella is enveloped by the quadriceps tendon-ligament confluence. Note also how the infrapatellar fat pad serves to help prop the patella such that it lies recessed along the supratrochlear surface located within the intercondylar femoral groove. (From Tria AJ, Klein KS: *An illustrated guide to the knee.* New York, 1992, Churchill Livingstone.)

eration in which the organization of collagen fibers comprising the soft tissue is lost. Subsequently, regeneration is attempted by way of fibroblast regeneration. If the quadriceps tendon or patellar ligament is further stressed then tissue necrosis and degeneration may set in. Following 6 months of symptoms, the site of injury may undergo cartilage calcification. When symptoms have lasted more than 1 year, bone spicules may be present at the original site of injury. Rupture of the quadriceps tendon or patellar ligament from indirect injury represents the end stages of jumper's knee and is a result of severe degeneration that has evolved into a chronically weakened tendon. This pathologic sequence highlights the importance of timely diagnosis and intervention of tendinitis. Indeed, jumper's knee is not a benign, self-limiting condition. It is a progressive condition that, if not adequately managed in a timely fashion, may result in irreversible pathologic change and the eventual failure of conservative treatment.[10]

6. What is the mechanism of injury?

The mechanism of injury often involves repeated landings from an elevated platform or from jumping activities[45] performed with slight flexion of the knee so as to dampen the force of impact. The excessive forces generated here derive from the mass of body weight multiplied by the speed of the descent. The impact from landing in this posture will tug on both the patellar ligament and patellar retinaculum and, following chronic abuse, result in laxity of these structures. These forces are normally minimized by eccentric quadriceps muscle contractions and, as an injury-sparing strategy, act to absorb potentially injurious forces imparted to the musculoskeletal system.

In sporting activities, the repetitive actions of acceleration, deceleration, jumping, and landing, most commonly occurring in basketball and volleyball, may concentrate enormous stress upon the extensor mechanism at the knee (Fig. 38-4). Alternately, injury may occur from leaping during ballet. A critical level is reached in which the tendon's inherent tensile capacity is exceeded by both the magnitude and repetition of applied stress during the jump landing in which the effect of body weight and gravity multiply the forces to the extensor mechanism. An acute stretching or tearing of the superior fibers of the patellar tendon just inferior to the inferior patellar pole will occur when the quadriceps pulls explosively during a leap or jump. Eventually, an inflammatory process manifests as tendinitis, characterized by thickening and contracture of the sheath as well as adhesion between the tendon and sheath.[40] Unabated tendon stress causes the condition to become chronic as nodules of granulated tissue form in the tendon. If the predisposing stress continues, the condition may progress to full thickness rupture of the distal aspect of the extensor mechanism.

If the magnitude of forced flexion incurred during injury is large, then the patellar ligament may rupture. Rarely, the tendon may pull a fragment of bone from the lower pole of the patella. A forced flexion injury involves falling with the flexed knee under the body or stepping upon a nonexistent step. This type of injury may also cause ruptures of the extensor mechanism above the patella, including the patellar tendon and the quadriceps expansions on either side of the patella (Fig. 38-5). Moreover, this same mechanism of indirect violence may cause a transverse fracture of the patella. Left untreated, the patellar fragments split widely and result in loss of quadriceps function and extensor lag.

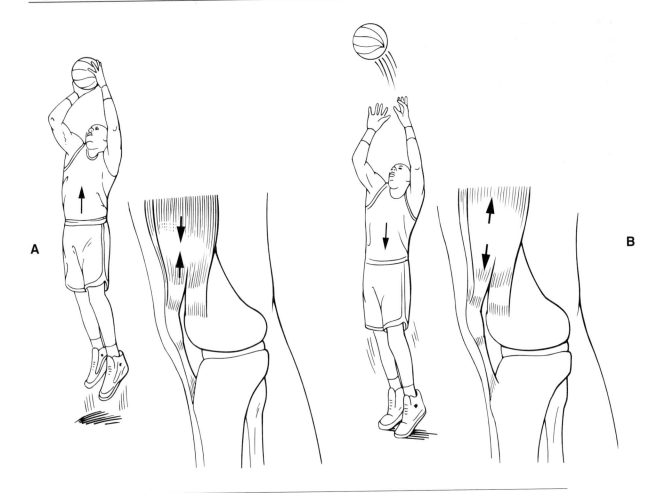

FIG. 38-4 A, Jumping up high toward the basket involves enormous concentric forces generated within the quadriceps muscle that quickly extend the knee by way of the distal aspect of the extensor mechanism pulling upon the tibia. **B,** During the jump landing, the quadriceps cushion the force of impact by eccentrically contracting. During the jump landing the forces directed through the extensor mechanism are magnified to at least 1½ times the body weight secondary to the effect of gravity. It is the enormous magnitude of distractive force during the jump landing that stresses the extensor mechanism to near its critical level of tolerance and may result in injury.

The same effect occurs if a full thickness defect of the extensor mechanism is not repaired.

7. What is the Q angle, how does it normally bias patellar ligament excursion laterally, and how does this bias minimize the length-tension of the extensor mechanism?

The architectural inequality between the anteroposterior projection of the two condyles, which favors a longer medial condyle, imparts a valgus angulation to the normal knee in the erect standing posture. The two femoral condyles diverge at an intercondylar angle of 28° from each other.[57] An anterior view of the extended knee shows a lateral angle between the shafts of the femur and tibia. This angle is due to the body's attempted to narrow down the base of support of the lower extremities. This is accomplished by an adducted femoral shaft and a corresponding compensatory rotation of the tibial shaft so that weight is transmitted perpendicularly to the ground. The size of the angle is variable, although the maximal values are 13° for males and 18° for females, the latter due to the relatively wider diameter of the female pelvis.

The *extensor mechanism* of the knee involves a

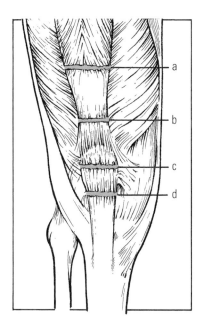

FIG. 38-5 Sites of rupture of the extensor mechanism: *a*, rectus femoris; *b*, quadriceps tendon; *c*, patella; *d*, patellar tendon. (From Dandy DJ: *Essential orthopaedics and trauma*, ed 2, Edinburgh, 1993, Churchill Livingstone.)

delicate and complex balance among the many forces converging upon the knee. Deviation due to weakness or other cause will readily disturb this balance and may cause a host of biomechanical deviations at the knee, as well as both up and down the kinetic chain. The impact of this deviation in the direction of quadriceps pull will reconfigure converging forces at the knee so as to bias *excessive lateral pull* of the extensor mechanism. This lateral bias is responsible for medial facet wear in chondromalacia as well as predisposing the patella towards lateral instability. Lateral patellar tracking is magnified in the presence of an increased Q angle. The biomechanical implications of femoral anteversion are such that the Q angle is substantially increased. The kinesiologic effect upon patellofemoral mechanics is one that increases the valgus force to the patella by way of imparting a valgus angulation to the quadriceps *tendon*. This increases the *pinnation angle* between the superior patellar pole and the quadriceps muscle and represents a proximally originating lateral or valgus vector force to the patella (see Fig. 41-14, *A*). This lateral glide at the inferior patellar pole biases extensor mechanism balance in favor of vastus lateralis by increasing the

mechanical advantage of that muscle over the vastus medialis. Moreover, lateral patellar ligament excursion represents a deviation of the extensor mechanism optimal length-tension relationship. The resultant macrophysiologic alteration places the quadriceps-extensor tendon unit at mechanical disadvantage and predisposes the patellar ligament towards injury.

8. How may an excessive Q angle or over-pronated foot result in jumper's knee due to excessive frontal plane excursion of the extensor tendon?

Infrapatellar tendinitis may occur at the superior posterior aspect of the patellar tendon secondary to excessive tibial torsion.[4] Excessive medial torsion is consistent with over-pronation of the foot whereas excessive lateral torsion is consistent in the foot that does not pronate. Torsion in turns manifests as a quasi-valgus or varus force at the knee that will adversely affect the angle between the inferior patellar pole and the anterior tibial tubercle. This may aggravate the patellar tendon at its superior insertion onto the inferior patella. For example, excessive internal tibial rotation will manifest in the leg secondary to compensatory foot movements such as over-pronation in the closed kinetic chain. Thus medial torsion, whether stemming from over-pronation of the foot or due to a structural tibial deformities serves to tauten the suprapatellar tendon and infrapatellar ligament by introducing a pathomechanical valgus stress that increases the Q angle at the knee (see Fig. 41-14, *C*). These already tight structures are primed for injury as they are now structurally approximated to their elastic limit.

Thus proximal and distal causes of unbalanced extensor mechanism function may result in excessive patellar excursion. A proximal origin of dysfunction derives from femoral anteversion, which in turn, causes an increase of the pinnation angle of the quadriceps tendon. The biomechanical implications of femoral anteversion are such that the Q angle is substantially increased. The kinesiologic effect would be the same as described in the previous section. This increases the pinnation angle between the superior patellar pole and the quadriceps muscle and represents a proximally originating lateral or valgus vector force to the patella. A distal origin of patellofemoral dysfunction stems from excessive pronation of the subtalar joint. A foot that over-pronates as a compensatory mechanism is accompanied by excessive obligatory internal rotation or torsion of the tibia. By virtue of the lower extremity linkage, this excessive valgus torsion is imparted upward to the proximal tibia and increases the pinnation angle between the inferior patellar pole and the anterior tibial tubercle, hence the patellar *ligament.*

Thus regardless of whether the pinnation angles of either the patellar tendon or ligament are increased, the common denominator of both the proximal and distal origins of extensor mechanism imbalance is a medial glide of either the tendon or ligament (see Fig. 41-14).

9. How may asynchronous rotations occur along the tibial shaft?

The individual who has a pes planus deformity will maintain their foot in pronation after mid-stance would impart an internal tibial rotation moment proximally and acts to delay the normal external rotation of the femoral-tibial shafts at this stage of stance. During the interim between foot-flat phase of gait and mid-stance the knee joint moves toward full extension. Extension at the tibiofemoral joint is accompanied by obligatory external rotation of the proximal tibia as the screw home mechanism engages. Although internal tibial rotation occurs distally, the more proximal knee joint is undergoing external rotation and imparts a lateral torsion distally down the tibia. The sum of these two opposite torsion moments, instead of canceling, manifest as a valgus stress applied to the knee joint and cause a tracking deficit in the trochlear groove. The confluence of these opposing transverse plane torsions has potentially deleterious ramifications upon the adjacent soft tissue, namely, the extensor mechanism, and particularly the extensor tendon. As the point of confluence of opposing torsions spans the tibial shaft, the patellar ligament is most likely to absorb these forces (Fig. 38-6). This may account for why most jumper's knee involve the patellar ligament juncture with the inferior patellar pole. Correspondingly, a reduction in subtalar joint pronation has the effect of minimizing the magnitude of stress to the extensor tendon-ligament complex. This may be accomplished by a variety of interventions including the use of a functional orthoses at the subtalar joint and the institution of an appropriate stretching regimen to the tightened triceps surae distally, and the hamstring muscle group proximally.

Poor training in jumping sports may also be implicated as contributory to patellar tendinitis. Athletes who place their knee into a valgus and internally rotated posture during the acceleration phase before take-off alter their biomechanics so that their tibia undergoes an excessive and forceful excursion through its rotational range. This alteration in biomechanics results in a pathomechanic that may predispose the athlete to injury by increasing patellofemoral forces as well as torsion to the already overloaded patellar ligament.

10. How may a patella alta disorder predispose to other forms of knee dysfunction?

The length of the patellar ligament is normally equivalent to a 1:1 ratio with the diagonal length of the patella. An increase in ligament length greater than 20% results in abnormal patellar height due to an uncovering of the infrapatellar fat pad characteristic of patella alta.

Normally, the patella lies above and between the femoral condyles and is in contact with the suprapatellar fat pad in the extended knee posture. As the knee flexes, tension in the quadriceps tendon and patellar tendon compress the patella against the femoral condyle. As both bony surfaces are well covered with cartilage, there is a happy marriage of articulation.

However, in patella alta, the patella rides upward, over, and beyond the cartilaginous femoral surface and rubs against cortical bone, which may lead to patellofemoral arthritis, whereas the resultant ligamentous laxity may predispose lateral patellar subluxation.

11. What sporting activities are most often implicated in patellar alta syndrome?

Patella alta most commonly occurs in athletic activities that place short duration, high intensity stress of a repetitive nature upon the extensor mechanism. Athletes at risk include basketball players, weight lifters, as well as those engaged in volleyball, soccer, badminton, and athletes involved in repetitive running and, particularly, repetitive jumping activities. Patella alta may also present as an occupational disorder involving a great deal of squatting, kneeling, or climbing. These activities typically involve repetitive high loading of the quadriceps mechanism, causing the patellar tendon to succumb to internal disruption as a function of it being, potentially, the weakest link in the series of soft tissue structures negotiating the powerful knee extensor forces. External factors that correlate positively with the incidence of jumper's knee include hard playing surfaces (i.e., cement vs. softer parquet surfaces), and increased frequency of training sessions. Internal factors may be attributable to mechanical properties of the tendon such as resistance, elasticity, and extensibility at the bone-tendon junction as a direct function of aging.[10]

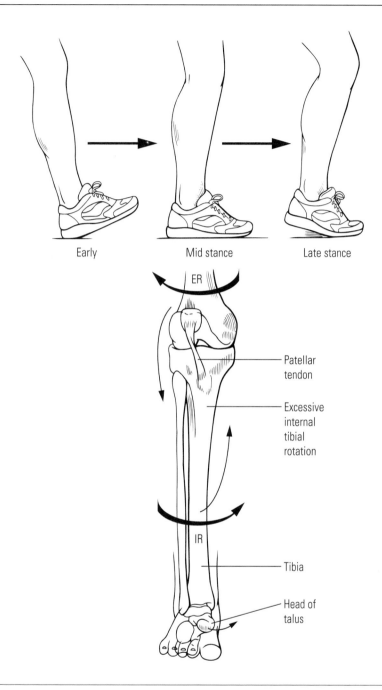

Early   Mid stance   Late stance

ER

Patellar
tendon

Excessive
internal
tibial
rotation

IR

Tibia

Head of
talus

FIG. 38-6 The extensor tendon below the patella may undergo torsion secondary to the conflicting confluence of distal and proximal torsions imparted to the tibial shaft. Subtalar joint over-pronation imparts a medial torsion up along the tibial shaft beyond mid-stance phase of gait when the requirements of the screw-home mechanism extend the knee by imparting an external torsion down the tibial shaft. The length of the patellar ligament corresponds to the locus of these asynchronous forces and may sustain injury.

12. What are the clinical stages of tendinitis?

Pathologic stages include:

- Pain after activity with no functional impairment. The patient rarely seeks medical attention at this early stage. Pain will usually resolve with rest in a few days to a week.[10]
- Pain at the beginning of activity that disappears after warm-up; satisfactory athletic performance followed by reappearance of pain after activity. Tendon disease will evolve into stage II with continued participation by the athlete who performs despite pain. The previously dull ache assumes a more sharp, stabbinglike quality. Athletes will often seek medical attention at this stage because of persistent symptoms.
- Pain during and after activity that impairs function and precludes athletic participation as performance is impaired. At this stage the athlete may become apprehensive about further sport participation. Histopathologic tendon changes such as mucoid degeneration and fibrinoid necrosis are characteristic of this stage and may represent an irreversibly compromised tendon. Tendon disease becomes progressively worse for those patients who have ignored previous warning of pain that has now become constant. Climbing stairs, jumping, landing, sitting for prolonged periods of time with the knee flexed, or in a more involved case, simply walking will exacerbate symptoms.
- Complete tendon rupture will occur if the knee is left untreated while intensive activity is permitted to continue unabated. Rupture may be experienced as a sudden painful traumatic event associated with immediate functional impairment and an inability to extend the knee. Stage IV represents the catastrophic end stage of jumper's knee. This will be radiographically demonstrable with traumatic patella alta visible upon a lateral radiograph (Fig. 38-7).

13. What is the clinical presentation?

A diagnosis of patellar tendinitis is established after acquiring a detailed history that closely correlates with the findings of a careful physical examination. The most likely site of symptomatic development of jumper's knee is the inferior patellar pole, superior patellar pole, and the insertion of the patellar ligament at the tibial tubercle, in that order. The patient may complain of pain or dull ache in the infrapatellar region at the beginning of athletic practice or a competitive event such as jumping, running, climbing, kicking, deceleration cutting maneuvers, or kneeling activities that abate after warming up. Pain may then reappear after activity or

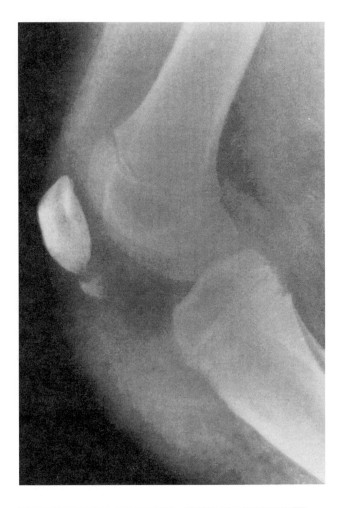

FIG. 38-7 Traumatic patella alta in patient with patellar tendon rupture. (From Scott WN: *The Knee,* St Louis, 1994, Mosby.)

competition. The onset may be insidious (that is, in a gradual and subtle manner), and the patient may have no recollection of a specific traumatic event. Patients may also complain of weakness or giving way, although true locking, clicking, or knee effusion are rarely seen.

Elicitation of tenderness to palpation localized to the patellar tendon insertion at the inferior patellar pole (Fig. 38-8) (or superior patellar pole in the case of quadriceps tendinitis), along the course of the patellar tendon, or to the tibial tubercle is the hallmark of patellar tendinitis. Palpatory examination should be performed with the knee in full extension; if the knee is flexed, tenderness will be difficult to elicit. The double hump characteristic of a camel sign is due to high-riding

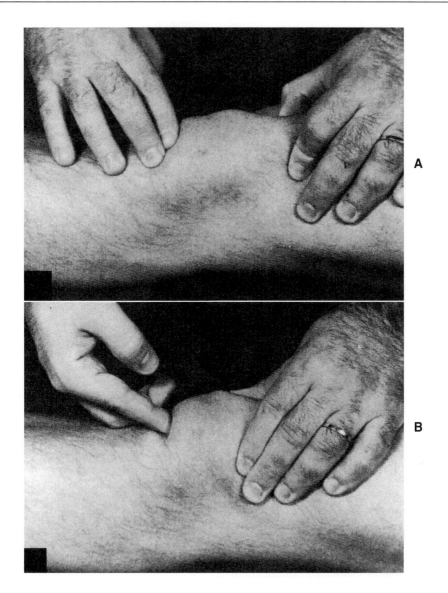

FIG. 38-8 The most typical form of jumper's knee involves the inferior pole. This sign is the hallmark of patellar tendinitis, and should be assessed with the knee in complete extension. **A,** To examine the patellar tendon for inflammation, the entire tendon must be palpated. Occasionally, there is no tenderness except at the junction of the tendon and inferior patellar pole **(B).** It is best to examine this area by displacing the patella distally and palpating the inferior patellar pole. Tenderness in this area confirms suspected patellar tendinitis. (From Grossman RB, Nicholas JA: *Orthop Clin North Am* 8[3]:619, 1977.)

patella superiorly and an uncovered infrapatellar fat pad inferiorly (see Fig. 41-15). Other associated patellar signs include ligamentous laxity, hypermobile patellae, chondromalacia patellae, quadriceps atrophy, patellar malalignment and tight hamstrings, tight triceps surae, but not meniscal or ligamentous derangement. Genu recurvatum or valgum, as well as retropatellar crepitus may be present; occasionally, swelling may be seen over the patellar tendon insertion. The presence of other intrinsic factors such as an increased Q angle value and excessive subtalar joint pronation represent an increased predisposition toward the development of extensor tendinitis.[4,9,47,54] In addition, diffuse weakness of the entire affected lower limb may set in because of disuse.[41] Roentgenographic findings are typically negative.

A visual assessment of patellar height with the knee flexed to 90° indicates any alteration of patellofemoral contact as a consequence of patella alta or baja. With the former, the patella will be aligned in the shallow portion of the proximal trochlear groove when the tibia is flexed on the femur. Clinical assessment may then be confirmed by a lateral radiograph with the knee at 45° of flexion in which the inferior pole of the patella may seem elongated. Radiographic evaluation may show a radiolucency or elongation of the involved patellar pole.[10] Other appropriate imaging techniques that help determine the area and extent of intratendon involvement include scintigraphy, ultrasonography, computerized tomography, and magnetic resonance imaging. Diagnosis, however, is based on the clinical presentation, whereas further diagnostic studies are only appropriate to those patients.

14. What is patella baja?

Patella baja (patella infera) is an abnormally low patellar posture that may result from one of three different causes: (1) an acquired congenital condition; (2) soft tissue contracture of the ligamentum patellae; or (3) quadriceps hypotonia following surgery or some other form of knee trauma. In the congenital form, this condition is frequently asymptomatic and requires no treatment. When patella alta results from the latter cause, the potentially catastrophic results make prompt recognition of utmost importance because early treatment can reverse muscle hypotonia. With patella baja, the patient exhibits a low patella and narrowing of the distance between the patella and the level of the tibial plateau.[22] Treatment consists of vigorous rehabilitation of the quadriceps muscles and mobilization of the soft tissue structures about the knee if the cause is soft tissue contracture. Failure to implement treatment may lead to significant long-term pain and stiffness around the knee. Jumper's knee involving the quadriceps tendon (suprapatellar tendon) at its junction with the superior patellar pole may also result in patella baja. This is because tendon disease, whether represented by tendon stretching or rupture, results in a loss of continuity of the extensor mechanism. This may result in caudal glide of the patella due to diminishment of, or in the case of full thickness rupture, an absence of cephalic pull upon the tendon. Over time, the distal patellar ligament may undergo retraction secondary to contracture as a direct function of discontinuity of the extensor mechanism.

15. How may inflammation of the infrapatellar fat pad result in patella baja?

Fat pad inflammation or *fibrosis* is a relatively common problem contributing to inferior knee pain in patients who have had previous knee surgery or in those who play sports or engage in vocations that directly traumatize this area. Injury to the fat pad may have caused bleeding (and hence, enlargement) of the fat pad at the time of initial trauma that, over time, has led to fat pad fibrosis and reduction of size. The patella, which is normally propped up into its normal posture in the recession of the intercondylar femoral groove, will migrate caudally. Pain is located immediately adjacent to the patellar ligament and stems from the richly enervated fat pad. If fibrosis is extensive as it may be following several knee surgeries or severe trauma to this site, the retropatellar tendon bursa as well as the infrapatellar tendon will eventually scar down to the proximal tibia. This will significantly alter the extensor mechanism mechanics and produce patella baja. Patients with an irritated infrapatellar fat pad stand with their knees locked back and typically exacerbate pain with knee extension.[44] Radiologically, the patella seems to descend lower and lower until it almost rests on the anterior aspect of the tibial plateau.

16. What is Sinding-Larsen-Johansson disease?

Sinding-Larsen-Johansson disease is an apophysitis of the inferior patellar pole, or less commonly the superior patellar pole, and may be thought of as the counterpart of Osgood-Schlatter's disease at the patellar poles (Fig. 38-9). It is not unusual to see tibia tubercle apophysitis develop synchronously with Sinding-Larsen-Johansson disease, although the latter condition typically occurs one to several years (age 8 to 13) before the former. This condition is most common to normal males at puberty, but may also occurs in spastic children. Quadriceps spasticity with hamstring spasticity associated with hamstring contracture and knee flexion deformity leads to similar anterior knee pain secondary to chronic extensor mechanism overloading.

Although considered an adolescent form of patellar tendinitis, Sinding-Larsen-Johansson disease is more accurately described as an osteochondritis of the inferior patellar pole in the skeletally immature. The etiology of Sinding-Larsen-Johansson syndrome is ascribed to excessive traction on the patellar tendon secondary to chronic extensor mechanism overloading. Apophysitis is exceeded by a history of chronic anterior knee pain that has an initially gradual onset related to activity such as jumping, running, ascending stairs, and pro-

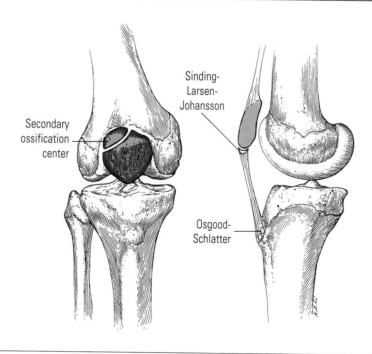

FIG. 38-9 Sites of tendon insertion (apophysis) represent susceptible sites to overuse injury. Distal patellar pole fragmentation is known as Sinding-Larsen-Johansson disease, whereas tibial tubercle fragmentation is known as Osgood-Schlatter disease. (From Tria AJ, Klein KS: *An illustrated guide to the knee,* New York, 1992, Churchill Livingstone.)

longed sitting. Repetitive loaded knee activity leads to a progression of extensor tendinitis, partial ligament avulsion, or stress fracture of the inferior patellar pole. Pain and swelling at either patellar pole as well as a relatively weak quadriceps mechanism are universally present. Tenderness is localized to the inferior patellar pole. Presentation to the primary care provider is often preceded by an acute trauma that amplifies ongoing symptoms to an intolerable level. Occasionally a prominence is present and is best viewed with the patient supine and the knee hyperflexed. Radiographic confirmation presents as inferior pole fragmentation of the patella.[10]

Lateral radiographic evaluation may frequently show irregularity or fragmentation at the distal patellar pole, superior patellar ossification, patellar elongation, or even bony avulsion. Pain and swelling at either the inferior or superior patellar pole in the absence of radiographic findings are suggestive of attritional partial ligament rupture. Full-thickness tendon rupture will be radiographically observed as traumatic patella alta (see Fig. 38-7).

Treatment consists of rest by way of activity restriction, followed by stretching of the hamstring mus-

culature and strengthening, particularly eccentric working, of the quadriceps musculature. When chronic symptoms are exacerbated by chronic symptoms, cylinder casting is used for 4 to 6 weeks before instituting an exercises program. Healing is often rapid, with symptom abatement after 3 to 4 weeks and complete radiologic healing in 6 to 8 weeks following onset of treatment. Typically, no residual disability occurs as the child returns to their pre-injury status. There is no evidence to suggest that children with this problem are more susceptible to the development of jumper's knee in early adulthood.

17. What therapeutic management is appropriate for patellar tendinitis?

Because jumper's knee is a progressive disease, early recognition is of paramount importance in providing an adequate and successful treatment program. It is essential to interrupt and attempt reversal of the pathologic progression of tendon disease before that critical point, beyond which, the likelihood of successful conservative management has diminished. Physical therapy represents the intervention of choice in the early stages of tendon disease. Surgical treatment does offer gratifying long standing results, but should only be considered in the event of failed conservative treatment. Management for stages I, II, and III patellar tendinitis is conservative. Stage I and II disease may generally respond well to therapeutic management, although they may require months to resolve even with the best conservative measures. A reliable indicator of inflammation in the early stage is the presence of inflammation. This sign should be periodically re-evaluated, and if tenderness and swelling persist, further rest and activity reduction are mandatory. Stage III involvement and outcome following physical therapy has an unpredictable course. This potentially irreversible stage is managed in the same way as the more benign forms of tendinitis, with the addition of a prolonged rest period from provocative activities. The patient with persistent symptoms, particularly with tenderness along the inferior patellar pole, should be evaluated with a bone scan to rule out potential stress fracture and thereby avoid potential catastrophic failure of the patella.[17,56] A conservative management program of 4 to 6 months should be undertaken before surgical intervention for stage III involvement

- *Modalities.* Modality application is helpful in the management of acute symptoms. The judicious use of modalities such as moist heat by way of hydrocollator packs, ice massage, ultrasound, and phonophoresis with a 10% hydrocortisone cream are appropriate modalities to effect symptomatic relief. Phonophoresis introduces hydrocortisone into tissue, thereby decreasing inflammation, providing pain alleviation, and increasing range of motion.[19,30] A 10% solution has be reported as more effective than a 1% solution.[30] Steroid injection of the patellar tendon is discouraged as it may result in tendon failure due to the degenerative intratendinous process as well as the adverse effect of corticosteroid on soft-tissue healing. Although the short-term benefits of steroid injection may bring deceptive relief, its use allows the athlete to continue to overload an already weakened tendon, leading to long-term loss and eventual rupture as the tendon is further damaged.[2,13,38]

- *Rest.* Rest is an essential element of the rehabilitative process. Prolonged immobilization, however, in a cast or a splint may prove deleterious. As with many other overuse syndromes, avoidance of the inciting activity with rest of the affected extremity almost universally yields complete symptom resolution. This may not be practical with the highly competitive athletes who attend college on athletic scholarships or

play professional sport. With this population, judicious selective rest is balanced with other treatment modalities.

Muscle rehabilitation is imperative to the treatment of patellar tendinitis and includes stretching of tightened musculature, particularly the hamstring muscles. Stretching exercises are performed slowly with sustained pull and rapid or ballistic motions are avoided because of the potential for microtear in the healing tissue and interruption of the repair process. The ratio of forces transmitted to the patellar tendon from the quadriceps muscles varies with flexion angle at the knee; thus, a tightened hamstring acts to multiply the amount of stress delivered to the patellar tendon during running, walking, and fully extending the knee joint. Stretching of the gastrocnemius and soleus muscle groups and their common distal tendon is important, as tightness of these structures may be associated with the development of extensor tendon disease. Increased extensibility of these structures results in increased dorsiflexion range of motion at the ankle joint, thereby reducing the need for compensatory subtalar joint pronation.[24] A reduction in subtalar joint pronation has the effect of minimizing the magnitude of stress to the extensor tendon-ligament complex.

- *Strengthening.* Strengthening of the quadriceps muscle group begins with quad sets and straight leg raising in the early phases of rehabilitation, and later progressing to isotonic and eccentric quadriceps strengthening. The range of knee motion exercises performed must initially be limited to knee flexion greater than 45°, as working the knee closer to the fully extended posture may excessively tense the patellar tendon. Initial strength training emphasizes high repetition with low weights. Strengthening exercises are initiated with pain-free isometrics and only progressed to isotonic forms of activity if the initial strength program does not cause recurrence of symptoms. Isotonic exercises may begin with terminal knee extension and straight leg raising activities, and may progress to one-quarter squats and leg extensions as symptoms decrease. Exercises may be initiated with 3 sets of 10 repetitions performed slowly, with rest periods of at least 1 minute in between each cycle. The speed by which the exercise is performed is increased as the patient progresses, but is slowed down as resistance is increased. Eccentric quadriceps strengthening, although emphasized at the end of the strengthening program is imperative to injury recurrence.[15,25,51] This is because the initial mechanism implicated in the onset of patellar tendinitis, according to some authorities, was an insufficient ability to muster adequate quadriceps eccentric contraction so as to minimize the excessive forces delivered to the patellar tendon during the jumping descent. Eccentric muscle contractions allow higher musculotendinous tension levels than concentric contractions, and unlike concentric contractions, the tension level rises with increases in angular joint velocity.[1] Eccentric ankle dorsiflexion exercises haven also been reported to reduced the symptoms associated with patellar tendonitis.[49] Isokinetic training are considered by some authorities to be safe only for end stage training because they may potentially cause high tissue stress and exacerbate tendinitis symptoms in the early stages.

- *Bracing.* Bracing by way of a simple elastic sleeve that circles the entire patella or provides a lateral buttress may prove an effective treatment adjunct in minimizing excursion of the quadriceps tendon and patellar ligament. A neoprene sleeve with a horseshoe or an infrapatellar strap may be used to relieve stress and reduce unwanted excursion of the patellar tendon, and provide compression to control edema. The Levine or infrapatellar strap[33] is applied over the patellar ligament midway between the patella and tibial tubercle. Its function may be analogous to that of the lateral counterforce brace used with tennis elbow, in that it attempts to change the direction of pull of the patellar ligament. A simple brace, such as an elastic sleeve with a patellar cutout and lateral buttress to prevent lateral patellar tracking, controls patellar excursion and reduces the incidence of repeated injury. The Palumbo uses straps to develop a dynamic medial force that better controls patellar alignment throughout the range of knee motion. It is designed with two "live" rubber straps and a pad that provides dynamic tension to the lateral patella. This brace may be particularly useful for patients with patellar tendinitis as it attempts to diminish traumatic tensile stresses at the bone-tendon junctions by absorbing and dissipating the forces generated during jumping and running.[43]

- *Orthoses.* Functional foot control is addressed by using an appropriate arch support to prevent abnormal pronation. Abnormal subtalar joint pronation increases tibial internal rotation, resulting in increased transverse plane forces at the knee joint.[8,23,24,34,35,36,46,55,58] Orthoses with varus posting have been found to decrease subtalar joint pronation in the frontal plane,[3,42,50,53] and thereby diminish injurious transverse plane forces transmitted up to the knee joint. The orthosis alters local biomechanics by imparting a supinatory bias to an over-pronated foot. This has far reaching implications upon the function of the entire lower limb. For every degree that the foot is supinated, the Q angle decreases 0.44°. Thus a prescribed foot orthosis may favorably and significantly alter lower limb kinesiology as proximally as the thigh and hip. Leg length discrepancies of approximately 4 cm or greater that are associated with microtrauma injuries may benefit from a heel lift.[52] The initial lift should attempt to correct no more than one half of the measured discrepancy.[5]

- *Patient education.* Activity modification is an essential component to management to preclude pathologic relapse. It is essential to educate the patient about the importance of adequate pre-athletic warm ups and postathletic cool downs. Warm-ups have the effect of increasing circulation in the muscle and tendon, thereby increasing cellular metabolism, and are believe to decrease the incidence of any associate muscle soreness.[16,32] Patients should be instructed in warming up before athletic participation by light jogging to the point of light perspiration, as well as application of ice to the knee following practice. Practice session should eliminate or attempt to reduce jumping and sudden deceleration, whereas the overall duration of the workout should be diminished. It is essential that patient activity be reduced to a level at which improvement continues to be clinically demonstrable.

Stages I and II disease may generally respond well to therapeutic management. Stage III involvement and outcome following physical therapy has an unpredictable course. This potentially irreversible stage is managed similarly to the more benign forms of tendinitis plus a prolonged rest period from provocative activities. A conservative management program of 4 to 6 months should be undertaken before surgical intervention for stage III involvement. In the event of surgery, it is important to slowly advance into the rehabilitation process because the area of involvement is located a point of relatively poor blood supply. Immobilization is typically 6 months and is followed by some 4 to 6 months before allowing the patient to proceed into more vigorous athletic activity.[6] In the event of patellar ligament rupture, excellent function may be obtained provided repair is performed early and normal tendon length is restored. Quadriceps tendon ruptures have a less favorable prognosis.[28]

REFERENCES

1. Albert M: Physiologic and clinical principles of eccentrics. In Albert M, editor: *Eccentric muscle training in sports and orthopedics,* New York, 1991, Churchill Livingstone.
2. Bassett FH, Soucacos P, Carr W: AAOS Instructional Course Lectures, 25:96-106, 1976.
3. Bates BT, Osternig LR, Mason B et al: Foot orthotic devices to modify selected aspects of lower extremity mechanics, *Am J Sports Med* 7:338, 1979.
4. Blazina ME, Kerlan RK, Jobe FW et al: Jumper's knee, *Orthop Clin North Am* 4:665, 1973.
5. Blustein SM, D'Amico JC: Leg length discrepancy, *J Am Podiatr Med Assoc* 75:200, 1985.
6. Boland AL, Hulstyn MJ: Soft-tissue injuries of the knee. In Nicholas JA, Hershman EB, editors: *The lower extremity and spine,* ed 2, vol 1, St Louis, 1995, Mosby.
7. Bradley EL: The anterior tibial compartment syndrome, *Surg Gynecol Obstet* 136:298, 1973.
8. Buchbinder MR, Napora NJ, Biggs EW: The relationship of abnormal pronation to chondromalacia of the patella in long distance runners, *J Am Podiatr Med Assoc* 69:159, 1979.
9. Clancey WG: Runner's injuries, *Am J Sports Med* 8:137, 1980.
10. Colosimo AJ, Bassett III FH: Jumper's knee-diagnosis and treatment, *Orthop Rev* 19(2), 1990.
11. Colson JH, Armour WJ: *Sports injuries and their treatment,* Philadelphia, 1975, JB Lippincott.
12. D'Ambrosia R, Drez D: *Prevention and treatment of running injuries,* Thorofare, NJ, 1982, Charles B Slack.
13. Ferretti A, Puddu G, Mariani PP et al: The natural history of jumper's knee. Patellar or quadriceps tendonitis, *Int Orthop (SICOT),* 8(4):239-242, 1985.
14. Fritschy D, de Gautard R: Jumper's knee and ultrasonography, *Am J Sports Med* 16:637, 1988.
15. Fyfe I, Stanish WD: The use of eccentric training and stretching in the treatment and prevention of tendon injuries, *Clin Sports Med* 11:601, 1992.
16. Gieck JH, Saliba EN: Application of modalities in overuse syndromes, *Clin Sports Med* 6:427, 1987.
17. Goodrich A, DeFiore RJ, Tippens JK: Bilateral simultaneous ruptures of the infrapatellar tendon, *Orthopedics* 6:1472, 1983.
18. Greenfield BH: *Rehabilitation of the knee: a problem-solving approach,* Philadelphia, 1993, FA Davis Company.
19. Griffin JE, Echternach JL, Price RE et al: Patients treated with ultrasonic driven cortisone and with ultrasound alone, *Phys Ther* 47(7):594-601, 1967.
20. Helfet AJ: *Disorders of the knee,* ed 2, Philadelphia, 1982, JB Lippincott.
21. Hendryson IE: *Injuries to the knee joint,* ed 5, Edinburgh, 1978, Churchill Livingstone.
22. Jacobson KE, Flandry FC: Diagnosis of anterior knee pain, *Clin Sports Med* 8(2):179-92, 1989.
23. James SL, Bates BT, Ostering LR: Injuries to runners, *Am J Sports Med* 6:40, 1978.
24. James SL: Chondromalacia of the patella in the adolescent, In Kennedy JC et al editors: *The injured adolescent knee,* Baltimore, 1979, Williams & Wilkins.
25. Jensen K, DiFabio RP: Evaluation of eccentric exercise in treatment of patellar tendinitis, *Phys Ther* 69:211, 1989.
26. Kalebo P, Sward L, Karlsson J et al: Ultrasonography in the detection of partial patellar ligament ruptures (jumper's knee), *Skeletal Radiol* 20:285-289, 1991.
27. Karllson J, Lundin O, Lossing IW et al: Partial rupture of the patellar ligament. Results after operative treatment, *Am J Sports Med* 19:403-408, 1991.
28. Kelly DW, Carter VS, Jobe FW et al: Patellar and quadriceps tendon ruptures—jumper's knee, *Am J Sports Med* 12:375-380, 1984.
29. King JB, Perry DJ, Mourad K et al: Lesions of the patellar ligament, *J Bone Joint Surg* 72B:46-48, 1990.
30. Kleinkort JA, Wood F: Phonophoresis with 1 percent versus 10 percent hydrocortisone, *Phys Ther* 55:1320, 1975.
31. Kujala UM, Aalto T, Osterman K et al: The effect of volleyball playing on the knee extensor mechanism, *Am J Sports Med* 17:766-769, 1989.
32. Kulund DW: *The injured athlete,* ed 2, Philadelphia, 1988, JB Lippincott.
33. Levine J: A new brace for chondromalacia patellae and kindred conditions, *Am J Sports Med* 6:137, 1978.
34. Lutter LD: Foot-related knee problems in the long distance runner, *Foot Ankle* 1:112, 1980.
35. Lutter LL: Injuries in the runner and jogger, *Minn Med* 63:45, 1980.
36. Mann RA: Biomechanics of running, In Mack R editor: *Symposium the foot and leg in running sports,* St. Louis, 1982, CV Mosby.
37. Martens M, Wouters P, Burssens A et al: Patellar tendinitis: pathology and results of treatment, *Acta Orthop Scand* 53:445-450, 1982.
38. Martens M, Wouters P, Burssens A et al: Patellar tendinitis: Pathology and results of treatment, *Acta Orthop Scand* 53:445-450, 1980.
39. Medlar RC, Lyne ED: Sinding-Larsen-Johansson disease, *J Bone Joint Surg* 60A:1113-1116, 1978.
40. Milan KR: Injury in ballet: a review of relevant topics for the physical therapist, *J Orthop Sports Phys Ther* 19(2):123, 1994.
41. Nicholas JA, Strizak AM, Veras GJ: A study of thigh muscle weakness in different pathological states of the lower extremity, *Am J Sports Med* 4:241, 1976.
42. Novick A, Kelley DL: Position and movement changes of the foot with orthotic intervention during the loading response of gait, *J Orthop Sports Phy Ther* 11:301, 1990.
43. Palumbo PM: Dynamic patellar brace: A new orthosis in the management of patellofemoral disorders—preliminary report, *Am J Sports Med* 9:45-49, 1981.
44. Pronsati MP: Australian PT introduces new treatment for patellofemoral pain. *Advance Phy Ther* Dec. 1991.
45. Puddu G, Ippolito E, Postacchini F: A classification of Achilles tendon disease, *Am J Sports Med* 4:145, 1976.
46. Ramig D et al: The foot and sports medicine: biomechanical foot faults as related to chondromalacia patellae, *J Orthop Sports Phys Ther* 9:160, 1987.

47. Roels J, Martens M, Mulier JC et al: Patellar tendinitis (jumper's knee), *Am J Sports Med* 6:362-368, 1978.

48. Scranton PE Jr., Farrar EL: Mucoid degeneration of the patellar ligament in athletes, *J Bone Joint Surg* 74A:435, 1992.

49. Shelton GL, Thigpen LK: Rehabilitation of patellofemoral dysfunction: a review of literature, *J Orthop Sports Phys Ther* 14(6): 243, 1991.

50. Smith LS, Clarke TE, Hamill CL et al: The effects of soft and semi-rigid orthosis upon rearfoot movement in running, *J Am Podiatr Med Assoc* 76:227, 1986.

51. Stanish WD, Rubinovich RM, Curwin S: Eccentric exercise in chronic tendinitis, *Clin Orthop* 208:65, 1986.

52. Subotnick SI: Limb length discrepancies of the lower extremity (the short leg syndrome), *J Orthop Sports Phys Ther* 3:11, 1981.

53. Taunton JE, Clement DB, Smart GW et al: A triplanar electrogoniometer investigation of running mechanics in runners with compensatory overpronation, *Can J Appl Sports Sci* 10:104, 1985.

54. Taunton JE, Clement DB, Smart GW et al: Non-surgical management of overuse knee injuries in runners, *Can J Appl Sports Sci* 12:11, 1987.

55. Tiberio D: The effect of excessive subtalar joint pronation on patellofemoral mechanics: A theoretical model, *J Orthop Sports Phys Ther* 9:160, 1987.

56. Tibone JE, Lombardo SJ: Bilateral fracture of the inferior poles of the patellae in the basketball player, *Am J Sports Med* 9:215, 1981.

57. Tria AJ, Klein KS: *An illustrated guide to the knee,* New York, 1992, Churchill Livingstone.

58. Weiss BD: Nontraumatic injuries in amateur long distance bicyclists, *Am J Sports Med* 13:187, 1985.

RECOMMENDED READING

Colosimo AJ, Bassett FH: Jumper's knee-diagnosis and treatment, *Orthop Rev* 19(2), 1990.

Ferretti A, Ippolito E, Mariani P et al: Jumper's knee, *Am J Sports Med* 11:58, 1983.

39

Painful, Red, Warm, Gross Prepatellar Swelling in the Absence of Direct Trauma with Pain at Either Extreme of Terminal Knee Motion

CASE 1: A 29-year-old carpet layer complains of insidious left knee pain of 4 weeks duration that was relieved by taking aspirin and occasional use of a kneepad. He reports no recollection of any trauma to the knee and screens negative for any family history. Pain was especially exacerbated when working in the quadruped position and was often severe unless the kneepad was used while working. The patient is also a varsity coach for a college football team, and yesterday sustained a direct fall onto his left knee. Today he presents with acute swelling and moderate pain of the left knee.

OBSERVATION   Grossly prominent swelling over left knee that does not proximally extend beyond the lower portion of the left vastus medialis muscle. The left knee joint appears to be postured in approximately 20° of flexion.

PALPATION   Yields tenderness over the entire swollen area of the left knee.

RANGE OF MOTION   Full range of motion is present in the left knee although uncomfortable at either extreme of terminal range. Terminal knee flexion is achievable, although painful.

STRENGTH   Untested secondary to pain.

SELECTIVE TENSION   Untested secondary to pain and tenderness.

SENSATION   Normal to light touch and pinprick on entire left lower extremity.

VASCULAR STATUS   Intact left pedal pulses.

SPECIAL TESTS   Negative patellar apprehension sign, and negative anterior/posterior draw signs.

RADIOGRAPHS   Anteroposterior, lateral, and tangential radiographs demonstrate an intact patella.

CLUE:

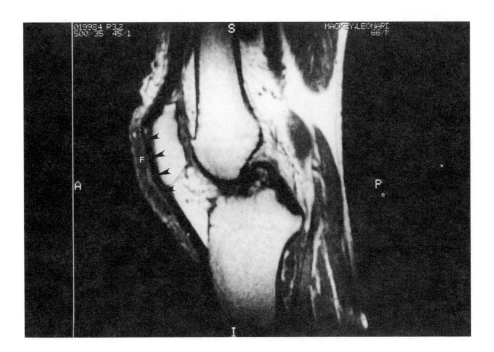

(From Scott WN: *The knee*, St Louis, 1994, Mosby.)

CASE 2: A 46-year-old nun spent the past 2 years working in a small rural community. She would spend at least 2 hours a day praying in the kneeling posture. On the previous evening, vandals had desecrated the house of worship by breaking many of the stained glass windows. She spent many hours the next day clearing the tiny shards of glass off the sanctuary floor. She now presents with a painful and swollen left knee, and nearly an identical presentation to the previous case with several notable exceptions. Swelling is somewhat inferiorly located than the latter case. In addition, skin dimples that are normally present on either side of the patellar ligament and typically most prominent upon full knee extension have been obliterated secondary to swelling. Moreover, terminal knee extension is more painful than terminal knee flexion. Finally, radiographs show a calcified avulsion fragment over the bilateral proximal tibial apohyses.

CLUE:

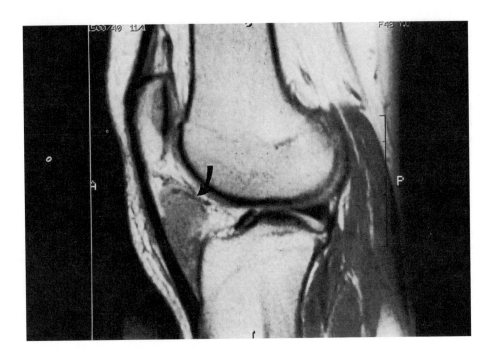

(From Scott WN: *The knee,* St Louis, 1994, Mosby.)

CASE 3: An obese 65-year-old male complains of right knee pain upon standing or walking during the past several weeks. He occasionally is awakened by nocturnal pain. Relief is found by sleeping on his left side with a pillow between his 2 knees. When asked, he reports no history of any trauma to either knee, or any recent fever. His significant medical history includes moderate osteoarthritis to the knees bilaterally. There are no complaints of giving way or locking.

OBSERVATION   The patient is observed to stand with bilateral flat feet and marked bilateral tibia vara that is more prominent in the right lower extremity.

PALPATION   Point tenderness is elicited in the area of the medial tibial collateral ligament, both anteromedially and posteromedially, and is excessive just 2 to 4 cm below the tibiofemoral joint line. There is no crepitus felt along the semimembranosus tendon during knee flexion or extension.

RANGE OF MOTION   Is grossly limited to three-quarter range in the knees, bilaterally.

STRENGTH   Left knee demonstrates good strength, whereas the right knee is graded G− for both flexion and extension.

FLEXIBILITY   Passive stretching of the semimembranosus muscle is tight, although painless.

SELECTIVE TENSION   Selective tension of the semimembranosus muscle is painless.

SENSATION   Normal.

SPECIAL TESTS   Negative McMurray and Apley tests. Valgus stress to the knee joint is painless. A positive leg length discrepancy finds the left lower extremity 2-cm longer.

RADIOGRAPHS   Show erosion of medial tibiofemoral joint of the right knee with erosion, cartilage erosion, and hypertrophic bone changes at the joint margins.

? Questions

1. **What is afflicting these patients?**
2. **What are bursae?**
3. **Between what types of tissue are bursae found at the knee joint?**
4. **What are adventitious bursae?**
5. **Where are the various bursae adjacent to the knee joint located?**
6. **What is the pathophysiologic response during the evolution of bursitis?**
7. **How does inflammatory prepatellar bursitis become septic arthritis?**
8. **What is the origin and presentation of prepatellar bursitis?**
9. **What is the origin and presentation of infrapatellar bursitis?**
10. **What is the relationship between the infrapatellar bursa and fat pad syndrome?**
11. **What is the functionally significant role of the medial insertion of the pes anserinus?**
12. **What is the etiology of pes anserinus bursitis?**
13. **What kind of distal and proximal articular functional deviations diminish the optimum macrophysiologic state of the pes anserine?**
14. **How may osteoarthritis of the knee joint predispose toward the development of pes anserine bursitis?**
15. **Are females more prone to the development of pes anserine bursitis and tendinitis?**
16. **What is the presentation of pes anserine bursitis?**
17. **What is the differential diagnosis of pes anserine bursitis?**
18. **What is Baker's cyst?**
19. **What is the natural history of this cyst?**
20. **How do popliteal cysts in children differ from those occurring in adults?**
21. **What therapeutic intervention best manages bursitis at the knee?**

1. What is afflicting these patients?

Prepatellar bursitis (housemaid's knee) in Case 1, *infrapatellar bursitis* (clergyman's knee) in Case 2, and *pes anserine bursitis* in Case 3.

2. What are bursae?

The human body contains an excess of 150 bursae,[29] with approximately 2 dozen located in the areas of the knee joint.[13] (Fig. 39-1) A *bursa* is a round, flattened sac occupying a potential space, that is loosely tethered to joint capsules, tendons, ligaments, or beneath overlying skin,[31] and therefore capable of a limited yet significant range of motion along these structures. Composed of synovial membrane, the two inner walls of the bursa are separated by a thin layer of synovial fluid acting as a lubricant allowing bone, tendon, or skin to which the bursa is tethered, to move on adjacent structures and thereby reduce friction. Thus bursae represent a friction reducing strategy in much the same fashion that a water balloon compressed by two moving structures prevents contact or excessive rubbing between those two structures. As such, the location of bursae at

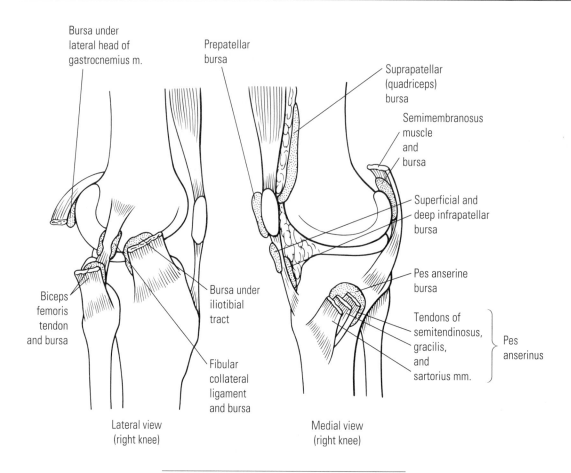

FIG. 39-1 Location of common bursae at the knee joint.

potentially high friction areas permit virtually friction-free movement between adjacent moving body tissue and thereby minimize irritation.

3. Between what types of tissue are bursae found at the knee joint?

Bursae are situated throughout the musculoskeletal system at potential sites of high friction between soft and osseous tissue or between differing types of soft tissue. The *prepatellar bursa* lies between skin and the kneecap, the *deep infrapatellar* and *pes anserine bursae* lies between bone and tendon, the *semitendinosus bursa* lies between tendon and tendon, the *popliteus bursa* lies between ligament and tendon, whereas the *semimembranosus bursa* lies between tendon and joint capsule.

4. What are adventitious bursae?

Bursae are synovial lined sacs that normally occur at genetically predetermined areas throughout the body.

Adventitious bursae, however, may evolve when excessive forces accumulate along an interface within the musculoskeletal system due to excessive, repetitive, or unusual activity. These bursae arise from connective tissue cells secondary to bony protuberances such as hallux valgus, or from protruding parts of metallic inserts.[33] Adventitious bursae may also occur as a complication of chronic bursitis of a normally present bursa. Here, the collagen fibers and ground substance adjacent to the chronically inflamed bursa become a fibrous, culminating in a cystic structure filled with cellular debris, extracellular fluid, and inflammatory exudate.[4]

5. Where are the various bursae adjacent to the knee joint located?

Anterior to the knee joint, there are 4 major bursae, which serve to reduce friction throughout the quadriceps extensor mechanism. Most superficial are the subcutaneous *prepatellar bursa,* which lies between the skin and the patella, as well as the *superficial infrapatellar bursa* located between the skin and the patellar tendon as its insertion on the tibial tubercle. The *deep infrapatellar bursa* also known as the *retropatellar tendon bursa* resides between the posterior aspect of the distal portion of the patellar tendon and proximal tibia. During knee extension, the two infrapatellar bursae facilitate gliding between the tibia and infrapatellar tendon, respectively. The *suprapatellar bursa* is a large pouchlike extension of the knee joint cavity that lies between the quadriceps femoris muscle tendon and the distal femur.[19]

Laterally, there are 4 significant bursae. One lies between the lateral head of the gastrocnemius and the knee joint capsule. Two bursae are associated with the fibular collateral ligament. The first resides between the ligament and the biceps femoris tendon, while the second lies between the ligament and the popliteus tendon.[31] The latter may either be separate from, or communicate with a fourth bursa located between the popliteus tendon and the lateral femoral condyle. The latter bursa is often an extension of the synovial membrane at the knee joint.[4] Although several other bursae may be found laterally, they are not commonly associated with microtrauma type injuries.

Several bursae may be found along the medial aspect of the knee joint. The *pes anserinus bursa* may be found between the tibial collateral ligament and the pes anserinus. A bursa is present deep to the medial collateral ligament between the joint capsule, the tibia, the medial meniscus, and the anterior extension of the semimembranosus tendon. A bursa exists within the medial head of the gastrocnemius muscle belly that communicates with the knee joint.[30] This is not to be confused with the adjacent bursa located between the medial head of the gastrocnemius muscle belly and the semimembranosus tendon. Some individuals may have a bursa located between the semimembranosus tendon and the medial femoral condyle and joint capsule.[4]

6. What is the pathophysiologic response during the evolution of bursitis?

Repetitive or excessive microtrauma to a bursa causes bursal irritation, to which the bursa responds by producing more fluid to lubricate adjacent tissues as a friction-reducing strategy. If microtrauma continues, however, a point is reached when the now larger bursa protects adjacent tissue from injury and inflammation at the expense of absorbing friction. Eventually, the price

of unrelenting friction results in inflammation of the bursa. Whether the mechanism of injury was *macrotraumatic* (direct blow) as may occur to the anteriorly located bursae, or *microtraumatic* due to biomechanical malalignment in the more deeply located bursae, the common pathophysiologic response is an inflammatory response.[1,11,21,32] The initial (acute) reaction to gross trauma is a vascular one, in which there is emigration (diapedesis) of red blood cells from ruptured vessels during which the local vessels vasoconstrict briefly. This is followed by vasodilation that ushers serous exudate into the area, resulting in a bursa that is distended with a watery mucoidlike fluid. As the condition progresses to become chronic, the bursal walls become thickened and distended with excessive exudate. Eventually, the inner wall lining become filled with gritty calcific precipitates.[4]

7. How does inflammatory prepatellar bursitis become septic arthritis?

Individuals who return to the activity that provoked bursitis prematurely or without adequate prophylaxis frequently develop recurrent bursitis. With the advent of a second episode the likelihood of both multiple recurrences and prolonged disability increase significantly. Of even greater concern is the increased likelihood for the progression of inflammatory bursitis into the less benign complication known as septic bursitis.

The vector whereby bacterial organisms, most commonly staphylococcus,[6,7,16,26] are introduced into the prepatellar bursa is via repeated trauma to the anterior knee. As staphylococcus is indigenous to the surface of skin, abrasions to the knee allow bacteria to penetrate the skin and seed the underlying bursa (Fig. 39-2). Because the fluid in the swollen bursa is an excellent medium for bacterial growth, it may lead to a condition known as *septic bursitis* in which an infective state is superimposed upon an inflammatory bursitis. Infection may lead to extensive cellulitis characterized by heat, swelling, marked local tenderness, and loss of range of motion of the adjacent joints.[29] At the knee, however, clinical signs of infection may be very misleading and easily overlooked for a variety of reasons. Because the bursal walls are thickened in chronic bursitis, the usual rubor associated with infection is rarely seen in septic bursitis at the knee. Moreover, septicemia with chills, fever, and positive blood cultures are uncommon because the infection is usually contained by the thick bursal walls. To confuse matters even more, local warmth and swelling are typically signs of inflam-

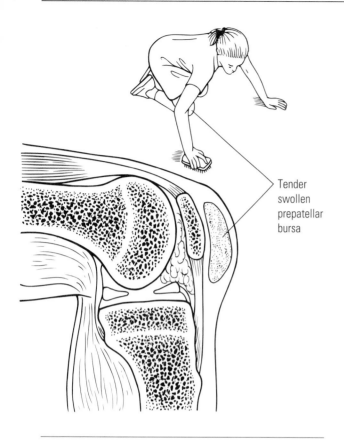

FIG. 39-2 Mechanism for the development of *septic arthritis* at the knee joint. Repetitive trauma to the anterior knee, as may occur from constant kneeling of bare skin against the floor, may cause small punctures in the prepatellar bursa. Bacterial contamination in the form of staphylococcus, which is indigenous to the outer surface of human skin, may be introduced beyond the protective layers of skin and result in septic arthritis, which must be differentiated from arthritis of the knee joint.

matory bursitis as well as septic bursitis.[4] Because of this, diagnosis of persistent bursitis is accurately made by needle aspiration and culture of bursal fluid, administration of antibiotics, and continuous application of warm, moist compresses, rest, and immobilization. Treatment may be prolonged as the thickened bursal walls may impede transport of antibiotics into the bursa, and may require the physician to incise and drain the bursa.[29]

8. What is the origin and presentation of prepatellar bursitis?

Prepatellar bursitis is the most common type of sports related bursitis[31] at the knee as it is most likely injured secondary to acute trauma owing to its subcutaneous

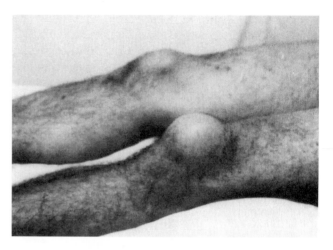

FIG. 39-3 Prepatellar bursitis. (From Magee DJ: *Orthopedic physical assessment*, Philadelphia, 1997, WB Saunders.)

location. Also known as *housemaid's knee*, it is an occupational hazard of domestic cleaning services or any type of manual labor that requires spending excessive time in the quadruped posture. Thus this type of bursitis commonly occurs in plumbers, carpet layers, as well as surfers who kneel on surfboards and wrestlers, who must also spend considerable time kneeling on all fours. Football players may incur prepatellar bursitis secondary to repetitive falling on their knees on artificial turf.[22,26,38] Because of its superficial location, prepatellar bursitis should be treated with utmost care so as to prevent the possibility of multiple recurrence or septic bursitis.

Clinical presentation of prepatellar bursitis (Fig. 39-3) usually includes anterior knee pain of insidious onset, although acute or posttraumatic inflammation is not uncommon. In the latter two scenarios, sudden onset of severe pain occurs owing to bleeding secondary to trauma within the prepatellar bursa. Over time, blood formation within the bursa will clot and form loose bodies, which may be a source of inflammation, effusion, and severe pain.[9] The clinician should note whether or not swelling is localized to the bursa or, in more severe cases, extend proximally over the lower portion of the vastus medialis. If swelling extends beyond the confines of the bursa, the examiner should be alert to the possibility of an *intraarticular joint injury* with associated joint effusion. Prepatellar bursitis is characterized by *extraarticular swelling* that is very prominent. *Intracapsular swelling* occurs within the knee joint capsule and is referred to as a *primary joint effusion*[37] and may occur secondary to rupture of an anterior cruciate ligament or patellar dislocation.* This effusion causes the knee joint to assume a posture of 15° to 25° of flexion known as the *resting* (or, *loose packed*) *position of the knee* as this posture permits the synovial cavity to contain a maximal volume of fluid. Moreover, a true hemarthrosis or synovitis of the knee joint typically shows a significant limitation of terminal flexion *and* extension of the knee joint. In contradistinction, acute or even severe prepatellar bursitis presents a knee range of nearly full flexion. The last several degrees, however, are often painful as this endrange elicits pressure, hence pain, to an already sensitive prepatellar bursa.[4]

An astute clinician must also be alert to the possibility of other knee injuries accrued by a fall in the kneeling posture, namely ligamentous strain or transverse patellar fracture. The latter may occur from a direct blow to the patella with the knee joint in flexion, or as a secondary result of violent contraction of the quadriceps mechanism. Because of this, radiographs taken in the anteroposterior, lateral, and tangential planes are appropriate following a violent fall onto the knee(s).

9. What is the origin and presentation of infrapatellar bursitis?

Both the suprapatellar and infrapatellar bursae relate to friction reduction of the quadriceps extensor mechanism. Whereas the former permits friction-free gliding of the quadriceps tendon over the proximal tibia, unhindered by overlying skin, the latter allows the same in relation to the quadriceps (i.e., patellar) ligament. Like prepatellar bursitis, subcutaneous *infrapatellar bursitis* is a trauma-related bursitis following direct injury due to kneeling along the skin surface overlying the tibial tuberosity. Also known as *clergyman's bursitis,* this condition differs from prepatellar bursitis in having a slightly different mechanism as a result of biped kneeling (Fig. 39-4). Infrapatellar bursitis typically occurs in carpet layers, roofers, floor tilers, miners, plumbers, and carpenters. Clinical presentation is very similar to superficial prepatellar bursitis with the exception that the reactive enlargement is more inferiorly located, and often obliterates those normally present dimples located

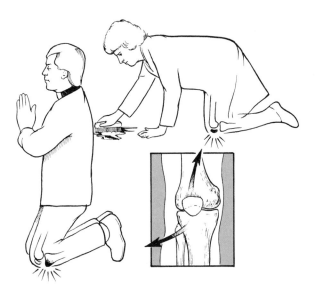

FIG. 39-4 *Housemaid's knee* affects the prepatellar bursa and is associated with excessive time spent in the quadruped posture. *Clergyman's knee* affects the infrapatellar bursa and occurs from excessive kneeling. (From Dandy DJ: *Essential orthopaedics and trauma,* ed 2, Edinburgh, 1993, Churchill Livingstone.)

on each side of the patellar ligament that are most pronounced during leg extension.[25] Bursitis of the deep infrapatellar bursa is characterized by pain upon terminal knee extension which compresses the bursa. Both forms of anterior bursitis are common to football, soccer, baseball, and wrestling.[37] Occasionally, patient may exhibit clinical signs of chronic Osgood-Schlatter disease and demonstrate radiographic signs of calcified avulsion fragment in the area of the proximal tibial apophysis.[4]

10. What is the relationship between the infrapatellar bursa and fat pad syndrome?

In the same way that the fat pad beneath the heel bone acts as a cushion to dampen the concussive force of heel strike, the fat pad at the knee serves to dampen the impact of the inferior aspect of the patella from concussive collision with the tibiofemoral joint during knee extension. Moreover, the fat pad also functions to maintain patellar posture. The *infrapatellar fat pad* is located between the patellar tendon and the underlying synovial tissue and bone.[14] The kinesiologic function of the patella is to increase the leverage of the quadriceps muscle by increasing the lever arm of the patella ten-

*The patellar-femoral articulation shares the same joint capsule as the tibio-femoral joint.

don. This ability is compromised in the event of fat pad atrophy due to loss of normal patellar posture, resulting in an alternation in the angle of insertion of the patellar tendon and subsequently, an alteration in patellofemoral biomechanics. Fat pad inflammation, bleeding, and eventual fibrosis may occur following multiple blows that traumatize this area. Alternately, the fat pad may undergo inflammation and fibrosis following multiple surgical procedures to the knee. If fibrosis is extensive, the retropatellar bursa and patellar tendon may scar down to the proximal tibia, resulting in a *patella baja.* On lateral radiograph, the patella has the appearance of lying so low as to almost rest upon the anterior aspect of the tibial plateau. The fat pad is richly innervated with contributions from the femoral, tibial, recurrent, common peroneal, and obturator nerves.[15] Also known as *Hoffa's disease, fat pad syndrome* clinically presents as tenderness both medial and lateral to the patellar tendon[10] as well as jabs of pain at the anterolateral joint line[8] especially during terminal knee extension[23] as the fibrotic pad is caught between the patella and femur.[10] It may also be associated with thickening of the peritendinous area.[15] The patient may experience pain during weight bearing as well as sudden knee buckling secondary to an altered quadriceps mechanism. Internal derangement is ruled out as locking does not occur.[10] Conservative management is often successful and involves use of antiinflammatory medication and a patella-restraining device, as well as restricted terminal knee extension for approximately three months.

Infrapatellar contracture syndrome is an exaggerated pathologic fibrous hyperplasia of the fat pad beyond that associated with normal healing. This will occasionally occur in the presence of prolonged knee joint immobilization, which leads to excessive fibrosis of the fat pad that interferes with the normal patellar gliding during knee motion. Pain is elicited during attempted knee extension owing to entrapment of the fibrotic pad between the articulating surfaces of the tibiofemoral joint. Restoration of full knee joint motion may necessitate surgical removal of the fat pad.[4]

11. What is the functionally significant role of the medial insertion of the pes anserinus?

The *pes anserinus* is a triplex of tendons derived from large and powerful muscles on the anterior, medial, and posterior compartments of the thigh. The confluence of these tendons join to course around the side of the tibial metaphysis where they are separated from it and the medial collateral ligament by the pes bursa. The tendons insert upon the medial tibial plateau, which primarily ascribes to them both knee flexion function as well as a rotary capacity with regard to the tibiofemoral joint. Normally, the tibia has a slight valgus angulation in relation to the femur that is commonly more pronounced in females.[17] By virtue of their medially located insertion, the pes anserinus tendons support the medial side of the knee, which is normally under considerable tension owing to the valgus angle inherent to the tibiofemoral joint. Thus in addition to providing a medial restraint to excess knee valgus, the pes anserine tendons (providing an internal rotary knee torque[4]) work together with the lateral hamstrings to cancel the opposite rotatory moment imparted to the knee by the quadriceps muscle group.

12. What is the etiology of pes anserinus bursitis?

The pes anserinus bursa is located between the medial collateral ligament and the tendons of the sartorius, gracilis, and semitendinosus (Fig. 39-5). This form of bursitis often presents either in long distance runners[4,12] or in middle aged, overweight females having a history of osteoarthritis at the knees. In the former, an angular protuberance may occur at the precisely balanced knee joint due to a disturbance of the frontal plane alignment either proximally or distally along the lower extremity linkage. Another mechanism that may contribute toward the development of pes anserine bursitis in runners is tightness of the medial hamstring muscle group, inadequate preactivity stretching of the hamstrings, and excessive mileage.[4] Pes bursitis may also occur in sports that involve pivoting, jumping, and deceleration.

13. What kind of distal and proximal articular functional deviations diminish the optimum macrophysiologic state of the pes anserine?

A distally originating cause of pes anserine bursitis may be attributable to either excessive or diminished *pronation*[37] of the ipsilateral subtalar joint with concomitant excessive tibial torsion that manifests as distraction or approximation of the medial tibiofemoral joint, respectively. The macrophysiological consequences of distraction or approximation of the medial tibiofemoral joint upon length-tension relationships of the tendons comprising the pes anserine are such that their contractile ability may be placed at mechanical disadvantage.

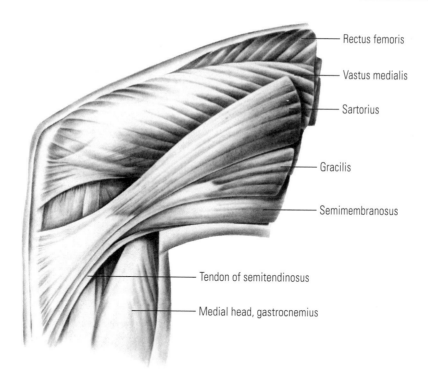

Rectus femoris

Vastus medialis

Sartorius

Gracilis

Semimembranosus

Tendon of semitendinosus

Medial head, gastrocnemius

FIG. 39-5 The muscles of the anterior aspect of the knee. Note the goose's foot confluence of tendons known as the pes anserinus upon the anterior medial tibial plateau. Pes anserine means "three toes," and resembles a goose's foot because of connective tissue webbing between the distal tendon attachments. The pes anserine tendons are a composite structure comprised of muscles from the anterior, medial, and posterior compartments of the thigh. These tendons, by virtue of their wrap-around insertion upon the anterior medial tibial plateau, provide a counter-rotational torque that dynamically dampens excessive engagement of the screw-home mechanism at knee joint extension, thereby preventing abnormal stress to the articular surfaces. (From Houghston JC: *Knee ligaments: injury and repair,* St Louis, 1993, Mosby.)

This macrophysiologic relationship is demonstrated by the Blix curve (Fig. 39-6).

The foot that functions by way of compensatory over-pronation will also demonstrate, by way of the proximal linkage system, excessive internal torsion of the tibial shaft. The proximal consequences of this excessive transverse plane motion of the tibia manifests as a valgus force at the knee and patellofemoral joints. A knee valgus force has the effect of distracting the medial tibiofemoral hemi-joint (while approximating the lateral tibiofemoral joint line). Distraction of the knee joint will mechanically disadvantage the pes anserine tendons by placing them on slight tension, thus subjecting their associated bursa to excessive friction. The relative convexity of the tibiofemoral joint in valgus may also causes excessive friction to the pes anserine tendons owing to their anatomic approximation to the medial tibial plateau and possibly rubbing of those tendons against that ridge of bone. Thus an individual with a *genu valgus* deformity may also sustain a pes anserine bursitis.

Conversely, the individual with the *supinated* or cavus foot posture is characterized by an excessive external tibial torsion[31] during stance phase, which acts to impart a varus force to the medial tibiofemoral joint line. The effect of varus angulation to the knee joint has the effect of approximating the medial tibiofemoral hemi-joint. Both the pronated or supinated subtalar joint (intrinsic) mechanisms may be (extrinsically) mimicked by running along a banked surface. This occurs because a nonlevel surface topography forces excessive medial sole contact of the higher foot, and di-

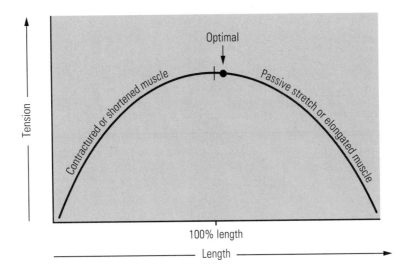

FIG. 39-6 Macrophysiologic function of muscle with regard to length and tension parameters. The Blix curve demonstrates the relationship between length of a muscle and its ability to generate tension. The bell curve demonstrates that when muscle is at rest length it can generate the most amount of tension. Rest length of a muscle represents an ideal microphysiologic milieu of muscular tissue in which there is optimum binding, that is, cross bridging of actin and myosin. Any other length represents a deviation from ideal muscle length and produces diminished tension production. This diminishment of muscular tension is represented by either slope on either side of the apex of the curve.

minishment of medial sole contact of the lower foot. The cavus (or supinated) foot is characterized by decreased weight bearing area, whereas the planus (or pronated) foot is characterized by increased surface contact. The foot along the elevated surface undergoes excessive pronation, while the foot along the lower ground undergoes diminished pronation. Running on a banked surface, like hill running, represents external factors that mechanically force the foot into postures-deviant from subtalar joint neutral because of nonhorizontal terrain.

These subtalar joint deviations may also occur from downhill or uphill running. Downhill running is characterized by pronation beyond midstance phase of gait, whereas uphill running is characterized by a diminishment of pronation such that supination begins prior to midstance. The combination of downhill running on a banked surface represents a compounding pronatory effect upon the lower subtalar joint, whereas uphill running compounds the supinatory effect upon the subtalar joint of the higher foot. An alteration of knee biomechanics may stem from a proximal extrinsic deformity such as excessive femoral anteversion.[4] Femoral anteversion represents excessive internal femoral torsion. This has the effect of slackening the pes anserine and represents, in contrast to the subtalar joint, a macrophysiologic disadvantage due to a proximal articular deviation.

14. How may osteoarthritis of the knee joint predispose toward the development of pes anserine bursitis?

Degenerative joint disease of the tibiofemoral joint classically affects the medial femoral condyle as a function of the larger magnitude and hence greater weight bearing of the medial column. Consequently, the more extensively damaged medial knee undergoes excessive joint erosion that culminates in narrowing of the medial compartment, widening of the lateral compartment, and a varus deformity of the involved knee.[9] A varus inclination of the knee results in approximation of the medial tibiofemoral hemi-joint. Subsequently, the pes anserine insertion is slackened. This slackening has the macrophysiologic effect of diminishing the tension generating capacity of the entire muscle-tendon unit comprising the pes anserinus. Consequently, these tendons will have to overwork to yield the same contractile output and become candidates for premature fatigue and tendon failure. Pes anserine bursitis is also associated with a *genu varum* deformity[5] owing to an alteration of the normal biomechanical milieu at the knee.[27] This structural deformity results in a medial convexity of the knee joint that approximates the medial aspect of the tibiofemoral joint. Consequently, the pes anserinus tendons are mechanically disadvantaged by virtue of their newly acquired slackened posture, resulting in potentially excessive friction to the site derived from inefficient mechanical function of these tendons. Thus pes anserine bursitis may be an indirect, if not direct function, of angular deformities superimposed upon the knee joint, and must be appreciated against the backdrop of frontal plane rotation along the tibiofemoral linkage. Pes anserine bursitis may uncommonly occur in children during the teen years[34] and may be related to pathologic tibia vara.

15. Are females more prone to the development of pes anserine bursitis or tendinitis?

The skeletal characteristics of females differ from males in several respects, among which include narrower shoulders, shorter leg length, smaller articular surfaces, smaller bone size, and a lower center of gravity. Pelvic differences include the wider gynecoid type in females compared to the android (male) pelvis resulting in increased hip varus angulation* and knee valgus in the former.[18] The consequences of an increased quadriceps angle (see Fig. 41-2) value may anatomically predispose females toward the development of a

---

*The deformities of varus and valgus refer to abnormal angulation within a limb that manifests as deformity in a particular joint, a bone near that joint, and even through an adjacent shaft of long bone.[33] This is precisely what occurs at the knee. *Genu varus* and *valgus* are generic terms for those structural deformities of the knee colloquially known as *bowleg* and *knock knee*. More specific terms exist that describe the origin of bowleg and knock knee positions and include tibial varum and valgum, as well as tibia vara and valga. The former terms designate the angular alignment or deformity of the leg with respect to the floor during quiet standing in growing children or young adults once the growth process is complete. Thus tibial varum refers to physiologic bowlegs, and is accompanied by compensatory internal tibial torsion and a cavus foot profile. *Tibial valgum* refers to physiologic knock knees, and is accompanied by compensatory external tibial torsion and a planus foot profile. In contrast, *tibia vara* also refer to the pathologic knock knee and bowleg deformities deriving from diseases to the proximal growth plate in children or disease of the knee joint in adults. Thus these terms refer to these deformities deriving from pathological conditions such as rickets, Blount's disease, or osteoarthritis, and are also accompanied by compensations in tibial torsion and the subtalar joint identical to physiologic bowleg and knock knee.

number of overuse syndromes occurring at the hip and knee, including pes anserine bursitis. Similarly, these differences in the female skeletal system may lower the fatigue threshold of the pes anserine tendons by way of an inherent mechanical disadvantage, and thereby exposing their knees to a higher incidence of pes anserine tendinitis as compared with males.

16. What is the presentation of pes anserine bursitis?

Pes anserine bursitis presents as insidious-onset pain perceived over the proximal anteromedial[31] or posteromedial[27] tibial metaphysis approximately 2 to 4 cm below the tibiofemoral joint line. The patient often reports discomfort in this area of pain, or to just posterior to the medial collateral ligament,[4] and extending superiorly to the medial joint line. Pain may radiate along the joint line and extend along the course of the hamstring tendons posteromedially.[4] Tenderness is similarly located over the proximal tibial metaphysis extending along the posteromedial corner of the knee to the attachment of the semimembranosus tendon. When the originating mechanism is osteoarthritis, patients may often complain of painful morning stiffness, as well as night pain that may awaken them but is relieved by turning on their sides and placing a pillow between their thighs. Radiographs of the knee are appropriate to detect for bony lesion, fracture, or the presence of bone spurs in the region of the pes anserinus that may resemble osteochondroma.[36]

17. What is the differential diagnosis of pes anserine bursitis?

A differential diagnosis of medial knee pain must always include pes anserine bursitis, but may also derive from a number of other conditions:

- *Hamstring tendinitis.* The medial hamstring tendon may develop an inflammation as it winds around the medial tibial metaphysis known as *semimembranosus tendinitis.* A host of extrinsic and intrinsic factors may contribute to pes anserine tendinitis due an alteration of the macrophysiologic state of these tendons. These factors include leg length discrepancy, excessive foot pronation, external tibial torsion, or an external cause such as running along a banked surface. The clinical presentation is nearly identical to pes anserine bursitis, with the exception that hamstring tendinitis imparts crepitus along the course of the semimembranosus tendon to the therapist's hand as well as positive sign for resisted flexion of the hamstring muscles[4] as well as passive stretching of the semi-membranosus. Also, semimembranosus tendinitis manifests as maximal tenderness in the posteromedial corner of the knee.

- *Tibial collateral ligament bursitis.* This is yet another cause of medial knee pain. The tibial collateral ligament bursa lies between the capsule and ligament adjacent to the medial meniscus. The proximity of the tibial collateral ligament bursa to the medial meniscus is a source of potential misdiagnosis. Positive findings for bursitis include medial joint line pain exacerbated by valgus stress of the medial collateral ligament and relief following a trial of conservative treatment. This may help avoid unnecessary diagnostic tests or arthroscopic surgery.[4]

- *Tibial stress fracture.* Because the tibia transmits approximately five-sixths of the body's weight, stress fractures of the tibia are much more problematic than fibular stress fractures. The most common location for tibial stress fracture is the proximal metaphysis.[20] Stress fractures occurring at the *posteromedial tibial plateau* are commonly misdiagnosed as sprain of the medial collateral ligament or pes anserine bursitis. Stress fractures just distal to the tibial tubercle most frequently manifest in young runners and may be confused with patellar tendinitis or malignancy by those unfamiliar with this problem.[2]

- *Degenerative joint disease.* Degenerative joint disease of the tibiofemoral joint is the articulation most commonly affected by osteoarthritis.[28] Because of the asymmetry of the femoral condylar size, the medial compartment of the knee is more seriously damaged than the lateral compartment, and is often accompanied by erosion of the tibial plateau. Structural damage causes much pain, crepitation, and motion restriction, with subluxation and angular deformity as late sequelae. Pain is often subjectively reported to focus at the medial joint line or just distal to it.

- *Pseudogout.* Pseudogout is also known as chondrocalcinosis and has a pathogenesis whose cause is unknown[24] but is hypothesized to result from a host response to pathologic (calcium pyrophosphate) crystal deposition into systemic joint cavities and adjacent tendons, ligaments, articular capsules, meniscus, cartilage, and synovium. The bursae at the knee may become involved by undergoing thickening that resolves in approximately 1 month.[10] Pseudogout affects men more often than women; typically occurs in the middle aged or elderly in the larger peripheral joints; most often appears in the knee; reaches peak intensity more slowly (1 to 2 weeks); is somewhat less painful than urate gout,[4] and may, like hyperuricemic gout, manifest as pain along the dorsal aspect of the first metatarsophalangeal joint. Pseudogout and classic gout may co-exist simultaneously. Symptoms include intermittent attacks of acute arthritis and fever. Diagnosis is made upon rectangular shaped crystal identification* from aspirated joint fluid as well as well as radiographic appearance of crystalline arrangement parallel to the cartilaginous surface.[5] With proper treatment, the prognosis of this condition is excellent.[2]

- *Meniscal injury.* Because pain derived from pes bursitis frequently extends up towards the medial joint line, it is important to rule out medial meniscal damage by way of screening for positive provocative tests and a history of knee locking. *Tumors* of the knee may be considered in the presence of night pain or when provocative examination has ruled out all other causes. Diagnosis is confirmed by biopsy after initial imaging findings. Bilateral bursitis of the knee joints is an occasional manifestation of *tertiary syphilis.*[10]

18. What is Baker's cyst?

Two significant bursae located along the posterior aspect of the knee joint are the subpopliteus and gastrocnemius bursae. The *gastrocnemius bursa* lies deep to the tendon of the medial head of the gastrocnemius muscle (and adjacent to the semimembranosus insertion on the tibia) and separates the muscle tendon from the femur, whereas the *subpopliteus bursa* lies between the tendon of the popliteus muscle and the lateral tibial condyle. The former bursa may become inflamed from activities such as rowing, which requires repeated contraction of both the gastrocnemius-soleus muscle group as well as the hamstring muscles.[3] The patient typically complains of pain and swelling behind the knee.

Because the gastrocnemius and subpopliteus bursae often communicate with the knee joint capsule, they may become effused. This may occur following synovitis secondary to gout, pseudogout, rheumatoid arthritis,[4] osteoarthritis, polymyalgia rheumatica, infectious arthritis, tuberculosis, pigmented villonodular synovitis, or chondromalacia patella. In the adult population,[27] these posterior bursae communicate with the knee joint

---

*Gout crystals are needle shaped. (Case stud. rheum.)

via what may be described as a weakening or defect of the posterior joint capsule. The most common site of such defect lies beside the semimembranosus tendon[9] in the posteromedial aspect of the knee. Posterior distention of these bursae[19] through this defect secondary to tuberculosis was first described by William Baker in 1877 and subsequently named for him. *Baker's* (or *popliteal*) *cyst* (Fig.39-7) produced a massive swelling in the popliteal fossa that extended distally to the ankle, but is rare today. Presently, this condition manifests as a round swelling in the region of the semimembranosus tendon and the medial gastrocnemius muscle belly[27] usually the size of a golf ball, although sometimes as large as a tennis ball. Cysts are comprised of distended bursae filled with synovial-like fluid that herniate posteriorly via a hollow and narrow stalk (defect) secondary to synovial fluid pressure rise within the knee joint, (primer) and will occasionally bulge medially.

Popliteal cyst in childhood more frequently occur in males and commonly present in children between the ages of 6 and 8, and again between the ages of 12 and 14 following that period corresponding to the rapid growth spurt. Baker's cysts are best palpated with the knee in full extension. In contrast to those seen in adults, popliteal cysts in childhood do not communicate with the joint capsule, but originate instead in the semimembranosus bursa[35] located inferior to the semimembranosus tendon, presumably because of chronic irritation.

19. What is the natural history of this cyst?

The evolution of a popliteal cyst in the adult may occur along one of several routes. The cyst may disappear gradually. Alternately, it may grow so large and extend so inferiorly as to interfere with function and cause compression of the popliteal artery decreasing distal pulses. In addition, painful thrombophlebitis may result from venous obstruction due to a particularly large cyst. Either of these latter cases is managed by surgical cyst excision.[9] An athlete may return to sporting activity approximately 8 to 12 weeks following surgery. An alternate possibility includes spontaneous rupture of the cyst, which may occur because of venous obstruction known as *pseudothrombophlebitis*. Most ruptures occur downward, although a proximal rupture into the thigh may also occur. Clinical manifestations of a ruptured cyst include leg swelling, positive Homans' sign, a *lack of* bruits, fever, sweat, rash, or skin redness. In addition, a *crescent sign* appearing as a curved discoloration in the ankle area may be present and suggests the diagno-

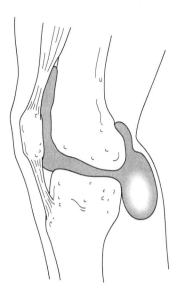

FIG. 39-7 Baker's cyst. The posterior bursae, which include the gastrocnemius and subpopliteus bursae, often communicate with the knee joint capsule a defect of the posterior joint capsule adjacent to the semimembranosus tendon located at the posteromedial aspect of the knee. Baker's cyst represents posterior herniation of synovial fluid and distension of the potential space provided by the popliteal fossa. (From Magee DJ: *Orthopedic physical assessment*, Philadelphia, 1997, WB Saunders.)

sis of cyst rupture. The clinician must differentiate a ruptured popliteal cyst from *deep vein thrombosis,* in which the calf is hot, red, and tender. Doppler ultrasound or a venogram may be used to help exclude deep vein thrombosis. *Arterial aneurysm* is ruled out by an excessive pulsation in the popliteal space. *Soft tissue tumor* must also be ruled out. The use of arthrograph, computed tomography, or magnetic resonance imaging may help delineate the extent of rupture.

Medical management for the patient with the ruptured popliteal cyst includes joint aspiration, elevation, heat, elastic bandage wrap, and oral nonsteroidal antiinflammatory medication. In those patients whose cysts have not ruptured it is important to ensure that a stretching program of the hamstrings and gastrocnemius muscles are adequately performed so as to fend off development of a knee flexion contracture. Short-arc hamstring activity exercises are also helpful. A physician may elect to aspirate the knee joint and then inject it with a corticosteroid injection. Excision of a Baker's cyst is rarely indicated.[8]

20. How do popliteal cysts in children differ from those occurring in adults?

Popliteal cysts in children occur most frequently in males between 5 and 10 years of age, and differ from the adult form in that the popliteal cysts of children do not generally communicate with knee joint capsule.[27] Instead, they are simply an inflammation of the semimembranosus and popliteal bursae presumably due to chronic irritation.[27] Evaluation is typically sought because of a recently noted, and sometimes large, painless swelling in the popliteal space. A particularly large cyst may interfere with knee flexion.[27] It is very important to assuage a parent's fear of malignancy, and is accomplished by transilluminating the lesion via an arthrogram and demonstrating that it consists of fluid only.[9] Popliteal cysts are benign in children, often resolve over time, and may be followed without surgical intervention as long as it does not increase in size.[27]

21. What therapeutic intervention best manages bursitis at the knee?

The treatment of acute bursitis of the knee is conservative and depends on the degree of swelling within the bursa. If only mild to moderate bursal distention is present, the management strategy focuses on reduction of inflammation by way of ice, compression, elevation, and (rest via) immobilization using a knee splint. The use of oral antiinflammatory medications, as well as phonophoresis to introduce an antiinflammatory agent directly to the area, are appropriate. Once the acute inflammatory process abates (i.e., following the first 48 to 72 hours) isometric activity may be cautiously introduced along with gentle range of motion in the non-painful range, and progression to concentric, eccentric, and resistive exercises when symptoms allow to prevent residual weakness and contractures. Stretching of the adjacent musculature is particularly important in the therapeutic exercise program. It is essential to protect the area with prophylactic padding to reduce incidence of recurrent trauma. With pes anserine bursitis it is essential to correct the biomechanical origin of pathology by the use of an inner heel wedge in individuals with genu valgus or excessive heel valgus. Here, concentric medial hamstring strengthening and eccentric lateral hamstring work is appropriate. An orthosis properly addresses a subtalar joint that deviates from neutral. When running or other sport activity commences, patients should be encouraged to reduce their mileage, shorten their stride, gain adequate flexibility in their hamstrings, allow for appropriate warm ups and cool downs, and allocate sufficient periods of rest between workouts. During the recovery period, the uninvolved leg and upper body, as well as cardiopulmonary fitness must be addressed and maintained. For patients with contractures of the quadriceps mechanism or patellofemoral malalignments, an elastic knee support with a felt patella-restraining pad may be of help in controlling abnormal forces.[4]

REFERENCES

1. Aegerter E, Kirkpatrick JDJ: *Orthopedic disease: physiology, pathology, radiology,* Philadelphia, 1963, WB Saunders.
2. Bachner EJ, Friedman MJ: Injuries to the leg. In Nicholas JA, Hershman EB, editors: *The lower extremity and spine,* ed 2, vol 1, St Louis, 1995, Mosby.
3. Boland AL, Hosea TM: Rowing and the older athlete, *Clin Sports Med* 10(2):245, 1991.
4. Boland AL Jr, Hulstyn MJ: Soft-tissue injuries of the knee. In Nicholas JA, Hershman EB, editors: *The lower extremity and spine,* ed 2, vol 1, St Louis, 1995, Mosby.
5. Brody DM: Clinical symposia: running injury-prevention and management, 39(3). Summit, NJ, 1987, CIBA-GEIGY.
6. Canosa JJ, Sheckman PR: Septic subcutaneous bursitis: report of 16 cases, *J Rheumatol* 6:196, 1979.
7. Canosa JJ, Yood RD: Reaction of superficial bursae in response to specific disease stimuli, *Arthritis Rheum* 22:1361, 1979.
8. Cyriax J: *Textbook of orthopedic medicine,* ed 8, vol 1, London, 1982, Bailliere Tindall.
9. Dandy DJ: *Essential orthopedics and trauma,* Edinburgh, 1989, Churchill Livingstone.
10. Fochios D, Nicholas JA: Football injuries. In Nicholas JA, Hershman EB, editors: *The lower extremity and spine,* ed 2, vol 2, St Louis, 1995, Mosby.
11. Gardner DL: *Pathology of the connective tissue diseases,* London, 1965, Edward Arnold.
12. Girgis FG, Marshall JL, Almonajem RS: The cruciate ligaments of the knee joint: anatomical, functional, and experimental analysis, *Clin Orthop* 106:216, 1975.
13. Gray H: *Gray's anatomy,* Philadelphia, 1974, Lea & Febiger.
14. Greenfield BH: *Rehabilitation of the knee: a problem-solving approach,* Philadelphia, 1993, FA Davis.
15. Henry JH: The patellofemoral joint. In Nicholas JA, Hershman EB, editors: *The lower extremity and spine,* ed 2, vol 1, St Louis, 1995, Mosby.
16. Ho G, Tice AD, Kaplan SR: Septic bursitis in the prepatellar and olecranon bursae, *Ann Intern Med* 89:21, 1978.
17. Hoppenfeld S: *Physical examination of the spine and extremities,* Norwalk, Conn, 1976, Appleton-Century Crofts.
18. Hunter-Griffin LY: Aspects of injuries to the lower extremity unique to the female athlete. In Nicholas JA, Hershman EB, editors: *The lower extremity and spine,* ed 2, vol 1, St Louis, 1995, Mosby.
19. Kessler RM, Hertling D: *Management of common musculoskeletal disorders,* Philadelphia, 1983, JB Lippincott.
20. Kimball PR, Savastano AA: Fatigue fractures of the proximal tibia, *Clin Orthop* 70:170, 1970.

21. King DW, Fenoglio CM, Lefkowitch JH: *General pathology, principles, and dynamics,* Philadelphia, 1983, Lea & Febiger.
22. Larson RL, Osternig LR: Traumatic bursitis and artificial turf, *J Sports Med* 2:183, 1974.
23. Lynch MA, Henning CE: Physical examination of the knee. In Nicholas JA, Hershman EB, editors: *The lower extremity and spine,* ed 2, vol. 1, St Louis, 1995, Mosby.
24. *Merck Manual,* ed 15, Rahway, NJ, 1987, Merck, Sharp, & Dohme Research Laboratories.
25. Moore KL: *Clinically oriented anatomy,* ed 2, Baltimore, 1985, Williams & Wilkins.
26. Mysnyk MC, Wroble RR, Foster DT et al: Prepatellar bursitis in wrestlers, *Am J Sports Med* 14:46, 1986.
27. Netter FH: *The Ciba Collection of Medical Illustrations,* vol 8 Part I, Summit, NJ, 1990, CIBA-GEIGY.
28. Netter FH: *The Ciba Collection of Medical Illustrations,* vol 8 Part II, Development disorders, tumors, rheumatic diseases and joint replacement, Summit, NJ, 1990, CIBA-GEIGY.
29. Netter FH: *The Ciba Collection of Medical Illustrations,* vol 8 Part III, Musculoskeletal system: trauma, evaluation, and management, Summit, NJ, 1993, CIBA-GEIGY.
30. Pagnani MJ et al: Anatomy of the knee. In Nicholas JA, Hershman EB, editors: *The lower extremity and spine,* ed 2, vol 1, St Louis, 1995, Mosby.
31. Reilly JP, Nicholas JA: The chronically inflamed bursa, *Clin Sports Med* 6:345, 1987.
32. Robbins SL, Cotran RS: *Pathologic basis of disease,* Philadelphia, 1979, WB Saunders.
33. Salter RB: *Textbook of disorders of the musculoskeletal system,* ed 2, Baltimore, 1983, Williams & Wilkins.
34. Staheli LT: *Fundamentals of pediatric orthopedics,* New York, 1992, Raven Press.
35. Tria AJ, Klein KS: *An illustrated guide to the knee,* New York, 1992, Churchill Livingstone.
36. Ugai K, Sato S, Matsumoto K et al: A clinicopathologic study of bone spurs on the pes anserinus, *Clin Orthop* 231:130, 1988.
37. Wallace LA, Mangine RE, Malone TR: The knee. In Gould JA III, editor: *Orthopedic and sports physical therapy,* ed 2, St Louis, 1990, Mosby.
38. Waters P, Kasser J: Infection of the infrapatellar bursa, *J Bone Joint Surg* 72A:1095, 1990.

RECOMMENDED READING

Boland AL, Hulstyn MJ: Soft tissue injuries of the knee. In Nicholas JA, Hershman EB, editors: *The lower extremity and spine in sports,* ed 2, vol 1, St Louis, 1995, Mosby.

Reilly JP, Nicholas JA: The chronically inflamed bursa, *Clin Sports Med* 6:345, 1987.

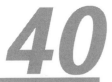

40

Retropatellar Pain, Crepitus, Mild Swelling, Slight Quadriceps Atrophy, Facet Tenderness, and Stiffness After Sitting, and an Occasional Sensation of Giving Way

CASE 1: A 31-year-old professional baseball catcher complains of dull ache in both knees, especially the right knee, that is most acute during sport, after sitting for long periods, and a day before a significant weather change. When squatting during a long inning he complains of moderate stiffness when attempting to stand, which has become progressively more pronounced. Pain is localized to the medial retropatellar area. Driving for long periods also provokes pain and stiffness. The patient complains of a painless grinding sensation when extending his right knee. He reports that taking aspirin twice per day has afforded some relief. Upon probing, you discover that the patient had bilateral metatarsus adductus during childhood.

OBSERVATION Patella alta is present and both patellae appear to face outward (grasshopper eyes). When asking the patient to extend the knee in the short sitting posture, a dimple appears over the superomedial patellar border as extension is approached. When viewed from behind, a calcaneal valgus posture is present in both feet. The patient appears to present with a combination deformity of pronated feet, knock knees (genu valgum), external tibial torsion, and femoral anteversion.

PALPATION Tenderness upon palpation of the medial patellar facet, and the medial retinacular structures. Pain is present during patellar compression. A dimple over the right superior-medial patellar border is palpated upon full knee extension. Vastus lateralis muscles seem hypertrophied bilaterally. Firm palpation of the vastus medialis muscle during a quadriceps setting exercise imparts a relatively soft muscle mass relative to the vastus lateralis.

RANGE OF MOTION Range of motion is full and painless in the open kinetic chain.

STRENGTH Right resisted terminal knee extension requires less applied external force than the contralateral knee. Moreover, it is painful from 30°-knee flexion to full extension.

FLEXIBILITY Tightness is present in both hamstring, triceps surae, and tensor fasciae latae muscles.

JOINT PLAY There is excessive lateral patellar mobility during joint glide assessment.

GIRTH MEASUREMENT There is approximately 1 cm less girth of the right quadriceps muscle when measured at the superior patellar pole.

SPECIAL TESTS A positive leg length discrepancy of ¼ inch is present in the right lower extremity. The Q angle for the right lower limb measures 4° greater than the contralateral lower extremity. Negative apprehension, McMurray, Apley, Lasagues, and prone knee bend tests. Squat test is positive for pain. A normal Thomas test is demonstrated. Positive Ober test, and excessive femoral anteversion is present, right greater than left.

RADIOGRAPHS An anteroposterior, lateral, and infrapatellar view confirm the clinically determined patellar tilt, height, and presence of a low lateral femoral condyle, respectively. Radiographs also reveal a shallow sulcus angle bilaterally and a Wiberg II patella. There is no evidence of fracture, tumor, or arthritis.

CLUE:

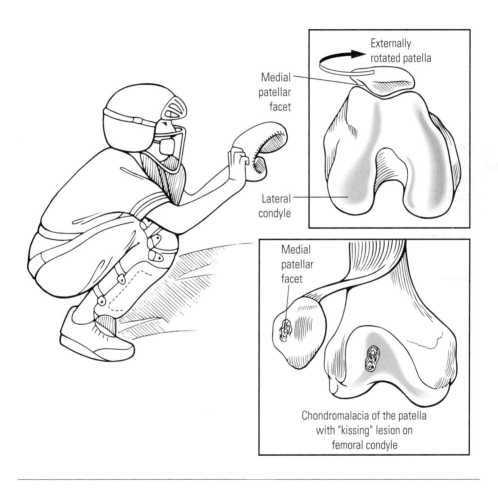

CASE 2: An overweight 19-year-old woman complains of vague ache in her right anterior knee following a freshman semester of running track at her university. She reports a grinding sensation in her knee, as well as stiffness and pain in the morning hours that occur following her film class during which she sits for 3 hours twice per week. She reports feeling better after she begins running, although soreness sets in towards the end of her activity. Walking downhill and stairs is more painful than ascent. Also, she occasionally experiences a "giving way" sensation during descent, as if she cannot rely on her right leg as much as she does on her left leg. Kneeling is uncomfortable. There is no history of trauma to her knee or back, although her mother has osteoarthritis of both hips and knees. Both her sensation and deep tendon reflexes are normal during examination. When asked, she reports that a grinding sensation is felt during knee flexion.

OBSERVATION   Patella infera of both patellae is observed and accompanied by a squinting patellae profile. Patellar tilt is observed to be more pronounced in the right patella. Mild physiologic knock knees (genu valgum) is observed in both lower extremities, right greater than left. As expected, compensatory pronation of both feet accompanies the proximal angular knee deformity. Rotational deformities observed include bilateral femoral anteversion, right greater than left, and compensatory external tibial torsion. The right subtalar joint is more prominently postured in over-pronation. She appears to ambulate with the mild toe-in gait and slight antalgia.

PALPATION   There is tenderness upon palpation of the medial patellar facet, and the medial retinacular structures. Pain is present during patellar compression. A dimple over the right superomedial patellar border is palpated upon full knee extension. Both vastus lateralis muscles appear hypertrophied. Firm palpation of the vastus medialis muscle during a quadriceps setting exercise imparts a relatively soft muscle mass relative to the vastus lateralis.

RANGE OF MOTION   Range of motion is full and painless in the open kinetic chain.

STRENGTH   Right resisted terminal knee extension requires less applied external force than the contralateral knee. Moreover, it is painful from 30°-knee flexion to full extension. Right hip flexion strength is graded at G+.

FLEXIBILITY   Tightness is present in the posterior soft-tissue structures of the entire right and left lower extremities including the tendo Achillis.

JOINT PLAY   There is excessive lateral patellar mobility during joint glide assessment.

GIRTH MEASUREMENT   There is approximately 1 cm less girth of the right quadriceps muscle when measured at the superior patellar pole.

SPECIAL TESTS   There are negative apprehension, McMurray, Apley, Lasègue, and prone knee bend tests. Squat test is positive for pain. A normal Thomas test is demonstrated. Positive Ober test. The right Q angle measures 22°.

RADIOGRAPHS   An anteroposterior, lateral, and infrapatellar view confirm the clinically determined patellar tilt, height, and presence of a low lateral femoral condyle, respectively. Radiographs also reveal a shallow sulcus angle bilaterally and a Wiberg III patella. There is no evidence of fracture, tumor, or arthritis.

CLUE:

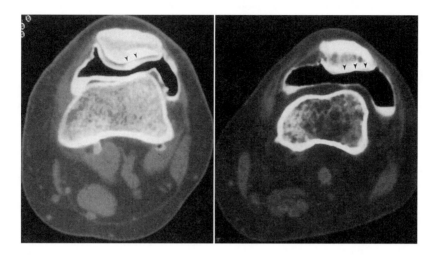

(From Nicholas JA, Hershman EB: *The lower extremity and spine in sports medicine*, ed 2, St Louis, 1995, Mosby.)

? Questions

1. What is the most probable cause of both patients' symptoms?
2. What is chondromalacia patellae?
3. What controversy surrounds the nomenclature of chondromalacia?
4. What is the spectrum of anterior knee pain?
5. What is the anatomy of the patella?
6. What is the nerve and blood supply to the patella?
7. What is the patellofemoral articulation?
8. How do the points of contact change during the arc of motion?
9. In addition to simple glide, what is the rotational component of patellar motion?
10. Is patellofemoral motion determined by open or kinetic chain function of the lower extremity?
11. What are the biomechanical functions of the patella in relation to the quadriceps muscle?
12. Is patellar contribution to the mechanical advantage of the quadriceps muscles constant throughout the arc of knee motion?
13. What is the biomechanical function of the patella in relationship to the joint reaction force at the patellofemoral joint?
14. What other functions does the patella serve?
15. What are the four stages describing histologic change associated with chondromalacia patellae?
16. What is the etiology of chondromalacia?
17. How does imbalance in the quadriceps extensor mechanism and/or the static patellar stabilizers contribute to degenerative wear of the patellar surface?
18. What is the relationship between the predominantly valgus force afforded the patellofemoral joint by the osseous, dynamic, and static patellar stabilizers and excessive patellar cartilage stress?
19. How do laterally dominating forces at the patellofemoral joint cause excessive wear of the extreme medial facet?
20. What is patellar tilt and how does it increase stress to the medial odd patellar facet?
21. Which areas of the patellar surface typically experience wear associated with chondromalacia?

22. **What is the effect of excess or deficiency of pronation at the subtalar joint upon patellar facet wear?**
23. **What is the effect of patella alta or baja on patellofemoral instability or pain?**
24. **What are the signs and symptoms associated with chondromalacia?**
25. **What is the differential diagnosis?**

26. **What is patellar overload syndrome?**
27. **What is retropatellar pain syndrome?**
28. **What radiographs are appropriate when evaluating the patellofemoral joint?**
29. **What physical therapy is appropriate in management of patellofemoral dysfunction?**
30. **What are the surgical options or alternatives to management of recalcitrant patellofemoral pain?**

1. What is the most probable cause of both patients' symptoms?

Chondromalacia patellae falls under the category of patellofemoral disorders, and is implicated as the cause of symptoms in both Cases 1 and 2. This pathologic condition is commonly encountered in joggers and long-distance runners, and has subsequently been called *runner's knee*.[65] However, chondromalacia patellae is far from clinically apparent in runners only. Nevertheless, with the increasing interest in sports among the general population, patellofemoral pain has been identified as the primary complaint of knee pain.[53] Adolescent females are often susceptible to developing chondromalacia as well as patellofemoral instability.[61] The clue following Case 2 depicts a CT arthrogram used to view chondromalacia. *A*, in the figure for the clue in Case 2 shows increased uptake of contrast in articular cartilage of the lateral facet consistent with a grade I chondromalacia. *B*, in this figure shows nearly total absence of articular cartilage on both the medial and lateral facets consistent with a grade III chondromalacia *(arrowheads)*.

2. What is chondromalacia patellae?

Difficulty encountered in analysis of patellofemoral joint dysfunction stems from an ambivalence of nomenclature describing patellofemoral disorders. Chondromalacia is literally a pathologic description that means "softening" of the articular cartilage located along the underside of the patella, and is commonly the diagnosis given to patients with anterior knee pain. Chondromalacia is a degenerative process believed to result from *excessive loading* of articular cartilage lining the patellar facets. Articular cartilage is loaded by compressive forces that may be exceeded resulting in decreased diffusion of nutrients and eventual *malacia** of the

involved facet. If significant disruption of hyaline cartilage has occurred, the release of chondral debris serves as an antigenic stimulus to the synovial lining, resulting in secondary synovitis of the knee as well as recurrent effusions.[36] Classic physical symptoms of chondromalacia include retropatellar pain, recurrent effusion, retropatellar crepitation, patellofemoral grinding during knee flexion or extension, and tenderness upon palpation of the patellar facets.

3. What controversy surrounds the nomenclature of chondromalacia?

Considerable criticism has historically been leveled at the appellation *chondromalacia,* reducing it to a "wastebasket term" or a clinical diagnosis at best. Confusion stems from a lack of authoritative consensus about the meaning and usage of this term. Some authorities believe that chondromalacia is a primary condition with signs and symptoms in and of itself. Other authorities maintain that chondromalacia, at best, is a secondary disorder resulting from some other patellofemoral dysfunction; at worst, chondromalacia may merely be a description rather than an attempt to describe the etiology of pain. Attempts to correlate the pathologic changes on the patellar surface to clinical presentation have proven frustrating. This is because many patients who have no patellofemoral symptoms show arthroscopic changes associated with chondromalacia.[79] On the other hand, some patients complain of significant peripatellar or retropatellar pain in the absence of visible patellar changes. Alternative terms have been alternately suggested and include anterior patellar pain syndrome[74] or patellofemoral pain syndrome, or patellalgia. However, the established terminology persists as most surgeons refer to the symptoms that result from pathologic changes along the posterior patellar surface as chondromalacia patellae.[90]

---

*Malacia means morbid softening of tissue in Greek.

4. What is the spectrum of anterior knee pain?

The myriad sources of anterior knee pain is often confined, but not limited to, dysfunction of the extensor mechanism at the knee (Fig. 40-1). The various disorders the patellofemoral joint falls subject to are many and often age specific. Congenital dislocation of the cartilage anlage (i.e., primordium) occurs in infants. The older child with Osgood-Schlatter disease is initially seen with tenderness and swelling of the tibial tubercle usually associated with a high and unusually mobile patella.[67] Alternately, the pubescent child demonstrates symptoms localized to the inferior patellar pole that is often accompanied by patella alta in Sinding-Larsen-Johansson syndrome.[59] In addition, the rapidly growing adolescent may exhibit a growth differential between the bones of the leg and the adjacent soft tissues in patellar overload syndrome.[62] Active children and young adults between 10 and 25 years of age may damage the articular surface of their patella (chondromalacia) owing to excessive involvement in sporting activities, particularly in the presence of dysplasia or anatomic malalignment. Adolescent girls and young women are particularly vulnerable towards patellar instability secondary to increased hip varus and knee valgus characteristic of the gynecoid (i.e., wider) pelvis.[64] Young adults are also affected by patellar tendinitis and overuse syndromes of the superior lateral patellar pole following repeated stress.[14] The primary manifestations of adult patellofemoral disease are changes in the retropatellar hyaline cartilage known as chondromalacia[91] that may, in later years, progress to patellofemoral arthritis.

5. What is the anatomy of the patella?

The *patella* (Fig. 40-2) is a large sesamoid bone that lies in the substance of the quadriceps tendon. The in-

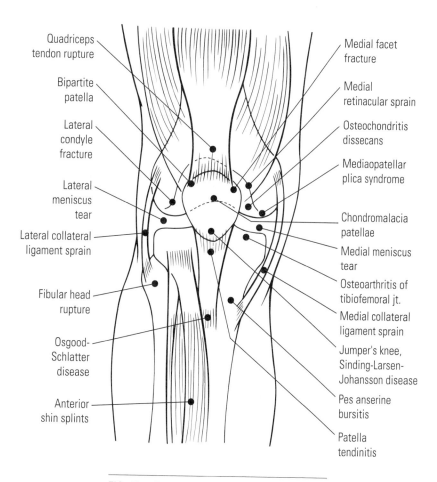

FIG. 40-1 The many causes of anterior knee pain.

Quadriceps tendon rupture
Bipartite patella
Lateral condyle fracture
Lateral meniscus tear
Lateral collateral ligament sprain
Fibular head rupture
Osgood-Schlatter disease
Anterior shin splints

Medial facet fracture
Medial retinacular sprain
Osteochondritis dissecans
Mediaopatellar plica syndrome
Chondromalacia patellae
Medial meniscus tear
Osteoarthritis of tibiofemoral jt.
Medial collateral ligament sprain
Jumper's knee, Sinding-Larsen-Johansson disease
Pes anserine bursitis
Patella tendinitis

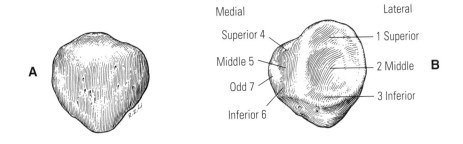

FIG. 40-2 A, Anterior view of the patella. **B,** Posterior view showing the seven facets of the articular surface. Note the central vertical ridge separating the medial and lateral facets. This ridge is alternately known as the median ridge as it is asymmetrically placed closer to the medial aspect of the patella. (From Tria AJ, Klein KS: *An illustrated guide to the knee*, New York, 1992, Churchill Livingstone.)

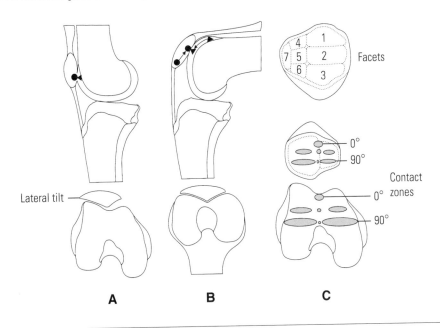

FIG. 40-3 As flexion increases the patella moves more medially and the contact zones shift proximally and to the medial and lateral facets. **A,** In extension the patella sits slightly lateral in the femoral sulcus, and the distal patellar articular surface is in contact with the femur. **B,** As flexion progresses, the patella reduces into the sulcus of the femur, and the contact zone on the patella shifts proximally. **C,** As the knee flexes, the patellar surface contact spreads medially and laterally onto the femoral surfaces. (From Tria AJ, Klein KS: *An illustrated guide to the knee*, New York, 1992, Churchill Livingstone.)

ferior one-third of the patella is extraarticular. The patella's nonarticular anterior surface is shaped like a rounded inverted triangle with a superior base and inferior apex, and the primary tendinous and ligamentous attachments are at the superior and inferior poles. The posterior patellar surface is oval and covered by the thickest layer of articular cartilage in the human body. The upper two thirds of the posterior patellar surface may be divided into seven different articulating facets corresponding to different portions of the patellar sur-

face that articulate with the distal femur at different points in knee range of motion (Fig. 40-3). The location of the facets is symmetrical with three located medially and three located laterally. The facets may also be categorized proximodistally as *superior, middle,* and *inferior* for both the medial and lateral facets. Thus six out of seven facets may be described as mediolateral and superior–inferior pairs. A seventh *odd* or *medial vertical* facet is located above the medial facet, specifically on the far medial border of the middle portion of the

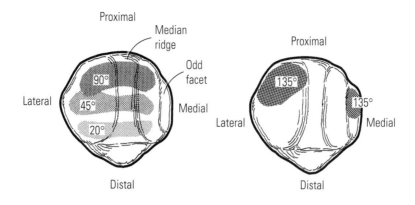

FIG. 40-4 Patellofemoral contact area with degree of flexion. (From Scott WN: *The knee,* St Louis, 1994, Mosby.)

patella and separated from the medial facet by a small ridge of subchondral bone. The magnitude of size of the medial facets is generally smaller than the lateral facets. In addition, the medial facets are more convex than concave whereas the lateral facets may be either concave or convex. All facets are covered by *hyaline cartilage,* which receives nutrition from the surrounding synovium.[68] The purpose of hyaline cartilage is to facilitate ease of motion between the two articular surfaces owing to its low coefficient of friction.

The medial and lateral facets are divided by a significant longitudinal ridge of subchondral bone known as the *median* or *central ridge* that is located lateral to midline (but never medial) and articulates with the center of the femoral sulcus. Thus the location of the central ridge asymmetrically divides the posterior patellar surface such that the lateral facet has a larger surface area.[58] A second vertical ridge isolates the odd facet.

6. What is the nerve and blood supply to the patella?

The four geniculate arteries and the recurrent anterior tibial arteries form an arterial circle around the patella that directly enter the patella and do not rely upon the fat pad as was once believed.[91] Two systems of vessels feed the patella, the principal being the polar vessels that enter inferiorly at the distal pole (apex) of the patella.[80,81] Thus, a transverse fracture may result in avascular necrosis of the proximal portion.[91] The midpatellar vessels enter the middle third of the nonarticular patellar surface. Both systems arborize in the patella and anastomose one with the other.

Innervation to the knee is by way of the distal branches of the femoral nerve, which is formed from the posterior divisions of the anterior rami of L2, L3, and L4 spinal nerve root segments, with L4 contributing most significantly.[73] The knee is also innervated by branches of the obturator and sciatic nerves.[43] No nerve fibers are found in the substance of the patella and so patient complaints of pain must be extrapolated along a different route.[91] Pain is the most outstanding symptom associated with chondromalacia and is generally inexplicable as *articular cartilage has no nerve fibers.*[65] It is hypothesized that subjective pain is derived from the disruption of the normal passage of fluids to surrounding tissues. This change in local metabolism may be a result of increased pressure to abnormal patella tracking.[68,72] This may explain why chondromalacia is so often seen clinically as a secondary complication to long term long-leg cast immobilization.[16] Also, because the patellar periosteum is innervated from the three vasti muscles, it may be that patellar pain originates from these sites by mechanical stresses in rotation, tilt, shear, and traction.[65]

7. What is the patellofemoral articulation?

The *patellofemoral articulation* consists of the distal femoral condyles in contact with the patellar facets. This occurs by way of the posterior patellar facets articulating with the medial and lateral trochlear facets at the supratrochlear region of the femoral condyles throughout varying degrees of knee flexion and extension (Fig. 40-4). The patella maintains a shifting contact with the femur in all positions of the knee as it glides over the distal femur. As the knee shifts from a fully flexed to a fully extended posture, first the superior, then the middle, and finally the inferior portions of the patellar articular surface are brought into contact with the patellar surfaces of the distal femur. Correspondingly, the area of femoral contact throughout the arc of knee motion begins with the patella recessed into the intercondylar femoral groove during flexion. As extension commences the patella slides up and out of that groove and migrates proximally along the uneven slopes of the femoral sulcus. At full extension, the patella rests in the trochlear fossa. The total distance traversed during patellofemoral joint slide is approximately 7 cm.[25]

As 20° to 30° of knee flexion is approached, the patella is lowered into the trochlear groove and drifts laterally as a function of unlocking of the tibiofemoral joint. This causes compressive force across the medial and lateral facets as well as to the median ridge. The combined motions of lateral drift and cephalad migration characterizing flexion of the knee joint may be called lateral patellar rotation. During extension, this process is reversed and mediopatellar rotation occurs as the patella migrates in a caudad fashion. However, at the end of extension, a lateral patellar displacement is again observed.

8. How do the points of contact change during the arc of motion?

Patellofemoral joint movement occurs by way of cephalo-caudal *glide* between the posterior patellar facets and the supratrochlear region of the femoral condyles. As the knee joint flexes and extends, the contact points of the patellofemoral joint undergo changes in contact area and joint reaction force. During full knee extension the patella lies in the supratrochlear fossa in a bed of fat and synovium, which makes the patella so amenable to manual motion and palpation. In this position, it is the inferior facet that contacts the femur. Here, the median patellar ridge and the lateral facet articulate with the lateral side of the femoral sulcus.[91] As flexion commences, the patellar surface articulates with the trochlear patellar surface in a distal to proximal manner. Simultaneously, the patella migrates centrally in a lateral to medial fashion. Thus early flexion begins with inferior facet engagement, proceeds to middle facet articulation, and reaches 90° with superior facet engagement. Moreover, in full extension to 90° of flexion both the medial and lateral facets of the patellar articulate with the femur. Beyond 90° of flexion the patella externally rotates and only the extreme medial (odd) facet articulates with the medial trochlear patellar facet on the femur. At terminal flexion the patella moves into the intercondylar groove. The total amount of proximodistal patel-

lar glide along the femoral condyles is approximately 7 cm (see Fig. 40-3).[24]

Although the points of contact along the posterior surface of the patella move proximally and medially with progressive flexion, the corresponding points of contact along the trochlear facets move in opposite direction, namely distally and laterally. In other words, as the knee flexes, the contact point of the patellofemoral joint moves proximally on the patella and distally on the femoral intercondylar sulcus.[8,34]

9. In addition to simple glide, what is the rotational component of patellar motion?

It is essential to understand that patellofemoral joint motion involves both a *translational* and *rotational* component of motion. The dual nature of patellar motion in relation to the distal femur is related to the dual nature of motion that is also present in the tibiofemoral articulation. Because of the architectural disparity between the lengths of the articular surfaces of the femoral condyles, the tibiofemoral joint is characterized by two types of motion during flexion and extension. The tibiofemoral joint possesses features characteristic of both the ginglymus (hinge joint) and a trochoid (pivot joint) articulation. The tibiofemoral articulation undergoes flexion and extension in the sagittal plane as well as some degree of internal and external rotation when the joint is flexed.[9]* Thus, the biomechanics of patellofemoral joint motion are inextricably linked with, and may be considered dependent upon the kinesiology of the tibiofemoral joint.

As 20° to 30° of knee flexion is approached, the patella is lowered into the trochlear groove and drifts laterally as a function of unlocking of the tibiofemoral joint. This causes compressive force across the medial and lateral facets as well as to the median ridge. The combined motions of lateral drift and cephalad migration with flexion of the knee joint may be called lateral *patellar rotation*. During extension, this process is reversed and mediopatellar rotation occurs as the patella migrates caudally; however, at the end of extension, a lateral patellar displacement is again observed. Thus the patella, in addition to sliding over the distal femur, also undergoes a helical motion comprised of mediolateral drift as a function of a size differential between the femoral condyles comprising the articular surface. From full extension to 90° of flexion both the medial and lateral facets of the patella articulate with the femur. Beyond 90° of flexion the patella externally rotates

---

*No rotation is possible when the knee is in full extension.

and only the medial (odd) facet articulates with the medial trochlear patellar facet on the femur. At terminal flexion the patella moves into the intercondylar groove.[24] The direction of rotation is reversed during the arc of motion from full flexion to extension as the patella correspondingly internally rotates at its point of contact and migrate superiorly, while the patellar body is recessed into the intercondylar femoral groove.

10. Is patellofemoral motion determined by open or kinetic chain function of the lower extremity?

The relationship between the femur and patella is affected by whether or not the lower limb functions in the open or closed kinetic mode of function. In the open kinetic chain the tibia moves on a stationary femur, and the patella slides on the femoral condyles. However, although the femur is relatively stationary, it still undergoes sagittal plane motion as the femoral condyles glide backward and forward along the tibial plateau with extension and flexion of the tibiofemoral joint. Moreover, rotation of the femoral condyles also occur in the transverse plane.

In contrast, in the closed kinetic mode, characterized by the femur moving on a fixed tibia, the femoral condyles slide under a stationary patella. This difference between the two articulating surfaces of the patellofemoral joint occurs as a direct function of patellar attachment to both the femur (via the quadriceps tendon) and the tibia (via the patellar ligament).

11. What are the biomechanical functions of the patella in relation to the quadriceps muscle?

A primary function of the patella is to increase the mechanical *leverage* afforded by the quadriceps muscle group. The patella acts to lengthen the moment arm, of the quadriceps anteriorly from the center of rotation at the tibiofemoral joint during extension (Fig. 40-5).[18,41] The contribution of the patella to the *mechanical advantage* of the quadriceps muscle varies from full extension to full flexion of the knee joint.[52,71] At full tibiofemoral flexion the patella is recessed into the concavity of the intercondylar groove of the femur and is thus adjacent to the axis of motion. As such, the patella yields little anterior quadriceps tendon displacement, and contributes only 10% to the torque of the quadriceps. As the knee is extended, the patella follows the contour of the distal femur to rise out of the intercondylar groove to glide proximally and upon full extension, to lie an average of 1.5 cm proximal to the knee joint.[68] This patellar position results in significant anterior displacement of the quadriceps tendon and length-

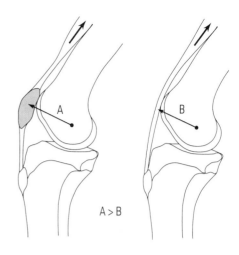

FIG. 40-5 The patella increases the moment arm of the quadriceps mechanism, thus improving its mechanical advantage. (From Tria AJ, Klein KS: *An illustrated guide to the knee,* New York, 1992, Churchill Livingstone.)

ens the quadriceps lever arm by approximately 30% at 45° of flexion.

12. Is patellar contribution to the mechanical advantage of the quadriceps muscles constant throughout the arc of knee motion?

Following patellectomy the quadriceps tendon lies closer to the instant center of the tibiofemoral joint than in the normal knee. During terminal extension, the quadriceps' mechanical advantage is decreased due to a reduction in lever arm length. Additional force during this terminal arc may also result from the magnification of transverse plane motion as a function of engagement of the screws home mechanism of the knee.

13. What is the biomechanical function of the patella in relationship to the joint reaction force at the patellofemoral joint?

The patella serves as a *simple pulley* in much the same way as the fabella posterolaterally* or the sesamoid beneath the metatarsal head of hallux. Tensile forces from the quadriceps muscles are delivered to the patella via the quadriceps tendon and routed to the tibial tubercle

---

*The *fabella,* present in approximately one-fifth of the population, lies at the site of high intersecting tensile stress along the posterolateral corner of the knee joint in the lateral head of the gastrocnemius muscle. Biomechanically it serves as a pulley to redirect forces and equalize stress along the posterior lateral knee joint capsule.

via the patellar ligament. In the process of transferring this extensor force the patella sustains compressive forces to its superior and inferior surfaces from the quadriceps tendon superiorly and the patellar ligament inferiorly. The result of these two forces is called the *patellofemoral joint reaction force.* Thus the tensile forces originating in the quadriceps mechanism is converted into compressive patellofemoral joint force.

As the knee flexes and extends, the patellofemoral joint undergoes changes in contact area and hence joint reaction force. Stress is defined as force divided by area over which the force is applied. Thus increased forces will increase the magnitude of stress delivered, while increasing area will decrease stress. The magnitude of these compressive forces approaches zero[57] at full extension of the knee as a function of a quiescent quadriceps muscle group during quiet standing. This is because the forces of both the tendon and ligament are minimal secondary to being in an almost straight line one with the other.[47]

In contrast, progressive amounts of flexion* of the knee joint necessitate increased contractile force output by the quadriceps muscle group to overcome the moment created by body weight. The quadriceps must therefore generate forces that exceed body weight and transmit those forces to the patellofemoral surface. As 90° of knee flexion is approached the patellofemoral compressive joint forces are distributed among both the medial and lateral facets, and consequently minimized by increased patellofemoral contact. Flexion activities such as walking or stair climbing will increase patellofemoral compressive joint forces 0.5 to 3.3 times body weight. Beyond 90°, as in a deep knee bend, stress is narrowly focused along the odd facet and results in patellofemoral compressive joint forces 7 to 8 times normal body weight.[51]† Thus, for a person weighing 170 lbs, about 1190 lb of compressive force are imposed upon the patellofemoral joint during squatting activities.

The patella functions to help distribute the magnitude of patellar forces across as wide a surface as possible along the patellofemoral articulation. The patellar surface must be prepared to sustain forces approximately 500 pounds per square inch. This magnitude of force helps explain why the hyaline cartilage of the patellar surface is the thickest in the human body and may range from anywhere between 3 and 12 mm thick. With the passage of time, the patellofemoral articulating surface sustains forces during normal activity that far exceed body weight and are thus subject to eventual microtrauma and its concomitant degeneration. The early stages of degeneration manifest as cartilage softening known as chondromalacia, and if unabated, progress to patellofemoral osteoarthritis.

14. What other functions does the patella serve?

By virtue of being the intermediary attachment between the quadriceps tendon and the patellar ligament, the patella has the important function of transmitting the quadriceps force to the tibia. In the absence of a patella, a strong contraction of the quadriceps muscle may result in anterior displacement of the femur on the tibia. The patella serves as a retainer for the femur by acting as an osseous bearing surface to prevent anterior femoral displacement.[41] The patella also functions as an osseous shield protecting the anterior aspect of the knee joint. Finally, the patella serves a cosmetic purpose. Patellectomized knees have a flat shape of the femoral condyles when the flexed, and this area may be subject to damage should contusion occur.

15. What are the four stages describing histologic change associated with chondromalacia patellae?

Chondromalacia refers to degenerative *softening* of the hyaline cartilage, may occur in any joint in the body, but has a predilection for the posterior patella. This predilection for the patellofemoral joint is extremely common to all peoples except the Chinese in whom the condition rarely presents.[54] Gradations of articular cartilage pathology (Fig. 40-6) begin with (stage I) localized softening (malacia) and inflammation of the articular joint surface known as patellofemoral chondrosis corresponding to no visible arthroscopic damage.[6] This leads to eventual breakdown of the surface covering of the hyaline cartilage known as the lamina splendens,‡ resulting in loss of water content and loss of resilience.[50,71] Breakdown is frequently viewed as blister-

---

*In the closed kinetic chain, but not when sitting with the leg hanging freely over the edge of a table or a chair.

†As flexion proceeds, the force upon the patella gradually increases as the quadriceps vector becomes more perpendicular. This is not the case regarding the valgus force vector delivered to the patella via the extensor mechanism. In the latter, the lateral force vector gradually increases with increased extension. An inverse relationship may be said to define the relationship between the quadriceps and extensor vectors in relation to the patella throughout the arc of flexion and extension.

---

‡This refers to the *gliding zone* of the articular cartilage. The chondrocyte cells comprising the *lamina splendens* lie horizontally, and are shiny and perfectly smooth.

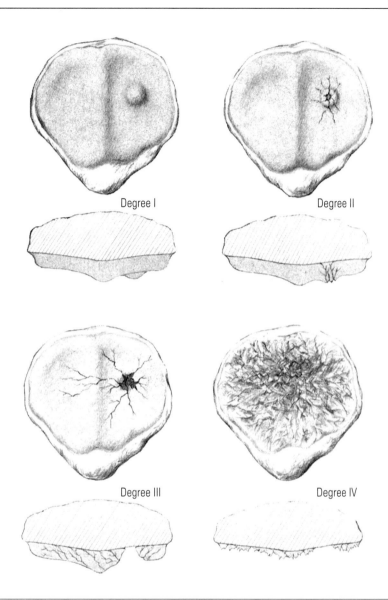

FIG. 40-6 *Degree I,* Softening and blistering. *Degree II,* Fissures. *Degree III,* Fissures widen and deepen to extend to underlying subchondral bone, and have the appearance of crabmeat. *Degree IV,* Patellofemoral arthrosis—total destruction of articular cartilage known as full cartilage defects in which the subchondral bone is exposed. (From Peterson L, Renstrom P: *Sports injuries: their prevention and treatment,* Chicago, 1983, Yearbook Medical Publishers.)

like marring of the hyaline surface. These blisters progress to fissures (stage II) that gradually widen and deepen, and take on the appearance of crabmeat (*crabmeat changes*-stage III). Degeneration finally progresses to full cartilage defects in which *denudation* (i.e., extend down to) of the underlying subchondral bone has occurred. The final stage is really one of osteoarthritis as the subchondral bone has become exposed. At this point in the degenerative process articular cartilage has been stripped away and bone on bone rubbing, or *eburnation* occurs. Dead cartilage may calcify and form spurs, or it may break off and become lodged in surrounding synovium causing inflammation and pain. Unlike chondromalacia, radiographs of patellofemoral arthritis show narrowing of joint space, sclerosis, as well as spurring.[74]

16. What is the etiology of chondromalacia?

The etiology of *chondromalacia* is controversial and may be traced to 1 of 4 schools of thought. Anatomic malalignment of the patella in the femoral sulcus leads to oblique lateral tracking that may focus pressure over the medial aspect of the posterior patellar surface and cause pain.[33,60] This results from an architectural asymmetry between the trochlea of the distal femur as well as the medial and lateral underside of the patella that favors lateral glide. An additional factor may stem from a low lateral femoral condyle. A second explanation ascribes the disorder to derive from an anatomic imbalance in the static ligamentous as well as muscular mediolateral restraints in favor of excess lateral pressure, again causing pain from excessive medial patellar wear.[55] A third explanation implicates quadriceps dysplasia or atrophy, particularly of the medial side, resulting in a dynamic imbalance of the quadriceps extensor mechanism causing lateral tracking due to lateralis overpull.[20] A fourth explanation involves the biochemistry of the underside of the patella, and ascribes a cascade of events initiated by surface changes progressing to more significant defects.[11] Chondromalacia may also occur following trauma from a direct blow to the patella, for example, during a motor vehicle accident in which the patella is forcefully and suddenly pressed against an automobile dashboard.[65]

17. How does imbalance in the quadriceps extensor mechanism and/or the static patellar stabilizers contribute to degenerative wear of the patellar surface?

The confluence of anatomic contractile and noncontractile structures on the patella play a key role in offsetting the laterally displaced valgus force superiorly derived from the quadriceps tendon. Dynamic patellar stabilizers are particularly active when the loaded knee moves into extension. The most significant dynamic stabilizer of the patellofemoral joint is the *vastus medialis obliquus* (VMO), as the horizontal fiber orientation of this muscle restricts excessive lateral movement of the kneecap.

In addition to VMO, other dynamic influences upon patellar stabilization include the pes anserinus[46] indirectly, medial hamstring muscles medially and the iliotibial band and short head of biceps laterally through its relationship to the iliotibial tract.[83] Static stabilizers include the medial and lateral patellar retinacula. Injury and atrophy, or tightness of either side will alter the dynamic balance of the patellofemoral joint and result in overpull and maltracking. Tightness of the medial structures favors lateral compression and subluxation, whereas tightness of the medial structures favors medial compression and subluxation.[10] The magnitude of excessive soft tissue on the lateral side is more likely to develop shortening or contracture of the lateral structures and subsequent overpull of the medial structures in the individual, such as the arm-chair executive, who must spend much time in the knee flexed posture. The domination of laterally displaced forces may contribute to patellofemoral joint dysfunction and cause a tracking deficit of the joint. Ultimately, this may culminate in anterior knee pain syndrome,[19,89] with a predilection for lateral subluxation or lateral compression causing wear of the medial border of the medial facet.

18. What is the relationship between the predominantly valgus force afforded the patellofemoral joint by the osseous, dynamic, and static patellar stabilizers and excessive patellar cartilage stress?

Both osseous and dynamic factors favor lateral instability of the normal patellofemoral joint. From an osseous perspective, the incline (slope) of the lateral aspect of the femoral sulcus angle is less acute than the medial side. This results in a diminished surface contact between the patella and femur and is magnified in those individuals with a femoral sulcus angle approaching 150°. Moreover, the location of the central ridge along the posterior patellar surface is asymmetrically located lateral to midline in the normal patella. This asymmetry contributes to a geometric fit into the asymmetric basin of the femoral sulcus that, from a geometric standpoint, is poorly designed for stability despite any anterior abutment provided by a prominent anterior lateral femoral condyle. Instead, the combined asymmetries of the patellar and femoral surfaces magnify, rather than cancel, the likelihood for lateral patellar instability. This effect is magnified in the event of an excessively shortened lateral retinaculum or atrophy of the VMO secondary to immobilization following injury or surgery.

The *quadriceps mechanism* represents the dynamic component contributing to patellar imbalance. The line of pull of the quadriceps muscles parallels the shaft of the femur (i.e., with the anatomic axis and not with the mechanical axis). Thus the combined force vector of the rectus femoris, vastus intermedius, and vastus lateralis pull represents a significant overpull that overwhelms the medialis vector and thereby favoring lateral distraction of the patella. The tibiofemoral joint, however, is normally in slight valgus with respect to the joint line due to the longer medial femoral condyle.[92] This directly impacts upon the direction of the quadriceps force vector and imparts a lateral or valgus force on the patella away from the midline. This effect is magnified by the presence of *hypoplasia* of the oblique head of the vastus medialis, a common problem in patellofemoral disorders of children and adolescents.[85]

Thus normal patellofemoral mechanics is characterized by a lateral force vector that pulls the patella laterally when the knee joint is fully extended causing the patella to sit lateral to the trochlea.[73] This inherent imbalance in the quadriceps mechanism favoring lateral patellar tracking derives from osseous, dynamic, and ligamentous factors that may lead to excessive cartilage stress[21] and wear of the medial facet, or lateral patellar subluxation.[90]

19. How do laterally dominating forces at the patellofemoral joint cause excessive wear of the extreme medial facet?

If the patella is pulled too far laterally during loaded knee extension the posterior articular surface is pulled such that it predominantly articulates with the lateral femoral condyle. Because of the asymmetrical surface topography of the patellar articular surface, a valgus force applied to the entire patella will cause it to undergo excessive rotation in the transverse plane, bringing the odd medial facet into contact with the femoral condyle. This occurs during loaded knee extension, although the extreme medial facet, under more balanced conditions typically undergoes contact during extreme flexion of the knee. Because stress is defined as force per unit area, the enormous quadriceps-extensor forces that come to bear upon the small medial facet are amplified. With repetition and time, the thick hyaline cartilage of the medial facet[28] is worn away and the capacity of the relatively weak subchondral bone beneath the medial facet is exceeded by the loads imposed. Trabecular microfracturing occurs and incites a low-grade, painful inflammatory response. Trabecular breakdown is often focused along the medial border of the medial facet that separates the medial facet from the extreme medial odd facet. Despite the fact that articular cartilage is thickest along this border, the effect of rotation results in shear stress delivered to this juncture that further enhances the degenerative process.[65,90]

20. What is patellar tilt and how does it increase stress to the medial odd patellar facet?

Discussion of patellar tilt must be prefaced by an analysis of the static patellar stabilizers (Fig. 40-7). The tendinous expansions of the medial and lateral vasti insert onto the medial and lateral aspects of the patella and are termed the *medial* and *lateral patellar retinacula*.[65] Secondary transverse thickenings (condensations) of the superior retinacula are anatomically discernible as the *patellofemoral ligaments,* whereas oblique condensations of the inferior retinacula are termed the *patellotibial ligaments*. The patellofemoral ligaments originate from the epicondylar[64] and condylar[91] protuberances of the femur and insert into the superomedial and superolateral facets[91] of the patella, respectively. The function of the retinacular ligaments is to centralize patellar tracking. Although the medial restraints oppose lateral patellar displacement, the lateral restraints oppose medial patellar displacement.

On the lateral side, static stabilization of the patellofemoral joint is provided by the lateral retinaculum augmented by support from interdigitation of the ilio-

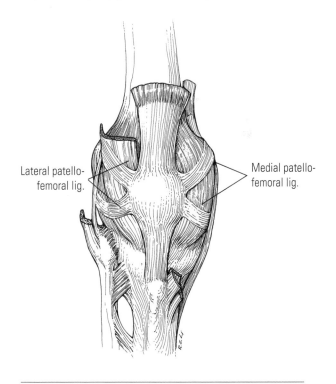

Lateral patello-
femoral lig.

Medial patello-
femoral lig.

FIG. 40-7 The *patellofemoral ligaments* are comprised of medial and lateral patellofemoral and patellotibial ligaments. (From Tria AJ, Klein KS: *An illustrated guide to the knee,* New York, 1992, Churchill Livingstone.)

tibial band known as the *iliopatellar band* as well as the lateral *meniscopatellar ligament.*[19,40] Beneath these are found an even deeper layer of supporting ligamentous structures namely, the transverse band, patellar tibial band, and the epicondylar patellar ligament.[21] The lateral meniscopatellar and patellotibial band provide inferior support to the patella. These lateral structures, by virtue of their iliotibial band and lateral intermuscular septal attachment, passively draw the patella posteriorly and laterally during knee flexion.[89] In contrast, the medial side restraints are characterized by a paucity of structures that include the vastus medialis oblique muscle and two capsular condensations known as the *patellofemoral* and medial *meniscopatellar ligaments.* These ligaments insert into the patella and attach to the femoral condyles and medial meniscus, respectively. The medial patellofemoral ligament may be substantial and comprise a formidable checkrein to lateral displacement whereas in some individuals it may be thin.[73]

The ligamentous imbalance between the medial and lateral retinacula has clinical implications with regard to patellar tilt,[7] and may be of particular clinical significance in the individual who spends much of their time in the sitting position. As the retinacula are tensed during knee flexion, the tug of war on the patella between the medial and lateral retinacula favors the lateral side as it is more heavily reinforced with static and dynamic interdigitations. Tightness of the lateral structures may result in lateral tilting of the patella, such that excessive stress is delivered to the medial side of the articulating surface as it abuts against the lateral femoral articulating surface. This causes abnormal positioning of the patella characterized by excessive lateral glide and external rotation of the patella with respect to its inferior pole. Moreover, the disproportionate articulation of the wider lateral retropatellar surface and central ridge with the distal femur has the effect of levering the medial patella upward such that it appears more prominent. If a line extending from the lateral articular patellar facet is parallel to or converges with a line from the lateral condyle of the patellofemoral groove, an abnormal condition exists and is indicative of increased pressure.[43]

21. Which areas of the patellar surface typically experience wear associated with chondromalacia?

The pathologic areas of degenerative wear are located in a *horizontal zone*[91] across the patellar facets, with the primary area being the *medial border of the medial facet.* Ironically, as this area corresponds to the thickest

articular cartilage in the body (0.08 cm),[2] this area is most prone to deficiency of nutrients from adjacent synovium as well as being vulnerable to repetitive shearing stress.[21] Cartilage is less resistant than bone in attenuating the destructive effects of shear and torsional stress. The secondary area of degenerative wear occurs on the lateral facet, and a lesser area exists between the two facets along the vertical medial (i.e., central ridge)[91] located just lateral to midline and separating the two halves of the articulating patellar surface.

22. What is the effect of excess or deficiency of pronation at the subtalar joint upon patellar facet wear?

The presentation of chondromalacia is often accompanied by a pronated foot.[37,38] To understand the relationship between pronation and patellofemoral wear, it is necessary to appreciate the significance of synchronized joint motion, particularly transverse plane rotation of the tibia. When the subtalar joint pronates during weight bearing, the tibia rotates internally. In contrast, subtalar joint supination causes external rotation. Rotation at the knee joint is attributable to the difference in femoral condylar length (screw-home mechanism). In the foot, rotation occurs as a function of the subtalar and transverse tarsal joints. The connecting link between these proximal and distal sources of rotation is the tibial shaft spanning from the knee to the ankle. Concerted synchronous function of these two sources of rotation is obligatory for normal function. The talus and tibia always rotate together. Excessive pronation imparts internal torque on the tibial shaft at a time when the knee is externally rotating, as during engagement of the screw-home mechanism during knee extension. The confluence of these two opposing torques disrupts patellofemoral mechanics such that the medial patellar facet is excessively compressed along the width of the lateral femoral condyle beyond the articular area on the lateral trochlear facet. With repetition and the passage of time, this results in wearing down of the patellar articular surface as well as stretching the static and dynamic medial patellar stabilizers. Overpronation may therefore be implicated as contributory patellar maltracking and culminate in patellofemoral arthritis and/or subluxation.

Similarly, a subtalar joint that shows inadequate pronation is dominated by excessive external rotation of the talus and hence the distal tibia. Such a rigid foot shows an inability to absorb the ground reaction forces following heel strike. The resultant external torsion is imparted proximally along the tibial shaft to the knee at a time when the knee internally rotates. Immediately following heel strike, the knee joint disengages the screw-home mechanism and internally rotates into tibiofemoral flexion. The opposing torques are absorbed by the largest adjacent structure to their point of confluence at the proximal tibia—the patellofemoral joint. In contrast to the over-pronated foot, the excessively supinated foot may theoretically cause lateral patellar wear and medial patellar subluxation.

23. What is the effect of patella alta or baja upon patellar instability or pain?

The vertical orientation of the patella may be abnormally high (alta) or low (baja or infera). *Patella alta* represents a disruption of the knee extensor mechanism because of an abnormally high-riding patella on the femur both during standing and sitting postures. Patella alta results from *patellar tendon disease* that may include tendinitis or even partial rupture of the *infrapatellar tendon* (patellar ligament) at the patella bone-patellar tendon junction (i.e., the proximal posterior portion of its origin). Patella alta is but a symptom of chronic overloading of the knee extensor mechanism. Midsubstance patellar injury or distal failure may also occur. Patella alta may also result from stretching or tearing of the patellar retinaculum bilaterally.

The vertical position of the patella is radiographically determined by a comparison of patellar length with patellar tendon length. The length these two determinants is normally equivalent in a 1:1 ratio. An increase in ligament length greater than 20% results in abnormal patellar height due to an uncovering of the fat pad characteristic of patella alta (see Fig. 38-1), whereas a lower ratio indicates patella baja.[30] Both extremes of patellar vertical posture have potentially adverse consequences.

Normally, the patella lies above and between the femoral condyles and is in contact with the suprapatellar fat pad in the extended knee. As the knee flexes, tension in the quadriceps tendon and ligamentum patellae compress the patella against the femoral condyle. As both bony surfaces are well covered with cartilage, there is a happy marriage of articulation.

However, in patella alta the patella rides upward, over, and beyond the cartilaginous femoral surface and lies against cortical bone. This may lead to patellofemoral arthritis, whereas the resultant ligamentous laxity may predispose lateral patellar subluxation and dislocation.[84] During clinical assessment for patellar height, patella alta typically presents as the so-called *grasshopper* or *frog eyes*[30] in which the patellae are

pointed toward the ceiling, and, frequently tilted laterally. The opposite presentation of *squinting patellae,* in which the patellae face inward, is characterized by patella baja. A low riding patella may cause anterior knee pain due to increased patellofemoral contact force. This is because the patella sits lower in the trochlear groove such that bony contact occurs earlier as the knee is flexed.[30,19]

24. What are the signs and symptoms associated with chondromalacia?

The hallmark of chondromalacia is vague aching or soreness of insidious onset in the vicinity of the anterior aspect of the patella or adjacent to the patella and often increased with activity. *Pain* is most commonly present on the undersurface (i.e., retropatellar surface) or underneath (i.e., retropatellar) the patella, most often at the medial facet.[6] Pain is provoked by periods of prolonged knee flexion, such as sitting in a theater or following a long automobile drive or pushing the clutch during driving,[87] kneeling, climbing or descending stairs, or hill running. Typically, walking downhill will be more painful owing to more compressive force acting on the patellofemoral joint. There may be an antalgic gait observed on the affected side.[91]

Retropatellar *crepitus* upon extension or flexion is a common finding in patients with chondromalacia, although the degree of crepitus does not correlate with the magnitude of chondromalacia present. Crepitus is often found in the normal knee[56] and should not be the basis for diagnosis because, without concomitant pain, swelling, or giving way, it may not be significant.[77] Mild swelling of the knee may also be present. Stiffness is often present after sitting.[6] The patient may also have a subjective feeling of instability or giving way owing to reflex inhibition of the quadriceps when ascending or descending stairs or when walking down an incline.[53]

Signs that typically present in patients with chondromalacia, include facet *tenderness* (Fig. 40-8) beneath the patella, or over the medial retinaculum, pain upon patellar compression, or during resisted knee extension from 30° of knee flexion, mild *effusion, excessive patellar mobility,* a *positive apprehension sign, squinting patella, patella alta,* and *quadriceps muscle atrophy.* The latter is the most consistent sign in patellofemoral pain and instability. As little as 20 to 30 ml of saline experimentally injected into knees to simulate mild effusion has been shown to inhibit the VMO.[77,94] Even small reductions in girth measurements as little as 1 cm represent significant quadriceps *atrophy.*[15] *Loss of tone* of the VMO muscle is best assessed by placing a hand or

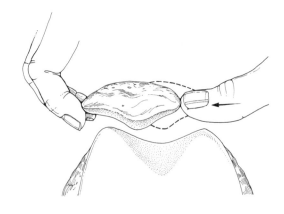

FIG. 40-8 Checking for medial and lateral facet tenderness. Note that tenderness may be related to structures other than patellar surfaces beneath the examining finger. (From Scuderi GR, McCann PD, Bruno PJ: *Sports medicine: principles of primary care,* St Louis, 1997, Mosby.)

towel in the popliteal space with the patient supine on the examining table with the knees extended. Observation of the quadriceps during a quadriceps setting exercise may give the appearance of an adequate VMO contraction, whereas firm palpation during the exercise may reveal a soft, ineffective muscle mass.[36] *Dysplasia* of VMO is revealed by asking the patient to extend his or her knee while in the sitting position. A dimple will become readily apparent where the VMO should normally be owing to the greater than 55° pinnation angle of insertion for the VMO. This dimple may be palpated medially. The vastus lateralis is often hypertrophied and may show a *hyperactive electromyographic* pattern.[70]

25. What is the differential diagnosis?

The temptation to cut corners and proceed directly to a diagnosis of patellofemoral pain is common. This diagnostic trap represents a significant clinical error and must be avoided. As with every condition facing the clinician, there is no substitute for a complete history, physical examination, radiographic evaluation, and systematic differential diagnosis before starting the treatment regimen.[92] This is especially so owing to the multifactoral cause of patellofemoral pain syndrome.

- *Plica syndrome.* Synovial plica (see Chapter 47) are embryologic remnants presenting as folds of tissue adjacent to the patella. They are a rare source of pain

and dysfunction at the knee and may present a challenge to differentiating from chondromalacia. Similar to the latter, synovial plica may prove symptomatic and manifest as knee stiffness following sitting with the knee bent for any length of time. Stiffness may be experienced when attempting to get up out of this position. In plica syndrome this occurs because the plica is pulled tightly over the femoral condyles when the knee is flexed for any great length of time. The key, however, to differentiating between plica and chondromalacia derived pain is by historically determining when the patient experiences pain. Pain *during* activity is generally seen with patellar tracking abnormalities such as chondromalacia or patellar instability, whereas pain *after* activity is typical of inflammatory disorders such as synovial plica irritation.[23,92]

- *Fat pad inflammation.* Fat pad inflammation, or fibrosis, is a relatively common problem contributing to inferior knee pain in patients who have had previous knee surgery or in those who play sports or engage in vocations that directly traumatize this area. Injury to the fat pad may have caused bleeding at the time of initial trauma which, over time leads to fat pad (enlargement and) fibrosis. Pain is located immediately adjacent to the patellar ligament and stems from the richly innervated fat pad. If fibrosis is extensive, as it may be following several knee surgeries or severe trauma to this site, the retropatellar tendon bursa as well as the infrapatellar tendon will eventually scar down to the proximal tibia. This will significantly alter the extensor mechanism mechanics and produce patella baja. Patients with an irritated infrapatellar fat pad stand with their knees locked back and typically exacerbate pain upon knee extension.[73] Radiologically, the patella appears to descend lower and lower until it almost rests on the anterior aspect of the tibial plateau.

- *Pes anserine bursitis.* The pes anserinus (see Fig. 39-5) represents the confluence of the sartorius, gracilis, and tendinosis muscles of the thigh on the anteromedial proximal tibia. The triple redundancy from the anterior, medial, and posterior thigh musculature serves as a buttress to excessive valgus force to the knee, assists the anterior cruciate ligament and the popliteus muscle in preventing excessive external knee rotation, and assists the VMO in providing centralized patellar tracking. Chondromalacia may be differentiated from anserine bursitis by the location of tenderness.[82] Chondromalacia presents an anterior knee pain, especially when the patella is firmly compressed against the femur. Pes anserine bursitis is characterized by medial knee pain 2 to 4 cm below the joint line.[49]

- *Patellofemoral osteoarthritis.* Patellofemoral osteoarthritis represents the end sequelae of chondromalacia and presents with symptoms similar to chondromalacia. However, the articular surface involvement is more advanced with subchondral bone exposure and often has a poorer prognosis.[91] Unlike chondromalacia, radiographs of patellofemoral osteoarthritis show narrowing of the joint space, scleroses, and spurring.[73] These patellofemoral osteophytes typically form on the marginal areas of the femur and may be palpated during physical examination and viewed on infrapatellar radiographs. These osteophytes may result in catching and popping sensations from synovial catching, entrapment, and irritation from these bone spurs. Patellofemoral arthritis may show a relatively short onset following traumatic injury or may have a more insidious onset in patients with long standing patellofemoral complaints. The latter typically occurs in patients who endure abnormal forces to the knee, such as may be incurred from rough sports or heavy work, over many years.

The differential diagnosis of patellofemoral pain must also include ligamentous injury, tumors such as osteoid osteoma of the patella, inflammatory or degenerative arthritis, osteochondritis dissecans of the medial femoral condyle, Sinding-Larsen-Johansson syndrome, collateral and cruciate ligamentous injury, synovitis of the knee joint, high lumbar disc pathology, patellar fracture, patellar tendinitis or prepatellar bursitis, retropatellar bursitis, and pes anserine bursitis.[2,6,33,45,75]

26. What is patellar overload syndrome?

During childhood, growth increases steadily until the onset of puberty, when hormonal factors set off a tremendous increase in the rate of growth.[42,68] Rapidly growing adolescents may show a growth differential between the rate of growth of bone and adjacent soft tissue. At the knee, the rapid longitudinal skeletal growth outstrips the rate of growth of the adjacent soft tissues and results in tightness of the quadriceps and hamstring muscles. In *patellar overload syndrome,* tightness of the quadriceps causes tightness throughout the extensor mechanism as well as the medial and lateral patellar retinacula. This results in increased contact pressure between the patella and femur during knee flexion and may cause irritation. Rapid growth is sug-

gested by the boy who enters the clinic wearing "high water pants." On visual inspection, muscle tone appears tight as the muscles have not kept pace with bone growth. The child may run with a short stride and slightly flexed knees because of muscle tightness. Straight leg raising scores bilaterally positive for tightness as pain at the distal hamstrings behind the knee.[64] Similarly, a prone knee bend is uncomfortable and may be accompanied by rising buttocks as a substitution strategy. Trauma may also contribute to development of this condition, especially if followed by immobilization. The ensuing disuse may lead to soft-tissue contracture and a tight patellofemoral joint. The child may complain of a "toothache-like" pain over the anterior surface of the knee, particularly over the lateral patellar border. Management includes stretching of the hamstrings and calf musculature while strengthening the quadriceps in the extension range and avoiding acute flexion. Riding a bicycle with an elevated seat stretches both the quadriceps and hamstrings while strengthening the quadriceps and avoiding acute flexion. Eccentric quadriceps strengthening may also prove helpful.[64] An external patellofemoral support may be helpful in protecting the patella from further irritation.

27. What is retropatellar pain syndrome?

Retropatellar pain, parapatellar pain, and patellofemoral stress syndrome all describe an overuse injury characterized by peripatellar pain following acutely or slowly from repetitive knee flexion-extension activities such as jumping, running, or kicking. This type of patellar disorder differs from chondromalacia in that arthroscopic evaluation of the retropatellar surface does not reveal the typical fibrillated cartilage surfaces associated with chondromalacia or degenerative changes following an acute blow to the patella. Instead, the articular surface is smooth and without irregularity. In contrast, the patient shows many of the same signs and symptoms as chondromalacia, as well as presenting with positive malalignment of the lower extremity such as increased Q angle, or dysplasia of the VMO. The exact pathologic mechanism that produces pain in patellofemoral stress syndrome is unknown. Some authorities maintain that the pain occurs from stretching of the parapatellar retinaculum as the patella tracks laterally.[22] Others maintain that pain is secondary to increased forces on the retropatellar cartilage (minus cartilage softening) causing pressure on the subchondral bone below and, hence, pain.[31] Management is similar to that of chondromalacia.

28. What radiographs are appropriate when evaluating the patellofemoral joint?

Radiographs will help to rule out arthritic involvement, the presence of fractures or tumors, and the visualization of any malalignment. Roentgenographic views should include an anteroposterior standing view, a lateral view in 30° to 45° of knee flexion, and a patellar axial view at approximately 30° and 60° of knee flexion.[19] Visualization permits the following determinations to be made: (1) the relationship of the patella to the knee joint from an anterior/posterior perspective to determine presence of patellar tilt by gauging patellar orientation. Conclusions about the presence of lateral subluxation, however, may only be drawn if the contralateral asymptomatic knee does not have a similar orientation.[36] (2) Measurement of patellar height and relative patellar height from a lateral view to determine if patella alta is present[4]; and (3) measurement of sulcus angle.[36,60] The infrapatellar, or sunrise, view is helpful as it best demonstrates the patellofemoral articulation. The presence of a shallow notch or particular low lateral femoral condyle offers much less of a sulcus available for centralized patellar tracking.[23,36,92] Radiographic evaluation is also helpful in ruling out avulsion fracture, and secondary patellar ossification center at the superolateral aspect of the patella. MRI enhances evaluation of cartilage on the posterior aspect of the patella and is useful in confirming diagnosis of patellofemoral subluxation.

29. What physical therapy is appropriate in management of patellofemoral dysfunction?

Approximately 95% of patients with patellofemoral pain improve following a conservative treatment approach. The initial goals of patellofemoral dysfunction management are to reduce pain, diminish atrophy, and improve function. No one program will suit all patients. Rather, the rehabilitation program should be based upon the clinician's examination and tailored to the specific needs of each patient. Exercises comprise the first line of defense in patellofemoral dysfunction and should not be substituted with bracing or medication alone. A multifaceted approach to management of chondromalacia and instability is advocated as being more likely to address the many aspects of patellofemoral dysfunction. The key to patellar realignment is strengthening the VMO as it is the only direct dynamic medial stabilizer during knee extension in which valgus forces dominate and attempt to abduct the patella laterally. Thus the focus of early rehabilitation is geared toward VMO strengthening, while keeping compressive forces on the patellofemoral joint to a minimum. Although many rehabilitation protocols emphasize the quadriceps muscle, the literature also supports a hamstring protocol[13] of strengthening as a therapeutic regimen of patellofemoral rehabilitation. The absence of patellofemoral symptoms is the essential guide to determining the rate of progression in the therapeutic regime. As the patient's pain and swelling reduce, and range of motion and strength increase, higher level activities are indicated. Weight loss in the obese patient is an essential ingredient in the overall rehabilitation of patellofemoral pain.

- *Strengthening.* The key to realignment of the patella in the femoral sulcus is strengthening of the entire quadriceps group, and the vastus medialis oblique in particular. Strengthening exercises comprise the primary treatment approach in patellofemoral dysfunction. The traditional mode of strengthening exercises has been pain-free quadriceps exercises, which are intended to strengthen the VMO.[39] This may be accomplished by performing *straight leg raising exercises* (Fig. 40-9) and *isometric quadriceps sets in terminal*

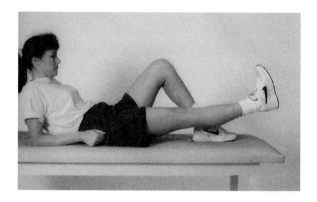

FIG. 40-9 *Straight leg raising* activates the hip flexor muscles. The patient tightens the quadriceps muscles and holds for 2 seconds, and then lifts the entire lower limb until the heel is some 6 to 8 inches above the mat. The extremity is held in that posture for 2 seconds, and then lowered for 2 seconds. This exercise may be repeated for two sets of ten repetitions. As the patient progresses, resistance may be added in the form of a cuff weight at the ankle. Weight until three repetitions of ten are accomplished. Weight may be progressively added and increased every 2 to 3 days as the patient tolerates the increased weight. The goal is to attempt to lift up to one-third of body weight until three repetitions of ten are accomplished. (From Brotzman SB: *Clinical orthopaedic rehabilitation,* St Louis, 1996, Mosby.)

extension (Fig. 40-10). Moreover, these exercises are often performed in various degrees of hip rotation and adduction so that a stronger contraction of the VMO may be recruited by way of contractile overflow from a D1 or D2 proprioceptive neuromuscular facilitation (PNF) technique.[88]

However, research suggests that straight leg raises and isometric quad sets are not exercises specific for strengthening the VMO. The VMO has been shown not to be the primary extensor in the last 15° of extension, and is rather active throughout the range of knee motion. In contrast, other studies have shown the opposite, namely that the VMO is most active during terminal knee extension.[19] Conflicting data as to the selectivity of VMO contraction supports the need to design therapeutic programs for the specific needs of the patient and to adjust the program when appropriate. Certainly, the advantage of working the quadriceps muscles during the last 30° of knee extension includes minimizing patellofemoral joint contact forces. Electromyographic analysis of the quadriceps muscle during varying degrees of hip rotation has not been shown to increase muscle activity during isometrics or straight leg raising, and may not support the use of PNF patterns. Thus while traditional resisted exercises in the painless range of motion may

prove beneficial, they are not specific to strengthening of the VMO; consequently, recovery time may be extended.

Short arc knee extension is usually performed in the open chain mode with the patient extending the knee against gravity from 0° to 30° of extension. Known as the *short arc quadriceps exercise,* these exercises are incorporated into the treatment regimen once the patient can tolerate 2 pounds of resisted straight leg raising. With the patient in the long sitting posture, a firm bolster is placed under the knee to flex it to approximately 40° to 45°. The patient extends the knee and raises the heel for 10 seconds and slowly lowers it.[86] Knee extension is accompanied by simultaneous cocontraction of the hamstring muscles in which the back of the thigh is pressed into the pad. The patient may complete two sets of ten repetitions. Patients usually tolerate terminal knee extension exercises early in the rehabilitative program, possibly due to low compressive forces at the patellofemoral joint (i.e., only 1½ times body weight).[68] By keeping the knee in complete extension, the patella is not in full contact with the femoral condyles. At this range the patella sits above the slopes of the femoral sulcus in a bed of fat in the (supra) trochlear fossa, resulting in near zero patellofemoral forces.[19] Terminal knee extension exercises may also be performed in the closed kinetic mode by using surgical tubing or varied resistance Thera-Band (Hygenic Corp., Akron, OH). The patient is instructed to stand with the tubing behind the knee and attached to an immovable object behind them. The knee is slowly flexed while the foot maintains ground contact. The knee is subsequently allowed to extend against the chosen resistance. Alternately, the patient may perform minisquats while leaning his or her back against a wall.

Straight leg raises may be performed in a variety of postures including supine, prone, or side lying on either side. Hip abduction of the involved limb in the lateral decubitus position, according to some authorities, may be contraindicated because strengthening of the dynamic lateral thigh muscles may further tighten the already tight lateral structures and thereby prove counterproductive to patellar tracking.[88] In contrast, ipsilateral hip adduction (Fig. 40-11) may be helpful in recruitment of the VMO. Most of the oblique fibers of the VMO arise off the tendon of the adductor magnus and off the tendon of the adductor longus muscle.[5] Whereas selective targeting of VMO contraction may not be achieved via terminal knee exten-

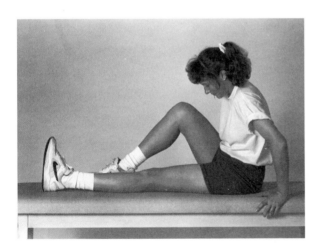

FIG. 40-10 *Quadriceps setting exercises* involve actively contracting the quadriceps muscle, while dorsiflexing the foot and toes and pushing the heel away from the body. This helps initiate contraction of the vastus medialis obliquus, which is held maximally for 10 seconds, followed by 5 seconds of relaxation, and repeated for two sets of ten. (From Brotzman SB: *Clinical orthopaedic rehabilitation,* St Louis, 1996, Mosby.)

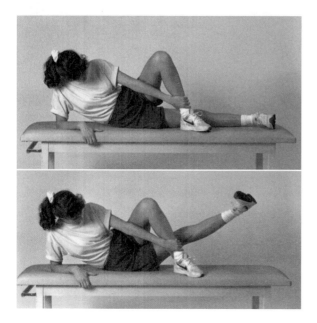

FIG. 40-11 Isometric right hip adduction may be performed with maximal contraction, which are held for 10 seconds and relaxed for 5 seconds. (From Brotzman SB: *Clinical orthopaedic rehabilitation*, St Louis, 1996, Mosby.)

sion or straight leg raising, the electrical activity of the VMO is significantly greater than that of the vastus lateralis during ipsilateral adductor strengthening. This provides the clinician with the ability to selectively target the VMO for strengthening. Isotonic adduction exercises may be incorporated by simple straight leg raising in the side-lying posture, or via the adduction ball squeeze performed supine, sitting, or standing. The advantage of performing this exercise in the closed kinetic mode leads to recruitment of the other knee stabilizers to maintain this position. An advantage of performing this exercise in the standing position is that the VMO is strengthened with minimal compressive forces at the patellofemoral joint. Resistive isotonic hip adduction is possibly the hardest exercise for the patient to accomplish, and the most common error made is lack of full knee extension. If the knee is not extended, then adductor tendinitis may occur as progressive resistance (with a cuff at the ankle) is obtained.[27]

As symptoms subside and increases are made in range and strength, higher level activities are incorporated into the rehabilitation program. Progression to full range of motion activities, low knee squats, and bicycle riding with a low seat may be added as per patient tolerance. Exercises should be designed to suit the particular needs of the athlete so that skill-specific activities are incorporated into the program. Running, lifting, and climbing activities may be added to the program as symptoms permit.[95]

The use of *isokinetics* in the management of patellofemoral dysfunction is now a topic of controversy in rehabilitation. Some authorities are reluctant to advocate use of this modality because of its high compressive forces as slow speeds and its lack of functional application. In contrast, some clinicians report documented success with speeds as low as 20° or 60°.[29]

- *Stretching.* Stretching exercises comprise an integral and important component of the rehabilitation of patellofemoral dysfunction as restrictions in length of both thigh and tibial muscles are directly and indirectly linked to patellar maltracking. This group includes the hamstrings, quadriceps, tensor fascia latae, triceps surae muscles, and the Achilles tendon. It is essential to determine which muscle group(s) are tight so that appropriate stretching may be initiated. Proprioceptive neuromuscular facilitation techniques including contract-relax and reflex inhibition may be helpful in gaining flexibility. The application of passive stretching, soft tissue mobilization, friction massage, moist heat, and ultrasound may be helpful to implementing stretching. Passive stretching may help ease patellofemoral pain by increasing knee joint motion to normal.[45]

- *Orthoses.* The individual with femoral anteversion, external tibial torsion, genu valgus, a laterally placed tibial tubercle, an increased Q angle, a toed-in gait, a longer leg, and pronated feet requires more than an exercise program in the management of their patellofemoral dysfunction. The presence of one or more of these malalignments may contribute to patellofemoral maltracking, facet wear, and instability. When the source of malalignment is the subtalar joint, the use of an arch support and/or heel wedge may minimize the excessive rotation directed proximally to help realign the patella more centrally. For every degree that the foot is supinated, the Q angle decreases 44°.[66] It is thus advantageous to impart supination to the over-pronated foot in the attempt to realign the subtalar joint closer to neutral.[17] The use of soft foot orthotics are particularly effective in decreasing patellofemoral pain. If the hindfoot is postured in valgus, a 5° to 9° medial hindfoot wedge with a 1-mm heel height may be indicated. If the hindfoot is in neutral, then a 0° hind foot wedge, and a 5° medial forefoot wedge with a 1-mm heel height is appropriate.[76]

- *Biofeedback.* Recruitment of the VMO muscle may be enhanced using biofeedback (Fig. 40-12), and consequently reduce the rate of recovery time. The VMO is innervated from a single branch of the femoral nerve and may therefore be activated as a single motor unit. By supplementing a selective strengthening program, the VMO may be consciously targeted for contractile recruitment using tactile cues or an electric stimulator. Normal subjects have a 1:1 ratio of VMO to vastus lateralis strength.[56] Patient with patellofemoral dysfunction fall short of this ratio, with greater vastus lateralis than VMO strength.[95] The patient is instructed to place one hand on the VMO and the other along the vastus lateralis. It is essential to instruct patients in the exact location of these muscles and their function so that they may better understand the technique. Once the patient feels the muscle contracting and relaxing, they are asked to attempt to maintain a VMO contraction while relaxing the vastus lateralis. Positive feedback is imparted to the palm of the patient's hand or may be heard or viewed using an electrical biofeedback unit. In this fashion, *neuromuscular education* allows the reassertion of VMO muscle control while keeping vastus lateralis activity to a minimum.

- *Electrical stimulation.* Patients may show difficulty during the early phases of rehabilitation at producing a voluntary muscle contraction, particularly following surgery. Electrical stimulation may be helpful during the muscle re-education process. High-frequency stimulation of the VMO in conjunction with the patient's own voluntary contraction may prove a helpful adjunct in increasing muscle strength. The use of ice massage before electrical stimulation may increase patient pain tolerance for electric stimulation, and thereby increase a maximum voluntary contraction.[56] When tolerance to electric stimulation is low for desired therapeutic effects the following method may be helpful. A 10-minute period of stimulation at an amplitude between sensory and motor thresholds of the quadriceps femoris muscle group results in an increased tolerance for high amplitude stimulation, which, in turn, results in increased torque production by the quadriceps.[93]

- *Bracing.* The patella brace provides external realignment and thereby reinforces centralization of the pa-

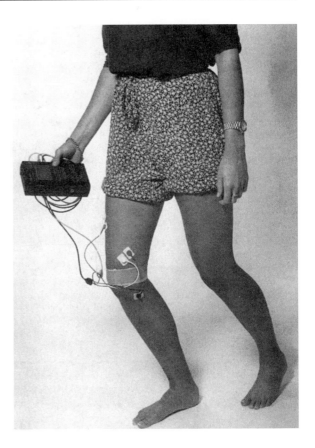

FIG. 40-12 EMG biofeedback of vastus medialis oblique (VMO) muscle to improve quality of contraction. (From Zachazewski JE, Magee DJ, Quillen WS: *Athletic injuries and rehabilitation,* Philadelphia, 1996, WB Saunders.)

tella, leading to better patellar tracking.[56] The patellar brace directs a medial directed force that negates the valgus vector force causing malalignment and allows the patient to perform painless exercises as well as daily functional activities. A brace may also be used as a therapeutic trial in the differential diagnosis of patellofemoral problems.[27] Simply, braces consist of an elastic sleeve with a patellar cutout and a buttress, which may be on the lateral side of the patella or may encircle the entire kneecap while avoiding direct pressure. A makeshift brace is easily fabricated using only felt horseshoes and an ace bandage. The therapist may cut out a horseshoe shaped piece of felt ½ inch thick, and large enough to partially envelop the kneecap with the open side pointing downward. This is then held snugly in place using an Ace bandage; alternatively, it may be covered or sutured

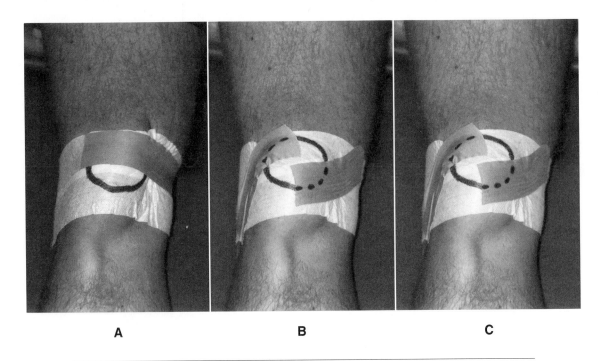

A   **B**   **C**

FIG. 40-13 McConnell taping is based on assessment of patellar position and maltracking. Three abnormal patellar orientations are examined: **A,** patella glide, **B,** patella rotation, **C,** patella tilt. (From Maxey L, Magnusson J: *Rehabilitation of the postsurgical orthopedic patient,* St Louis, 2001, Mosby.)

into an elastic sleeve. Additions of metal struts or hinges are superfluous as they do not help the patellofemoral mechanism and at most, support ligamentous injuries.[95]

The *Levine infra patellar strap* is applied beneath the patella but over the patellar tendon midway between the patella and the tibial tubercle such that it changes the direction of pull of the patellar ligament.[48] The infra patellar strap alters patellofemoral mechanics and relieves pain by slightly elevating the patella. The *Palumbo patella stabilizer* (Dynorthotics, Vienna, VA) uses straps to develop a dynamic medial force to provide improved patellar alignment. It is designed with "live" rubber straps and a pad that provides dynamic tension to the lateral patella. The intent of these dynamic straps is to provide effective tension throughout the range of motion.[69]

The use of bracing provides the patient with the added psychologic benefit that the knee is secure and protected, and may facilitate earlier return to activity as patients often report symptomatic relief using braces. However, if the devices are used for a significant period of time, or as the sole treatment of patellofemoral dysfunction, they may lead to atrophy of the extensor mechanism and aggravation of the problem they are designed to relieve. Thus bracing is secondary to exercise[70] and should always be accompanied by a concurrent exercise program.

- *Taping.* Taping is another means of external support forcing the patella to track medially, thereby decreasing pain and dysfunction. Ms. Jenny McConnell, an Australian physiotherapist, proposed that pain inhibits muscle function and initiated a taping technique that realigns the abnormally positioned patella out of the *glide, tilt,* and *rotation* components that cause pain and lateral tracking (Fig. 40-13). Appropriate taping increases the normal articular surface contact area while minimizing contact over nonarticular areas. With patellofemoral pain relieved, quadriceps muscle training becomes more effective.[56] This was borne out by studies demonstrating improved quadriceps and hamstring torque output as measured by isokinetic testing.[56] Taping is preceded by shaving the knee and covering the anterior knee surface with a water repellent underwrap to protect the skin. Abnormal patellar tilt is corrected by extending the tape from the mid-patellar region to the medial femoral condyle. Abnormal patellar glide is corrected by a second tape placed along the lateral patellar border and pulled across to the medial femoral condyle. Abnormal external rotation of the patella is corrected by placing tape on the distal patellar pole and pulling it such so as to rotate the patella to the opposite patellar direction. Once the VMO is sufficiently re-educated so that it provides an adequate dynamic medial patellar support, the patient is weaned off tape during functional activity. The problems with taping include skin compromise and allergic reaction. The effect on the vastus lateralis may be passively inhibited by the use of firm taping at the superolateral aspect of the knee. Taping may also act to stretch the lateral retinaculum and iliopatellar band, and enhance VMO muscle contraction.

- *Mobilization.* Mobilization of the patella by way of patellar gliding techniques (Fig. 40-14) may be helpful in managing cases of lateral tracking and patella infera. Medial patellar glide are particularly appropriate for stretching the lateral soft tissue structures adjacent to the patella.[25,78]
- *Activity modification.* Certain activities and positions of the knee increase patellofemoral contact stress and pain. Running, biking, and knee flexion above 90° may increase symptoms by way of increasing forces across the patellofemoral joint contact surface. It is essential that the patient be educated about the avoidance of certain activities and positions.
- *Endurance training.* Endurance training is essential to maintenance of the patient's cardiopulmonary sta-

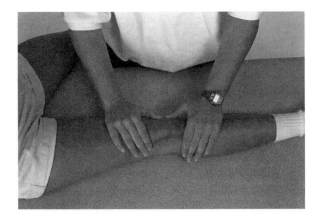

FIG. 40-14 The patella is mobilized medially, laterally, and especially, superiorly. (From Brotzman SB: *Clinical orthopaedic rehabilitation*, St Louis, 1996, Mosby.)

tus and general strengthening, and should be performed with a minimal of patellofemoral compressive stress. Bicycling and swimming are advocated owing to their low impact force upon the lower extremities. Single limb stance bicycling with the involved limb on the floor may be performed. Alternately, patellofemoral joint reaction force may be minimized by using a high saddle position during biking activities.[7] Stair climbing activities may improve endurance, but caution must be exercised against increasing patellofemoral symptoms. The use of *aquatic therapy* may be incorporated into a range of motion, strength, and endurance program. Proprioception activities may include use of the BAPS board (Camp Jackson, MI) by patients with partial or full weight bearing strength, and combine proprioceptive skill with strength and speed (Fig. 40-15). Specific emphasis may be place upon those leg muscles responsible for pronation deceleration. The use of the mini-trampoline is helpful as it combines proprioceptive function with strength, speed, endurance, eccentric, isometric, and concentric loading.[95]

- *Modality.* Modality use is beneficial to the patellofemoral rehabilitative regimen. Both pain and the presence of even slight effusion causes joint distension and inhibits the VMO muscle via a local spinal reflex.[62] Because of this, the reduction of both pain and swelling is essential in reestablishing control of the VMO. The application of cryotherapy in the form of ice is easily applied and effective in reducing pain, inflammation, and swelling.[7] Warm soaks may prove beneficial during the chronic stage.
- *Medication.* Studies have shown that although the use of salicylates retarded cartilage degeneration, steroid accelerated it.[25,78] The retarding effect of salicylates appears beneficial only before setting in of fibrillation changes characteristic of chondromalacia.[12] Phenylbutazone has been found to be helpful in addressing the inflammatory response around the soft tissues of the knee.[3] The use of steroids in reducing the inflammatory response in patellofemoral pain is not popular as the side effects and potential complications of systemic steroids outweigh the potential benefit derived. Local steroid use in the form of intraarticular injection is reserved for patients with advanced osteoarthritis of the tibiofemoral joint rather than chondromalacia.[92] Medications are not to be used as the sole treatment for patellofemoral disease, but only as adjuvant therapy in conjunction with an eclectic rehabilitative approach.

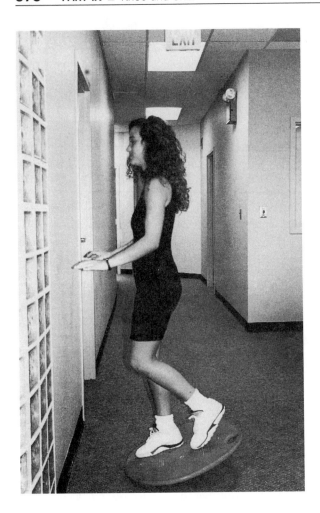

FIG. 40-15 Proprioception with BAPS board. (From Scott WN: *The knee*, St Louis, 1994, Mosby.)

- *Rest.* As many forms of patellofemoral pain result from overuse, rest is recommended as part of the treatment algorithm. Relative rest is recommended and refers to avoiding or modifying the offending activity, or by selection of other activities to reduce symptoms. Complete rest is only recommended in the event of failure of conservative treatment.
- *Patient education.* The patient is educated to avoid prolonged flexion, squatting, kneeling, running, and stair negotiation when possible during the rehabilitative period. One of the most difficult challenges in conservative rehabilitation of patellofemoral dysfunction is patient compliance.[70] The patient with patellofemoral pain my demonstrate high levels of frustration due to the insidious onset of pain rather than a specific traumatic event. It is helpful to the clinician to appreciate the psychologic impact of persistent patellofemoral dysfunction because it will greatly influence the relationship established between the therapist and patient during rehabilitation. It is essential to explain the condition and its causative factors as well as the plan for recovery so that the patient is made into a full participant in his or her own rehabilitation. By allowing the patient to become an active participant in their own therapy, they are empowered with their own healing and thereby motivated to comply with the rehabilitation program.[95]

When dealing with the professional athlete, the therapist should not open the discussion of treatment by telling the patient to cease the pain-provoking activity. Athletes do not seek professional advice to simply to be told to stopping running or playing tennis. These patients already know that stopping their sporting activity will alleviate the problem. Rather, they seek treatment that will allow them to continue their sporting activity despite their limitations. The challenge for the therapist is to devise a rehabilitation protocol that best suits the needs of his or her patient. The more positive aspects of the treatment program should first be presented to the athlete, followed by the gentle introduction of modified rest to the injured area.[23,36,92]

30. What are the surgical options or alternatives to management of recalcitrant patellofemoral pain?

Arthroscopic shaving of the inner patellar surface does little to improve the long-term prognosis as it does not address the cause of patellofemoral pain and dysfunction. The short-term benefits of this procedure include decreased crepitation and synovial effusion. Fifteen months following surgery, fibrocartilage may fill the defect caused by the initial shaving if the subchondral bone is perforated during surgery and if motion is instituted following surgery. This fibrocartilage is not as durable as normal articular cartilage. Because of this, surgical procedures should be reserved for truly recalcitrant cases in which pain interferes with daily activities.[6]

REFERENCES

1. Basmajian JV: Re-education of the vastus medialis: a misconception, *Arch Physical Med Rehab* 51:245-247, 1970.
2. Bentley G, Dowd G: Current concepts of etiology and treatment of chondromalacia patella, *Clin Orthop* 189:209-228, 1984.

3. Black HM, Straughn WR: Use of phenylbutazone in sports medicine: understanding the risks, *Am J Sports Med* 8:270, 1980.

4. Blackburne JS, Peel TE: Measuring patellar height, *J Bone Joint Surg* 59(B):241-242, 1977.

5. Bose K, Kanagasuntheram R, Osman MBH: Vastus medialis oblique: an anatomic and physiological study, *Orthopedics* 39:880-883, 1980.

6. Brody DM: *Clinical symposia: running injuries—prevention and management,* Summit, NJ, 1987, CIBA-GEIGY.

7. Brontzman SB: *Clinical orthopaedic rehabilitation,* St Louis, 1996, Mosby.

8. Caillet R: *Knee pain and disability,* Philadelphia, 1983, FA Davis.

9. Canale ST, Campbell WC: *Campbell's operative orthopaedics,* St Louis, 1998, Mosby.

10. Ceder LC, Larson Rl: Z-plasty lateral retinaculum release for the treatment of patellar compression syndrome, *Clin Orthop* 144: 110-113, 1979.

11. Chrisman OD, Ladenbauer-Bellis IM, Fulkerson JP: The osteoarthritic cascade and associated drug actions, *Arthritis Rheum* 145 (suppl), 1981.

12. Chrisman OD, Snook GA: Studies on the protective effect of aspirin against degeneration of human cartilage: a preliminary report, *Clin Orthop* 56:77, 1968.

13. De Haven DE, Dolan WA, Mayer DJ: Chondromalacia patella in athletes: clinical presentation and conservative management, *Am J Sports Med* 7:5-11, 1979.

14. Devas MB: Stress fractures of the patella, *J Bone Joint Surg* 42B:71, 1960.

15. Doxey GE: Assessing quadriceps femoris muscle bulk with girth measurements in subjects with patellofemoral pain, *J Orthop Sports Phys Ther* 9:5, 1987.

16. Eftimiades J: Anatomy, etiology and treatment of patellofemoral dysfunction examined, *Adv Phys Ther* 1991.

17. Eng JJ, Pierrynowski MR: Evaluation of soft foot orthotics in the treatment of patellofemoral pain syndrome, *Phys Ther* 73(2):62-67, 1993.

18. Ferguson AB, Jr: Elevation of the insertion of the patellar ligament for patellofemoral pain, *J Bone Joint Surg* 64(A):766-771, 1982.

19. Ficat PR, Hungerford DS: *Disorders of the patellofemoral joint,* Baltimore, 1977, Williams & Wilkins.

20. Ficat RP, Philippe J, Hungerford DS: Chondromalacia patellae: a system of classification, *Clin Orthop* 144: 55-62, 1979.

21. Fulkerson JP, Grossling HR: Anatomy of the knee joint lateral retinaculum, *Clin Orthop* 153: 183-185, 1980.

22. Fulkerson JP: Evaluation of the peripatellar soft tissues and retinaculum in patients with patellofemoral pain, *Clin Sports Med* 8(2):197, 1989.

23. Garrick JJ: Anterior knee pain (chondromalacia patellae), *Phys Sports Med* 17(1), January 1989.

24. Goodfellow J, Hungersford DS, Zindel M: Patellofemoral joint mechanics and pathology. I. Functional anatomy of the patellofemoral joint, *J Bone Joint Surg* 58B:287, 1976.

25. Greenfield BH: *Rehabilitation of the knee: a problem-solving approach,* Philadelphia, 1993, FA Davis.

26. Reference deleted.

27. Henry J: Conservative treatment of patellofemoral subluxation, *Clin Sports Med* 8(2):261-278, 1989.

28. Herthing D, Kessler RM: *Management of common musculoskeletal disorders—physical therapy principles and methods,* ed 2, Philadelphia, 1990, JB Lippincott.

29. Hilty BE, Silver RA, Wilkinson JK: The use of the KinCom for the treatment of patellofemoral dysfunction, *Athletic Training* 21:3, 1986.

30. Hughston JC, Walsh WM, Puddu G: *Patellar subluxation and dislocation,* Philadelphia, 1984, WB Saunders.

31. Hunter L, et al: *Common orthopaedic problems of the female athlete,* American Academy of Orthopaedic Surgeons Instructional Course Lectures, vol 31, St. Louis, 1892, Mosby.

32. Reference deleted.

33. Insall JN: Patella pain syndromes and chondromalacia patellae, *Instr Course Lect* 30:342- 356, 1981.

34. Insall JN: *Surgery of the knee,* New York, 1984, Churchill Livingstone.

35. Reference deleted.

36. Jacobson KE, Flandry FC: Diagnosis of anterior knee pain, Hughston Orthopaedic Clinic 8(2), Columbus, GA, April 1989.

37. James SL, Bates BT, Osternig CR: Injuries to runners, *Am J Sports Medicine* 6:40-50, 1978.

38. Jernick S, Heifitz NM: An investigation into the relationship of foot pronation to chondromalacia patellae. In Rinaldi RR, Sabia ML editors: *Sports medicine,* Mt. Kisco, NY, 1979, Futura.

39. Johnson D: Electrical stimulation for treatment of chondromalacia patella, *Clin Management* 4:44-45, 1984.

40. Kaplan EB: Surgical approach to the lateral (peroneal) side of the knee joint, *Surg Gynecol Obstet* 104:346, 1957.

41. Kaufer H: Patellar biomechanics, *Clin Orthop* 144:51-54, 1979.

42. Kempe C, Silver H, O'Brien D: *Current pediatric diagnosis and treatment,* Los Altos, 1984, Lange Medical Publications.

43. Kennedy JC, Alexander LJ, Hayes KC: Nerve supply of the human knee and its functional importance, *Am J Sports Med* 10:329, 1982.

44. Kramer PG: Patella malalignment syndrome: rationale to reduce excessive lateral pressure, *J Orthop Sports Phys Ther* 8(6):301, 1986.

45. Kummel B: The treatment of patellofemoral problems, *Primary Care* 7:217-229, 1980.

46. Larson RL: Problems of the extensor mechanism, *Athletic Training,* 13:4, 1978.

47. Lehinkuhl LD, Smith LK: *Brunstromm's clinical kinesiology,* ed 4, Philadelphia, 1989, FA Davis.

48. Levine J: A new brace for chondromalacia patella and kindred, *Am J Sports Med* 6:137-139, 1978.

49. Lillegard WA, Rucker KS: *Handbook of sports medicine: a symptom oriented approach,* Boston, 1993, Andover Medical Publishers.

50. Lindahl O, Movin A: The mechanics of extension of the knee joint, *Acta Orthop Scand* 38:226, 1967.

51. MacDonald DA, Hutton JF, Kelly IG: Maximal isometric patellofemoral contact force in patients with anterior knee pain, *J Bone Joint Surg* 71(B):296-299, 1989.

52. Magee DJ: *Orthopedic physical assessment,* ed 3, Philadelphia, 1997, WB Saunders.

53. Malek MM, Mangine RE: Patellofemoral pain syndromes: a comprehensive and conservative approach, *J Orthop Sports Phys Ther* 2(3), 1981.

54. Marar BC, Pillay UK: Chondromalacia of the patella in Chinese: a postmortem study, *J Bone Joint Surg* 57A:342, 1973.

55. Marian PP, Caruso I: An electromyographic investigation of subluxation of the patella, *J Bone Joint Surg* 61(B):169-171, 1979.

56. McConnell J: The management of chondromalacia patella: a long term solution, *Australian J Physiother* 32:4, 1986.

57. McLeod WD, Hunter S: Biomechanical analysis of the knee primary functions as elucidated by anatomy, *Phys Ther* 60:12, 1972.

58. McMinn RMH, Hutchings RT: *Color atlas of human anatomy,* Chicago, 1997, Year Book Medical Publishers.

59. Medlar R, Lyne E: Sinding-Larsen-Johansson disease, *J Bone Joint Surg* 60(A):1113, 1978.

60. Merchant AC, Mercer Rl, Jacobsen RH et al: Roentgenographic analysis of patellofemoral congruence, *J Bone Joint Surg* 56(A):1391-1396, 1974.

61. Micheli, LJ: Special considerations in children's rehabilitation programs. In Hunter LY, Funk FJ, Jr editors: *Rehabilitation of the injured knee,* St Louis, 1984, Mosby.

62. Netter FH: *The Ciba collection of medical illustration,* vol 8, Part II, Developmental disorders, tumors, rheumatic diseases and joint replacement, Summit, NJ, 1990, CIBA-GEIGY.

63. Netter FH: *The Ciba collection of medical illustrations,* vol 8 Part III, Musculoskeletal system: trauma, evaluation and management, Summit, NJ, 1993, CIBA-GEIGY.

64. Netter FH: *The Ciba collection of medical illustrations,* Musculoskeletal system, vol 8, Summit, NJ, 1990, CIBA-GEIGY.

65. Nicholas JA, Hershman EB: *The lower extremity and spine in sports medicine,* ed 2, St Louis, 1995, Mosby.

66. Olerud C, Rosenthal Y: Torsion—transmitting properties of the hindfoot, *Clin Orthop* 214:285, 1987.

67. Osgood RB: Lesions of the tibial tubercle occurring during adolescence, *Med Sci J* 148:114, 1903.

68. Outerbridge RE, Dunlop JA: The problem of chondromalacia patellae, *Clin Orthop* 110:177, 1975.

69. Palumbo PM: Dynamic patella brace: a new orthosis in the management of patellofemoral disorders: a preliminary report, *Am J Sports Med* 9:1, 1981.

70. Parkes, A: Ischemic effects of external and internal pressure on the upper limb, *Hand* 5:105, 1973.

71. Perry J, Norwood L, House K: *Knee posture and biceps and semimembranosis muscle action in running and cutting (an EMG study).* Transactions of the 23rd Annual Meeting of the Orthopaedic Research Society, Las Vegas, Feb 1-3, 1977.

72. Pevsner DN, Johnson JR, Blazina ME: The patellofemoral joint and its implication in the rehabilitation of the knee, *Phys Ther* 59:869-894, 1979.

73. Pronsati MP: Australian PT introduces new treatment for patellofemoral pain, *Adv Phys Ther* 16:6-7, 1991.

74. Radin EL: A rational approach to the treatment of patellofemoral pain, *Clin Orthop* 144:107-109, 1979.

75. Reider B et al.: The anterior aspect of the knee joint, *J Bone Joint Surg* 63(A):351-356, 1981.

76. Reiley MA: *Guidelines for prescribing foot orthotics,* Thorofare, NJ, 1995, Slack.

77. Rintala P: Patellofemoral pain syndrome and its treatment in runners, *Athletic Training* 25:2, 1990.

78. Roach JE, Tomblin W, Eyring EJ: Comparisons of the effects of steroids, aspirin, and sodium salicylate on articular cartilage, *Clin Orthop* 106:350, 1975.

79. Royle SG, Noble J, Davies DR et al: The significance of chondromalacic changes on the patella, *Arthroscopy* 7(2):158, 1991.

80. Scapinelli R: Blood supply to the human patella, *J Bone Joint Surg* 49(B): 563, 1967.

81. Scapinelli R: Studies on the vasculature of the human knee joint, *Acta Anat* 70:305, 1968.

82. Schumacher HR, Bomalaski JS: *Case studies in rheumatology for the house officer,* Baltimore, 1990, Williams & Wilkins.

83. Sheath RS: The insertion of the biceps femoris, *J Anat* 89:550-553, 1955.

84. Smillie IS: *Injuries of the knee joint,* London, 1978, Churchill Livingstone.

85. Spencer JD, Hayes KC, Alexander IJ: Knee joint effusion and quadricep reflex inhibition in man, *Arch Phys Med Rehab* 65:171, 1984.

86. Staheli LT: *Fundamentals of pediatric orthopedics,* New York, 1992, Rowen Press.

87. Subotnick SI: *Pediatric sports medicine,* Mt. Kisco, NY, 1975, Futura.

88. Sullivan PE, Markos PD, Minor MD: *An integrated approach to therapeutic exercise, theory and clinical application,* Reston, VA, 1982, Reston.

89. Thabit G III, Micheli LJ: Patellofemoral pain the pediatric patient, *Orthop Clin North Am* 23(4):568, 1992.

90. Townsend PR, Rose RM, Radin EL et al: The biomechanics of the human patella and its implications for chondromalacia, *J Biomech* 10:403-407, 1977.

91. Tria AJ, Klein KS: *An illustrated guide to the knee,* New York, 1992, Churchill Livingstone.

92. Tria AJ, Palumbo RC, Alicea JA: Conservative care for patellofemoral pain, *Orthop Clin North Am* 23(4):545, 1992.

93. Underwood FB et al: Increasing voluntary torque production by using TENS. *J Orthop Sports Phys Ther* 12:3, 1990.

94. Wittenbecker NL, Dinitto LM: Successful Treatment of patellofemoral dysfunction in a dancer, *J Orthop Sports Phys Ther* 10:7, 1989.

95. Zappala FG, Taffel CB: Rehabilitation of patellofemoral joint disorders, *Orthop Clin North Am* 23(4):559, 1992.

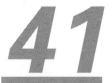

Anterior Knee Instability, Pain, Swelling, and Pseudolocking After Injury

CASE 1: An 18-year-old overweight young woman spent much of her time away from her first desk job, sitting reading books in her favorite easy chair. Once every week she participated in a game of basketball with her parents and siblings. Last week the ball was passed to her beyond her reach, forcing her to suddenly decelerate and pivot on her right foot to prevent the ball from going out of bounds. She felt a sudden pain and sensation that something had "gone out" in her right knee. On inspection, her knee appeared normal although she experienced soreness and tenderness when touching her kneecap. She thought nothing of it and continued playing, only to experience a recurrence later during the game. Later that evening she noted swelling in her right knee.

OBSERVATION   The patient exhibits a high riding, type III patella. A dimple is present where vastus medialis obliquus inserts into the patella, suggesting dysplasia of this muscle. Patellar tilt is present bilaterally. Postural deformities include femoral anteversion, secondary external tibial torsion and bilaterally pronated feet. Both patellae face each other during quiet standing.

PALPATION   Palpation provokes tenderness peripherally, around, and behind the patella. The right lateral patellar retinaculum appears tight when compared with the medial supporting structures. There is no crepitus present.

RANGE OF MOTION   Range of motion is in functional limits bilaterally with the exception of a 5° flexion contracture in both knees.

STRENGTH   Terminal knee extension is mildly weaker than the contralateral knee joint.

FLEXIBILITY   Flexibility reveals bilateral tightness in the hamstrings (particularly the short head of biceps), the tensor fascia latae, and the gastrocnemius muscle groups, right greater than left. Both heel cords are moderately tight.

GIRTH MEASUREMENTS   No effusion present in the right knee. Girth was measured bilaterally at the knee joint line and at 5 cm proximal to the superior patellar border.

JOINT PLAY   Reveals excessive lateral patellar glide.

SPECIAL TESTS   The Ober test and patellar tilt test are positive; there is a positive patellar glide test into the third quadrant; positive camel-back sign and positive apprehension sign. The right Q angle is 19°. No leg length discrepancy noted. Normal Thomas test.

RADIOGRAPHS   Patellofemoral radiograph imaging the lateral patellofemoral angle shows no evidence of osteoarthritis of the patellofemoral joint. A type III patella, with a *jockey-cap* contour, is observed. There is no evidence of osteochondral avulsion fracture of either the patella or distal femur.

ELECTROMYOGRAM   Electromyogram reveals a hyperactive pattern in the right vastus lateralis muscle and disuse atrophy of the vastus medialis oblique (VMO).

CLUE:

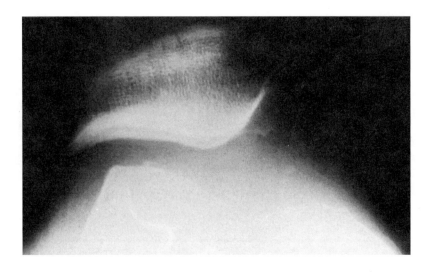

(From Nicholas JA, Hershman EB: *The lower extremity and spine in sports medicine,* ed 2, St Louis, 1995, Mosby.)

CASE 2:   A young athletic woman went jogging every morning and decided to jog several days ago despite the mild rain that began falling early that dawn. When rounding a corner she collided with a cyclist who could not stop owing to wet brakes. She tumbled to the ground unhurt except for a valgus injury to her right anterior knee. As she cradled her knee she noted that her kneecap appeared laterally deviated when compared with her uninjured knee. She somehow maneuvered her knee back to normal and walked back home. Later that day she experienced recurrent pain and increasing swelling. Over the next several days she had bouts of recurrent instability and "catching" in her right knee.

OBSERVATION   Bilateral patellar tilt and patella alta present. There is evidence of long standing Osgood-Schlatter disease. A small scar is observed along the right medial retinacula. Postural deformities include mild genu recurvatum and genu valgum as well as subtalar over-pronation present bilaterally.

PALPATION   Palpation provokes tenderness peripherally, around, behind the patella, and along the medial retinaculum. A relatively larger fat pad is felt beneath the right patella. No crepitus is present.

RANGE OF MOTION   Range of motion is within functional limits.

STRENGTH   Terminal knee extension is moderately weaker than the uninvolved knee.

FLEXIBILITY   Flexibility testing reveals tight lateral knee structures bilaterally including the iliotibial bands, the lateral hamstrings, and the triceps surae; tightness is greater on the right than on the left. Both heel cords are moderately tight.

JOINT PLAY   Joint play reveals excessive lateral patellar glide.

GIRTH MEASUREMENTS   Girth measurements reveal mild to moderate effusion that peaked at 12 hours following injury. Girth was measured bilaterally at 5 cm and 20 cm proximal to the superior patellar border.

SPECIAL TESTS   The Ober test and patellar tilt test was positive; there was a positive patellar glide test into the third quadrant; positive camel-back sign and positive apprehension sign. A right Q angle of 17° is measured. No leg length discrepancy noted. Valgus stress testing of the right knee joint revealed no medial opening at the knee joint. Normal Thomas test.

RADIOGRAPHS   A sunrise view reveals hypoplasia of the lateral femoral condyle. Degenerative changes associated with chondromalacia were absent. There was no concomitant osteochondral fracture. Merchant-view radiographs reveal a loss of central patellar tracking.

ARTHROCENTESIS   Arthrocentesis demonstrates serosanguiness joint aspirate.

CLUE   Merchant radiographs taken of bilateral patellofemoral joints during a subsequent loss of knee stability:

Merchant radiographs taken of bilateral patellofemoral joints during a subsequent loss of knee stability. (From Nicholas JA, Hershman EB: *The lower extremity and spine in sports medicine,* ed 2, St Louis, 1995, Mosby.)

? Questions

1. What is the probable cause of the knee disorders in both cases?
2. Patellar instability demonstrates a preference for which age and gender group?
3. What are the many variables that impact on patellofemoral joint function?
4. How does the architectural asymmetry of the distal femur predispose for lateral patellofemoral joint instability?
5. What is the femoral trochlear sulcus angle, and how does it relate to patellofemoral instability?
6. What are the variations of patellar shape and facet configuration, and what is their clinical significance?
7. What key role does the patella serve in relation to the quadriceps extensor mechanism at the knee?
8. What is the patellofemoral articulation?
9. How do the points of articular contact change during the arc of knee motion?
10. Is patellofemoral motion determined by open or closed kinetic chain function of the lower extremity?
11. What are the dynamic stabilizers of the patellofemoral joint?
12. How do the angles of attachment of the quadriceps muscles predispose for lateral patellar tracking?
13. What is the VMO muscle and what is its function?
14. What is the effect of knee effusion on function of the VMO muscle?
15. What is the role of the VMO during knee extension?
16. What is developmental dysplasia at the knee?
17. What is the effect of lower limb musculature tightness upon patellofemoral tracking?
18. Which lower extremity muscle groups indirectly affect patellofemoral tracking by virtue of their attachment to the knee joint capsule?
19. Which osseous and dynamic patellofemoral stabilizers contribute to lateral patellar tracking?
20. What are the static stabilizers of the patellofemoral joint?
21. Is there an imbalance in the static restraints along the medial and lateral patellar borders?
22. How do static patellar restraints negate dynamic patellar rotation imparted by the quadriceps tendon and ligament?
23. How is tightness of the medial and lateral patellar retinacula clinically assessed?
24. What is the most commonly accepted clinical and radiographic determinant of patellar position with respect to the femur and tibia?
25. How is the Q angle a biomechanical determinant of the hip or subtalar joint in relation to the patellofemoral joint?
26. How may proximal or distally originating malalignment increase the Q angle by virtue of the lower extremity linkage?
27. What is tibial torsion; how may it affect patellar tracking at the knee joint; and how is its lateral pull on the patella amplified by the presence of an excessively prominent tibial tubercle?
28. What is femoral neck anteversion and how does it affect patellar tracking at the knee?
29. What is a common noncontact mechanism for lateral patellar subluxation?
30. What is the mechanism of direct trauma to the patellofemoral joint, and how may associated effusion result in lateral patellar tracking?
31. What is the clinical presentation?
32. What is the differential diagnosis?
33. What therapeutic intervention is appropriate to management of patellar instability?
34. What is the surgical management of patellar dislocation and when is it appropriate?

1. What is the probable cause of the knee disorders in both cases?

The disorder in Case 1 is caused by *lateral subluxation of the patella* due to a noncontact mechanism of injury and lateral patellar dislocation (Fig. 41-1). Case 2 is caused by a strain of the right vastus medialis muscle following a contact mechanism of injury. Patellar subluxation refers to partial loss of contact between the articular surfaces of the patella and femur, whereas patellar dislocation refers to complete loss of contact, that

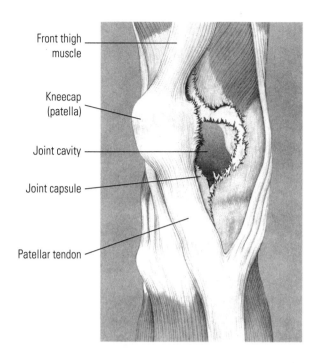

FIG. 41-1 Lateral dislocation of the patella may be accompanied by extensive soft tissue injury to the knee capsule and medial retinaculum. (From Peterson L, Renstrom P: *Sports injuries: their prevention and treatment*, Chicago, 1983, Yearbook Medical Publishers.)

Labels on figure:
- Front thigh muscle
- Kneecap (patella)
- Joint cavity
- Joint capsule
- Patellar tendon

may be accompanied by a tear of the medial capsule[10] or retinacula. Patellar dislocations are most commonly lateral and occur in the first 30° from full knee extension.[71]* The previous history of surgery to the medial static supporting structures predisposed the involved patella to *static lateral overpull*. The presence of even mild effusion may serve to distend the articular capsule and inhibit the femoral nerve and result in inhibition and atrophy of the VMO muscle. This represents a loss of dynamic medial restraint whose imbalance results in *dynamic lateral overpull*. Osseous stability of the patellofemoral joint in both patients was compromised by poor patellar contact owing to *patellar dysplasia* in the form a small and convex medial facet in Case 1 and a lack of lateral buttress in the form of lateral *femoral condylar hypoplasia* in Case 2. The patella was subsequently more at risk for instability before injury.

The origin of patellofemoral instability, similar to degenerative patellofemoral wear of the medial articu-

lar patellar surface, results from an alteration in patellar kinesiology. Normal patellar motion necessitates proper alignment within the trochlear groove of the femur. The capacity for normal tracking is predicated upon a complex dynamic and static balance among all the patellofemoral stabilizers. Patellar malalignment caused by altered mechanics may result in patellofemoral joint wear and pain with chondromalacia, or instability, as in patellar subluxation or dislocation. Lateral patellar instability often occurs as a function of insufficiency of the extensor mechanism at the knee joint. This may occur in the knee with normal anatomic alignment as the disparity in the topography of the human knee and patellofemoral joint may themselves be considered a risk factor for patellar instability. Given the inherent osseous and soft-tissue asymmetries favoring lateral tracking, it is perhaps surprising that patellofemoral pathology does not occur more often than it does.[58]

2. Patellar instability demonstrates a preference for which age and gender group?

Patellar problems, particularly instability, are more often than not the affliction of adolescent girls and young women.[51] The predilection of females for patellar instability may be derived from the excessive valgus forces to the patella (genu valgum) owing to a greater Q angle (Fig. 41-2).[67] Instability may also occur in males or females in the presence of predisposing factors, such as femoral anteversion, excessive external tibial rotation, excessive subtalar pronation, vastus medialis dysplasia, hypoplasia of the lateral femoral condyle, patella alta, patellar tilt, insufficiency of the VMO muscle, genu valgum, tight lateral retinaculum, obesity, or generalized ligamentous laxity (such as may occur in the Down syndrome population or in individuals with Ehler-Danlos syndrome).[7] In addition, the repeated stresses applied to the patellofemoral joint in deceleration maneuvers[41] are the most common cause of traumatic injury to this joint. Subluxation and dislocation of the patella rarely, if ever, occur in older persons with patellofemoral osteoarthritis because arthritic byproducts such as bone spurring tend to limit joint motion and hence stabilize the patellofemoral joint.[30]

3. What are the many variables that impact on patellofemoral joint function?

The patellofemoral joint is significantly influenced by the quadriceps muscle, the shape of the trochlear sulcus, patellar shape, the magnitude and location of ligamentous restraints, the biomechanics of the hip and foot joints,[40] as well as the pathologic presence of condi-

---

*Medial dislocations are rare and are most commonly iatrogenic due to extensor mechanism realignment in which medial reefing has been overdone (Tria).

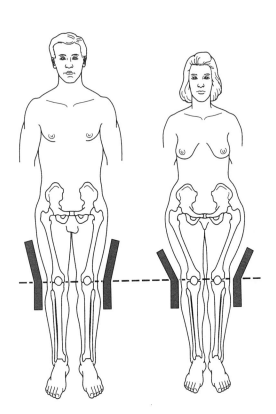

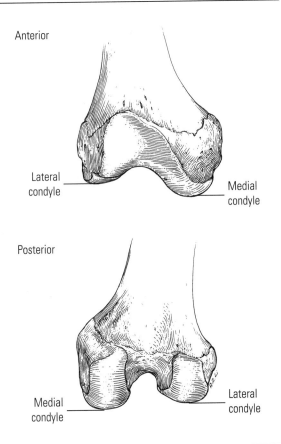

FIG. 41-2 Quadriceps (Q) angle difference between males and fe-males. Because of the broader pelvis in the female, and hence, greater varus at the hips, the femur must compensate by angling in-ward at a higher angle in order that the distal end of the femoral condyles are postured parallel with the ground and thereby articu-late with the tibial plateau. This is accomplished by a relatively greater valgus at the knees, when compared with males. The quad-riceps, patella, and patellar tendon make an angle centered at the patella. As the quadriceps contracts, the angle tends to straighten, which forces the patella laterally. (Redrawn from O'Donoughue, DH: *Treatment of injuries to athletes,* ed 4, Philadelphia, 1984, WB Saunders. In Magee DJ editor: *Orthopedic physical assessment,* Philadelphia, 1997, WB Saunders.)

FIG. 41-3 Anterior and posterior view of the right distal femur. (From Tria AJ, Klein KS: *An illustrated guide to the knee,* New York, 1992, Churchill Livingstone.)

tions such as femoral anteversion, over-pronation, tibia varum, and genu recurvatum. In addition to these vari-ables, a key orienting factor in understanding dysfunc-tion is the quadriceps-extensor mechanism. This mechanism provides a balance of the many forces about the knee. Alteration of even a single force variable in the patellofemoral joint may disrupt a delicately bal-anced mechanism and result in abnormal patellar track-ing. It is imperative for the clinician to appreciate the multiple factors contributing to patellar tracking dys-

function, as well as the anatomy and kinesiology of the region to effectively manage patellofemoral disorders.

4. How does the architectural asymmetry of the distal femur predispose for lateral patellofemoral joint instability?

The osseous structures that form articulations at the knee include the femur, tibia, and patella. The knee is a diarthrodial, tricompartmental articulation consisting of a medial and lateral tibiofemoral and an anterior patel-lofemoral articulation. Although the tibiofemoral and patellofemoral joints are anatomically separate articu-lations, they are functionally related. The distal femur is formed by medial and lateral condyles that are shaped like thick rollers diverging inferiorly and posteriorly (Fig. 41-3). The medial condyle is longer and larger than the lateral femoral condyle (Fig. 41-4), and has a larger circumference, although the lateral condyle at the level of the tibiofemoral articulation is slightly higher when viewed in the sagittal plane. This is clinically sig-

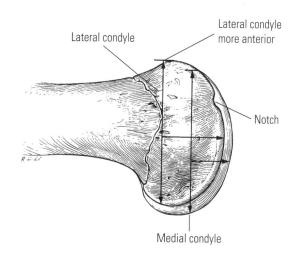

FIG. 41-4 Lateral view of the right knee shows the *medial condyle* larger in the sense that it protrudes distally and has a greater circumference when compared with the lateral femoral condyle. The lateral condyle, however, rises slightly anteriorly above the level of the medial femoral condyle. Note the horizontal notch unique to the lateral femoral condyle. The area above the notch is referred to as the *supratrochlear region* and corresponds to the surface area of the patellofemoral articulation; whereas the femoral surface inferior to this notch is part of the tibiofemoral articulation. (From Tria AJ, Klein KS: *An illustrated guide to the knee,* New York, 1992, Churchill Livingstone.)

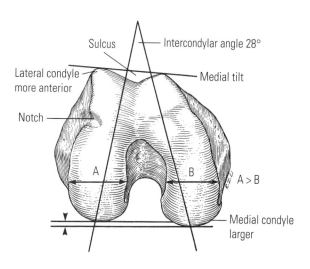

FIG. 41-5 Flexion view of the distal aspect of the right femur. (From Tria AJ, Klein KS: *An illustrated guide to the knee,* New York, 1992, Churchill Livingstone.)

nificant as this added height affords an added measure of osseous stability by acting as a *buttress* discouraging lateral patellar migration and subluxation; moreover, this prominent lateral condylar height better accommodates the large lateral facet of the patella.[23] In contrast, the medial condyle has a more symmetric radius of curvature. This variation in architectural configuration between the two femoral condyles accounts for kinesiologic divergence of function between the medial and lateral tibiofemoral joints.

The architectural inequality between the anteroposterior projection of the two condyles that favors a longer medial condyle imparts a valgus posture to the normal knee in the erect standing posture. This slight genu valgum is referred to as the *tibiofemoral angle* and permits the tibia to remain essentially vertical and the feet close together while the femurs diverge to articulate with the pelvis. The two femoral condyles diverge at an *intercondylar angle* of 28° from each other (Fig. 41-5). Although the distal bulbous protuberances of the femoral condyle comprise one-half of the tibiofemoral joint, the proximal and anterior aspect of both condyles, known as the *supratrochlear* region,

comprise the articulating surface of the patellofemoral joint known as the trochlear facets. Indeed, this is anatomically demarcated along the lateral femoral condyle by a horizontal notch located between the anterior one-third and the posterior two-thirds of the circumference. This notch, lacking at the medial condyle, separates the patellofemoral articulation from the tibiofemoral articulation.

The medial and lateral trochlear facets of the anterodistal femur also possess an architectural asymmetry that markedly influences the kinesiology of the patellofemoral joint, just as the different lengths of the distal femoral condylar affect the biomechanics of the tibiofemoral joint. The lateral trochlear facet projects further anteriorly and proximally than its medial counterpart. Proximally, these two facets slope inward to form a valley, or central *sulcus* whose low point is known as the *trochlear groove.* The entire sulcus is slightly internally rotated with respect to the femoral shaft, partly due to the higher prominence of the lateral condyle. Simply speaking, the sulcus may be thought of as a valley with divergent slopes. Although the lateral slope is longer it is less acute, whereas the more acute medial slope is shorter. The femoral sulcus is angled slightly medially, with the lateral femoral condyle higher than the medial. This variation directly impacts upon the increased likelihood for lateral patellar instability and subluxation, and offsets stability offered by the more anteriorly prominent lateral femoral condyle.

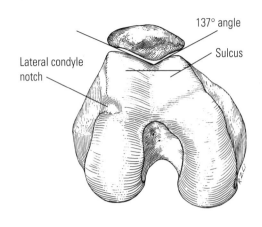

137° angle

Sulcus

Lateral condyle
notch

FIG. 41-6 Right patellofemoral articulation. The femoral-trochlear *sulcus angle* is normally 137°. (From Tria AJ, Klein KS: *An illustrated guide to the knee*, New York, 1992, Churchill Livingstone.)

5. What is the femoral trochlear sulcus angle, and how does it relate to patellofemoral instability?

The *femoral-trochlear sulcus angle* (Fig. 41-6) (note the *trochlear groove* whose *medial longitudinal ridge* proceeds vertically down the center of the sulcus) is defined as the angle formed by a line drawn from the deepest point of the femoral groove or sulcus to the highest point along the lateral femoral condyle and a second line from the deepest point of the femoral sulcus to the top of the medial femoral condyle.[25] The apex of this sulcus is defined by a vertical trochlear groove that proceeds distally to terminate as the intercondylar notch. The *medial longitudinal ridge* is seated within the center of the femoral sulcus or groove. The femoral sulcus is angulated slightly medially, with the lateral femoral condyle higher than the medial. Thus the static stabilization offered the patellofemoral joint by the distal femur favors lateral subluxation[72] such that normal anatomy may itself be considered a risk factor in patellar instability. The posterior continuation of the sulcus ends in a hollow known as the *intercondylar notch* that houses both cruciate ligaments and serves as their attachment site.

In addition to the trochlear depth of the distal femur, another osseous factor determining the stability of patellofemoral surface contact is the facet anatomy along the undersurface of the patella. The normal angle of the sulcus is 137°, although an obtuse or shallow sulcus angle may predispose towards instability of the patellofemoral joint and possible subluxation or dislocation because of poor osseous stability. Conversely,

the more acute the sulcus angle, the greater osseous stability is afforded to the patellofemoral joint during knee range of motion. The only osseous stabilization of the patellofemoral joint, in addition to patellar shape, derives from the depth of the intercondylar notch of the femur, which is minimal at best and is extremely variable from person to person.[41] In summation we may conclude that the patellofemoral joint is inherently predisposed towards lateral subluxation.[25] This anatomic predisposition for patellar instability is magnified in those individuals having a shallow intercondylar groove known as a *tabletop femur*,[58] a dysplastic lateral femoral condyle, or a dysplastic patella with a *jockey-cap contour*. In addition to sulcus angle, other determinants of patellofemoral congruence include the congruence angle, the lateral patellofemoral angle, and the patellofemoral index.

6. What are the variations of patellar shape and facet configuration, and what is their clinical significance?

The morphology of both the shape (convex or concave) of the posterior patellar surface as well as facet configuration derives from constitutional anatomic predisposition, as well as physiologic patellofemoral forces from patellofemoral insult. These factors model the developing patella into a variety of patella shapes and may also cause topographic asymmetry of the articular facet surfaces. A *type I patella* refers to a normal patella whose cartilage has not been subjected to maltracking[70] because of the relative balance amongst the many lower extremity osseous and soft-tissue components. This type of patella is characterized by symmetry of its articular surfaces such that its size is roughly equal in magnitude whereas the shape of the posterior articular surface is concave. A *type II patella* is characterized by a smaller medial facet, and a concave or flat posterior patella surface. A *type III patella* is characterized by an even smaller medial facet, and a convex posterior patella surface (Fig. 41-7).[73]

Patellar types that deviate from the type I patellar configuration are said to represent dysplastic patellar and facet anatomy that lead to incomplete surface contact and resultant patellofemoral pain and dysfunction. Several authorities postulate that patellofemoral pain and instability are predisposed in individuals with a type III patella. This is thought to derive from a lack of balanced force distribution to the asymmetric slopes of the medial and lateral facets, causing unequal stress and leading to lateral subluxation or dislocation.

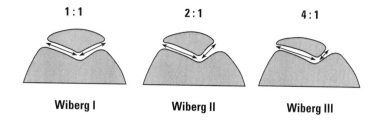

| 1 : 1 | 2 : 1 | 4 : 1 |
| Wiberg I | Wiberg II | Wiberg III |

FIG. 41-7 Classification of variations of patellar shape, particularly as they relate to the ratio between the medial and lateral facet vis-a-vis the surface of the trochlea of the distal femur. **A,** Type I has equal facet sizes and is considered normal and the most stable. **B,** Type II represents a less stable patellofemoral articulation as the majority of surface contact is confined to the lateral facet. Here the medial facet is concave, and thereby lends an element of stability to the articulation. **C,** Type III variation has minimal medial facet contact as well as a convex medial facet. Both of these factors create an unstable patellofemoral articulation that is more likely to sustain subluxation or dislocation. (From Tria AJ, Klein KS: *An illustrated guide to the knee,* New York, 1992, Churchill Livingstone.)

7. What key role does the patella serve in relation to the quadriceps extensor mechanism at the knee?

The patella serves as a locus for the delicately balanced interaction of the various osseous, tendinous, and soft tissues comprising the quadriceps mechanism (Fig. 41-8). We may conceptualize the patellofemoral joint as centrally balanced by a hexagonal system of guy supports consisting of the quadriceps tendon and ligament superoinferiorly and the patellofemoral and patellotibial ligaments transversely and obliquely. The purpose of this system is to precisely anchor the articulating patellar surface to the femoral articular surface such that the intercondylar notch receives the central patellar ridge. An alternation in balance between components of this system may significantly alter the biomechanics of the patellofemoral joint and, indeed, the entire extensor mechanism. A thorough understanding of this delicate system of dynamic-static balanced restraint is necessary to appreciate both normal kinesiology of the extensor mechanism as well as patellofemoral dysfunction.

8. What is the patellofemoral articulation?

The *patellofemoral articulation* consists of the trochlear facets of distal femoral condyles in contact with the patellar facets. This occurs by way of the posterior patellar facets articulating with the medial and lateral trochlear facets at the supratrochlear region of the femoral condyles throughout varying degrees of knee flexion and extension. The patella maintains a shifting contact with the femur in all positions of the knee as it glides over the distal femur. As the knee moves from a fully flexed to a fully extended posture, first the superior, then the middle and finally the inferior portions of the patellar articular surface are brought into contact with the corresponding trochlear facets of the distal femur. During maximal knee extension the patellofemoral contact area occurs between the posterior patellar facets and the supratrochlear region of the femoral condyles. In contrast, the area of femoral contact throughout the arc of knee motion begins with the patella recessed into the intercondylar femoral groove during flexion. In fact, flexing the knee beyond 90° allows the patella to drop into the lower femorotrochlear groove; the femoral condyles are then palpable at sites normally covered by the kneecap.[14]

9. How do the points of articular contact change during the arc of knee motion?

During knee extension the patellofemoral contact area occurs between the posterior patellar facets and the supratrochlear* region of the femoral condyles. As the knee joint flexes and extends, the contact points of the patellofemoral joint undergo changes in contact area and joint reaction force. Between full extension and 90° of flexion both the medial and lateral facets of the patellar articulate with the femur. Beyond 90° of flexion the patella externally rotates and only the medial (odd) facet articulates with the medial trochlear patellar surface on the femur.[57]

Trochlea means pulley, and refers to the pulleylike curve of the femoral condyles.

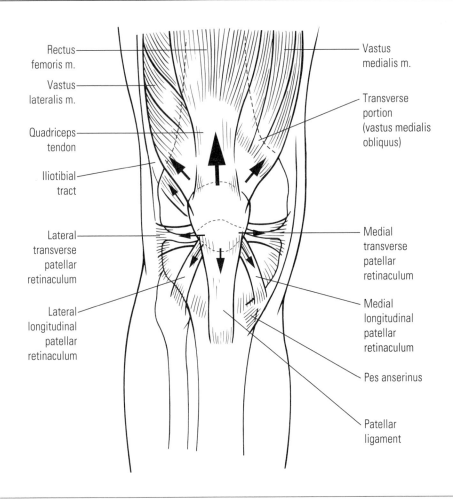

Rectus femoris m.

Vastus lateralis m.

Quadriceps tendon

Iliotibial tract

Lateral transverse patellar retinaculum

Lateral longitudinal patellar retinaculum

Vastus medialis m.

Transverse portion (vastus medialis obliquus)

Medial transverse patellar retinaculum

Medial longitudinal patellar retinaculum

Pes anserinus

Patellar ligament

FIG. 41-8 Anterior view of the knee joint demonstrating the *extensor mechanism*. Resolution of the many dynamic and static restraint forces illustrates the precise and delicately balanced factors necessary to maintaining patellofemoral stability and normal function. Alteration of one or more of these variables will result in an imbalance of the extensor mechanism and result in patellofemoral maltracking.

During full knee extension the patella lies in supratrochlear fossa in a bed of fat and synovium, which makes the patella amenable to manual motion and palpation. In this position, it is the inferior facet that contacts the femur. Here, the median patellar ridge and the lateral facet articulate with the lateral side of the femoral sulcus. As flexion commences, the patellar surface articulates with the trochlear patellar surface in a distal to proximal manner. Simultaneously, the patella tilts centrally, with respect to the frontal plane, in a lateral to medial fashion. Patellar tilt is normal and results from the asymmetric surface topography of the distal femur owing to the divergence in size between the medial and

lateral femoral condyles. Thus early knee flexion begins with inferior facet engagement, proceeds to middle facet articulation, and reaches 90° with superior facet engagement.

At terminal flexion the patella moves into the intercondylar groove.[22] The total cephalo-caudal patellar glide along the femoral condyles is approximately 7 cm.[14] Although the points of contact along the posterior surface of the patella move proximally and medially with progressive flexion, the corresponding point of contact along the trochlear facets move in opposite direction, namely distally and laterally. As the knee flexes, the contact point of the patellofemoral joint moves proximally on the patella and distally on the femoral intercondylar sulcus.[8]

10. Is patellofemoral motion determined by open or closed chain function of the lower extremity?

The relationship between the femur and patella is affected by whether or not the lower limb functions in the open or closed kinetic modes of function. In the open kinetic chain the tibia moves on a stationary femur, and the patella slides on the femoral condyles. However, although the femur is relatively stationary, it still undergoes sagittal plane motion as the femoral condyles glide backward and forward along the tibial plateau with extension and flexion of the tibiofemoral joint. Moreover, rotation of the femoral condyles also occurs in the transverse plane. In contrast, in the closed kinetic mode, characterized by the femur moving on a fixed tibia, the femoral condyles slide under a stationary patella. This difference between the two articulating surfaces of the patellofemoral joint occurs as a direct result of patellar attachment to both the femur (via the quadriceps tendon) and the tibia (via the patellar tendon.)

11. What are the dynamic stabilizers of the patellofemoral joint?

The four muscles comprising the *quadriceps muscles* are the largest muscle unit in the body and capable of generating significant intraarticular force (that may be in excess of 1000 lb of internal force.) These muscles include the *rectus femoris* and the three vasti muscles— the *medialis, intermedius,* and *lateralis.* While rectus femoris spans both the hip and knee joint, the vasti are one-joint muscles. Although the rectus femoris originates from the anterior inferior iliac spine, the vasti take origin from the anterior and posterior surface of the femur. A common distal attachment of all four quadriceps muscles occurs by way of a trilaminar insertion on the superior pole of the patella. The rectus femoris occupies the superficial layer, the vastus medialis and lateralis in the middle layer, and the vastus intermedius comprises the deepest layer. Superiorly, the portion of the quadriceps attaching to the proximal patella is called the quadriceps tendon whereas the tendinous structure emerging from the inferior patellar pole is called the patellar ligament (ligamentum patellae). The quadriceps muscles comprise the extensor mechanism at the knee and exert pull by way of a common distal tendon. In addition to providing dynamic stability to the patellofemoral joint, the quadriceps muscles prevent

the knee from collapsing during activities such as walking, running, or landing from a jump.[43]

12. How do the angles of attachment of the quadriceps muscles predispose for lateral patellar tracking?

The fibers of the rectus femoris run nearly parallel to the long axis of the femur and continue over the anterior patella surface confluent with the quadriceps tendon and merging into the patellar ligament to ultimately insert on the proximal tibia. Most of the fibers of the vastus intermedius run parallel to the long axis of the femur to insert upon the superior patellar pole. Although the rectus femoris approaches the patella at an angle of 10°, the vastus intermedius approaches at angle of 0°;[30] both muscles exert an essentially cephalad pull. The two lateral and medial vasti approach the patella at divergent angles of attachment known as *pennation angles.* The pennation angle of the vastus lateralis is oriented in a slightly lateral direction of 15° as it approaches the patella. Most fibers of the vastus medialis consist of a longitudinal head attached to the patella from a slightly medial direction of 20°. However, a small but significant portion of the distal vastus medialis, known as the oblique head called the VMO, deviates at an angle of 50° to 60° as it inserts into the superomedial portion of the patella. The divergence of pennation angles of the vasti accounts for the inherent dynamic imbalance of the extensor mechanism that results in uneven pull of the patella, which may result in a tracking deficit of the patella that favors lateral patellar distraction. Thus *the quadriceps mechanism favors lateral distraction of the patella.** Although the vastus lateralis is also augmented by a vastus lateralis obliquus muscle, the pinnation angle of this latter muscle slip is not nearly as acute as that of the vastus medialis obliquus. Moreover, the lateralis inserts higher up on the patella. The acute pennation angle of VMO may

---

*Lateral patellar distraction also occurs because of the osseous asymmetry of the patella. When the patella is viewed as a wedge on a skyline view, the distance between the medial border and apex spans a smaller dimension than does the distance between the lateral border and patellar apex, The relatively higher insertion of the lateralis on the patella, as well as the increased distance between the lateral patellar border and patellar apex, bias the force vectors at the knee laterally. The asymmetry between the medial and lateral aspects of the patella, and indeed, of other osseous components such as the femoral condyles and tibial plateau may derive as an accommodation to lateral tibial rotation.

represent a "design" strategy that attempts to offset the anatomic imbalance that favors lateral patellar overpull.

13. What is the VMO muscle and what is its function?

The *vastus medialis muscle* may be divided into the vastus medialis longus (VML) and the VMO. The superior longitudinal fibers of the VML are directed 15° to 18° medially from their attachment on the patella.[8] Originating from the medial aspect of the distal femur and running almost horizontally to insert along the medial aspect of the patella, the prominent inferior fibers of the VMO play a critical stabilizing role that centers the patella in the intercondylar groove. Following the principle that form follows function, the singularly unique pennation angle of the VMO may be viewed as a dynamic counter balance offsetting a predisposed tendency towards lateral patellar deviation. Although the VMO is innervated independently from the other quadriceps by a branch of the femoral nerve it is not a separate muscle, but is a continuous extension of the vastus medialis.[74] Some authorities maintain that a substantial portion of the VMO arises from the adductor magnus tendon and the adductor longus muscle.[5] As VMO inserts on the patella it shares the common function of cephalic patellar glide with the other three muscles of the quadriceps mechanism. Its primary function, however, is to exert a medial directed pull on the patella and thereby realigns the patella in the femoral sulcus. In such fashion, the VMO represents a dynamic restraint preventing lateral patellar tracking.

14. What is the effect of knee effusion on function of the VMO muscle?

The vastus medialis fibers insert into the medial and distal aspect of the patella, providing dynamic medial patella support preventing lateral overpull. From a dynamic standpoint, the checkrein function preventing lateral maltracking is provided by the vastus medialis, a muscle that is phylogenetically the weakest of the quadriceps group and appears to be the first to atrophy and last to rehabilitate.[18] The VMO muscle is further disadvantaged because even a relatively minimal amount of effusion at the knee may result in reflex inhibition of the VMO[75] and subsequent lateral maltracking. Edema in excess of 55 cc of fluid causes mechanical pressure on capsular receptors, especially medially and posteriorly[63] Activated receptors reflexively inhibit the quad-

riceps mechanism, which is usually most profound in the VMO[44,56]

15. What is the role of the VMO during knee extension?

VMO is active throughout the entire range of knee extension[3,42] and is not the primary extensor during terminal knee extension.[13] Moreover, during knee extension, the VMO is the least active of the quadriceps muscles as it takes a proportionately lesser role with increased resistance.[15] This is clinically relevant as the terminal arc of knee extension corresponds to that time when a peak valgus vector dominates patellofemoral biomechanics. Ironically, the patella is most vulnerable to lateral tracking in a range when VMO is least active and subsequently least capable in providing a counterbalanced medial force that would centralize the patella.

16. What is developmental dysplasia at the knee?

Patellofemoral dysplasia refers to an abnormality of development, particularly with relation to size and orientation of the extensor mechanism. Histologically, dysplasia represents an alteration, specifically a disorganized state of the cartilage cells in the case of the patella or the muscle fibers of the VMO. Developmental dysplasia (i.e., hypoplasia) of the VMO exists when the oblique portion fails to develop properly, demonstrating an abnormally high pinnation angle of 65° or greater.[41] This causes a lateral deviation of the resultant quadriceps force and compromises patellofemoral balance and stability.[68] Some persons may have an additional lack of lateral osseous restraint, resulting in lateral drift, owing to a poorly developed lateral condyle known as *femoralcondylar hypoplasia*.[64] *Patellar dysplasia* is yet another factor in the equation that defines stability of the patellofemoral joint.

The natural history of untreated patellofemoral dysplasia is that, if left untreated, continued disruption of knee pathomechanics will lead to an increased likelihood of pain, disability, and progressive arthrosis.[59] In contrast to the poor regenerative response of adult articular cartilage to mechanical insult, the immature chondrocytes in the pediatric population appear to be capable of satisfactory cartilage repair. Thus findings suggesting patellofemoral dysplasia in the immature knee mandate early intervention at a time when the reparative powers of cartilage are optimal, but before initiation of intervening degenerative changes.[58]

17. What is the effect of lower limb musculature tightness upon patellofemoral tracking?

Normal patellofemoral joint motion is characterized by vertical tracking of the patella between the femoral condyles. For centralized patellofemoral sulcus tracking to occur there must be an equal balance among the soft-tissue structures attaching to the kneecap. Imperative to this balance, is the dynamic stabilization of the patellofemoral joint afforded by the quadriceps mechanism. The knee extensors, directly attaching on the patella, are often weak in patients with chondromalacia, and may be accompanied by overpull of the antagonistic hamstring muscles. Posteriorly, excessive hamstring overpull occurs secondary to hamstring tightness, opposes quadriceps function, and causes greater loading of the patellofemoral joint.[38]

18. Which lower extremity muscle groups indirectly affects patellofemoral tracking by virtue of their attachment to the knee joint capsule?

Other muscles indirectly affect patellofemoral dynamics because of their attachments to the knee joint capsule. Laterally, a tight iliotibial band may be a contributing factor in patellofemoral pain. At the knee, the iliotibial tract sends a slip to the patella known as the *iliopatellar band* [69] that partially interdigitates with the superficial, and primarily, with the deep fibers of the lateral retinaculum and joint capsule, and hence, the patella. Thus as the knee flexes, the iliotibial band is pulled posteriorly, causing the patella to track laterally. This lateral overpull is magnified in the presence of a tight iliotibial band.[74] Medially, expansions from the semitendinosus and sartorius muscles (comprising the pes anserine tendinous insertion) fuse with the capsule.[26] Posteriorly, the gastrocnemius and semimembranosus muscles blend with the capsule. Tightness of these muscles would unilaterally restrict capsular mobility and bias patellofemoral tracking toward the direction of tightness.

19. Which osseous and dynamic patellofemoral stabilizers contribute to lateral patellar tracking?

Both osseous and dynamic factors favor lateral instability of the normal patellofemoral joint. From a bony perspective, the incline (slope) of the lateral aspect of the femoral sulcus angle is less acute than the medial side. This results in diminished surface contact between the patella and femur and is amplified in those individuals with a femoral sulcus angle approaching 150°. More-

over, the location of the central ridge along the posterior patellar surface is asymmetrically located lateral to midline in the normal patella. This asymmetry contributes to a fit into the asymmetric basin of the femoral sulcus that, from a geometric standpoint, is poorly designed for stability despite any anterior abutment provided by a prominent anterior lateral femoral condyle. Instead, the combined asymmetries of the patellar and femoral surfaces magnify the likelihood for lateral patellar instability. This effect is enhanced in the event of an excessively shortened lateral patellar retinaculum or atrophy of the VMO secondary to immobilization following injury or surgery.

Some persons may have an additional lack of lateral osseous restraint to lateral tracking due to a poorly developed lateral condyle known as *condylar hypoplasia*.[15] Here, a lack of lateral condylar prominence accommodates lateral patellar migration which, over time, distorts the patella into a "jockey cap contour."[6] Deficiency of the lateral femoral condyle as well as patellar deformation may be viewed on a tangential (i.e., sunrise) radiographic view.

The *quadriceps mechanism* represents the dynamic component contributing to patellar imbalance. The line-of-pull of the quadriceps muscles parallels the shaft of the femur (i.e., with the anatomic axis and not with the mechanical axis.) Thus the combined force vector of the rectus, intermedius and lateralis pull represents a significant lateral overpull that overwhelms the medialis vector and thereby favoring lateral distraction of the patella. The tibiofemoral joint, however, is normally in slight valgus with respect to the joint line due to the longer medial femoral condyle.[25] This directly impacts upon the direction of the quadriceps force vector and imparts a lateral force on the patella away from the midline.

Normal patellofemoral mechanics are characterized by a lateral force vector that pulls the patella laterally when the knee joint is fully extended causing the patella to sit lateral to the trochlea.[71] This inherent imbalance in the quadriceps mechanism derives from osseous, dynamic, and ligamentous factors and may lead to a tracking deficit manifesting as excessive cartilage stress[20] and wear of the medial border of the medial patellar facet, or lateral patellar subluxation.[8] Other dynamic influences upon patellar stabilization include the pes anserine[74] medial hamstring muscles, and the iliotibial band and short head of biceps femoris laterally through its relationship to the iliotibial tract.[62] Injury and atrophy, or tightness of either side will alter the dynamic balance of the patellofemoral mechanism and result in overpull and maltracking. Tightness of the medial structures and/or laxity of the lateral structures favor lateral compression and subluxation, whereas tightness of the lateral structures and/or laxity of the medial structures favor medial compression and subluxation.[13]

20. What are the passive stabilizers of the patellofemoral joint?

Although the bony configuration of the patellofemoral joint provides passive osseous stability, passive static restraint is augmented by the noncontractile soft-tissue restraints surrounding the anterior patellofemoral joint. A description of these various interconnected static restraints may be explained by beginning peripherally and ending centrally. The tendinous expansions of the medial and lateral vasti insert onto the medial and lateral aspects of the patella respectively, and are termed the *medial* and *lateral patellar retinacula*.[14] Secondary transverse thickenings (condensations) of the superior retinacula are anatomically discernible as the patellofemoral ligaments, whereas oblique condensations of the inferior retinacula are termed the *patellotibial ligaments*. The patellofemoral ligaments originate from the epicondylar[49] and condylar protuberances of the femur and insert into the superomedial and superolateral facets of the patella. The function of the ligaments is to centralize patellar tracking. Although the medial restraints oppose lateral patellar displacement, the lateral restraints oppose medial patellar movement. Deviation from this narrow parameter of motion may stem from imbalance and may express as pathologic dysfunction of the patellofemoral joint. Excessive patellar displacement in either direction will either manifest as excessive wearing of bone, subluxation, or both.

21. Is there an imbalance in the static restraints along the medial and lateral patellar borders?

Inherent to the anatomy of the confluence of tendons and ligaments stabilizing the patellofemoral joint is a soft-tissue imbalance that may be considered an anatomical predisposition for patellofemoral dysfunction. On the lateral side, the patellofemoral joint supports are fairly well designed as the lateral retinaculum is augmented by support from interdigitation of the iliotibial band known as the *iliopatellar band* as well as the *lateral meniscopatellar ligament*.[17,39] Beneath these are found an even deeper layer of supporting ligamentous

structures: the transverse band, patellar tibial band, and the epicondylar patellar ligament.[6] The lateral meniscopatellar and patellotibial band provide inferior support to the kneecap. These lateral structures, by virtue of their iliotibial band and lateral intermuscular septal attachment, passively draw the patella posteriorly and laterally during knee flexion.[58] In contrast, the medial patellofemoral restraints are characterized by a paucity of structures that include the VMO muscle and two capsular condensations known as the *patellofemoral* and *medial meniscopatellar ligaments*. These ligaments insert into the patella and attach to the femoral condyles and medial meniscus, respectively. The thin medial retinaculum is only one layer thick[71] in some persons whereas in others, the medial patellofemoral ligament may be substantial and form a substantial and formidable checkrein to lateral displacement.

22. How do static patellar restraints negate dynamic patellar rotation imparted by the quadriceps tendon and ligament?

In addition to cephalocaudal glide during knee extension and flexion, patellar motion is also characterized by rotation of the patella. During its helical arc of motion beginning with extension and ending with flexion, the point of contact along the patella begins laterally and migrates medially to terminate on the odd facet. The magnitude of this normal mediolateral patellar rotation ranges between 5.6° to 6.5° and is attributed to the medial condyle being larger than the lateral condyle.[19] When the tibiofemoral joint is in full extension the patella lies above the trochlear groove in a slightly lateral position because of the externally rotated end point of the tibia during extension. Thus patellofemoral rotation may be attributable to the same cause of rotation as the tibiofemoral joint. Patellar movements are thus considerably influenced by the magnitude of tibial[41] or femoral rotation. Whereas femoral rotation is transmitted to the patella via the quadriceps tendon, tibial rotation is transmitted superiorly to the patella via the patellar ligament. An additional function of the static ligamentous restraints of the patella may be to absorb and thereby minimize rotational patellar displacement from above or below the knee.

23. How is tightness of the medial and lateral patellar retinacula clinically assessed?

A *passive patellar tilt test* determines the presence or absence of an excessively tight lateral retinaculum. This is done with the knee extended and the quadriceps muscle relaxed. The examiner then lifts the lateral edge of the patella from the lateral femoral condyle (Fig. 41-9). An excessively tight lateral retinaculum is discovered by the presence of a neutral or negative angle to the horizontal and is referred to as a *negative passive patellar tilt.*

The *patellar glide test* demonstrates either medial or lateral retinacular integrity or tightness. The quadriceps is relaxed by placing the knee joint in 10° to 30° of flexion. The examiner attempts to displace the patella in the medial and then lateral direction using his/her index finger and thumb. By subdividing the patella into four longitudinal quadrants, the examiner may roughly gauge the magnitude of retinacular incompetence. A medial glide of one quadrant is consistent with a tight lateral retinaculum and often correlates with a negative passive patellar tilt test. A medial glide of three to four quadrants suggests a hypermobile patella. A lateral glide of three quadrants suggests an incompetent me-

dial restraint, whereas a lateral glide of four quadrants is consistent with patellar dislocation.[67]

24. What is the most commonly accepted clinical and radiographic determinant of patellar position with respect to the femur and tibia?

The kinesiology of the patellofemoral joint is such that it is easily altered by transverse plane motion deriving either proximally at the hip joint or distally at the subtalar joint. *Patellar malalignment* in relation to the trochlear groove may stem from an altered kinesiology that may be quantified as an excessive quadriceps Q angle. Before understanding the significance of the patellotibial Q angle, it is necessary to appreciate the difference between the anatomic and mechanical axes of the lower limb. The lack of symmetry among these parameters translates into an alignment differential between the quadriceps tendon and patellar ligament.

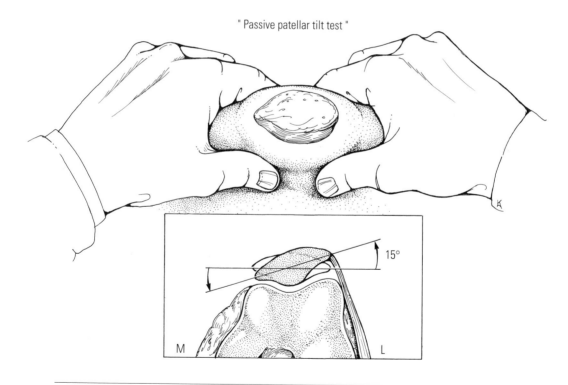

" Passive patellar tilt test "

FIG. 41-9 Passive *patellar tilt* test. Normally, one should be able to lift the lateral border of the patella beyond the horizontal. An excessively tight lateral restraint (lateral retinaculum) is demonstrated by a neutral or negative knee angle to the horizontal. This test is performed with the knee fully extended and the quadriceps relaxed. (From Scuderi GR, McCann PD, Bruno PJ: *Sports medicine: principles of primary care,* St Louis, 1997, Mosby.)

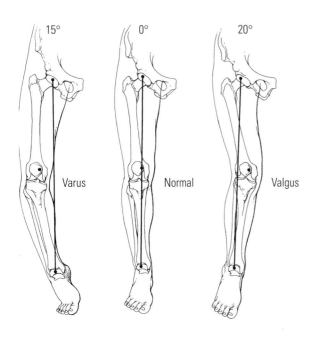

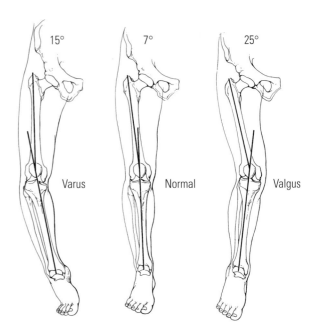

FIG. 41-10 The *mechanical axis* of the leg is measured in the standing position with an imaginary plumb line dropped from the femoral head to the ground. This angular measurement gives the best functional evaluation of the lower extremity alignment. (From Tria AJ, Klein KS: *An illustrated guide to the knee,* New York, 1992, Churchill Livingstone.)

FIG. 41-11 The *anatomic axis* of the lower limb is measured by drawing lines parallel to the long axis of the femur and the tibia and measuring the intercepting angle. (From Tria AJ, Klein KS: *An illustrated guide to the knee,* New York, 1992, Churchill Livingstone.)

The *mechanical axis* of the lower extremity (Fig. 41-10) is measured in the standing posture with an imaginary plumb line dropped from the femoral head to the ground. The value of this type of measurement is that it best demonstrates whether the lower extremity alignment is in varus or valgus, or plain normal. The anatomic axis determines the clinical alignment of the lower limb and measures the femorotibial angle. The *anatomic axis* of the leg (Fig. 41-11) is ascertained by drawing lines parallel to the long axis of the femur and the tibia and measuring the intercepting angle.

The quadriceps mechanism pulls the patella on the mechanical axis of the femur and not on the anatomic axis of the leg. This is because the functional distal insertion of the quadriceps is the tibial tubercle which, by virtue of the slight valgus at the knee joint, is 6° more laterally displaced than the mechanical axis of the femur.[41] Although the direction of quadriceps (tendon) pull is in line with the shaft of the femur, the pull of the patellar tendon is in line with the long axis of the tibia.[32] The differential between the proximal (quadriceps tendon) and distal aspect (patellar ligament) of the

quadriceps mechanism forms an angle known as the Q angle (Fig. 41-12).

One may determine the Q angle to gauge *patellofemoral joint alignment* by drawing a line from the center of the patella proximally toward the anterior superior iliac spine, followed by a second line from the center of the patella to the tibial tubercle with the foot in the subtalar neutral posture and the knee extended and weight bearing. The angle subtended by the intersection of these two lines is (identical to the femorotibial angle) the Q angle. The effect of the Q angle value on patellofemoral biomechanics may be appreciated by resolving the vastus lateralis force into longitudinal (extensor) and lateral vectors components. The longitudinal vector derives from the lateralis and quadriceps vector sum of force delivered via the quadriceps tendon to the superior patellar pole. The lateral vector component derives from the lateral displacement of the tibial tubercle, and hence the patellar ligament insertion some 6° lateral to the shaft of the femur, owing to the pull of the lateralis. The higher the Q angle, the greater the magnitude of the lateral vector. A larger Q angle will bias this traction differential upon the superior and inferior patellar poles during loaded knee extension in

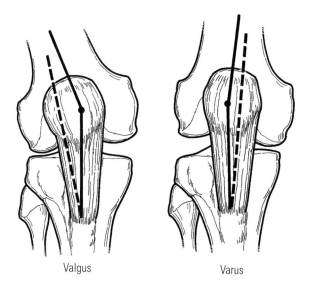

Valgus   Varus

FIG. 41-12 The Q angle is the angle subtended by lines drawn from the anterior superior iliac spine to the patella, and from the patella to the tibial tubercle. Patients with patellofemoral subluxation commonly have Q angle values >15°. (From Scott WN: *The knee,* St Louis, 1994, Mosby.)

favor of the lateral direction. The patella, by virtue of its location, is at the focus of these diverging forces and absorbs them during loaded knee extension by deviating laterally. Moreover, the patella is naturally displaced laterally as it anatomically lies more medial to the line of pull between the quadriceps tendon and the tibial tubercle.[48] Thus quasi-valgus forces are imparted to the patella by normal lower limb alignment in addition to other variables such as bony anatomy, muscular force, and ligament balance.

The normal Q angle values differ in males and females owing to the wider pelvis in women. The normal femur for men is angled and ranges 8° to 14° from the midline, and for women an average of 11° to 20°.[1,31] The mean Q angle for men is approximately 12.7° in the supine position and 13.6° in the standing position. The mean Q angle for women is approximately 15.8° in the supine posture and as high as 17° while weight bearing. The increased Q angle during standing may derive from a more pronounced knee valgus due to engagement of the tibiofemoral joint in extension.[41] *Q angle values greater than 14° to 16° are considered to be pathologic as they result in excessive lateral vector force upon the patella as the knee is extended.* Such a knee may exhibit a propensity for patellar tracking dys-

function or a subluxing/dislocating patella. Moreover, a knee with an excessive Q angle may suggest structural abnormalities such as excessive femoral anteversion, increased lateral tibial torsion,[67] or the presence of metatarsus adductus.[25]

The value for the Q angle varies during the arc of knee motion. As the knee progresses from full extension to flexion in the open kinetic chain, the Q angle decreases with internal rotation of the tibia on the femur. During closed chain flexion, the Q angle will also decrease as the femur externally rotates on a fixed tibia.[13] For both the open and closed kinetic modes the Q angle approaches 0° with flexion of the normal knee as the differential between the pull of the quadriceps tendon and patellar ligament are equalized. An individual with a high Q angle may manifest in the knee flexed posture as when the patient is short sitting.

25. How is the Q angle a biomechanical determinant of the hip or subtalar joint in relation to the patellofemoral joint?

The knee is the central link of the lower extremity connecting osseous, musculotendinous, and fascial tissues extending distally from the hip, and coursing distally towards the ankle and foot.[27] The biomechanical significance of this linkage is nowhere more apparent than when we examine the relationship between the Q angle and corresponding lateral patellar tracking, and how both of these parameters are directly affected by the hip joint proximally and the subtalar joint distally.

Hyperextension at the knee (or genu recurvatum) represents an angular malalignment, which alters the screw-home mechanism at the tibiofemoral joint such that excessive external tibial rotation occurs. This results in compensatory medial femoral rotation that causes an increase in the Q angle and the increased likelihood for patellofemoral dysfunction. Although the medial femoral condyle angles away from the femoral shaft in line with the mechanical axis of the lower limb, the lateral femoral condyle is more closely oriented to the femoral shaft.

Insall et al[35] define a Q angle of 14° as normal and above 20° as abnormal, whereas as Hughston[33] defines a Q angle >10° as abnormal. Hyperextension at the knee (or genu recurvatum) alters the screw-home mechanism at the tibiofemoral joint such that excessive external tibial rotation occurs. This results in compensatory medial femoral rotation that causes an increase in the Q angle and the increased likelihood for patellofemoral dysfunction.

26. How may proximal or distally originating malalignment increase the Q angle by virtue of the lower extremity linkage?

Altered patellofemoral mechanics may originate proximally or distally. The classic presentation is the *miserable malalignment syndrome* (see Chapter 52) characterized by internally rotated hips (femoral anteversion) that causes the following compensatory malalignments: knock knees (genu valgum), external tibial torsion, and pronated feet. This syndrome is characterized by both rotatory and angular malaligments of the lower extremity. This combination of postures may be initiated by a single malalignment (proximally) and cause further compensatory malalignments distally. The reverse may occur in the individual with abnormally pronated feet that impart an internal rotary torque to the tibia resulting in knock knees (genu valgus) and a compensatory femoral anteversion. In this case the initiating factor stemmed distally from the foot and altered patellar tracking in a distoproximal direction. Regardless of whether the initiating malalignment originated proximally or distally, the compensatory malalignments may reinforce the original initiating malalignment in a vicious cycle. Another common pattern of malalignment may originate from gastrocnemius or hamstring tightness in which excessive tightness of the posterior leg musculature will restrict talocrural dorsiflexion, producing compensatory pronation at the subtalar joint. This may migrate proximally to create internal femoral rotation, which manifests as an increase in the dynamic Q angle.[25]

27. What is tibial torsion; how may it affect patellar tracking at the knee joint; and how is its lateral pull on the patella amplified by the presence of an excessively prominent tibial tubercle?

Excessive tibial rotation is a proximal transverse plane motion accompanying subtalar joint pronation or supination at the foot. During stance phase of gait, deviation from subtalar neutral during stance along either extreme along the spectrum of intrinsic foot deformities may manifest as excessive pronation and supination. During quiet standing as well as during stance phase, the normal foot exerts no significant torsion to the most distal component of the quadriceps mechanism (i.e., the patellar ligament). At heel strike, the tibia is externally rotated and the patellar tendon is slightly medially angulated, and the Q angle is reduced. When the foot pronates following heel strike, the patellar tendon is slightly angulated into valgus and the Q angle is increased correspondingly. However, the foot that over-

pronates as a compensatory mechanism is accompanied by excessive obligatory internal rotation of the tibia. By virtue of the lower extremity linkage, this excessive quasi-valgus force is imparted upward to the proximal tibia and increases the angle between the inferior patellar pole and the anterior tibial tubercle, hence the patellar *ligament*. This effectively increases the Q angle and represents a distally originating lateral vector force to the patella.[67] Regardless of whether the source of lateral patellar tracking is proximal or distal, the common denominator of both mechanisms is a medial glide of either the quadriceps tendon or patellar tendon. This will result in a valgus force imparted to the patella as it increases the mechanical advantage of the vastus lateralis. This effect may be magnified by the presence of long standing Osgood-Schlatter disease as the patellar ligament, now further away from the knee, represents increased leverage that heightens the distally originating lateral overpull derived from internal tibial torsion.

28. What is femoral neck anteversion and how does it affect patellar tracking at the knee?

Femoral anteversion (Fig. 41-13) is a gradually acquired torsional deformity[61] in which femoral neck points more anteriorly than normal[46] resulting in an excessively internally rotated femur. Femoral anteversion

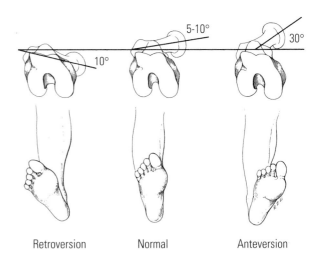

FIG. 41-13 Femoral neck *anteversion* measures the angle between the neck and shaft of the femur. Anteversion causes internal rotation of the lower limb that distally manifests as in toeing of the foot. In contrast, *retroversion* externally rotates the lower limb, and results in toeing out of the foot. (From Tria AJ, Klein KS: *An illustrated guide to the knee*, New York, 1992, Churchill Livingstone.)

is twice as common in girls compared boys,[45] and results in a gait deviation described as a *toe-in gait*. Femoral anteversion is a transverse plane deformity that is often accompanied by compensatory rotations of the tibia and talus such as external tibial rotation and over-pronation of the subtalar joint. The biomechanical implications of femoral anteversion are such that the Q angle is substantially increased, which imparts a valgus angulation to the quadriceps *tendon*. This increases the pennation angle between the superior patellar pole and the quadriceps muscle and represents a proximally originating lateral or valgus vector force on the patella (Fig. 41-14).

29. What is a common noncontact mechanism for lateral patellar subluxation?

An acute cause of patellar instability in the absence of trauma derives from deceleration maneuvers.[41] This presents as a complaint of the knee giving way while cutting away from the affected side such that the foot is planted and the femur internally rotates upon a laterally rotating, but fixed, tibia. This mechanism involves no direct contact but imparts a severe and sudden valgus force to the patellofemoral joint.

30. What is the mechanism of direct trauma to the patellofemoral joint, and how may associated effusion result in lateral patellar tracking?

Direct trauma to the patella or surrounding structures occurs because of a severe twist or valgus blow to the patella. Also included in this category is trauma secondary to knee surgery. An incision that weakens the medial capsule predisposes the patella to lateral overpull.[36] Associated effusion may distend the articular capsule such that inhibition of the femoral nerve occurs,[11] resulting in *neurogenic quadriceps atrophy*. The ensuing imbalance of stabilizing forces upon the patellofemoral joint derived from diminishment of medial quadriceps pull, biases the lateral contractile and noncontractile stabilizing structures towards lateral patellar deviation. A noncontact mechanism of injury may include a sharp twisting movement of the lower limb.

31. What is the clinical presentation?

The physical presentation of patients with patellofemoral instability is consistent. The signs of patellar instability include concomitant presence of patella alta, and an enlarged patellar fat pad apparent on lateral view as the knee approaches full extension with the patient in the short sitting posture. When both of these signs present simultaneously, the enlarged fat pad protrudes upward equal to the patella and presents as two humps similar to double-hump camel and designated as the *camel-back sign* (Fig. 41-15). Other signs include lateral patellar tilt, evidence of long-standing Osgood-Schlatter disease, dysplastic vastum medialis obliquus, hypoplasia of either the lateral femoral condyle or of the patella, a Wiberg II or III patella, dysplastic VMO as evidenced by a medially observed and palpated dimple, positive apprehension sign, vastus lateralis hypertrophy, excessive patellar mobility, and tenderness peripherally but especially along the medial patellar border as well as behind the patella (subpatellar tenderness).[41] Electromyographic testing of the VMO may reveal disuse atrophy.[28]

Other signs include obesity,[58] the presence of other knee malalignments such as genu recurvatum, genu valgum, an increased Q angle, femoral neck anteversion, and excessive pronation of the subtalar joint. A marked increase in the Q angle value may present as a *positive bayonet sign* in which the alignment of the quadriceps, patellar tendon, and tibial shaft resembles a French bayonet (Fig. 41-16). These postural deformities may present individually, or in groupings such as the miserable malalignment syndrome consisting of internal femoral rotation and compensatory external tibial rotation and subtalar joint pronation. Miserable malalignment syndrome[52] (Fig. 41-17) results in *squinting patellae* that almost face each other at termination of stance phase and during quiet standing.

With the patient short sitting with both hips and knees flexed to 90°, one may observe the presence of the patella pointing laterally and superiorly. This *lateral patellar tilting* is referred to as a *grasshopper eye*[34] or *owl eye*[58] patella and indicates lateral overpull of the patella. This type of lateral patellar tilt is obviated during short sitting only in those individuals who do not have a genu valgum deformity at the knee, but who sustained an injury to the knee. In contrast, individuals with a lateral patellar tilt during quiet standing derive their tilt from a genu valgum deformity. The end result of a long standing unresolved genu valgum deformity is stretching of the medial structures and tightening of the lateral structures at the knee that predisposes the patella to instability.

Many patients with patellar instability complain of a *giving-way sensation* that usually occurs when the patient decelerates by cutting away from the affected side. The patient may occasionally remember that the patella "slid over" or that a "click" was felt and interpreted as

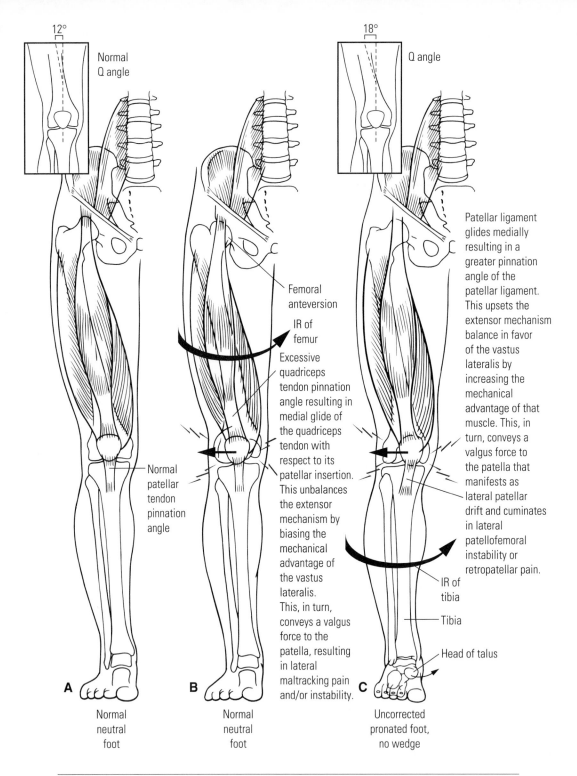

FIG. 41-14 Proximal and distal causes of patellar instability and retropatellar pain owing to unbalanced extensor mechanism function. **A,** A proximal origin of dysfunction derives from femoral anteversion, which in turn, causes an increase of the pennation angle of the quadriceps tendon. **B,** A distal origin of patellofemoral dysfunction stems from excessive pronation of the subtalar joint. The concomitant obligatory internal tibial torsion increases the pinnation angle of the patellar ligament. Regardless of whether the pennation angles of either the patellar tendon or ligament are increased, the common denominator of both the proximal and distal origins of extensor mechanism imbalance is a lateral glide of either the tendon or ligament. This lateral glide, either at the superior or inferior patellar poles, biases extensor mechanism balance in favor of vastus lateralis by increasing the mechanical advantage of that muscle over the vastus medialis.

The following labels appear within the figure:

12° — Normal Q angle
18° — Q angle

Normal patellar tendon pinnation angle

A Normal neutral foot

Femoral anteversion
IR of femur
Excessive quadriceps tendon pinnation angle resulting in medial glide of the quadriceps tendon with respect to its patellar insertion. This unbalances the extensor mechanism by biasing the mechanical advantage of the vastus lateralis. This, in turn, conveys a valgus force to the patella, resulting in lateral maltracking pain and/or instability.

B Normal neutral foot

Patellar ligament glides medially resulting in a greater pinnation angle of the patellar ligament. This upsets the extensor mechanism balance in favor of the vastus lateralis by increasing the mechanical advantage of that muscle. This, in turn, conveys a valgus force to the patella that manifests as lateral patellar drift and cuminates in lateral patellofemoral instability or retropatellar pain.

IR of tibia
Tibia
Head of talus

C Uncorrected pronated foot, no wedge

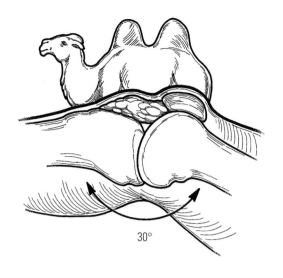

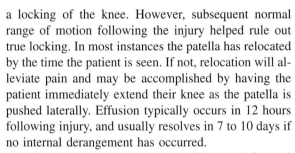

FIG. 41-15 Patients with patellofemoral subluxation often have high patellae known as patella alta. As the knee approaches extension, the enlarged fat pad becomes prominent. Fat pad prominence and a high riding patella appear as two humps known as the "camel back sign." (From Scott WN: *The knee*, St Louis, 1994, Mosby.)

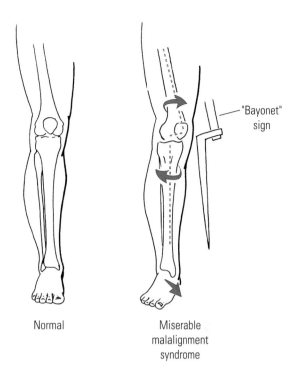

Normal

Miserable malalignment syndrome

"Bayonet" sign

FIG. 41-16 Bayonet sign observed in the standing posture of an individual with a markedly increased Q angle deriving from tibia vara of the proximal third. Alignment of the quadriceps, patellar tendon, and tibial shaft resembles a French bayonet. (From Shankman GA: *Fundamental orthopedic management for the physical therapist assistant*, St Louis, 1997, Mosby.)

a locking of the knee. However, subsequent normal range of motion following the injury helped rule out true locking. In most instances the patella has relocated by the time the patient is seen. If not, relocation will alleviate pain and may be accomplished by having the patient immediately extend their knee as the patella is pushed laterally. Effusion typically occurs in 12 hours following injury, and usually resolves in 7 to 10 days if no internal derangement has occurred.

The only independent motion of the patellofemoral joint is proximal migration for approximately 2 cm by the contracting quadriceps muscle with the knee fully extended. This motion is eliminated by placing the knee in as little as 30° of flexion. The presence or absence of a hypermobile patella may be gauged by attempting to laterally subluxate the patella manually at this angle of knee motion. The normal patella may be manually displaced 25% to 50% the width of the patella either medially or laterally. Greater deviation represents a laxity of the medial or lateral patellar restraints. Apprehension noted on the patient's face during this maneuver indicates a positive *apprehension test* and is considered a sign of recurrent subluxation.[16] This test is best performed in the *prone position* as this posture short-circuits protective quadriceps contraction that may skew the results, and facilitate quadriceps relaxation.[41]

Pseudolocking represents a common symptom associated with patellar instability. Patients may complain of a knee locking sensation, when they, in fact, are referring to pseudolocking. Pseudolocking refers to a ratchet-rhythm sensation in which the knee catches but does not require any particular maneuver (unlike true locking) to achieve full restoration of range of motion.[65] Pseudolocking may result from reflexive inhibition of the quadriceps mechanism, and may often manifest as an unstable knee when negotiating stairs.[44,56]

An associated injury that may occur simultaneously with lateral patellar dislocation includes *sprain of the medial retinacula* in which the *medial patellofemoral ligament* may undergo stretching or rupture. This clinically presents as tenderness along the medial retinaculum. Sometimes, the vastus medialis muscle is strained or avulsed from the medial intermuscular septum, causing pain in the medial region of the knee that may be confused with sprain of the medial collateral

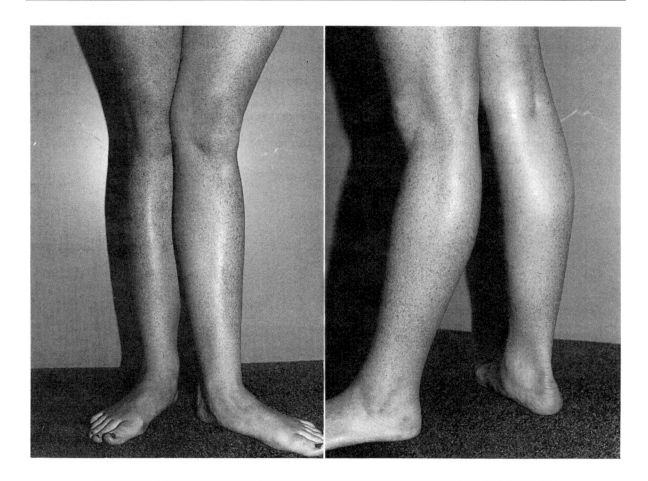

FIG. 41-17 "Miserable malalignment syndrome" of the lower extremities is characterized by excessive internal femoral rotation due to femoral anteversion, causing compensatory external tibial rotation and pronation of the feet. The patellae almost face each other at termination of stance phase. (From Griffin LY: *Rehabilitation of the injured knee,* ed 2, St Louis, 1995, Mosby.)

ligament.[50] Sprain of the medial retinacula is associated with negative frontal plane testing of the knee joint. In addition, patellar dislocations are commonly associated with avulsion fracture of either the lateral femoral condyle or the medial patellar facet.

32. What is the differential diagnosis?

The diagnosis of patellofemoral instability by radiologic evaluation alone is difficult[41] and should be discouraged.[36] Ancillary testing via CT and MRI are helpful in diagnosing patellofemoral instability.[41] Similarly, the use of thermograms can show a rise in temperature, indicating inflammation, along the medial side of the patella at the insertion of the vastus medialis. Despite the availability of ancillary testing, a diagnosis of patel-

lofemoral instability is usually based on the history and clinical presentation.

The history following patellar dislocation is one in which the patient felt or even saw the patella slide laterally. If the patella dislocated, then the diagnosis is more obvious than when evaluating cases of subluxation. As such, determination of patellar subluxation represents a challenge to the clinician and requires a higher degree of suspicion, especially as subluxation may be easily confused with plica syndrome.

- *Plica syndrome* (see Chapter 47). The synovial plicae are vestigial remnants of the septum that, in the embryonic knee, divided the joint capsule into three distinct parts. Plicae are crescent-shaped folds of tissue that extend medially from the infrapatellar fat pad to loop around the femoral condyle, cross under the quadriceps tendon, and pass laterally over the lateral femoral condyle to the lateral retinaculum. Because they are adjacent to the patella and palpable over the medial and lateral retinacular regions, symptomatic plica may be confused with patellar subluxation. Moreover, the patterns of innervation of the structures of the knee are such that the afferent feedback that signify patellar dislocation is cross-innervated with those same nerves that innervate the synovial plica. Thus patients with synovial plica fibrosis or hypertrophy may sustain plica interposition and impingement in the patellofemoral joint during quadriceps contraction. The afferent impulse the patient receives is similar to that which would have occurred in true subluxation.[64] With medial collateral ligament sprain following acute patellar dislocation, gentle manual patellar subluxation will produce discomfort, a finding not seen with primary injury to the medial collateral ligament.[41] In addition, sprain of the medial collateral ligament is characterized by positive valgus stress testing of the knee joint.

- *Medial meniscus injury* (see Chapter 42). Meniscus pathology is characterized by true locking of the knee joint, and locking in extension and flexion. In contrast, patellar instability is characterized by pseudolocking, and a blockage of flexion range in the event of a nonrelocated patella.[10] Moreover, patellar dislocation occurs before the age of meniscus rupture.[9] Finally, provocative stress testing for meniscal injury will yield negative results in the patient with patellar instability.

- *Osteochondral fracture of the patella or distal femur.* Tangential superoinferior (skyline) radiographic views are essential following suspected lateral patellar dislocation to rule out an associated osteochondral avulsion[15] fractures of either the medial patellar edge or the lateral lip of the patellar groove (i.e., the site of impact during lateral dislocation—Salter). Effusion collects much more rapidly following osteochondral fracture—in 2 hours compared with the typical 12 hours associated with subluxation/dislocation. Moreover, osteochondral fracture is suggested by aspiration that yields hemarthrosis with fat droplets, whereas dislocation yields serosanguinous fluid.[4] The presence of such a fracture is an indication for surgery and removal of smaller fragments while affixing the larger fragment(s)[10] as well as repair of any soft-tissue disruption secondary to dislocation.[33]

33. What therapeutic intervention is appropriate to management of patellar instability?

Therapeutic intervention follows relocation of the displaced patella, which is accomplished by manual pressure in full knee extension. Surgical intervention is only necessary in the event of a displaced fragment. Otherwise, the simple dislocation is managed with immobilization followed by physical therapy beginning after 4 to 6 weeks. The dislocation recurrence rate is approximately 30% in individuals younger than 20 years of age, and decreases to 5% in those over 40 years old.[25]

Conservative management of patellar dislocation is recommended in patients whose postreduction Merchant-view radiographs show central tracking of the patella, an absence of underlying anatomic predisposition for dislocation, and those patients lacking evidence of osteochondral fracture.[67] It is imperative to institute treatment of patellar subluxation as the condition will worsen if left untreated. If ignored, the lateral retinaculum gradually becomes contracted, exacerbating abnormal patellofemoral tracking.[58] The rehabilitative approach to patellofemoral instability, like the management of chondromalacia, includes strengthening and stretching exercises, bracing, modality use such as cryotherapy and electrical stimulation, biofeedback, molded in-shoe orthoses, weight reduction, activity modification, and medications. The benefit of immobilization following dislocation remains unproven.[67]

Conservative management of patellofemoral joint instability carries a success rate of approximately 80%.[12,24,29] More than 90% of patient who attain the ability to perform three sets of ten repetitions of 12 pounds of weight achieve excellent clinical results. However, patient compliance is essential to a successful rehabilitation program that precludes future instability. During therapy, athletic activities that helped precipitate symptoms, such as performing duck walks or running stadium stairs, are strongly discouraged and eliminated in the athlete's program. Other athletic activities may be done provided that the patient adheres to his/her therapeutic regimen.[36]

- *Exercise.* Exercise in the form of progressive resistive exercise and appropriate muscle stretching exercise remain the foundation of a comprehensive rehabilitation program in the management of patellofemoral instability. The cornerstone of this treatment strategy is directed towards centralizing the patella. Exercises should be done 3 times per day. Weights may be progressed at approximately 2.5 lbs every 3 to 4 days depending upon patient tolerance and provided that no pain or extensor lag accompanies the increase.

- *Quadriceps setting exercises.* Quadriceps setting exercises are done with the patient supine and the contralateral hip and knee flexed to support the pelvis low back. The ipsilateral quadriceps is contracted and held for 8 seconds as the foot is dorsiflexed.[2] Straight leg raises are done in the same position to a height of 12 inches and held for a count before slowly lowering the limb downward. Hip flexor strength may also be done in the short sitting posture. To strengthen the ipsilateral hip abductors, the patient lies on his or her contralateral side with the contralateral knee flexed to stabilize the pelvis as the hip is abducted to 30°. This strengthens the gluteus medius, gluteus minimus, tensor fascia femoris, as well as the peroneals of the foot. It is important to prevent the pelvis from rocking anteriorly or posteriorly and, thereby substitute by way of the hamstrings or the adductors. Weights are progressed at approximately 2.5 lb every 3 to 4 days depending on patient tolerance. Hip adductor work is done by first placing the contralateral flexed hip behind the pelvis, thereby providing clearance for the upward adductor antigravity swing of the ipsilateral hip. The most common error committed with this particular exercise is lack of full ipsilateral knee extension so as to preclude adductor tendinitis. All exercises are begun with 1 set of 10 repetitions. Resistance may be added to all these exercises by the attachment of the cuff weight at the ipsilateral ankle. Weights are progressed at approximately 2.5 lb every 3 to 4 days depending on patient tolerance.

The inclusion of terminal knee extension exercises, which, according to some, is specific for VMO strengthening, is controversial because this range may reproduce or increase the patient's symptoms and signs. Perhaps an alternate VMO strengthening strategy would incorporate the use of biofeedback and electric muscle stimulation

- *Stretching.* Flexion contractures of the knee secondary to tight hamstrings commonly present in patients with patellofemoral joint problems.[36] This is because tight hamstrings increase patellofemoral joint contact forces. The hamstrings, gastrocnemius, and quadriceps muscles are two jointed muscles that may be optimally stretched by posturing both joints across their span such that they are placed in *passive insufficiency.* Hamstring stretching is crucial in any conservative treatment program for patellofemoral dysfunc-

tion as tight hamstrings increase patellofemoral contact forces. The Ober position may be used to stretch the iliotibial band (see Chapter 48). Stretch may be maintained for 20 to 30 seconds followed by a 5-second rest, and repeated up to 10 times daily.

- *Modalities.* Modalities in the form of heat before exercise and ice following activity will relieve pain derived from the inflammatory state. Judicious use of antiinflammatory medication may be helpful. VMO strengthening may be augmented by biofeedback in which the patient learns how to isolate VMO contraction. VMO strengthening may also be facilitated by using electrical stimulation, which recruits more muscle fibers in conjunction with patient contraction. External support in the form of bracing may be used as a therapeutic trial in the differential diagnosis of patellofemoral instability.[55] The most simple, yet effective, external support consists of cutting out a horseshoe-shaped felt pad and wrapping it snugly to the patient's knee with an Ace bandage or an elastic sleeve. Braces minimize the load on the patellofemoral joint, prevent atrophy of the quadriceps muscle,[47] and represent a buttress to lateral dislocation.

- *Orthosis.* The inclusion of an appropriate orthotic is an indispensable component of the rehabilitation program as it compensates for the malalignment that initiated the biomechanical imbalance that resulted in pathokinesiology at the knee. For every degree the over-pronated foot is supinated the Q angle will diminish 0.44°.[53,60] The individual experiencing excessive valgus force to the patellofemoral joint owing to an increased pinnation angle as a function of excessive subtalar joint pronation will clearly benefit from an orthosis that restores subtalar joint balance. The application of a 5° or 9° medial hindfoot wedge[60] (i.e., rearfoot posts) will help restore balance to the extensor mechanism at the knee by diminishing the magnitude of internal tibial torsion, and thereby reduce the Q angle (Fig. 41-18).

- *Home exercise program.* Given the degree of compliance decreases after the symptoms improve, patients often pose the question, "Do I have to do these boring exercises for the rest of my life?" It is imperative that the therapist communicates with patients and empowers them with the belief that a continuous home maintenance exercise regimen will best prevent future dislocation. A maintenance program may be defined as that point when the addition of more exercise or weight causes an increase in symptoms.[36] Those patients who, despite warning, will not continue a maintenance program following a successful response to physical therapy, are urged to perform exercises, at the very least, when their knees become symptomatic.

- *Activity alteration.* Various activities should be eliminated in patient's who have sustained subluxation of the patellofemoral joint. A common high school coaching technique used to build lower extremity strength is running up stadium stairs. In similar fashion, "frog walking" involved squatting down to the ground with the hip and knees fully flexed and walking some 40 to 50 yards. Both of these activities may produce patellofemoral problems by way of impacting upon the extensor mechanism and tracking of the patella within the femoral groove and should be eliminated in patients who have experienced subluxation of the patellofemoral joint.

34. What is the surgical management of patellar dislocation and when is it appropriate?

Following dislocation, the knee should be palpated medially for a possible tear in the distal substance of the vastus medialis, a tear of the vastus medialis from its attachment at the medial femoral condyle, or a tear of the vastus medialis into the patella. If the latter is discovered, then the patient ought to promptly be referred to an orthopaedic surgeon for surgical repair.[41] Also, the medial patellar facet or the lateral femoral condyle may be injured during dislocation, leading to an intraarticular loose body requiring excision.[25]

Patellofemoral surgical realignment is recommended only when a minimum of 4 to 6 months of physical therapy has been unsuccessful.[21] This procedure is intended to correct any dysplastic features and establish muscle balance and bony alignment. Approximately 5% of patients do not respond to conservative measures; approximately half of these patients live with their discomfort as it remains, and the other half (2% to 3%) go on to surgical intervention.[25] Surgery is also indicated for recurrent and chronic patellar dislocation. *Percutaneous lateral retinacular release* for patellar instability, done arthroscopically, detaches the patella from the tight lateral soft-tissue structures, including the lateral retinaculum fibers, from the tensor fasciae latae muscle, and joint capsule. The lateral retinacular release acts to diminish the valgus overpull towards the lateral side so that more centralized patellar tracking may occur. Moreover, repair of the lax medial joint capsule may be attempted, as well as redirection of the line of pull of the patellar tendon by way of the semitendinosus tendon may be appropriate.[33]

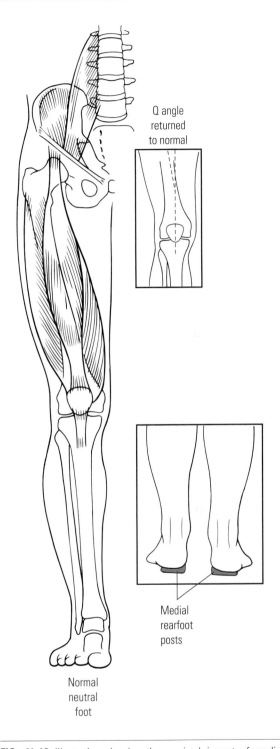

Q angle returned to normal

Medial rearfoot posts

Normal neutral foot

FIG. 41-18 Illustration showing the proximal impact of medial rearfoot posts upon the biomechanics of the knee and hip. Medial wedging has a supinatory effect upon the over-pronated foot. This diminishes the excessive medial tibial torsion that accompanies excessive subtalar joint pronation. This, in turn, reduces the pinnation angle of the patellar ligament, diminishes the valgus force to the patella, and thereby reduces the value of the Q angle.

Following release, rapid mobilization of the joint is important to prevent scarring and tightening along the released lateral structures. Also, intense strengthening of the vastus medialis muscle is required.[41] If the lateral release procedure fails, a formal patellofemoral reconstruction is considered in which operative realignment of the extensor mechanism is done. Patellofemoral realignment procedures may include medial plication of the vastus medialis, patellar tendon hemitransfer, and a semitendinosus check rain.[15] Overenthusiastic lateral release may result in more problems than it solves, particularly in the pediatric population, which is more flexible and whose muscle balance is in a constant state of flux.[66]

REFERENCES

1. Aglietti P, Insall JN, Cerulli G: Patellar pain and incongruence. I. Measurements of incongruences, *Clin Orthop* 176:217-224, 1983.
2. Antich TJ, Brewster CE: Modification of quadriceps femoris muscle exercises during knee rehabilitation, *Phys Ther* 66(8):1246-1251, 1986.
3. Basmajian JV: Re-education of the vastus medialis: a misconception, *Arch Phys Med Rehab* 51:245-247, 1970.
4. Bassett FH: Surgery of the patellofemoral joint: acute dislocation of the patella, osteochondral fractures, and injuries to the extensor mechanism of the knee, *Am Acad Orthop Surg* (Instructional Course Lectures), 25:40, 1976.
5. Bose K, Kanagasuntheram R, Osman MBH: Vastus medialis oblique: an anatomic and physiological study, *Orthopedics* 39:880-883, 1980.
6. Brody DM: *Clinical symposia: running injury: prevention and management,* Summit, NJ, 1987, CIBA-GEIGY.
7. Brontzman SB: *Clinical orthopedic rehabilitation,* St Louis, 1996, Mosby.
8. Caillet R: *Knee pain and disability.* Philadelphia, 1983, FA Davis.
9. Cyriax J: Diagnosis of soft tissue lesions. In *Textbook of orthopedic medicine,* Vol 1, ed 8, London, 1982, Bailliere Tindall.
10. Dandy DJ: *Essential orthopedics and trauma,* Edinburgh, 1989, Churchill Livingstone.
11. DeAndrade JR, Grant C, Dixon AJ: Joint distention and reflex muscle inhibition in the knee, *J Bone Joint Surg* 47A:313-322, 1965.
12. DeHaven K, Dolan W, Mayer P: Chondromalacia patellae in athletes, *Am J Sports Med* 7:5, 1979.
13. DePalma FA: *Management in medicine and surgery,* Philadelphia, 1954, JB Lippincott.
14. DiStefano VJ: Skeletal injuries of the knee. In Nicholas JA, Hershman EB editors: *The lower extremity and spine,* ed 2, vol 1, St Louis, 1995, Mosby.
15. Eftimiades J: Anatomy, etiology and treatment of patellofemoral dysfunction examined. In *Advance for physical therapists,* King of Prussia, 1991, Merion Publications.
16. Fairbanks HAT: Internal derangement of the knee in children and adolescents, *Proc R Soc Med* 30:427, 1937.
17. Ficat PR, Hungerford DS: *Disorders of the patellofemoral joint,* Baltimore, 1977, Williams & Wilkins.
18. Fox TA: Dysplasia of the quadriceps mechanism, *Surg Clin North Am* 55:199-226, 1975.
19. Fujckawan K, Dredham B, Wright V: Biomechanics of the patellofemoral joint, a study of the congruity of the patellofemoral compartment and movement of the patella, *English Medicine* 12:3-11, 1983.
20. Fulkerson JP, Grossling HR: Anatomy of the knee joint lateral retinaculum, *Clin Orthop* 153:183-185, 1980.
21. Fulkerson JP, Schutzer SF: After failure of conservative treatment for painful patellofemoral malalignment: lateral release or realignment? *Orthop Clin North Am* 17:283, 1986.
22. Goodfellow J, Hungersford DS, Zindel M: Patellofemoral joint mechanics and pathology. I. Functional anatomy of the patellofemoral joint, *J Bone Joint Surg* 58B:287, 1976.
23. Gould JA III: *Orthopedic and sports physical therapy,* ed 2, St Louis, 1990, Mosby.
24. Grana WA, Krieghauser SF: Scientific basis of extensor mechanism disorders, *Clin Sports Med* 4(2):247-257, 1985.
25. Greenfield BH: *Rehabilitation of the knee: a problem-solving approach,* Philadelphia, 1993, FA Davis.
26. Gross M: *Gray's anatomy,* ed 29, Philadelphia, 1973, Lea & Febiger.
27. Grossman RB, Nicholas JA: Common disorders of the knee, *Orthop Clin North Am* 8:619, 1977.
28. Henry JH: Conservative treatment of patellofemoral subluxation, *Clin Sports Med* 8(2):263, 1989.
29. Henry JM, Crossland JW: Conservative treatment of patellofemoral subluxation, *Am J Sports Med* 7:12, 1979.
30. Henry JH: The patellofemoral joint. In Nicholas JA, Hershman EB editors: *The lower extremity and spine,* ed 2, vol 1, St Louis, 1995, Mosby.
31. Horton MG, Hall TL: Quadricep femoris muscle angle: normal values and relationships with gender and selected skeletal measures, *Phys Ther* 69:11, 1989.
32. Hertling D, Kessler RM: *Management of common musculoskeletal disorders: physical therapy principles and methods,* ed 2, Philadelphia, 1990, JB Lippincott.
33. Hughston JC: Subluxation of the patella, *J Bone Joint Surg* 50:1003-1026, 1968.
34. Hughston JC, Walsh WM, Puddu G: *Patellar subluxation and dislocation: Saunders monographs in clinical orthopedics,* Philadelphia, 1984, WB Saunders.
35. Insall JN, Aglietti P, Tria AJ: Patella pain and incongruence. II. Clinical application, *Clin Orthop* 176:225-232, 1983.
36. Insall JN, Falvo KA, Wise DW: Chondromalacia patellae: a prospective study, *J Bone Joint Surg* 58A:1-8, 1976.
37. Insall JN: *Surgery of the knee,* New York, 1983, Churchill Livingstone.
38. Jacobson KE, Flandry FC: Diagnosis of anterior knee pain, *Clin Sports Med* 8(2):183, 1989.
39. Kaplan EB: Surgical approach to the lateral (peroneal) side of the knee joint, *Surg Gynecol Obstet* 104:346-356, 1957.
40. Kaufer H: Mechanical function of the patella, *J Bone Joint Surg)* 53A:153, 1971.
41. Kettelkamp DB: Current concepts review management of patellar malalignment, *J Bone Joint Surg* 63A:1344, 1981.

42. Knight KL, Martin JA, Londodee BR: EMG comparison of quadriceps femoris activity during knee extension and straight leg raises, *Am J Phys Med* 58:57-69, 1979.

43. Lehmkuhl LD, Smith LK: *Brunstromm's clinical kinesiology,* ed 4, Philadelphia, 1989, FA Davis.

44. Lieb FJ, Perry J: Quadriceps function: an anatomical and mechanical study using amputated limbs, *J Bone Joint Surg* 50A:1535-1548, 1968.

45. Magee DL: *Orthopedic physical assessment,* Philadelphia, 1987, WB Saunders.

46. Meals RA: *One hundred orthopedic conditions every doctor should understand,* St Louis, 1992, Quality Medical.

47. Moller BN, Krebs B: Dynamic knee brace in treatment of patellofemoral disorders, *Arch Orthop Trauma Surg* 104:377-379, 1986.

48. Moore KL: *Clinically orientated anatomy,* Baltimore, 1980, Williams & Wilkins.

49. Netter FH: *The Ciba collection of medical illustrations,* vol 8, Part I, Summit, NJ, 1990, CIBA-GEIGY.

50. Netter FH: *The Ciba collection of medical illustrations,* vol 8, Part II, Development disorders, tumors, rheumatic diseases and joint replacement, Summit, NJ, 1990, CIBA-GEIGY.

51. Netter FH: *The Ciba collection of medical illustrations,* vol 8, Part III. Musculoskeletal system: trauma, evaluation, and management, Summit, NJ, 1993, CIBA-GEIGY.

52. Nicholas JA: The lower extremity and spine, ed 2, vol 1, St Louis, 1995, Mosby.

53. Olerud C, Rosendahl Y: Torsion-transmitting properties of the hindfoot, *Clin Orthop* 214:284-294, January 1987.

54. Pagnani MJ et al: Anatomy of the knee. In Nicholas JA, Hershman EB editors: *The lower extremity and spine,* ed 2, vol 1, St Louis, 1995, Mosby.

55. Pearson CY: After treatment of lateral dislocation of the patella by a new form of knee cap, *Lancet* 1, 1984.

56. Perry J: *Gait analysis: normal and pathological function,* Thorofare, NJ, 1992, Slack.

57. Pitman MI, Frankel VH: Biomechanics of the knee in athletes. In Nicholas JA, Hershman EB editors: *The lower extremity and spine,* ed 2, vol 1, St Louis, 1995, Mosby.

58. Pronsati MP: Australian PT introduces new treatment for patellofemoral pain. In *Advance for physical therapists,* Pennsylvania, 1991, Merion.

59. Reilly DT, Martens M: Experimental analysis of the quadriceps muscle force and patellofemoral joint reaction force for various activities, *Acta Orthop Scand* 43:126-137, 1972.

60. Reiley MA: *Guidelines for prescribing foot orthotics,* Thorofare, NJ, 1995, Slack.

61. Salter RB: *Textbook of disorders of the musculoskeletal system,* ed 2, Baltimore, 1983, Williams & Wilkins.

62. Sneath RS: The insertion of the biceps femoris, *J Anat* 89:550-553, 1955.

63. Spencer JD, Hayes KC, Alexander IJ: Knee joint effusion and quadricep reflex inhibition in man, *Arch Phys Med Rehabil* 65:171, 1984.

64. Staheli LT: *Fundamentals of pediatric orthopedics,* New York, 1992, Raven.

65. Stanitski C: *Getting a jump on anterior knee pain,* Pittsburgh, 1988, Sportcare & Fitness.

66. Strizak AM: Knee injuries. In Nicholas JA, Hershman EB editors: *The lower extremity and spine,* ed 2, vol 2, St Louis, 1995, Mosby.

67. Subotnick SI: *Podiatric sports medicine,* Mt. Kisco, NY, 1979, Futura.

68. Terry GC: The anatomy of the extensor mechanism, *Clin Sports Med* 8(2):174, 1989.

69. Terry SC, Hughston JC, Norwood LA: The anatomy of the iliopatellar band and iliotibial tract, *Am J Sports Med* 14:139, 1986.

70. Thabit G III, Micheli LJ: Patellofemoral pain in the pediatric patient, *Orthop Clin North Am* 23(4):568, 1992.

71. Tria AJ, Klein KS: *An illustrated guide to the knee,* New York, 1992, Churchill Livingstone.

72. Tria AJ, Palumbo RC, Alicea JA: Conservative care for patellofemoral pain, *Orthop Clin North Am* 23(4):547, 1992.

73. Wiberg G: Roentgenographic and anatomic studies of the patellofemoral joint, *Acta Orthop Scand* 12:319, 1941.

74. Wickiewicz T, Roy RR, Powell PL et al: Muscle architecture of the human lower limb, *Clin Orthop* 179:275, 1983.

75. Zappala FG, Taffel CB, Scuderi GR: Rehabilitation of patellofemoral joint disorders, *Orthop Clin North Am* 23(4):557, 1992.

RECOMMENDED READING

Henry JH: Conservative treatment of patellofemoral subluxation, *Clin Sports Med* 8(2), April 1989.

Zappala FG, Taffel CB, Scuderi GR: Rehabilitation of patellofemoral joint disorders, *Orthopedic Clin North Am* 23(4), October 1992.

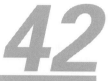

Knee Catching and Locking in Both Flexion and Extension, Accompanied by Joint-Line Tenderness, Giving Way, Pain, Swelling, and Clear Joint Fluid during Arthrocentesis

CASE 1: A 27-year-old fireman wearing full gear descended down the last step of a flight of basement stairs with his right foot and felt his right knee twist as the left side of the stairwell collapsed underneath him. He presented the next day with effusion, and arthrocentesis yielded serosanguinous fluid. He describes a sensation of giving way or impending collapse, particularly when attempting to negotiate stairs. On 3 occasions since the injury the knee actually buckled painfully while ascending and descending stairs. There is pain present during active knee joint flexion. There is no previous history of knee injury, and the patient ambulates into your office with crutches.

OBSERVATION Neither patella baja nor alta are viewed from the lateral knee posture. Mild to moderate effusion noted during ballottement testing. No atrophy observed in the right quadriceps femoris muscle and vastus medialis obliquus (VMO).

PALPATION Yields point tenderness along the medial joint line.

RANGE OF MOTION Full range of motion is present during knee extension, although pain increases beyond 70° flexion and locks in the vicinity of 90°. An empty end-feel is imparted to the examiner's hand as the upper range of right knee flexion is approached.

STRENGTH Normal strength between 0° and 60° of knee flexion.

GIRTH MEASUREMENT Girth measurement for the right quadriceps and vastus medialis oblique muscles are normal when compared with the uninvolved knee.

SPECIAL TESTS Positive Apley, McMurray, and "bounce home" tests. Negative tests for anterior or posterior draw, and valgus or varus stress tests.

RADIOGRAPHS Radiographs are negative for loose bodies, tumors, and fracture.

CLUE:

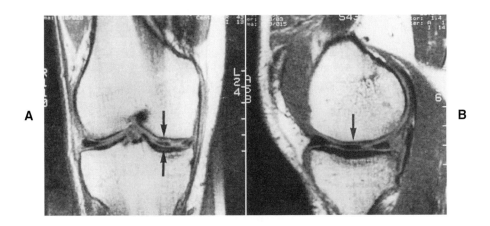

Clue. Coronal **(A)** and **(B)** sagittal plane MRI of the knee. (From Nicholas JA, Hershman EB editors: *The lower extremity and spine in sports medicine,* ed 2, St Louis, 1995, Mosby.)

CASE 2: A 49-year-old armchair executive and recreational athlete was playing tennis with his brother and reports a click in his right knee and a sensation of locking at some point during the game. When asked to describe the moment he explains that he suddenly reached laterally to his right to hit the oncoming ball with a forward stroke with his right leg still planted and pointing forward. You interpret this description as a lateral femoral rotation on a (medially rotated) fixed tibia. Effusion at the knee joint gradually developed over 1 to 3 days following injury. The patient complains of pain at the extremes of extension and often feels a sudden locking sensation just short of full extension. He also admits to a history of earlier acute episodes that have been recurring with increasing frequency over the past several years. Each episode is followed by gradual abatement of symptoms, although not as quickly or completely with the last 2 episodes. Gradual onset of symptoms will recur if he "doesn't take it easy." Although pain was worse during activity it was still present at rest. Joint aspiration following this last injury showed serosanguinous fluid. Medially rotating the tibia consistently reproduces symptoms. The patient reports no night pain.

OBSERVATION   Lateral view of the knee shows normal patellar height. A dimple is viewed at the area where the vastus medialis obliquus muscle normally inserts into the patella. Slight hypertrophy of the vastus lateralis. No atrophy observed in the right quadriceps femoris muscle and vastus medialis obliquus. Mild effusion is observed during ballottement testing.

PALPATION   Point tenderness localized to the lateral joint line.

RANGE OF MOTION   Locking tends to occur between 10° and 20° of full extension, although full and painless toward the higher range of knee flexion. An empty end-feel is imparted to the examiner's hand as terminal knee extension is approached.

STRENGTH   Normal strength between 40° and 135° of knee flexion (relative to full extension).

GIRTH MEASUREMENT   Girth measurement reveals a 2.2-cm deficit, and a 1.4-cm deficit at 20 cm and 5 cm above the base of the patella, respectively, as compared with the uninvolved side.

SPECIAL TESTS   A valgus stress applied to the right knee during flexion and extension between 0° and 90° results in both pain and a "clicking" sensation. Negative tests for anterior/posterior draw or valgus/varus stress testing of the knee joint.

RADIOGRAPHS   Radiographs are negative for tumor, loose bodies, and fracture.

? Questions

1. What is most likely causing symptoms in these patients' knees?
2. What is the history of meniscal injury management?
3. Is the tibiofemoral articulation a simple hinge joint?
4. What is the role of the menisci in enhancing the contact of the femorotibial articulation?
5. Is the helical motion of the knee joint during terminal knee extension a result of architectural osseous asymmetry between the medial and lateral femorotibial joints?
6. What are the biomechanics of the screw-home locking mechanism at the femorotibial articulation?
7. What is the difference between the open and closed kinetic chain function in relation to the screw-home mechanism at the knee?
8. Why are injuries to the meniscus more likely to occur during closed kinetic chain function?
9. What is the structure of the menisci?
10. What are the meniscal functions?
11. What kinds of lubrication strategies are used at the tibiofemoral joint, and what role do the menisci play in joint lubrication?
12. What is the nerve supply to the meniscus?
13. What is the developmental anatomy of the menisci?
14. What gross anatomy is shared by the medial and lateral menisci?
15. What is the anatomy of the medial meniscus?
16. What accounts for the different shape of the medial and lateral menisci?
17. What is the anatomy of the lateral meniscus?
18. What is the function of the meniscofemoral ligaments of Wrisberg and Humphry?
19. Which ligament attaching to the medial meniscus is endowed with a dynamic ability not present in the lateral meniscus?
20. What is the relationship between the ACL and the menisci?
21. What determines the direction of meniscal motion?
22. What is the direction of femoral condylar displacement during the initial 100° of knee flexion range?
23. Are the directions of motion of the tibia and femur concurrent during terminal knee extension?
24. What mechanism of injury frequently injures the meniscus?
25. What area of which meniscus is most often injured, and what range of knee motion places the menisci at greater risk for sustaining injury?
26. Why is the medial meniscus most often injured in lateral cutting movements?
27. What is the classification of meniscal tears?
28. What is the prognostic classification of meniscal injury?
29. What is the clinical presentation of meniscal tears?
30. What physical signs are present during patient examination?
31. What imaging techniques are appropriate following suspected meniscus tear?
32. What is the differential diagnosis of meniscal lesions?

33. How do meniscal injuries in children differ from adults?
34. What are the different management strategies for a meniscus injury?
35. What therapeutic intervention is appropriate for a conservative management program of a torn meniscus?
36. What is the medical management of a locked knee?
37. What postoperative rehabilitative management is appropriate following partial meniscectomy or repair?
38. What are future trends in meniscal management?

---

1. What is most likely causing symptoms in these patients' knees?

The signs and symptoms of Case 1 suggest an acute peripheral tear of traumatic origin, of the bucket handle variety (see Clue), to the periphery of the *posterior horn of the medial meniscus.* Medial meniscus involvement is suggested by a mechanism of injury that involves medial femoral rotation on a (laterally rotated) planted tibia. The posterior meniscal horn is most likely involved as pain elicited upon knee flexion translates the femoral condyles posteriorly and causes anteroposterior deformation of the intact posterior horns or impingement of a loose posterior horn fragment. Joint aspiration yielded bloody synovial fluid as the lesion occurred in the vascularized peripheral rim. Case 2 suggests a chronic meniscal tear, most likely of the radial type, occurring on the central portion of the *anterior horn of the lateral meniscus.* An anterior horn injury is suggested by the presentation of pain and mechanical symptoms. Pain and locking elicited during knee extension implicate the anterior horns. During knee extension, the femoral condyles translate anteriorly and cause mediolateral deformation of the intact anterior horns or impingement of a loose anterior fragment. Arthrocentesis yielded clear and yellow (straw-colored) joint fluid suggesting the lesion occurred along the avascular central aspect of the meniscus. Atrophy of the quadriceps muscle, particularly the VMO muscle, is indicated by a dimple effect as the latter muscle inserts into the patella at an angle greater than the usual 55°.[37] This will occur in patients who cannot achieve full extension, causing subsequent atrophy of the VMO.

2. What is the history of meniscal injury management?

The history of our understanding of meniscal function spans two opposite approaches. The first advocated meniscal removal and was popular some 50 years ago, whereas today preservation of the meniscus is encouraged as often as is practically possible. The mammalian meniscus has been present for some 320 million years.[22] Relegated to the status of a vestigial organ,[91] as the tonsils or the appendix, the menisci were once routinely excised because of a short sighted approach that derived from an inability to understand the role of the menisci in knee biomechanics. The passage of time and clinical studies[15,24,38,39,92] have borne out the folly of this approach. Investigations into the biomechanical function of the menisci have revealed their importance in knee mechanics. Today, a preservationist attitude toward the menisci with attempts to save as much meniscal tissue as possible predominates. Partial arthroscopic meniscectomy with retention, when possible, of an intact peripheral rim preserves the normal biomechanics of the knee and has better long-term results owing to the absence or minimization of degenerative changes to articular cartilage[64] and reduced operative morbidity.

Any appreciation of meniscal function must occur in the context of the knee joint's complex function. An introduction to the anatomy and biomechanics of the knee joint is therefore necessary to fully appreciate the role of the meniscus.

3. Is the tibiofemoral articulation a simple hinge joint?

The knee joint, more properly known as the *tibiofemoral articulation,* bears the body's superincumbent weight and is situated as a fulcrum between the two longest bones or levers in the body. The knee joint is subject to bending and torsional stresses and may be considered the body's most vulnerable articulation.[21] The motion of the tibiofemoral joint is complex and includes anteroposterior translation of the femur in relation to the tibial plateau by way of arthrokinematic *gliding* and *rolling.*[99] The possibility of a simple equivalent 1:1 ratio of gliding is precluded by an inequity of articular surface between the femoral condyles and the tibial plateau. Because the lengths of the femoral condyles are twice as great as the anteroposterior dimensions of the corresponding tibial plateaus, joint play in the form of *slide* accompanies rolling in the joint during flexion and extension.

Because of the asymmetrical architectural configuration of the medial and lateral tibiofemoral joint, flexion and extension are accompanied by transverse plane motion, or *rotation* of the tibia and femur during normal function. By way of analogy, motion of the tibiofemoral joint may, in part, be likened to the triplanar motion at the subtalar joint, which also has components of anterior/posterior talar translation as well as talar rotation. This analogy is appropriate, particularly as transverse and sagittal plane components of both the subtalar and tibiofemoral joints cooperatively move together with respect to the tibial shaft spanning the distance between them. Thus motion of the tibiofemoral articulation may be said to occur in all three planes[94] and may appropriately be referred to as a rolling, gliding, and rotating hinge joint, or *modified hinge joint*[98] with 2 degrees of freedom. These movements include rolling during flexion and extension in the sagittal plane around a mediolateral axis and rotation in the transverse plane around a superior-inferior axis. More recent analysis shows the femorotibial joint to be an even more complex articulation with 3 rotational and 3 translational movements for a total of 6 degrees of freedom.[30] Best described by an *orthogonal coordinate system*, the 6 degrees of freedom include anteroposterior translation, mediolateral translation, internal-external rotation, flexion-extension, and varus-valgus movement.

4. What is the role of the menisci in enhancing the contact of the femorotibial articulation?

The elbow is the upper extremity analogue of the knee joint, and more classically fits the description of a hinge joint. A joint of any kind permits a union between 2 opposing surfaces of contact such that the 2 components may engage harmoniously by allowing cooperative movement. This is accomplished by a precise fit between two diverse shapes, which is conceptually most easily understood in terms of a hinge joint. Although one articulating surface protrudes as a convexity, the opposing female articulation is a concave receiver. The geometric shape of the tibiofemoral articulation is poorly designed for stability, and as such, is an unhappy marriage of osseous instability (Fig. 42-1). The menisci serve as extensions of the tibial plateau that augment the convex-concave relation by enhancing the concavity of the tibial plateau. Although the inferior meniscal surfaces are flattened in relation to the tibial surface, they are concave with respect to their superior surface so as to receive the convex femoral con-

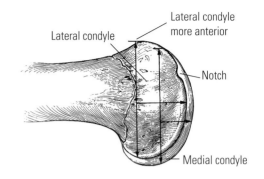

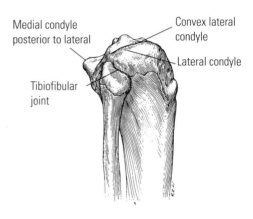

FIG. 42-1 The distal femur and proximal tibia (particularly the lateral convex tibial plateau) poorly articulate and lack stability without the presence of the menisci. (From Tria AJ, Klein KS: *An illustrated guide to the knee,* New York, 1992, Churchill Livingstone.)

dyles (Fig. 42-2). The meniscal system is therefore a stabilization-enhancing strategy that converts the tibial shelf into a concave articular surface capable of normal articulation. Strategic evolution of ligamentous placement about the knee joint cooperates with spiral motion during locking and unlocking of the screw-home mechanism.[94]

5. Is the helical motion of the knee joint during terminal knee extension a result of architectural osseous asymmetry between the medial and lateral femorotibial joints?

The kinematics of the tibiofemoral articulation are such that the areas of contact of the femur in relation to the tibia varies according to the direction of motion. As knee motion proceeds from full extension to flexion, the contact point of the femur on the tibia moves posteriorly. As the knee flexes the contact point of the femur on the tibia moves anteriorly (Fig 42-3). The key to appreciating tibiofemoral joint biomechanics is the helicoid or *spiral* figure-eight motion[32] so necessary to

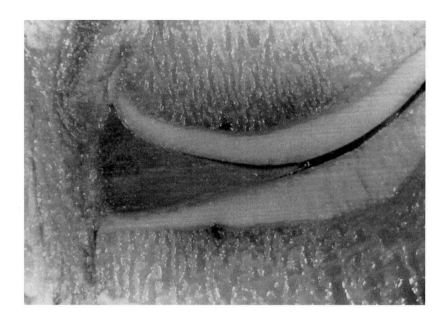

FIG. 42-2 The menisci function as joint fillers, compensating for the gross incongruity between the femoral and tibial articulating surfaces, thereby converting the articular relationship from a convex-convex incongruency to a convex-concave congruency. (From Nicholas JA, Hershman EB: *The lower extremity and spine in sports medicine,* ed 2, St Louis, 1995, Mosby.)

understanding the *screw-home locking mechanism.* Screw-home movement at the knee joint is an angular motion that occurs during the last 15°[93] to 30°[31] of full extension and is known as *terminal knee extension.* This mechanism, as well as the concurrent helical motion, occurs as a direct function of the architectural asymmetry of the medial versus lateral tibiofemoral joint. These differences are derived from the divergent length and orientation between the two femoral condyles. The ability of the human knee to engage this mechanism allows the conversion of a potentially unstable joint into a locked pillar necessary to vaulting body weight over the stance leg during foot-flat phase of stance. During late swing phase, a locked knee prepares for landing during subsequent heel-strike. Thus, the screw-home mechanism provides the knee with a higher degree of stability than would be attainable if the femerotibial joint were a pure hinge joint.[71]

6. What are the biomechanics of the screw-home locking mechanism at the tibiofemoral articulation?

Terminal knee extension and concomitant engagement of the screw-home mechanism at the knee joint occurs in the open and closed kinetic chains, that is, during late swing and stance phase (between foot-flat and mid-stance phases) of gait, respectively. The tibiofemoral motion during the arc of flexion and extension is described by way of a railroad car-to-track analogy as femoral condylar tracking atop the tibial plateau in the closed kinetic chain, or the tibial plateau riding under the contour of the femoral condyles (upside down railroad analogy). As terminal knee extension is approached, the smaller lateral femoral condyle may be thought of as riding along a track and runs out of track as a function of the smaller anteroposterior surface area of the lateral tibial plateau.[94] Moreover, the lateral femoral condyle, unlike its medial counterpart, has a small ridge known as the *impressio terminalis*[90] (Fig. 42-4) that impinges on the tibia and thus acts as a brake to halt further anterior glide[61] owing to termination of motion at the lateral hemi-joint. The medial femoral condyle, however, continues unhindered but may only undergo an angular motion beyond this point in the range of motion. The medial hemi-joint still rides the track, but like a train riding along a single track, veering (rotates) away from the track. This angular motion, aptly described as helical or spiral, allows engagement of the tibiofemoral joint such that the articulation is screwed home into the closed packed position. This mechanism serves to convert the lower limb into a weight-bearing pillar capable of bearing as much as

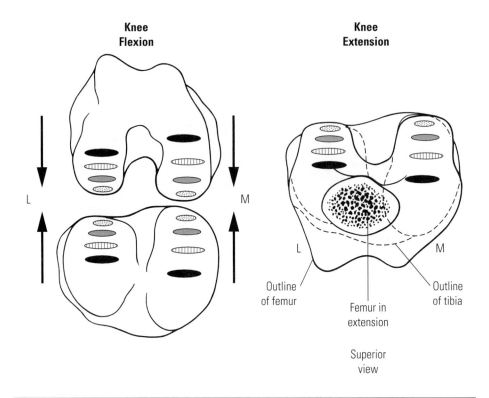

FIG. 42-3 Posterior and anterior shift of the tibiofemoral contact points with flexion and extension of the knee, respectively. There is a larger distance traversed on the medial side than on the lateral side because the components of the lateral tibiofemoral hemi-joint are correspondingly smaller than the medial tibiofemoral joint.

1½ times body weight during stance phase of gait. Thus the screw-home mechanism occurs during terminal knee extension as a consequence of the osseous configuration of the tibiofemoral joints. This process is dynamically augmented by the hamstrings, and the iliotibial band insertion into Gerdy's tubercle,[94] and statically guided by the antagonistic interplay between the cruciate and collateral ligaments.

One may visualize this sequence of events by referencing spin in relation to a stationary anatomic post, that is, the intercondylar eminence (tibial spine) located between the medial and lateral femorotibial joints and separating the medial and lateral tibial plateaus. Closed kinetic chain engagement of the screw-home mechanism (in the right knee) occurs by way of external medial condylar rotation toward the tibial spine as full extension is approached. Disengagement of the locked position occurs by way of internal rotation (or, counterclockwise rotation) of the medial femoral condyle away from the tibial spine. Because the focus of helical motion occurs in the

medial tibiofemoral joint, a greater magnitude of rotation occurs at that hemi-joint, and the axis of transverse plane rotation is said to reside in the medial joint.

In the closed kinetic chain, the medial femoral condyle (of the right knee) laterally winds or rotates approximately 15° externally (clockwise) along its long axis around the fixed tibia.[33] Rotation is terminated when the medial femoral condyle runs out of "track" along the medial tibial plateau. At this point the (right) medial meniscus has reached the limit of anteroposterior as well as mediolateral deformation and acts as a wedge, a function of its wider periphery, to terminate motion of the femoral condyle. Moreover, motion is further prevented by tensing of the cruciate ligaments, which prevent any further rotation between the femur and tibia. Rotation at the lateral hemi-joint has already ceased because of the smaller lateral condyle "running out of track," as well as because of the brakelike engagement of the impressio terminalis with the lateral tibial plateau.

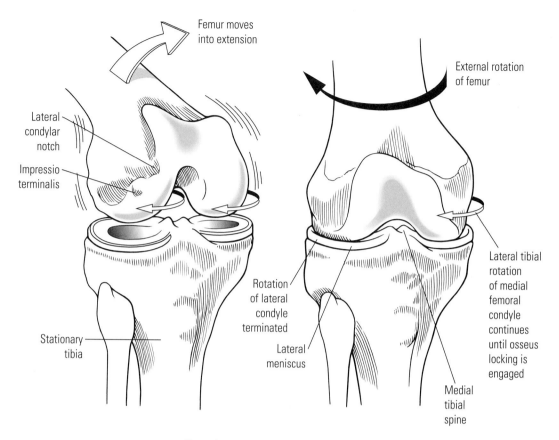

Femur moves
into extension

Lateral
condylar
notch

Impressio
terminalis

External rotation
of femur

Stationary
tibia

Rotation
of lateral
condyle
terminated

Lateral
meniscus

Lateral tibial
rotation
of medial
femoral
condyle
continues
until osseus
locking is
engaged

Medial
tibial
spine

Screw-home mechanism of the knee joint

FIG. 42-4 Screw-home mechanism of the tibiofemoral joint. Motion is terminated in the lateral hemi-joint before the medial hemi-joint because of the smaller anteroposterior surface area offered by the lateral tibial condyle, as well as because of the *impressio terminalis*. This small ridge of bone, present on the lateral condyle only, is located beneath the lateral condylar notch and acts like a brake to halt the lateral condyle from translating beyond the rim of the lateral tibial plateau during knee extension. Diminishment of anterior femoral translation is also facilitated by the wedgelike function of the menisci.

7. What is the difference between the open and closed kinetic chain function in relation to the screw-home mechanism at the knee?

Closed kinetic chain terminal knee extension involves movement of the femur on a tibia that is held stationary by ground reaction forces working through the foot. Engagement of the screw-home mechanism in the closed kinetic chain occurs by way of lateral femoral rotation on a fixed tibia. Thus the medial femoral condyle rotates externally (in clockwise manner) as the knee joint engages the screw-home mechanism to lock into closed packed extension. In contrast, during open kinetic chain terminal knee extension the same process

occurs, albeit with rotation of the distal articulating segment (tibial spine) in the same direction of external rotation. Open chain motion at the knee joint is characterized by the tibia moving relative to a fixed femur. As full extension is approached, the screw-home mechanism is engaged by external tibial rotation such that the tibial spine(s) externally rotate in relation to the femoral condyles (in a clockwise manner). The end result of terminal knee extension, whether done in the closed or open kinetic mode of function, is engagement of the screw-home locking mechanism of the knee (Fig. 42-5). The direction of transverse plane rotation has not changed. However, the articulating surfaces undergo

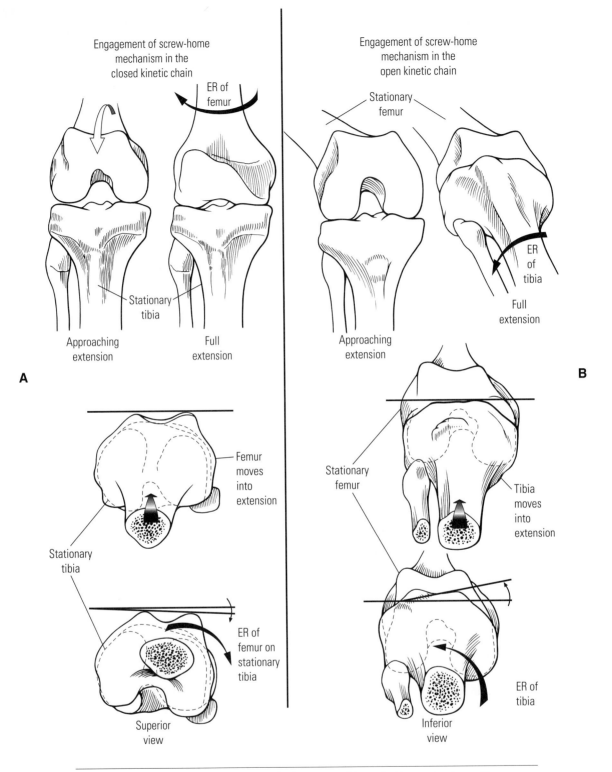

FIG. 42-5 Engagement of the *screw-home mechanism* occurs with terminal knee extension and is accompanied by lateral rotation of a moving segment upon a fixed segment. **A,** In the closed kinetic chain mode screw-home engagement into extension occurs by way of external femoral condylar rotation on a fixed tibia. **B,** In the open kinetic chain mode engagement occurs by external rotation of the tibia upon the femur. Thus, the lateral rotary component of screw-home mechanism engagement is independent of whether the lower limb functions in an open or closed kinetic mode. The only change occurs with regard to which of the articulating surfaces undergo lateral rotation. This is directly related to whether the femur or tibia assumes the role of stabilizer or mover.

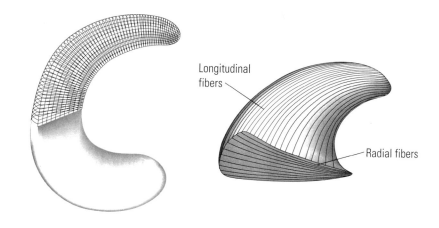

Longitudinal fibers

Radial fibers

FIG. 42-6 The dual architectural design of the collagen fibers comprising the meniscus are arranged in both a *radial* and *circumferential (longitudinal) pattern,* thereby providing resistance to *tensile* (rotational loading) as well as *compressive forces* (axial loading). (From Tria AJ, Klein KS: *An illustrated guide to the knee,* New York, 1992, Churchill Livingstone.)

transverse plane motion changes because the roles of the tibia and femur have alternated between stabilizer and mover.

8. Why are injuries to the meniscus more likely to occur during closed kinetic chain function?

The closed kinetic chain is a finite system that prohibits the function of one portion of the system (such as the foot for example) to the exclusion of the other portions (namely, the hip and knee joint.) Function in a closed kinetic chain introduces the concept of linkage between all the joints and tissues of the lower extremity. Closed chain function of the knee joint implies a biomechanical dependence between the hip joint proximally and the joints of the foot distally. Forces, especially rotary forces, are therefore not entirely dissipated as they migrate proximally along the kinetic chain. Dispersion must occur by way of transmission across as large a magnitude of tissue as possible as a strategy toward the diminishment of the potentially injurious capacity of these ground reaction forces. These forces may focus on interposed articular structures such as the menisci and ligaments and result in their ultimate failure. This mandatory absorption of abnormal forces accounts for the increased likelihood for injury during closed rather than open kinetic chain function.

9. What is the structure of the menisci?

The primary meniscal functions of load transmission and shock absorption of large compressive loads are di-

rectly related to meniscal structure. The menisci are comprised of mostly type I collagen fibers* that are oriented in a *circumferential* and *radial* pattern of alignment (Fig. 42-6). Although circumferential collagen orientation is primary and allows absorption of axial loading, the radial orientation allows for rotational loading.[94] Both types of tissue orientation are essential for resisting superincumbent body weight applied to the menisci through the femoral condyles. This tightly woven dual pattern of design provides both great elasticity and an ability to withstand compression. During flexion, femoral condylar compression on the posterior meniscal horns[19] causes anteroposterior spreading of the menisci. During knee extension, femoral condylar compression on the anterior horns causes mediolateral deformation of the menisci.[33]

The function of the meniscal circumferential fibers may be compared with metal hoops around a wooden barrel that resist elongation and thereby resist barrel expansion. The radial fibers serve as "ties" to provide structural rigidity that prevents longitudinal splitting resulting from excessive compression. Thus, the vertical compressive load of superincumbent body weight is imparted to the menisci whose fiber orientation absorbs centripetal load by translation of force into tensile or circumferential stresses.[11,12,65] In this fashion, *hoop*

---

*The presence of type I collagen fibers distinguishes fibrocartilage from hyaline cartilage, which contains predominantly type II collagen.[76]

tension generated in the menisci as a function of meniscal collagen fiber orientation represent an intraarticular meniscal constraint, like hoops on a barrel[17] preventing peripheral meniscal displacement. These hoop forces are then transmitted to the tibial plateau by virtue of the strong anterior and posterior meniscal horn[76] attachments, the intermeniscal ligament, the meniscofemoral ligaments of Wrisberg and Humphry, as well as extraarticular meniscal constraint including the collateral ligaments, joint capsule, and popliteus.[34] Thus instead of moving on the tibial plateau during compression, the circumferentially oriented collagen meniscal fibers elongate as the femur compresses down on the tibia.[17]

10. What are the meniscal functions?

- *Load transmission function* A primary meniscal function is transmission of superincumbent body load from the femur to the tibia, and thereby relieve stress transmitted through the articular cartilage and subchondral bone. The meniscus accomplishes this by virtue of its interposition between the tibiofemoral joint, and undergoes elongation as the femur compresses down upon the tibia. Although load transmission across the medial and lateral meniscus is approximately equal,[81,82,84] the posterior horns carry a greater proportion of load than the anterior horns, and the distribution of load depends upon the amount of knee flexion.[82,97] Although at least 50% of the compressive load at the knee joint is transmitted through the menisci in extension, 85% is transmitted during 90° of flexion.

  Load transmission function is appreciated by considering the profound alteration in load bearing at the knee joint following meniscectomy leading to joint space narrowing, osteophyte formation, flattening of the femoral condyles[24] persistent pain and effusion, ligamentous laxity, gait abnormality, and varus angulation.[3,38,39,41] Load may be described as force per unit area or pressure and is best understood by considering how a woman of average weight but wearing high heeled shoes exerts more pressure per unit area than an elephant foot. Similarly, the pressure in the normal knee is distributed over a wide area of the tibial plateau by the menisci. In contrast, the removal of a meniscus may increase the magnitude of contact (bone-to-bone) stress some two to three times higher than the normal knee.[81]

- *Shock absorption* Shock adsorption is another function of the menisci. The menisci absorb energy by

undergoing elongation[40] of their circumferentially oriented fibers during joint compression and extruding peripherally. In doing so, the viscoelastic menisci absorb energy and reduces shock that the underlying cartilage and subchondral bone might otherwise endure. Meniscectomy reduces the shock absorption capacity of the otherwise normal knee by 20%.[96]

- *Joint stability* The menisci serve to maintain the proper position of the femur relative to the tibia. Joint stability between the two articular surfaces is increased as the menisci serve to augment the concavity of the tibial plateau while filling the dead space that would otherwise exist at the periphery of the condyle.[87] The menisci also act as joint spacers that fill and contour the shape of the incongruous area between the convex femoral condyles and the relatively flat medial and lateral tibial plateaus.[20,86] Thus the menisci act as joint fillers, compensating for the gross incongruity between the femoral and tibial articulating surfaces.

- *Joint lubrication* The menisci contribute to knee joint lubrication by decreasing the coefficient of friction[94] by spreading a film of nutrient synovial fluid over the articular surfaces, and by limiting the space available within which fluid may pool. Following meniscectomy, the coefficient of friction in the knee joint is increased by 20%.[54–56]

- *Joint nutrition* The menisci may serve to compress the nourishing synovial fluid into articular cartilage during weight bearing. Loss of this function following meniscectomy may result in degenerative changes in the articular cartilage of the tibial plateau.[3,38,39,41]

11. What kinds of lubrication strategies are used at the tibiofemoral joint, and what role do the menisci play in joint lubrication?

Like any mechanical system, human joints must attenuate friction, which acts to minimize efficiency by impeding motion. Lubrication, like oil in a car, minimizes friction by decreasing contact between moving parts. Similarly, boundary lubrication makes use of graphite dust in which dry particles glide over each other and prevent contact of moving parts. Human joints use two different strategies, depending on whether the joint operates under slow or rapid conditions. The menisci contribute toward joint lubrication and thereby decrease the coefficient of friction in the knee joint up to 20%.

- *Elastohydrodynamic strategy* This is used by a joint during relatively slow movement in which synovial fluid in the joint is used as an elastohydrodynamic lubricant preventing contact while facilitating movement between the articulating surfaces.

- *Weeping and squeeze* Articular cartilage is normally imbibed with water. As the knee joint begins moving faster, the lubricating capacity of the synovial fluid is exceeded, as it can no longer maintain distance between the two joint surfaces. At that point the knee switches to the weeping and squeeze strategy of lubrication in which squeezing or compression of articular cartilage causes weeping of water from the cartilage. The emerging fluid permits friction reduced motion as the two joint surfaces slide forward on the fluid covering the opposing articular surface. This friction reducing strategy is so successful as to reduce the coefficient of friction of articular cartilage to some ten times less than steel on ice (ice skating).

12. What is the nerve supply to the meniscus?

In human menisci, free nerve endings involved in the transmission of pain stimuli, apparently innervate the peripheral portions of the meniscal bodies, particularly the anterior and posterior horns.[4] In addition, mechanoreceptors provide a proprioceptive function relating to joint position and may also be present in the anterior and posterior horns. The central third of the menisci are entirely devoid of innervation. The number of meniscal nerve fibers seems to diminish with advancing age.[6] Ironically, the most serious kinds of meniscal injuries are those that include tears of the poorly vascularized central two-thirds and are less likely to cause pain during the initial injury because of poor innervation of those areas. Subsequently, symptoms become apparent with knee locking or loss of stability.

13. What is the developmental anatomy of the menisci?

The menisci derive from differentiation of mesenchymal tissue* of the developing lower extremity limb bud in the eighth week of fetal gestation.[43] Although the lateral meniscus develops slightly earlier than the medial, both menisci take on an immediate semi-lunar shape.[94]

14. What gross anatomy is shared by the medial and lateral menisci?

The menisci are semicircular or crescent shaped slips of fibrocartilage when viewed from above, which fit between the tibiofemoral articulation like two door

---

Mesenchyme is that embryonic tissue that is the forerunner of all connective tissue, as well as vascular tissue in the body.

wedges when viewed sagittally. Thicker at their external margins and tapering to thin edges along their interior, they are firmly tethered in place to the tibial condyles at their outer borders by both static and dynamic restraints. Along their tapered interior, the menisci are similarly bound to their respective intercondylar eminences (also known as tibial spines). Peripherally, they are attached to the knee joint capsule, and are reinforced by a secondary thickening of the capsule known as the *coronary ligaments*. These ligaments proceed horizontally around the entire peripheral rim of the meniscus.[94] The coronary ligament is contiguous with the ligamentum patellae, and as such, is endowed with a dynamic ability to translate the anterior horns of both menisci during quadriceps contraction that accompanies knee extension.

The proximal end of the tibia is formed by two tibial plateaus known as *condyles*. Although the medial plateau is relatively concave, the lateral plateau is relatively convex.[94] Relative to the bulbous convexity of the femoral condyles, the tibial condyles are flat and make for a poor articular fit. The superior meniscal surfaces are concave to receive the convex femoral condyles whereas the inferior meniscal surfaces are flat to mold over the flattened surfaces of the tibial condyles.[98] Thus the menisci improve joint congruity by way of creating a socket[85] for the tibial plateau to properly articulate with the femur.

15. What is the anatomy of the medial meniscus?

The medial meniscus is *semicircular* in shape and has relatively broad posterior horns compared with its narrow anterior horns. Horn width is pathologically significant as a narrow meniscus is less likely to be injured than a broad one.[96] This may correlate with findings that over 70% of tears occur in the posterior horns.[94]

The key orienting clinical factors essential to understanding the medial meniscus are the peripheral and central meniscal attachments, as well as static and dynamic features. Central attachments of the anterior horn include the *transverse ligament,* which connects the anterior horns of both the medial and lateral menisci.[31] The posterior horn is centrally anchored to the posterior intercondylar fossa of the tibia just anterior to the insertion of the posterior cruciate ligament. The medial meniscus is continuously attached along its periphery to the joint capsule. At its peripheral midpoint, the medial meniscus is firmly tethered to the femur and tibia through a condensation of the joint capsule known as the *deep medial ligament.*[3,38,39,41] Additional support occurs at the meniscal midportion by way of the deep capsular layer of the medial collateral ligament.[98] Other capsular restraints include support in the form of the *coronary ligament,* which is comprised of the *meniscotibial* and *meniscofemoral ligaments,* and which may be thought of as the tibial and femoral portions of the continuous peripheral capsular meniscal attachment (Fig. 42-7).[31]

Dynamic attachments to the medial meniscus include no direct muscular attachments. However, indirect dynamic attachments occur in the form of a slip from the meniscopatellar ligament and hence, the *quadriceps muscle* indirectly,[19] to the anterior horn. Posteriorly, the medial meniscus receives a slip of the *semimembranosus* tendon by way of the capsule.[40,65,81] These two indirect dynamic attachments provide anterior translation during knee extension and meniscal retraction during knee flexion, respectively. However, despite these dynamic influences on the medial meniscus, relatively less anterior-posterior translation (5.1 mm)

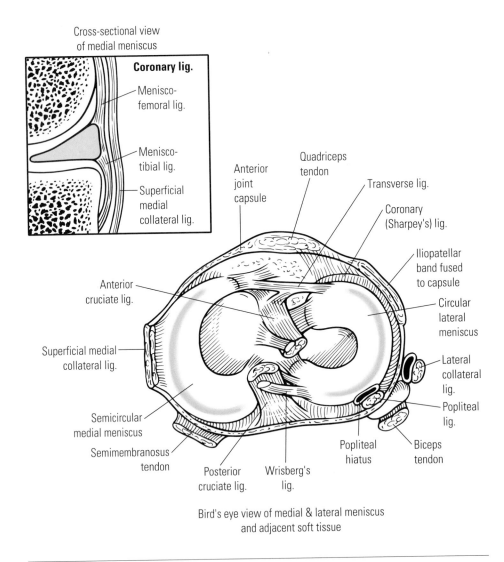

FIG. 42-7 The meniscoligamentous complex at the knee is comprised of a myriad of structures in continuous association with each other. Several ligaments are also endowed with a dynamic capability by virtue of association with adjacent tendons. The continuity of structure, and hence, function among the many soft-tissue structures at the knee accounts for why injury to a meniscus or cruciate ligament negatively affects knee biomechanics by way of association.

occurs during knee motion because of its extensive peripheral attachments compared with the lateral meniscus. Anteroposterior translation of the lateral meniscus is 11.2 mm during a 120° arc of knee motion.[28]

16. What accounts for the different shape of the medial and lateral menisci?

Although the lateral meniscus is described as nearly *circular,* the medial meniscus is more aptly described as *semi-circular.* This variation is attributed to the difference observed when comparing the anterior horns of both menisci. The anterior horn of the medial meniscus lacks the same wide, circular shape as its lateral counterpart and characteristically differs by virtue of its slim substance along the medial tibial plateau. This difference in meniscal horn architecture may be ascribed to the similar yet divergent biomechanics occurring at the knee when we compare the medial and lateral tibiofemoral joints. Engagement and disengagement of the screw-home mechanism introduces transverse plane rotation to the knee joint. The locus of this rotational axis occurs at the medial tibiofemoral joint as that hemijoint undergoes a greater magnitude of rotation owing to the architectural differences between the medial and lateral tibiofemoral joints. The relatively greater angular displacement or spinning of the medial femoral condyle along the medial tibial plateau may place the interposed meniscus at greater risk for impingement. A thinner meniscus may therefore represent an impingement prevention strategy while still serving to limit excessive medial rotation by acting as a stop wedge as the medial femoral condyle approaches the edge of the medial tibial condyle at terminal knee extension.

17. What is the anatomy of the lateral meniscus?

The lateral meniscus is almost *circular* in shape and both its anterior and posterior horns are consistent in width. The lateral meniscus differs from the medial meniscus in several respects. The most important difference is that the lateral meniscus is less firmly attached around its peripheral margin.[50] The clinical significance here is that the lateral meniscus is consequently endowed with *greater mobility.* Its total anteroposterior movement is approximately 12 mm.[98] The reason for this increased mobility may be derived from a hiatus in the static peripheral attachment where it is crossed by the popliteus tendon. Thus the popliteus tendon, passing posteroinferior to anterosuperior beneath the lateral collateral ligament and above the posterior lateral aspect of the lateral meniscus, creates a defect or *popli-*

teal hiatus in the capsular peripheral lateral meniscal restraints. Two synovial pillars both anterior and posterior to the defect enforce support of the capsular attachment to the meniscus so as to compensate for the defect and protect the defect area from rupture.[94] Increased mobility is also a result of less extensive attachment along the midportion of the lateral meniscus owing to an absence of attachment to the lateral collateral ligament.

The anterior horn of the lateral meniscus is attached to the proximal tibia in front of the intercondylar eminence whereas the posterior horn centrally attaches behind the intercondylar eminence,[66] The former blends into the anterior aspect of the ACL and the posterior horn often blends into the posterior aspect of the ACL.[17] The lateral meniscus receives the same anterior attachment of the quadriceps expansion from the patella, resulting in anterior translation of this structure during knee extension.[42,81] Along its posterior border, the lateral meniscus receives a slip of the popliteal tendon known as the superior popliteomeniscal fascicle that directly inserts onto the posterior horn, while an inferior popliteomeniscal fascicle blends into the midportion of the peripheral aspect of the lateral meniscus. Contraction of the popliteus muscle occurs as the knee flexes after terminal extension and provides dynamic posterior retraction of the lateral meniscus.[66]

In addition, the posterior horn of the meniscus may receive variable support by way of one of three possible structures: the meniscofemoral ligaments of Humphry and Wrisberg, or the posterior crucial ligament.

18. What is the function of the meniscofemoral ligaments of Wrisberg and Humphry?

The *meniscofemoral ligaments* (not to be confused with the meniscofemoral ligaments relating to the medial meniscus) consisting of the *ligaments of Humphry* and *Wrisberg,* pass from the anterior and posterior horns of the lateral meniscus, respectively, to the lateral aspect of the medial femoral condyle (Fig. 42-8). The posteriorly located ligament of Wrisberg passes just behind the origin of the posterior cruciate ligament, whereas the anterior ligament of Humphry just anterior to it. The meniscofemoral ligaments demonstrate the intimate relationship of the lateral meniscus to the posterior cruciate ligament (PCL), as the ligament of Wrisberg passes just behind the origin of the PCL and the ligament of Humphry passes in front of the PCL insertion. Together, both meniscofemoral ligaments connect the anterior and posterior horns of the lateral meniscus to the medial

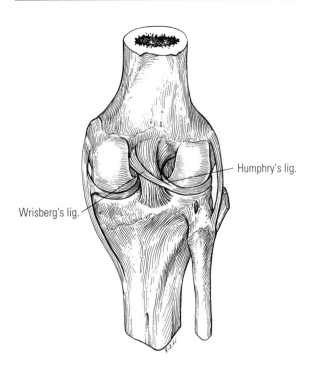

Wrisberg's lig.

Humphry's lig.

FIG. 42-8 The *meniscofemoral ligaments of Humphry* and *Wrisberg* in relationship to the posterior cruciate ligament. (From Tria AJ, Klein KS: *An illustrated guide to the knee,* New York, 1992, Churchill Livingstone.)

femoral condyle.[47] The medial meniscus has no such corresponding ligamentous attachments. Gray describes these common, but poorly understood structures[32] as giving support to the rotational movement of the tibia.[32]

Understanding the function of these posteriorly located meniscofemoral ligaments must occur against the backdrop of understanding both anatomy and function of the PCL (Fig. 42-9). The PCL, comprised of both anterior and posterior fascicles, serves as the primary restraint against posterior translation of the tibia on the femur. During extension of the knee joint the posterior band is made taut, whereas the anterior band tenses during knee flexion. The posteriorly located ligament of Wrisberg passes just behind the origin of the PCL, whereas the anterior ligament of Humphry passes just in front of the PCL. This is highly significant as the PCL may, indirectly, endow the meniscofemoral ligaments the role of "dynamic ligaments" that serve to limit the magnitude of anteriorposterior lateral meniscal mobility. During knee extension, when the femur rolls forward along the tibia, the posterior band of PCL

tenses, which retracts the ligament of Wrisberg, which, in turn pulls backward on the lateral meniscus. In contrast, knee flexion involves the femoral condyles rolling back along the tibial plateau, causing tightening of the anterior band of the PCL, which is tensed and pulls on the ligament of Humphry, which in turn pulls the lateral meniscus forward.

The medial meniscus has no equivalent posterior retractor analogue to the meniscofemoral ligaments of Wrisberg and Humphry as a function of its greater stability owing to uninterrupted peripheral meniscal restraints. In contrast, the lateral meniscus has greater mobility (up to 1 cm) due to an interruption of peripheral meniscal restraints. The lateral meniscofemoral ligaments represent a protective compensatory strategy that prevents excessive anteroposterior meniscal translation by limiting the magnitude of meniscal mobility. In this manner, the menisci precisely follow the displacement of the femoral condyles and avoid becoming impinged between the femur and tibia.

19. Which ligament attaching to the medial meniscus is endowed with a dynamic ability not present in the lateral meniscus?

Both the medial and lateral meniscus indirectly attach to the quadriceps mechanism by way of the *meniscopatellar ligaments* inserting on the anterior horns of both menisci. During knee extension, contraction of the quadriceps muscle indirectly pulls on the anterior horns of both menisci. However, the medial meniscus also has another mechanism ensuring anterior meniscal translation during quadriceps contraction due to blending of the quadriceps expansion with the coronary ligament. The *coronary ligament* is the tibial thickening of the joint capsule surrounding the periphery of the medial meniscus. The continuity of the ligamentum patellae and the coronary ligament endows this static restraint with a dynamic ability similar to the ligament of Humphry. Although morphologically different, the coronary ligament is a "dynamic ligament," which may be thought of as the functional equivalent of the ligament of Humphry.

20. What is the relationship between the ACL and the menisci?

The menisci are formed in the eighth embryonic week, along with the cruciate ligaments, from interposed mesenchymal tissue.[6] The common origin of both the menisci and cruciate ligaments suggests *coordinated function of the meniscoligamentous complex.*[27] In fact, the

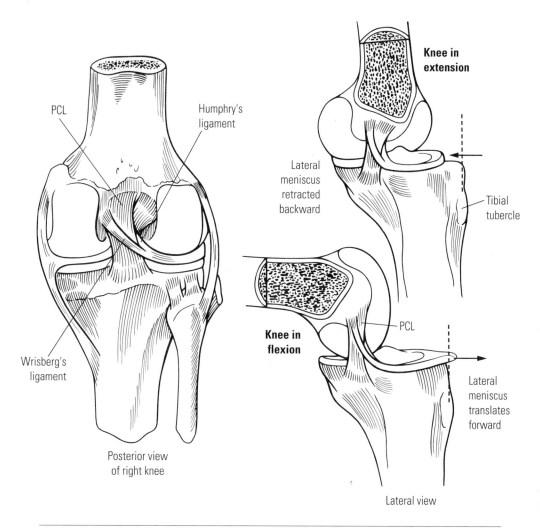

PCL

Humphry's
ligament

Knee in
extension

Lateral
meniscus
retracted
backward

Tibial
tubercle

Wrisberg's
ligament

Knee in
flexion

PCL

Lateral
meniscus
translates
forward

Posterior view
of right knee

Lateral view

FIG. 42-9 The *meniscofemoral ligaments* have the *dynamic retractor function*, not present in the medial meniscus, that serves to restrain the magnitude of anterior lateral meniscal translation during knee extension. This is probably a protective strategy that prevents excessive lateral meniscal translation that may cause meniscal impingement and injury.

anterior fibers of the ACL merge with the transverse ligament, which connects the anterior horns of the medial and lateral menisci.[31] An intimate association also exists between the posterior cruciate ligament and the lateral meniscus by way of the meniscofemoral ligaments of Wrisberg and Humphry. This close association highlights a continuity of structure and therefore function between the menisci and the cruciates that exemplifies the static and dynamic interrelationships amongst the myriad of soft and osseous structures comprising the knee joint. Hence, it is not surprising that tears of the medial meniscus may develop after an apparently isolated disruption of the ACL because of ab-

normal joint motion. For example, the medial meniscus serves as a secondary buttress to anterior displacement of the knee joint in the ACL deficient knee. This is because the firm fixation of the meniscus to the tibial plateau allows it to act as a wedge that restrains anterior translation of the femur on the plateau.[40,65,81] Thus removing a significant portion of the medial meniscus is equivalent to eliminating an important secondary stabilizer of the knee joint[17] preventing excessive anterior laxity. With time, the viscoelastic strength of the medial meniscus may be exceeded by the excessive anterior translational forces associated with knee extension and develop a tear. Conversely, various grades of cruciate or

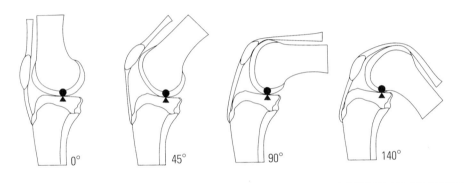

FIG. 42-10 As the knee flexes, the areas of contact on the femur and tibia move posteriorly. As the knee extends, the *tibiofemoral contact points* shift anteriorly. (From Tria AJ, Klein KS: *An illustrated guide to the knee,* New York, 1992, Churchill Livingstone.)

collateral ligament tears are often associated with meniscal tears.[94] Moreover, many of the mechanisms resulting in cruciate or collateral ligament injuries are similar if not identical to mechanisms resulting in meniscal injury.[94]

21. What determines the direction of meniscal motion?

The menisci undergo both anteroposterior translation as well as rotatory motion along the tibial plateau. Meniscal motion is determined in large part by the osseous configuration of the tibiofemoral joint as well as indirectly by way of contraction of the quadriceps, semimembranosus, and popliteus muscles.

As knee motion proceeds from full extension to flexion, the contact point of the femur on the tibia moves posteriorly (Fig. 42-10). As the knee flexes out of extension, the contact point of the femur on the tibia moves anteriorly. Meniscal motion *follows the direction of femoral condylar displacement* rather than the tibial plateau during knee movement solely because of the geometric shape of the meniscus. Although the inferior meniscal surface is relatively flat and rests upon the rather flat tibial plateau, the superior meniscal surfaces bear a concavity of architectural design. The consequences of this design differential between the superior and inferior surfaces of the meniscus dictate whether the femur or tibia controls meniscal movement. Tibial motion cannot significantly cause meniscal motion because the interface between the flat inferior meniscal surface and the flat tibial plateau (*inferior meniscal surface*) does not significantly engage. In contrast, the convexity of the medial femoral condyle readily engages the *superior meniscal surface*. As such, the superior meniscal inter-

face is described as convex on concave. Because of this, femoral motion during flexion or extension of the knee moves the menisci in the same direction as the movement of the femoral condyles, thus maintaining joint congruence throughout the range of knee motion (Fig. 42-11).[42]

22. What is the direction of femoral condylar displacement during the initial 100° of knee flexion range?

During the entire range of knee motion, but not including the last 20° or 30° of extension, the osteokinematic motion of knee flexion is characterized by arthrokinematic motion in which areas of contact on the femur and tibia move posteriorly. As the knee moves into *flexion*, the condyles *roll backward* onto the tibial plateau while the menisci deform mediolaterally. In contrast, knee *extension* is accompanied by the areas of contact on the femur and tibia moving anteriorly. Here, the femoral condyles *roll forward* along the tibial plateau while the menisci undergo anteroposterior deformation. The purpose of meniscal motion during movement of the tibiofemoral joint helps maintain a stable point of contact between the changing radii of curvature of the bulbous femoral condyles relative to the tibial plateaus. In this way the menisci help maintain joint congruity through knee joint range of motion.

Because meniscal motion follows the direction of the femoral condyles, posterior meniscal retraction occurs, in part, as a result of the direct force imposed by rolling back of the femoral condyles during knee flexion. Posterior meniscal retraction during knee flexion is aided by semimembranosus and popliteus attachment to the medial meniscus, as well as the meniscofemoral ligaments of Humphry and Wrisberg on the lateral me-

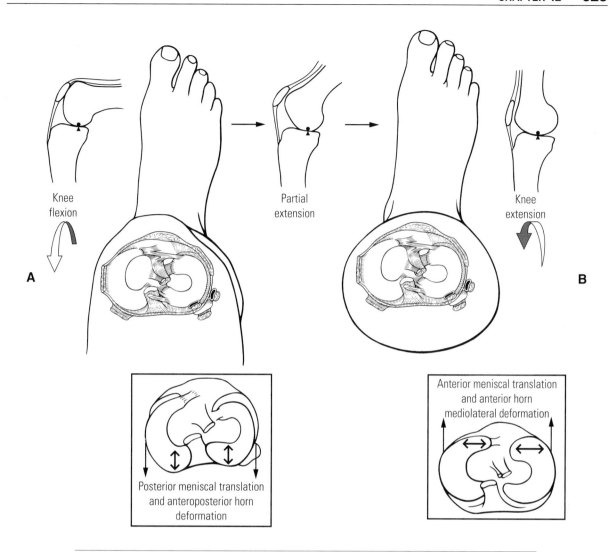

FIG. 42-11 Bird's eye view of right knee flexion and extension showing concomitant direction of meniscal motion and variation in the magnitude of translation. The direction of meniscal translation is dictated by the movement of the bulbous femoral condylar projections. The femoral contact points move posteriorly along the tibia during **A,** knee flexion, and **B,** anteriorly during knee extension. Hence, the menisci undergo anterior translation during knee extension as well as mediolateral deformation of their medial horns. In contrast, the menisci undergo posterior retraction during knee flexion, as well as anteroposterior deformation of their posterior horns. Although meniscal movement along the tibial plateau is principally defined by the motion of the femur, it is dynamically augmented by contraction of the quadriceps and hamstring musculature. Despite the smaller anteroposterior width of the lateral tibial plateau, the lateral meniscus moves to and fro in the anteroposterior direction more so than the medial meniscus. This is because the lateral meniscus has less extensive peripheral attachments, that is, the lateral popliteal hiatus, and unlike the medial collateral ligament in relation to the medial meniscus, has no direct or indirect continuity with the lateral collateral ligament.

niscus. Similarly, anterior meniscal translation occurs by way of the femoral condyles rolling forward along the tibial plateau and effectively "dragging the menisci along." Anterior meniscal translation is aided by the meniscopatellar ligament by way of the quadriceps ex-

pansion, which helps avoid entrapment of the meniscus in the joint space.

Although the menisci serve the knee by facilitating joint congruity through a wide arc of flexion and extension, they do so at the risk to the integrity of their structure. Should the menisci fail to follow the femoral condyles along the tibial plateau, they risk becoming trapped between the two articulating surfaces and sustain injury due to *compression*. Fortunately, this is unlikely to occur during pure flexion and extension as these motions are characterized by *concurrent motion* of the femoral and tibial articular surfaces. During knee flexion the areas of contact of both the femur and tibia move posteriorly, whereas during extension the areas of contact of both the femur and tibia move anteriorly. Thus regardless of whether the direction of knee is flexed or extended, the femur and tibia always move concurrently.

23. Are the directions of motion of the tibia and femur concurrent during terminal knee extension?

The last 20° to 30° of knee extension is known as *terminal knee extension* and introduces a rotational variable in knee joint kinematics. Motion occurring in this narrow range is accompanied by rotation of the femur and tibia, in opposite directions. The menisci, however, still follow the displacements of the femoral condyles and, consequently, move in directions *opposite* of the tibial plateau. It is here, therefore, that the menisci are at greatest risk for injury. The menisci avoid injury by virtue of the many static and dynamic restraints, both central and peripheral, that limit their motion within a narrow margin of safety between the femoral and tibial articulating surfaces. However, certain motions may exceed the meniscus capacity, and result in injury as the meniscus becomes trapped and torn. Thus the menisci may be said to have *2 degrees of motion* that include both anteroposterior translation as well as internal and external rotation.

During right terminal knee extension in the closed kinetic chain the direction of angular motion of both femoral condyles is equivalent as both rotate in the clockwise direction on the tibial plateau. However, their concomitant anteroposterior motions are opposite. As the medial femoral condyle rotates toward the tibial spine it approaches the anterior edge of the medial tibial plateau. In doing so, it translates the medial meniscus anteriorly. In contrast, rotation of the lateral condyle is also clockwise, but by virtue of its lateral location, translates the lateral meniscus posteriorly toward the posterior rim of the lateral tibial plateau (Fig. 42-12). These motions are reversed during disengagement of the screw-home mechanism upon knee flexion out of terminal extension. Thus, because meniscal movements

follow displacement of the femoral condyles they are said to move in directions opposite to the movement of the tibial plateaus.

24. What mechanism of injury frequently injures the meniscus?

The most frequent mechanism of meniscal injury is a *noncontact* stress resulting from *deceleration* or *acceleration* coupled with changing direction. These *cutting maneuvers* typically occur in running agility sports such as football and soccer. Meniscal lesions may also result from contact stress in which a violent varus, valgus, or hyperextension force is coupled with rotational motion yielding a meniscal tear. A collateral ligament sprain resulting from a varus or valgus force will involve the collateral ligament on the opposite side of the applied force as that side has been subjected to a distraction force. Jumping sports may result in meniscal lesions from the angular momentum and femoral tibial rotation that occur when the athlete lands.[40,65,81]

Cutting maneuvers involve knee flexion and the introduction of rotation of the femur and tibia. During the initial 120° of knee flexion, the areas of contact of the tibia and femur (and hence, menisci) move posteriorly in the same direction. A cutting maneuver typically involves medial femoral rotation as the player moves at an angle medial to the original direction of movement. The planted tibia undergoes an obligatory lateral rotation. Because the femur and tibia just before the cutting maneuver were moving concurrently, the introduction of rotation will subject the interposed meniscus to shear[40,65,81] or *spiral forces*. Shearing occurs when two uniplanar forces work in opposite directions with some distance between them. The interposed meniscus undergoes an oblique distortion and succumbs to injury. Thus an isolated medial meniscus tear may result from a marked external rotation load.[53]

Although sudden rapid actions characterizing contact sports are much less common in ballet,[29] acute bucket-handle type meniscal tears may occur in dancers attempting to assume the fifth position of classical ballet. Achieving the fifth classical dance posture is accomplished by externally rotating both hips and then crossing one's legs so that the left medial arch lies flush against the lateral aspect of the right foot. However, dancers with poor turnout have difficulty achieving this position at the barre, and attempt to force the position by "screwing the knees."[73] This commonly used compensation applies a high rotational shear force upon the

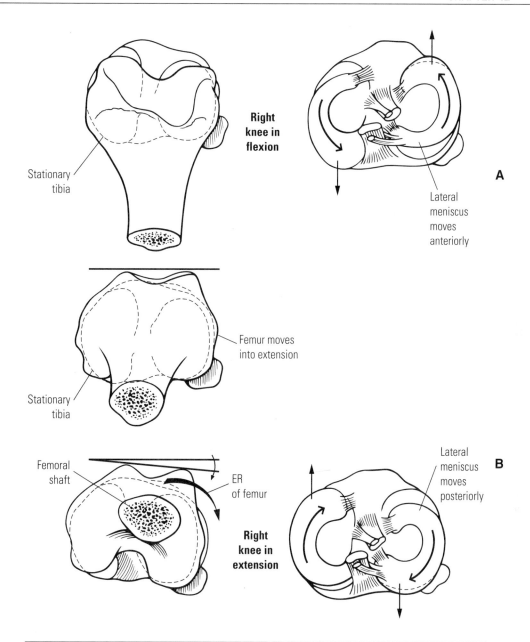

FIG. 42-12 The last 20° to 30° of tibiofemoral joint motion introduces transverse plane rotation. This results in *opposite* anteroposterior translation and rotation in the *same* direction. **A,** During terminal knee extension the medial meniscus undergoes anterior translation whereas the lateral meniscus undergoes posterior translation; both, however, rotate externally. **B,** During flexion out of terminal extension the medial meniscus translates posteriorly whereas the lateral meniscus translates anteriorly; both, however, rotate internally. Because meniscal movement follows displacement of the femoral condyles, the menisci move in directions opposite that of the tibial plateau. The menisci are therefore subject to shear and are more likely to sustain injury during this range of knee motion.

meniscus as the tibial plateau is forced against the femur, and may result in meniscal tear.[80]

25. What area of which meniscus is most often injured, and what range of knee motion places the menisci at greater risk for sustaining injury?

The medial meniscus is most commonly injured, although lateral meniscus injuries are by no means rare. Most injuries of the medial meniscus occur in that portion of the meniscus that is thicker and carries the brunt of superincumbent body weight—the posterior horn.[60] Moreover, the menisci are especially vulnerable to sustaining injury during the last 30° of terminal knee extension. During the 120° arc of motion before terminal knee extension, the menisci undergo anterior-posterior translation as they follow the femoral condyles along the tibial plateau. Flexion and extension during this range is characterized by arthrokinematic motion in which the tibiofemoral articulating surfaces move concurrently. During knee extension, the areas of contact of the femur and tibia move anteriorly as the femoral condyles glide and roll anteriorly along the tibial plateau. Correspondingly, the menisci undergo mediolateral elongation. During knee flexion the area of contact of the femur and tibia move posteriorly as the femoral condyles glide and roll posteriorly along the tibial plateau, and the menisci undergo anteroposterior elongation. If, however, the menisci deviate from their motion out from their synchronous motion with the femoral condyles they become interposed between the articulating surfaces and sustain a compressive or shear force leading to injury.

During the last 30° before full knee extension, rotation results in torsion of the femoral and tibial shafts. At the articulating surfaces, the femoral condyles, and hence the menisci, rotate in a direction opposite to the tibial plateau. Should the menisci be caught between the two articulating surfaces during this arc of motion, they will be subject to torsional forces. *Torsion** forces, like shear forces (uniplanar), work in opposite directions and cause distortion of the interposed meniscus that exceeds its viscoelastic capacity.

26. Why is the medial meniscus most often injured in lateral cutting movements?

Cutting movements typically occur medially rather than laterally so as to maintain the center of gravity in the base of support. In the weight-bearing posture this

occurs by planting the stance foot and twisting inward causing lateral displacement and lateral rotation of the tibia on the femur and relative medial femoral rotation. As the menisci follow displacement of the femoral condyles, the medial meniscus rotates medially along with the medial femoral condyle. This twisting of the two articulating surfaces in directions opposite to one another subjects the interposed meniscus to torsion, resulting in a longitudinal bucket handle tear. In contrast, a movement causing sudden lateral femoral (and hence medial tibial) rotation may cause injury to the lateral meniscus.

Twisting of the femoral and tibial articulating surfaces in opposite directions is also the mechanism of injury for knee sprains with concurrent meniscal injury. During a skiing injury, one ski may be caught in a snow bank resulting in ipsilateral femoral medial rotation and tibial lateral rotation. The direction of disruptive forces are similar to those occurring during cutting movement, although the magnitude of forces are considerably greater and may tear the cruciate ligaments, the medial collateral ligament, and pull the medial meniscus from its articulation. The latter occurs because of tearing of the meniscotibial and/or meniscofemoral parts of the middle third of the medial capsular ligament, permitting the medial meniscus to "float." This meniscocapsular separation results in shearing of the meniscus from the capsule that endows the meniscus with excessive mobility. Thus the outer meniscal edge may move excessively inward toward the central aspect of the joint or extrude outward beyond the tibiofemoral articular surface. This excessive mobility may render the susceptible meniscus more likely toward entering that range of movement in the tibiofemoral joint where it may sustain impingement.

27. What is the classification of meniscal tears?

Tears may occur in either structure or both menisci at the same time.[62] An *incomplete tear* partially extends across the body of a meniscus, whereas a *complete tear* extends across the entire meniscal body. Relative to the cross section of the meniscus, tears may be classified as either *vertical* or *horizontal* (Fig. 42-13). Relative to their long axis, meniscal tears may be classified as *longitudinal* or *transverse*.[2] Because a meniscus is a three dimensional tissue, every tear in its substance may be described relative to its cross section and long axis. Categorizing meniscal tears anatomically is simplified by assigning certain tears with descriptive names such as *parrot beak* or *bucket handle* (Fig. 42-14).

---

*Torsion involves multiplanar forces, is considerably less benign than shear forces, and may wreak havoc upon soft and osseous tissue.

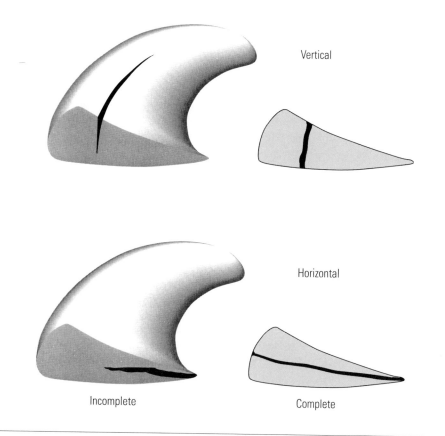

Vertical

Horizontal

Incomplete

Complete

FIG. 42-13 Meniscal tear classification relative to the cross section of the meniscus. (From Tria AJ, Klein KS: *An illustrated guide to the knee,* New York, 1992, Churchill Livingstone.)

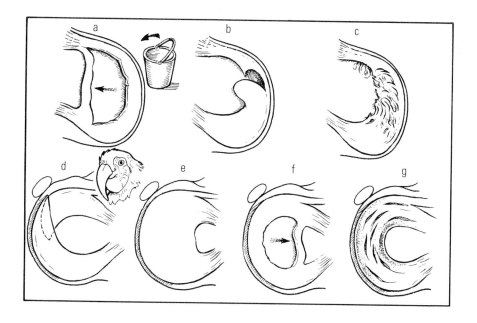

FIG. 42-14 The gross anatomic appearance of the common meniscal tears of the knee: **(a)** bucket handle tear; **(b)** flap tear; **(c)** degenerate tear of the medial meniscus; **(d)** oblique "parrot beak" tear of the lateral meniscus; **(e)** discoid lateral meniscus; **(f)** locked bucket handle tear of the lateral meniscus; **(g)** cystic or myxoid degeneration of the lateral meniscus. (From Dandy DJ: *Essential orthopaedics and trauma,* ed 2, Edinburgh, 1993, Churchill Livingstone.)

- *Horizontal tears.* These are most often the result of chronic degenerative change[21] associated with degradation of fibrocartilage and proteoglycan disruption of the meniscal ground substance.[94] These tears, typically occurring in the elderly population and manifest as a delamination of the meniscal substance. If neglected, they may progress to become flap tears.[80] These unstable flaps do not cause mechanical locking, although they may move in and out of the joint space[11,12,65] and cause other mechanical signs[80] such as palpable clicking or popping.
- *Vertical tears.* These are most often traumatic in origin[60] and are alternately described as longitudinal or circumferential, which consists of a long central fragment attached at each end to the meniscal horns. Over time, these tears may progress such that the long fragment migrates centrally into the intercondylar fossa of the joint. The movement of the fragment is likened to a bucket handle and these types of injury are known as **bucket-handle tears.** When the unstable bucket-handle fragment displaces into the intercondylar notch, it blocks full extension of the knee joint.[80]
- *Radial tears.* These may occur in either the medial or lateral menisci and cause few symptoms. These tears are characterized by tears in the central aspect of the meniscus that migrate inward toward the periphery. If untreated, they may progress to a deeper, more symptomatic **parrot beak tear.** This unstable beaklike flap of meniscal tissue may cause mechanical signs in the injured knee such as recurrent effusions, giving way, and a catching sensation.[11,12,66] Progression of a radial tear is more likely in the lateral meniscus.[11,12,65] This may be attributable to relatively greater width of the lateral meniscus owing to its more circular shape and subsequent likelihood for pathologic progression of a tear across the meniscal body.

28. What is the prognostic classification of meniscal injury?

Meniscal lesions are categorized according to a three-tier classification scheme in relation to likelihood for healing based on meniscal vascular supply.[5] Generally, the vascularity of the menisci decrease as one progresses from the capsular attachment to the leading edge. A *red-red tear* refers to a tear in which both sides of the torn tissue occur in the blood-rich peripheral margin of the meniscus; this type of lesion has a favorable prognosis for healing. A *red-white tear* refers to a tear in which one end of the torn lesion resides at the well supplied peripheral rim, whereas the other end is located along the central, hence less vascularized portion of the meniscus. A *white-white tear* is a lesion that entirely resides in the avascular central portion; here, the prognosis for healing is poor.

29. What is the clinical presentation of meniscal tears?

A meniscal tear becomes symptomatic if its torn portion is mobile and slides into an abnormal position between the articular surfaces of the femur and tibia. The clinician should bear in mind general guidelines about patient age when evaluating for a potential meniscus tear. Younger patients tend to have acute injuries resulting from trauma or sport whereas older persons tend to have a gradual onset of symptoms owing to the degenerative process. Meniscal tears commonly result in symptoms of *pain, swelling, and instability* such as locking in flexion, extension, or both,[80] as well as frank collapse, or a feeling of giving-way.

Knee locking occurs because a torn fragment becoming lodged in the joint and may be subjectively reported as a rubbery resistance during extension. **Medially displaced tears typically present as locking between 10° and 30° of knee flexion, whereas laterally displaced meniscal tears tend to lock in greater degrees of flexion (70° or more).**[94] Unlocking of the joint may be accompanied by a click or snap.[19] A sensation of giving way causes momentary lodging of the loose fragment resulting in a sensation of impending knee buckling. Onset of pain is usually immediate and may be localized to either the medial or lateral side of the knee.[94] Pain is usually aggravated by activity but may also be present at rest.[94]

Swelling, ecchymosis, and tenderness signify a significant knee injury. Soft tissue swelling should be distinguished from true effusion of the knee. The swelling associated with meniscal injury develops gradually over 1 to 3 days. Effusions occurring within hours of the injury resulting from bleeding in the joint (hemarthrosis) are indicative of an osteochondral fracture or rupture of either cruciate ligament. *A tear of the vascular periphery of the meniscus may cause an acute hemarthrosis as well.*[94] Arthrocentesis is a diagnostic tool in which aspirated fluid obtained from within the joint helps clarify the cause of swelling. Fluid that is bloody is most frequently associated with cruciate rupture; an effusion that yields blood and fat droplets indicates an intraarticular fracture; a lack of joint fluid upon aspiration occurs following a large tear of the capsular ligaments (such as the medial collateral ligament) because fluid leaks into surrounding tissues; aspiration of clear yellowish fluid is generally associated with meniscal tears. Meniscal injuries may result in recurrent effusion.[80]

Extracting a reliable *history* is important to the determination of whether or not meniscal injury has occurred. The patient may often describe a giving way of the involved knee at the moment of injury. Alternately, the knee may instantaneously lock short of full extension upon meniscal displacement. It is essential to ask the patient if it was possible to fully extend the knee immediately following injury. This is because lack of full extension often develops gradually with increasing pain of effusion even in the absence of a major meniscal injury.[94] In contrast, young patients such as children or adolescents may have a vague history of injury, and may even be afraid to recall their injury.[13]

As more people over the age of 40 participate in sporting activities, degenerative tears of the menisci may occur with increasing frequency. Individuals with chronic meniscal tears typically provide a history of an earlier acute episode followed by gradual improvement in function, albeit with persistent disability.

30. What physical signs are present during patient examination?

The physical examination of a knee with a suspected meniscal injury begins with search for the presence of any thigh atrophy indicating a more chronic problem. Careful palpation of the medial and lateral joint lines with the knee in various degrees of flexion may elicit tenderness corresponding to the side of meniscal injury. Limitations in range of motion, particularly limitations of full flexion or extension suggest a mechanical blocking typical of meniscal tear. **Pain may be elicited at the extremes of motion as the femoral condyle presses upon the anterior horns in extension or the posterior horns in flexion.** Atrophy of the quadriceps femoris muscle, especially the VMO segment, may be an indication of a long-standing meniscal injury. This is because the patient may be avoiding and unable to achieve full extension due to mechanical blockage, whereas it is at or near full extension that most tension is required of the VMO muscle.[52]*

---

*Atrophy may also be secondary to capsular swelling leading to reflex inhibition of the quadriceps. Mechanoreceptors in the joint capsule are stimulated by pressure exerted by fluid build-up. Afferents projecting from these receptors synapse with, and inhibit interneurons communicating with anterior horn efferents causing an aerogenic inhibition of the quadriceps muscle (McDonough and Wein 1996).

Many provocative stress tests for meniscal tears exist and have in common the goal of duplicating symptoms by attempting to trap abnormally mobile meniscal fragments between the femur and tibia, causing either pain or clicking. These findings are elicited by superimposing rotation upon flexion/extension of the knee by externally or internally rotating the (foot and) tibia. Alternately, one may apply a valgus stress to the knee joint while moving the knee through flexion/extension. Pain elicited during knee flexion implicates the posterior horns as the femoral condyles press on the posterior meniscal horns during flexion. Conversely, pain elicited during knee extension implicates the anterior horns as the femoral condyles press on the anterior meniscal horns. Internal rotation of the tibia tests the lateral meniscus while external tibial rotation tests the medial meniscus. Alternately, a valgus stress applied to the knee during gentle flexion and extension of the knee between 0° and 90° may result in a click or pain that implicates the anterior and middle portion of the lateral meniscus. This test is less helpful in diagnosing tears of the anterior medial meniscus (varus stress) because of the small size of the anterior medial horn.[49] Thus, the anterior medial horn is, by virtue of its size, is less likely to become trapped during a provocative maneuver. Provocative meniscal maneuvers that depend upon palpation to elicit tenderness or clicking include the palpation tests of Bragard, McMurray, and Steinmann's second sign (Fig. 42-15). Provocative meniscal maneuvers that depends upon symptoms of joint line pain with rotation are more numerous and include the tests of Apley, Apley grid, Bohler, Duck walking, Helfet, Merke, Payr, and Steinmann's first sign (Fig. 42-16).[94]

31. What imaging techniques are appropriate following suspected meniscus tear?

Because the menisci are soft-tissue structures, imaging techniques other than standard radiographs are used to aid detection of meniscal lesions. Radiographs are essential, however, before other types of imaging so as to rule out tumors, osseous loose bodies, and fractures within the knee.[94] Plain films include those taken in the anteroposterior, lateral, tunnel, and tangential patellofemoral (Merchant) projections. The traditional approach to detection of a meniscal lesion is the arthrogram in conjunction with contrast agents to outline the presence, location, and magnitude of the deficit. Although use of the arthrogram is less expensive than magnetic resonance imaging (MRI), the latter is nonin-

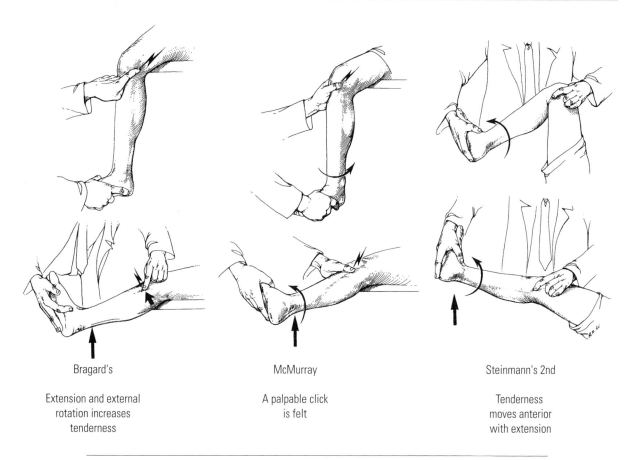

Bragard's

Extension and external
rotation increases
tenderness

McMurray

A palpable click
is felt

Steinmann's 2nd

Tenderness
moves anterior
with extension

FIG. 42-15 Provocative meniscal maneuvers that rely upon palpation to elicit tenderness or a clicking sound. (From Tria AJ, Klein KS: *An illustrated guide to the knee,* New York, 1992, Churchill Livingstone.)

vasive, painless, and yields excellent resolution of meniscal injuries (Fig. 42-17). The problem with MRI is that normal interface between two low density structures falsely implies the presence of a tear known as a *pseudotear.* An example of this would be the interface between the transverse meniscal ligament connecting the anterior horns of the medial and lateral meniscus and parallels their surfaces before attaching, or where the popliteal tendon sheath courses around the lateral margin of the lateral meniscus. Other areas include the posterior horn of the lateral meniscus and the meniscofemoral ligament, as well as the medial meniscal body and the medial collateral ligament. These commonly encountered imaging pitfalls may result in misdiagnosis by an interpreter lacking a detailed anatomic knowledge of the knee.[60] CT is excellent for bone detail but not especially helpful for meniscal imaging.[94]

32. What is the differential diagnosis of meniscal lesions?

A clinical diagnosis of meniscal injury is suspected certain if three or more of the following findings are made during examination. These findings include localized tenderness over the joint line, pain present at the joint line during hyperextension or hyperflexion of the knee joint, presence of positive findings upon provocative stress testing, and weakened or atrophied quadriceps musculature.[74] Invasive arthroscopy is the most certain way of confirming a diagnosis of meniscal injury. Notwithstanding, the clinician must be alert to the many other disorders that may have similar presentations. These pathologies must be ruled out and include:

- *Discoid meniscus.* In approximately 5% of the general population the lateral meniscus is congenitally abnormal, lacking its normal crescentic shape.[11,12,65] The meniscus in these patients is more circular or dis-

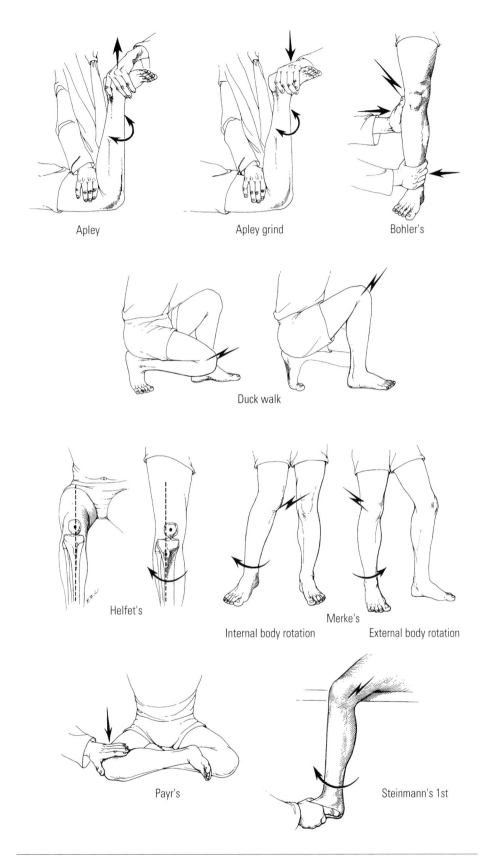

FIG. 42-16 Provocative meniscal maneuvers that rely upon symptoms and joint-line pain with rotation of the lower limb. (From Tria AJ, Klein KS: *An illustrated guide to the knee,* New York, 1992, Churchill Livingstone.)

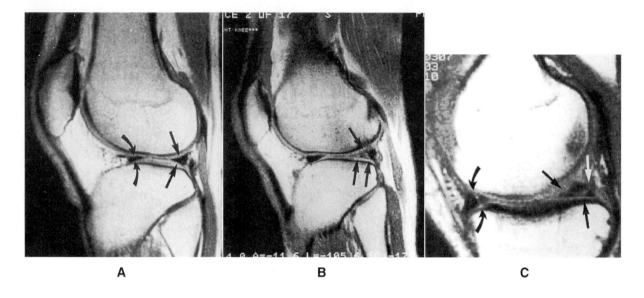

FIG. 42-17 Menisci. Sagittal T1-weighted scan. **A,** Normal lateral meniscus, anterior horn *(curved arrows),* and posterior horn *(straight arrows.)* **B,** Tear of the posterior horn on the lateral meniscus *(arrows).* **C,** Medial meniscal tears involving the anterior horn *(curved arrows)* and posterior horn *(straight arrows).* (From Nicholas JA, Hershman EB: *The lower extremity and spine in sports medicine,* ed 2, St Louis, 1995, Mosby.)

coid in shape and may also be thicker than normal. The etiology of these aberrantly formed menisci is controversial. Some authorities ascribe discoid meniscus to a developmental arrest in utero, whereas others ascribe its origin to a shortening of the ligament of Wrisberg that causes the meniscus to ride more posteriorly thereby deforming the meniscus into a circular shape.[94] Most meniscal disorders in patients under ten years of age are due to discoid menisci. The discoid meniscus is typically bulky along its periphery and may therefore sustain impingement with joint motion. Occurring more commonly on the lateral side of the knee, a tear of a discoid meniscus frequently precipitates onset of symptoms.[88] A discoid meniscus may thus become torn and cause mechanical symptoms like other meniscal tears. Clinical presentation includes a "snapping knee"[94] in which pain and popping, or a "clunk" at the lateral joint line may be felt or heard when the knee is straightened.[11,12,65] Occasionally, an effusion is present. The snapping may be difficult to distinguish from a symptomatic popliteus tendinitis[94] except that the latter presents no mechanical blocking. Diagnosis of discoid meniscus is made by arthrography, arthroscopy, or MRI. If a discoid meniscus is incidentally discovered during arthroscopic exploration, it may be left

alone with realization that there is an increased risk of a future tear developing compared with a normal meniscus.[94] Management of a torn and symptomatic discoid meniscus includes arthroscopically contouring the disc into a more C-like shape to render the patient less symptomatic.[94]

- *Cystic menisci.* These typically involve the lateral menisci, and most frequently afflict young adults[10] The etiology of meniscal cysts is thought to derive from infiltration of synovial fluid through a horizontal meniscal tear with the tear edge acting as a one way valve.[7,25] Presentation includes a dull aching pain on the lateral side of the knee, "like a toothache in the knee," often worse at night.[11,12,65] The cyst may herniate outside the capsule of the knee and be palpable during the examination.[94] Management involves arthroscopic partial meniscectomy that allows the cyst to recede back into the joint.[67,83]

- *Popliteus tendinitis.* The popliteus tendon crosses the lateral joint line adjacent to the lateral meniscus through a recess in peripheral capsular reinforcement known as the popliteal hiatus. Because of its oblique orientation of span from the medial proximal femur to the posterior tibia, popliteal contraction is involved in disengagement of the screw-home mechanism via a flexor-rotary function regardless of the open or closed kinetic mode of knee function. The popliteal hiatus is a potential stress riser that may result in increased friction to the muscle substance running adjacent to the lateral meniscus. This may result in inflammation and swelling of the muscle, which may be likened to a trigger finger phenomenon, in which the enlarged muscle is caught within the stricture of an unyielding tunnel. As such, popliteus tendinitis may result in painful popping. Diagnostic studies, including MRI may all be negative. The diagnosis is made clinically, with tenderness localized beneath the fibular collateral ligament and elicited by palpating with the knee in the "figure of 4" position (see figure on p. 722).

- *Plicae.* These are normally occurring folds in the synovium of the knee that embryologically derive from the fusion of the three separate synovial pouches comprising the fetal knee. Following birth, the synovium of the knee is structurally unified although telltale remnants of the fusion of the three original pouches are present in the knee and are known as plicae. Of all three plicae, the mediopatellar plicae is most commonly symptomatic.[63,68,79] When enlarged because of (unknown reasons, or) direct knee trauma such as twisting that causes associated hemorrhage, inflammation, and fibrosis, the mediopatellar plicae may become thickened and less flexible.[35,69,70] Because of its orientation of span, the mediopatellar plicae may bowstring across the anteromedial portion of the medial femoral condyle and result in distal impingement of that condyle. More superficial and proximally, the mediopatellar plicae impinges the medial patellar facet with increasing flexion of the knee. Thus repeated rubbing of the mediopatellar plica across the medial femoral condyle and the medial patellar facet may contribute to chondromalacia.[8] Clinically, the bowstring effect of a fibrous plical band may cause a snapping sensation mimicking medial meniscal pathology.[94] However, medial plica pathology is characterized by pain over the medial femoral condyle, as compared with medial meniscus injury with pain at the medial joint line. Mediopatellar plica injury may also present with giving way, while a thickened and tender band may be palpable beneath the medial retinaculum. Here, pseudolocking may occur as compared with true locking associated with meniscal tears. Provocative maneuvers for mediopatellar plica pathology reproduce medial pain and clicking, and include flexion of the knee, application of a valgus force, and alternating between internal or external rotation of the leg while the patient resists knee flexion from a position of maximal extension.[48] Arthrography helps to differentiate between a symptomatic plica and a torn meniscus. Arthroscopy is the best means of identifying abnormal plicae.

- *Osteochondritis dissecans.* This is an osseous lesion most often occurring on the lateral aspect of the medial femoral condyle, the medial aspect of the lateral femoral condyle, and the patella. Males with right leg dominance in the second decade of life are most affected,[1] although it may also occur in adults (particularly in the third decade) up to age 50.[78] The etiology of this lesion is controversial.[14] The ischemic theory proposes this lesion to be an avascular necrosis of a pressure epiphysis. The traumatic theory suggests either an external or an internal source of trauma that raises intraarticular osseous stress. The latter is postulated to derive as a function of tibiofemoral rotation[44,75] during engagement of the screw-home mechanism in which the lateral aspect of the medial femoral condyle impinges upon the tibial spine. In contrast, the lateral femoral condyle may sustain injury as a function of its impressio terminalis repetitively impinging upon the lateral tibial plateau during terminal knee extension. A constitutional theory suggests a preexisting bone abnormality as an etiologic factor. Affecting a fragment of articular cartilage and its underlying subchondral bone, the resulting fragment may remain attached, partially detached, or completely detached and free to roam in the joint cavity. Fragments colloquially known as "joint mice" may be as large as a hazelnut and are released into the knee joint to elusively flit from place to place in the synovial cavity and cause mechanical symptoms. Clinical findings include knee pain, joint effusion, giving way, catching, locking, and thigh atrophy. Osteochondritis dissecans may mimic medial or lateral meniscal pathology. Although meniscal lesions may result in locking in either flexion or extension, osteochondritis dissecans is characterized by mechanical locking or locking in extension.[16] Moreover, tests for meniscal impingement performed on the knee with osteochondritis dissecans alternate between positive and negative test results. This may be due to the relatively greater mobility of the bone fragment relative to the torn meniscal fragment, which endows it an ability to flit across the tibial plateau. In addition, unlike meniscal pathology, the knee with osteochondritis dissecans may be unlocked without the need for manipulation. Finally, loose bone fragments are readily identified on radiographs whereas menisci are not. Management consists of a protective regimen for children with the hope that the fragment will reattach to the physis. With adolescents and adults surgery involving reattachment or removal of the fragment will prevent degenerative changes to the articular cartilage.

- *Meniscotibial ligament sprain.* Partial[23] or complete disruption of the meniscotibial ligaments can occur as part of a medial collateral ligament sprain[72] and may be clinically indistinguishable from a medial meniscus tear. Patients typically present with medial joint line tenderness, hemarthrosis, clicking with McMurray's test, and no gross ligamentous instability. Diagnosis of meniscotibial ligament sprain is only confirmed at arthroscopy by the presence of an intact meniscus.[94]

- *Tibial spine avulsion fracture.* This type of fracture may be overlooked during radiographic review, especially if they are minimally displaced. In addition to the joint pain and swelling that may occur from the fracture itself, the medial meniscus may become entrapped beneath the fracture fragment.[94]

- *Fat pad syndrome.* The infrapatellar fat pad is located between the patellar ligament and the underlying synovial tissue and bone.[33] By serving to help maintain patellar posture, the fat pad has a direct bearing upon patellofemoral biomechanics. The kinesiologic function of the patella is to increase the leverage of the quadriceps muscle by increasing the lever arm of the quadriceps. This ability is compromised in the event of fat pad atrophy due to loss of normal patellar posture, resulting in an alteration in the angle of insertion of the patellar tendon and, subsequently, an alteration in patellofemoral biomechanics. Fat pad inflammation, bleeding, and eventual fibrosis may occur following several blows that traumatize this area, converting the fat pad into fibrocartilage. Alternately, the fat pad may undergo inflammation and fibrosis following several surgical procedures to the knee. If fibrosis is extensive, the retropatellar bursa and patellar tendon may scar down to the proximal tibia, resulting in a patella baja. On lateral radiograph, the patella has the appearance of lying so low as to almost rest upon the anterior aspect of the tibial plateau. The fat pad is richly innervated with contributions from the femoral, tibial, recurrent, common peroneal, and obturator nerves.[86] Also known as Hoffa's disease, fat pad syndrome clinically presents as tenderness both medial and lateral to the patellar ten-

don[26] as well as jabs of pain at the anterolateral joint line[1] especially during terminal knee extension[40,65,81] as the fibrotic pad is caught between the patella and femur.[1] It may also be associated with thickening of the peritendinous area.[94] The patient may experience pain during weight bearing as well as sudden knee buckling secondary to an altered quadriceps mechanism. Internal derangement is ruled out as locking does not occur.[1] Conservative management is often successful and involves use of antiinflammatory medication and a patella-restraining device, as well as restricted terminal knee extension for approximately 3 months. The prepatellar fat pad may undergo a similar process, after which impingement of its fibrotic bands and overlying synovium produce pain at the anteromedial joint line.[59]

33. How do meniscal injuries in children differ from adults?

The most common meniscal lesions in younger patients are longitudinal (vertical) tears and peripheral detachments[77] and most often involve the posterior meniscal horn.[45,58] Bucket handle tears typically occur in teenage patients. Most knee related problems in youths are due to meniscal problems. Not withstanding, meniscus tears in youths do occur, and are typically associated with *high-energy activities* such as sports. Meniscal injuries, occurring secondary to a twisting motion of the knee, more commonly occur in older adolescents than in younger children as the lower extremities are subject to high-energy activities.[94] The positive findings typical of meniscal injury in adults are frequently not present in children.[77] An example of why this is so is ascribed to the relatively greater ligamentous laxity in children, resulting in hypermobility that may yield a *false-positive McMurray's test.*[94] The most common signs of meniscal injury in children include joint line tenderness and effusion.[58] The child may also present *pain upon passive extension.*[95] Symptoms include pain, locking, intermittent swelling, clicking, and limping.[77,94]

34. What are the different management strategies for a meniscus injury?

Management of meniscal injury is determined by seeking an intervention that maintains the best long term results with the lowest possible risk for degenerative arthritis. Under these criteria, management strategies of meniscal lesions fall into one of three categories:

- *Meniscal tears that are better left alone.* The most frequent kind of tear that does not require surgical intervention is a *partial thickness tear oriented along the longitudinal meniscal axis when the inner segment is stable* to arthroscopic probing. These types of injuries are often seen in the posterior lateral horn of the lateral meniscus in association with an ACL lesion. In addition, *full thickness peripheral tears* ($<$5 mm) may be conservatively managed if they are stable to arthroscopic probing, as are *short radial tears* ($<$5 mm). The rationale justifying noninvasive management of these types of lesions is that damaged menisci continue to serve a useful biomechanical function if the peripherally located circumferential fibers remain intact,[9,36] especially when the extent of the tear is relatively small and the meniscus is stable. Moreover, from a pragmatic standpoint, more meniscus may always be removed in the future if this initial approach proves disappointing, whereas removed meniscal tissue cannot be replaced. Thus, management of these lesions involves observation of the patient over time while a full program of physical therapy is implemented.

- *Meniscus repair.* The definite criteria for suitability of meniscal repair include: (1) a lesion within 3 mm of the meniscosynovial junction and therefore within the vascular zone; (2) normal meniscal body contour; and (3) the tear should be of sufficient length ($>$7 mm) so as to make the meniscus unstable. Approximately 30% of isolated meniscal tears and 60% of meniscal tears associated with ACL tears in patients less than 30 years old are suitable for repair.[94] The geometric configuration of a meniscal tear is also an important factor in determining suitability for repair. The single longitudinal type tear is common in the younger active population, and when located in the vascularized outer third, responds well to percutaneous sutures. Attempted repair should be tempered by the presence of any associated ligamentous injury. For example, the ACL deficient knee is not appropriate for meniscal repair because the repair may be subject to abnormal anterolateral rotary instability. Similarly, a medial meniscus repair (ill advised in the older population) may be doomed to failure because of a preexisting varus deformity at the knee with resultant increased stress delivered to the side of repair. The failure rate of repair widely ranges between 10% and 50% and is dependent upon the experience of the surgeon, the age of the patient, as well as the age and location of the tear.[94]

- *Partial meniscectomy.* This involves operative resection that is limited to removal of the mobile portion, and is presently one of the most commonly performed surgical procedures. This type of surgery, reserved for irreparable types of lesions, is quickly and easily performed, often done under local anesthesia, and is associated with a low complication rate. However, although short-term patient satisfaction is often high, long term degenerative changes, although not nearly as high as those associated with total meniscectomy, may be deleterious to the long-term function of the knee. This is especially so in the patient with ligamentous instability of the knee such as the ACL deficient knee, in which the posterior horn of the medial meniscus functions as a secondary restraint to anterior-posterior translation by wedging between the femur and tibia.[51] Partial meniscectomy should not be performed in the patient with an axial malalignment. For example, a medial meniscectomy of a patient with a varus position of the knee will lead to increased varus and may increase the pain the surgeon wishes to alleviate.

- Performing a partial meniscectomy of a tear located in the outer one-third results in removal of 12% to 35% of the meniscus, resulting in joint contact force increasing by 300% to 400%. Open partial meniscectomy is indicated in the event that the surgeon cannot perform the excision arthroscopically. Unfortunately, arthrotomy of the knee results in protracted and often painful rehabilitation and leaves an obvious scar.[11,12,65]

35. What therapeutic intervention is appropriate for a conservative management program of a torn meniscus?

Approximately one-third of meniscal tears may be treated with conservative therapy consisting of exercises, bracing, and oral medications. With time and therapy the patient's symptoms may often improve and may completely resolve. The other two-thirds often require surgical intervention[94] because mechanical blocking to extension interferes with walking and activities of daily living, and necessitate surgery. Generally, older patients or athletes with suspected meniscal tears should undergo a trial of conservative management unless they have mechanical symptoms. Those unresponsive to physical therapy are then candidates for arthroscopic partial meniscectomy.[94]

Manipulative intervention typically involves maneuvering the knee joint such that the torn fragment is relocated and is often accompanied by a loud, palpable "clunk." This sound and the temporary resolution of symptoms indicate reduction of the mobile fragment into its anatomic position. Having removed a mechanical blocking toward extension, therapeutic exercises may commence without concern for knee motion that might mar the articular surfaces by way of forced flexion or extension in the presence of an unreduced meniscal fragment. Thus, provided there is no locking, a trial of physical therapy may be initiated that involves protection from full weight bearing, the use of a knee immobilizer, nonsteroidal antiinflammatory oral medications. Therapeutic exercises begin with range of motion, isometric, and straight leg raising activities and are initiated as soon as symptoms permit. *Therapeutic management focuses on progressive resistive exercises of the hamstrings and quadriceps musculature.* The anterior horns of both menisci are indirectly attached (via the meniscopatellar and coronary ligament) to the quadriceps muscle such that knee extension dynamically translates the menisci anteriorly. Moreover, the posterior horns are indirectly attached to the hamstrings (semimembranosus) so that knee flexion results in posterior meniscal retraction. *By strengthening these muscles the dynamic influence upon meniscal movement is enhanced such that the meniscus and/or its loose fragment follows the femoral condyles closely and is less likely to sustain impingement resulting in mechanical symptoms.* In this manner, the meniscal tear (if located along the periphery) is allowed to heal without undergoing reimpingement. Spontaneous healing of a peripheral meniscal tear has been documented in adolescents and arthroscopically demonstrated as scarring of the tear site.[46] During this rehabilitative period, athletic activity should be avoided. A favorable response is indicated by resolution of the signs and symptoms suggestive of a meniscal tear. Orthopaedic referral is indicated for joint locking, associated ligamentous or osseous injury, or failure of resolution of symptoms within 6 months. When an adequate trial of physical therapy yields no relief, arthroscopic evaluation may be indicated.[94]

36. What is the medical management of a locked knee?

When an unstable torn portion of the meniscus becomes lodged between the two articulating surfaces in the area of the intercondylar notch, the knee will lock. This occurs because the notch acts to tether the meniscal fragment and thereby interferes with its migration along the tibial plateau. The patient may attempt to unlock the knee by moving that joint back into its mobile range

and reattempt motion, with the intent of dislodging the fragment away from the intercondylar notch. However, this may not always be possible and a locked knee requires urgent intervention. If neglected, further attempts at motion or weight bearing upon a locked knee may cause severe, irreversible erosion of the opposing articular surfaces of the femur and tibia.[80] In this situation, prompt arthroscopic repair, or partial meniscectomy must be carried out to remove the interposed tissue. It is important for the clinician presented with a locked knee to differentiate true meniscal locking from hamstring spasm.

37. What postoperative rehabilitative management is appropriate following partial meniscectomy or repair?

The primary goal following meniscectomy and meniscal repair is to protect the remaining articular cartilage and underlying subchondral bone while strengthening the lower extremity musculature to reduce knee joint stresses.[19] A structured physical therapy program helps avoid postoperative complications such as meniscal reinjury or patellofemoral pain. The rehabilitation program for meniscus repair is similar to that following meniscectomy except that repair is characterized by more restricted weight bearing to protect the repair site. Moreover, the duration of each phase of rehabilitation following meniscal repair is relatively longer so as to allow for repair of the tear site and maturation of the fibrovascular scar.[18]

- *Phase I.* The initial phase of treatment focuses on overcoming any limitations to range of motion. This may be helped by way of modality application to decrease pain and swelling, and may include ice, heat/ice contrast baths, transcutaneous electrical nerve stimulation, electric galvanic stimulation, and phonophoresis. The patient uses crutches but is allowed to weight bear as tolerated on the operated extremity. The patient is encouraged to continually use crutches until they can ambulate without a limp.[94] The patient immediately begins a regimen of range of motion, straight leg raising, and quadriceps setting exercises. Wall slides may be performed to increase passive flexion range of motion for one set of 20 repetitions, while attempting to increase range gradually with repetition. Supine wall slides to increase flexion range may be implemented once the patient attains 110° to 115° range of motion.

  Gel slides, repeated 20 times, facilitates improved knee extension, and are performed by having the patients sit on a smooth surface with the uninvolved leg fully extended and the involved leg flexed. Then placing a lubricant, such as a gel or powder medium to reduce friction, under the heel of the involved foot the patient actively extends the knee for 5 to 10 seconds before releasing the stretch into flexion.

Isometric hip adduction exercises strengthen the adductor musculature and may enhance patellofemoral biomechanics. The horizontal fibers of these muscles originate from the medial intermuscular septum and distal hip adductor tendons and insert into the suprapatellar tendon.[74] Thus, strengthening of these muscles may help improve patellar tracking. Isometric quadriceps setting exercises are especially helpful in strengthening the VMO segment of the quadriceps muscle. The use of neuromuscular electrical stimulation may be used in conjunction to help facilitate contraction of a poorly contracting VMO. Short arc quadriceps femoral muscle extension exercises may be used to strengthen the quadriceps femoris muscle.

Strengthening and stretching of other lower extremity musculature is also important to the rehabilitative process. Isotonic hamstring muscle strengthening may begin when the patient can flex the knee to at least 80° to 90°. Hip abduction activities may begin when the VMO demonstrates adequate muscle contraction and strength. This is because lateral patellar tracking during hip abduction may occur in the presence of a weakened VMO. Stationary bicycling may be initiated when the knee attains 115° to 120° of knee flexion providing that soft tissue swelling and pain have subsided.[19]

- *Phase II.* This phase involves the continual use of modalities as needed as well as flexibility and strengthening exercises. The patient may progress to endurance and isokinetic strength training. Speeds performed at 300° per second for 30 to 60 seconds are recommended for endurance training, while speeds greater than 200° per second and six to nine sets of 10 repetitions for strength training. Exercises at higher resistance or lower speeds are not recommended owing to the high stresses resulting in the patellofemoral joint. Closed chain exercises may also be initiated during this phase.
- *Phase III.* During this phase, progress in strength training is continued as the patient gradually returns to sport related activities. When the patient is able to run on the treadmill for 10 to 15 minutes at a pace of 7 to 8 minutes per mile, track running may be initiated.

Agility drills and sport specific activities may begin once the patient can jog 2 to 3 miles on the track.[19]

38. What are future trends in meniscal management?

Several developments are now underway about management of meniscal injury, and include the use of a laser (light amplification by stimulated emission of radiation) scalpel to partially remove or smoothly contour an irregular meniscal tear.[57] Meniscal allograft transplantation[34,51] with perimeniscal synovium or fibrin clot may eventually become a management option for patients with previous meniscectomies who now demonstrate early degenerative symptoms. Vascularization of the inner portion of the meniscus may be possible via use of cell mediators, such as angiogenin—an angiogenesis inducing protein.[46] This may help preserve valuable meniscal tissue following injury and possibly preclude the need for partial or complete meniscectomies. Finally, replacement of absent or damaged menisci is now being researched using collagen-based scaffolds acting as biologic superstructures for meniscal regeneration[89] similar to the human ear that grew off the back of a living mouse in 1996 at the Massachusetts Institute of Technology.

RECOMMENDED READING

Weiss CB, Lundberg M, Hamberg P et al: Non-operative treatment of meniscal tears, *J Bone Joint Surg* 71A:811, 1989.

Rensstrom P, Johnson RJ: Anatomy and biomechanics of the menisci, *Clin Sports Med* 9(3), 1990.

REFERENCES

1. Aichroth P: Osteochondral fractures and their relationship to osteochondritis dissecans of the knee: an experimental study in animals, *J Bone Joint Surg* 53B:448, 1971.
2. Albert S et al: Imaging of the knee. In Nicholas JA, Hershman EB editors: *The lower extremity and spine,* ed 2, vol 1, St Louis, 1995, Mosby.
3. Appel H: Late results after meniscectomy in the knee joint. A clinical and roentgenographic follow-up investigation, *Acta Orthop Scand* 133(Suppl):1-111, 1970.
4. Arnoczky S et al: Meniscus. In Woo SY, Buckwalter JA editors: *Injury and repair of the musculoskeletal soft tissues,* Chicago, 1987, American Academy of Orthopedic Surgeons.
5. Arnoczky SP: Arthroscopic surgery: meniscal healing, *Contemporary Orthopedics* 10:31, 1985.
6. Assimakopoulos A, Katonis PG, Agapitos MV et al: The innervation of the human meniscus, *Clin Orthop* 275:232, 1992.
7. Barrie HJ: The pathogenesis and significance of meniscal cysts, *J Bone Joint Surg* 61B:184, 1979.

8. Boland AL Jr, Hulstyn MJ: Soft-tissue injuries of the knee. In Nicholas JA, Hershman EB editors: *The lower extremity and spine,* ed 2, vol 1, St Louis, 1995, Mosby.

9. Bourne RB, Finlay JB, Papadopoulos P et al: The effect of medial meniscectomy or strain distribution in the proximal parts of the tibia, *J Bone Joint Surg* 66A:1431, 1984.

10. Breck LW: Cysts of the semilunar cartilage of the knee, *Clin Orthop* 3:29, 1954.

11. Bullough PG, Munuera L, Murphy J et al: The strength of the menisci of the knee as it relates to their fine structure, *J Bone Joint Surg* 52A:564, 1970.

12. Bullough PG et al: The menisci of the knee. In Insall JN editor: *Surgery of the knee,* New York, 1984, Churchill Livingstone.

13. Busch MT: Meniscal injuries in children and adolescents, Georgia, *Clin Sports Med* 9(3), 1990.

14. Clanton TO, DeLee JC: Osteochondritis dissecans, *Clin Orthop,* 167:50, 1982.

15. Cox JS, Nye CE, Schaefer WW et al: The degenerative effects of partial and total medial meniscus in dogs knees, *Clin Orthop* 109:178, 1975.

16. Cyriax J: Textbook of orthopedic medicine. In *Diagnosis of soft tissue lesions,* ed 8, vol 1, London, 1982, Bailliere Tindall.

17. Dandy JJ: *Essential orthopedics and trauma,* Edinburgh, 1989, Churchill Livingstone.

18. DeHaven KE, Black KP, Griffiths HJ: Open meniscus repair: technique and two-to nine-year results, *Am J Sports Med* 17:788-795, 1989.

19. DeHaven KE, Bronstein RD: Injuries to the menisci of the knee. In Nicholas JA, Hershman EB editors: *The lower extremity and spine,* ed 2, vol 1, St Louis, 1995, Mosby.

20. DeHaven KE: The role of the meniscus. In Ewing JW editor: *Articular cartilage in knee joint function: basic science and arthroscopy,* New York, 1994, Raven Press.

21. DiStefano VJ: Skeletal injuries of the knee. In Nicholas JA, Hershman EB editors: *The lower extremity and spine,* ed 2, vol 1, St Louis, 1995, Mosby.

22. Dye SF, Via MW, Andersen C: An evolutionary perspective of the knee, *Orthop Trans* 10:70, 1986.

23. El-Khoury GY, Usta HY, Berger RA: Meniscotibial (coronary) ligament tears, *Skeletal Radiol* 11:191-196, 1984.

24. Fairbank TJ: Knee joint changes after meniscectomy, *J Bone Jint Surg* 30B:664, 1948.

25. Ferrer-Roca O, Vilalta C: Lesions of the meniscus. Part II. Horizontal cleavages and lateral cysts, *Clin Orthop* 146:301, 1980.

26. Fochios D, Nicholas JA: Football injuries. In Nicholas JA, Hershman EB editors: *The lower extremity and spine,* ed 2, vol 2, St Louis, 1995, Mosby.

27. Fowler PJ: Functional anatomy of the knee. In Hunter, LY, Funk FJ Jr. editors: *Rehabilitation of the injured knee,* St Louis, 1984, Mosby.

28. Fritz JM, Irrgang JJ, Harner CD: Rehabilitation following allograft meniscal transplantation: a review of the literature and case study, *JOSPI* 21(2), 1996.

29. Garrick J, Fillien D, Whiteside P: The epidemiology of aerobic dance injuries, *Am J Sports Med* 14:67, 1986.

30. Goodfellow J, O'Connor J: The mechanics of the knee and prosthesis design, *J Bone Joint Surg* [BR], 60:358, 1978.

31. Goss M: *Gray's anatomy,* ed 29, Philadelphia, 1973, Lea & Febiger.

32. Gray H: *Gray's anatomy,* Philadelphia, 1974, Lea & Febiger.

33. Greenfield BH: *Rehabilitation of the knee: a problem-solving approach,* Philadelphia, 1993, FA Davis.

34. Grood ES: Menisci function, *Adv Orthop Surg* 4:193, 1984.

35. Hardaker W Jr, Whipple TL, Bassett FH III: Diagnosis and treatment of the plica syndrome of the knee, *J Bone Joint Surg* 62A:221, 1980.

36. Hargreaves DJ, Seedholm BB: On the "bucket-hand" tear: partial or total meniscectomy? A quantitative study, *J Bone Joint Surg* 61B:381, 1979.

37. Henry JH: The patellofemoral joint. In Nicholas JA, Hershman EB editors: *The lower extremity and spine,* ed 2, vol 1, St Louis, 1995, Mosby.

38. Jackson JP: Degenerative changes in the knee after meniscectomy, *J Bone Joint Surg* 49B:584, 1967.

39. Johnson RJ, Kettelkamp PB, Clark W et al: Factors affecting late results after meniscectomy, *J Bone Joint Surg* 56A(4):719-729, 1974.

40. Johnson RJ, Pope MH: *Functional anatomy of the meniscus.* Symposium on reconstruction of the knee, American Academy of Orthopedic Surgeons, St Louis, 1978, Mosby.

41. Jones RE, Smith EC, Reisch JS: Effects of medial meniscectomy in patients older than forty years, *J Bone Joint Surg* 60A(6):783-786, 1978.

42. Kapandji IA: The physiology of joints. In *Lower limb,* ed 2, vol 2, New York, 1970, Churchill Livingstone.

43. Kaplan EB: The embryology of the knee joint, *Bull Hosp J Dis Orthop Inst* 16:111, 1955.

44. Kennedy JC, Grainger RW, McGraw RW: Osteochondral fractures of the femoral condyles, *J Bone Joint Surg* 48B:436, 1966.

45. King AG: Meniscal lesions in children and adolescents. A review of the pathology and clinical presentation, *Injury* 15:105-108, 1985.

46. King TV, Vallee BI, Rosenberg AE: Induction of angiogenesis in the knee meniscus using argiogenin, *Orthop Res Soc Trans* 14:206, 1989.

47. Kircher MT, Hershman EB: Arthroscopic cruciate reconstruction. In Nicholas JA, Hershman EB editors: *The lower extremity and spine,* ed 2, vol 1, St Louis, 1995, Mosby.

48. Koshino T, Okamoto R: Resection of painful shelf (plica synovialis mediopatellaris) under arthroscopy, *Arthroscopy* 1:136, 1985.

49. Kromer K: *Der verletzte meniskus,* Wien, 1942, Maydrich.

50. Levy M et al: The effect of lateral meniscectomy on motion of the knee, *J Bone Joint Surg* 71A:401-406, 1989.

51. Levy M, Torzilli PA, Warren RF: The effect of medial meniscectomy an anterior-posterior motion of the knee, *J Bone Joint Surg* 64A(6):883-888, 1982.

52. Lieb FJ, Perry J: Quadriceps function, *J Bone Joint Surg* [Am] 50:1535, 1968.

53. Lynch MA, Henning CE: Physical examination of the knee. In Nicholas JA, Hershman EB editors: *The lower extremity and spine,* ed 2, vol 1, St Louis, 1995, Mosby.

54. MacConaill MA: The function of intra-articular fibrocartilages, with special reference to the knee and inferior radioulnar joints, *J Anat* 66:210-227, 1932.

55. MacConaill MA: The movements of bones and joints III: the synovial fluid and its assistants, *J Bone Joint Surg* 32B:244, 1950.

56. MacConaill MA: Studies in the mechanics of synovial joints II: displacements on articular surfaces and the significance of saddle joints, *Ir J Med Sci* 6:223-235, 1946.

57. Meade TD: Meniscus tears: diagnosis and treatment. p. 56.

58. Medlar RC, Manidberg JJ, Lyne ED: Meniscectomies in children—report of long term results, *Am J Sports Med* 8:87-92, 1980.

59. Methany JA, Mayor MB: Hoffa disease: chronic impingement of the infrapatellar fat pad, *Am J Knee Surg* 1:134-139, 1988.

60. Milbauer DL, Patel SA: Radiographic examination of the knee. In Nicholas JA, Hershman B editors: *The lower extremity and spine,* ed 2, vol 1, St Louis, 1995, Mosby.

61. Muller W: *The knee: form, function, and ligament reconstruction,* New York, 1983, Springer-Verlag.

62. Netter FH: *The Ciba Collection of Medical Illustrations,* vol 8, Part III. Musculoskeletal system: trauma, evaluation and management. Summit, NJ, 1993, CIBA-GEIGY.

63. Nottage WN, Sprague NF, Auerbach BJ: Medial patellar plica syndrome, *Am J Sports Med* 11:211-214, 1983.

64. O'Connor R: *Textbook of arthroscopic surgery,* Philadelphia, 1984, Lippincott.

65. Oretorp N, Risberg B: *Studies on the fine structure of the medial meniscus and ligaments and their anatomical relations in the human knee.* Medical Dissertation 63, Sweden, 1978, Linkoping University.

66. Pagnani MJ et al: Anatomy of the knee. In Nicholas JA, Hershman EB editors: *The lower extremity and spine,* ed 2, vol 1, St Louis, 1995, Mosby.

67. Parsien JS: Arthroscopic treatment of cysts of the menisci: a preliminary report, *Clin Orthop* 257:154, 1990.

68. Patel D: Arthroscopy of the plica-synovial folds and their significance, *Am J Sports Med* 6:217-225, 1978.

69. Pipkin G: Lesions of the suprapatellar plica, *J Bone Joint Surg* 32A:363, 1950.

70. Pipkin G: Knee injuries: the role of the suprapatellar plica and suprapatellar bursa in simulating internal derangements, *Clin Orthop* 74:161, 1971.

71. Pitman MI, Frankel VH: Biomechanics of the knee in athletes. In Nicholas JA, Hershman EB editors: *The lower extremity and spine,* ed 2, vol 1, St Louis, 1995, Mosby.

72. Price CT, Allen WC: Ligament repair in the knee with preservation of the meniscus, *J Bone Joint Surg* 60A(1), 1978.

73. Quirk R: Knee injuries in classical dancers, *Med Prob Perf Art* 3(2):52, 1988.

74. Raskas D, Lehman RC: Meniscal injuries in athletes: pinpointing the diagnosis, *J Musculoskeletal Med* 5:18, 1988.

75. Rehbein F: Die enstehung der osteochondritis dissecans, *Arch Klin Chir* 265:69, 1950.

76. Renstrom P, Johnson RJ: Anatomy and biomechanics of the menisci. Vermont, *Clin Sports Med* 9(3):526, 1990.

77. Ritchie DM: Meniscectomy in children, *Aust NZ J Surg* 35:239-241, 1965.

78. Roberts JM, Kennedy JC: Osteochondritis dissecans. In Roberts JM, Kennedy JC editors: *The injured adolescent knee,* Baltimore, 1979, Williams & Wilkins.

79. Rovere GD, Adair DM: Medial synovial shelf plica syndrome, *Am J Sports Med* 13:382-386, 1985.

80. Sammarco GJ: Dance injuries. In Nicholas JA, Hershman EB editors: *The lower extremity and spine,* ed 2, vol 2, St Louis, 1995, Mosby.

81. Seedholm BB, Dowson D, Wright V: The load-bearing function of the menisci: a preliminary study. In Ingwersen OS et al editors: *The knee joint: recent advances in basic research and clinical aspects,* Amsterdam, Excerpta Academy of Orthopedic Surgeons. St Louis, 1978, Mosby.

82. Seedholm BB: Transmission on the load in the knee joint with special reference to the role of the menisci: I. Anatomy, analysis and apparatus, *Eng Med* 8:207-219, 1979.

83. Seger BM, Woods GW: Arthroscopic management of lateral meniscal cysts, *Am J Sports Med* 14:105, 1986.

84. Shrive N: The weight-bearing role of the menisci of the knee, *J Bone Joint Surg* 56B:381, 1974.

85. Simon WH, Friedenberg S, Richardson S: Joint congruence: a correlation of joint congruence and thickness of articular cartilage in dogs, *J Bone Joint Surg* 55A:1614, 1973.

86. Smillie IS: *Injuries of the knee joint,* London, 1978, Churchill Livingstone.

87. Smillie JS: *Injuries of the knee joint,* ed 4, Edinburgh, 1971, Churchill Livingstone.

88. Smillie IS: The congenital discoid meniscus, *J Bone Joint Surg* 30B:671-682, 1948.

89. Stone KR, Rodykey WG, Webber RJ et al: Future directions: collagen-based prosthesis for meniscal regeneration, *Clin Orthop* 252:129, 1990.

90. Strasser H: *Lehre der muskel-und gelenkmechanik,* Berlin, 1917, Springer-Verlag.

91. Sutton JB: *Ligaments. Their nature and morphology,* London, 1987, HK Lewis.

92. Tapper EM, Hoover NW: Late results after meniscectomy, *J Bone Joint Surg* 51A:517, 1969.

93. Trent PS, Walker PS, Wolf B: Ligament length patterns, strength, and rotation axes of the knee joint, *Clin Orthop* 117:263-270, 1976.

94. Tria AJ, Klein KS: *An illustrated guide to the knee,* New York, 1992, Churchill Livingstone.

95. Vahvanen V, Aalto K: Meniscectomy in children, *Acta Orthop Scand* 50:791-795.

96. Voloshin AS, Wosk J: Shock absorption of the meniscectomized and painful knees: a comparative in-vivo study, *J Biomed Eng* 5:157, 1983.

97. Walker PS, Erkman MJ: The role of the menisci in force transmission across the knee, *Clin Orthop* 109:184, 1975.

98. Wallace LA, Mangine RE, Malone TR: The knee. In Gould III JA editor: *Orthopedic sports physical therapy,* ed 2, St Louis, 1990, Mosby.

99. Weber W, Weber E: *Mechanik der menschlichen genverkzenge,* Gottingen, 1836.

43

Knee Injury with Rapid Swelling and Giving Way When Pivoting

CASE 1: A 22-year-old male college football player received a blow to the posterior right knee as he was tackled from behind. During the tackle, a player from the opposite team brought the patient to an immediate halt by grabbing his extended-stance lower leg during midgait and fixing it to the ground. This high-speed maneuver caused a forceful, momentary forward translation of the shinbone that was accompanied by an audible "pop" and was later vividly recollected by the patient. Pain was excruciating and localized to the posterolateral aspect of the proximal tibia. The patient, initially unable to stand without assistance, was evaluated by a physical therapist and athletic trainer on the playing field. Although capable of walking with difficulty the next day using crutches, the knee would experience frank collapse unless the patient took special care to point his right toes forward while bearing weight on the limb. Downhill walking was difficult if not impossible. Unless he ambulated "gingerly" on his right stance limb, taking pains not to turn his toes either externally or internally, the entire limb would suddenly buckle.

OBSERVATION The knee, accompanied by ecchymosis, appeared to be increasingly more swollen over time, and became maximally tense at 12 hours following the injury.

PALPATION The knee was becoming increasingly tense and hot, suggesting hemarthrosis. The hamstring muscles were tight and appeared to be in protective spasm.

RANGE OF MOTION Range of motion was grossly limited to the flexed open-packed position for the knee. Full extension was impossible.

STRENGTH Strength was at least fair plus, but generally untestable secondary to pain.

FLEXIBILITY Flexibility was not tested secondary to pain.

SPECIAL TESTS Tests for straight anterior instability show a positive anterior draw for anteromedial bundle accompanied by unequal anterior displacement of both tibial condyles in neutral rotation. When performing the anterior draw at 25° of flexion, the tibia momentarily subluxed forward and out from underneath the femur followed by immediate reduction. The magnitude of anterior draw during the Lachman test revealed a grade III

(1.0 to 1.5 cm) sprain that imparts an empty endpoint to the examiner's hand; rotational draw in 10° of external rotation was negative, but positive in internal rotation. A pivot shift test, which indicates anterolateral knee stability, showed anterior subluxation of the lateral tibial condyle out from under the lateral femoral condyle, and indicating concurrent injury to the anterolateral knee capsule. This was positive for only the first hour following the injury. Negative reverse pivot shift, McMurray, Apley, and Slocum tests. Provocative varus and valgus stress testing are negative in full knee extension indicating preservation of collateral ligamentous stabilizers. However, whereas valgus testing was negative with the knee in slight flexion, varus testing with the knee in 20° to 30° of flexion was positive when the right tibia is internally rotated confirming suspicion of anterolateral rotatory instability due to injury of the anterolateral capsule. Positive patellar tap test.[23]

RADIOGRAPHS   Radiographs indicated a positive lateral capsular sign showing avulsion of the inferior meniscocapsular attachment of the lateral meniscus. Both tibial spines were intact.

ARTHROCENTESIS   Arthrocentesis revealed bloody joint fluid aspiration without presence of fat droplets.

CLUE:

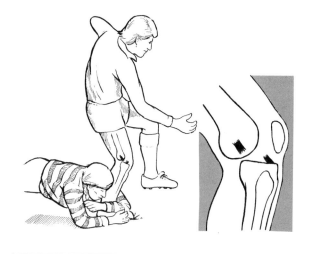

(From Dandy DJ: *Essential orthopaedics and trauma*, ed 2, Edinburgh, 1993, Churchill Livingstone.)

CASE 2: A 41-year-old female was on a business trip to the local metropolis and began her day by jogging around a 2-mile theater district in the early morning. After 20 minutes of jogging, she was startled by the sound of an automobile horn. In response, she decelerated and cut toward the sidewalk with her stance leg, only to land in a shallow pothole. Momentary hyperextension was severe enough to cause stabbing pain to her right knee, causing her to pitch forward and land on the tibial tubercle. A policeman rushed to her aid and called an ambulance, then she was taken to a local hospital. In the emergency room she was diagnosed with a knee sprain and released on crutches.

OBSERVATION   The right shin seems to sag backward on the femur compared with the contralateral knee when viewed laterally. Ecchymosis appeared several days following the injury.

PALPATION   Tenderness was provoked when palpating the right popliteal fossa. There was no tenderness to the patella.

RANGE OF MOTION   Range of motion was grossly limited to the flexed open packed position for the knee. Full extension was virtually impossible.

STRENGTH   Strength was at least fair plus, but generally untestable secondary to pain.

FLEXIBILITY   Not tested secondary to pain.

SPECIAL TESTS   A 3+ (1.0 to 1.5 cm) difference during posterior draw is detected during arthrometric testing, and a "mushy" rather than an abrupt end-feel was imparted to the examiner's hands during manual stress testing. Posterior draw in 10° of internal and external rotation was negative and indicated an intact knee joint capsule. Negative varus and valgus testing with the involved knee in full extension. Positive straight posterior instability was further suggested by a positive drop back test. Negative reverse pivot shift, McMurray, Apley, and Slocum tests.

RADIOGRAPHS   No previous evidence of Osgood-Schlatter's disease. Both tibial spines were intact.

ARTHROCENTESIS   Arthrocentesis shows bloody joint fluid aspirate; no evidence of fatty aspirate.

CLUE:

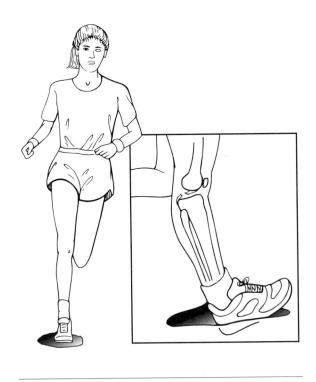

? Questions

1. What is the most likely cause of the patient's symptoms in Cases 1 and 2?
2. What are the cruciate ligaments?
3. What is the anatomy of the anterior cruciate ligament (ACL)?
4. What are the fascicular bundles comprising the ACL, and how are they functionally different?
5. What is the anatomy of the posterior cruciate ligament (PCL)?
6. What is the significance of the multifascicular cruciate structure in relation to the kinesiology of these ligaments?
7. How does the unique orientation of span of the cruciate ligaments endow them with restraining roles in multiple planes?
8. What are the synergistic and antagonistic functions of the cruciate and collateral ligaments at the knee?
9. What is the relative strength of the cruciate ligaments?
10. What is the relationship between the ACL and the menisci?
11. What is the nerve and blood supply to the cruciate ligaments?
12. Which gender is more likely to sustain a tear of the ACL?
13. What is a common noncontact mechanism of injury to the ACL?
14. What are contact mechanisms of injury to the PCL?
15. Why are ski injuries, derived from falls, well understood and result in predictable patterns of injury?
16. What are three common ski-related mechanisms of injury to the ACL?
17. What is the most common combined ligament sprain at the knee joint?
18. What is the presentation of multiple knee ligament disruption?
19. What is the worst consequence of combined ligament tear at the knee?
20. What are the clinical features of cruciate ligament rupture?
21. How are cruciate ligament injuries differentiated from meniscal injuries?
22. What type of fracture may result from distal detachment of the ACL?
23. What imaging is appropriate to the patient with a cruciate ligament injury?
24. What is the classification of cruciate ligament tears?
25. What are the benefits and disadvantages of arthrometric testing of cruciate integrity?
26. What provocative tests determine integrity of the ACL?
27. What are the three provocative tests for determination of PCL sprain?
28. What are the various straight and rotary instabilities about the knee?
29. What are combined straight and rotatory instabilities at the knee joint, and how are they most readily assessed?
30. How does the osseous design of the lateral tibiofemoral joint facilitate mechanical instability following rupture of the ACL?
31. What is the "pivot shift" phenomenon?
32. How is the pivot shift test performed?
33. What is anteromedial rotatory instability?
34. How is anteromedial instability assessed?
35. What tests indicate instability of the posterolateral corner of the knee?
36. What are the frontal plane stress tests for straight, medial, and lateral instabilities?
37. How may provocative stress testing falsely score negative in the event of PCL rupture?
38. What is the most commonly encountered combination of straight and rotatory instability of the knee joint?
39. What is the sequela of chronic isolated ACL rupture?
40. What factors determine whether ACL tear is conservatively or surgically managed?
41. How may the performance and grading of various provocative tests determine whether patients should undergo conservative or surgical management?

42. What are the soft and osseous tissue sequelae in surgical candidates for ACL repair who elect to forego operative management?
43. What is the pathologic process by which failure of the ACL leads to degenerative osseous changes of the tibiofemoral joint?
44. What are the two surgical options for operative management of the ACL?
45. What indirect evidence argues against dynamic ACL reconstruction?
46. What postoperative complications may follow cruciate ligament repair?

47. What is the medical management following acute rupture of the ACL?
48. What is the quadriceps-cruciate interaction, and how may it be used to dynamically compensate for sprain of the ACL?
49. What is the effect of closed versus open kinetic chain exercises with regard to ACL rehabilitation?
50. What physical therapy is appropriate following ACL repair?
51. What physical therapy is appropriate following postoperative PCL repair?

1. What is the most likely cause of the patient's symptoms in Cases 1 and 2?

Grade III midsubstance tear of the *anterior cruciate ligament* (ACL) as well as anterolateral capsule in Case 1 derived from a contact mechanism of injury, and isolated grade III interstitial sprain of the posterior cruciate ligament in Case 2 derived from a noncontact injury. The mechanism of injury, whether contact or noncontact in nature, may result in one of several patterns of injury for either cruciate ligament. The mechanism of injury from sprain of the posterior cruciate ligament (PCL) was due to straight posterior displacement of the tibia on the femur that occurred from extreme momentary hyperextension. This resulted in posterior translation of the tibia beneath the femur, causing tensing of both the proximal and distal attachments of the PCL to the point of rupture. The subsequent fall onto the tibial tubercle of the involved knee may have represented a secondary mechanism of injury to the PCL if the patient's foot was postured in plantarflexion.

2. What are the cruciate ligaments?

The *cruciate ligaments* (Latin: resembling a cross) are strong flattened ligaments that, by virtue of their oblique intraarticular orientation, twist along their longitudinal axis and take on the appearance of being cordlike. Both ligaments have broad areas of attachment along both the femur and tibia, and have an average length of 3.8 cm.[65] At approximately midway across their span they cross each other and form a cross or, more appropriately, an X. They are named anterior or posterior relative to their distal attachment at the anterior or posterior intercondylar aspect of the tibial plateau (Fig. 43-1). Thus the ACL inserts upon the

tibia anteriorly, whereas the PCL attaches to the tibia posteriorly.

The anterior and posterior cruciate ligaments lie within the intercondylar notch of the femur and possess an anatomic and functional mirror image relative to each other. The broad substance of these ligaments as well as their oblique orientation endows the cruciate ligaments with a spiral orientation of the fibers comprising these structures. In addition to the ligaments twisting on themselves en route their span across the tibiofemoral joint, they additionally cross each other's paths to form a cross as the knee moves through its range of motion. The term *cruciate* is thus descriptive of both their individual and collective anatomy. The an-

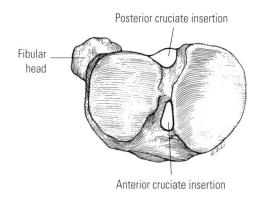

FIG. 43-1 Superior view of the insertions of the cruciate ligaments into the proximal tibial plateau. The cruciates are referenced as being either anterior or posterior relative to their tibial attachments. (From Tria AJ, Klein KS: *An illustrated guide to the knee*, New York, 1992, Churchill Livingstone.)

terior cruciate ligament runs from the lateral femoral condyle to the medial tibial plateau, whereas the posterior cruciate ligament runs from the medial femoral condyle to the lateral tibial plateau (Fig. 43-2).

3. What is the anatomy of the anterior cruciate ligament (ACL)?

The ACL distally arises from a 30-mm long fossa just anterior and lateral to the medial intercondylar eminence (also known as the tibial spine) along a nonarticular area of the tibia. This distal attachment originates between the anterior external attachments of the medial and lateral menisci[40] approximately 1 cm posterior to the anterior margin of the tibial plateau.[6] The ligament extends upward (superior), lateral (oblique), and backward (posterior) to proximally attach on the nonarticular posteromedial surface of the lateral femoral condyle, well posterior to the longitudinal axis of the femoral shaft.[17] Thus when describing its proximodistal course, the ligament is said to course anteriorly, medially, and distally in what may be described as a semicircular arc across the tibiofemoral joint as it passes from the femur to the tibia. In contrast to the tibial collateral ligament, the ACL is not a single ligamentous cord, but rather a collection of individual fascicles that fan out broadly across the tibiofemoral joint.[9,40,67,114] Because of the flattened nature of the fascicles comprising the ACL as well as its oblique orientation of span, the ligament is said to twist on itself

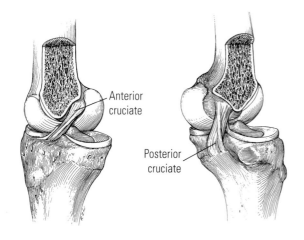

FIG. 43-2 Cutaway lateral view of the cruciate ligaments. The anterior cruciate ligament runs from the lateral femoral condyle to the medial tibial plateau, whereas the posterior cruciate ligament spans between the medial femoral condyle and the lateral tibial plateau. (From Tria AJ, Klein KS: *An illustrated guide to the knee,* New York, 1992, Churchill Livingstone.)

in a slight outward (lateral) spiral. Thus the unique form and span of this ligament endows it with a twisted configuration that imparts tension to the ligament throughout its range of knee motion.[40] When we compare the proximal and distal attachments of the ACL we note that the tibial attachment is wider and stronger, and hence more secure,[17] than the femoral attachment.[9,40] Radiographs should be inspected at the proximal and distal attachment points of the PCL for signs of avulsion.[78,91,95]

4. What are the fascicular bundles comprising the ACL, and how are they functionally different?

Complete agreement does not exist about the collagen orientation of the ACL and whether it exists as separate fiber bundles within the ligament. The notion that discrete subdivisions within the ACL exist, either on a gross or microscopic level has been challenged.[95] A three-bundle model for the ACL has been proposed, which recognizes an intermediate bundle that is held responsible for the straight anterior stability provided by the ACL.[91] Nevertheless, the concept of a functional differentiation of fibers within the ligament is widely accepted and seems necessary to explain the stability provided by the ligament through the full arc of knee motion.

Most authorities recognize a continuum of fibers that may functionally be divided into two principle bundles, known as the posterolateral and anteromedial bundles in reference to their tibial attachment. None of the bundles of the ACL attach onto the tibial spines.[17] These bundles are also anatomically discrete, although this is not readily apparent unless the synovial covering embracing the ACL is removed. The bulky *posterolateral bundle* is the more significant of the two and is comprised of fascicles inserting at the posterolateral aspect of the tibial attachment, while the smaller *anteromedial* bundle inserts upon the anteromedial aspect of the tibial insertion. The posterolateral bundle is taut during knee extension because of its posterior position and its relatively lengthened anatomic position. It is relatively longer than the anteromedial bundle because it comprises the convex surface of the semicircular arc as it spans across the tibiofemoral joint. In contrast, the anteromedial bundle is located along the shorter diameter concave aspect of this semi-arc, and therefore is endowed with a shorter orientation of span. Subsequently, the anteromedial bundle becomes most taut in knee flexion and less so during knee extension.[83] The clinical significance here is that a portion of the ACL is functionally active as a taut static restraint regardless of the position of the knee joint.[114] However, the greatest amount of laxity in both bundles comprising the ACL exists at approximately 40° of knee flexion,[36] whereas the greatest amount of tension occurs in both bundles during knee extension.

5. What is the anatomy of the posterior cruciate ligament (PCL)?

The PCL lies in the posterior region of the intercondylar femoral notch. Like the ACL femoral attachment, the proximal attachment of the PCL occurs in the form of an oval and originates from the posterolateral aspect of the medial femoral condyle. The ligament runs posteriorly (backward), laterally (oblique), and distally (inferiorly) to insert upon a 13-mm wide[65] midline depression in the tibial plateau located just behind the tibial eminence. The PCL is also comprised of two functionally distinct bundles known as the *anterolateral* and *posterior bands,* and named for their tibial attachment site. In extension the anterior bulk of the PCL is lax, whereas the smaller posterior band of fascicles is taut. During knee flexion, the posterior band becomes lax while the anterior bulk of this ligament tightens.[40]

As the PCL spans the tibiofemoral joint it crosses the medial side of the anterior cruciate ligament. The significance of the PCL running 90° offset from the ACL determines that the posterior bundle of the PCL becomes taut in flexion, whereas most fascicles comprising the anteromedial bundle become maximally stretched (hence, taut) during extension. The posterolateral bundle is the more vertical, bulky, and short than the anteromedial bundle, whereas the latter is thinner and longer.[17]

Thus different portions of both cruciate ligaments are taut throughout the arc of flexion and extension owing to bundle tension derived from respective tensing both the ACL and PCL. During knee flexion the anteromedial band of the ACL and the posterior band of the PCL sustains stretch and limit anterior and posterior tibial translation, respectively. Conversely, during knee extension, the posterolateral portion of the ACL and the anterolateral portion of the PCL undergo tensing and thereby check respective anterior and posterior tibial translation.

6. What is the significance of the multifascicular cruciate structure in relation to kinesiology of these ligaments?

A biomechanical analysis of cruciate ligament reveals most fibers comprising the ACL as slack when the knee is flexed and taut when the knee is fully extended. Similarly, most fibers comprising the PCL are taut during knee joint flexion except for the posterior portion, and are slack upon knee extension, except for the posterior portion, which is tight. This variation in tension of different portions of the ligaments throughout the arc of knee flexion and extension occurs as a direct function of the multifascicular nature of the cruciate ligaments.

7. How does the unique orientation of span of the cruciate ligaments endow them with restraining roles in multiple planes?

The cruciate ligaments work in static synergy to restrain anteroposterior translation, varus-valgus angulation, and internal rotation of the knee. The unique orientation of span of the cruciate ligaments endows them with a *restraining function in multiple planes.* Although the ACL is the primary restraint against anterior translation of the tibia on the femur or posterior translation of the femur on the tibia, the PCL acts as the primary buttress against posterior translation of the tibia on the femur or anterior translation of the femur on the tibia. This unique multi-planar span of both cruciate ligaments across the knee joint axes endow these ligaments the role of checkrein restraint preventing excess anteroposterior (sagittal plane) motion, as well as excessive degrees of rotation (transverse plane) and mediolateral (valgus-varus) motion in the frontal plane. This multifunctional role of the cruciate ligaments elevates their status to being considered the principal stabilizers of the knee joint.[1,32,53,56,57,66,93]

8. What are the synergistic and antagonistic functions of the cruciate and collateral ligaments at the knee?

The primary functions of the cruciate ligaments occurs as a direct result of the location of these ligaments in relation to the mechanical axis of the knee joint. Because the ACL is primarily anterior to the mechanical axis of the tibiofemoral joint, it serves as a primary restraint against anterior translation of the tibia on the femur. When the knee is flexed to a right angle, the tibia cannot be pulled anteriorly because it is held by the ACL.[85] The posterolateral band of the ACL also limits hyperextension of the knee.[36] Similarly, because both attachment sites of the PCL are posterior to the mechanical axis of the knee,[65] the PCL is the primary restraint against posterior translation of the tibia on the femur.[97] Thus the anteroposterior stabilizing function of the cruciate ligaments occur synergistically with the restraining function of the tibial and fibular collateral ligaments, and prevent excessive sagittal and frontal plane motion.

Because portions of each of the cruciate ligaments, by virtue of their oblique orientation of span, are contained in the medial and lateral compartments of the knee joint, the cruciate ligaments provide collateral stability role for their respective knee joint compartments. In the frontal plane, the PCL significantly contributes medial-lateral stability.[88] The PCL, in particular, plays a role in checking varus force in the presence of lateral collateral ligament disruption, and may serve as a secondary restraint to valgus stress when the medial collateral ligament is disrupted.[97] Both the ACL and PCL offer greater resistance for varus and valgus stress in full knee extension compared with partial flexion.[44] The PCL also limits excessive hyperflexion of the knee joint.[85]

With regard to transverse plane motion, however, the cruciate and collateral ligaments function antagonistically. During external tibial rotation, it is the collateral ligaments that tighten to inhibit excessive rotation by undergoing helical twisting along their longitudinal axis. In contrast, external tibial rotation promotes relaxation of the cruciate ligaments as these ligaments slacken and unwind from their helical long axis configuration. In neutral rotation, neither the cruciate ligaments nor the collateral ligaments are under unusual tension. During internal tibial rotation the collateral ligaments slacken as they become more vertical and lax, while the cruciate ligaments individually become more helically twisted along their longitudinal axis, while collectively becoming more coiled around each other as they come under strong tension.[86] A secondary function of the cruciate ligaments therefore includes *limiting the magnitude of internal rotation.*

Although the cruciate ligaments and collaterals work antagonistically with respect to the proximal tibia, they work in synergy with respect to the shaft of the tibia, particularly with regard to the distal tibia and the subtalar joint. Distally, subtalar joint pronation occurs during early stance and is consistent with internal rotation of the tibia; subtalar joint supination occurs during late stance and is consistent with external tibial rotation. Proximally, the cruciate ligaments tighten with internal tibial rotation while the collaterals tauten upon external tibial rotation. By limiting the magnitude of tibial rotation, the cruciate ligaments and collaterals synergistically insure that proximal tibial rotation occurs in tandem with and does not exceed the magnitude of rotation distally generated by the subtalar joint distally (Fig. 43-3).

9. What is the relative strength of the cruciate ligaments?

The ACL is the weaker of the two ligaments.[85] The ACL has about the same strength as the medial collateral ligament, and is approximately one half as strong as the PCL[17] The PCL is approximately 50% thicker than the ACL,[40] and requires twice as much force (80 kg) to rupture.[44] This difference in the relative strength of the cruciate ligaments may explain why the incidence of PCL tears is substantially less than ACL injury.

10. What is the relationship between the ACL and the menisci?

The menisci are formed in the eighth embryonic week along with the cruciate ligaments from interposed mesenchymal tissue.[64] The early embryonic appearance of the cruciate ligaments supports the notion that the cruciate ligaments are of great significance as essential stabilizers of the knee joint. The common origin of both the menisci and cruciate ligaments suggests *coordinated function of the meniscoligamentous complex.*[44] In fact, the anterior fibers of the anterior cruciate ligament merge with the transverse ligament, which connects the anterior horns of the medial and lateral menisci.[99] In addition, some fascicles along the posterior aspect of the tibial attachment of the ACL may blend with the posterior attachment of the lateral meniscus.[44] The capsuloligamentous complex formed between the anterior cruciate ligament and the menisci may, in part, account for the relatively high incidence of meniscal lesions that occur in the presence of acute injuries to the anterior cruciate ligament. An intimate association also exists between the posterior cruciate ligament as that structure sends a slip into the posterior horn of the lateral meniscus. Thus although the lateral menisci are understood as being more mobile than the medial menisci, they nevertheless have their anteroposterior translation influenced by tensing and relaxing of the cruciate ligaments.

These anatomic associations highlight a continuity of structure and function between the menisci and the cruciate ligaments that exemplifies the static and dynamic interrelationships among the myriad of soft and osseous structures comprising the knee joint. Hence, it is not surprising that tears of the medial meniscus may develop after an apparently isolated disruption of the anterior cruciate ligament because of abnormal joint motion. For example, the medial meniscus serves as a secondary buttress to anterior displacement of the knee joint in the ACL deficient knee. This is because the firm fixation of the meniscus to the tibial plateau allows it to

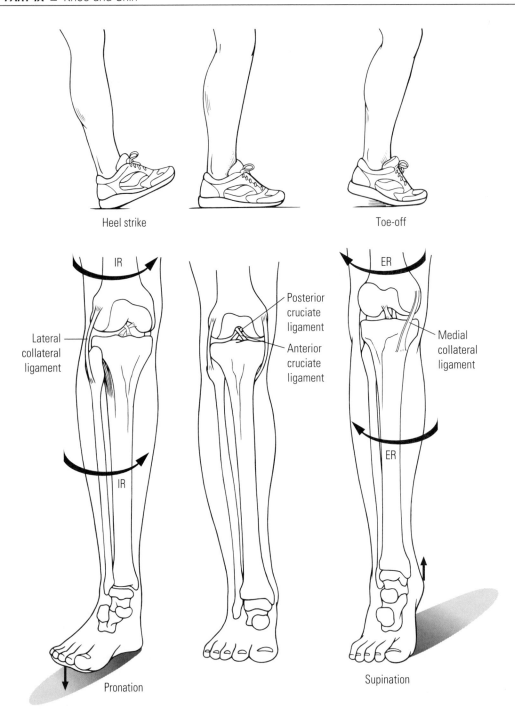

Heel strike

Toe-off

IR

IR

Lateral
collateral
ligament

Posterior
cruciate
ligament

Anterior
cruciate
ligament

ER

ER

Medial
collateral
ligament

Pronation

Supination

FIG. 43-3 The *antagonistic function of the cruciates and collateral ligaments* is apparent only in reference to the proximal tibia. Whereas the cruciate ligaments tauten upon and thereby check excessive internal tibial torsion, the collaterals tighten upon and prevent excessive external tibial portion. However, when we expand our focus beyond the knee joint to the distal tibial articulation, the collaterals and cruciates may be considered to work together as limiting the magnitude of tibial torsion and thus ensuring that the proximal and distal rotations occur in tandem one with the other.

act as a wedge that restrains anterior translation of the femur on the plateau.[99] Thus removing a significant portion of the medial meniscus is equivalent to eliminating an important secondary stabilizer of the knee joint[99] preventing excessive anterior laxity. With time, the viscoelastic strength of the medial meniscus may be exceeded by the excessive anterior translatory forces associated with knee extension and develop a tear. Conversely, various grades of cruciate or collateral ligament tears are often associated with meniscal tears.[26] Moreover, many of the mechanisms resulting in cruciate or collateral ligament injuries are similar if not identical to mechanisms resulting in meniscal injury.[9]

11. What is the nerve and blood supply to the cruciate ligaments?

The vascular supply to both cruciate ligaments arises from the ligamentous branches of the middle genicular artery and enters by way of the intercondylar notch near the femoral attachment of the cruciate ligaments. The adult ACL receives no significant blood supply from its bony attachments, but is entirely supplied by the vasculature of its synovial sheath.[9] Both cruciate ligaments are covered by a synovial membranous fold that forms an envelope about the ligaments. Although the cruciate ligaments are intracapsular, they are extrasynovial as they are enveloped in their own synovial sheath that prevents the synovial fluid bathing the tibiofemoral joint from contacting the cruciate ligament surface.[110] This meager vascular supply reaches the cruciate ligaments by way of this enveloping synovium and arborizes to form a weblike synovial plexus of vessels that ensheathe and penetrate both ligaments.[97] A significant vascular contribution to this synovial network also derives from the retropatellar fat pad.

The cruciate ligaments receive afferent innervation from the posterior articular branches of the tibial nerve, as well as medial articular branches from the saphenous, obturator, as well as lateral articular branches of the peroneal nerve.[87] The posterior articular nerve is the largest nerve supplying the knee joint and is a branch of the posterior tibial nerve. Most nerve fibers course along with the endoligamentous vasculature and penetrate the cruciate ligaments, although some fibers lie along among the many fascicles comprising the ligaments. These latter fibers may serve a proprioceptive function.[67] A decline in proprioceptive sensation has been clinically noted in patients with full thickness ACL rupture.[11] Mechanoreceptors, which respond to tension within ligaments, have also been found in the human ACL.[103] Mechanoreceptors such as Ruffini's endings include Pacinian corpuscles, which detect crude touch and pressure, whereas changes in ligament length/tension are detected by the Golgi tendon organ.[63] All three have been found to be present in the ACL.[103] As relatively few free nerve endings are found in the ACL, the ligament is relatively insensitive to pain.[97]

12. Which gender is more likely to sustain a tear of the ACL?

An increased incidence of ACL sprain is found in women, although the reason for this is not clear. Some authorities attribute this difference to females having less muscle mass per total body weight as compared with males. Thus if the balance of the osseous, dynamic, and other soft tissue components comprising the knee is disturbed by an awkward knee movement, their hamstrings and other dynamic restraints are less capable of compensating adequately. Subsequently, greater demand for maintenance of stability is shifted to their static restraints, particularly the anterior cruciate ligament. Other authorities theorize that woman's knees may be more subject to ACL injury due to peculiarities in bony contour of the tibiofemoral articulation.[42,77]

13. What is a common noncontact mechanism of injury to the ACL?

In sports, noncontact or just minimal contact mechanisms leading to cruciate ligament sprain are increasingly likely owing to the vast magnitude of forces generated through the linkage system.[35] Injury to the anterior cruciate ligament represents a major injury to the knee whom mechanism often involves a *noncontact* twisting injury from landing on the leg and suddenly changing direction at the same time, as in an off-balance landing following a basketball jump shot. The player descending from a basketball rebound may land a little off balance with one knee nearly straight and tear the ACL through a vertical deceleration mechanism (Fig. 43-4).[73] The most frequent combination of forces implicated in isolated ACL sprain include *deceleration, valgus, and external rotation.* Less common mechanisms include deceleration, valgus, and internal rotation, or hyperextension of the knee.[40,113] The former two mechanisms may occur during vigorous athletic participation when a player swerves and pivots his or her torso to the side of the planted leg, thus twisting the knee while the foot is firmly planted on the ground. A contact mechanism of injury to the ACL may be incurred from a tackle from behind that pushes the upper part of the tibia of the planted foot forward.[23] In American football, injury to the ACL may be sustained by a maximal effort plant-and-cut strategy in which a running back attempting to avoid a tackle may fake one way and tear the ACL while planting and cutting to go the opposite direction.[73]

14. What are contact mechanisms of injury to the PCL?

The most common mechanism of injury to the posterior cruciate ligament is the dashboard or bumper blow to the anterior tibia with the knee flexed to 90°. This same injury is reproduced when an individual forcefully falls directly upon a flexed knee (Fig. 43-5), striking the tibial tubercle against the ground with the foot plantarflexed.* The common denominator uniting these mechanisms is posterior translation of the tibia beneath

---

*When the foot is plantarflexed, the tibia is driven posteriorly, causing sprain of the PCL. However, if the same type of fall is incurred with the ankle in dorsiflexion, the force is redirected anteriorly to the patella causing patellar injury. (Clancy WG et al: Anterior cruciate ligament reconstruction using one-third of the patellar ligament, augmented by extra-articular tendon transfers, *J Bone Joint Surg* 64A:352, 1982.)

the femur that causes the PCL to tear. The posterior cruciate ligament may be injured secondary to extreme hyperextension of the knee joint, as may occur from quickly and forcefully stepping into a hole. The ACL, like the PCL, may sustain a sprain when receiving a blow to the anterior knee, although the force moves the femur back on the tibia. Severe varus or valgus stress to the knee following injury to the collateral ligament can also cause rupture of the PCL.[88]

15. Why are ski injuries, derived from falls, well understood and result in predictable patterns of injury?

The history of skiing traces its beginnings to mountain warfare and gradually was acquired as a sport by civilians in Scandinavia and Austria in the nineteenth century. In the United States, skiing as a form of sport did not gain popularity until after the Winter Olympics at

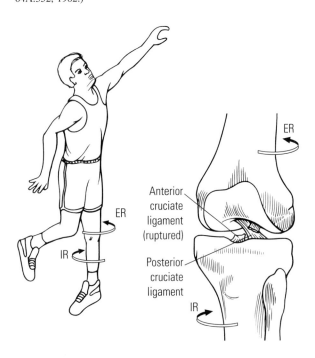

FIG. 43-4 Common cause of ACL injury in basketball players occurs following an off-balance landing upon the leg and attempted recovery in which the knee is hyperextended and the proximal (femoral) and distal (tibial) osseous shafts comprising the lower limb rotate in opposite directions.

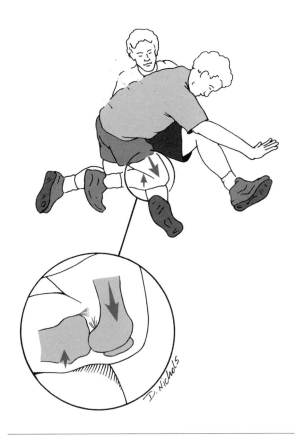

FIG. 43-5 Mechanism of posterior cruciate ligament injury. (From Shankman GA: *Fundamental orthopedic management for the physical therapist assistant,* St Louis, 1997, Mosby.)

Lake Placid, New York in 1932. Although a popular form of winter recreation, skiing can be a dangerous sport. Approximately 5% of all patients engaging in downhill (Alpine) skiing will descend the slopes in toboggans towed by members of the National Ski Patrol System. The number of injuries in novice skiers is three times more likely than the expert skier. The two basic kinds of accidents occurring in skiing are falls and collisions. Collisions may result from an almost unlimited number of factors, and produce and wide variety of injuries to any part of the body. Falls, however, occur in a fairly predictable manner, thereby lending themselves to study and definition. Thus the mechanisms involved in falls may be studied and the injury patterns predicted.[15]

16. What are three common ski-related mechanisms of injury to the ACL?

The anterior cruciate ligament is frequently sprained during skiing accidents by one of three mechanisms of injury. The *most common* mechanism of injury involves an *external rotation valgus moment* to the knee occurring when the skier catches a ski tip on a tree stump or snow bank. As the skier continues downhill on the opposite weighted limb, the moment arm caused by the unweighted ski places a larger torque across the knee joint. Here, the femur is medially rotated as the body falls to the opposite side. The knee is partially flexed and the tibia is moderately to markedly externally rotated and abducted by leverage from the ski (Fig. 43-6). This type of noncontact mechanism, similar to the

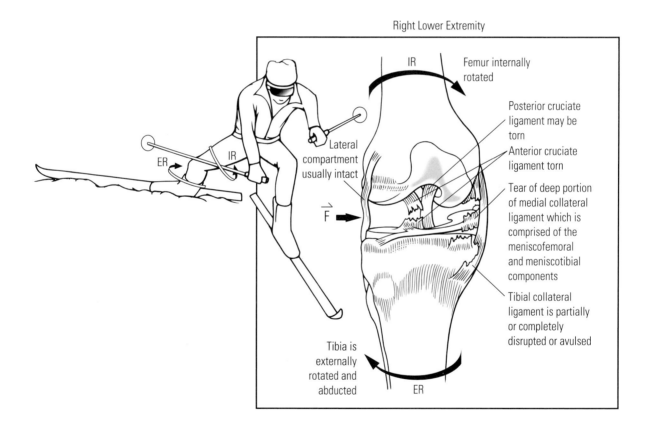

FIG. 43-6 The most common type of mechanism of ACL injury in skiing is an *external rotation valgus moment*. Here, the inner tip of one ski gets caught on ice or in a snow bank and turns outward. This forces the ipsilateral lower limb into internal femoral rotation and external tibial rotation that are magnified by the leverage of the ski and the contralateral lower limb and body moving forward. The knee of the unweighted ski undergoes enormous torque that may result in injury to the medial collateral ligament, the meniscus, the anterior cruciate ligament, and the posterior cruciate ligament in that order. The cruciates suffer injury because they are tensioned owing to internal femoral rotation beyond their tensile capacity as their proximal and distal attachments are distanced.

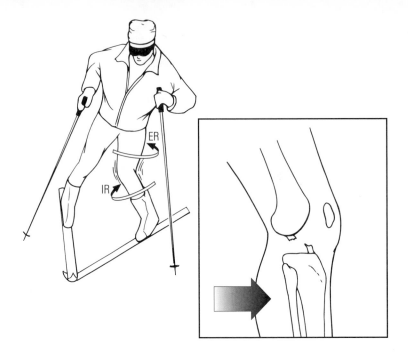

FIG. 43-7 *Deceleration-type injury* in which the femur undergoes external rotation while the tibia undergoes internal rotation, followed by hyperextension of the knee. The ACL is tensed by internal tibial rotation, and further stressed by hyperextension forces that exceed the tensile strength of the ACL and result in rupture.

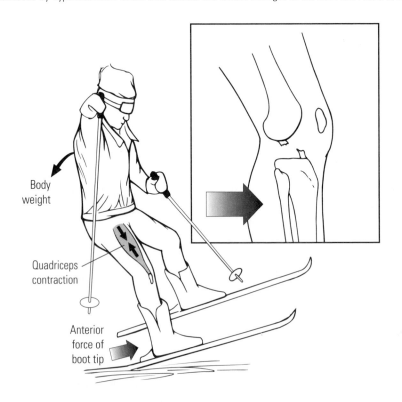

FIG. 43-8 A third mechanism occurs in more advanced skiers during landing from a mogul or jump as a result of direct anterior tibial translation on the femur. As the back of the ski hits the snow, the skier jackknifes backward. The nonyielding rigid boot covering the calf abuts against the calf and results in the tibia moving anteriorly relative to the femur. Moreover, the quadriceps provide a sudden and violent anterior tibial translation as they protectively contract in the attempt to right the body into extension in an attempt to regain balance. The cumulative effect of these two anterior tibial translatory forces results in rupture of the ACL.

unhappy triad of O'Donoghue associated with football clipping injuries, wreaks severe damage to the knee and involves rupture of the medial collateral ligament, rupture of the meniscotibial and/or meniscofemoral parts of the meddle third of the medial capsular ligament thereby causing the medial meniscus to "float," as well as tear of the ACL.[30]

Another common mechanism associated with skiing is *hyperextension and internal rotation* during a forward fall (Fig. 43-7). This deceleration-type injury may occur if the skier crosses the ski tips or catches the outer edge of one ski in the snow, resulting in sudden hyperextension and internal rotation of that knee. The internal rotation mechanism may also occur during the "phantom fall" seen in beginning skiers in which their skis curve inward and their weight falls backward. As their ski continues to internally rotate, the ACL is progressively tensed to the point of rupture. A third mechanism occurs in more advanced skiers during landing from a jump or mogul. As the backs of the skis hit the snow, the skier falls backward resulting in hyperflexion of the knee. The skier attempts to recover his or her

balance and, in the process, focuses anterior force from the posterior shell of the boot top on the calf together with anterior pull of the quadriceps muscle amounts to anterior translation of the tibia on the femur. This momentary anterior translation causes anterior subluxation and possible rupture of the ACL (Fig. 43-8).[106]

17. What is the most common combined ligament sprain at the knee joint?

Combined ligament disruptions may result from a single plane injury taken to an extreme. A severe contact mechanism for ACL rupture is laterally derived but medially directed *valgus stress* to the knee, derived from a posterolateral impact to the anchored foot (Fig. 43-9). This clipping-type injury, although against sport regulation, may occur in American football causing the player to sustain injury to a triad of knee structures including the medial collateral ligament, the anterior cruciate ligament, and the medial meniscus. Known as the *unhappy triad of O'Donoghue,* this type of combined ligament rupture wreaks severe damage to the knee and involves rupture of the medial collateral ligament and

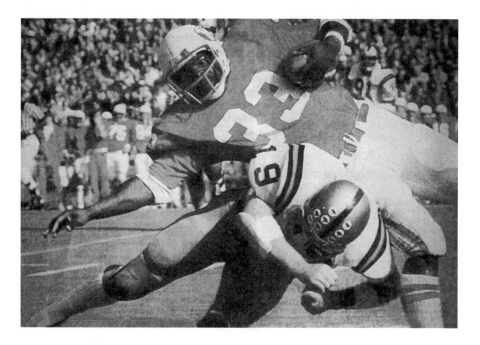

FIG. 43-9 *Clipping-type injury* represents an infraction of the rules of football because of its devastating consequences. The mechanism of injury includes a severe valgus force to the knee with the foot of the involved leg fixed to the ground with the knee semiflexed. The force of impact internally rotates the femur, while the tibia is forced into abduction and internal rotation. The severe combined ligamentous injury may result in the *unhappy triad of O'Donoghue.* (From Nicholas JA, Hershman EB: *The lower extremity and spine in sports medicine,* ed 2, St Louis, 1995, Mosby.)

meniscotibial and/or meniscofemoral parts of the middle third medial capsular ligament causing the medial meniscus to "float," and the ACL to tear.[15] The valgus force initially tears the medial collateral ligament and, if of sufficient magnitude, continues to tear the medial meniscus and then the ACL. A second pattern of single plane injury occurs at the extreme of hyperextension after the anterior cruciate and posterior capsule sustain sprain, in which the PCL ruptures, the neurovascular structures are torn and the tibiofemoral joint has dislocated. The difference between two and three ligament injuries may be that the knee has dislocated. If dislocation has occurred, there is a 50% probability of an associated neurovascular injury.

18. What is the presentation of multiple knee ligament disruption?

Disruption of several knee ligaments represents a severe knee injury and is highly suggestive of tibiofemoral dislocation, which may have spontaneously reduced. A severe knee injury often appears less swollen and less painful on stress testing than a knee with a less severe ligament injury. This is ascribed to the extreme magnitude of joint displacement associated with multiple joint disruption that concomitantly ruptures synovium and capsule, allowing blood inside the joint to dissipate into surrounding soft tissue. In addition to an absence of tense hemarthrosis, an empty end-feel is imparted to the examiner's hand upon provocative stress testing. A marked valgus deformity may be readily apparent during stress testing.[116]

19. What is the worst consequence of combined ligament tear at the knee?

Traumatic dislocation of the knee joint is an uncommon injury that represents a dire emergency that, if not quickly addressed, may result in loss of limb distal to the dislocation. This type of injury involves severe forces, which may occur from an automobile accident, in which all four principal knee ligaments are ruptured, resulting in trauma to the popliteal nerves and vessels. The popliteal artery runs behind the knee and is normally so flexible as to tolerate repeated collapse during normal flexion of the knee joint. The most serious immediate complication is tearing or kinking of the popliteal artery which, in the latter, may lead to clot formation along the injured inner arterial surface. The incidence of popliteal artery injury has been reported greater than 50%.[52] Because of this, a dislocated knee should be assumed to have sustained popliteal artery

compromise until proven otherwise. It is the therapist's obligation to evaluate the condition of such a patient to the status of a medical emergency and seek out immediate physician care. The evaluation of pulses and neurologic function is mandatory and can be limb saving. Popliteal artery involvement is ruled out by injecting dye into the artery and taking radiographs (femoral arteriogram.) Medical management of this condition involves joint reduction and secondary determination of pulse and neurological status. Immediate arteriogram is indicated if pulses are absent or even diminished. If an arteriogram is unavailable for greater than a 6 hour period, immediate exploration is considered. If neurovascular status is adequate, the knee is place in a brace set at 30° of flexion, the extremity is elevated, and monitoring of neurovascular status is continued for 3 to 7 days to rule out the presence of swelling or neurovascular occlusion. Range of motion between 15° to 30° is permitted as well as quad sets and electric stimulation to maintain muscle tone across the joint and encourage fluid mobilization.[30] If this potentially devastating condition is overlooked, the leg may require amputation due to gangrene setting in distal to the knee joint.[23]

20. What are the clinical features of cruciate ligament rupture?

Patients with ACL instability typically present a characteristic history, beginning with a violent injury during which the patient feels something break in the knee and is often accompanied by an audible pop. The mechanism usually accompanies *high speed twisting motions* of the lower extremity with the knee postured closer to the full extension range than the flexion range of motion in which the player swerves, twisting the knee while the foot is firmly planted on the ground. The pain is often excruciating, causing immediate knee collapse, and is often so acute as to be remembered vividly many years after the injury. The player may not be able to continue playing, and the knee may feel unstable during weight bearing. Indeed, after the acute phase has subsided, the knee may collapse whenever the patient puts weight through it or twists it, or walks over uneven ground or a cobblestone road. Although some patients may report being able to resume running fast in straight lines beyond the subacute phase, he or she must slow down to turn corners. Ambulating or running downhill is difficult and produces the highest magnitude of strain along the already injured ligament. Pain and tenderness are most often reported at the posterolateral aspect of the proximal tibia.

Swelling occurs immediately and is most pronounced within 12 hours following injury. A knee joint effusion consisting principally of blood (hemarthrosis) following arthrocentesis and is most frequently associated with rupture of the ACL.[88] The *patellar tap test* (Fig. 43-10) indicates the presence of a large effusion, and pushes fluid up into the suprapatellar pouch so that the patella may be bounced against the femur. This is to be differentiated from a small effusion (5 to 10 ml), which only fills the hollows of either side of the patella. A small effusion is detected by stroking fluid into and out of a parapatellar gutter; this is accomplished by moving fluid manually into the opposite gutter of the knee and then pushing it back to the other side.

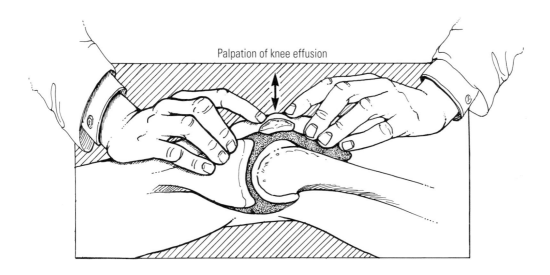

Palpation of knee effusion

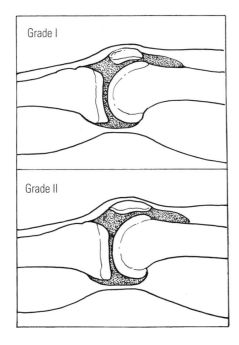

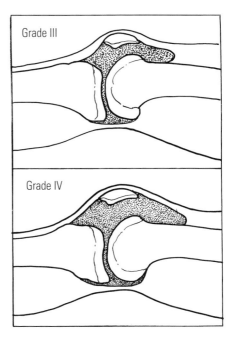

FIG. 43-10 Effusions of the knee are graded from one to four. (From Scuderi GR, McCann PD, Bruno PJ: *Sports medicine: principles of primary care,* St Louis, 1997, Mosby.)

Unfortunately, patients with cruciate ligament rupture are often told they merely have a "sprained knee" after radiographs appear negative in the emergency room.[65] Moreover, diagnosis may be difficult following acute ACL disruption and may go undetected as stress testing is next to impossible owing to pain and muscle spasm. Because of this, it is essential to examine the patient immediately after injury before assessment is precluded or masked by pain and protective muscle spasm. If delay is unavoidable, then specialized diagnostic aids such as arthrography, arthroscopy, or examination of the knee with the patient under anesthesia are appropriate. *Unless detected within the first few days following acute injury, the opportunity for primary repair of acute anterior cruciate ligament ruptures may be lost.*[17,31] It is therefore imperative to maintain a high index of suspicion for ACL injury if the history and clinical examination is suggestive of sprain. Diagnostic accuracy as high as 85% may be achieved by history and clinical presentation with four essential ingredients—a pop at the time of injury, inability to continue participation, gross swelling of the knee, and maximal swelling within 12 hours after injury.[32] Typically, adjuncts such as MRI, arthroscopy, and examination under anesthesia are not carried out unless the diagnosis is not clear from the patient history and clinical examination.[15]

The clinical presentation of sprain of the PCL may include swelling and tenderness in the popliteal fossa. The hemarthrosis may be smaller than expected as blood tends to dissect into the popliteal space rather than inside the knee, and the ecchymosis may appear several days after injury.[15] Regardless of mechanism of injury, the athlete who sustains a sprain of the PCL is usually able to continue competition and may only experience minimal swelling. The effusion does not become tense within the first 24 hours, and the patient does not experience the pseudolocking associated with ACL injury.[65]

21. How are cruciate ligament injuries differentiated from meniscal injuries?

The history of ACL injury is different from that of a meniscus lesion. Although cruciate ligament injuries are typically caused by high speed twisting injuries when the tibiofemoral joint is near extension, meniscus lesions are often sustained by low speed low limb motions with the knee bent into flexion.[118] Also, whereas ligamentous injuries often follow a memorable injury, meniscal injuries are seldom memorable to the patient. Moreover, finally, meniscal injuries often lock the knee and block (i.e., true locking) extension, whereas liga-

mentous injuries result in pseudolocking of the knee, and frank collapse of the knee joint.[23]

22. What type of fracture may result from distal detachment of the ACL?

Tibial spine fracture is usually caused by hyperextension of the knee or a sudden twisting motion, and indicated partial or complete detachment of the ACL from the tibia. Arthrocentesis of the knee joint may consist of a hemarthrosis with a few fat droplets.[88] Nondisplaced fractures and those that reduce anatomically when the knee is in full extension may be managed by casting the knee in extension and waiting for rehabilitation to commence after union has occurred some 5 to 6 weeks following injury. In contrast, complete and displaced fractures as well as those fracture types which are complete, displaced, and rotated out of position may represent a loose fragment that may block motion and cause severe swelling and hemarthrosis. Any mechanical block to full extension is an indication for surgery.

23. What imaging is appropriate for the patient with a cruciate ligament injury?

Following isolated injury of the ACL, radiographs may be normal or may present with effusion (hemarthrosis). Avulsion fracture of the lateral tibial cordyle, known as the *lateral capsular sign,*[2,115] or *Segond's fracture,* has a high association with ACL injury, and typically occurs by forced internal tibial rotator with the knee flexed.[115] This mechanism places enormous force on the middle portion of the lateral capsule.[25] The presence of this sign indicates a possible anterolateral rotation injury with a resultant avulsion fracture of the distal attachment of the lateral capsular ligament.[115] This small avulsion fracture from the lateral margin of the superior tibial condyle can be seen on an anteroposterior or tunnel view adjacent to the lateral tibial plateau. Presence of this elliptical fragment implies avulsion of the meniscotibial portion of the mid-third lateral capsule (lateral meniscotibial ligament) from the tibia. When this finding is discovered, a high index of suspicion (75% to 100%)[25] is held for possible ACL injury. Larger avulsion fractures of the tibial attachment of the ACL are often visible on routine anteroposterior views. The possibility of concomitant injury of the medial collateral ligament, which may be confirmed by stress films.[79] Similarly, a small avulsion fracture may also be found on lateral radiograph as a bony fragment superior and anterior to the tibial spines, or of the tibial spine. Avulsion from the proximal attachment is less common, and the avulsed fragment is best seen on the tunnel view su-

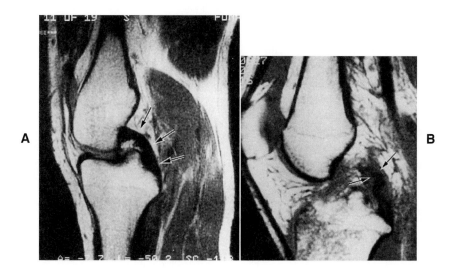

FIG. 43-11 Posterior cruciate ligament. Sagittal T1-weighted scans. **A,** Normal PCL *(arrows).* **B,** Ruptured PCL *(arrows).* (From Nicholas JA, Hershman EB: *The lower extremity and spine in sports medicine,* ed 2, St Louis, 1995, Mosby.)

periorly within the intercondylar notch. Radiographs also rule out tibial plateau fractures and loose bodies. Magnetic resonance imaging (MRI) is extremely accurate in detecting ACL injury[60] and has been found to be 96% specific for disruption to that ligament.[81] The use of MRI is helpful in determining whether the ligament is formed from its femoral or tibial attachments, or whether a midsubstance tear has occurred, or if there is only an intrasubstance change (grade I sprain) of the midsubstance representing a stretching of the ligament. Chronic ACL tears may differentiated from acute tears by a lack of adjacent edema or hemorrhage.[112] Moreover, with chronic ACL tears the ligament appears lax and frequently fused to the PCL. Following injury to the PCL, standard lateral radiographs of the acutely injured knee may demonstrate posterior tibial subluxation on the femur if taken with the knee in 90° of flexion. As with injury to the ACL, sprain of the PCL usually involves an interstitial tear. Hence standard radiographs rarely display an avulsion of one or the other of its bony attachments.[65] Injuries to the PCL are easily demonstrated using sagittal MRI[82] as the PCL is significantly thicker than the ACL (Fig. 43-11).

24. What is the classification of cruciate ligament tears?

One classification of cruciate ligament tear is based upon the site of ligament disruption. *Midsubstance* (interstitial) tears of the ACL account for 75% of injuries;

20% are from the femoral attachment; and the remaining 5% are from the tibial side. Occasionally, the femoral or tibial disruptions may be accompanied with an avulsed periosteal sleeve or bone flake. Seventy percent of PCL tears occur on the tibial side and are similarly associated with a fleck of bone or larger fragment; 15% of tears occur on the femoral side, whereas another 15% of PCL tears occur in the midsubstance.* Disruption of the synovial sleeve covering the ligament may lead to loss of vascularity from the middle geniculate and ligament compromise of one or more bundles comprising the cruciates.[110]

Anterior cruciate ligament compromise may alternately be classified according to the magnitude of fiber disruption, and clinically correlates with the magnitude of translational draw upon anterior and posterior stress

---

*Midsubstance tears of the ACL rarely occur in children or adolescents. This population more readily sustains avulsion of the tibial attachment with a bone fragment, or a physeal injury. The tibial attachment is elevated and displaced, and open reduction and internal fixation of the tibial spine is recommended. (Meyers MH, McKeever FM: Fracture of the intercondylar eminence of the tibia, *J Bone Joint Surg* 52A:1677, 1970.) *Congenital absence* of the ACL may occur but is unusual. It should be suspected in the skeletally immature individual where the adolescent complains of sensation of instability and even pivot shift, but no pain, swelling, and often no history of classical injury of mechanisms. It may either present as an isolated finding or as part of a combination of lower limb anomalies. (Strizak AM: Knee injuries. In Nicholas JA, Hershman EB editors: *The lower extremity and spine,* ed 2, vol 2, St Louis, 1995, Mosby.)

testing. With *first degree sprains (minor tear)* there is little forward glide, and return to near premorbid level of function within a few days provides symptomatic relief via rest, ice, elevation, and compression. Grade I sprain is characterized by microscopic tearing or stretching of the ligament, with no loss of function. With second-degree sprains *(partial tear)* of the ACL there is forward glide of limited magnitude that has an abrupt stop. Here, the strength of the ligament is considerably impaired and, although the ligament still acts to limit anterior draw of the tibia, premature return to full activity, especially athletics, may lead to complete rupture. Grade II sprain involves partial macroscopic disruption of the ligament and partial loss of function that may lead to gross disruption in which the stretched, nonfunctional ligament is still grossly intact. These patients require protection either in a long leg cast, cast brace, or, preferably, a restriction motion brace with the knee flexed between 30° to 40° for 4 to 6 weeks. This degree of knee flexion is ideal for immobilization as it places the least amount of tension upon the ACL, whereas facilitating foreshortening of the ligament during functional weight bearing activities. Little, if any, residual laxity may be expected upon completion of the rehabilitation program. With *third degree sprains* (complete tear) forward glide ends secondary to muscle tension (no *endpoint*) suggesting a full thickness ACL rupture. A grade III sprain is characterized by complete tearing of the ligament and complete loss of function. Alternately, the third degree ACL sprain may correspond to a ligament that is still in continuity, but becomes so stretched as to retain no restraining function.[15]

25. What are the benefits and disadvantages of arthrometric testing of cruciate integrity?

Mechanical testing with arthrometric devices have been useful but not diagnostic.[24,110] Knee arthrometers are most commonly used to measure anterior tibial displacement relative to the femur following ACL injury. They may also be used to measure posterior tibial displacement on the femur. Arthrometric measurement seeks to quantify the magnitude of integrity of cruciate ligament sprain. Instrumented testing quantitates the anterior translation of the tibia on the femur relative to the uninjured knee. The test position for arthrometric testing is identical to that of the Lachman test. A key variable in the use of instrumented arthrometry is obtaining muscle relaxation. The arthrometer is positioned on the knee, and anterior and posterior displace-

ment loads are applied. A side-to-side difference in anterior translation of greater than 2 mm at 89 N (20 lb) is considered positive for ACL injury with 94% accuracy.[24] Although the Lachman test assigns an ordinal value to the magnitude of knee laxity, instrumented testing provides an absolute numeric value. The Lachman test is, nevertheless, considered to provide superior diagnostic accuracy than arthrometric testing as it imparts the presence or absence of an endpoint to the examiner's hands.[29] Some authorities ascribe a false-negative test result in as much as 20% of instrumented testing.[74] Accurate quantitation noting the difference between the suspected involved and uninvolved knees is essential. Thus arthrometric testing is of limited use when bilateral ACL compromise is suspect. Another drawback of arthrometric testing is that measurements are operator dependent and require significant technical expertise.[7]

26. What provocative tests determine integrity of the ACL?

Despite the availability of mechanical testing, physical examination of the knee is still the best diagnostic approach for cruciate ligament injury.[110] In evaluating the knee joint, the therapist conducts a laxity examination of the normal and injured knees to determine the presence of an anatomic lesion. Anterior instability is the most controversial of the instabilities because there are several types of anterior draw and a lack of unanimous agreement on the interpretation of pathology that produces each type. A multitude of examinations exists for determination of ACL integrity. The anterior draw and Lachman tests are two of the most common. Both involve the application of anterior stress to the tibia at 90° and 25° of flexion, respectively. The *anterior draw test* is thought to be more sensitive for testing integrity of the anteromedial bundle, whereas the *Lachman test* is considered more specific for testing for the integrity of the posterolateral bundle of the ACL. Others differentiate between these two tests by claiming the anterior draw useful for detecting complete ruptures of the ACL, but not as sensitive as the Lachman test for detecting partial ACL injuries.[88] The examiner must bear in mind that often, the first observation will be the only valid one because pain caused by the procedure may yield voluntary or involuntary spasm.[88] Thus provocative stress tests should be performed deliberately and carefully. The magnitude of injury is numerically graded as 0, 1+, 2+, or 3+. A grade of 1+ indicates that the degree of anterior draw in the injured knee is less than 0.5 cm greater than in the uninjured knee, 2+ indicates a difference of 0.5 to 1.0 cm, and 3+ represents more than a 1.0-cm difference between the injured and noninjured knee.

ANTERIOR DRAWER

During the *anterior draw test* (Fig. 43-12), the examiner's thumbs are placed on the tibial crest overlying the knee joint line while the index fingers are placed posteriorly to gauge the presence of excessive hamstring tension. With his/her index fingers, the examiner palpates the hamstrings to be certain these muscles are relaxed. The patient's foot is stabilized during the test in neutral rotation and may be held in place by the seated therapist's thigh; alternately, the examiner partially sits on the dorsum of the patient's foot. The therapist then grasps the patient's calf near the popliteal fossa with both hands and strongly but gently pulls forward on the tibia in symmetrical fashion. Forward displacement of 2 to 3 mm is considered normal, whereas a 6 to 8 mm anterior tibial draw greater than the contralateral knee indicates a torn ACL. The drawback of the anterior draw test is that this provocative stress test often yields a false-negative result because of either hamstring muscle spasm, the presence of hemarthrosis, or because of the ball-valve action of the medial meniscus.[29,108]

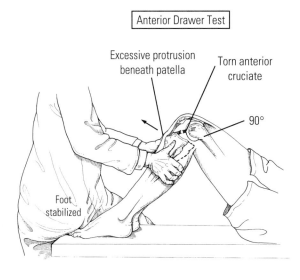

Anterior Drawer Test

Excessive protrusion
beneath patella

Torn anterior
cruciate

90°

Foot
stabilized

FIG. 43-12 The *anterior drawer test* is performed with the knee flexed to 90° and with the anterior force applied to the proximal tibia. (From Scuderi GR, McCann PD, Bruno PJ: *Sports medicine: principles of primary care*, St Louis, 1997, Mosby.)

The latter effect result from the posterior horn of the medial meniscus having a "door stopper" effect that minimizes tibial translation on the femur during anterior draw.

LACHMAN TEST

The *Lachman test* is universally recognized as the best method for assessing ACL integrity because it minimizes the stabilizing effects to the knee joint from the bony contour of the femoral condyles and the posterior horns of the menisci. Sensitivity for possible tear has been reported between 87% to 98%.[29] In addition, the position of slight flexion (in contrast to the anterior drawer test) is more comfortable for the patient with acute injury and hemarthrosis. This position, in turn, is less likely to elicit hamstrings spasm and places the hamstrings at mechanical disadvantage should they spasm and attempt to skew test results. An additional advantage of performing anterior draw at 25° flexion derives from isolating the ACL as a primary resistance to anterior tibial translation. Also, when testing for ACL integrity at 25° flexion, tibial subluxation occurs anteriorly with reference to the femur. If the joint is loaded during the testing, this subluxation/reduction phenomenon becomes more noticeable.[51] The Lachman test is positive when the tibia can be subluxated forward without the presence of an end-feel.* The resultant tibial displacement is primarily a translocation rather than a rotation phenomenon such that both the medial and lateral tibial surfaces slide forward on the femoral condyles and back again.[93]

One of the therapist's hands grasps the distal femur while the other hand grasps the proximal tibia. The tibia is alternately pulled forward on the femur (Fig. 43-13). An intact ACL prevents the tibia from sliding forward. If the ligament is injured, the tibia may be moved beyond its normal excursion and even subluxated anteriorly during this stress test. Imperative to proper performance of this provocative test is adequate determination of the quality of the end point of this stress test. Whereas a solid mechanical stop at the most anterior extent of tibial motion indicates only a partial ACL tear, a soft and spongy end point or end-feel signifies a full thickness ACL rupture. However, before a positive Lachman test is pronounced valid, the integrity of the posterior cruciate ligament must first be ascertained. A

---

*Or, *with* the presence of a "mushy" end-feel. In the uninjured knee, the examiner experiences a solid end-feel.

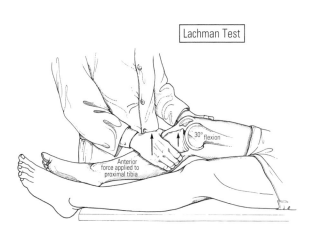

FIG. 43-13 The *Lachman test* is performed in 30° of flexion with anterior force exerted on the proximal tibia. (From Scuderi GR, Mc-Cann PD, Bruno PJ: *Sports medicine: principles of primary care*, St Louis, 1997, Mosby.)

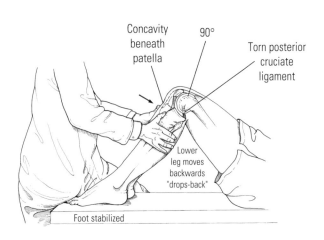

FIG. 43-14 The *posterior drawer test* is performed in 90° of flexion with posterior force on the proximal tibia. (From Scuderi GR, Mc-Cann PD, Bruno PJ: *Sports medicine: principles of primary care*, St Louis, 1997, Mosby.)

false positive sign for ACL rupture may be incorrectly interpreted by the novice evaluator when a PCL rupture is really the injury responsible for instability. In the event of a PCL rupture, the proximal tibia sags posteriorly, and the Lachman test will appear falsely positive as the posterior subluxation is reduced.[88,108] A *false negative sign* may result from a displaced bucket handle tear of the meniscus, blocking anterior translation.[108] Thus it is mandatory that posterior instability be excluded by the appropriate test before making a diagnosis of anterior instability.

27. What are the three provocative tests for determination of PCL sprain?

POSTERIOR DRAW

The procedure for determining PCL integrity is identical to the anterior draw test, except that the *tibia is pushed backward* (posteriorly) instead of forward with both hands so as to displace the proximal tibial relative to the distal femur (Fig. 43-14). At the same time, the therapist may alternately push and pull the tibia so as to determine if the ACL is intact or was injured as well. However, the therapist must be aware that it is possible to confuse straight posterior insta-

bility with anterior instability. This is particularly so if the posterior draw test is done from an anterior subluxated position to neutral. Hence, a tear of the PCL is occasionally misdiagnosed as an ACL tear because the tibia is already in the posteriorly displaced position and the examiner is merely pulling the tibia forward to the neutral position.[73] Because of this possibility, it is essential to accurately recognize the neutral starting point of the drawer test by relying upon a lateral radiograph.[15] Clinical confirmation of suspected PCL injury may be ascertained by asking the patient with a posteriorly sagging tibia to extend his or her knee. The resulting quadriceps extensor contraction obliterates the posterior sag by anteriorly displacing the tibia into a neutral position until the ACL tautens and prevents further anterior displacement (Fig. 43-15). The posterior drawer sign may also be obscured if there is an associated ACL tear as it becomes even more difficult to determine a neutral reference point in the sagittal plane.[15]

POSTERIOR LACHMAN TEST

This test (Fig. 43-16) is performed in 30° of knee flexion and the tibia is forced back posteriorly.[110]

POSTERIOR SAG SIGN

Posterior *sag* or *dropback* involves visual inspection or palpation of the anterior aspect of both knees at 90° of knee and hip flexion. With the patient supine and relaxed and the heel of the involved knee resting upon the examining table, a pad is placed under the distal thigh of the involved extremity. Alternately, the patient is supine, with hips and knees flexed at 90° and ankles supported by the examiner. The weight of the tibia of the involved leg causes posterior displacement (Fig. 43-17). The test may be enhanced by having the patient actively flex the knees against resistance, using the hamstrings as additional posterior displacement force and displacing the tibia even further posteriorly.[73] The therapist views the knee from the side to discover a drop-back of the involved tibia if the PCL is torn, representing proximal tibial subluxation. Unlike ACL injury, a posterior sag sign is not masked by muscle spasm. However, reliable posterior sag may be obscured if the patient has a previous history of Osgood-Schlatter's disease. This is suspected by visual asymmetry in the prominence of the tibial tubercles.

28. What are the various straight and rotary instabilities about the knee?

Any combination of knee instability may occur, including complete dislocation of the knee with 360° circumduction.[88] Terminology describing knee instability underwent major changes in the 1970s and still has not become entirely resolved.[89] With their classic article in 1968 Slocum and Larson[105] introduced the concept of rotary instability. In 1973 Nicholas introduced terms describing the direction of abnormal motion of the tibia in relation to the femur such as "anteromedial, anterolateral," and " posterolateral," as well as the characteristics of simple, complex, and combined instabilities.[90] In 1976 Hughston also described rotary and straight instabilities.[56,57] Losee et al[71] and Jakob et al[62] introduced the concept of the reverse pivot shift as a sign of posterolateral rotatory instability. The complexity of nomenclature describing cruciate instability is unique and derives from the unique orientation of span of these ligaments across all three planes within the knee joint. Although benefit and value may be derived from the use of a complex classification of knee instability, we can certainly appreciate Apley's "plea for plain words"[8] in describing lesions of the cruciate ligaments.

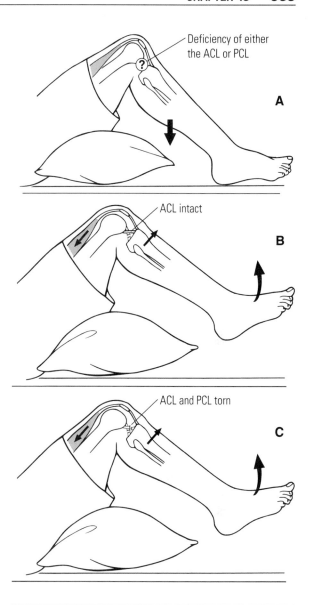

FIG. 43-15 A, Observed *posterior sag sign.* Clinical confusion regarding whether an observed sag represents deficiency of the anterior or posterior cruciate ligament may be resolved by **B,** asking the patient to raise the foot off the examining table. The resulting quadriceps contraction obliterates the lag in the posterior cruciate ligament-deficient knee as the pull of the quadriceps displaces the tibia anteriorly into the neutral position until the anterior cruciate ligament is tight. **C,** If the tibia further displaces anteriorly, then both cruciates have sustained injury.

Posterior Lachman Test

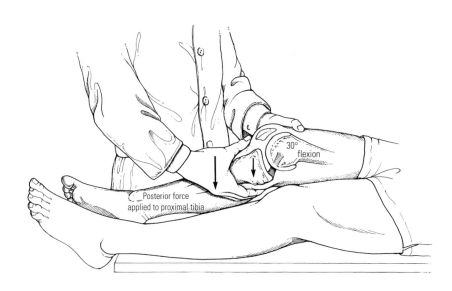

FIG. 43-16 The *posterior Lachman test* applies posterior force to the proximal tibia with the knee flexed 30°. (From Scuderi GR, McCann PD, Bruno PJ: *Sports medicine: principles of primary care,* St Louis, 1997, Mosby.)

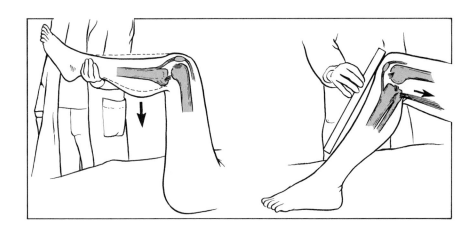

FIG. 43-17 Posterior cruciate rupture. The tibia sags backward when the foot is lifted. A ruler run from the patella to the front of the shin shows the tibia sagging backward. (From Dandy DJ: *Essential orthopaedics and trauma,* ed 2, Edinburgh, 1993, Churchill Livingstone.)

29. What are combined straight and rotatory instabilities at the knee joint, and how are they most readily assessed?

The knee joint should not simply be thought of as a hinge joint. To do so is misleadingly oversimplistic and erroneous. Various rotations in the transverse plane occur at the knee joint, and soft tissue surrounding and moving the knee joint is designed to facilitate and maintain this rotatory capability. The cruciate ligaments, by virtue of their unique span across the knee joint cross all three planes and play a principal role in the rotary function of the tibiofemoral joint. Because of this, virtually any possible pathologic combination of instability may occur following injury to the knee joint.

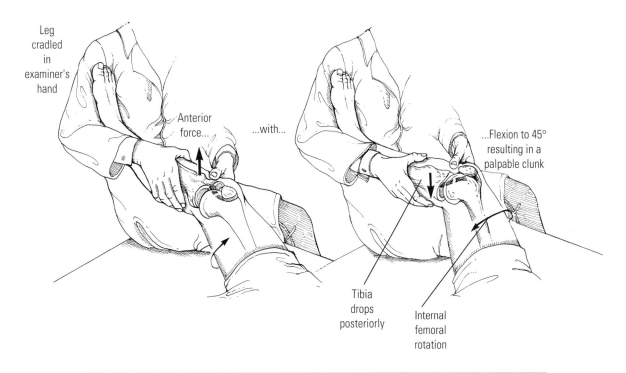

Flexion-Rotation Drawer Test

Leg cradled in examiner's hand

Anterior force...

...with...

...Flexion to 45° resulting in a palpable clunk

Tibia drops posteriorly

Internal femoral rotation

FIG. 43-18 The *flexion-rotation drawer test* cradles the tibia in the examiner's hands and flexes the knee to demonstrate tibial reduction and internal femoral rotation. (From Scuderi GR, McCann PD, Bruno PJ: *Sports medicine: principles of primary care,* St Louis, 1997, Mosby.)

When performing the *simple anterior draw test* in neutral rotation, it is essential to focus on the movement of both the medial and lateral tibial condyles to gauge whether or not an asymmetric rotatory component accompanies the anterior tibial excursion. Provided the patient is cooperative, the *rotational elements* of the anterior drawer should then be assessed by alternately applying pure rotational force to the fibular head and the lateral tibial condyle (internal rotation), followed by an external rotatory torque to the medial tibial condyle. This assessment is known as the *flexion-rotation drawer test* (Fig. 43-18). The importance of constant comparison with the normal knee cannot be overemphasized. Thus once the neutral anterior drawer test has been performed, the test should be repeated at intervals of approximately 10° of external tibial rotation as well as internal tibial rotation to assess the *posteromedial capsule* and rule out *anteromedial rotatory instability,* as well as assess the *posterolateral capsule* to rule out *anterolateral rotatory instability,* respectively.

30. How does the osseous design of the lateral tibiofemoral joint facilitate mechanical instability following rupture of the ACL?

An osseous asymmetry exits between the medial and lateral tibial plateau that results in less than adequate stable articulation between the articulating surfaces comprising the knee joint. The odd design of the tibial plateau is such that although the medial tibial plateau is concave, the lateral plateau is flat or convex (Fig. 43-19). Moreover, the lateral femoral condyle is rounder and shorter in the anteroposterior direction compared with the larger, longer medial femoral condyle. Thus although the bulbous medial femoral condyle is received by a shallow dish that is the medial tibial plateau, the convex lateral condyles articulate

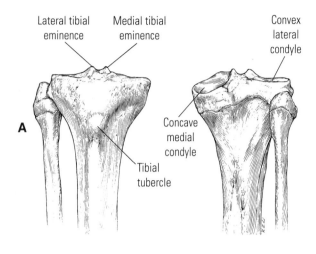

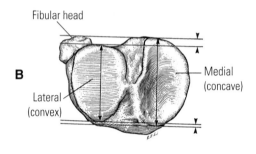

FIG. 43-19 A, Anterior and posterior view of the right proximal tibia. **B,** Superior view of the right tibial plateau. (From Tria AJ, Klein KS: *An illustrated guide to the knee,* New York, 1992, Churchill Livingstone.)

with a convex lateral plateau. The articulation of two convex surfaces is the anathema of an articulation resulting in one or both articulating surfaces sliding off each other when the compartment is loaded unless the anterior cruciate is intact.[23],* If the lateral capsular restraints are stretched in additional to an ACL sprain, the observed lateral tibial subluxation may be even more apparent.[15]

31. What is the "pivot shift" phenomenon?

Mild anterior tibial subluxation may be a physiologic event, such as in loose jointed persons endowed with ligamentous laxity. However, following an ACL injury,

---

*In addition, the presence of the lateral meniscus also provides more stability by converting the convex lateral tibial plateau into a concave shelf that better seats the lateral femoral condyle.

patients often complain that their knee shifts or "gives out" when they turn right or left with their stance foot planted (as may occur when decelerating or attempting to cut). This shifting reflects the lateral tibial condyle subluxating anteriorly and rotating medially[88] out from under the lateral femoral condyle, and occurs an involuntary reaction of the patient's own muscles. Despite the essential *medial rotatory component* of this event that incites instability due to *medial tibial rotation,* this type of instability is known as *anterolateral rotatory instability* and is named for momentary subluxation and reduction of the *lateral knee compartment.* Thus the pivot shift test is a confirmatory test of the ACL deficient knee.[33,37,38,70,72] Anterolateral rotatory instability is particularly suspect in the individual with an acute third degree ACL sprain, as studies have shown that ACL deficiency and anterolateral rotatory instability are associated with the development of degenerative arthritis.[61,105]

The lateral pivot shift test reproduces this functionally unstable event associated with sudden directional changes by replicating the shift the patient feels when performing pivoting motions. The Lachman test and the pivot shift test both result in the same phenomenon of anterior tibial subluxation on the femur, except that the pivot shift test also results in a dramatic reduction following forward tibial displacement.[15] This is because the pivot shift test involves loading of the knee by way of axial compression, valgus stress (which loads the lateral compartment) and internal rotation. Moreover, in addition to straight translation, the lateral pivot shift test is also characterized by a *rotatory component* such that it yields an anterior internal rotational subluxation of the lateral tibial condyle on the femur, thereby testing for *anterolateral rotary instability* of the knee joint.[15] The anterolateral rotation of the tibia is a secondary component of subluxation indicating injury to the ACL as well as the lateral capsular structures and demonstrated as anterolateral motion of the tibia beneath the femur. The portion of the lateral capsule identified as torn is the middle third of the lateral capsular ligament.

32. How is the pivot shift test performed?

The pivot shift test for anterolateral knee instability reflects ACL rupture and sprain of the lateral capsule, and is performed with the patient supine and the knee fully extended. The key elements of a positive lateral pivot shift test are *internal rotation* of the lower leg on the femur, lateral compartment compression by way of a

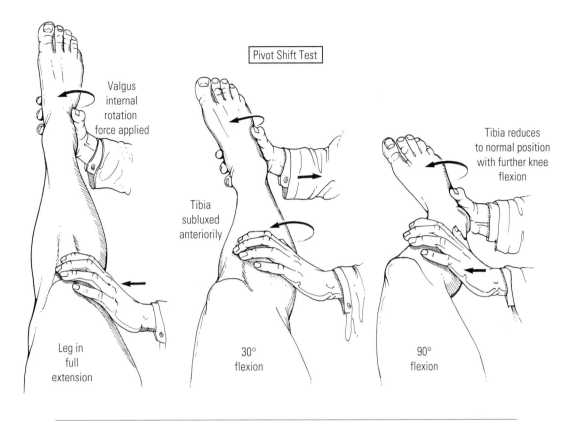

Pivot Shift Test

Valgus internal rotation force applied

Tibia subluxed anteriorly

Tibia reduces to normal position with further knee flexion

Leg in full extension

30° flexion

90° flexion

FIG. 43-20 The *pivot shift test* begins with the knee in full extension and simultaneously imparts an internal tibial rotation and valgus stress to the knee to demonstrate anterolateral subluxation in a positive test. In this position the tibia is subluxed anteriorly. As the knee is flexed, the tibia subluxes posteriorly to its normal position, and a "clunk" is seen and felt by the examiner. (From Scuderi GR, McCann PD, Bruno PJ: *Sports medicine: principles of primary care,* St Louis, 1997, Mosby.)

manually applied valgus force, and excursion of the knee from an extended to a flexed position (Fig. 43-20).[88] The test is performed with the patient supine and the knee in full extension. The examiner applies a medially rotated torque to the tibia and fibula so as to internally rotate the lower leg on the femur. At the same time, the examiner imparts an anterior translation of the tibia. The superimposition of these two motions upon the lower leg cause the lateral tibial plateau to sublux anteriorly out from under the lateral femoral condyle, and indicate positive anterolateral instability. With the knee in this extended posture, the iliotibial band is located anteriorly to the instantaneous center of rotation of the knee joint, thereby converting it into an extensor. This replicates the functional mechanism during cutting movements of the injured stance limb that causes anterior pull on the tibia through the extending quadriceps mechanism direction. Thus subluxation occurs

indirectly through the iliotibial band being converted from a flexor to an extensor in relation to the knee joint axis as it passes anterior to the lateral femoral condyle (Fig. 43-21).*

The knee is then allowed to slowly flex to 20°, and the subluxation becomes more apparent. At some point between 20° to 40° of flexion the iliotibial band is now located posterior to the instant center of knee rotation, and thereby converting into a knee flexor. This effect is heightened by compressing the lateral compartment by way of a valgus force that causes

---

*Demonstration of anterolateral instability is not as evident at 90° of knee flexion because of the powerful stabilizing effect of the iliotibial band when the knee is flexed and the tibia is internally rotated. (Lynch MA, Henning CE: Physical examination of the knee. In Nicholas JA, Hershman EB editors: *The lower extremity and spine,* ed 2, vol 1, St Louis, 1995, Mosby.) Because of this the pivot shift test begins with the knee in full extension.

maximum tension upon the iliotibial tract. At this range subluxation can no longer be maintained. If ACL rupture has occurred, and especially if the lateral capsule is torn, the anteriorly displaced tibial plateau will spontaneously reduce with a sudden visible, audible, and palpable thud.

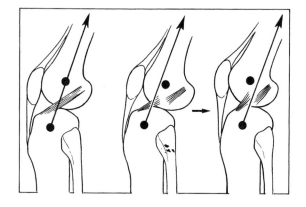

FIG. 43-21 Mechanism of the *pivot shift phenomenon*. If the anterior cruciate ligament is ruptured, the short arched tibial plateau can slip in front of the femoral condyle. As the knee is flexed, the iliotibial tract moves behind the line of rotation and bone bones reduce with a thud. (From Dandy DJ: *Essential orthopaedics and trauma*, ed 2, Edinburgh, 1993, Churchill Livingstone.)

Although almost always positive during the first several minutes to approximately 1 hour following acute injury, the pivot shift test is frequently negative for 6 weeks following ACL tear.[91] This may be a result of muscle spasm and edematous thickening of the capsular ligament from the hemarthrosis. The test becomes more positive in the chronic ACL deficient knee as the secondary stabilizers relax and the menisci either degrade or suffer a tear.[73]

Several other tests including the jerk (Fig. 43-22), Losee (Fig. 43-23), anterolateral rotatory instability test, and flexion-rotation-drawer test all test the same pivot shift phenomenon. The anterolateral rotatory instability test is a modification of the lateral pivot shift test. Controversy surrounds the use of the jerk test as it is similar to the McMurray maneuver for meniscus pathology.[88]

33. What is anteromedial rotatory instability?

Anteromedial rotatory instability, the first rotatory instability to be described, is the best understood and the least controversial. Skiing injuries often result from this kind of instability, which is caused by the most commonly pathologic force in skiing: *external rotation-abduction of the lower leg on the femur.* Severity of injury is dependent on several variables including the magnitude of force, speed of the skier, and position of

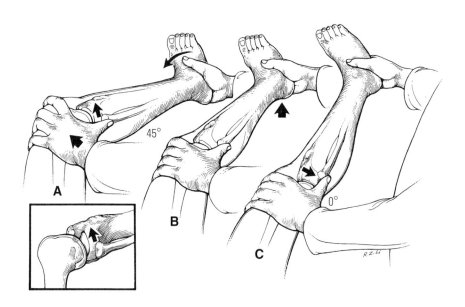

FIG. 43-22 The *jerk test* begins **(A)** with the knee in flexion and applies internal tibial rotation and a valgus stress. The knee is then extended **(B** and **C)**. A positive test demonstrates anterolateral subluxation of the tibia. (From Scott WN: *Ligament and extensor mechanism injuries of the knee: diagnosis and treatment,* St Louis, 1991, Mosby.)

the joint at the time of injury. Following rupture of the capsular ligament, progress external rotation-abduction causes a tear of the superficial portion of the medial collateral ligament. More force will then involve the deep layer of the medial collateral ligament (MCL), thereby tearing the meniscotibial or meniscofemoral portion of the middle third of the MCL. With still more abduction, a tear of the ACL may ensue. Even more force absorbed during injury will result in rupture of the *posteriormedial corner of the knee capsule* if the injury is incurred with the knee in extension. Alternately, if the force is absorbed with the knee in flexion, as is less common, the anterior third of the capsular ligament and quadriceps retinaculum may sustain damage.

34. How is anteromedial instability assessed?

Known as the *Slocum test,* the anterior drawer test for anteromedial rotatory instability involves superimposing external rotation of the lower leg upon an anterior drawer test (Fig. 43-24). The test is always performed on both legs; the normal knee is always tested first, and compared with the injured knee. The hip and knee are flexed to approximately 45° and 80°, respectively. It is helpful to have the patient lean back against the examining wall table so as to relax the hamstrings and qua-

driceps muscle groups. The tibia is externally rotated by externally rotating the foot followed by the examiner sitting on the patient's forefoot to stabilize the rotation during the subsequent examination. External tibial rotation causes the posteromedial capsule to tighten and permit less anterior excursion than the drawer test in neutral rotation. In the event of a torn posteromedial capsule, the Slocum test demonstrates a relative increase in the anterior translation of the tibia as the medial tibial condyle "rolls out" from under the medial femoral condyle. It is best to perform the anteromedial rotatory instability test with application of small load so as to prevent inadvertent locking of a torn medial meniscus that might otherwise occur from the application of high loads. This may present difficulty for the examiner who may then be unable to unlock the knee; because of this, a high load Slocum test is better performed under anesthesia (Henning CE: Unpublished data). Anteromedial rotatory instability indicates possible rupture of the ACL, although the likelihood of ACL sprain is increased in the presence of injury to the MCL and the medial meniscus. In the normal knee, the first 10° to 20° of external tibial rotation during simultaneous anterior draw owes to an unwinding of the cruciate ligaments. Thereafter, the amount of anterior draw

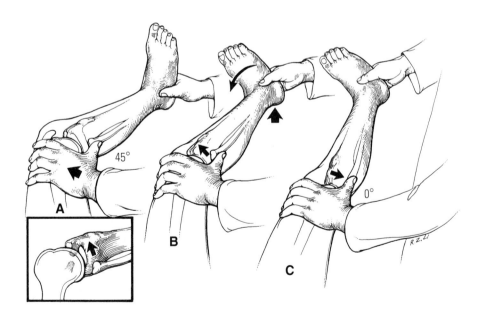

FIG. 43-23 The *Losee test* begins **A,** with the knee in flexion while the foot is externally rotated. **B,** The tibia (via the foot) is then internally rotated as a valgus stress is applied to the knee. **C,** The knee is then extended. (From Scott WN: *Ligament and extensor mechanism injuries of the knee: diagnosis and treatment,* St Louis, 1991, Mosby.)

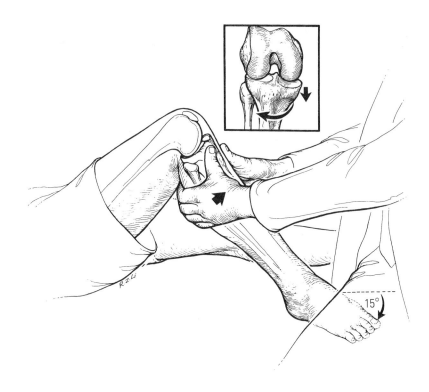

FIG. 43-24 The *Slocum test* is performed in 90° of knee flexion with the foot externally rotated. Anterior proximal tibial force is applied to test the posteromedial capsule. (From Scott WN: *Ligament and extensor mechanism injuries of the knee: diagnosis and treatment,* St Louis, 1991, Mosby.)

becomes progressively more difficult to elicit as the tibial rotation on the femur tightens the posteromedial ligamentous capsular sleeve. However, if the medial structures, including the medial meniscus, MCL, and posteromedial capsule have been compromised, the test will prevent anterior draw beyond 20° of external rotation. Thus in the absence of intact medial restraints, the medial tibial condyle externally rotates out from under the medial femoral condyle excessively, when compared with the uninjured knee. However, it is possible for a positive anteromedial stability test to exist with a completely intact ACL as the ACL unwinds its helical coil along its longitudinal length, as well as from its wound position with the PCL. This is particularly so at 20° of external tibial rotation. At this arc of rotational motion, the results of the test will be more dramatically positive when the ACL is also torn. The test is thus repeated in progressively greater intervals of 10° of external rotation.[88] If anterior draw is unhindered at even greater degrees of external rotation, the examiner may then conclude that the ACL has also been compromised.

35. What tests indicate instability of the posterolateral corner of the knee?

As the knee has four corners, a third instability involves the posterior portion of the lateral capsular ligament known as the *arcuate ligament complex.* If the posterolateral capsular sleeve is torn, the knee will demonstrate *posterolateral rotatory instability.* In addition, the popliteus muscle is torn, although the PCL is intact.[10,27,55,]* Injury to the arcuate ligament complex may occur from a direct blow to the anteromedial tibia[27] and may commonly leave the ACL and PCL intact. However, if the blow was to the medial knee (varus force) with the knee in extension, then the ACL and PCL are commonly injured in addition to the arcuate

*A final instability at the knee is posteromedial rotary instability that results from tearing of the posteromedial capsule complex. This is determined by holding the knee in extension and applying a valgus stress. A positive test correlates with apparent knock knee of the medial side of the knee. This is rare in the absence of a PCL injury. (Lynch MA, Henning CE: Physical examination of the knee. In Nicholas JA, Hershman EB: *The lower extremity and spine,* ed 2, vol 1, St Louis, 1995, Mosby.)

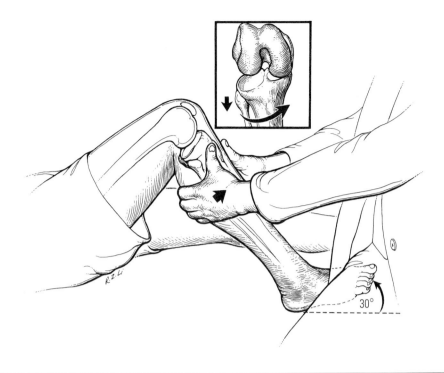

FIG. 43-25 Integrity of the posterolateral capsule is tested with the knee flexed to 90°. Anterior proximal tibial force is applied with the tibial internally rotated. (From Scott WN: *Ligament and extensor mechanism injuries of the knee: diagnosis and treatment,* St Louis, 1991, Mosby.)

ligament complex.[73] The posterolateral capsule may be tested with the knee flexed to 90°, followed by the application of force to the anterior proximal tibia with the tibia internally rotated (Fig. 43-25).

Previously, we learned that the pivot shift test scores positive for tear of the lateral capsular ligaments, causing anterolateral rotatory instability as evidenced by the lateral tibial condyle subluxating anteriorly and rotating medially[88] out from under the lateral femoral condyle.

The pivot shift test begins with the knee in full extension and undergoes flexion and valgus as the test commences. In contrast to the pivot shift test, which assesses the anterolateral corner of the knee, the *reverse pivot shift test* known as the *Jakob test*[62] is performed with the knee flexed and the tibia externally rotated. Subluxation occurs posteriorly at 20° to 30° of flexion. As the knee is extended, the tibia reduces (if the ACL is intact) with a palpable "clunk," indicating that the *posterolateral capsule* is deficient.[110] A positive Jakob test is indicative of a slightly lax PCL.

In contrast to the Slocum test for postero*medial* capsular integrity assessed with the tibia in external rotation, assessment of the tibia in *internal rotation superimposed upon the anterior draw* also tests the postero*lateral* capsule. If the posterolateral capsule is sprained, the drawer test with internal rotation will demonstrate an increase in the anterior motion versus the drawer test in neutral, and the tibia will tend to "roll in." If, in addition to posterolateral capsular damage, the PCL is torn, the tibia will sublux posteriorly in addition to posterolateral rotation.

The *hyperextension recurvatum test* also correlates with injury to the posterolateral capsule (arcuate complex), as well as to tear of the anteromedial and intermediate fibers of the ACL.[55] If the great toes of both feet are held in full extension off the examining table, the knee hyperextends and the tibia externally rotates due to the absence of an intact posterolateral capsule and supporting structures.[110] The knee will show an apparent bowleg.

36. What are the frontal plane stress tests for straight medial and lateral instabilities?

In the acutely injured knee, tests for straight medial (valgus) and straight lateral (varus) instabilities should be initially performed with the knee in 20° to 30° of knee flexion because full extension is often impossible to achieve. Even if full extension is achieved, it is best to conduct these tests with the knee flexed. This is because knee extension may cause pain resulting in muscle spasm, and thus distort any valid information to be obtained by subsequent tests.

Instability is pronounced even in the presence of one positive test.[88] A straight frontal plane instability is indicated only if valgus and varus tests are *positive in full extension;* moreover, a grossly positive varus or valgus test indicates disruption of both the ACL and PCL. In contrast, if these tests are negative in extension *but positive in flexion,* a rotatory instability exists and signifies cruciate ligament compromise, although a collateral ligament injury is ruled out.

Valgus testing with knee flexion assesses the antero*medial* and postero*medial* knee joint capsule, whereas *varus* testing of the flexed knee assess the anterolateral and posterolateral knee capsule. We may advance provocative testing to an even higher degree of sensitivity by adding a *rotatory component* to this stress test. By alternately superimposing internal and external tibial rotation upon frontal plane testing with the knee in partial flexion, the examiner may hone onto the portion of the knee capsule that suffered injury from the same mechanism that caused cruciate ligament injury. *With varus testing, the anterolateral capsule is selectively stressed and thereby tested for integrity if the tibia is internally rotated during the exam; whereas the posterolateral capsule is stressed if the tibia is externally rotated during frontal plane varus testing with knee flexion. In contrast, with valgus testing and partial knee flexion, the anteromedial capsule is selectively stressed if the tibia is simultaneously internally rotated; whereas integrity of the posteromedial capsule is selectively assessed if external tibial rotation is superimposed upon a valgus stress test to the partially flexed knee.*

The large magnitude of forces yielding straight medial or lateral instabilities are often severe enough to cause lesions to the medial and/or lateral menisci. Injuries may also result in disruption of the medial or lateral head of the gastrocnemius, the semimembranosus, the biceps femoris, and the patellar retinacula.

Straight medial instability obviated by a valgus or abduction stress test to the knee indicates a lesions of the tibial collateral ligament, the deep portion of the medial collateral ligament (the meniscofemoral and meniscotibial portions of the medial capsular ligament), and the posteromedial corner of the posterior oblique ligament or posterior capsule itself. Straight medial instability is a severe knee injury that, if positive in the

internally rotated leg, is indicative of both anterior and posterior cruciate, as both ligaments are normally tautened on internal tibial rotation. However, in the chronically injured knee, a valgus stress applied in full extension is not a reliable indicator for PCL injury because the medial structures may be healed or scarred. In these knees, more reliance should be placed on the posterior drawer test for diagnosis.

Straight lateral instability determined by a positive adduction (varus) stress test in full extension is also indicative of severe injury to the ligamentous complex of the knee joint. The involved structures here include the meniscotibial or meniscofemoral portions of the lateral capsular ligament, the posterolateral corner of the arcuate ligament, as well as both the ACL and PCL. Additionally, the fibular collateral ligament, the popliteus muscle, and the peroneal nerve may also be injured.

37. How may provocative stress testing falsely score as negative in the event of PCL rupture?

Straight instability of the knee, with the exception of straight anterior instability, is *ipso facto* evidence of PCL deficiency. Straight posterior instability certainly indicates a deficit of the PCL and is most reliably tested by a posterior sag or posterior drawer sign.[84,111] However, both tests are less reliable following a valgus external rotation injury or a varus internal rotation type injury with a posteriorly directed force. In both mechanisms of injury there may be complete rupture of the PCL even though the posterior draw test is negative.[15] This is because the posteroinferior obliquity of the fibers of the intact posterior oblique and arcuate ligaments prevent posterior displacement of the tibia on the femur. A positive abduction or adduction stress test in complete knee extension is clinically helpful, as they strengthen the suspicion of PCL injury.[89] Thus in the acutely injured knee, a negative posterior drawer sign indicates an intact PCL only if valgus and varus stress testing of the involved limb is negative in full extension. Although the popliteal artery is uncommonly injured following sprain of the PCL, a thorough examination for signs of neurovascular compromise is appropriate if tear of the PCL is suspected.[15]

38. What is the most commonly encountered combination of straight and rotatory instability of the knee joint?

Although any combination of straight and rotary instabilities may occur, the one most clinically encountered is known as *anteromedial-anterolateral combined instability.* This combined instability typically involves a triad lesion to the medial side of the knee joint and may result from the application of noncontact external rotation-abduction forces that stress the medial joint stabilizers, or from a contact mechanism in which laterally applied valgus forces disrupt the medial aspect of the knee. In the presence of this combined instability, the ACL has invariably lost its integrity. Diagnosis of the various injured structures is fairly straightforward following total disruption of one entire compartment, as might result from as overwhelming varus force that involves virtually every anterolateral and posterolateral element. However, the clinical challenge inherent in the presentation of this combined instability is recognition that capsular and meniscal injury accompanied by sprain of the ACL may be present in both the medial and lateral compartments of the knee joint even in the presence of an intact PCL.*

Special consideration during the evaluation is mandated in such a knee so that the examiner may discover all of those injured structures, and subsequently initiate appropriate management and restoration. In the acutely injured knee with an intact PCL, there will be instability in full extension and internal rotation. However, if the knee presents with a negative abduction stress test in extension, but positive signs of anteromedial rotatory instability, all structures from the patellar tendon to the posterior cruciate ligament should be suspect and repaired if torn.[88]

39. What is the sequela of chronic isolated ACL rupture?

Genu recurvatum refers to an excessive hyperextension at the knee joint that develops from weight bearing on an unstable knee. This malalignment may result from injury to the ACL, muscle paralysis of the quadriceps femoris, or limitation of ankle motion as may occur from spasticity of the plantarflexors.[68] Alternately, the individual with a leg length discrepancy may demonstrate recurvatum in the longer leg caused by chronic stretch of the posterior ligaments and the posterior knee capsule. Because a principal function of the ACL is limitation of hyperextension, the individual with ACL deficiency will sustain a secondary gradual stretching out of the PCL and posterior capsule. It is essential to appreciate the relationship between the ACL and genu recurvatum as the examiner may draw an erroneous conclusion during the course of the evaluation of an injured knee if leg length measurement for possible discrepancy is omitted.

This highlights the interrelated relationship among the many structures comprising the knee joint that results in eventual failure of residual supporting structures when any of the principal stabilizing structures fail. Instability is thus a dynamic phenomenon and may easily progress to a failing unstable knee if unhindered by the implementation of early physical therapy, which attempts to provide compensatory support *before* the knee's other supporting ligaments fail. A correctly implemented therapeutic management early on is far more successful than an attempt to replace a ligament after continuity has been destroyed.[15,18,19,59,76]

In chronic anterior cruciate deficiency, the incidence of meniscal pathology has ranged between 85% to 91%.[18,19,59,76] In both the acute and chronic settings, the peripheral posterior horns are at the greatest risk for tearing and account for over half of the meniscal pathology encountered. The medial meniscus is twice as frequently damaged as the lateral.[59] Moreover, the articular cartilage of the medial and lateral compartments is also at risk for chondral fracture or articular surface erosion in both acute and chronic ACL deficiency.

40. What factors determine whether ACL tear is conservatively or surgically managed?

Suffice it to say that the approach to management of the ACL tear is fraught with controversy. Determining whether or not a given patient should or should not undergo ACL repair depends on a host of factors including patient age, associated knee injury, past history of knee injury, the demands of work, athletic activity level, as well as patient motivation. Factors to consider in the management of ACL injury include age, activity level, secondary restraint integrity, meniscal status articular cartilage status, rehabilitation potential, and patient goals and expectations. Age is

---

*Because of its relatively larger size and stronger resistance to selective tension testing, the PCL is considered the key stabilizer of the knee, (Hughston JC, Norwood LA: The posterolateral drawer test and external rotary recurvatum test for posterolateral rotary instability of the knee, *Clin Orthop* 147:82, 1980. And Hughston JC, Andrews JR, Cross MJ et al: Classification of knee ligament instabilities. Part I. The medial compartment and cruciate ligaments, *J Bone Joint Surg* 58A:159, 1976.) and acts as its rotational center. (Brody DM: *Clinical symposia: running injury—prevention and management,* vol 39, no. 3, Summit, NJ, 1987, CIBA-GEIGY.) Hughston et al (Hughston JC, Andrews JR, Cross MJ et al: Classification of the ligament instabilities. Part I. The medial compartment and cruciate ligaments, *J Bone Joint Surg* 58A:159, 1976.) considers the PCL to be the primary stabilizer of the knee in flexion, extension, and rotation. During knee motion the tibial plateaus move anteriorly and posteriorly by rotating around the axis of the PCL.

the most important single factor in determining mode of treatment. Patients who are less than 25 years old at the time of injury generally have a poor prognosis if treated nonoperatively compared with a good prognosis for patients older than age 35.[15] Thus patients younger than 25 years of age are best managed by a more aggressive surgical approach, as this group tends to be more active and more likely to sustain reinjury. Some patients have anterior cruciate ligament–dependent knees[17,39,92,96]; that is, their secondary stabilizers are ineffective. Loss of the ACL in such patients has devastating effects and mandate surgery. In contrast, some patients who rupture the ACL have excellent secondary stabilizers that may be effective over a lifetime if activity modifications are accepted and bracing is used during athletics.

Another deciding factor for or against surgery is the type of instability caused by the injury. Simple straight instabilities may be more benign than the more complex rotatory instabilities, which are more likely candidates for surgery so as to prevent residual rotational instability. The magnitude of injury is also a significant deciding factor in management of ACL injury. Partial tears, reported to occur between 24%[39] and 39%[92] of all injuries, have a more favorable prognosis, with good and excellent results being the rule rather than the exception in nonoperatively treated cases.[96]

Following ACL injury, few high caliber athletes can function without causing more pathologic changes to the knee, especially in sports such as basketball, football, gymnastics, or soccer which commonly require quick deceleration and directional changes. The presence or absence of injury to the medial and lateral stabilizers of the knee has direct bearing on the treatment choice in athletes. In American football, offensive linemen, particularly tacklers and centers, cover a limited area and require a lesser ability than wide receivers, defensive backs, and linebackers to perform lateral cutting movements. Adequate management for these patients may be procured with the less invasive extraarticular repairs of the posteromedial capsule and meniscal complex, especially as these athletes have adequate hamstring strength that serve to protect the tibia from anterior displacement. In contrast, for those patients whose professional athletic requirements involve a great deal of cutting movements, or in any athlete with a grossly unstable knee, the treatment of choice is primary operative intervention.[35]

On the other side of the spectrum, older patients with isolated ACL injury who are willing to modify their activities and avoid running, jumping, and cutting movements will do well without surgery. Conversely, any patient who finds activity modification too restrictive or troublesome is a suitable candidate for surgery. Because of the different needs and lifestyles of patients, each case must be considered individually. The decision to operate or to conservatively manage an ACL sprain is shared by the physician and the patient. Some authorities prefer to treat ACL injury aggressively with early reconstruction in females rather than early protection followed by rehabilitation and activity modification. This is particularly so in the woman athlete showing mild physiologic laxity in the medial-lateral plane, as well as slight hyperextension, because it is believed that such an athlete already has significant physiologic laxity.[58]

Clearly, those patients with partial injuries of the ACL, as evidenced by instrumented measurements, with no more than 3 mm of side-to-side comparison, minimal or absent pivot shift, minimal MRI visualization, and minimal injury upon arthroscopic visualization and probing are generally treated conservatively or by arthroscopy, which creates a fracture or a healing response at the anatomic site of partial fiber avulsion. Those patients who are neither athletes nor senescent, but who do not plan on continuing athletics or who plan to have a lifestyle that is relatively sedentary should not be encourage to undergo reconstruction. Both of the aforementioned patient populations are best managed by undergoing a rehabilitation program that emphasizes strengthening of the active knee restraints as a compensatory strategy for the compromised passive restraints. This is coupled by a life long commitment to the use of a functional knee brace during vigorous activity or work.[30]

Nonoperative management for PCL sprain is generally recommended for tears with mild to moderate posterior instability, in which there is posterior tibial displacement of less than 1 cm.[15] Surprisingly, and in contrast to ACL management, football players who have undergone surgical management following PCL rupture have shown a dismal return to function following surgery. Even surgery for a simple avulsion of the PCL of the femoral condyle has proven deficient in restoring high performance to football players with a running position. In contrast, conservative management of PCL sprain has yielded surprisingly satisfactory results.[35]

41. How may the performance and grading of various provocative tests determine whether patients should undergo conservative or surgical management?

The magnitude of functional instability following ACL injury is defined by anterior tibial subluxation due to sagittal translational laxity and seems to directly correlate with various tests for the pivot shift phenomenon. This may be used as a prognosticator of the kind of intervention that best manages this type of injury. If the knee displays a (grade I) mild anterior tibial subluxation with a slightly positive Lachman and flexion-rotation-drawer tests, but other tests are negative, the patient may be expected to have little or no functional instability. Indeed, this degree of laxity may be physiologic, as in loose-jointed individuals. Generally, this group does well with a nonoperative program of management. A second group refers to patients having moderate (grade II) anterior tibial subluxation exhibited by positive Lachman, flexion-rotation-drawer test, as well as a positive pivot "slide" or "slip" in the absence of pivot shift phenomenon or jerk tests. These patients usually have little short-term functional impairment, but are certainly at a higher risk for reinjury as the secondary restraints undergo compensatory stretching. This group may be managed nonoperatively provided there are no injuries to other ligaments such as the medial collateral ligament, or a repairable meniscal tear. On the other hand, patients in this group showing general ligamentous laxity with perform less well with a nonoperative approach, especially those whose activities place high demands upon their knees. Finally, patient showing a grade II or IV anterior tibial subluxation as evidence by a markedly positive pivot shift and jerk tests usually have functional instability manifested by giving way of the knee. For this patient population, operative treatment is usually indicated, especially for those patients in the high-risk categories.[15]

42. What are the soft and osseous tissue sequelae in surgical candidates for ACL repair who elect to forego operative management?

The anterior cruciate ligament is an essential stabilizer of the knee in the sense that its absence initiates a cascade of relentless deterioration of the knee joint that culminates in both clinical and functional instability.[34] An ACL rupture has been heralded as "the beginning of the end of the knee joint."[17] Although a knee may function satisfactorily for a short time with an incompetent or deficient ACL, the secondary stabilizers are eventually overwhelmed by the sheer magnitude of rotational and other forces routed through the knee, both up and down the kinetic chain, and succumb to progressive deterioration. The entire knee joint may slowly fail pending secondary attritional degeneration following a severe ACL injury, if surgery is discarded as a management option. This is clinically borne out by the draw test, which is minimally positive at 3 to 6 months following injury and progresses to grossly positive following 18 to 24 months. This occurs by way of gradual deterioration in the form of capsular stretching, meniscal injury, and osseous insult.

The natural history of a knee with a torn ACL is one of increasingly repeated episodes of "giving way," especially upon pivoting or twisting motions. A common casualty in such a knee is the meniscus. Forward tibial subluxation (pivot shifting) of the tibia underneath the femur imparts compression, shear, and torsional forces to the posterior horns of the lateral meniscus should it become wedged between the femoral and tibial condyles. As the tibia subluxates forward on the femur, the lateral meniscus is carried forward and may become trapped between the lateral femoral condyle and the posterior edge of the lateral tibial plateau.[88] Hence the lateral femoral condyle moves relatively backward as the lateral tibial condyle moves forward. The interposed posterior horn of the lateral meniscus follows along with the bulbous convexity of the lateral femoral condyle and may be pulled apart by shear forces. Alternately, meniscal injury may occur during the subsequent spontaneous reduction typically manifesting as circumferential (vertical longitudinal) tears.[117] If the torn central part of the meniscus remains forward of the femoral condyle when the tibia reduces, a displaced "bucket handle" type tear of the meniscus may result.[15] Alternately, if sudden tearing does not occur, gradual erosion of the meniscus may occur and lead to knee locking and eventual osteoarthritis of the knee joint.[88] The prevalence of meniscal tears associated with an acutely torn ACL is as high as 60% to 70%. If the meniscus is repaired but the instability is not corrected, then the meniscus may retear for the same reason it tore originally.[15] The same shear forces causing meniscal injury cause further deterioration, possibly in the form of chondral fractures of the femoral condyles that eventually result in degenerative changes. Degenerative arthritis of the lateral compartment of the knee joint has been shown to be a long-term sequela of loss of the ACL[61,75] in those individuals who are candidates for operative management, but either refuse surgery or do not have access to it.

43. What is the pathologic process by which failure of the ACL leads to degenerative osseous changes of the tibiofemoral joint?

To fully appreciate the mechanism by which an ACL deficient knee leads to degenerative changes of the femoral condyles, it is essential to comprehend the function of the screw-home mechanism at the knee joint and how malfunction of that mechanism may result in arthritic wear of the femoral condyles. The key to understanding tibiofemoral joint biomechanics is the helical or *spiral* figure-eight motion[43] so necessary to appreciating the *screw-home locking mechanism.* Screw-home movement at the knee joint is an angular motion that occurs during the last $15°^{41}$ to $30°^{109}$ of flexion to full extension of the knee known as *terminal knee extension.* This mechanism, as well as the concomitant helical motion, occurs as a direct function of the architectural asymmetry of the medial versus lateral tibiofemoral joint. These differences are derived from the divergent length and orientation between the two femoral condyles. The ability of the human knee to engage this mechanism allows the conversion of a potentially unstable joint into a locked pillar necessary to vaulting body weight over the stance leg during foot-flat phase of stance.

Terminal knee extension and concomitant engagement of the screw-home mechanism at the knee joint occurs in the open and closed kinetic chains, that is, during swing and stance phase of gait, respectively. As terminal knee extension is approached, the smaller lateral femoral condyle, to borrow a locomotive analogy, may be thought of as riding along a track, runs out of track as a function of the smaller anteroposterior surface area of the lateral tibial plateau.[110] Moreover, the lateral femoral condyle, unlike its medial counterpart, has a small ridge known as the *impressio terminalis*[107] that impinges upon the tibia and thus acts as a brake to halt further anterior glide.[86] The medial femoral condyle, however, continues unhindered but may only undergo an angular motion beyond this point in range. This motion, aptly described as helical or spiral, allows engagement of the tibiofemoral joint such that the articulation is screwed home into the closed packed position.

Thus the screw-home mechanism is an obligatory occurrence during terminal knee extension as a consequence of the osseous configuration of the tibiofemoral joints. This process is dynamically facilitated by the popliteus muscles, the hamstrings, and the iliotibial band insertion into Gerdy's tubercle.[110] The end result of terminal knee extension, whether performed in the closed or open kinetic mode of function is engagement of the screw-home locking mechanism of the knee. The direction of transverse plane rotation changes when comparing the open and closed kinetic modes of function because the roles of the tibia and femur have alternated between stabilizer and mover.

Torsional motion or rotation of the bones of the lower extremity in the transverse plane represent part of the repertoire of strategies evolved to diminish and absorb the potentially disruptive forces inherent to locomotion. The femoral condyles represent the potential locus of endogenous trauma due to torsion forces, as a function of engagement of the screw-home mechanism during forceful terminal knee extension. The medial femoral condyle is particularly vulnerable as the medial tibiofemoral hemi-joint contains the center for the rotational axis of rotation at the knee joint.

An alteration from the precise sequence of rotations comprising the screw-home mechanism represents an alteration in the normal kinesiology of terminal knee extension, whose consequences may be injurious to the knee. For example, repeated blows of the lateral aspect of the medial femoral condyle amount to impingement of the *intercondylar eminence,* and has been postulated as a mechanism of injury in osteochondritis dissecans, and may be causative of degeneration in the ACL deficient knee. Eventually, subchondral bone undergoes fatigue failure resulting in minute subchondral fractures that grow with repeated insult. *Torsional impaction* is postulated to derive as a function of tibiofemoral rotation[28] during engagement of the screw-home mechanism in which the lateral aspect of the medial femoral condyle impinges upon the tibial spine. In contrast, the lateral femoral condyle may sustain injury as a function of its *impressio terminalis* repetitively impinging upon the lateral tibial plateau during terminal knee extension.

The cruciate ligaments fine-tune the precision of the screw-home mechanism as the knee joint approaches terminal extension.[44] How this occurs is understood if we appreciate that although both cruciate ligaments relax during external tibial rotation, they tense during internal tibial rotation. If we shift our frame of reference from the open to the closed kinetic mode of function, we may repeat the latter by stating that the cruciate ligaments collectively relax during internal femoral rotation (relative to a fixed tibia) and come under strong tension upon external femoral rotation. As terminal knee extension is approached during stance phase of gait the distal femur medially rotates relative to the stationary tibia as screw-home mechanism engagement is initiated. Both the magnitude and speed of this rotation may be guided by the presence of an intact ACL that precisely navigates the femoral condylar rotation atop the tibial plateau.

An ACL deficient knee represents a diminishment of this motion-guidance system, resulting in a minimal tendency for the distal femur to internally rotate. This minimal internal rotatory moment, compounded by hard use or length of time eventually stretches the lateral knee joint capsular structures and may culminate as a subluxation of the anterolateral tibial plateau in the case of ACL deficiency. In the event of PCL deficiency, the medial knee joint capsular structures may be compromised, resulting in eventual anteromedial tibial plateau subluxation of functional pivot shift. Alternately, the medial femoral condyle may undergo excessive external rotation without the presence of an ACL acting as a tether to limit its motion. Here, the medial femoral condyle may suffer repeated blows against the intercondylar eminence. The cumulative effect of cruciate deficiency upon the femoral condyles may be a more rapid wearing away of articular cartilage and eventual chondral fractures of the condyles typical of arthritis[15]

44. What are the two surgical options for operative management of the anterior cruciate ligament?

Because of the meager blood supply to the cruciate ligaments, anatomic repositioning or surgical repair of the residual ligament does not result in healing. Operative management of ACL injury is technically difficult because the ligament crosses the synovial cavity of the knee. Its torn ends, having the appearance of soggy string, are revitalized at the moment of injury and rapidly retract.[20,23] Despite this, patients with significant associated injury including capsular, collateral ligament, meniscal, or articular surface defects are best managed by surgery, which attempts to reproduce the position and function of the native ligament as precisely as possible. Reconstructive procedures utilizing autogenous, allographic, xenographic, or synthetic tissue may be performed via a wide variety of techniques that may be described as extraarticular, intraarticular, and combined intra- and extraarticular procedures. *Intracapsular surgery* involves replacement of the ACL with natural tissue, and is classified as a *static repair.* Typi-

cally, reconstruction is performed via a *patellar tendon autograft* or *allograft* in which the central third of the patellar tendon substitutes for part of the patellar ligament and its bony attachment as a bone-tendon-bone autograft. Autografts are alternately harvested from the semitendinosus and gracilis tendons, or the iliotibial band. *Extracapsular dynamic reconstruction* typically involves a pes anserine transfer in which the distal attachment of the sartorius muscle is reattached, thereby converting the line of pull of that muscle from primarily a knee flexor to an internal rotator of the tibia. Following surgery, patients may still show a positive anterior draw sign, although the leg is considerably stabilized. Alternately, dynamic reconstruction may be performed via the iliotibial band. Cadaveric allograft tissues most frequently used for anterior cruciate ligament substitution have been the patellar and Achilles tendons.[20] Bovine xenografts consist of animal tendon. Recently, synthetics such as carbon fiber or knitted Dacron, have included stents for biological tissue, or as complete substitutes for the ACL. Synthetic stents protect the biologic tissue from disruption or stretching until collagenization and reorganization have occurred.

Primary repair of the PCL is usually less successful than repairs of the ACL. Instability often recurs following surgery, and full extension range of motion may be lost, particularly due to prolonged immobilization in a flexion splint for up to 8 weeks. Thus only patients who have high-demand knees and severe instability are candidates for PCL reconstruction.[88] Operative treatment of the PCL injury may involve *direct repair,* which yields questionable results,[53,84] *transfer of the medial gastrocnemius,*[54] or using a *free graft of the patellar tendon.*

45. What indirect evidence argues against dynamic ACL reconstruction?

The validity of dynamic repairs is of questionable efficacy and may only provide a passive static restraint to the knee joint for several reasons. a transferred muscle or tendon loses one entire strength grade upon being transferred.[80] Second, knee injury occurs with such rapidity that there is insufficient time for the reflex arc to initiate protective muscle contraction.[100] Moreover, advancing a musculotendinous insertion weakens its muscle by elongating the muscle beyond its optimal length, and thereby minimizing its mechanical efficiency. In addition, the transferred tendon has a tendency to scar to adjacent tissues, thereby reducing its restraint capability from dynamic to one of a static restraint. Finally, the mechanical advantage of musculo-tendinous units about the knee is stronger at 90° of flexion than in full extension. Thus as the knee approaches extension the tendons will assume a more parallel orientation to the knee joint, and the mechanical advantage of those muscle-tendon units will be correspondingly diminished. This is clinically significant as knee injuries more commonly occur in the relatively extended position than in the knee flexion posture.[15]

46. What postoperative complications may follow cruciate ligament repair?

- *Arthrofibrosis.* This refers to loss of motion, and is one of the most common postoperative complications following ACL reconstruction. Arthrofibrosis is defined as a knee flexion contracture of more than 10° and/or knee flexion range of motion less than 125°.[16] The results of several studies indicate an increased incidence of arthrofibrosis after reconstruction of an acutely injured ACL, possibly due to aggravation of the already inflamed and painful synovium. Because of this, delaying surgery some 3 weeks following injury or until the patient has regained full range of motion with minimal or no pain is justified. With respect to the tibiofemoral joint, it is important to initiate passive full knee extension exercises early in the rehabilitation regimen so as to prevent scar tissue formation in the intercondylar notch. These exercises may take the form of prone leg hangs and towel extensions, and should be performed until full knee extension is achieved and assured. Mobilization of the tibiofemoral joint may also be of help in promoting knee flexion and extension. Patients with unacceptable motion are initially managed with aggressive physical therapy. A helpful conservative adjunct to therapy is the Dynasplint, which produces a low-load prolonged force on restricted soft tissues to restore range of motion. Patients are surgically managed when conservative measures fail. Closed manipulation of the knee is accompanied by arthroscopic lysis of adhesion and debridement of the intercondylar notch at less than 6 months postoperatively. Open debridement is recommended at more than 6 months after surgery. With regard to the patellofemoral joint, patellar mobilization in the form of superior glide should be initiated without delay to prevent shortening of the patellar tendon and decreased patellar mobility.
- *Patellar tendinitis.* (see Chapter 12) This may be avoided by meticulous harvest of the patellar tendon graft, as well as immediate motion and weight bearing, patellar mobilization, and quadriceps strengthening. However, it is important to take care to avoid initiation of overaggressive quadriceps strengthening as this may stimulate development of patellar tendinitis. If detected, it is essential to initiate treatment during the acute phase which generally includes ice-cup massage, flexibility exercises, the use of nonsteroidal antiinflammatory medications, reduction and/or modification of quadriceps strengthening exercises, as well as eccentric versus concentric quadriceps work. If initially undetected or ignored, an acute patellar tendinitis may well progress into a chronic condition that is harder to manage and may hinder the patient's progress with ACL rehabilitation[16]
- *Patellar entrapment syndrome.* This is more likely to be encountered with autogenous bone-patellar tendon-bone grafts; patellar entrapment is clinically diagnosed by decreased mediolateral and superoinferior mobility of the patella. This specifically limits patellar mobility and generally limits mobility of the knee.[98] Extensor mechanism tightness also magnifies contact patellofemoral pressure and may lead to patellofemoral chondrosis. Clinical presentation includes induration of the peripatellar tissues, painful range of motion, restricted patellar mobility, extensor lag, and the presence of a "shelf sign."[16] If allowed to progress without appropriate intervention, patellar entrapment syndrome may evolve into its most serious form known as *infrapatellar contracture syndrome* resulting in fibrous hyperplasia of the anterior soft tissues of the knee. Here, permanent shortening of the patellar tendon known as *fibrous hyperplasia* that entraps the patella and limits both flexion (more than 25°) and extension (more than 10°) of the knee. Here, the fibrous hyperplasia entraps the patella and limits knee motion such that the entire extensor mechanism undergoes pathologic tightening. Severe cases typically require numerous operations. Thus *the best treatment for this debilitating condition is prevention by way of* **early patellar mobilization,** *including medial, lateral,* **but especially superior glide,** *incorporated into the postoperative rehabilitation program.*
- *Edema.* Early edema control is necessary to prevent induration of the peripatellar soft tissues. Induration of these tissues may result in decreased patellar mobility with resulting loss of motion. An overaggressive strengthening program may also lead to joint effusion. In this case, modification of the rehabilitation

program, nonsteroidal antiinflammatory medications, cryotherapy, distoproximal massage, electrical stimulation, limb elevation, and distoproximal isotonic contraction may be necessary until the effusion can be controlled.

- *Articular cartilage defects.* These are often associated with ACL tears and may deleteriously alter the program of rehabilitation. These defects are surgically managed by attempting to stimulate ingrowth of fibrocartilage into the site of defects[102] in a manner analogous to the culturing of pearls. By causing multiple microfractures through the subchondral plane at the area of the defect, blood is allowed to pool. The subsequent clot provides a medium for fibrocartilage to form. Therapy involves continuous passive motion, beneficial to healing cartilage, is applied for 8 weeks while the patient does not bear weight on the involved extremity. Water exercise and gentle bicycling may begin during the first 2 weeks following the procedure.[30]

47. What is the medical management following acute rupture of the ACL?

Roughly 75% of knee effusions secondary to hemarthrosis have a major ligament injury, usually the anterior cruciate ligament. Swelling typically occurs quickly and reaches maximal effusion at 12 hours following injury. Blood contains lysosomal enzymes from phagocytic white cells that endow it with a hemolytic digestive effect upon articular cartilage. If not quickly aspirated, blood may cause an intense synovitis that may require weeks to resolve. Moreover, blood in the knee acts like a SuperGlue causing blood clots inside the joint that results in intraarticular adhesions that may limit mobility. If arthroscopy is not available, then blood should be aspirated from the joint and examined for fat globules. The presence of fat suggests a serious injury as fat can only enter the knee from a fracture site or a contused area of subcutaneous fat communicating with the knee.[23]

48. What is the quadriceps-cruciate interaction, and how may it be used to dynamically compensate for sprain of the ACL?

The cornerstone of a conservative intervention for cruciate ligament injury is based on the idea that increasing strength of specific muscles adjacent to the knee joint may have a dynamic effect that compensates for the static stabilizing role of the cruciate ligaments in the event of ligamentous injury.

Several studies[24] have demonstrated an interaction between the contraction of the quadriceps muscle and the loading of the ACL through the anterior shear force of the tibia. In 1956 DeLorme hypothesized that quadriceps contraction may be antagonistic to the stability of the ACL and discovered that contraction causes anterior displacement of the tibia, thereby increasing the tensile load through the ACL. (Moreover, as the quadriceps function as extensors of the knee, the closer to full extension the knee is postured, the greater the magnitude of this anterior shear effect upon the tibia.* We may extrapolate from this concept that it is in the interest of the ACL deficient knee to minimize the anterior translation so as to prevent further sprain and instability. Minimizing the *quadriceps-cruciate interaction* may be accomplished by negating the contractile effect of the powerful quadriceps group by selectively working the hamstrings. By working the antagonist muscle of the quadriceps, and avoiding quadriceps group, we may effectively limit the anterior translatory force delivered to the tibia during function.[46,69,104]

In contrast, an intact PCL limits the magnitude of posterior tibial displacement. The PCL deficient knee is likely to sustain instability in the form of excessive posterior tibial displacement when the hamstring muscles contract. A good strategy to negate this posterior translatory shear is to work the quadriceps muscle group. In such a manner, the destabilizing effect of the hamstrings upon the knee joint will be minimized by an over abundance of antagonistic quadriceps muscle tone that works to neutralize the hamstrings effect upon the knee.

Initial management consists of cryotherapy, immobilization with an external splint, and partial weight bearing during gait while utilizing crutches. With the diminishment of pain and hemarthrosis resolution over the subsequent 2 to 3 weeks, gentle range of motion may be initiated. As the patient regains full range of motion, muscle strength, and functional ability, an external brace may be introduced. *(For a more complete management strategy of the conservatively managed cruciate ligament injury, the reader is referred to the subsequent discussion of postoperative therapy following ACL repair, as many of the same treatment strategies are employed for both patient populations.)*

---

*The anterior translatory shear of the tibia is particularly acute from 45° of knee flexion to full extension. (Jonsson T, Althoff B, Peterson L, et al: Clinical diagnosis of ruptures of the anterior cruciate ligament: a comparative study of the Lachman test and the anterior drawer sign, *Am J Sports Med* 10:100, 1982.)

49. What is the effect of closed versus open kinetic chain exercises with regard to ACL rehabilitation?

The types of knee exercise that may be used to following knee injury may be categorized into the open and closed kinetic chains. *Open kinetic chain* (OKC) activities of the lower extremity is described as motion of the knee is independent of motion at the hip and ankle, such that the distal segment is free to move on the more proximal segment. Functionally, open kinetic chain movements correspond to the swing leg motions during stance. Moreover, open kinetic chain movement is characterized by motion only distal to the axis of the joint, is predominantly a concentric muscle contraction, typically occurs in one of the cardinal planes of motion, provides action and less reaction to movement, and typically requires no balance and little coordination during activity. With regard to cruciate ligament rehabilitation, the use of OKC exercises may cause excessive stress to the graft site if performed early on as it isolates quadriceps activity. Biomechanical analysis has shown that an inverse relationship exists between ACL load and knee flexion angle.[46,69] Because of this, OKC quadriceps strengthening increases anterior tibial translation and thereby stress the reconstructed ACL, particularly from 30° flexion to full knee extension, and should be avoided.[16] However, active quadriceps contraction beyond 60° is permissible as it does not strain the ACL.

The *closed kinetic chain* (CKC) or mode of function occurs to the stance limb during ambulation and refers to a combination of several successively arranged joints in which the terminal joint meets with enough resistance that prohibits or restrains it from movement. Here, motion at the knee is accompanied by motion at the hip and ankle. Closed kinetic chain motion differs from and offers several benefits not offered from open kinetic chain motion. With CKC motion, the motion is both proximal and distal to the joint axis, the type of muscular work may include concentric, eccentric, or isometric. Moreover, with CKC motion, muscles work more functionally, in unison, and not in isolated fashion. With regard to stress and strain, CKC motion involves biomechanically consistent stress and strain within tissues and joints; stabilization is provided through normal postural means; combination of motion occurs in all three planes, consistent with motion of joints and structures; CKC also provides both action and reaction to certain movements, and requires both balance and coordination during activity.[30] In addition,

CKC exercises promote cocontraction and increase stability through increased joint compressive loads. Anterior translation of the tibia on the femur occurs with increased compressing loads, but is minimized by cocontraction. Thus *CKC has the advantage of reducing shear forces on the joint and strain on the ACL.* Primarily because of the reduced strain on the ACL, closed kinetic chain exercises may be incorporated early in the rehabilitation program to strengthen the quadriceps muscle group.

50. What physical therapy is appropriate following ACL repair?

Management of the patient who is a surgical candidate has two parts: phase I—the actual operation and phase II—the subsequent rehabilitation. Both are equally important.[14] For the benefit of the patient it is imperative that an open line of communication be made available between the therapist and surgeon. Failure of appropriate communication represents a failure in patient advocacy that minimizes patient welfare and may result in an incompletely rehabilitated knee, which is ultimately at greater risk for reinjury.

The three principal goals of knee rehabilitation are to: (1) decrease swelling and pain; (2) restore full range of motion, and (3) restore adequate strength and endurance. Therapeutic management of the cruciate compromised knee involves three phases—initial, intermediate, and advanced phases. Patients progress into the next phase once the goals of the previous level are achieved. This is known as a *criteria-based progression* from one level or phase to the next one. Phases may overlap, although one phase does not need to be entirely completed before proceeding to the next level. Throughout the rehabilitation it is imperative to convey to the patient the importance of reporting any pain or swelling experienced during of after exercise so that the therapist may appropriately modify, substitute, or discontinue an exercise. A supervised daily therapy session may be ideal and appropriate for the professional or college level athlete but may be impossible for most other patients because of temporal and economic restraints. Thus many patients undergo a supervised physical therapy regimen three times per week that is accompanied by a home exercise program during the off days. With proper management intervention a patient with a cruciate ligament injury may be returned to a preinjury level of activity.

Returning the patient's knee to a premorbid level of function is accomplished by a proper balance between protection of the reconstructed ligament and prevention of decompensation secondary to disuse. Certainly, rigid immobilization in a long leg cast represents an outdated management approach as the deleterious effects of joint immobilization such as disuse muscle atrophy, severe changes in articular cartilage and ligaments, patellofemoral crepitus and pain, profound quadriceps weakness, selective atrophy of type I slow-twitch muscle fibers,[47] and loss of joint range from formation of intraarticular adhesions, outweigh any potentially derived benefits.

Today, an **accelerated rehabilitation management strategy** has been widely adopted as the preferred treatment approach. These accelerated protocols have emerged following the observation that patients who did not comply with the restrictions imposed by traditional protocols have better range of motion, strength, and function without compromising joint stability than did those who complied.[16] The challenge to the therapist in applying aggressive physical therapy is to do so while avoiding excessive loading of the reconstructed ligament as well as minimizing inflammation, while maximizing desirable components of therapeutic intervention. The cornerstone of accelerated rehabilitation is the early initiating of range of motion and weight bearing through knee, as well as the long-term maintenance of full knee extension. Motion, which was once discouraged during the early period of rehabilitation, has been found to be helpful for ligament healing, articular cartilage nutrition, as well as prevention of capsular and soft tissue contraction.[3,4,5,94] In this fashion, early motion and weight bearing provide desired stress to the reconstructed ligament in a functional manner without deformation, and stimulates collagen formation along the lines of stress. Early motion and weight bearing causing controlled stress to the healing ligament, as well as the application of closed kinetic chain exercises have considerably improved the outcome of ACL reconstruction.

Rehabilitation takes the form of early motion of full passive range of motion, as well as full weight bearing. A hinged knee brace permitting full extension and preventing hyperextension or hyperflexion is achieved by permitting no more than a setting of 10° to 90° of motion so as to avoid stretching or rupturing the graft. This type of brace is recommended for the first 6 weeks postoperatively. Double-leg and one-third knee bends may be initiated on the first postoperative day. **Aquatic exercise** in the form of deep water running with a buoyancy vest is an excellent vehicle for aerobic exercise

and range of motion, the minimizing the adverse effects of concussive impact of gravity, and may be initiated approximately 2 weeks postoperatively.[30] The criteria for discharge from physical therapy for the athlete are determined by isokinetic testing. The athlete may return to full sport activity when strength, power, and endurance* values are 80% to 85% of the normal leg.[102]

- *Edema control management.* Joint effusion primarily interferes with knee function and rehabilitation by having an inhibitory effect on the quadriceps muscles that may result in significant muscle atrophy. This is borne out by the fact that an infusion of as little as 60 cc of saline injected results in inhibition of voluntary muscle contraction by as much as 30% to 50%. Increasing joint pressure stimulates types I and II mechanoreceptors which, in turn, increase the threshold of the spinal reflex arc by Hoffman's reflex, resulting in neuromuscular inhibition. Because of this inhibitory effect, it is imperative to minimize joint effusion as soon as possible following ACL reconstruction so as to minimize the neuromuscular inhibitory effects and subsequent rapid atrophy of the quadriceps muscles. Edema control techniques are of primary importance and include the application of cryotherapy, compression, limb elevation, high volt galvanic stimulation, active quadriceps sets, ankle pumps, as well as the commercially available cooling/compression devices such as the CryoCuff (Aircast Inc., Summit, NJ).[16]

- *Proprioceptive retraining.* The intact uninjured ACL is endowed with mechanoreceptors that may play a role in detecting joint position, as well as sudden or slow joint position changes. Joint perception at the knee is minimized or lost following disruption of the ACL that is not restored from surgical reconstruction of the ligament. A compensatory rehabilitative strategy involves *neuromuscular reeducation,* in which the knee's remaining proprioceptive structures are "taught" to compensate by learning to better detect joint position as well as rate of change of position. The advantage of using a simple elastic bandage for support, in addition to reminding the patient to be caution when pivoting on the leg, is the beneficial effect of facilitating proprioception by sensory cutane-

---

Strength is defined as the peak torque developed at speeds to 200°, 240°, and 275° per second; *power* is defined as the time taken to develop this torque. *Endurance* is recorded at 300° per second and is performed for 30 seconds. (Brewster CE, Seto JL, Shields Jr, CL et al: Rehabilitation of the knee. In Nicholas JA, Hershman EB editors: *The lower extremity and spine,* ed 2, vol 1, St Louis, 1995, Mosby.)

ous feedback.[15] Additionally, use of the BAPS board may further help stimulate proprioceptive awareness of those mechanoreceptors located in those soft tissue structures adjacent to the ACL.

- *Continuous passive motion (CPM).* This involves initiating early movement and was introduced by Salter et al in 1970,[16] and is believed to counter many of the deleterious effects of immobilization. The many physiologic benefits of CPM upon joint surfaces and soft tissue includes nutrition of the articular cartilage, retardation of intraarticular adhesions and joint stiffness, improvement of articular cartilage nutrition, accelerating clearance of hemarthrosis, improving matrix formation by stimulation of chondrocytes, and providing early controlled forces acting upon collagenous tissues. In addition, CPM may accelerate clearance of blood and fluid from the joint, which may facilitate mobility of the joint. Some clinicians prefer to initiate early movement by utilizing passive, active assisted, and active range of motion that is initiated by the patient rather than the use of a CPM device. Judicious use of CPM is recommended, particularly with regard to possible damage to the reconstruction site if the range of motion settings are incorrectly set. This may result in graft damage incurred by cyclic fatigue at the notch margins, or the development of a knee flexion contracture or an extensor lag because the CPM is set such that it does not permit terminal knee extension. Finally, the use of a CPM device may not be available throughout the socioeconomic population distribution because of its significant financial cost.

- *Electomyogram* (EMG) *biofeedback.* This facilitates neuromuscular reeducation of the quadriceps muscle group, particularly the vastus medialis obliquus (VMO), by transforming myoelectric signals produced by the muscle into visual and/or auditory signals for the patient. A threshold or preset goal is set by the therapist for the patient to attempt to master. If the muscle contraction is strong enough to exceed a threshold level, the auditory and/or visual signals will occur; stronger contractions elicit stronger feedback. A higher threshold is then determined to elicit an even stronger contraction by the patient.[16]

- *Electric muscle stimulation* (EMS). Electric muscle stimulation following ACL reconstruction is controversial owing to conflicting results of various investigations. Some studies indicate significant clinical benefits such as more rapid gains in range of motion, decreased strength loss during the postoperative pe-

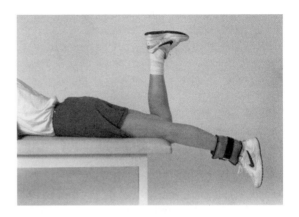

FIG. 43-26 *Prone leg hangs* to increase knee extension in patients with restricted knee extension. Gravity is allowed to gently pull the knee down into extension as the patient relaxes. This posture is maintained for some 5 minutes as tolerated. A cuff weight around the distal ankle may be added. (From Brotzman SB: *Clinical orthopaedic rehabilitation,* St Louis, 1996, Mosby.)

riod, augmentation of oxidative enzyme activity in muscle,[102] and increased overall rate of return to sporting activities. The results of other studies are less optimistic, reporting that the use of EMS is no more effective than volitional exercise in maintaining quadriceps strength.[16]

- *Stretching exercises.* These should include the gastrocnemius muscle, the soleus muscle, the Achilles tendon, the Iliotibial band, the hamstring muscles, the quadriceps muscles, the adductor muscles, and the hip flexors. Knee extension range of motion may be restricted. Gaining an increase in knee extension may be performed by *prone leg hangs* (Fig. 43-26), with a cuff weight around the distal ankle. To gain knee flexion, passive knee flexion (Fig. 43-27) may be accomplished by short sitting over the edge of the plinth and gently lowering the involved leg with the uninjured leg to 90°. Once 80° to 90° of knee flexion has been accomplished, the patient may initiate increased knee flexion by beginning wall slide activities. *Wall slides* aid in gaining increased knee flexion by utilizing gravity to assist flexion. The patient slowly slides the foot down the wall until a sustained stretch is felt in the knee. Once flexion range of knee motion has progressed to 115° to 120°, *heel slides* may be substituted for wall slides

- *Strengthening exercises.* Exercises of the appropriate muscle group provide improved joint stability and represents a dynamic strategy that compensates for

quadriceps work is used early, as soon as the patient can tolerate them.[102]

- *Isometric exercises.* Although not as dramatically beneficial as isotonic exercises, static isometric quadriceps exercises are practical as they can produce strength gains,[45,101] when performed as isometric hip adduction on the exercise mat in the long sitting posture. A bolster or rolled up towel is placed between the thighs just above the knee to avoid any medial knee incisions, and followed by maximal adductor contractions. Quadriceps setting exercises are better performed if they immediately follow isometric adductor strengthening, possibly because of overflow from the VMO having an attachment to the adductor tendon.[50]

- *Quadriceps setting.* Only certain types of quadriceps strengthening may used following ACL sprain. Quadriceps setting exercises are an isometric type contraction of the quadriceps muscle group that should be encouraged early on to improve neuromuscular control and prevent quadriceps shut down owing to inactivity and atrophy. Quadriceps setting also aids in the resorption of joint effusion and provides a dynamic superior patellar mobilization, thereby staving off the likelihood of infrapatellar contracture syndrome and knee flexion contracture. Performed in the long sitting posture, the patient actively contracts the quadriceps muscle while actively dorsiflexing the foot. The latter is helpful in initiating contraction of the VMO muscle.[102]

- *Hamstring setting.* These exercises are particularly helpful in maintaining hamstring muscle tone and staving off hamstring atrophy following PCL sprain, while eliminating the potentially destabilizing effects of isotonic hamstring work to the PCL deficient knee. Hamstring setting exercises are performed with the patient sitting in 40° to 50° of knee flexion. The patient isometrically works the hamstring by attempting to dig the heel into the mat while pulling downward on the leg.

- *Isotonic exercises.* In contrast to hamstring setting activities, which involve isometric exercises for the PCL compromised knee, OKC **hamstring curls** are an isotonic form of muscular exercise that is beneficial to the ACL compromised knee. OKC hamstring curls may be performed early in the rehabilitative course of therapy because they decrease the level of strain on the ACL throughout the entire range of knee motion. Early initiation of hamstring strengthening in the ACL compromised knee is emphasized especially

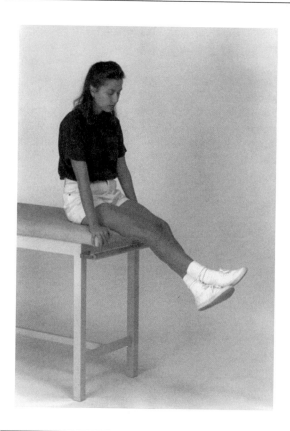

FIG. 43-27 Passive flexion of the knee. (From Brotzman SB: *Clinical orthopaedic rehabilitation*, St Louis, 1996, Mosby.)

loss of static cruciate stabilization. The strengthening of the hamstring or quadriceps muscle group, respectively, depends on which of the cruciate ligaments sustained injury. When managing a sprain of the ACL, it is appropriate to minimize the quadriceps-cruciate interaction by strengthening the hamstring musculature so as to minimize the anterior shear of the tibia upon the femur and hence strain to the already compromised ACL. Hamstring work, both concentric and eccentric, is helpful in negating the destabilizing role of the quadriceps muscles. When managing a sprain of the PCL, it is appropriate to minimize the hamstring-cruciate interaction by strengthening the quadriceps musculature, thereby minimizing the posterior shear of the tibia upon the femur and decrease strain of the sprained PCL. Thus improved tone of the quadriceps musculature in the form of quadriceps hypertrophy helps negate the destabilizing effect of the hamstrings upon the PCL by pulling the tibia forward on the femur. Eccentric

as the hamstrings muscle group represent the *primary dynamic stabilizers of the knee.*

- *Cross over effect.* This is a neurophysiologic concept in which vigorous exercise of the contralateral (uninjured) extremity has been shown to cause a "cross over" strengthening effect by as much as 30%[48,49,50] in the injured knee, even if that knee were immobilized. This effect may be used early in the rehabilitation program with isometric quadriceps strengthening to induce a stronger quadriceps contraction in the involved knee.[16]

Open kinetic chain isolated quadriceps exercise, although ordinarily deleterious to the ACL deficient knee, may be used in a restricted manner to allow for restoration of normal strength and girth to the quadriceps muscle if the exercise avoids the last 30° to 45° of knee extension. Straight leg raising exercises, like quadriceps setting exercises, are another form of allowable OKC exercise permitted in the rehabilitation of the ACL deficient knee. Straight leg raising involves isometric contracture of the quadriceps muscle group and simultaneous isotonic contraction of the iliopsoas that lifts the entire lower limb 6 to 8 inches above the plinth.

- *Resisted exercises.* These exercises, in the form of isotonic **concentric** free weight exercises, may be incorporated into the rehabilitation program. The utilization of Universal or Nautilus Gym equipment, particularly the leg press, may be helpful. Exercises may also include **eccentric** strengthening of musculature. Calf exercises, by way of *toe raises* performed in either the sitting or standing posture represent a combination of both *concentric* (triceps surae contraction) during the rise and *eccentric* (pretibial) muscle work during lowering of the heel. **Isokinetic** strength training may be incorporated into the rehabilitation regimen provided that the resistance generated is never greater than the produced muscle tension. Isokinetic training has been demonstrated to result in hypertrophy of type II muscle fibers and glycolytic enzyme enhancement.[21,22]

- *Bracing.* A number of braces are available to the injured knee and are classified as prophylactic, rehabilitative, and functional. However, with the trend toward more aggressive rehabilitation, the difference between the different categories of braces may merely be one of semantics.[13] The purpose of the brace includes protection of the graft from stress in the early postoperative period. Thus the brace protects the healing knee by controlling the amount of

motion allowed and thereby deflecting excessive loads away from the knee ligaments. proceeds. The biomechanical purpose of a knee brace is to mimic function of those ligaments for which the brace attempts to compensate over a broad range of loading conditions. The ACL is estimated to endure loads as high as 2160 N before failing.[116] A brace must either shield or share such a load while permitting for normal knee kinematics and protecting against pathologic laxity. To accomplish these tasks the structural stiffness of the brace must be greater than or equal to that of the knee. The characteristics of the ideal brace include: reasonable cost, possessing durability, good fit and comfortable, allow normal activity, no increased risk of additional injury, and have documented decrease in risk or severity of knee ligament injury. It is incumbent upon the therapist to counsel the patient against developing a false sense of security or becoming dependent upon the brace. The beneficial effect of any brace however, is diminished with increasing load.*

Although custom made braces incorporate a rigid shell manufactured according to patient measurements, non–custom-made braces use a soft shell with Velcro strapping that deforms so as to mold to the contour of the wearer's knee. With the off-the-shelf variety of brace, no effort is made to precisely fit the brace to the contour of the patient's leg. The literature comparing these two varieties of bracing does not support the belief that a custom made brace, despite its presumably better fit to the patient's leg, provides any greater stability than the off-the-shelf model.[12] In fact, a distinct disadvantage of the custom made brace is that the patient does not fit into the brace during the postoperative course of management owing to the changing girth of thigh muscle as rehabilitation proceeds. The biomechanical purpose of a knee brace is to mimic function of those ligaments for which the brace attempts to compensate for over a broad range of loading conditions. The ACL is estimated to endure loads as high as 2160 N before failing. A brace must either shield or share such a load while permitting for normal knee kinematics and protecting

---

*Although less supporting than bracing, the use of a simple elastic bandage provides the unique benefit of providing proprioception enhancement by way of sensory cutaneous feedback, thereby reminding the patient to be cautious when pivoting on the leg. (Zarins B, Fish DN: Knee ligament injury. In Nicholas JA, Hershman EB editors: *The lower extremity and spine,* ed 2, vol 1, St Louis, 1995, Mosby.)

against pathologic laxity. To accomplish these tasks the structural stiffness of the brace must be greater than or equal to that of the knee. It is incumbent upon the therapist to counsel the patient against developing a false sense of security or becoming dependent upon the brace. The beneficial effect of any brace however, is diminished with increasing load.

Although it is commonly held as fact that prophylactic knee braces decrease the risk of knee injury, this belief is not entirely supported by either epidemiologic or basic science literature.[16] This is because the studies reporting on the efficacy of these braces in minimizing knee injury have not been in agreement. Nevertheless, American football players serving as tight end, linebacker, as well as offensive and defensive lineman, are believed to be at highest risk for reinjury may be advised to wear prophylactic braces because a reinjury may end their athletic career. Patients typically respond positively to brace use as they feel a subjective sense of improvement from wearing it.

- *Functional exercises.* These are important to incorporate into a rehabilitation program and include forward and lateral *(pliometric)* step-ups and step-downs, stair climbing activities, and lunges. *Lunges* represent a form of CKC exercises that strengthen the lower extremity. *Agility drills* include backward running, rope skipping, vertical jumping, lateral running, crossovers (carioca), and figure-eight running. Before initiating a running program, the patient begins jogging on a *min-trampoline* as this minimizes stress to the injured knee compared with actual jogging. Mini-trampoline jogging is initiated only if the involved knee is free of pain and swelling with exercise.[102] *Upper body strengthening* in the form of rowing exercise is a form of **aerobic activity** necessary to maintain the athlete's cardiopulmonary conditioning. Well-leg bicycling may be initiated within a few days following surgery. Finally, the implementation of *sport-specific drills* allow the athlete to regain confidence in the injured extremity.

51. What physical therapy is appropriate following postoperative PCL repair?

Following surgery, the patient is placed in a knee brace locked at 0° of extension. Weight bearing as tolerated is allowed while using two crutches. Hip strengthening exercises, straight leg raises, isotonic knee extension, and isometric quadriceps are allowed, whereas isometric hamstring exercises are contraindicated because of

the possible increases to posterior stress on the knee. At 3 weeks after surgery the brace may be adjusted to allow 0° to 90° of knee flexion. Stationary bicycling is permitted when the patient has attained 115° of knee flexion. The patient then progresses to resistive quadriceps exercises, but avoidance of gastrocnemius stretching. The brace may be adjusted to full range of motion at 6 weeks after surgery. Toe raises may be initiated. Active knee flexion exercises in the form of hamstring curls may not be incorporated into the rehabilitation program until 2 months postoperatively.

RECOMMENDED READING

Bessette GC, Hunter RE: The anterior cruciate ligament, *Orthopedics* 13(5), 1990.

REFERENCES

1. Abbot LC, et al: Injuries to the ligaments of the knee joint, *J Bone Joint Surg [Am]* 26:503, 1944.
2. Abdalla FH, Tehranzadeh J, Horton JA: Avulsion of lateral tibial condyle in skiing, *Am J Sports Med* 10:368, 1982.
3. Akeson WH, Amiel D, Mechanic DL et al: Collagen cross-linking alterations in joint contractures, *Connect Tissue Res* 5:15, 1977.
4. Akeson WH, Amiel D, Woo SL: Immobility effects on synovial joints: the pathomechanics of joint contracture, *Biotechnology* 17:95, 1980.
5. Akeson WH: An experimental study of joint stiffness, *J Bone Joint Surg* 43(A):1022, 1961.
6. Albert S, Katz R, Schneider M et al: Imaging of the knee. In Nicholas JA, Hershman EB editors: *The lower extremity and spine,* ed 2, vol 1, St Louis, 1995, Mosby.
7. Anderson AF, Snyder RB: "Instrumented evaluation of anterior knee laxity: a comparison of five devices." Paper presented at the Special Day Meeting of the American Orthopaedic Society for Sports Medicine. San Francisco, 1990.
8. Apley AG: Instability of the knee resulting from ligamentous injury: a plea for plain words, *J Bone Joint Surg* 62B:515, 1980.
9. Arnoczky SP: Anatomy of the anterior cruciate ligament, *Clin Orthop* 1983;172:19-25. And: Arnoczky SP: Blood supply to the anterior cruciate ligament and supporting structures, *Orthop Clin North Am* 16(1):15-28, 1985.
10. Baker CL, Norwood LA, Hughston JC: Acute combined posterior cruciate and posterolateral instability of the knee, *Am J Sports Med* 12:204, 1984.
11. Barrack R, Skinner H, Buckley S: Proprioception in the anterior cruciate ligament deficient knee, *Am J Sports Med* 17:1, 1989.
12. Beynnon BD, Pope MH, Wertheimer CM, et al: The effect of functional knee-braces on strain on the anterior cruciate ligament in vivo, *J Bone Joint Surg* 74A:1298, 1992.
13. Black KP, Raasch WG: Knee braces in sports. In Nicholas JA, Hershman EB editors: *The lower extremity and spine,* ed 2, vol 1, St Louis, 1995, Mosby.

14. Brewster CE, Seto JL, Shields CL Jr et al: Rehabilitation of the knee. In Nicholas JA, Hershman EB editors: *The lower extremity and spine,* ed 2, vol 1, St Louis, 1995, Mosby.

15. Brody DM: *Clinical symposia: running injury-prevention and management,* vol 39, no. 3, Summit, NJ, 1987, CIBA-GEIGY.

16. Brotzman SB: *Clinical orthopaedic rehabilitation,* St Louis, 1996, Mosby.

17. Campbell's Orthopedics-Mosby.

18. Clancy WG: Anterior cruciate ligament functional instability, *Clin Orthop* 1172:102-106, 1983.

19. Clancy WG, Nelson DA, Reider B et al: Anterior cruciate ligament reconstruction using one-third of the patellar ligament, augmented by extra-articular tendon transfers, *J Bone Joint Surg* 64A:352-359, 1982.

20. Corsetti JR, Jackson DW: Failure of anterior cruciate ligament reconstruction, *Clin Orthop Related Res* 323:42-49, 1996.

21. Costill DL, Coyle EF, Fink WF et al: Adaptations in skeletal muscle following strength training, *J Appl Physiol* 46:96, 1979.

22. Coyle EF, Feiring DC, Rotkis TC et al: Specificity of power improvements through slow and fast isokinetic training, *J Appl Physiol* 51:1437, 1981.

23. Dandy DJ: *Essential orthopaedics and trauma,* Edinburgh, 1989, Churchill Livingstone.

24. Daniel DM, Malcolm LL, Losse G et al: Instrumented measurement of anterior laxity of the knee, *J Bone Joint Surg* 1985; 67A:720-726.

25. Davis DS, Post WR: Segond fracture: lateral capsular ligament avulsion, *J Orthop Sports Phys Ther* 25(2):103-106, 1997.

26. DeHaven KE, Bronstein RD: Injuries to the menisci of the knee. In Nicholas JA, Hershman EB editors: *The lower extremity and spine,* ed 2, vol 1, St Louis, 1995, Mosby.

27. DeLee JC, Riley MB, Rockwood CA: Acute posterolateral rotary instability of the knee, *Am J Sports Med* 11:199, 1983.

28. DiStefano VJ: Skeletal injuries of the knee. In Nicholas JA, Hershman EB editors: *The lower extremity and spine,* ed 2, vol 1, St Louis, 1995, Mosby.

29. Donaldson WF, Warren RF, Wickiewicz T: A comparison of acute anterior cruciate ligament examinations: initial versus examination under anesthesia, *Am J Sports Med* 13:5, 1985.

30. Ellison AE: *Clinical symposia: skiing injuries,* vol 29, no. 1. U.S.A., 1977, Ciba Pharmaceutical.

31. Feagin JA, Curl WW: Isolated tear of the anterior cruciate ligament: five-year follow-up study, *J Orthopaedic Sports Phys Ther* 12:6, 1990.

32. Feagin JA, Walton WC: Isolated tears of the anterior cruciate ligament: 5-year follow-up study, *Am J Sports Med* 4:95, 1976.

33. Fetto JF, Marshall JL: Injury to the anterior cruciate ligament producing the pivot shift sign: an experimental study on cadaver specimens, *J Bone Joint Surg* 61A:710, 1979.

34. Fetto JF, Marshall JL: The natural history and diagnosis of anterior cruciate ligament insufficiency, *Clin Orthop* 147:29, 1980.

35. Fochios D, Nicholas JA: Football injuries. In Nicholas JA, Hershman EB editor: *The lower extremity and spine,* ed 2, vol 2, St Louis, 1995, Mosby.

36. Furman W, Marshall JL, Girgis FG: The anterior cruciate ligament: a functional analysis based on postmortem studies, *J Bone Joint Surg* 58A:179, 1978.

37. Galway HR, Beaupre A, MacIntosh D: Pivot shift: a clinical sign of symptomatic anterior cruciate insufficiency, *J Bone Joint Surg* 54B:763, 1972.

38. Galway HR, MacIntosh DL: The lateral pivot shift: a symptom and sign of anterior cruciate ligament insufficiency, *Clin Orthop* 147:45, 1980.

39. Gilquist J, Hagberg G, Oretorp N: Arthroscopy in acute injuries of the knee joint, *Acta Orthop Scand* 48:190-196, 1977.

40. Girgis FG, Marshall JL, Monajem ARS: The cruciate ligaments of the knee joint: anatomical, functional, and experimental analysis, *Clin Orthop* 106:216, 1975.

41. Goss M: *Gray's anatomy,* ed 29, Philadelphia, 1973, Lea & Febiger.

42. Grana WA, Muse G: The effect of exercise on laxity in the anterior cruciate ligament-deficient knee, *Am J Sports Med* 16(6):586, 1988.

43. Gray H: *Gray's anatomy,* Philadelphia, 1974, Lea & Febiger.

44. Greenfield BH: *Rehabilitation of the knee: a problem-solving approach,* Philadelphia, 1993, FA Davis.

45. Grimby G, Gustafsson E, Peterson L, et al: Quadriceps function and training after knee ligament surgery, *Med Sci Sports Exerc* 12:70, 1980.

46. Grood ES, Noyes FR, Butler DL: Biomechanics of the knee extension exercise, *J Bone Joint Surg* 65A:725-734, 1984.

47. Haggmark TN, Eriksson E: Cylinder or mobile cast brace after knee ligament surgery, *Am J Sports Med* 7:48, 1979.

48. Hellebrandt FA et al: Influence of bimanual exercise on unilateral work capacity, *J Appl Physiol* 2:452, 1950.

49. Hellebrandt FA et al: Tonic neck reflexes in exercises of stress in man, *Am J Phys Med* 35:144, 1956.

50. Hellebrandt FA, Waterland JC: Indirect learning: the influence of unimanual exercise on related muscle groups of the same and the opposite side, *Am J Phys Med* 41:45, 1962.

51. Hey-Grooves EW: The crucial ligaments of the knee joint: their function, rupture, and the operative treatment of the same, *Br J Surg* 7:505, 1920.

52. Hoover NW: Injuries of the popliteal artery associated with fractures and dislocations, *Surg Clin North Am* 41:1099, 1961.

53. Hughston JC, Bowden JA, Andrews JR et al: Acute tears of the posterior cruciate ligament, *J Bone Joint Surg* 62A:438, 1980.

54. Hughston JC, Degenhardt TC: Reconstruction of the posterior cruciate ligament, *Clin Orthop* 164:59, 1982.

55. Hughston JC, Norwood LA: The posterolateral drawer test and external rotatory recurvatum test for posterolateral rotary instability of the knee, *Clin Orthop* 147:82, 1980.

56. Hughston JC, Andrews JR, Cross MJ et al: Classification of knee ligament instabilities. I. The medial compartment and cruciate ligaments, *J Bone Joint Surg* 58A:159, 1976.

57. Hughston JC, Andrews JR, Cross MJ et al: Classification of knee instabilities. II. The lateral compartment, *J Bone Joint Surg* 58A:173, 1976.

58. Hunter-Griffin LY: Aspects of injuries to the lower extremity unique to the female athlete. In Nicholas JA, Hershman EB editors: *The lower extremity and spine,* ed 2, vol 1, St Louis, 1995, Mosby.

59. Indelicato PA, Bittar ES: A perspective of lesions associated with ACL insufficiency of the knee. A review of 100 cases, *Clin Orthop* 198:77-80, 1985.

60. Jackson DW et al: Magnetic resonance imaging of the knee, *Am J Sports Med* 16(1):29, 1988.

61. Jacobsen K: Osteoarthritis following insufficiency of the cruciate ligaments in man: a clinical study, *Acta Orthop Scand* 48:520, 1977.

62. Jakob RP, Hassler H, Staeubli H-U: Observations on rotatory instability of the lateral compartment of the knee: experimental studies on functional anatomy and the pathomechanism of the true and reversed pivot shift sign, *Acta Orthop Scand* (suppl 191) 52:1, 1981.

63. Kapit W, Macey RI, Meisami E: *The physiology coloring book,* New York, 1987, Harper & Row.

64. Kaplan EB: The embryology of the knee joint, *Bull Hosp J Dis Orthop Inst* 16:111, 1955.

65. Keene JS: Ligament and muscle-tendon-unit injuries. In Gould JA III editor: *Orthopaedic and sports physical therapy,* ed 2, St Louis, 1990, Mosby.

66. Kennedy JC, Granger RW: The posterior cruciate ligament, *J Trauma* 7:367, 1967.

67. Kennedy J, Weinberg H, Wilson A: The anatomy and function of the anterior cruciate ligament as determined by clinical and morphological studies, *J Bone Joint Surg* 56A:223, 1974.

68. Lehmkuhl LD, Smith LK: *Brunstromm's clinical kinesiology,* ed 4, Philadelphia, 1989, FA Davis.

69. Lindahl O, Movin A: The mechanics of extension of the knee joint, *Acta Orthop Scand* 38:226-234, 1967.

70. Losee RE: Concepts of the pivot shift, *Clin Orthop* 172:45, 1983.

71. Losee RE, Johnson TR, Southwick WO: Anterior subluxation of the lateral tibial plateau, *J Bone Joint Surg* 60A:1015, 1978.

72. Lucie RS, Wiedel JD, Messner DG: The acute pivot shift: clinical correlation, *Am J Sports Med* 12:189, 1984.

73. Lynch MA, Henning CE: Physical examination of the knee. In Nicholas JA, Hershman EB editors: *The lower extremity and spine,* ed 2, vol 1, St Louis, 1995, Mosby.

74. Magnusson SP, McHugh MP: Current concepts on rehabilitation in sports medicine. In Nicholas JA, Hershman EB editor: *The lower extremity and spine,* ed 2, vol 1, St Louis, 1995, Mosby.

75. Marshall JL, Olsson SE: Instability of the knee: a long-term experimental study in dogs, *J Bone Joint Surg* 53A:1561, 1971.

76. McDaniel WJ, Dameron TB: Untreated ruptures of the anterior cruciate ligament, *J Bone Joint Surg* 62A:696-705, 1980.

77. McNair PJ, Marshall RN: Important features associated with anterior cruciate ligament injury, *N Z Med J* 103:537, 1990.

78. Meyers MH: Isolated avulsion of the tibial attachment of the posterior cruciate ligament of the knee, *J Bone Joint Surg* 57A:669, 1975.

79. Milbauer DL, Patel SA: Radiographic examination of the knee. In Nicholas JA, Hershman EB editors: *The lower extremity and spine,* ed 2, vol 1, St Louis, 1995, Mosby.

80. Milford L: The hand. In Crenshaw AH editor: *Campbell's operative orthopaedics,* vol 1, St Louis, 1971, Mosby.

81. Mink JH, Levy T, Crues JV: Tears of the anterior cruciate ligament and menisci of the knee: MR imaging evaluation, *Radiology* 167:769, 1988.

82. Mink JH, Reicher MA, Crues JV: *Magnetic resonance imaging of the knee,* New York, 1987, Raven Press.

83. Monaco BR, Noble HB, Bachman DC: Incomplete tears of toe, anterior cruciate ligament and knee locking, *JAMA* 247:1582, 1982.

84. Moore HA, Larson RL: Posterior cruciate ligament injuries: results of early surgical repair, *Am J Sports Med* 8:68, 1980.

85. Moore KL, *Clinically oriented anatomy,* ed 2, Baltimore, 1985, Williams & Wilkins.

86. Muller W: *The knee: form, function, and ligamentous reconstruction,* New York, 1983, Springer-Verlag.

87. Munuera L, Reinoso F, Martinez-Moreno E: "The innervation of the anterior cruciate ligament and the patellar ligament of the knee," thesis, Madrid, Universidad Autonoma, 1992.

88. Netter FH: *The Ciba collection of medical illustrations,* vol 8, Part III. Musculoskeletal system: trauma, evaluation and management. Summit, NJ, 1993, CIBA-GEIGY.

89. Nicholas JA: Report of the committee on research and education, *Am J Sports Med* 6:295, 1978.

90. Nicholas JA: The five-one reconstruction for anteromedial instability of the knee, *J Bone Joint Surg* 55A:899, 1973.

91. Norwood LA, Cross MJ: Anterior cruciate ligament: functional anatomy of its bundles in rotatory instabilities, *Am J Sports Med* 7(1):23-26, 1979.

92. Noyes FR, Bassett RW, Grood ES et al: Arthroscopy in acute traumatic hemarthrosis of the knee. Incidence of anterior cruciate tears and other injuries, *J Bone Joint Surg* 62A:687-695, 1980.

93. Noyes FR, et al: The three dimensional laxity of the anterior cruciate deficient knee as determined by clinical laxity tests, *Iowa Orthop J* 3:32, 44, 1983.

94. Noyes FR, Mangine RE, Baber S: Early motion after open and arthroscopic anterior cruciate ligament reconstruction, *Am J Sports Med* 15(2):149, 1987.

95. Odensten M, Gillquist J: Functional anatomy of the anterior cruciate ligament and a rationale for reconstruction, *J Bone Joint Surg* 67A:257-262, 1985.

96. Odensten M, Lysholm J, Gillquist J: The course of partial anterior cruciate ligament ruptures, *Am J Sport Med* 13(3):183-186, 1985.

97. Pagnani MJ, Warren RF, Arnoczky SP et al: Anatomy of the knee. In Nicholas JA, Hershman EB editors: *The lower extremity and spine,* ed 2, vol 1, St Louis, 1995, Mosby.

98. Paulos LE, Wnoroski DC, Greenwald A: Infrapatellar contraction syndrome, diagnosis, treatment, long-term follow-up, *Am J Sports Med* (in press).

99. Peterson L, Renstrom P: *Sports injuries—their prevention and treatment,* Chicago, 1986, Yearbook Medical Publishers.

100. Pope MH: The role of the musculature in injuries to the medial collateral ligament, *J Bone Joint Surg* 61A:398, 1979.

101. Rasch PJ, Morehouse LE: Effect of static and dynamic exercises on muscular strength and hypertrophy, *J Appl Physiol* 11:29, 1957.

102. Rodrigo JJ et al: Improvement of full-thickness chondral defect healing in the human knee after debridement and microfracture by the use of continuous passive motion, *Am J Knee Surg* (in press).

103. Schutte M, Dabezies EJ, Dimny ML et al: Neural anatomy of the human anterior cruciate ligament, *J Bone Joint Surg* 69A:243, 1987.

104. Shoemaker SC, Markolf KL: In vivo rotatory knee stability: ligamentous and muscular contributions, *J Bone Joint Surg* 64A:208, 1982.

105. Slocum DB, Larson RL: Rotatory instability of the knee, *J Bone Joint Surg* 50A:211, 1968.

106. Steadman JR, Scheinberg RR: Skiing injuries. In Nicholas JA, Hershman EB editors: *The lower extremity and spine,* ed 2, vol 2, St Louis, 1995, Mosby.

107. Strasser H: Lehre der muskel-und gelenkmechanik, Berlin, 1917, Springer-Verlag.

108. Torg JS, Conrad W, Kalen V: Clinical diagnosis of anterior cruciate ligament instability in the athlete, *Am J Sports Med* 4:84, 1976.

109. Trent PS, Walker PS, Wold B: Ligament length patterns, strength, and rotation axes of the knee joint, *Clin Orthop* 117: 263-270, 1976.

110. Tria AJ, Klein KS: *An illustrated guide to the knee,* New York, 1992, Churchill Livingstone.

111. Trickey EL: Injuries to the posterior cruciate ligament: diagnosis and treatment of early injuries and reconstruction of late instability, *Clin Orthop* 147:76, 1980.

112. Vahey TN, Broome DR, Kayes KJ et al: Acute and chronic tears of the anterior cruciate ligament: differential features of MR imaging, *Radiology* 181:251, 1991.

113. Wang JB, Rubin RM, Marshall JL: A mechanism of isolated anterior cruciate ligament rupture, *J Bone Joint Surg* 57A:411, 1975.

114. Welsh R: Knee joint structure and function, *Clin Orthop* 147:7, 1980.

115. Woods GW, Stanley RF, Tullos HS: Lateral capsular sign: x-ray clue to a significant knee instability, *Am J Sports Med* 7:27, 1979.

116. Woo SL, Hollis JM, Adams DJ et al: Tensile properties of the human femur-anterior cruciate ligament-tibia complex, *Am J Sports Med* 19:217, 1991.

117. Zarins B, Fish DN: Knee ligament injury. In Nicholas JA, Hershman EB editors: *The lower extremity and spine,* ed 2, vol 1, St Louis, 1995, Mosby.

118. Zarins B, McInerney VK: Lesions of the meniscus. In Cassells SW editor: *Arthroscopy: diagnostic and surgical practice,* Philadelphia, 1984, Lea & Febiger.

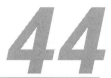

44

Severe Force to the Lateral Knee Joint, or Medial Foot, with and without a Planted Foot Resulting in Excessive Valgus Angulation of Knee During Knee Extension Evaluation

CASE 1: A friend who is an athletic trainer by profession has invited you to a preseason training game of an Olympic soccer team and you eagerly accept. Midway through the game, 2 players from opposite teams attempt to intercept and divert the soccer ball to fellow members of their own team. Each player rushes up to the ball and, with an inward oblique leg swing, attempts to kick the ball in opposite directions. Although both appear to strike the ball simultaneously, one of the contenders for the ball has misjudged its distance and has struck the ground with the medial aspect of his foot just before contacting the ball. The ball flies straight up into the air while the latter player falls to the grass clutching his right knee. Your friend runs onto the playing field to quickly examine the injured athlete before excessive swelling precludes a conclusive evaluation. The player says that he felt considerable pain to the area of his right knee before contacting the ball. After observing the entire evaluation first hand, your opinion is consulted regarding the possibility of injury. After about 5 minutes, the player can stand up and walk off the playing field with some assistance.

SUBJECTIVE The patient reports feeling something "give way" at the time of injury and denies hearing any popping or snapping sound at the moment of injury. When asked to walk several yards, the patient reports no locking, clicking, or giving way at the knee.

OBSERVATION Effusion is moderate. There is no gross deformity.

PALPATION Palpation yields hot and painful tenderness at the right adductor tubercle, and slight tenderness at the posteromedial aspect of the joint line. There is no tenderness present at any of the ipsilateral patellar facets. A painful gap in the soft-tissue continuum of the aspect of the right knee joint is perceived just below the right medial femoral condyle and above the right knee joint line.

RANGE OF MOTION This was decreased in both flexion and extension to an arc of 30° to 85°.

STRENGTH This was untested secondary to pain.

NEUROVASCULATURE Neurovasculature was intact.

SPECIAL TESTS   Valgus stress test performed at 0° is negative, while at 25° knee flexion yields a 2+ grade (3 to 5 mm opening) with a relatively firm and painful end point, although slight give is present. Negative varus stress testing. Negative patellar apprehension and lateral glide test of the patella. Negative Apley compression test. Negative Lachman test with a firm end point. Negative drawer test, although the patient complains of pain when the knee is flexed to 90°. McMurray's test was not performed owing to painful knee flexion. Negative pivot shift test.

RADIOGRAPHS   These show mild medial soft-tissue effusion.

CLUE:

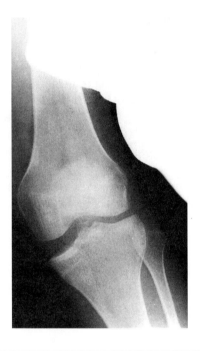

(From Nicholas JA, Hershman EB: *The lower extremity and spine in sports medicine*, ed 2, St Louis, 1995, Mosby.)

CASE 2: A 36-year-old female teacher went skiing during her winter vacation and was beginning to advance to a slope of intermediate difficulty. She reported that, as she was going downhill, she lost some control and veered off the trail toward her right only to impale the tip of her right ski in a snow bank. Although the right portion of her body had come to a relative stop, her left ski continued to move her forward down the slope. Contorted into a wide leg split, her stuck right limb is turned to the outside and she fell backward. The ski binding did not release. Down at the lodge infirmary she complains of a tearing sensation without any audible pop as well as immediate soreness just following the injury with no accompanying swelling. She was unable to ski again for the remainder of her trip and complains of soreness upon activity, and an inability to straighten or bend her knee fully because of pain. When asked, she admits to using a cane in her contralateral hand to relieve symptoms.

SUBJECTIVE   The patient reported a sharp pain to the medial side of her knee. When asked she admitted to being able to extricate herself out of her contorted posture, release her bindings, and gingerly walk down the slope.

OBSERVATION   Observation of gait shows decreased stance time to the involved foot characteristic of a slightly antalgic gait. No swelling or redness is observed.

PALPATION   There is point tenderness at the ipsilateral adductor tubercle and mild tenderness on the medial but particularly of the lateral (superior and middle) patellar facets.

RANGE OF MOTION   Motion is limited in *both* flexion and extension of the involved knee in a range of arc no greater than 25° to 90°.

STRENGTH   At least fair + but untested secondary to pain.

SPECIAL TESTS   Positive lateral patellar glide test, positive (1+) valgus stress test at 25° knee flexion with a painful firm endpoint, trace positive and painful patellar apprehension. Negative Lachman test with a firm endpoint. Negative valgus stress test at 0° flexion; negative painful drawer test, and varus testing both at 0° and at 25°. Unable to perform McMurray's test as extremes of knee flexion are painful. Pivot shift test was not attempted.

RADIOGRAPHS   These show mild medial soft tissue effusion.

GIRTH MEASUREMENTS   Measurements indicate no swelling or effusion.

? Questions

1. What knee structure(s) have most likely sustained injury in these patients?
2. What is the anatomy of the medial static and dynamic knee stabilizers?
3. What are the 3 distinct soft-tissue layers along the medial aspect of the knee?
4. What is the functional anatomy of the medial collateral ligament (MCL)?
5. What kinesiologic role is assumed by the anterior parallel fibers of the tibial collateral ligament?
6. What is the role of reflex muscle contraction in preventing injury to the knee joint?
7. What is the pathology of MCL sprain?
8. What is the classification of MCL sprain?
9. What is the contact mechanism of injury to the MCL?
10. What patterns of injury are derived from incrementally increasing varus and valgus forces to the knee?
11. What is the noncontact mechanism of injury to the MCL?
12. What is the clinical presentation?
13. What is the significance of the valgus stress test in determining the extent of injury?
14. What imaging techniques are appropriate to management of this injury?
15. What is the differential diagnosis?
16. What therapeutic management is appropriate to the patient with an isolated sprain of the MCL?
17. What potential sequelae may occur from an unresolved third-degree sprain of the MCL?
18. What are the histologic stages of healing of the MCL?
19. What sequelae may occur in the untreated MCL sprain, where the rupture site is at the medial femoral condyle?
20. Describe mechanism and management of the fibular collateral ligament.
21. How is a nonisolated injury of the MCL best managed?

1. What knee structure(s) have most likely sustained injury in these patients?

Isolated tear or *sprain* of the *medial collateral ligament* (MCL) and capsular complex in the absence of injury to other knee restraining mechanisms for both cases. The clue provided in Case 1 showed a positive valgus stress film to the involved knee. Medial collateral ligament sprain occurs more frequently than sprain of other knee ligaments. The mechanism of injury to the MCL is caused by a severe valgus force imparted to the lateral knee joint with or without a secured foot; alternately, injury may be incurred from a severe varus force to the medial foot. The common denominator to either mechanism results in disruptive force delivered to the medial knee restraining structures that normally check excessive medial gapping of the tibiofemoral joint. In contact sports such as American football, sprain of the MCL is the most common injury. In noncontact sports such as skiing, sprain of the MCL represents approximately 35% of all skiing injuries. Injury may also be sustained in such sports as wrestling, soccer, basketball, and tennis.

Based on the mechanism of injury and results of the manual examination, the first patient probably sustained an isolated grade II sprain, tearing both the superficial and the meniscofemoral portion of the deep MCL. The cause of injury involved a direct-contact mechanism of injury. There is no concurrent injury to the medial patellofemoral ligament, cruciate ligaments, or medial meniscus as evidenced by provocative testing. The second patient probably sustained a grade I sprain of the superficial MCL due to a noncontact type injury, as well as minor trauma to the medial patellofemoral ligament minus injury to the medial meniscus or the cruciate ligaments.

2. What is the anatomy of the medial static and dynamic knee stabilizers?

The medial stabilizing structures at the knee consist of both dynamic and static components. The MCL provides static support to the medial aspect of the knee joint. It is a strong, flat, two-layered band that runs inferoanteriorly and extends between the medial condyles of the femur and tibia. The MCL is actually composed of a superficial layer called the *tibial collateral ligament,* as well as deeper component of the *posteromedial joint capsule* and is firmly attached to the periphery of the medial meniscus. The *dynamic medial knee stabilizers* consist of the insertions of the semimembranosus and the pes anserine muscle group,

namely, the gracilis, sartorius, and semitendinosus muscles.

3. What are the 3 distinct soft tissue layers along the medial aspect of the knee?

The medial static restraints at the knee joint are divided into 3 basic layers (Fig. 44-1) each of which is comprised of deep meniscofemoral and meniscotibial components, as well as a superficial tibial collateral ligament. *Layer I* is the most superficial and consists of *fascia* overlying the vastus medialis, MCL, and sartorius tendon proximal to the pes anserine insertion on the anteromedial tibia. This fascia is continuous with the deep fascia of the thigh and leg, and extends from the extensor apparatus (including the patella) anteriorly to the popliteal fossa posteriorly. Posteriorly, this fascial layer is contiguous with the fascia of the lower leg, where it overlies the medial head of gastrocnemius.

Layer II contains the triangle shaped *superficial MCL,* which arises from the medial femoral epicondyle, and is composed of *anterior parallel fibers* and *oblique posterior fibers.* The anterior parallel fibers originate from the medial femoral condyle at the adductor tubercle and narrow as they descend distally to insert on the medial tibial metaphysis, that is, the anteromedial tibia 4 to 5 cm distal to the knee joint line and just posterior and deep to the pes anserinus.

The posterior oblique fibers converge toward the posteromedial corner of the knee joint from above and below and joins with the deep portion of the MCL to form a thickened pouch that envelops the medial femoral condyle known as the *posteromedial capsule* or *posterior oblique ligament.* The posteromedial capsule is the convergence of fibers from the posterior obliquely oriented fibers of the superficial MCL and the deep MCL, and represent a thickening of the posteromedial knee joint capsule.

Layer III consists of the knee joint capsule including the deep MCL fibers that firmly attach to the medial meniscus and the posterior fibrous capsule of the knee joint. The *deep MCL* consists of the vertical *meniscofemoral* and *meniscotibial ligaments,* which, across their span, join with the posterior oblique superficial fibers to form the *posteromedial capsule.* The deep layer of MCL originates from the medial femoral condyle slightly below the adductor tubercle and proceeds distally to attach to the superior aspect of the medial meniscus; this proximal segment of deep ligament is referred to as the *meniscofemoral ligament.* The deep ligament then takes leave of the inferior aspect of the medial meniscus to travel distally and blend into the

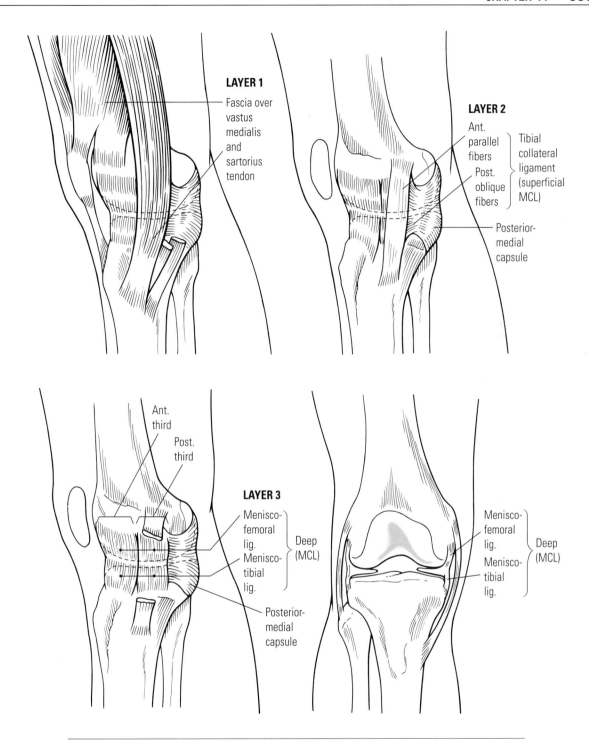

FIG. 44-1 The *medial static knee restraints* are divided into three layers (anterior, middle, and posterior), each of which is comprised of a *deep meniscofemoral* and *meniscotibial* components, as well as a *superficial tibial collateral ligament*.

superficial ligament along the proximomedial tibia; this distal stretch of deep ligament is known as the *meniscotibial ligament.*

4. What is the functional anatomy of the medial collateral ligament (MCL)?

The kinesiology of the MCL is determined by its origin and insertional span between the medial femoral and tibial condyles, as well as the anteroinferior orientation of the superficial aspect of that ligament. Thus the tibial collateral ligament, by virtue of its location, provides the primary restraint to medial joint valgus stress with the knee in 30° to 40° of flexion. The deep MCL serves as a secondary restraint to valgus stress and may be torn with more force necessary to tear the superficial MCL alone. Restraint to valgus opening at the knee joint is dynamically provided by the pes anserine insertion.

5. What kinesiologic role is assumed by the anterior parallel fibers of the tibial collateral ligament?

The anterior parallel fibers do not act as a single homogeneous unit. Instead, different portions of the parallel fibers take up tension as the position of the knee changes. This phenomenon occurs because the anterior border of the femoral insertion of the superficial MCL rotates cephalad with knee flexion and caudad with knee extension. Although the anterior leading edge of the superficial MCL tightens with knee flexion and relaxes with extension, the posterior leading edge tenses with knee extension and relaxes with flexion. Both the anterior and posterior portions of the superficial MCL tense in unison as they assume a major role in preventing excessive external rotation of the tibia on the femur (as during swing, with the foot free) or medial rotation of the femur on the tibia (as during stance, when the foot is planted.) As such, the superficial MCL may be thought of as a passive antagonist to the popliteus tendon by acting to dampen excessively forceful lateral locking of the knee joint during terminal knee extension. A third function of the superficial MCL is the role it plays as a secondary restraint preventing anterior tibial translation on the femur in the absence of an anterior crucial ligament.

6. What is the role of reflex muscle contraction in preventing injury to the knee joint?

Receptors in the MCL, anterior cruciate ligament, and posterior horn of the medial meniscus can, in theory, initiate a protective muscular contraction response to stave off knee injury (Fig. 44-2). In actuality, however, this does not occur. This is because knee injury occurs so quickly that the rapidity of injurious forces, aided by gravity, outstrip the ability of the reflex arc to initiate protective muscle contraction. Also, knee injuries commonly occur in the relatively extended position rather than flexion.[19] This posture represents a mechanically disadvantaged position for the knee muscles that may spring into protective flexion and extensor inhibition.[13]

7. What is the pathology of MCL sprain?

As excessive valgus torque is created at the knee, the MCL will undergo tension along its length. Persistent disruptive force causes ligament elongation and the tensile limit of the ligament is soon reached as rupture commences. During a slow rate of load, avulsion failure at the weakest link in the ligament will occur, namely, at the ligament insertion onto bone. Thus the tear may occur on the femoral side (65%), the tibial side (25%), or at the level of the joint line (10%.) On occasion, the ligament may tear on both sides of the joint. Preference for the weakest link (femoral tear) in the ligament-bone complex is bypassed during a rapid rate of loading in which a midsubstance tear is common.[1] A valgus force of greater severity will also result in sprain of the deep MCL. On occasion, the meniscotibial ligament may avulse off the distal insertion along with its tibial attachment—the tibial spine. The associated anteroposterior radiographic finding is known as the *lateral capsule sign.* A positive sign has great clinical significance as it is indicative of concomitant insult to the anterior cruciate ligament. As the severity of impact to the medial knee increases the anterior cruciate ligament is loaded and may thus sustain tearing; this may be accompanied by medial meniscus injury resulting in that *unhappy triad* described by O'Donoghue. If the valgus force is extremely forceful, the posterior cruciate ligament may also tear, resulting in anteroposterior as well as mediolateral knee instability.

8. What is the classification of MCL sprain?

GRADE I

First degree sprain involves stretching and possible microscopic tearing of the ligament. Such an injury may cause mild point tenderness anywhere along the length of MCL, slight hemorrhage, swelling, and erythema; the latter may develop over the painful area but usually resolves in 2 to 3 weeks following the injury. Joint laxity is absent both at 0° and 30° and there is no loss of

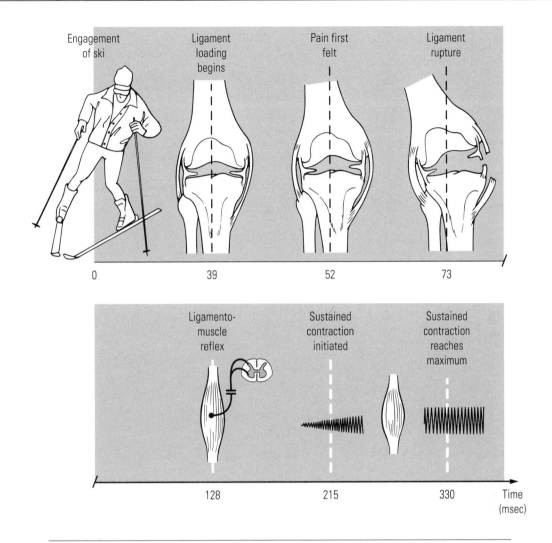

Engagement of ski · Ligament loading begins · Pain first felt · Ligament rupture

0 · 39 · 52 · 73

Ligamento-muscle reflex · Sustained contraction initiated · Sustained contraction reaches maximum

128 · 215 · 330 · Time (msec)

FIG. 44-2 Sequence illustrates how protective muscle contraction is outpaced by the speed of injury.

function. In addition, there is no valgus opening greater than 2 mm, and a firm end point is imparted to the examiner's hands.

GRADE II

Second degree sprain involves partial tearing of the ligament resulting in localized pain, tenderness, swelling, and joint laxity; the latter is particularly noticeable when a provocative valgus stress is applied to the knee resulting in valgus laxity of 3 to 5 mm compared with the contralateral knee. The examiner will feel a firm endpoint with slight give. The sum total of this clinical presentation most probably indicates tear of the deep tibial collateral ligament (known as the meniscotibial

and meniscofemoral portion of the medial capsular ligament) only without concomitant injury to the superficial MCL (Fig. 44-3).

GRADE III

Third degree sprain produces complete rupture of both the superficial and deep portions of the MCL ligament, thereby resulting in an unstable knee joint. Tenderness, pain, severe ecchymosis, and instability may be present. A valgus stress test equal to or greater than 5 mm accompanied by the presence of a soft end point are hallmarks of complete MCL tear. Usually, a complete tear of the MCL presents little tenderness initially, over the first 15 minutes following injury, and occa-

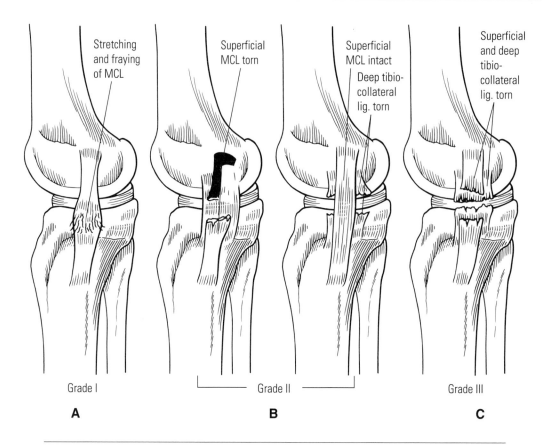

FIG. 44-3 Classification of medial collateral ligament sprains. **A,** Grade I sprain involves ligament stretch and microtearing; **B,** Grade II sprain is a partial thickness tear of either the deep or superficial portions of the medial collateral ligament; **C,** Grade III sprain involves a full thickness tear of the medial collateral ligament.

sionally over the ensuing several days, although instability and puffiness readily establish the diagnosis.[9]

9. What is the contact mechanism of injury to the MCL?

The most frequent mechanism of injury to the MCL is a contact-induced valgus stress to the knee with the foot fixed. This may occur in various sporting situations such as American football or soccer. With the former, MCL sprain typically occurs in rushing defensive linemen, who may sustain a blow to the outside aspect of their knee; this *clipping injury* is inflicted by members of the opposite team in an attempt to knock their legs out from under those linemen. Several factors determine which and how many structures sustain injury. These include fixation of the foot, the degree of femoral and tibial rotation, and the angle of flexion of the knee. Thus it is a simple matter to predict what will be spared with a given injury and what will not. It is certain though that excessive fixation with (femoral and

tibial) rotation in (knee) flexion may result in additional injuries such as torn cruciate ligaments, patella subluxation, as well as lateral tibial plateau compression fracture.[11]

10. What patterns of injury are derived from incrementally increasing varus and valgus forces to the knee?

A clipping type injury in American football is an infraction of the rules, and is due to contact-induced valgus stress to the knee with the foot fixed to the ground (see Fig. 43-9). The *posterolateral* side of the tackler's stance knee receives a valgus blow by the lineman's hip and suddenly forces the tackler's knee into abduction. Because the foot is anchored to the ground, the valgus blow is absorbed by knee flexion with obligatory internal femoral torsion and external tibial torsion. The collateral ligaments are collectively tautened by external rotation while the cruciate ligaments are collectively tautened by internal rotation. Both types of rotation are present as the stance knee receives a valgus directed stress. The external rotatory component tenses both collateral ligaments. However, as the force was valgus in nature, the medial collateral ligament absorbs the brunt of injury. If the magnitude of force is sufficient, then the cruciate ligaments, normally taut by internal torsion, succumb to injury in the form of anterior cruciate ligament sprain due to the internal femoral torsion. The cruciate ligament succumbs to failure before the posterior cruciate ligament because of the *posterior* force component accompanying the lateral blow. This posterior force component imparts an anterior draw to the tibia that further stresses the anterior cruciate ligament. If the magnitude of valgus force is sufficient enough, then injury to a third structure will occur in the form of medial meniscal detachment or tearing. Meniscal injury will occur because of the intimate anatomic attachment between the medial collateral ligament and the medial meniscus, as well as because of the attachment of the medial meniscus to the anterior cruciate ligament via the transverse ligament. The posterior cruciate may also suffer injury if the magnitude of injury is sufficient (Fig. 44-4). This triad injury involving the collateral and cruciate ligaments, as well as the meniscus is known as the *unhappy triad of O'Donoghue.*

The reverse type of injury (Fig. 44-5) involves a varus blow to the medial side of the knee and injures the lateral collateral ligament and possibly the cruciate ligaments as well. The obligatory rotations are reversed, as the force is varus in nature, resulting in external femoral rotation and internal tibial torsion. The lateral meniscus remains unharmed because, unlike the medial meniscus, it has no anatomic continuity with the lateral collateral ligament. In soccer, a common mechanism of injury to the ligament occurs when an inside kick is interrupted by striking another player or a blocked ball or inadvertently inflicting self-injury by accidentally missing the ball and instead hitting the ground with the foot. The injured player will report pain that occurred just before making contact with the ball corresponding to the excessive valgus torque created at the knee.

11. What is the noncontact mechanism of injury to the MCL?

In noncontact injuries, the MCL is usually spared and the anterior cruciate ligament is commonly injured. A skiing injury is the exception to this rule. Consider downhill skiers who gets the tip of their right ski caught in snow while gravity pushes the rest of their mass forward. The caught ski inevitably turns progressively outward causing the body to be contorted into a wide leg split.

This results in external rotation of the tibia and internal rotation of the femur. The patient, now off balance, falls backwards resulting in a valgus stress to the knee. If the ski binding does not release, then the kinetic energy of downhill motion will be converted into strain energy tensing the MCL as the knee is forced into valgus angulation. Note that the anteroinferior span of the MCL prevents rotation of the tibia laterally or the femur medially. The skier's knee, however, is in a predicament that rotates both femur and tibia such that the intervening ligament is maximally stretched at its proximal and distal attachment. The components of external tibial rotation, medial femoral rotation, extension, and abduction are magnified due to the leverage of the long ipsilateral ski.

A similar mechanism may result when a tennis player quickly attempts to hit a low ball, or when the player suddenly twists and falls away from the planted foot. This results in a valgus and external rotation force to the knee that may lead to disruption of the MCL, anterior cruciate ligament, or extensor knee mechanism. Another noncontact mechanism of gradual MCL compromise may be seen during swimming when using the breast stroke.

12. What is the clinical presentation?

The patient usually feels "something give" or experiences a sudden pain or cracklike sensation at the inner side of the knee during the instant of injury. Tearing of the MCL rarely produces a "poplike" sound similar to ACL rupture.[16] Range of motion is decreased to approximately 90° of flexion and the knee demonstrates an inability to perform terminal knee extension. In the closed kinetic chain, that is, during stance phase of gait, loss of terminal knee extension may manifest as pseudolocking of the knee joint. Unlike a displaced meniscus that prevents terminal knee extension due to true locking, the muscles surrounding the joint protectively spring into action to prevent the last 10° to 15° of extension as that range triggers pain by placing the MCL on maximal stretch.

If the deep MCL is also injured, the knee joint will rapidly fill with blood and is warm to the touch. Acute pain and tenderness, present over the palpated course of the ligament, is accentuated by valgus stress testing. Provocative valgus testing is difficult if not performed immediately following injury and may require anesthesia. With first- and second-degree sprains of the MCL an athlete may be able to hobble off the playing field unaided, but may require assistance. With third-degree sprains, the complete disrup-

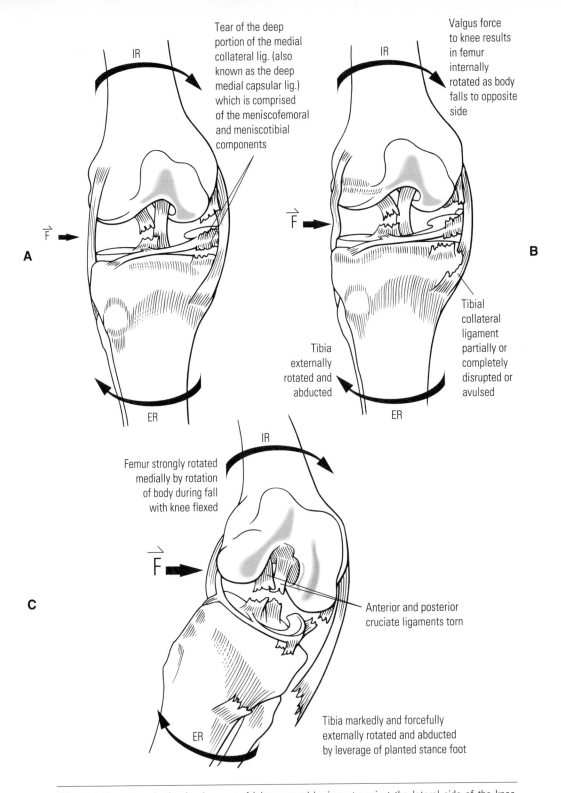

FIG. 44-4 The stages in the development of injury caused by impact against the lateral side of the knee. **A,** If the impact is moderate, then the deep portion of the medial collateral ligament ruptures first; the medial meniscus may become unattached to the medial collateral ligament and allowed to "float." If the impact is more violent, the superficial portion of the medial collateral ligament will rupture as well. **B,** An even more violent impact results in anterior tibial translation and in sprain of the anterior cruciate ligament. If the medial meniscus is still tethered to the deep portion of the medial collateral ligament, it may now sustain a tear due to the intimate association between the anterior cruciate ligament and medial meniscus via the transverse ligament. **C,** An extremely violent impact will cause injury to the posterior cruciate ligament as well.

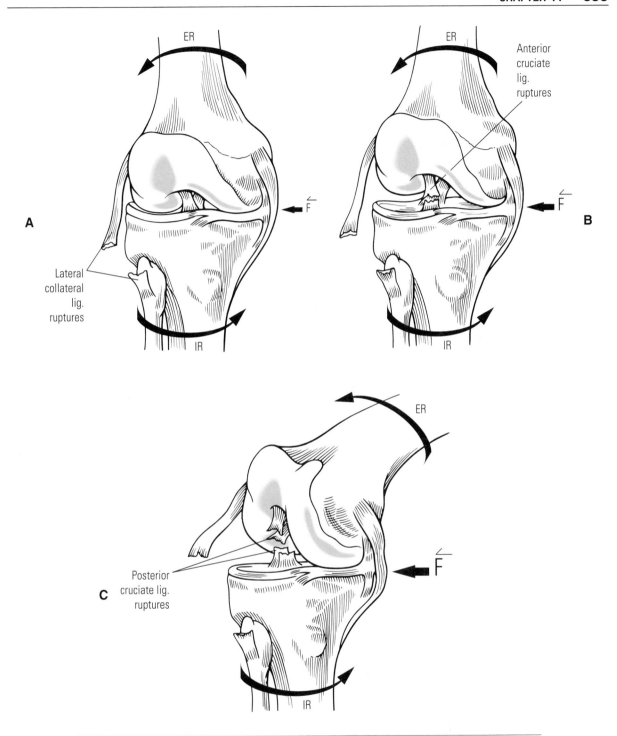

FIG. 44-5 A varus blow to the anchored knee results in injury to the lateral collateral ligament as well as cruciate ligaments, depending upon the magnitude of delivered force. Because of the varus nature of the force, the fixed knee bends into an opposite pattern of obligatory femoral external rotation and internal tibial torsion. **A,** If the impact is moderate, the lateral collateral ligament ruptures. A posteromedial-derived force will injure the anterior cruciate ligament before the posterior cruciate ligament, **B,** and will occur if the force is more violent. **C,** An extremely violent impact will damage the lateral collateral ligament as well as both cruciate ligaments.

tion of both ligament and capsule allows blood to run out of the joint and thereby lessen both swelling and pain. Medical management of sprains of lesser magnitude mandates hemarthrosis aspiration to preclude hemolytic lysis of the joint surface.

Following injury, examination shows localized swelling and tenderness over the site of injury, as well as a palpable defect at the sprain site. Tenderness is maximal at 24 to 36 hours following injury. Tenderness may so diminish over the ensuing days following injury (that is, after the acute stage) that a valgus stress applied to a knee with a complete isolated MCL rupture causes no pain to the patient. A click may even be heard as the medial femoral and tibial condyles approximate at the conclusion of the test. It is important to palpate along the entire span of the ligament. Palpating for the defect may be easier in the slim patient, particularly during valgus testing. The injured patient will often report pain that occurred just *before* a subsequent tearing sensation. If only the tibial collateral ligament sustained injury, the patient can usually continue to walk and may be able to temporarily continue the activity that precipitated injury. As the tibial collateral ligament portion of the MCL is entirely extracapsular, an effusion or hemarthrosis is indicative of injury to other structures in addition to the superficial MCL.

13. What is the significance of the valgus stress test in determining the extent of injury?

Integrity of the MCL complex is tested by applying an abduction stress (valgus force) to the knee in full extension (0° flexion), and at 30° of flexion. Serial testing of the medial knee in these positions helps the clinician identify whether or not an isolated MCL injury and sparing of other ligamentous restraints occurred (Fig. 44-6). A positive valgus (and varus) test in extension will be positive in flexion as well, whereas a positive test in flexion may, or may not, be positive in extension.

The MCL provides approximately three-quarters resistance to valgus opening of the knee joint when the knee is flexed at 30°. However, as the knee approaches full extension, the MCL contribution toward resisting medial opening is diminished to approximately one half, while resistance is increasingly assumed by the posterior and posteriomedial aspects of the capsule, and possibly the cruciate ligaments as well. Thus a false negative for MCL tear may result if the test is only performed in full knee extension. This is because the fully extended knee is stable to both valgus and varus testing even if the MCL is torn due to tautening of the posterior capsular and cruciate ligaments.[8] Hence, valgus testing in full ex-

tension may mask MCL deficiency owing to tightening of the posterior capsule and cruciate ligaments.

By placing the knee joint in 30° of flexion, the clinically distracting contributors toward mediolateral stability are eliminated to all but the medial collateral ligament. This knee posture slightly relaxes the cruciate ligaments and markedly relaxes the posterior capsular ligament. Thus this posture knocks the other structures "out of play" so that isolated testing of the MCL may ensue. The examiner places one hand upon the lateral side of the distal thigh and the other hand at the medial distal ankle and applies a valgus stress to the knee. The leg is initially supported against gravity to allow the condyles to come together before the application of valgus force. The degree of mobility is compared with that of the uninjured side, which is tested first. During this test, the amount of joint opening is visually estimated and the end point or end-feel is palpably estimated. Lack of end point is significant and suggests significant injury. The test is then repeated at full extension. If the knee is stable in full extension but unstable to valgus stress at 30° flexion, then an isolated sprain of the MCL is pronounced. Marked opening of the medial knee joint indicates a complete tear of both the superficial and deep portions of the MCL. Excessive laxity (compared with the opposite knee) in hyperextension signifies complete disruption of the MCL, posteromedial capsule, and both cruciate ligaments. Concomitant cruciate disruption associated with grade II injury may be ruled out clinically, or via stress testing under anesthesia or arthroscopy. For a varus stress test, the direction of pressure is reversed.

Laxity is graded on a 1 to 4 scale, and is subjective from one examiner to another. A 1+ grade equals 5 mm of medial joint space opening with a firm but abnormal end point. A 2+ grade is the equivalent of a 10 mm (1 cm) medial opening with a soft end point, and is suspect for concomitant cruciate ligament injury. When there is a 3+ or 4+ grade (15 mm and 20 mm, respectively) and medial instability at 20° of flexion, the examiner must check for cruciate ligament instability because of near certainty for simultaneous injury.[9]

14. What imaging techniques are appropriate to management of this injury?

Plain radiographs may show nothing more than soft-tissue swelling, whereas stress radiographs filmed under anesthesia reveal the degree of medial joint instability. To rule out bone avulsion, anteroposterior radiographs should routinely be taken. When present, this is most commonly seen at the femoral attachment. Adolescents, who by definition are skeletally immature,

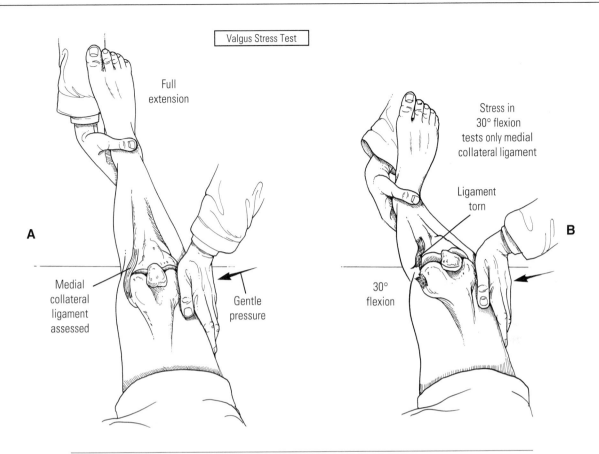

FIG. 44-6 The valgus stress test in **(A)** extension tests the medial collateral ligament and posteromedial capsule. If positive, the results of this test indicate a severe lesion and indicate that the posterolateral force upon the knee is of sufficient magnitude as to injure the cruciate ligaments and perhaps the medial meniscus as well. If positive, the clinician will then follow up by performing anterior and posterior Lachman tests, as well as provocative testing for meniscal integrity. **B,** Stress testing in 30° of knee flexion tests only the medial collateral ligament. (From Scuderi GR, McCann PD, Bruno PJ: *Sports medicine: principles of primary care,* St Louis, 1997, Mosby.)

may sustain excessive medial knee joint opening due to separation the distal femoral epiphyseal plate. Epiphyseal plate closure represents the "weak link" in the skeletally immature. Therefore a stress film is necessary in the young patient to demonstrate that laxity to valgus stress is caused by separation at the joint line or at the epiphyseal plate. On the other hand, an older person with osteoporosis is more likely to demonstrate excess laxity valgus opening due to a lateral tibial plateau fracture. Magnetic resonance imaging may differentiate between a sprain of the superficial and deep aspects of the MCL as well as identify the actual site of tear.

15. What is the differential diagnosis?

The same mechanism of injury that causes tear of the MCL may also result in several types of osseous injury

that the astute clinician must be aware of (Fig. 44-7). Generally, the differential diagnosis for sprain of the MCL includes:

- *Detached meniscus.* The menisci usually tear when subjected to compression and shear forces. As such, the medial meniscus is not usually torn when the knee sustains a valgus stress that sprains the MCL. However, the medial meniscus may be *torn away* from its tibial attachments when the meniscotibial ligament tears and is viewed as a detached rather than a torn meniscus. Meniscal pathology requires surgical intervention.

- *Medial meniscus tear.* The firm attachment of the deep medial collateral ligament to the medial meniscus is of considerable clinical significance because injury to that portion of the MCL complex may result in con-

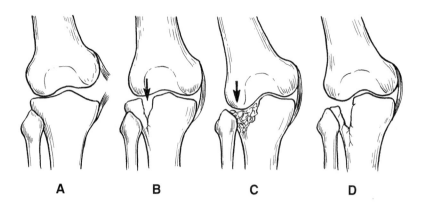

FIG. 44-7 Injuries from a force to the lateral side of the knee: **(A)** MCL rupture; **(B)** vertical split in the lateral plateau; **(C)** crush fracture of the lateral plateau; **(D)** crush and split of the lateral plateau. (From Dandy DJ: *Essential orthopaedics and trauma,* ed 2, Edinburgh, 1993, Churchill Livingstone.)

comitant injury to the medial meniscus. Medial tear is approximately 20 times more likely to occur than lateral meniscus tear mainly because the former is relatively larger and less mobile owing to its attachment to the MCL. Injury to the medial meniscus results from a sudden twisting strain to the flexed knee joint during a weight-bearing activity such as may occur during a cutting maneuver while running. A second-degree sprain of the MCL may result in tearing of the medial meniscus. The fragment of torn cartilage may become displaced toward the center of the joint and lodge between the tibial and femoral condyles. This "locks" the knee in the flexed posture and may prevent the patient from fully extending the knee. A more benign form of this condition only causes "clicking." Localized tenderness and pain, unlike MCL sprain, are elicited in the flexed knee posture on the medial side of the patellar ligament, just proximal to the medial tibial plateau. Whereas a medial meniscus tear in soccer may appear right after striking the ground while attempting an inside kick on a ball, the player with a sustained MCL sprain complains of pain just before making contact with the ball.[18]

- *Unhappy triad of O'Donoghue.* This is classically considered to include injury to the MCL, ACL, and tear of the peripheral medial meniscus. At present, it is believed that the injury often involves the lateral meniscus. This injury follows an infraction of football rules known as *clipping.* Such patients are encouraged to undergo magnetic resonance imaging and arthroscopic examination of the knee to determine extent of injury, with particular attention paid to these triad structures.

- *Common peroneal nerve injury.* The peroneal nerve derives from the bifurcation of the sciatic nerve at the proximal margin of the popliteal fossa. It then runs in an exposed fibro-osseous tunnel in the region of the fibular neck before dividing into its three terminal divisions. It is at its superficial exposure at the fibular neck that it may be subjected to excessive momentary compression from a valgus force to the outer knee joint. Alternatively, the nerve may sustain overstretching from a varus force at the knee that simultaneously sprains the lateral collateral ligament.[12] The common peroneal nerve supplies the dorsiflexors of the ankle and evertors of the foot, and sensation from the distolateral surface of the leg and dorsum of the foot.

- *Patellar subluxation.* This may occur from the same mechanism of injury that causes MCL sprain, namely, knee flexion between 25° and 30°, external tibial rotation, and the body force moving to cause a valgus stress. This mechanism may also cause injury to both the MCL and medial patellofemoral ligament. Hence, point tenderness at the adductor tubercle may indicate sprain of the superficial MCL (the TCL) as this site serves as the origin of that ligament; however, because the adductor tubercle also serves as an origin of the medial patellofemoral ligament, tearing of this ligament owing to lateral patellar subluxation will similarly cause point tenderness at the adductor tubercle. Thus point tenderness at the adductor tubercle raises a high index of suspicion for the possibility of isolated or concomitant sprain on the medial patellar restraints. Differentiating between these two different sprains is accomplished by several clinical tests. The *lateral patellar glide test* produces a stretch of the medial patellofemoral ligament. If injury to this structure has occurred, the test results include pain and increased patellar translation as compared contralaterally. Also, tenderness of the lateral patellar facets scores positive following lateral patellar subluxation. Range of motion (ROM) is a clear indicator of sprain to either ligament as is limited in both flexion and extension when only the MCL is involved; whereas with patellar subluxation, only one motion is limited. Finally, following patellar subluxation, there appears to be more knee joint effusion than in the presence of grade I sprain of the MCL.

16. What therapeutic management is appropriate to the patient with an isolated sprain of the MCL?

In the past, most MCL injuries were treated by cylindrical cast immobilization or surgical repair and postoperative cast immobilization for 6 to 10 weeks. The latter approach was supported by belief that if a primary repair were not performed, the torn ligament ends may not remain in closed apposition and result in prolonged and biomechanically inferior healing. The recent trend in management philosophy has veered diametrically toward promoting early motion and purporting that surgery has no role in the treatment of isolated MCL injury.[18] This is directly attributable to recent studies proving that tensile strength and biomechanical properties are maximized following injury if immediate motion and early exercise without surgical intervention were implemented. Investigators also reported that the longer the immobilization period, the lower the load to failure. Subsequently, the mainstay of current management to MCL sprain advocates minimizing immobilization by way of immediate motion and exercise without overstressing healing tissue in a program that is adaptable to each patients individual needs. This rehabilitative approach serves to provide a stimulus to the medial capsule toward earlier and better healing. The essential concepts in MCL rehabilitation are motion and controlled stress to the torn ligament that serves to accelerate regeneration and remodeling of the injured ligament.

The only drawback of nonsurgical management may occur in the knee with marked instability to valgus stress. Such a knee has slightly more residual valgus laxity when treated nonoperatively as compared to the repaired MCL. On the other hand, valgus laxity alone rarely causes functional instability except in highly competitive athletes or in the patient with physiologic genu valgum. Surgical management is appropriate in the event of double tears, or third-degree sprains in which both the cruciate ligaments have torn and the meniscus has avulsed (detached) following knee dislocation.

PHASE I—WEEK I

The goal of phase I MCL management is the initiation of *immediate motion* in a nonpainful arc to prevent the deleterious effects of immobilization while simultaneously facilitating acceleration of collagen synthesis and organization. Overaggressive stretching or painful motion may retard the healing process by stressing the injured ligament.[16] The rate of rehabilitation is determined by the degree of pain and the amount of restricted motion.[19]

Full weight bearing is immediately encouraged for the first-degree injury, while second-degree injuries are initially only permitted partial weight bearing. When in doubt as to the weight-bearing status in the grade I type injury, it is best to conservatively recommend painless ambulating via partial weight bearing because walking through the pain, even with crutches, may contribute toward retraumatization of the ligament. The patient may progress to full weight bearing as soon as swelling and pain subside. The exception to the former injury is the patient who has physiologic genu varum, and is therefore best placed on partial weight bearing. If a patient demonstrates significant valgus alignment (greater than 10° to 15°), the medial compartment will sustain excessive distractive forces that may actually retard healing. Ambulation with an *assistive device* is employed for several days or until acute symptoms subside with a first-degree sprain, and up to 2 weeks for a second-degree sprain. The beneficial physiologic benefits of weight bearing include nourishment to the articular cartilage and subchondral bone.[16]

The application of ice for 20 minutes every 2 waking hours, compression with an elastic wrap, elevation and rest are indicated to decreasing inflammation. A knee immobilizer *brace* may be used to protect the healing knee ligament,* particularly at night.

Because the quadriceps femoris muscle, particularly the vastus medialis oblique, atrophies at a faster rate than other muscles surrounding the knee joint following knee injury,[5,6,15] or quadriceps femoris shutdown may occur. The latter is defined as the patient's inability to perform an isometric quadriceps femoris

---

*The use of prophylactic knee bracing in sports has not been proven to reduce the number or severity of injury. The use of hinged knee bracing is forbidden in most organized soccer games.

muscle contraction or to exhibit quadriceps femoris muscle control,[16] particularly terminal knee extension. This is staved off by the implementation of immediate quadriceps femoris muscle strengthening exercises. Voluntary contraction may be augmented by the use of muscle reeducation through neuromuscular electrical stimulation.[16]

Passive range of motion activities are immediately initiated followed by *active assistive exercises* in non-painful ranges. *Active range of motion* is then permitted in a cold whirlpool bath and warm water after several days until 0° to 120° range is achieved. The patient then progresses to *isometric quads,* quadsets, and straight leg raises (SLR). As the acute condition subsides, the patient may perform hamstring setting and well leg exercises. Short arc (30° to 40°) or De Lorme quad isotonic exercises may be performed until the patient can actively and painlessly flex 0° to 90°. Eccentric quad work, bicycling, initial hip abduction and extension, balance drills in the seated position, and maintenance of cardiovascular condition are initiated in the latter half of the first week following injury. The patient may swim for up to 3 to 40 minutes per day with a flutter kick only. Resistive SLR with the maximum weight the patient can raise is performed 12 times and performed for hip abduction and extension; no hip adduction should be attempted at this time.

PHASE II—WEEK II

The goals of phase II management include reestablishment of full painless ROM, restoration of muscle strength, and normalization of gait by weaning the patient off the use of assistive devices. The criteria for progression include no increase in swelling, instability, the presence of minimal tenderness, and passive range of motion (PROM) of 10° to 100°.

Strengthening activities include implementation of *progressive resistive exercises* (PREs) that emphasize multiangle quadriceps muscle extension by way of a leg press machine. Hamstring curls as well as hip adduction are emphasized. *Isokinetic exercises* should begin with submaximal velocities and progress to maximal fast contractile velocities. *Closed kinetic chain exercises* include minisquats, step-ups, and the use of a stair climber machine, stationary ski track, and rowing machine. Proprioception drills using a balance device are performed to assist in the rehabilitation of balance and agility and to facilitate neuromuscular control. Participation in an aquatic training program by way of pool exercises and running (both forward and backward)

helps improve cardiovascular as well as local knee strengthening with minimal joint stress. This low-load activity serves as a prerequisite before initiation of normal running. Stationary cycling at 60 rpm for up to 15 minutes and high velocity tubing exercises are performed. Stretching activities to facilitate improved flexibility of the hamstrings, quads, and iliotibial band are appropriate.

PHASE III—WEEK III

The goals of phase III management include increasing patient strength, power, and endurance as well as the initiation of a gradual return to functional activity. The criteria for progression include no swelling, tenderness, or instability, and the presence of full painless ROM.

In the third phase of management, exercises are progressed with a focus on closed chain exercise, balance activity, endurance, and high velocity training. Exercises are the same as for phase II but are increased in intensity. Agility drills such as lateral shuffle, carioca, figure-of-eights, and cutting movements are begun to enhance coordination, balance, and neuromuscular control. Once full painless ROM is present the athletic patient may begin running while wearing a derotation type brace.[19]

PHASE IV

The last phase of management prepares the patient to return to sport-specific activities as well as a maintenance program. During this phase the patient continues to improve strength, endurance, coordination, and skill. Return to competition is predicated on full ROM, nontenderness, instability, presence of effusion, muscle strength at 85% of contralateral knee, quad strength = body weight (60%), and satisfactory demonstration of proprioceptive ability. Patients should be cautioned that they might feel slight pain along the MCL for up to 1 year following injury, particularly during excessive valgus stress at the knee joint, which may occur during cutting motions.

The treatment of isolated third-degree sprains of the MCL is controversial with the current trend in favor of a *nonoperative approach*. A complete rupture is kept nonweight bearing on crutches for 3 weeks, and the knee brace is kept locked at 45° flexion for 2 to 3 weeks, followed by no more than 90° of motion. During the period of immobilization isometric exercises (such as the straight leg raise and quadsets) are performed; gentle active range of motion exercises may be performed in the brace as tolerated, although restricted weight bearing is continued for 3 months.[3]

17. What potential sequelae may occur from an unresolved third-degree sprain of the MCL?

Chronic MCL instability manifests as persistent laxity to valgus stress in the absence of other knee laxity. Such a knee rarely demonstrates significant functional instability. If the ACL is intact, the knee is stable in the anterior direction and demonstrates a negative pivot shift. If instability is present, an anterior draw sign may implicate injury to the ACL. If chronic instability interferes with function, reconstruction is done using the semimembranosus tendon (Slocum procedure) or advancing the tibial MCL (Mauck procedure).

18. What are the histologic stages of healing of the MCL?

The uninjured MCL is composed of well organized (type I) *dense regular connective tissue* demonstrating a polarity of fiber orientation. Collagen is comprised of three polypeptide protein chains, each of which has a tropocollagen core and together are bound into a triple helix. A first-degree sprain of the MCL involves stretching of the collagen fibers beyond their tensile limit. This causes an unwinding of the ligament's helical configuration. Collagen is stretch resistant and is said to possess the tensile strength of steel. However, once the tensile modulus is surpassed, the unwound helix remains stretched as collagen lacks recoil properties. A macroscopic tear of the MCL results in an injury that is eventually filled with randomly oriented *loose connective tissue,* similar to scar tissue that is progressively organized over time. This process is accelerated by motion and controlled stress to the torn ligament.[16]

Four phases of the healing process of the MCL following sprain have been described including the inflammatory, reparative, remodeling, and maturation phases.[2,14] The earliest phase of healing, the acute or *inflammatory phase,* begins immediately after the injury and lasts anywhere from 48 to 72 hours to 1 week. During this time period, the space created by retraction of tendon ends is filled with blood. Subsequently, necrotic tissue is phagocytosed and is followed by migration of fibroblasts, ground substance, and collagen fibers to the wound site. This extracellular matrix is present in a random pattern within the wound and converts the original blood between the torn ligament ends into a clotted collection of blood known as a hematoma. A *proliferative* or *reparative phase* follows and involves the metamorphosis of the hematoma into a ma-

trix by way of collagen production over a 6-week period. The third phase of healing, the *remodeling phase,* begins at approximately 6 weeks following injury and is characterized by matrix organization. The *maturation phase* involves solidification of the matrix by way of increasing organization. Immobilization has proven detrimental to the biomechanical organization of many soft tissues surrounding joints. After 1 year following a complete MCL rupture, the tensile strength of the medial collateral ligament is approximately two-thirds of its pre-injury state.[17]

19. What sequelae may occur in the untreated MCL sprain where the rupture site is at the medial femoral condyle?

The *Pellegrini-Stieda sign* occurs as a complication of an ignored and untreated first-degree sprain of the MCL at its proximal origin (Fig. 44-8). Instead of a decrease in pain and increase in range of motion over time, the

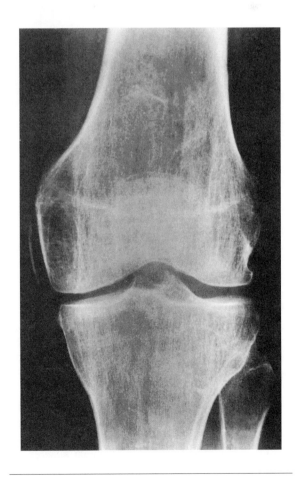

FIG. 44-8 *Pellegrini-Stieda disease.* Ossification of the MCL can be seen. (From Scott WN: *The knee,* St Louis, 1994, Mosby.)

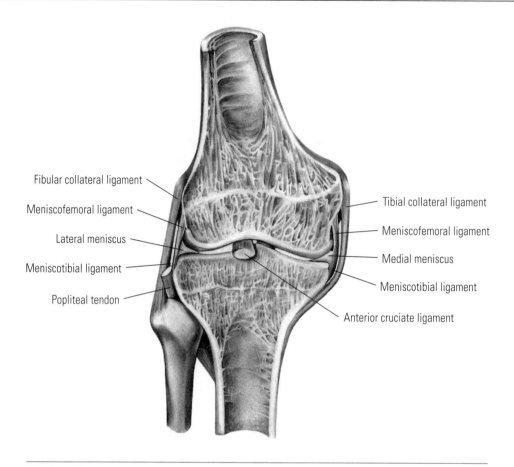

Fibular collateral ligament

Meniscofemoral ligament

Lateral meniscus

Meniscotibial ligament

Popliteal tendon

Tibial collateral ligament

Meniscofemoral ligament

Medial meniscus

Meniscotibial ligament

Anterior cruciate ligament

FIG. 44-9 When comparing the medial and lateral collateral ligaments, note that the lateral ligament, unlike the medial ligament, has no direct connection to its adjacent meniscus. (From Houghston JC: *Knee ligaments: injury and repair,* St Louis, 1993, Mosby.)

opposite occur and become more noticeable some 4 to 6 weeks following the initial injury. A subtle knee contracture may be found. Radiographic changes taken 2 to 3 months following the sprain show that ossification present in the ligament fibers are the actual sign and may be viewed on routine anteroposterior views. Because periosteum was initially torn off the femoral condyle by ligamentous avulsion, the body responds by way of bone ingrowth to fill in the vacant space until build-up reaches the adjacent periosteal fragment still attached to the ligament.

Physical therapy management includes mobilization and usually eliminates symptoms. Recalcitrant cases may receive a local corticosteroid injection, followed by mobilization to regain terminal knee extension. Activity is appropriately modified to eliminate significant valgus stress from the MCL.[19]

20. Describe mechanism and management of the fibular collateral ligament.

The fibular collateral ligament is seldom sprained as most incoming injurious forces approach the lateral rather than medial aspect of the knee. Its thin, cordlike, posterior-inferior span is taut on full extension and, together with the MCL, prevents excessive lateral tibial rotation and medial femoral rotation. Its pencil-like architecture is ascribed to the knee's attempt to provide lateral stability while not interfering with and possibly confounding lateral rotation during terminal knee extension that may be heightened by a broader ligament. The radiographic features, mechanism of injury, as well management of lateral collateral ligament (LCL) sprains are compared to its companion medial knee ligament with the sides reversed. Thus the mechanism of injury resulting in isolated TLC is a contact or non-

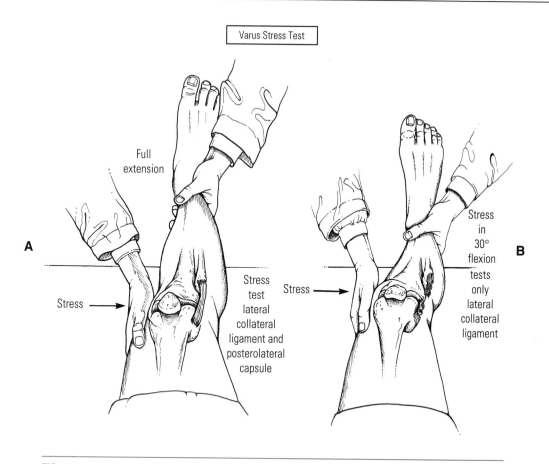

Varus Stress Test

A

Full
extension

Stress →

Stress
test
lateral
collateral
ligament and
posterolateral
capsule

Stress →

Stress
in
30°
flexion
tests
only
lateral
collateral
ligament

B

FIG. 44-10 A positive *varus stress test* of the knee in **(A)** full extension indicates a severe injury that may include compromise of one or both cruciate ligaments, the meniscotibial or meniscofemoral portions of the lateral capsular ligament, the posterolateral corner of the knee known as the arcuate ligament, the popliteus, and the peroneal nerve. **B,** Varus stress testing in 30° flexion tests only the lateral collateral ligament. (From Scuderi GR, McCann PD, Bruno PJ: *Sports medicine: principles of primary care,* St Louis, 1997, Mosby.)

contact hyperextension varus stress. An anteromedial originating force will simultaneously translate the tibia forward and cause concomitant injury to the anterior cruciate ligament (ACL); in contrast, a posteromedial originating force will translate the tibia posteriorly and result in tautening and possible sprain of the posterior cruciate ligament (PCL) given a malevolent force of sufficient magnitude. Sprain is usually associated with a pop, whereas as little or no swelling occurs afterwards. The latter is true because TLC is entirely extraarticular, so that an effusion or hemarthrosis is absent in isolated tears. If an effusion is present, it is suggestive of capsular tearing and possibly tearing of intraarticular structures as well. The LCL is less intimately attached to the joint when compared with the medial ligament, and hence, the clinical signs are less severe.

Thus although a sprain of the LCL will result in warmth and swelling, range of motion is almost full from the outset. Similarly, the lateral meniscus, smaller and more freely movable than the medial meniscus, is less likely to tear, mainly because it is not attached to the LCL (Fig. 44-9).[10] Lateral collateral ligament sprain occurs most commonly on the fibular side in association with a small bone fragment. Palpation reveals tenderness at the posterolateral aspect of the knee that is most marked over the site of injury. The ligament is best palpated with the knee in the figure-of-four position, while simultaneously applying a varus force (Fig. 44-10).[19] The LCL may also sustain injury due to a direct laceration. A complication of LCL sprains includes a traction injury of the lateral (popliteal) nerve. If the knee is unstable to varus stress in full extension, coexisting injury to the posterior crucial ligament is likely present.[4,7] Slower healing of the LCL compared to the MCL requires a longer period of brace protection. Complete tears of the LCL are often managed by surgical repair, with or without augmentation of the biceps tendon.[19]

21. How is a nonisolated injury of the MCL best managed?

In the unstable knee in which ACL compromise has occurred with concomitant to total rupture of the MCL, operative management is appropriate for athletes and young persons. Treatment by immobilization or therapy may be an acceptable alternative to surgery to nonactive middle-aged and elderly persons. However, these patients may eventually complain of occasional momentary instability as when playing tennis or performing other sports related activities. This may occur secondary to momentary forward subluxation of the inner tibial condyle when the tibia is fully laterally rotated while the knee is slightly flexed.

REFERENCES

1. Akeson WH, Amiel D, Lee Jet al: Cartilage and ligament: physiology and repair processes. In Nicholas JA, Hershman EB editors: *The lower extremity and spine,* ed 2, vol 1, St Louis, 1995, Mosby.
2. Andriacchi T et al: Ligament: injury and repair. In Woo SL-Y, Buckwalter JA editors: *Injury and repair of the musculoskeletal soft tissues,* Park Ridge, Ill, 1988, AAOS.
3. Brotzman SB: *Clinical orthopaedic rehabilitation,* St Louis, 1996, Mosby.
4. DeLee JC, Riley MB, Rockwood CA: Acute straight lateral instability of the knee, *Am J Sports Med* 11:404, 1983.
5. Eriksson E, Haggmark T: Comparison of isometric muscle training and electrical stimulation supplementing isometric muscle training in the recovery after major knee ligament surgery, *Am J Sports Med* 7(3):169, 1979.
6. Hastings DE: Non-operative treatment of complete tears of the knee joint, *Clin Orthop* 147:22, 1980.
7. Hughston JC, Bowden JA, Andrews JR et al: Acute tears of the posterior cruciate ligament, *J Bone Joint Surg* 62A:438, 1980.
8. Hughston JC, Andrews JR, Cross MJ et al: Classification of knee ligament instabilities. Part I. The medial compartment and cruciate ligaments, *J Bone Joint Surg* 58A:159, 1976.
9. Lynch MA, Henning CE: Physical examination of the knee. In Nicholas JA, Hershman EB editors: *The lower extremity and spine,* ed 2, vol 1, St Louis, 1995, Mosby.
10. Moore KL: *Clinically oriented anatomy,* ed 2, Baltimore, 1985, Williams & Wilkins.
11. Nicholas JA, Hershman EB: *The lower extremity and spine,* ed 2, vol 1, St Louis, 1995, Mosby.
12. Saunders HD: *Evaluation, treatment and prevention of musculoskeletal disorders,* Minneapolis, 1985, Viking Press.
13. Skoglund ST: Joint receptors and kinesthesis. In Iggo A, editor: *Handbook of sensory physiology: somatosensory system,* vol 2, New York, 1973, Springer-Verlag.
14. vann der Meulen JC: Present state of knowledge on processes of healing in collagen structures, *Int J Sports Med* 3(suppl 1):4, 1982.
15. Wilk KE, Corzatt RD: "Non-operative rehabilitation of grade I and II sprains of the medial collateral ligament in athletes." Paper presented at Combined Sections Meeting, American Physical Therapy Association, Washington, DC, Feb 1988.
16. Wilk KE: Rehabilitation of medial capsular injuries. In Greenfield BH editor: *Rehabilitation of the knee: a problem-solving approach,* Philadelphia, 1993, FA Davis.
17. Woo SL, Inoue M, McGurk-Burleson E et al: Treatment of the medial collateral ligament injury. II. Structure and function of canine knees in response to differing treatment regimens, *Am J Sports Med* 15:22, 1987.
18. Xethalis JL, Lorei MP: Soccer injuries. In Nicholas JA, Hershman EB editors: *The lower extremity and spine,* ed 2, vol 2, St Louis, 1995, Mosby.
19. Zarins B, Fish DN: Knee ligament injury. In Nicholas JA, Hershman EB editors: *The lower extremity and spine,* ed 2, vol 1, St Louis, 1995, Mosby.

RECOMMENDED READING

Fetto JF, Marshall JL: Medial collateral ligament injuries of the knee: a rationale for treatment, *Clin Orthop* 132:206, 1978.
Holden DL, Eggert AW, Butler JE: The non-operative treatment of grade I and II medial collateral ligament injuries to the knee, *Am J Sprts Med* 11:340, 1983.

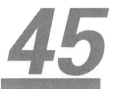

45

Obese, Early Adolescent, with Insidious Onset of Mechanical Obstruction in Knee Extension that is Accompanied by Knee Swelling, and Pain that Varies in Location, in the Absence of Acute Trauma or Giving-Way

An obese and active 12-year-old male is brought to your clinic by his mother complaining of vague and insidious onset intermittent and poorly localized medial knee ache of 4 weeks duration. Symptoms typically intensified with exercise and persisted for a while following exercise. Last week the symptom presentation began to include sudden locking of the left knee in extension that halted his gait midstride pitching him forward. Upon getting up, he found that his knee would bend quite well and so he begins walking and running again until the episode repeats itself. Otherwise, there are periods of aching and swelling that last up to several days. The pain occasionally shifts from the medial to a more central or even lateral side of the knee joint. Although the knee feels as if it might give way, careful questioning as to whether buckling had ever occurred reveals that the patient never experienced a giving-way sensation.

OBSERVATION　An antalgic limp is noted. The left foot appears to be postured in mild to moderate external rotation in relation to the ipsilateral lower extremity. Mild swelling is observed over the left anteromedial knee.

PALPATION　The left knee is warm to touch, and a loose body is inconsistently felt moving within the involved knee cavity. Pinpoint tenderness is confined to the area of the medial femoral condyle.

RANGE OF MOTION　Both passive and active knee extension are inconsistently blocked, whereas knee flexion is normal. Slight tenderness is reported at the left intercondylar notch of the knee during acute flexion.

STRENGTH　Strength of the left quadriceps muscle is one entire grade less then that of the uninvolved knee.

GIRTH MEASUREMENTS　Measurements of both knees indicate mild swelling of the left knee.

SPECIAL TESTS　Negative McMurray sign, positive Apley test initially and negative results when repeated. Forcible compression of the knee joint elicits crepitus during knee flexion and extension. Positive Wilson's sign.

RADIOGRAPHS　A well circumscribed area of subchondral bone separated from the remaining femoral condyle is viewed by a crescent-shaped radiolucent line.

CLUE:

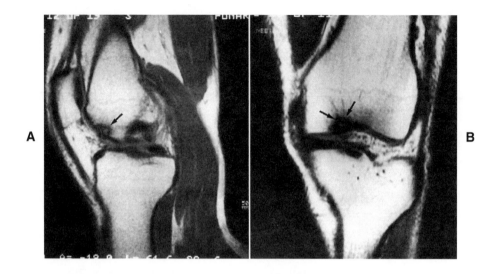

(From Nicholas JA, Hershman EB: *The lower extremity and spine in sports medicine,* ed 2, St Louis, 1995, Mosby.)

? Questions

1. **What is most likely wrong with this boy's knee?**
2. **What is osteochondritis dissecans?**
3. **What are the osteochondroses?**
4. **Where else do the osteochondroses manifest?**
5. **What is the evolution of osteochondritis dissecans in the knee?**
6. **Why are rotations in the transverse plane necessary to the repertoire of body motion?**
7. **What are the various forces contributing to bone fracture, and why is bone least able to withstand torsional forces?**
8. **What is the proposed traumatic etiology of this lesion?**

9. **Why is compressive force greatest in the medial tibiofemoral joint, and how may this account for the greater likelihood of osteochondritis dissecans in obese children?**
10. **What is the proposed ischemic etiology of this lesion?**
11. **What are the clinical features?**
12. **What are the radiographic features?**
13. **What is the differential diagnosis?**
14. **What is the prognosis of this disease?**
15. **What is the conservative management of osteochondritis dissecans and when is it an appropriate intervention strategy?**
16. **When is surgical management appropriate?**

1. What is most likely wrong with this boy's knee?

Osteochondritis dissecans of the left knee. Magnetic resonance imaging (see Clue) shows a sagittal T1 *(A)* and coronal T1 *(B)* scan demonstrating a lesion of the medial femoral condyle *(arrows).*

2. What is osteochondritis dissecans?

Osteochondritis dissecans is an osseous lesion most often occurring on the *posterolateral* aspect of the medial femoral condyle (75% to 85%), the posteromedial aspect of the lateral femoral condyle (15% to 20%), atypically at the lateral trochlear margin of the femur,[45] and the proximal one-half of the patella (5% or less).[16,22,32,35,39] Males with right leg dominance in the second decade of life are most affected,[2] although it may also occur in adults (particularly in the third decade) up to age 50.[36] In females this condition typically presents unilaterally.[25] When occurring in childhood and early adolescence, bilateral pathology for this disease ranges between 25% and 30%. There may be a positive association in obese adolescents with a short or tall body type.[46]

Osteochondritis dissecans literally means a loss of blood supply to an area of bone that is adjacent to a joint surface.[28] The dead subchondral bone and overlying articular cartilage evolves into a separate bone fragment that may either remain attached, partially detached, or completely detached and free to roam within the joint cavity. Fragments colloquially known as "joint mice" may be as large as a hazelnut and are released into the knee joint to elusively move about the synovial cavity[41] and cause mechanical symptoms. The etiology of this lesion is unknown but is postulated to derive from trauma, vascular insult, or genetic predisposition. Although the bony lesion is often the center of attention owing to its visibility on radiographs, maintenance of a smooth overlying articular weight-bearing surface is the significant prognostic factor.[15,30]

3. What are the osteochondroses?

Osteochondritis dissecans is categorized as a type of *osteochondroses,* referring to a disease of the growth or ossification centers.[15] The osteochondroses do not have a simple genetic basis[29] although there must be hereditary predisposition, as several joints of the same patient or several members of the same family may be affected.[28] This suggests a preexisting abnormality in the osseous tissue of some individuals predisposing development of osteochondritis dissecans, and is known as the *constitutional etiologic theory.* Morphologically, osteochondritis dissecans is an avascular necrosis of a pressure epiphyses. Osteochondroses refers to a group of disorders affecting the epiphyses or apophyses during childhood, and are characterized by noninflammatory, noninfectious derangement of the normal process of bony growth occurring at various ossification centers throughout the body at the time of their greatest developmental activity. In the developing child, growth cartilage is present at the *pressure epiphysis* (i.e., the articular cartilage between the tibia and femur), as well as at the *apophyseal tendinous insertions.*[3]

4. Where else do the osteochondroses manifest?

Although most commonly occurring at the medial femoral condyle of the knee as osteochondritis dissecans, osteochondroses may also occur in the capitulum of the distal humerus as Panner's disease, the proximal femur as Legg-Calve-Perthes disease, the dome of the talus, the head of the second metatarsal head as Freiberg's disease, the carpal lunate as Kienbock's disease, the tibial tuberosity Osgood-Schlatter's disease, the vertebra as Scheuermann's disease, the carpal scaphoid as Preiser's disease, the tarsal navicular as Kohler's disease, or at the calcaneus as Sever's disease. Notably, most, if not all osteochondroses involving pressure epiphyses, occur on *convex surfaces,*[28] and many involve joints or bones undergoing *torsional motion* in the transverse plane.

5. What is the evolution of osteochondritis dissecans in the knee?

The evolution of osteochondritis dissecans may be classified by three stages (Fig. 45-1). The convex surface of the distal femur, particularly the subarticular bone beneath the lateral aspect of the medial femoral condyle is susceptible to avascular necrosis and undergoes separation (i.e. dissection*). This represents a stage I lesion in which the defect is evident on radiographs as a bulge on the medial femoral condyle although the articular cartilage is still intact. The overlying cartilage continues to receive nourishment from the synovial fluid and grow larger, while the subchondral bone undergoes circulatory insufficiency and avascular necrosis from the disruption of its blood supply. Thus the fragment not only remains viable but also grows ever larger as the epiphysis matures and may either reunite with its bed or evolve pathologically. Although healing may occur at this stage, excessive activity such as joint motion or repeated impact may prevent capillary ingrowth into the necrotic bone fragment. This results in a stage II lesion in which the fragment is radiologically demarcated by separation of the articular cartilage.

If the ensuing defect is small or located along a different topographical site over the femoral condyle that is nonweight bearing, the consequences are considerably less significant. However, if the defect is large and present over a significant weight-bearing locale such as the lateral aspect of the medial femoral condyle, the medial tibiofemoral joint may become incongruous. In stage III, the overlying hyaline cartilage loosens and separates together with the necrotic fragment of sub-

---

*Dissection of the fragment occurs, not desiccation (drying up).

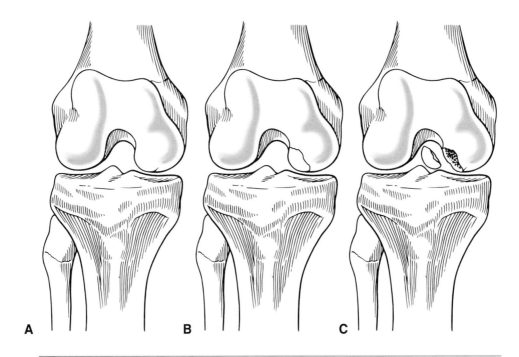

FIG. 45-1 Stages in the evolution of osteochondritis dissecans. **A,** *Stage I.* A bulge forms on the lateral aspect of the medial femoral condyle due to partial separation of the bone fragment. While the articular cartilage is intact, the defect is evident on radiographs. **B,** *Stage II.* The fragment is radiologically demarcated by separation of the articular cartilage. **C,** *Stage III.* The fragment of cartilage and bone have completely separated from the medial condyle. The resultant loose body (joint mice) migrates to the medial or lateral gutter of the knee.

chondral bone from the medullary bone and is free to migrate throughout the tibiofemoral joint. The knee, like an oyster, attempts to compensate for the freely roaming fragment by laying cartilage around it so as to minimize its irregular surfaces, and thereby prevent marring of the articular surface. The fragment will cause no problems if it migrates behind the knee or in the suprapatellar area. It typically migrates into the medial or lateral gutter of the knee joint.[30] The focus of attention following separation and migration of the fragment is not the fragment, but rather the residual defect or crater on the convex articular surface that will continue to bear weight unprotected, resulting in degenerative joint disease. Moreover, should the loose fragment become caught between the condyles, it may result in damage of other portions of the articular cartilage.

6. Why are rotations in the transverse plane necessary to the repertoire of body motion?

During the stance phase of the gait cycle the mechanical linkage comprised of the weight-bearing bones are subject to enormous forces. These forces include super-

incumbent body weight moving rostrocaudal and ground reaction force moving caudorostral. The body moves in all 3 planes during locomotion while minimizing the harmful cumulative effects of these forces. To this end, the many rotations of the body, particularly the lower extremity comprise a *force dissipating strategy* to attenuate the great forces incurred through interaction with the external environment.

7. What are the various forces contributing to bone fracture, and why is bone least able to withstand torsional forces?

Any discussion of pathologic forces causing bone disruption must be prefaced with a discussion of bone structure. The internal structure of bone matrix incorporates a protein fiber called *collagen* that is impregnated with calcium and mineral salts that endow osseous tissue with strength. Although the presence of insoluble calcium salts endow bone with *compressive strength,* the collagen fibrils running through bone withstand *tensile force.* Bone may thus be compared to reinforced concrete in which the concrete provides compressive strength, while the steel bars running through the concrete endow that material with tensile strength.[8,*]

Bone withstands compressive force better than tensile forces. Excessive tension causes the bone cement linking osteons to be exceeded and may result in a bone fracture. A *transverse type fracture* stems from bending on bone causing tensile (distractive) force along the convex surface and compressive (contractive) forces along the concave surface. The fracture invariably begins along the convex surface, as bone is less capable of attenuating tensile forces. In contrast, uniform vertical loading of bone will distort bone by pushing or compressing osteons rather than distracting them away from each other, resulting in a short and squat bone that succumbs to comminution. A *comminuted fracture* typically occurs during a vertebral compression fracture.

The application of shear forces to osseous tissue involves two uniplanar forces moving on the bone in opposite directions with some distance between them. This typically occurs in a ski-boot type of injury in which the downhill skier gets a ski caught in a snowbank. Although the distal tibia is not moving, the proximal tibia—carried forward by the momentum of the superincumbent body weight—continues to move forward. The tibia will thereby undergo an oblique distortion as a function of the imposed shear and sustain an *oblique fracture.*

Torsional stress involves rotation and is defined as a multiplanar force that is, by definition, force that occurs in more than one plane. Torsion forces are serious as bone can least attenuate spiral forces resulting from rotation. The tensile component of torsional force has the potential to exceed the adhesive capacity of the mucopolysaccharides cementing osteons together. This process of pulling osteons apart is referred to as *delamination.* Torsional forces typically result in a spiral pattern of fracture. Internally generated torsional motion or rotation of the bones of the lower extremity in the transverse plane represent part of the repertoire of strategies to diminish and absorb the potentially disruptive forces inherent to locomotion. The femoral condyles represent the potential locus of endogenous trauma due to torsion forces, as a function of engagement of the screw-home mechanism during forceful terminal knee extension. The medial femoral condyle is

particularly vulnerable as the medial tibiofemoral hemi-joint contains the center for the rotational axis of rotation at the knee joint. The epiphyseal growth plate is particularly vulnerable to the application of torsional stress.[3] The collagen tissue comprising the articular cartilage of adolescents demonstrates a greater capacity for plastic deformation while having the benefit of a better blood supply than adults and vastly improved healing ability. However, the rapidly growing porous bone in children demonstrates poorer tensile strength and is less capable of tolerating compressing force. Both of these factors may predispose the articular cartilage covering to the epiphyseal growth plate in the adolescent knee to pathologic development of osteochondritis dissecans.

8. What is the proposed traumatic etiology of this lesion?

Any traumatic mechanism favoring injury to the medial tibiofemoral joint must account for why that hemi-joint is singled out for pathology. The architectural inequality between the anteroposterior projection of the two condyles that favors a longer medial condyle imparts a valgus posture to the normal knee in the erect standing posture. An analogy may be drawn from a Colles fracture of the wrist. During a fall on an outstretched hand, although both the distal radius and ulna may sustain fracture, the radius is the first to sustain injury as it projects more distally than the ulna and is the principal link with the carpus. An analogous situation exists with respect to the medial and lateral tibiofemoral hemi-joints. The medial femoral condyle is longer and larger than the lateral femoral condyle. Because of its relatively greater role in weight bearing, more load is borne by the medial compartment,[11] specifically the lateral aspect of the medial femoral condyle. It is for this reason than osteoarthritis of the knee most typically evolves in the medial tibiofemoral hemi-joint.

In the traumatic etiologic mechanism, osteochondritis dissecans may be thought of as a stress fracture of the subchondral bone of the weight-bearing surface of the femoral condyle. The theory of *torsional impaction*[23] suggests that repeated blows to the lateral aspect of the medial femoral condyle amount to impingement of the *intercondylar eminence* (Fig. 45-2). Torsional impaction is postulated to derive as a function of tibiofemoral rotation[17] during engagement of the screw-home mechanism in which the lateral aspect of the medial femoral condyle impinges upon the tibial spine. The focus of delaminating forces owing to torsion generation may reside in the lateral aspect of the medial femoral condyle. Moreover, as the medial hemi-joint

---

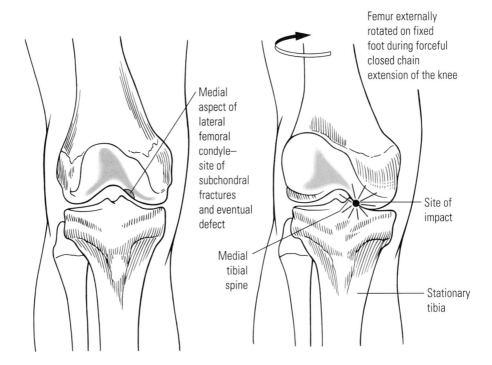

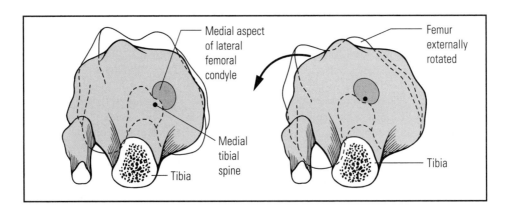

FIG. 45-2 Traumatic etiologic mechanism for osteochondritis dissecans by way *torsional impaction.* This may occur from repetitive and excessively forceful knee extension. Knee extension is accompanied by obligatory torsion at the tibiofemoral joint as the screw-home mechanism is engaged. In the closed kinetic chain the femur laterally rotates on a fixed tibia during engagement of the screw-home mechanism into terminal knee extension. At this end range of transverse motion the locus of torsional delaminating force resides at the lateral aspect of the medial femoral condyle. An additional contributing factor is the concussive force delivered to the lateral aspect of the medial femoral condyle impinges upon the medial tibial spine during full engagement of the screw-home mechanism into knee extension.

contains the center of rotation at the knee, the locus of torsional force may occur at the nonweight-bearing lateral aspect of the medial femoral condyle. Both factors may account for the increased likelihood of osteochondritis dissecans developing in the medial femoral condyle. In contrast, the lateral femoral condyle may sustain injury as a function of its *impressio terminalis* repetitively impinging upon the lateral tibial plateau during terminal knee extension. Eventually, subchondral bone undergoes fatigue failure resulting in minute subchondral fractures that grow with repeated insults.

9. Why is compressive force greatest in the medial tibiofemoral joint, and how may this account for the greater likelihood of osteochondritis dissecans in obese children?

The variation in architectural configuration between the medial and lateral tibiofemoral joints renders the medial condyle more vulnerable to the effects of compressive force in erect posture. Because the medial femoral condyle is larger it may sustain the brunt of superincumbent body weight compared with the shorter lateral femoral condyle. This may account for why approximately one fifth of all medial femoral condyle lesions extend medially to include the weight bearing portion of the medial femoral condyle.[14] Moreover, the knee joint is normally subjected to forces up to 6 times body weight. Obese children may be more prone towards development of osteochondritis dissecans because of increased load on their joints. An additional 30 pounds of body weight can add as much as 180 lbs. in forces to the knee joint.[15,30] Although the classic site for lesion development in osteochondritis dissecans involves the nonweight-bearing side of the medial femoral condyle in normal standing, it may be that twisting motions of the knee bias stress delivery toward the lateral border of the medial femoral condyle. Thus whereas this area is normally nonweight bearing, it may become the focus of repetitive stress due to excessively forceful torsion at the knee that accompanies terminal knee extension and engagement of the screw-home mechanism.

10. What is the proposed ischemic etiology of this lesion?

The blood supply of many bones provides nourishment and has the capability to allow for repair and remodeling in the event of a fracture. *Avascular necrosis* is an occasional but severe complication of high velocity fractures that causes destruction of the blood supply to a segment of bone causing bone cell death. This may occur to bones having a good blood supply that underwent a high velocity injury that stripped away soft tissue and vasculature from the osseous tissue at the time of injury.

Certain bone sites such as the femoral head, talar body, or the proximal pole of the scaphoid are at greater risk to undergo avascular necrosis because of their tenuous blood supply. It is unlikely that the femoral condyles succumb to osteochondritis dissecans as a direct function of dysvascularization as the subchondral area of the distal femur is supplied with a large network of anastomotic vessels.[38] An ischemic etiology is hypothesized to be due to *circulatory insufficiency* deriving from thrombosis or embolization of an end artery as the causative insult[28,33] at the pressure epiphyses of the knee. Such a vascular event may stem from repetitive loading and may result in an obstruction of the blood supply resulting in hypovascularity of the region.

Management consists of a protective regimen for children with the hope that the fragment will reattach to the physis. With adolescents and adults surgery involving reattachment or removal of the fragment will prevent degenerative changes to the articular cartilage.

11. What are the clinical features?

Patients classically present in their early teenage years during the adolescent growth spurt when they are athletically active. Osteochondritis dissecans affects a fragment of articular cartilage and its underlying subchondral bone, and the resulting fragment may remain attached, partially detached, or completely detached and free to roam within the joint cavity. Fragments colloquially known as "joint mice" may grow as large as a hazelnut,[33] are released into the knee joint to elusively flit from place to place within the synovial cavity[41] and cause mechanical symptoms. Clinical findings include intermittent and poorly localized knee pain or ache, occasional joint effusion, giving-way, catching, locking, anterior knee tenderness, antalgic limp, and thigh atrophy. Sometimes tenderness is reported at the intercondylar notch upon knee flexion. The patient may walk with the foot of the affected extremity in *external rotation* in an attempt to ease pain; subsequently, pain may be occasionally elicited with internal rotation of the leg on the thigh.[37,46] Mechanical obstruction such as locking and *catching in knee extension is the hallmark of osteochondritis dissecans,*[37] although giving-way or buckling is absent. Pain may vary in location due to mobile fragments floating within the knee.[10] Symp-

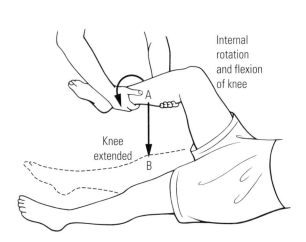

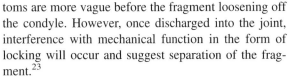

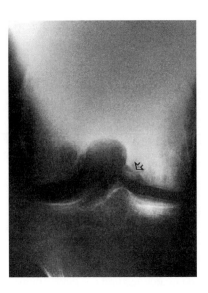

FIG. 45-3 Wilson's Test. In patients with osteochondritis dissecans, pain is subjectively perceived and reported by the patient as the knee is extended.

FIG. 45-4 Osteochondritis dissecans in its "classic" location on the lateral aspect of the medial femoral condyle. (From Scott WN: *The knee,* St Louis, 1944, Mosby.)

toms are more vague before the fragment loosening off the condyle. However, once discharged into the joint, interference with mechanical function in the form of locking will occur and suggest separation of the fragment.[23]

Clinical presentation of osteochondritis dissecans of the patella is ill-defined and resembles chondromalacia patellae with peripatellar and retropatellar knee pain aggravated by activity, especially activities involving weight bearing on a flexed knee. Symptoms are vague with intermittent pain made slightly worse by athletic participation, which may be provoked by patellofemoral compression with the knee in flexion. Retropatellar crepitus, joint effusion, and quadriceps muscle atrophy, and protective hamstring spasm (occasionally) may also be present.

Wilson's diagnostic test involves internal rotation and flexion of the ipsilateral knee to 90°. Pain is subjectively perceived and reported by the patient as the knee is extended (Fig. 45-3). This reaction is explained by abutment of the anterior cruciate ligament from its tibial attachment with the lesion on the medial femoral condyle.[47] Wilson's test *may* score positive for osteochondritis dissecans.

12. What are the radiographic features?

The classic site for osteochondritis dissecans at the knee is at the nonweight-bearing lateroposterior aspect of the medial femoral condyle in the region of the intercondylar notch that is best seen via the tunnel view (Fig. 45-4), although the lateral view helps estimate the size of the lesion. A notch view (anteroposterior view with the knee flexed to 90°) is also helpful in delineating the lesion.[15,30] The lateral femoral condyle and tibial plateau are less frequent sites of involvement.[13] The lesion classically presents as an elliptical, sharply defined area of subchondral bone separated from the medial femoral condyle by a *crescent-shaped radiolucent line corresponding to a secondary ossification center.* When present, loose bodies containing sufficient bone to be radiolucent may be found in the lateral gutters, notch, or posterior compartment. Other forms of adjunct imaging that may prove helpful in identifying osteochondritis dissecans include arthrography, scintigraphy, magnetic resonance imaging, or arthroscopy.[23] A bone scan helps differentiate an acute process from a chronic one.[15,30] Osteochondritis dissecans of the patella typically occurs along the distal portion of the patella and is best viewed on the lateral radiograph, whereas a skyline view may help localize a lesion of the medial or lateral facet. The open physes of juvenile patients may cause difficulty in establishing a radiographic diagnosis because of the normal variations in the distal contour of the epiphysis.[23] The use of bone scans or magnetic resonance imaging is of great value in diagnosis when radiographic changes are subtle.

13. What is the differential diagnosis?

- *Meniscal lesions.* These also manifest clinically as mechanical obstructions towards knee extension as well as knee flexion, whereas osteochondritis dissecans only locks in extension. Thus osteochondritis dissecans may be confused with meniscal impingement of the anterior horn(s). Meniscopathology, however, is uniquely characterized by giving-way or buckling of the knee. This does not occur with osteochondritis dissecans. Moreover, the locking associated with osteochondritis dissecans is of a different quality, and may be said to be more benign than that of meniscopathology. This is because the osteochondral fragment, unlike the meniscal fragment, is not tethered to its original source, but is free to roam about the knee joint. Consequently, provocative tests for meniscal pathology will inconsistently score positive. Moreover, unlike the knee that is locked because of meniscus related pathology, the knee may be unlocked without the need of manipulation.[41] Osteochondritis dissecans may mimic medial or lateral meniscal pathology. Finally, loose bone fragments are readily identified on radiograph whereas menisci are not.

- *Osteochondral fracture.* This fracture of the adolescent knee is very similar to osteochondritis dissecans as it typically involves the subchondral bone of the femoral condyles, as well as the patella. The pathogenesis of osteochondral fracture is derived from trauma that may either be endogenous or exogenous. Endogenous trauma stemming from torsional and compressive forces derived from a partially flexed weight-bearing knee may damage the centrally located portions of one or both condyles.[21] Direct exogenous trauma may include by falling upon a flexed knee or striking a firm object. Lateral femoral condylar exogenous injuries are usually the result of a direct blow, such as a kick to the lateral aspect of the knee, causing an acute subchondral fracture of the anterior and inferior weight-bearing surface of the lateral femoral condyle. Medial femoral condylar exogenous injuries are also incurred from a direct blow to the knee, typically a dashboard injury, causing injury to the medial aspect of the medial femoral condyle.[44]

Osteochondral fractures in adolescents demonstrate hemarthrosis with fat droplets during arthrocentesis whereas adults present a bloodless effusion. The clinical presentation of adolescent osteochondral fracture dramatically differs from osteochondritis dissecans, although strongly resembling injury to the anterior cruciate ligament in the adult. Osteochondral fracture is often accompanied by a history of trauma, typically resulting from torque to the knee. It is rapidly followed by a bloody effusion, pain, and mechanical block. Although osteochondral fracture resembles osteochondritis dissecans both histologically and radiographically, the former does not occur at the classic site of osteochondritis dissecans at the lateral side of the medial femoral condyle.[7] Moreover, the history of osteochondritis dissecans is much less dramatic. A history of trauma may or may not be elicited, or the trauma may have occurred many weeks or even months before the patient is seen. Osteochondral fractures require prompt surgical management[23] as the accompanying locking may cause further injury to the articular cartilage in the event of a delay. Following fracture debridement, an exercise rehabilitation program is preferable to allowing the adolescent to "run it out."

- *Osteonecrosis.* Idiopathic osteonecrosis may involve the medial,[1] or lateral[26] femoral condyles, medial tibial plateau,[12,19] and patella.[24] The etiology of this disease process is controversial and is thought to be either vascular or traumatic in nature. Alcoholism may play a role in etiology due, in part, to fat emboli or to marrow fat deposition with increased marrow pressure.[31,43] Other postulated causes include high dose corticosteroid therapy, vasculitis, atherosclerotic disease, pancreatic disease, radiation therapy to bones, or decompression sickness with nitrogen bubble emboli.[43] The historical presentation includes sudden, constant, and occasionally severe, medial knee pain without history of antecedent trauma or strenuous exertion. Pain in some patients does not begin with bone infarction, but is rather felt only after bone collapse and distortion. While in the acute phase, pain is frequently worse at night and may remain severe for 6 to 8 weeks. Recumbency offers partial relief. Medial tibial osteonecrosis may yield tenderness that is easily confusion with pes anserine bursitis, and is suspected following lack of relief from steroid injection to that area.[43] The incidence of osteonecrosis is three times higher in elderly woman.[26] Although the result of the physical examination are similar to osteochondritis dissecans, osteonecrosis differs in several respects.

Osteochondritis dissecans occurs in much younger patients, presents with a more insidious onset, demonstrates positive radiographic findings on initial presentation, and affects the posterolateral aspect of the medial femoral condyle as opposed to the more centrally located weight-bearing portion. Radiographic findings associated with osteonecrosis are seen as a flattened oval defect over the weight-bearing aspect of the medial femoral condyle whose long axis is aligned in the sagittal plane, some 3 weeks to 2 months after onset of pain. A crescentic line at the right medial condyle is often diagnostic. The differential diagnosis for osteonecrosis includes osteochondritis dissecans, osteoarthrosis, infection, diabetic derived Charcot neuropathy, neoplasm, and other causes of osteonecrosis such as Caisson disease,[27] sickle cell anemia,[34] Gaucher's disease,[4] systemic lupus erythematosus,[40] or following immunosuppression.[5,9,20] Patients with a small osteonecrotic lesion are nonoperatively managed by protected weight bearing, antiinflammatory medications, analgesics, and isometrics.[23] Arthroscopic debridement is indicated if a loose osteonecrotic fragment causes knee locking and refractory pain.[43]

14. What is the prognosis of this disease?

Important factors affecting the prognosis of osteochondritis dissecans include chronological and skeletal age, status of the physis (open or closed), the location of the lesion (in relation to the weight-bearing region) and radiographic appearance of a second ossification center. In young persons (under age 15 years) the damaged fragment often does not separate from the condyle, allowing for spontaneous healing to frequently occur within a year or more. The size of the lesion has prognostic significance such that larger lesions tend to be unresponsive to conservative therapy.[6] A child older than 12 years of age with a lesion greater than 1 cm in size should be treated surgically.[18] In older individuals, lesions are less likely to heal after closure of the growth plate and, unless very small, will traumatize the delicate articular surface. This will result in joint irregularity and lead to premature (secondary) osteoarthritis.

The difference between the juvenile and the young adult forms of osteochondritis dissecans lies in their different prognoses. Unlike the prognosis for the young adult, the outlook in adolescent osteochondritis dissecans is good. Few adolescent require surgery for defect excision or replacement, although an operation may be necessary if symptoms of locking, pain, and swelling persist.[46] Before skeletal age 11 for girls and 13 for boys, juvenile patients still have open physes. Once the diagnosis has been established for the juvenile patient, provided the fragment has not detached, *a race between lesion healing and closure of the femoral epiphysis begins.*[21] Healing is fostered by the initiation of a conser-vative management program and strict adherence to it. If the race against time is won, then the long-term prognosis is excellent and normal knee function is expected in adulthood. Detached lesions, large lesions, and loose bodies have the greatest propensity for nonunion. If the race is lost and juvenile osteochondritis dissecans evolves into adult osteochondritis dissecans with the potential for a permanent nonunion, the favorable prognosis is lost.

15. What is the conservative management of osteochondritis dissecans and when is it an appropriate intervention strategy?

The focus of conservative treatment is *protection* of the involved knee joint. For some children, all that is needed is several weeks rest (that is, restriction of vigorous exercise) followed by activity modification with avoidance of symptom-related activities. This is facilitated by minimizing weight bearing via crutch use. Aspirin may be prescribed. In children who cannot minimize their level of activity a crutch is necessary along with cast immobilization or splinting, although excessive or extended casting or rigid splinting should be avoided owing to the detrimental effect of immobilization upon articular cartilage.[42] Traction is rarely needed to control discomfort and secondary hamstring spasm. In the early adolescent child, exercises include isometric and slight resisted straight leg raising in flexion, abduction, and extension so as to improve tone of the hip and knee musculature. When symptoms permit, swimming and stationary bicycle riding may be introduced and may then progress to a standard resisted exercise program. Some 6 to 12 months are usually required for healing.[23]

Females from skeletal age 12 and males from skeletal age 14, and onward to age 20 possess physes that exhibit minimal vertical growth. This patient population demonstrates the physical maturation changes generally associated with adulthood. Nevertheless, nonprogressive lesions are treated as a healing fracture, with rest and observation similar to the juvenile group if the fragment has not separated from the femoral condyle.

16. When is surgical management appropriate?

A surgical approach is appropriate in juveniles with detached lesions greater than 1 cm[18] in young adults who do not respond to rest and observation, as well as with adult patient. When the fragment represents a large portion of the weight-bearing region, internal fixation is considered because of the degenerative effects of weight bearing upon the craterlike articular surface of the femoral condyle. If the overlying cartilage is still relatively intact reattachment may be accomplished by using headless screws or pins countersunk into the cartilage in the hope of inducing a new blood supply.[8] Otherwise, the loose or detached fragment is removed with arthroscopic forceps, followed by drilling through areas of poorly vascularized bone to induce a vascular healing response.[15,30]

REFERENCES

1. Ahlback S, Bauer GC, Bohne WH: Spontaneous osteonecrosis of the knee, *Arthritis Rheum* 11:705, 1968.
2. Aichroth P: Osteochondral fractures and their relationship to osteochondritis dissecans of the knee: an experimental study in animals, *J Bone Joint Surg* 53B:448, 1971.
3. American Physical Therapy Association: *Ped Orthop* 25, 1992.
4. Amstutz HC, Carey EJ: Skeletal manifestations and treatment of Gaucher's disease, *J Bone Joint Surg* 48A:670, 1966.
5. Bravo JF, Herman JH, Smyth CH: Musculoskeletal disorders after renal homotransplantation, *Ann Intern Med* 66:87, 1967.
6. Cahill B, Berg B: 99m-technetium phosphate compound joint scintigraphy in the management of juvenile osteochondritis dissecans of the femoral condyles, *Am J Sports Med* 11:329-335, 1983.
7. Cahill B: Treatment of juvenile osteochondritis dissecans and osteochondritis dissecans of the knee, *Clin Sports Med* 4(2):369, 1985.
8. Cormack DH: *Introduction to histology,* Philadelphia, 1984, JB Lippincott.
9. Cruess RL et al: Orthopaedic complications of renal homotransplantation, *J Bone Joint Surg* 50A:833, 1968.
10. Cyriax J: Textbook of orthopaedic medicine, *Diagnosis of soft tissue lesions,* ed 8, vol 1, London, 1982, Bailliere-Tindall.
11. Dandy DJ: *Essential orthopaedics and trauma,* Edinburgh, 1989, Churchill Livingstone.
12. D'Anglejean G, Ryckewaert A, Glimet S: Osteonecrosis du plateau tibial intern, *Extr Rheumat* 8:253, 1976.
13. De Smet AA, Fisher DR, Graff BK et al: Osteochondritis dissecans of the knee: value of MR imaging in determining lesion stability and the presence of articular cartilage defects, *AJR* 155:549, 1990.
14. DiStefano VJ: Skeletal injuries of the knee. In Nicholas JA, Hershman EB editors: *The lower extremity and spine,* ed 2, vol 1, St Louis, 1995, Mosby.
15. Dorland's *Illustrated medical dictionary,* ed 27, Philadelphia, 1988, WB Saunders.
16. Edwards DH, Bentley G: Osteochondritis dissecans patellae, *J Bone Joint Surg* 59B:58, 1977.
17. Fairbank HAT: Osteochondritis dissecans, *Br J Surg* 21:67, 1933.
18. Guhl J: Arthroscopic treatment of osteochondritis dissecans, *Clin Orthop* 167-65-74, 1982.
19. Houpt JB, Alpert B, Lotem M et al: Spontaneous osteonecrosis of the medial tibial plateau, *J Rheum* 9:81, 1982.
20. Irby R, Hume DM: Joint changes observed following renal transplants, *Clin Orthop* 57:101, 1968.
21. Kennedy JC, Grainger RW, McGraw RW: Osteochondral fractures of the femoral condyles, *J Bone Joint Surg* 48B:436, 1966.
22. Kleinberg S: Bilateral osteochondritis dissecans of the patella, *J Bone Joint Surg* 31A:185, 1949.
23. Langer F, Percy E: Osteochondritis dissecans and anomalous centres of ossification: a review of 80 lesions in 61 patients, *Can. J. Surg* 14:208, 1971.
24. Lotke PA, Ecker ML: Osteonecrosis-like syndrome of the medial tibial plateau, *Clin Orthop* 176:148, 1983.
25. Lynch MA, Henning CE: Physical examination of the knee. In Nicholas JA, Hershman EB editors: *The lower extremity and spine,* ed 2, vol 1, St Louis, 1995, Mosby.
26. Marmor L: Osteonecrosis of the knee: medial and lateral involvement, *Clin Orthop* 185:195, 1984.
27. McCallum RJ, Walder DN: Bone lesion in compressed air workers, *J Bone Joint Surg* 48B:207, 1966.
28. Meals RA: *One hundred orthopedics conditions every doctor should understand,* St Louis, 1992, Quality Medical Publishing.
29. *Merck manual,* ed 15, Rahway, NJ, 1987, Merck, Sharp, & Dohme Research Laboratories.
30. Netter FH: *Developmental disorders, tumours, rheumatic diseases and joint replacement,* vol 8, part II, Summit, NJ, 1990, CIBA-GEIGY.
31. Nicholas JA, Hershman EB editors: *The lower extremity and spine,* ed 2, vol 1, St Louis, 1995, Mosby.
32. Pautazopoulos T, Exarchou E: Osteochondritis dissecans of the patella, *J Bone Joint Surg* 53A:1205, 1971.
33. Peterson L, Renstrom P: *Sports injuries: their prevention and treatment,* Chicago, 1986, Yearbook Medical Publishers.
34. Reynolds J: *The roentgenological features of sickle cell disease and related hemoglobinopathies,* Springfield, IL, 1966, Charles C Thomas.
35. Rideout DG, Davis S, Navain SV: Osteochondritis dissecans patellae, *Br J Radiol* 39:673, 1966.
36. Roberts JM, Kennedy JC: Osteochondritis dissecans. In Roberts JM, Kennedy JC editors: *The injured adolescent knee,* Baltimore, 1979, Williams & Wilkins.
37. Rodnan GP, Schumacher HR, Zvaifler NJ: *Primer on the rheumatic diseases,* ed 8, Atlanta, GA, 1983, Arthritis Foundation.
38. Rogers WM, Gladstone H: Vascular foramina and arterial supply of the distal end of the femur, *J Bone Joint Surg* 32A:867, 1950.
39. Rombold C: Osteochondritis dissecans of the patella, *J Bone Joint Surg* 18:230, 1936.
40. Ruderman M, McCarty, Jr. DJ: Aseptic necrosis in systematic lupus erythematosus: report of a case involving six joints, *Arthritis Rheum* 7:709, 1964.
41. Salter RB: *Textbook of disorders of the musculoskeletal system,* ed 2, Baltimore, 1983, Williams & Wilkins.
42. Salter R, Field P: The effects of continuous compression on living articular cartilage: an experimental investigation, *J Bone Joint Surg* 42A:31, 1960.

43. Schumacher HR, Bomalaski JS: *Case studies in rheumatology for the house officer,* Baltimore, 1990, Williams & Wilkins.
44. Smillie IS: *Injuries of the knee joint,* ed 5, New York, 1978, Churchill Livingstone.
45. Smith JB: Osteochondritis dissecans of the trochlea of the femur, *Arthroscopy* 6(1):11, 1990.
46. Strizak AM: Knee injuries. In Nicholas JA, Hershman EB editors: *The lower extremity and spine,* ed 2, vol 2, St Louis, 1995, Mosby.
47. Wilson JN: A diagnostic sign in osteochondritis dissecans, *J Bone Joint Surg* 49A:477, 1967.

RECOMMENDED READING

Cahill B: Treatment of juvenile osteochondritis dissecans and osteochondritis dissecans of the knee, *Clin Sports Med* 4(2), 1985.
Smith JB: Osteochondritis dissecans of the trochlea of the femur, *Arthroscopy* 6(1):11, 1990.

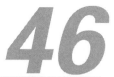

Posterolateral Exertional Knee Pain Immediately after Knee Extension Phases of Gait After Downhill Running Along Banked Surface

A 27-year-old actuary studying for his tenth actuarial examination spent 3 hours per day in preparation for a local marathon run. He ran for 3 miles every morning and evening for 3 consecutive months along a stretch of beach owned by the life insurance company for whom he was employed. In anticipation of his last exam his company offered him special dispensation over the upcoming summer months during which he was free to spend his days studying at home. He spent his summer in the Adirondack mountain region during which time he increased his training to 5 runs of 3 miles per day along a banked road. After 6 weeks of this regimen he enters your office with complaints of posterolateral exertional pain in the right knee noted at the end of workouts, particularly following a downhill run. When asked, he admits to running with the left foot on the upper side of the road crown. The patient reports no complaints of buckling, catching, or swelling. There is no history of injury.

OBSERVATION A moderate forefoot varus with compensatory rearfoot valgus is observed in both feet. The left knee appears to be in slight valgus. No swelling is present at the knee.

GAIT This appears normal, although the patient reports severe pain immediately following early stance phase of gait.

PALPATION This reveals point tenderness at the posterolateral aspect of the left knee, just posterior to the fibular collateral ligament. There is no tenderness at the left lateral femoral condyle, or at the left lateral tibial plateau at the tibiofemoral joint line upon slight knee flexion.

ACTIVE RANGE OF MOTION Active range of motion is normal.

PASSIVE RANGE OF MOTION Passive range of motion yields vague discomfort deep within the popliteal fossa upon full knee extension.

MUSCLE STRENGTH Normal muscle strength to the extrinsic evertors, dorsiflexors, and inverters of the upper ankle joint. Normal strength is present to all muscle groups of the left lower extremity.

SELECTIVE TENSION Selective tension yields no pain on resisted lateral hamstring contraction.

FLEXIBILITY Flexibility shows moderate tightness to both the left hamstrings and quadriceps muscle group.

721

SPECIAL TESTS   Negative Ober, McMurray, and Apley tests. Positive bilateral Thomas tests. Varus testing of the knee joint is negative for pain and yields no increase in valgus opening.

SENSATION   Sensation is intact to light touch to the left peronei sensory distribution.

CLUE:

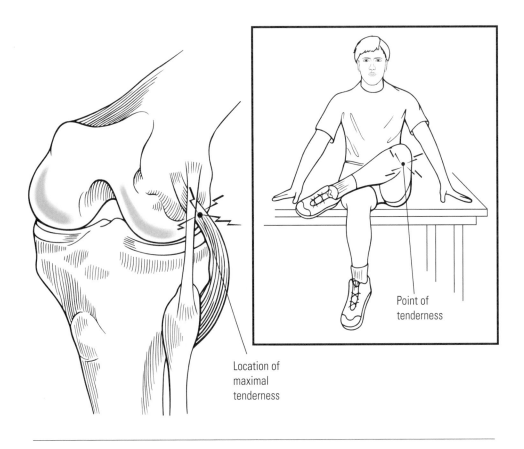

Location of maximal tenderness

Point of tenderness

? **Questions**

1. What is most likely the cause of this man's lateral knee pain?
2. What is the anatomy of the popliteus muscle?
3. When is popliteus most active during the gait cycle?
4. What is the screw-home mechanism of the knee joint?
5. What is the function of the popliteus in relation to the screw-home mechanism at the knee joint?
6. What is the role of the pes anserine during engagement of the screw-home mechanism at the knee?
7. How do extrinsic factors such as running on a hill or banked surface impose deviations from subtalar joint neutral upon the foot?
8. What is the significance of the popliteus having the same alignment as the posterior cruciate ligament?

9. **What synergetic relationship does the popliteus have with the lateral collateral ligament (LCL) at the knee?**

10. **What is the relationship between the popliteus and the lateral knee meniscus?**

11. **What is the clinical presentation of this disorder?**

12. **What is the differential diagnosis?**

13. **What therapeutic intervention may best manage this patient?**

1. **What is most likely the cause of this man's lateral knee pain?**

Popliteus tendinitis of the left knee. This disorder is a common clinical entity due to the rise in popularity of jogging and competitive distance running.

2. **What is the anatomy of the popliteus muscle?**

The *popliteus muscle* is a thin, flat, and short muscle of triangular shape located deeply in the popliteal fossa and forming the floor of that fossa (Fig. 46-1). Although the origin-insertional span of many skeletal muscles

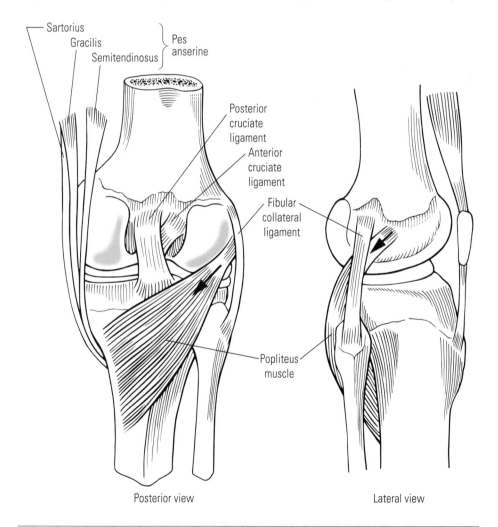

Sartorius
Gracilis
Semitendinosus
} Pes anserine
Posterior cruciate ligament
Anterior cruciate ligament
Fibular collateral ligament
Popliteus muscle

Posterior view   Lateral view

FIG. 46-1 Anatomic locale of popliteus. Posterior and lateral views. Popliteus works in the capacity of a dynamic ligament, together with the lateral collateral ligament in restraining excessive varus opening at the knee. It also works together with the pes anserinus as a dynamic checkrein against excessive valgus at the knee.

runs proximodistal along a straight course, the popliteus has a distinctly *oblique* orientation of span that endows it with a rotational action at the knee. Popliteus bears a synergetic relationship with several static knee stabilizers including the lateral collateral and cruciate ligaments, as well as an antagonistic relationship with the pes anserinus.

Popliteus, spanning the posterior aspect of the tibiofemoral joint, runs *proximal lateral to a distal medial* course. Popliteus is additionally unusual in that its tendinous attachment is proximal instead of distal. The muscle proximally originates from the posterolateral femoral condyle by way of a stout tendon. It angles medially across the posterior tibia to separate the lateral collateral ligament from the lateral meniscus before inserting fleshy fibers into the triangular portion of the proximal medial portion of the posterior tibia (just above the soleal line) adjacent to the medial tibial condyle. The relationship of popliteus to the lateral meniscus known as the *popliteus hiatus* is biomechanically significant to the lateral meniscus as it endows it with greater anteroposterior mobility than the medial meniscus (see Fig. 42-7). It is the tendinous route of this muscle that courses between the fibular collateral ligament and lateral meniscus. This tendinous span is surrounded by a synovial bursa that separates it from these structures as well as the femoral condyle and knee joint capsule. The bursa may also become inflamed resulting in bursitis as well as popliteal tendinitis.[1]

3. When is popliteus most active during the gait cycle?

Popliteus is an intrinsic knee muscle that runs intraarticularly between its proximal origin (lateral femoral condyle) and its distal insertion (medial tibial condyle). Although its line-of-pull falls behind the knee joint, anatomically categorizing it as a knee flexor, its leverage is poor for this motion. The oblique fiber orientation of this muscle suggests its primary function is rotating the knee medially between 10° and 14° (Mann R, 1992: personal communication) out of the lateral locked knee posture that occurs with engagement of the screw-home mechanism just after terminal knee extension.[11] Thus although anatomically considered a knee flexor, popliteus is actually a kinesiological *medial tibial derotator.* This is borne out by electromyographic studies that indicate greater popliteus activity surrounding knee extension than during knee flexion.[5] Popliteus also functions as a static checkrein to restrain anterior displacement of the femur on the tibia when the knee flexes or during downhill running (Fig. 46-2).[2]

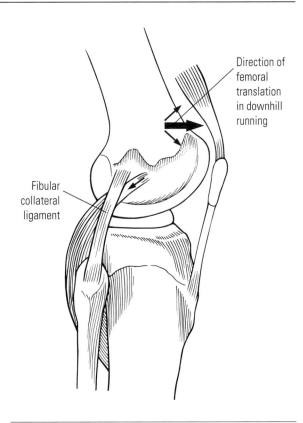

FIG. 46-2 Popliteus also functions as a static checkrein to restrain anterior displacement of the femur on the tibia when the knee flexes or during downhill running. Force vector summation represented by large arrow indicating forward displacement of distal femur.

4. What is the screw-home mechanism of the knee joint?

Any discussion of the *terminal locking* or *screw-home mechanism* at the knee joint must be prefaced with an understanding of the tibiofemoral joint. This joint is composed of the articulation between the medial and lateral femoral condyles with the corresponding medial and lateral tibial condyles (Fig. 46-3). Two "compartments" are formed by the juxtaposition of these two sets of condyles. The lateral tibiofemoral hemi-joint occupies the lateral knee compartment while the medial tibiofemoral hemi-joint occupies the medial compartment of the knee.

There is an inherent anterior/posterior asymmetry in the architectural configuration when comparing the medial and lateral femoral condyles. Had both condyles been designed symmetrically, the knee articulation would have functioned as a pure hinge joint. However, knee joint motion is characterized by sub-

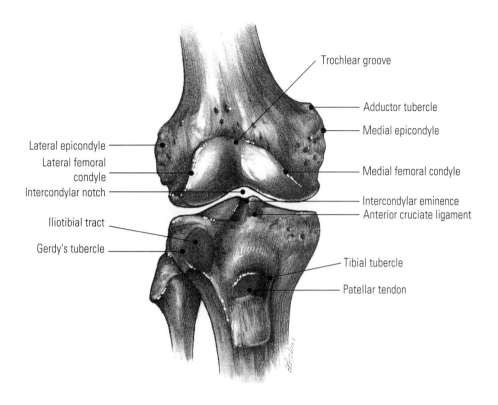

Trochlear groove

Adductor tubercle

Medial epicondyle

Lateral epicondyle

Lateral femoral condyle

Medial femoral condyle

Intercondylar notch

Intercondylar eminence
Anterior cruciate ligament

Iliotibial tract

Gerdy's tubercle

Tibial tubercle

Patellar tendon

FIG. 46-3 Anteroposterior view of the knee. The knee joint is composed of the articulation between the medial and lateral femoral condyles with the corresponding medial and lateral tibial condyles. The differing architectural configuration of these two hemi-joints accounts for asymmetric motion between the two hemi-compartments and endows the knee with gliding and sliding motion as well. (From Scott WN: *The knee*, St Louis, 1994, Mosby.)

stantial gliding (rolling and sliding) and is accounted for by the relatively larger (1.7 cm) medial femoral condyle. The medial condyle is also more symmetric in terms of its radius of curvature, whereas posteriorly the lateral condyle has a curve of decreasing radius. Hence a second degree of freedom is attributed to the knee joint.

As the femur and tibia move from flexion into extension, the tibial plateaus ascend and descend as they follow the convexity of the femoral condyles symmetrically. As the knee straightens, extension is blocked laterally while extension of the medial tibial condyle proceeds unhindered anteriorly along the longer medial condyle so that the knee joint veers or rotates laterally. Lateral blocking of motion occurs because that small ridge of bone the *impressio terminalis* (which traverses the lateral condyle just distal to the intercondylar notch) impinges on the tibia (see Fig. 42-4). This description aptly describes terminal knee extension during late *swing* phase of gait as the

tibia laterally rotates upon a relatively fixed femur. The locking mechanism occurs once during *stance* phase just before foot flat phase when the requirements of locomotion necessitate a locked rigid knee to elevate the body's center of gravity and vault it over a weight-bearing pillar. Complete engagement of the locking mechanism does not occur as the knee does not completely extend during stance (i.e., about 3° flexion; the knee never fully extends during midstance). Nevertheless, the screw-home mechanism endows the knee joint with a higher degree of weight-bearing stability than would be attainable if the tibiofemoral articulation was a pure hinge joint.

In addition to passive locking at the knee occurring as a function of bony architecture, external rotation of the tibia is dynamically aided by the *biceps femoris* muscle. This lateral hamstring muscle is composed of a short and long head that distally attaches on the fibular head and lateral tibial condyle. As such, contraction of the biceps femoris acts an-

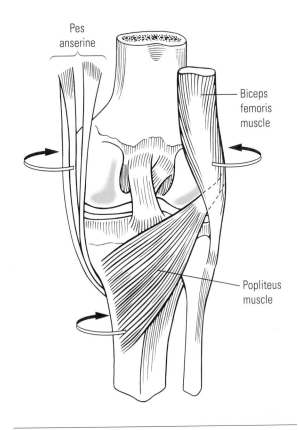

Pes anserine

Biceps femoris muscle

Popliteus muscle

FIG. 46-4 Although the four tendinous slips of pes anserine synergistically assist popliteus in rotating the knee medially, the lateral hamstring (biceps femoris) works in antagonism to externally rotate the knee.

tagonistically to popliteus and the pes anserinus by providing a minimal lateral rotary action of the tibia relative to the femur (Fig. 46-4).

5. What is the function of the popliteus in relation to the screw-home mechanism at the knee joint?

Disengagement of the screw-home mechanism primarily occurs owing to internal rotation of the knee that accompanies knee flexion. The rotations of the femoral condyles reverse themselves on the tibial plateau as the locking mechanism is disengaged. Popliteus, whose line of pull is ideal as an internal tibial rotator, is recruited to help disengage the locked extension posture of the tibiofemoral screw-home mechanism by derotating the knee joint medially out of extension just after heel strike. Popliteus is therefore being worked throughout those portions of the gait cycle corresponding to flexion following full or near full extension of the

knee. This is borne out by peak electromyographic intensity of popliteus muscle activity, which indicates maximal concentric contraction corresponding to terminal swing through early stance. Immediately following heel strike a flexion moment is realized at the knee joint to dissipate the force of impact. The only time that popliteus is quiescent is during early and mid swing[9] during which the knee joint is exclusively preoccupied with flexion vis-à-vis ground clearance.

6. What is the role of the pes anserine during engagement of the screw-home mechanism at the knee?

The confluence of the distal tendons of sartorius, gracilis, and semitendinosus on the anteromedial tibial flare is known as the pes anserinus (e.g., goose's foot). Normally, the tibia has a slight valgus angulation in relation to the femur that is commonly more pronounced in females.[3] Anatomically, these tendons support the knee's medial side, which is under considerable tension owing to the normal valgus angle inherent to the tibiofemoral joint.

The medial condyle is longer and larger than the lateral femoral condyle in the sense that it protrudes distally and has a greater circumference when compared to the lateral femoral condyle. In contrast, the medial condyle has a more symmetric radius of curvature (see Fig. 42-1). This variation in architectural configuration between the two femoral condyles accounts for kinesiologic divergence of function between the medial and lateral tibiofemoral joints. Moreover, the architectural inequality between the anteroposterior projection of the two condyles that favors a longer medial condyle imparts a *valgus posture* to the normal knee in the erect standing posture.

In addition to providing for medial stabilization at the knee by acting as a restraint to excessive valgus opening, these muscle provide a counter-rotary torque function to the knee joint. Despite its similar oblique orientation of span to popliteus, the pes anserine has an *eccentric* role during *engagement* of the screw-home mechanism that dampens the effect of excessively forceful lateral rotation that may accompany terminal knee extension.* The pes anserine is dynamically assisted by the other medial hamstring muscle (semimembranosus).

---

*If the pes anserine functioned concentrically, which they do not, they would work in synergy with popliteus.

7. How do extrinsic factors such as running on a hill or banked surface impose deviations from subtalar joint neutral upon the foot?

Popliteus tendinitis is frequent in runners who run downhill, or alongside a beach or other banked surfaces, which acts to increase pronation of the foot on the higher part of the slope. Both the pronated or supinated subtalar joint (intrinsic) mechanisms may be (extrinsically) mimicked by running along a banked surface. This occurs because a nonlevel surface topography causes diminishment of medial sole contact of the lower foot, and excessive medial sole contact of the higher foot. The cavus (or supinated) foot is characterized by decreased weight bearing area, whereas the planus (or pronated) foot is characterized by increased surface contact. The foot along the elevated surface undergoes excessive pronation, while the foot along the lower ground undergoes diminished pronation. Thus the topography of the terrain may mechanically force the foot into postures that deviate from subtalar joint neutral and thereby magnify or diminish pronation. These subtalar joint deviations may also occur from downhill or uphill running.

Downhill running is characterized by pronation beyond midstance phase of gait, whereas uphill running is characterized by a diminishment of pronation such that supination begins before midstance. The combination of downhill running on a banked surface represents a compounding pronatory effect upon the subtalar joint of the lower foot, whereas uphill running compounds the supinatory effect upon the subtalar joint of the higher foot.

8. What is the significance of the popliteus having the same alignment as the posterior cruciate ligament?

Human locomotion consists of repetitively throwing ourselves off balance by unilaterally falling forward and then catching ourselves before we fall by moving the ipsilateral foot forward into a new position under our center of gravity. If not for the dynamic and static restraints binding the femur to the tibia, the superincumbent body weight thrown forward with each step would cause the femur and body above it to shear right off the tibial plateau. This, in fact, is the noncontact mechanism of injury to the posterior cruciate ligament during stance as when one steps into a pit and does not extricate him- or herself before excessive hyperpronation of the femur on the fixed tibia.

The posterior cruciate ligament travels from the medial femoral condyle to the upper posterior surface of the tibia, whereas popliteus traverses an *opposite* diagonal course. In contrast, the alignment of popliteus runs parallel with the anterior cruciate ligament. The common denominator to these structures is that their diagonal and posterior placement in relation to the knee joint axis for flexion and extension prevents forward sliding of the condyles in weight bearing on flexed knees, particularly with the knee in 75° to 90° of flexion.[7] Popliteus synergistically assists the posterior cruciate ligament to retard forward displacement of the femur on the flexed tibia. In addition, similar to a twisting mechanism resulting in posterior cruciate disruption, rupture or avulsion of the popliteus tendon may occur with twisting injuries to the knee. Thus popliteus functions in the capacity of a *dynamic ligament* providing a passive checkrein against excessive femoral excursion on the tibia during knee flexion activities such as squatting, sitting, walking down an incline, or just plain walking. This is borne out by increased electromyographic activity in popliteus during squatting. Thus popliteus, like the posterior cruciate ligament, represents a restraint that checks posterior tibial translation as well as anterior femoral translation. In addition, because of its parallel orientation with the anterior cruciate ligament, popliteus acts a restraint to check anterior tibial translation as well as posterior femoral translation.

9. What synergetic relationship does popliteus have with the lateral collateral ligament (LCL) at the knee?

In addition to preventing anterior/ posterior translation of the femur on the tibia, as well as rotation of the femur in relation to the tibia, popliteus shares an important burden with the lateral collateral ligament at the knee. Both structures serve as a *primary restraint to varus* opening at the knee. Indeed, a larger portion of the popliteus tendon passes deep to the LCL to insert directly on the anterolateral femur. However, because of the oblique span of popliteus, it also serves (together with the pes anserinus) as a *restraint to valgus opening* at the knee. In addition, the lateral collateral ligament, by virtue of its orientation acts together with popliteus to provide a static checkrein in controlling excessive external rotation of the tibia on the femur as well as excessive internal rotation of the femur on the tibia. This may occur between mid swing and late swing phase of gait characterized by external tibial rotation and internal femoral rotation during which the popliteus and LCL are passively tautened. During stance phase of gait, these active and passive restraints are tensed during knee extension and prevent excessive lateral rotary force exerted during the screw-home locking mechanism.

10. What is the relationship between the popliteus and the lateral knee meniscus?

The lateral meniscus is less firmly attached around its peripheral margin[10] and is endowed with relatively *greater mobility* when compared to the medial meniscus as a direct function of the popliteus tendon. Increased mobility is attributed to a hiatus in the static peripheral meniscal attachments where it is crossed by the popliteus tendon. The popliteal tendon courses anteriorly beneath the lateral collateral ligament and adjacent to the lateral meniscus. It creates a defect in the capsular peripheral lateral meniscal restraints known as the *popliteal hiatus* in the capsular peripheral lateral meniscal restraints en route its distal insertion on the medial tibial condyle (see Fig. 42-7). Two synovial pillars, both anterior and posterior to the defect, support the capsular attachment to the meniscus so as to compensate for the defect and protect the area from rupture.[12] It is perhaps due to this relative mobility of the lateral meniscus that it seldom tears as compared with the fixed medial meniscus.

When carefully considering the complex distal insertion of this muscle, the dynamic role of popliteus in relation to lateral meniscal motion becomes more evident. Before inserting on the tibia, a portion of popliteus tendon (the superior popliteomeniscal fascicle) inserts directly onto the posterior horn of the lateral meniscus, while an inferior popliteomeniscal fascicle blends into the middle segment of the lateral meniscus. Thus popliteus, while unlocking the extended knee following terminal knee extension, simultaneously rotates the femoral condyles *as well as the lateral meniscus laterally* (in the closed kinetic chain). The role of popliteus in *external rotational meniscal movement* occurs synchronously with rotation of the lateral femoral condyle so as to avoid meniscal impingement between the tibiofemoral articulating surfaces during disengagement of the screw-home mechanism at the knee. Although meniscal motion follows the convexity of the femoral condyles and not the tibial plateau, popliteus facilitation of this motion may represent a strategy that fine tunes meniscal motion and thereby diminishes the likelihood of entrapment.

11. What is the clinical presentation of this disorder?

Signs and symptoms of popliteal tendinitis include exertional pain over the posterolateral aspect of the knee that is noted at the end of workouts, particularly following downhill running. Palpation yields tenderness localized over the popliteus tendon, just posterior to the fibular collateral ligament. Occasionally, crepitus is noted over the course of the tendon. Patients often report discomfort when sitting in a cross-legged position with subsequent stretch of the popliteal tendon. When placing the hip in (the Hardy posture of) flexion, abduction, and external rotation with the knee flexion and leg crossed over the opposite extremity, the posterolateral corner of the knee is best exposed for palpation of the popliteus tendon.

12. What is the differential diagnosis?

- *Iliotibial band tendinitis.* This is characterized by tenderness over the lateral femoral condyle. Popliteal tendinitis demonstrates pinpoint tenderness along the posterolateral aspect of the knee, just posterior to the fibular collateral ligament. The site of tenderness in iliotibial band tendinitis is located more proximally over the lateral femoral condyle as compared with popliteus tendinitis.[1]
- *Biceps femoris tendinitis.* This is differentiated from popliteus tendinitis by scoring positive during selective resistance of this lateral hamstring muscle. Selective tension of this muscle may also be accomplished by placing its two-jointed span on passive insufficiency by the combined posture of anterior pelvic tilt, internal hip rotation, and knee extension in that order.[4] Absence of muscle function will manifest in the case of tendon rupture.[10] The biceps femoris tendon becomes prominent where it crosses the knee joint before inserting into the fibular head. It may be palpated near its insertion when the knee is flexed as the patient is in the short sitting posture. Tenderness may be elicited by strumming over the biceps tendon or at its insertion.
- *Lateral meniscus tear.* This is characterized by symptoms of buckling, true locking, lateral joint line pain[6] or recurrent effusions. Tearing of the lateral meniscus will yield point tenderness as the clinician probes firmly into the lateral joint space to palpate the anterior margin of the meniscus. This is best assessed with the patient's knee in slight flexion.[1]

- *Common peroneal nerve entrapment.* This may also cause lateral knee pain and is associated with weakness or sensory changes in running athletes. This nerve is palpable where it crosses the fibular neck just slightly inferior to the insertion of the biceps femoris muscle. This neuropathy is differentiated from popliteus tendinitis by the presence of muscle weakness in the anterior compartment (dorsiflexors) musculature as well as the peronei (evertors), decreased sensation over the peroneal nerve topography, positive Tinel sign, and electromyographic studies, which help aid diagnosis of this condition.[8]

13. What therapeutic intervention may best manage this patient?

The management of popliteus tendinitis consists of rest, oral nonsteroidal antiinflammatory medications, local ice followed by heat, and ultrasound. Cortisone injections into the tendon are to be discouraged. When running is resumed, the individual should modify his/her activity by avoiding excessively long workouts as well as running along hills and banked surfaces. Treatment for popliteal tendinitis closely follows management of that other disorder of the lateral knee, that is, iliotibial band tendinitis (see chapter by this title). *Strengthening* of the muscles contributing to the tendinous pes anserine insertion effectively unloads the burden of a strained popliteus. The pes anserine tendinous insertion is a composite structure whose triple redundant insertion originates from the sartorius (anterior compartment), gracilis (medial femoral compartment), and the medial hamstring, the semitendinosus (posterior femoral compartment.) A strategy to selectively strengthen each of these muscles may facilitate a stronger collective pes anserine synergistic rotational unlocking of the screw-home mechanism at the knee.[10]

As popliteus is normally active immediately following terminal knee extension as flexion begins to predominate, a strategy that may unload the rate at which popliteus must operate to unlock the screw-home mechanism would include eccentric quadriceps strengthening. During stance phase of gait, and immediately following heel strike, derotation of the knee out of extension occurs extremely rapidly, as the ground reaction force is located behind the knee joint. The knee joint normally buckles into flexion, but does so in a controlled, noninjurious manner due to contraction of muscle located on the opposite side of the joint. The internally generated eccentric tension generated by the quadriceps muscle works to extend the knee and thereby counters the external ground reaction force generating a flexion moment that attempts to flex the knee. Eccentrically working the quadriceps muscle may serve to unload the popliteus by way of minimizing the speed with which it must respond to knee flexion out of extension.

Shortness of the hamstring muscles may approximate the origin and insertion of popliteus and thus result in shortening of that muscle. A muscle in its shortened state may exhibit decreased mechanical efficiency and sustain subsequent fatigue and injury in the presence of high muscle activity. Quadriceps shortening may also result in that muscle's decreased ability to generate sufficient tension to minimize the contractile load to a fatigued or injured popliteus tendon. As such, hamstring as well as quadriceps stretching is appropriate when shortness of these muscle groups is present.

The use of an orthosis to correct a foot-fault deformity is essential in the over-pronated foot. The use of an arch support will help support a foot with a sagging medial longitudinal arch. This may be augmented by the use of a lateral hindfoot wedge, which holds the tibia in an internally rotated position. This helps to decrease tension at the posterolateral corner of the knee and thereby diminishes the stress on the popliteus.[7]

REFERENCES

1. Boland AL, Hulstyn MJ: Soft-tissue injuries of the knee. In Nicholas JA, Hershman EB editors: *The lower extremity and spine in sports medicine,* St Louis, 1995, Mosby.
2. Brody DM: Clinical Symposia, 39(3):23, Summit, NJ, 1987, CIBA-GEIGY.
3. Hoppenfeld S: *Physical examination of the spine and extremities,* Norwalk, Conn, 1976, Appleton Century Crofts.
4. Kendall FP, McCreary EK: *Muscles—testing and function,* ed 3, Baltimore, 1983, Williams & Wilkins.
5. Lehmkuhl LD, Smith LK: *Brunstromm's clinical kinesiology,* ed 4, Philadelphia, 1989, FA Davis.
6. Lillegard WA, Rucker KS: *Handbook of sports medicine: a symptom-oriented approach,* Boston, 1993, Andover Medical Publishers.
7. Pagnani MJ, Warren RF, Arnoczky SP et al: Anatomy of the knee. In Nicholas JA, Hershman EB editors: *The lower extremity and spine,* ed 2, vol 1, St Louis, 1995, Mosby.
8. Patten J: *Neurological differential diagnosis,* ed 2, London, 1995, Springer.
9. Perry J: *Gait analysis: normal and pathological function,* Thorofare, NJ, 1992, Slack.

10. Peterson L, Renstrom P: *Sport injuries: their prevention and treatment,* Chicago, 1986, Year Book Medical Publishers.
11. Soderberg GL: *Kinesiology: Application to pathological motion,* Baltimore, MD, 1986, Williams & Wilkins.
12. Tria AJ, Klein KS: *An illustrated guide to the knee,* New York, 1992, Churchill Livingstone.

RECOMMENDED READING

Basmajian JV, Lovejoy JF Jr: Functions of the popliteus muscle in man, *J Bone Joint Surg* 53A:557, 1977.
Mann RA, Hagy JL: The popliteus muscle, *J Bone Joint Surg* 59A:924, 1977.
Mayfield GW: Popliteus tendon tenosynovitis, *Am J Sports Med* 5:31, 1977.

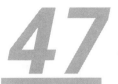

47

Painful Snapping, Give-Way Sensation, and Stiffness after Prolonged Sitting at the Right Medial Tibiofemoral Joint Line

A 36-year-old male stockbroker visits your office complaining of a dull aching pain along the right medial patella and tibiofemoral joint line that developed 1 week ago. He reports that pain is worse in the morning hours and that his right knee swells intermittently. He complains that his right knee occasionally feels as if it will "give way," as well as a snapping or "clunking" sensation when attempting to squat. There is a subjective feeling of stiffness and "tightness" within the knee. Sitting for any length of time is painful, as is stair climbing or squatting. When questioned, the patient admits to trying to stay in shape by doing calisthenics involving knee squatting exercises; this is occasionally followed by mild knee swelling. While at work he must often stand up quickly and yell bids across the commodities floor. After some probing questions he admits that his right leg never actually buckled although it often felt weak, as if it might give way, and as if "something came out of place." When questioned about his kneecap, he admits that he did not see it "come out of place." He also complains of severe stiffness when trying to get up out of position of knee flexion after riding in his automobile for an extended period of time. Pain and stiffness are most acute for the first 8 to 10 steps and then improve as he walks further.

OBSERVATION   There appears to be no swelling of the involved knee upon examination.

PALPATION   At 90° of knee flexion, a thickened band of tissue is palpated anterior to the medial femoral condyle and superior to the medial joint line. The knee does not feel warm to the touch.

RANGE OF MOTION   This is normal.

STRENGTH   This is normal.

FLEXIBILITY   Patient demonstrates mild tightness to both hamstring muscles.

GIRTH MEASUREMENT   There is no quadriceps atrophy present.

SPECIAL TESTS   Positive McMurray's sign, Stutter test, and O'Conner's sign. Negative Apley's compression test and patellar apprehension test.

RADIOGRAPHS   Radiographs show no evidence of knee pathology.

? Questions

1. What is most likely wrong with this man's knee?
2. What is plica syndrome?
3. What is the embryology of the knee joint?
4. At which locations do redundant plical tissues most likely occur?
5. Which one of these embryonic remnants is most often implicated in this disorder?
6. What is the pathophysiologic etiology of plica syndrome?
7. What is the function of the articularis genu muscle?

8. What are the clinical findings of this disorder?
9. How is the diagnosis of plica syndrome made?
10. Which special tests help diagnose this condition?
11. How does the clinical presentation of plica syndrome differ from derangement of the extensor mechanism or the menisci?
12. What therapeutic management is appropriate?
13. What therapeutic management is appropriate in the postsurgical patient?

1. What is most likely wrong with this man's knee?

Plica syndrome of the right mediopatellar plicae.

2. What is plica syndrome?

Plica syndrome is an uncommon pathology that goes by many synonyms including plica synovialis, medial shelf syndrome, suprapatellar plica synovitis, and medial plica synovitis. This syndrome most commonly occurs in adolescent athletes participating in running and jumping sports. Although rarely found in pre-adolescent children,[2,5] plicae may become symptomatic following puberty because the accompanying rapid growth and concurrent extensor mechanism elongation during adolescent growth spurt may relate to the prevalence of this syndrome in adolescent and adults.[15]

Synovial plicae are intraarticular folds of synovial membrane that are embryonic remnants of tissue. During embryologic development, synovial septa divide the knee into suprapatellar, medial, and lateral pouches that compartmentalize the intraarticular knee into three separate divisions. Failure of septal recession leads to the persistence of suprapatellar, medial patellar, and infrapatellar synovial folds.[10,11] The synovium of the knee joint is the largest in the human body and develops into three separate pouches in the mature knee. Persistent remnants of these synovial septa variably occur in the adult knee as seams within the synovial membrane comprising the knee joint capsule. These seams or plicae occur adjacent to the patella and are therefore termed the mediopatellar, suprapatellar, and infrapatellar plicae. Thus plicae represent vestigial remnants of

normal embryologic septa that have persisted into the mature knee in 20% of the adult population.[2,5] These partitions normally degenerate during the fifth month of fetal development so that the knee joint develops into a single cavity. However, incomplete degeneration and recession of these membranes results in persistence of vestigial remnants called plicae that may be found anywhere in the knee joint. Plicae are not present in every knee, and when present, are innocuous in the sense that they do not represent pathologic entities. The presence of a plica is not indicative of symptomatic disease. Normally, these elastic bands of tissue track freely and silently during knee motion.[15] However, when acute or chronic trauma occur, inflammatory changes in the synovium may spread to associated inflammation to a plical base.[17] This may lead to signs and symptoms in which case they may symptomatically mimic loose bodies, torn menisci, or lateral patellar subluxation.[16]

Mediopatellar plica is the most commonly symptomatic and the one usually implicated in symptoms describing plica syndrome. The infrapatellar plica rarely causes symptoms, although traumatic rupture has been cited as a rare cause of posttraumatic hemarthrosis in young patients. The suprapatellar plica may result in a suprapatellar bursitis, or demonstrate symptoms similar to chondromalacia patellae.

3. What is the embryology of the knee joint?

The knee joint is formed during the fourth fetal month of embryologic development. Two small medial and lateral compartments form beneath a relatively larger superior pouch within the developing limb bud. Anatomically, these septa correspond to the respective knee compartments, with the superior pouch forming the suprapatellar compartment. As growth commences, these primitive synovial cavities become separated by thin synovial membranes which, in many people, are eventually resorbed so that the entire knee becomes a singular chamber. Synovial resorption may be incomplete so that remnant vestigial synovium persists during fetal development and thus project into the joint. Remnants that survive into adult life are called plicae and may be present as thin synovial membrane or as strong fibrous walls of tissue.[9,12]

4. At which locations do redundant plical tissues most likely occur?

Although vestigial plicae may occur anywhere in the knee joint, they are most likely to occur in three distinct locations (Fig. 47-1).

MEDIAL PATELLAR PLICA (*PLICA SYNOVIALIS MEDIOPATELLARIS*)

This is found along the medial wall of the knee joint. It originates from the medial capsule at the level of the superior margin of the femoral condyle and loops around the outer border of the medial femoral condyle and across the medial joint space before distally attaching onto the synovial lining of the infrapatellar fat pad.

SUPRA PATELLAR PLICA (*PLICA SYNOVIALIS SUPRAPATELLARIS*)

This is crescentlike in appearance and courses from the inferior surface of the lateral quadriceps tendon (vastus lateralis oblique) to attach upon the rectus intermedius at the proximal patellar pole. It then curves around the medial patella, turning distally to insert onto the medial fat pad distally.[14] Less commonly, a similar lateral suprapatellar plica may be present. Together, both su-

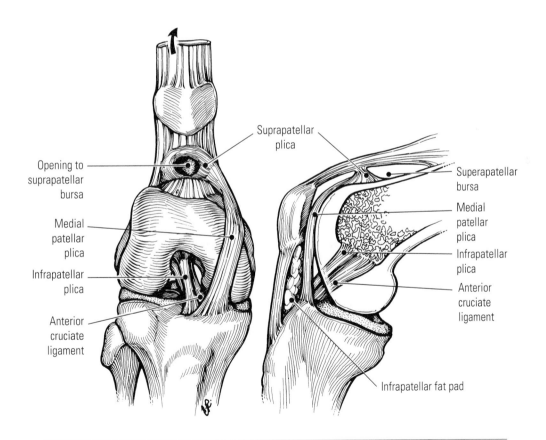

FIG. 47-1 Anatomy of plica. (From Scott WN: *Ligament and extensor mechanism injuries of the knee: diagnosis and treatment,* St Louis, 1991, Mosby.)

prapatellar plicae may rarely close off the suprapatellar pouch from the remainder of the knee joint.[17]

INFRA PATELLAR PLICA *(LIGAMENTUM MUCOSUM)*

This runs parallel with the anterior cruciate ligament. It originated from the roof of the intercondylar notch and widens as it crosses to insert on the infrapatellar fat pad. This plica, the most commonly found, is the most frequently encountered during arthroscopy[16] as it may be confused with the anterior cruciate ligament.[17] This plica is of little clinical significance except during arthroscopy where it may obscure portal entry sites and interfere with visualization of the anterior cruciate ligament.

5. Which one of these embryonic remnants is most often implicated in this disorder?

The *medial patellar plica,* located over the longer (medial) femoral condyle, is most often implicated in plica syndrome. When the knee is extended, the patella rides up between and over the femoral condyles. Protection to the anterior aspect of the femoral condyles from abrasion from the underside of the patella is afforded by the plica remnant rising up tentlike as a barrier that acts to distance the bone surfaces (Fig. 47-2). This hoodlike function occurs during the first 15° of knee flexion only, after which the medial plica provides surrogate protection by descending downward to contact the medial femoral condyle. At 30° of knee flexion the medial plica sweeps across the medial condyle. At 90° of knee flexion, a thickened tender band of tissue may be palpated anterior to the medial femoral condyle and superior to the medial joint line.

If the plical remnant is extensive it is referred to as medial synovial shelf formation. The synovial fold is wide enough as to be analogous to a "shelf" spanning the anterior aspect of the medial tibiofemoral hemijoint as well as the medial patellofemoral joint, and may become displaced during knee motion. Moreover, the extensor mechanism at the knee is characterized by dynamic as well as static stabilization resulting in a tracking deficit that favors lateral distraction of the patella. Lateral patellar distraction may promote formation of a medial synovial shelf as the medial plica,[15] by way of its approximation to the patella, is pulled centrally toward the lateral knee. This displacement may cause mechanical obstruction that interferes with patellofemoral and/or tibiofemoral joint motion. Thus whereas a normal medial patellar plical fold affords protection to the femoral condyles from abrasion, ex-

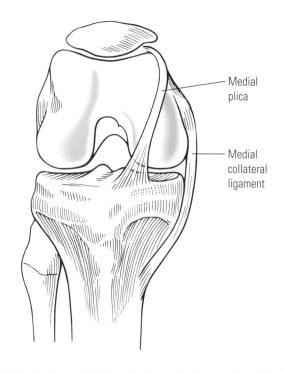

FIG. 47-2 Anterior view of the medial plica. The medial plica prevents abrasion from the convex medial patellar facet to the medial femoral articulating surface during knee extension.

cessive residual of this plica hinders normal patellofemoral as well as tibiofemoral joint function.

6. What is the pathophysiologic etiology of plica syndrome?

The rationale for why certain plicae become symptomatic while others remain quiescent remains a subject of controversy. Most injury to the plicae occurs because of intrinsic causes including athletic injuries, which may directly traumatize the plicae as they drape over the femoral condyles. Alternately, plicae injury may occur during a motor vehicle accident in which they may suffer contusion as the knee impacts against the dashboard.[6]

The *impingement theory* maintains that any of a variety of factors, including direct trauma, strenuous exercise, loose bodies, osteochondritis dissecans, or even meniscal pathology may impinge upon the plicae thereby initiating inflammation and hemorrhage within the synovium of the knee joint. Even if the plicae are not initially impinged upon, the chronic synovitis from aforementioned conditions create histologic changes within the adjacent synovial tissue comprising the plicae including fibrosis, hyalinization, and calcification. Thus the plicae are metamorphosed from pliant tissue (composed of elastin and areolar tissue) into tight, inelastic, thickened, and fibrotic bands that undergo impingement as they mechanically interfere with knee motion. Impingement of the mediopatellar plica occurs on the medial femoral condyle during knee flexion. This has been observed as articular cartilage wear or groove formation along the medial femoral condyle[3] owing to the mediopatellar plica repetitively sweeping across the condyle due to repeated knee flexion. With increasing flexion of the knee joint, impingement may occur by way of bowstringing of the mediopatellar plica across the medial patellar facet. The impingement theory identifies the offending entity as the mediopatellar plica with underlying secondary articular cartilage and bony changes of the medial femoral condyle. The end result of this repetitive rubbing across the medial patellofemoral articular surfaces may result in chondromalacia of the knee.[1]

Impingement as a pathological mechanism, is not operative with regard to the suprapatellar plica. Pipkin[12,13] postulated an underlying pathophysiology relating to the simulation of internal knee derangement as a function of the suprapatellar plica relative its relation to the suprapatellar bursa. In this theory, the suprapatellar plica is identified as the offending entity. The knee may be likened to a hydraulic system in which the suprapatellar plica acts as a one-way valve trapping fluid in the suprapatellar bursa. The patellar fat pad acts as a plunger forcing fluid into the suprapatellar bursa with each knee movement cycle. In the event that the suprapatellar plica becomes inflamed, the plica will reactively thicken, thereby accentuating the pistonlike force with which fluid is forced into the suprapatellar bursa. A vicious cycle is established that culminates with an enlarged suprapatellar bursa interfering with normal knee motion.

The presence of a symptomatic mediopatellar plica may also play a role in the development of abnormal biomechanics of the patellofemoral joint. This may be attributable to the bowstring effect[3] of this fibrous band interfering with the abnormal excursion of the quadriceps mechanism.[10] It is because of this that a rehabilitation program for mediopatellar plica pathology is directed at improving patellofemoral mechanics by way of quadriceps muscle strengthening, particularly vastus medialis obliquus.[1]

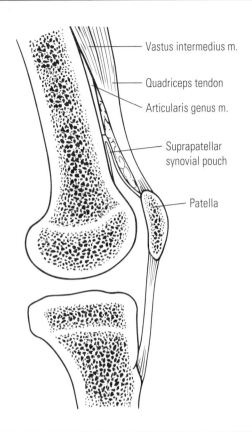

FIG. 47-3 Function of the articularis genu muscle. During knee extension, the plicae may undergo impingement within the patellofemoral articulation if not for the articularis genu, which contracts to draw the articular capsule superiorly and thus avoid abrasive injury to the synovial capsule.

7. What is the function of the articularis genu muscle?

The *articularis genu* (or, *subcrureus*) muscle is a small flat muscle that is highly variable and whose function is understood in relation to both the patella and synovium of the knee. The articularis genu arises from the supratrochlear region of the anterior femur (adjacent to the vastus intermedius) and inserts into the synovial joint capsule, which lines the suprapatellar synovial pouch.[9] During knee extension, the plicae may undergo impingement within the patellofemoral articulation if not for the articularis genu that contracts to pull the synovial capsule superiorly (Fig. 47-3). Moreover, during knee extension the anterior superior capsule moves with and must pleat so as to avoid injury to the capsule.[7] The articularis genu functions to draw the articular capsule proximally and thus avoid abrasive injury to the synovial capsule.

As the knee extends the articularis genu muscle normally pulls up on the plica and prevents it from becoming impinged within the patellofemoral joint. Prolonged sitting in acute knee flexion causes an aching discomfort owing to considerable tension in the synovial plicae as they are tightly draped over the femoral condyles. In cases of atonia of the articularis genu, the muscle is slow in responding to a sudden change in knee position that accompanies standing up after prolonged sitting. As the patient stands up and begins walking severe pain may be experienced, which may last some 8 to 10 steps and then feel better as walking continues. This is because the atonic muscle requires a greater time period to retract the plica into sufficient elevation to avoid entrapment within the patellofemoral joint.[6]

8. What are the clinical findings of this disorder?

The patient with mediopatellar plica syndrome may report pain over the medial femoral condyle. This is in sharp contrast to a medial meniscal tear, in which pain and tenderness are commonly localized to the medial tibiofemoral joint line. It is helpful to remember that a disorder of the plica only *feels as if* the knee will give way, but does not whereas meniscus pathology actually may cause the knee to buckle. Likewise, medial patellar pain is more likely related to patellofemoral maltracking. The latter two disorders are the most common misdiagnoses.

The patient may complain of pain brought on by activity, or may simply follow long periods of sitting with the knee in the flexed posture such as may occur after watching a show in a theater. The patient may also report a snapping sensation corresponding to the plica sweeping across the femoral condyle. Other nonspecific symptoms include locking, weakness, crepitus, loss of motion, quadriceps atrophy, stiffness, a sensation of "tightness," and intermittent or exercise-related swelling. A positive McMurray's sign may be present. There may also be tender bands or cords palpable along the medial condyle. Progressive fibrosis of a medial patellar plica may lead to a palpable snapping sensation as the knee is flexed and extended.[15]

9. How is the diagnosis of plica syndrome made?

A diagnosis of plica syndrome is made by the history alone and is supported by the physical examination. Routine radiographs are only useful in eliminating other causes of knee pain. Although computerized tomography and ultrasonography are helpful in aiding diagnosis, magnetic resonance imaging (MRI) is the only noninvasive procedure that clearly shows plicae. MRI is also useful in ruling out other causes of internal derangement. Arthroscopy is considered the gold standard for the diagnosis of plica syndrome. However, the mere presence of plica does not warrant invasive intervention. Plicae that appear wavy, soft, vascularized, and have synovial-covered edges are best left alone, whereas plicae with white inner borders should be considered pathologic. In addition, there may be articular cartilage wear of the medial femoral condyle corresponding to impingement of the plica as the knee is flexed from an extended position. The white inner borders of the pathologic plica correspond to excessive rubbing of the plica upon the underlying medial femoral condyle. The corresponding area of the condyle may show irritation or erosion of the underlying hyaline cartilage.[16]

10. Which special tests help diagnose this condition?

The synovial plicae are palpable in the medial and lateral parapatellar regions over both the medial and lateral retinacular ligaments. The presence of a palpable plica is, in the vast majority of cases, a normal finding. If they become inflamed or fibrotic, reproduction of pain will occur as they are palpated and compressed under the examiner's finger. Provocative tests that implicate the plicae may be painful and include:
- *Stutter test.* With one finger on the patella the patient is asked to extend the involved knee while sitting on the edge of the table with legs dangling. At some point in the range between 45° to 60° extension the examiner's fingers will feel the patella "jump" as it passes over the medial plica instead of the normally expected smooth movement. Indeed the finger may even be thrown off the patella.[18]
- *O'Conner's sign.* This yields point tenderness at the location of one finger's breadth above the medial knee joint line.
- *Mediopatellar plica test.* The examiner flexes the involved knee to 30° while the patient lies supine. The patient will complain of pain if their patella is manually moved medially (Fig. 47-4). Pain is indicative of a positive test result due to pinching of the mediopatellar plica between the patella and medial femoral condyle.[8]
- *Hughston plica test.* With the patient lying in the supine position the examiner will flex the knee and medially rotate the tibia with one arm and hand so that the foot and knee complex are held in internal rotation (Fig. 47-5). The patella is then medially dis-

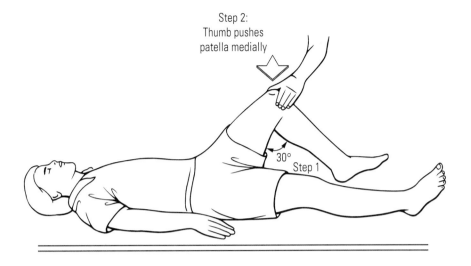

FIG. 47-4 *Impingement test* of the left medial patellar plica. Pain indicates a positive test and derives from the edge of the plica becoming pinched between the medial femoral condyle and the patella.

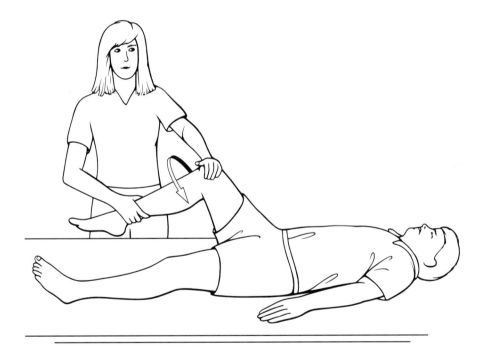

FIG. 47-5 *Hughston test* for suprapatellar plica pathology. The foot and tibia are held in internal rotation. The patella is displaced slightly medially with the fingers over the course of the suprapatellar plica. The knee is then passively flexed and extended. A positive test is pronounced if these motions elicit a "pop" and associated tenderness. A positive test may rule out suspected injury of the medial meniscus.

placed with the heel of the other hand simultaneously palpating the medial femoral condyle along the course of the plica with fingers of the same hand. The patient's knee is then passively flexed and extended so as to elicit a "pop" of the plica imparted to the examiners hand while confirming tenderness at that locale.

11. How does the clinical presentation of plica syndrome differ from derangement of the extensor mechanism or the menisci?

The signs and symptoms of plicae syndrome may mimic derangement of the extensor mechanism, that is, lateral patellar subluxation. The patterns of innervation in the structures about the knee are such that the afferent feedback that would signify a patellar dislocation is cross-innervated with nerves that innervate the synovial plica. As the quadriceps contract during gait the plica, if fibrosed, may become interposed within the patellofemoral joint. The afferent impulse the patient perceives is similar to that which would have occurred with true patellar instability.[6] Patellofemoral syndrome and tracking abnormalities of the patellofemoral joint are much more common than plica syndrome. Most clicking or snapping arising from the anterior knee compartment derives from maltracking of the patellofemoral joint, whereas most medial femoral condyle-derived pain occurs secondary to retinacular pain or pain deriving from the medial patellar facet. Accompanying clinical findings of patellofemoral dysfunction often include patellar malalignment, increased Q angle, genu valgum, femoral anteversion, and subtalar joint pronation. Pain following resistance against knee flexion or extension as well as patellar compression against the femoral condyle is also suggestive of patellofemoral joint abnormalities and not plicae involvement. Pain *during* activity is generally seen with patellar tracking disorders such as subluxation, whereas pain *after* activity is typically seen in inflammatory disorders, such as synovial plica irritation. Although stiffness presents in a variety of patellofemoral disorders, it is more often than not present in synovial plicae irritation because the plica is pulled tightly over the femoral condyles when the knee is acutely flexed for a significant time period. Radiographic changes typical of patellofemoral syndrome or malalignment demonstrate increased femoral sulcus angle, lateral patellar tilt or subluxation, or an underdeveloped lateral femoral condyle. With plica syndrome, unlike meniscus injury, there is no history of intermittent knee buckling or locking. An injury to the plica may only feel as if it will give way; a meniscus injury may actually give way and buckle underneath the patient.

12. What therapeutic management is appropriate?

Once synovial plicae syndrome is suspected, the initial treatment regimen during the acute phase includes rest from excessive knee movement; especially knee flexion that may irritate the plica. Cryotherapy may help relieve pain. Nonsteroidal antiinflammatory medications may be beneficial. Phonophoresis facilitates decreasing the acute inflammatory reaction, whereas activity modification helps reduce the inciting activity that caused synovial inflammation. After the acute phase, therapeutic exercises may be instituted to strengthen the quadriceps muscle group by way of quad sets and terminal knee extension exercises. During these exercises, the patient is instructed to concentrate on the sensation of drawing upward via the action of vastus intermedius so as to work the articularis genus muscle; this deep portion of the vastus intermedius attaches on the synovial membrane of the knee and acts to prevent it from becoming pinched. Selective strengthening of the vastum medialis obliquus is also appropriate. Stretching of both the quadriceps and hamstring muscle groups is appropriate, particularly if tightness is detected upon patient evaluation. Progressive resistive exercises should only be performed through the pain free range initially. An eclectic regimen of knee rehabilitation usually alleviates symptoms associated with plicae syndrome.[15]

Generally, patients who are younger and whose symptoms are associated with less than 3 months duration are more likely to respond to these measures. Patients with a chronic plica disorder are less likely to respond to conservative intervention, at which point surgical intervention may be appropriate. If significant fibrosis or adhesions are present, the plica may be scarred down so that it remains entrapped and cannot be retracted even after adequate muscle rehabilitation.[6] Arthroscopic plica resection is only recommended for plicae that are symptomatic or pathologic and not simply because they are present. Most plicae observed during arthroscopy are incidental findings. Relegation of the plicae to the role of appendix of the knee must be avoided because route resection is not a panacea and may, in fact, lead to significant complications.[4] Operative management is not an innocuous procedure as postsurgical complications may occur. Postoperatively, significant bleeding may occur, resulting in a large hemarthrosis and prolonged recovery period.

13. What therapeutic management is appropriate in the postsurgical patient?

Following arthroscopy, full knee extension is not permitted postoperatively until 7 to 10 days. During this time the patient must refrain from stair climbing or running, and should perform straight leg raises, quad sets, and hamstring stretching for 8 sets of 10 repetitions, 3 times a day. Once full knee extension is allowed, progressive resistive exercises may be initiated.

REFERENCES

1. Boland AL, Hulstyn MJ: Soft-tissue injuries of the knee. In Nicholas JA, Hershman EB editors: *The lower extremity and spine,* ed 2, vol 1, St Louis, 1995, Mosby.
2. Hardaker T, Whipple TL, Bussett FH: Diagnosis and treatment of the plica syndrome of the knee, *J Bone Joint Surg* 62(A):221, 1980.
3. Hughston JC, Stone M, Andrews JR: The suprapatellar plica: its role in internal derangement of the knee, *J Bone Joint Surg* 55(A):1318, 1973.
4. Hughston JC: Subluxation of the patella, *J Bone Joint Surg* 50(A):1003, 1968.
5. Hughston JC, Whatley GS, Dodelin RA et al: The role of the suprapatellar plica in internal derangement of the knee, *Am J Orthop* 5:25, 1963.
6. Jacobson KE, Flandry FC: Diagnosis of anterior knee pain, *Clin Sports Med* 8(2):187, 1989.
7. Lehmkuhl LD, Smith LK: *Brunstromm's clinical kinesiology,* ed 4, Philadelphia, 1989, FA Davis.
8. Mital MA, Hayden J: Pain in the knee in children: the medial plica shelf syndrome, *Orthop Clin North Am* 10:713, 1979.
9. O'Conner RL: *Arthroscopy,* Philadelphia, 1977, JB Lippincott.
10. Pagnani MJ, Warren RF, Arnoczky SP et al: Anatomy of the knee. In Nicholas JA, Hershman EB editors: *The lower extremity and spine,* ed 2, vol 1, St Louis, 1995, Mosby.
11. Patel D: Arthroscopy of the plica: synovial folds and their significance, *Am J Sports Med* 6:217, 1978.
12. Patel D: Plica as a cause of anterior knee pain, *Orthop Clin North Am* 17:273, 1986.
13. Pipkin G: Knee injuries: the role of the suprapatellar plica and bursa simulating internal derangement, *Clin Orthop* 74:161, 1971.
14. Pipkin G: Lesions of the suprapatellar plica, *J Bone Joint Surg* 32(A):363, 1950.
15. Terry GC: The anatomy of the extensor mechanism, *Clin Sports Med* 8(2), 1989.
16. Thabit III G, Lyle JM: Patellofemoral pain in the pediatric patient, *Orthop Clin North Am* 23(4):581, 1992.
17. Tindel NL, Nisonson B: The plica syndrome, *Orthop Clin North Am* 23(4):613, 1992.
18. Tria AJ, Klein KS: *An illustrated guide to the knee,* New York, 1992, Churchill Livingstone.

RECOMMENDED READING

Broom MJ, Fulkerson JP: The plica syndrome: a new perspective, *Orthop Clin North Am* 17:279, 1986.
Tindel NL, Nisonson B: The plica syndrome, *Orthop Clin North Am* 23(4), 1992.
Vaughan-Lane T, Dandy DJ: The synovial shelf syndrome, *J Bone Joint Surg* 64(B): 475, 1982.

PART X

HIP, THIGH, AND KNEE

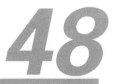

Painful Snapping over Greater Trochanter While Running Downhill on a Banked Surface

CASE 1: A 29-year-old tall, slender female presents with a 6-day history of right lateral thigh pain. She celebrated the oncoming of spring by donning her running shoes and running 6 miles per day for the past 2 weeks. She reports insidious onset of pain after 2 miles into her run, almost always beginning after a 600-yard downhill sprint. She reports that pain has been steadily increasing throughout her run, and when walking or descending a flight of stairs. As of late, symptoms are heightened in the morning hours although they tend to subside if she takes it easy. The patient reports hearing an audible "snap" at the hip that is often painful. She offers to show what she means by placing her right leg in front of her body in a semiflexed hip and knee posture. She then internally and externally rotates her hip, while bearing most of her weight on her unaffected left leg she reproduces the snap. As she does this you observe a flitting movement over the right greater trochanter. She denies any numbness, tingling, or any history of injury to that area. Pain does not extend to the groin or midthigh. When asked, she admits to running along the right side of a cambered road. She also admits to not warming up or stretching before running.

OBSERVATION Bilateral cavus foot posture is observed. A side profile view shows a flat-back posture.

PALPATION There is local tenderness over the greater trochanter. Callous foot patterns are located over the lateral plantar surface. Moderate right knee crepitus is noted.

RANGE OF MOTION Range of motion is full and painless.

MUSCLE STRENGTH G− muscle strength to her right quadriceps muscle. Good muscle strength to right hip abductors.

FLEXIBILITY Flexibility shows tightness in bilateral hamstring muscles.

SELECTIVE TENSION Discomfort reported at the left greater trochanter when right hip extension and lateral rotation were performed against resistance.

LOWER EXTREMITY ALIGNMENT This is normal.

SPECIAL TESTS These indicate a right Q angle measure of 20°. There is no leg-length discrepancy. Negative Faber and Trendelenburg tests. Negative Erichsen's sign. Positive Thomas test.

CASE 2: A 38-year-old male cyclist prepares for an upcoming diathelon race by riding 15 miles per day over the past month. Riding included several miles on steep hilly surfaces. He complains of rhythmic lateral left knee pain with each pedaling stroke that interfered with his ability to transfer power to the pedal. Pain radiates from the lateral knee up the lateral thigh and down to the proximal lateral tibia. When asked, he admits to using a new bike with a higher seat. He also runs along a long crested hill and back for a distance of 5 miles per day. His symptoms are replicated during running after approximately covering the same distance each time.

OBSERVATION   When observing him mounted on the bicycle you notice that his feet are placed externally rotated on the foot pedals. A slight skin dimpling is noted along the midline of the lateral length of the left thigh. An area of mild swelling is noted over the left lateral femoral condyle. A side profile view shows a "military-type" posture.

PALPATION   Point tenderness noted above the left tibiofemoral joint line at the left lateral femoral condyle, especially while extending the knee from 30° to 0° of flexion. Slight crepitus is felt over the left lateral femoral condyle.

ACTIVE RANGE OF MOTION   Active range of motion was full, although knee extension reproduced the patient's pain within a painful arc at approximately 30° of knee flexion.

MUSCLE STRENGTH   Normal bilateral quadriceps strength; good hamstring strength bilaterally.

FLEXIBILITY   Testing indicates tightness in the quadriceps bilaterally.

SELECTIVE TENSION   Discomfort is reported at the left lateral distal femoral condyle when left hip extension and lateral rotation were performed against resistance.

LOWER EXTREMITY MALALIGNMENT   A leg length discrepancy is noted on the left (1 inch shorter). Leg-heel and heel-forefoot relationships were normal.

CLUE   The following maneuver provoked painful reproduction of symptoms for both Cases 1 and 2:

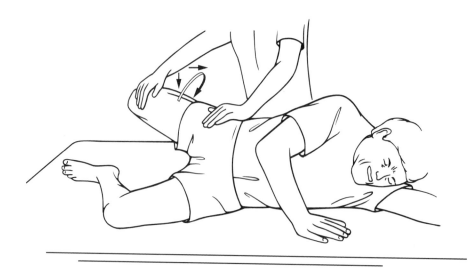

? Questions

1. What is probably wrong with these patients?
2. What is iliotibial band (ITB) friction syndrome?
3. What is the relevant anatomy of the tensor fasciae latae (TFL) muscle?
4. What bone-sparing strategy does the tensor fasciae latae muscle offer the proximal femur?
5. What is the anatomy of the longitudinal thickening of fascia lata known as the iliotibial band?
6. What is the kinesiology of the TFL-ITB complex?
7. What patterns of muscle weakness may contribute to ITB tendinitis?
8. When does distal ITB anteroposterior excursion across the lateral femoral condyle occur in the gait cycle?
9. Which site along the course of ITB-TFL is more commonly irritated in females?
10. What foot deformities are associated with the development of ITB tendinitis?
11. How does running along a crested surface relate to development of ITB tendinitis?
12. What is the relationship between leg length discrepancy and ITB tendinitis?
13. How is hill running contributory to development of ITB tendinitis?
14. How does ITB tendinitis occur in cyclists?
15. What is the classification of ITB tendinitis?
16. What provocative stress tests best reproduce the patient's symptoms?
17. Rotations of the lower limb result in a snapping sensation of which proximal structures?
18. What is the clinical presentation of ITB tendinitis?
19. What is the differential diagnosis?
20. What therapeutic management is appropriate for the treatment of ITB tendinitis?

---

1. What is probably wrong with these patients?

Case 1 is a result of right *snapping hip syndrome;* Case 2 is a result of left *runner's knee.* The former and latter are, respectively, proximal and distal forms of iliotibial band friction syndrome. Renne initially described this condition in the United States in 1975.[23]

The Clue shows a positive Ober test indicating tightness in the iliotibial tract and tensor fasciae latae muscle. A positive test is indicated if the ipsilateral lower limb remains abducted and does not adduct toward the examining table surface.

2. What is iliotibial band friction syndrome?

Iliotibial band friction syndrome (Fig. 48-1) is a repetitive stress injury caused by excessive friction anywhere along the course of this long strip of fascia. Irritation may occur proximally owing to a too-tight iliotibial band (ITB) pulling either at its origin on the ilium, or distally at the band's insertion on *Gerdy's tubercle* on the anterolateral portion of the proximal tibia. Intrinsic etiologic factors associated with this condition include an anatomically prominent lateral epicondyle, a tight iliotibial band, excessive subtalar joint pronation, excessive genu varum,[6,5,11,16] diminished flexibility, and prominence of the lateral femoral condyle.[27] Extrinsic factors associated with ITB tendinitis in runners include training errors such as sudden increases in mileage, training on transverse grades, excessive downhill running, running in shoes with excessive lateral heel wear, overstriding, and running on hard surfaces.[16,*] Although most iliotibial band friction syndromes have been reported in distance runners,[5,11,16,24] virtually anyone engaging in activity requiring repeated knee flexion and extension such as downhill skiing, circuit training, weight lifting, jumping sports, or cycling, is prone to developing this pathology.[10,19] In soccer, goalies are particularly vulnerable to the distal form of ITB irritation as they suffer from repeated contusions of this area during diving saves.[19]

When painful irritation occurs proximally between the origin and insertion proximally over the greater trochanter it is referred to as *snapping hip syndrome.* When pathology manifests distally over the lateral femoral condyle it is known as *runner's knee.* The former may occur from overload of the tensor fascia latae muscle and possibly inflame the bursa lying between the trochanter and the iliotibial band.

---

*Hard surfaces include paved roads, but not dirt roads.

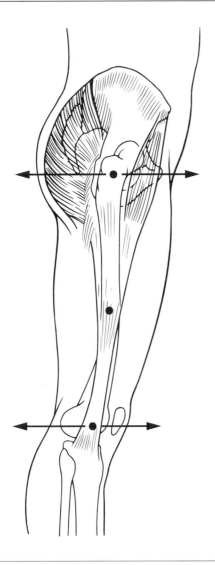

FIG. 48-1 *Iliotibial band friction syndrome* may occur proximally, distally, or at the midsubstance of that structure. The arrows indicate the direction of motion the iliotibial tract may translates as it moves across the bony protuberances of the greater trochanter proximally and lateral femoral epicondyle distally.

Runner's knee represents the *most common form of* ITB friction syndrome.[30] This distal form of ITB pathology most commonly involves the posterior fibers of the ITB as they are especially susceptible to friction irritation as they more closely contour to the lateral femoral condyle than do the anterior fibers. Patients with runner's knee often have a history of poor training techniques, lack an appropriate stretching regimen, run long distances without gradually building up to that level, exhibit excessive stride lengths, or run along irregular surfaces. Runner's knee may also occur in cyclists or skiers.

Middle and long distance runners may also develop "hot spots" of inflammation and tenderness at the junction of the tensor fascia latae (TFL) muscle and ITB. The structures comprising the TFL-ITB complex are composed of contractile and fascial tissue, respectively. Hot spots may arise owing to the differential capacity of contractile and fascial tissue in negotiating tensile stress. The confluence of these two structures represents a weak link that may be subject to stress rise.

3. What is the relevant anatomy of the tensor fasciae latae (TFL) muscle?

Tensor fasciae latae (TFL) is a fusiform muscle[4,5,11,15,16,23,24,26] originating from the tubercle at the anterior ridge of the iliac crest immediately superior to the anterior superior iliac spine and inserting into the proximal anterolateral iliotibial tract. This muscle, encased between two layers of fascia lata,[14] relates to the 3 axes of the hip joint so as to abduct, forward flex, and rotate the femur in either direction. *Contraction of this muscle simultaneously flexes the hip and extends the knee by tensing the iliotibial tract.* In addition to its leverage role in the musculoskeletal system, TFL also provides a dynamic vascular return mechanism of the lower extremity. Most lower-extremity veins are surrounded by musculature that help milk venous blood proximally. The greater saphenous vein is subcutaneous and thus is covered by muscle only on one side. Tensor fascia latae plays a role in venous return such that tension of this structure acts to tense the skin overlying the great saphenous vein, thus helping to return blood back toward the heart.

4. What bone-sparing strategy does the TFL muscle offer the proximal femur?

The superior portion of the femur is composed of a nearly spherical head mounted on an angulated shaft. The neck is approximately 5 cm long and forms an angle with the shaft that varies between 115° and 140° in the normal individual. Inherent to the proximal femoral architecture is a convex curve laterally and concavity medially. The consequences of this architecture results in *eccentric* (i.e., off-center) *loading* of the femur. Evidence for this type of loading is demonstrated in the bony trabeculae in the cancellous (spongy) bone, which demonstrate organizational alignment (Wolff's law) consistent with these stresses. As such, although the lateral side is subjected to tensile bending forces during loading, the medial concave aspect is subjected to compressive force. Correspondingly, trabecular organization of the cancellous bone comprising the proximal femur is perpendicular to the long axis of the femoral shaft along the medial convex aspect of the femur in response to compressive force. In contrast, trabecular organization runs parallel along the lateral concave aspect of the femur in direct response to tensile force. Bone lacks the inherent capacity to attenuate distractive tensile force as compared to compressive forces.

The TFL muscle may provide a bone sparing strategy to the lateral side of the femur that acts to absorb or cancel excessive tensile forces that may result in bone fracture (Fig. 48-2). The muscle concentrically contracts and in so doing provides a compressive force propagated through the ITB and acting as TFL's *surrogate tendon*. The compressive force generated by TFL counteracts the tensile forces realized in the femur secondary to eccentric hip loading. In this manner TFL unloads excessive lateral forces that develop along the convex aspect of the proximal femur and thereby avoid injury.

5. What is the anatomy of the longitudinal thickening of fascia lata known as the iliotibial band?

The *iliotibial band* or *tract* is a nonelastic, collagenous, dense, longitudinal thickening of fascia lata that connects the ilium to the tibia[13] by extending from the pelvis across the lateral aspect of the knee. The *fascia lata* is a complete stockinglike investment of the thigh. The fascia lata is strong, although thicker where it has tendinous contributions and thinner in the gluteal region. The proximal aspect of the ITB is held posterior to the hip axis at the level of the greater trochanter by the combined pull of the gluteus maximus posteriorly, the TFL muscle anteriorly, and by its deep attachment into the linea aspera of the femur. Distally, the tract's anterior border may be palpated as a strong band over the lateral aspect of the knee immediately lateral to the superior border of the patella during the last 30° of knee extension, or where it inserts into the lateral tibial tubercle.[8]

Tightness of the ITB may be due to its long orientation of span across both the hip and knee joints serving as a lateral stabilizer of both those articulations. Proximally originating from the tubercle of the iliac crest, the ITB receives tendinous attachment primarily from the TFL muscle as well as the gluteus maximus

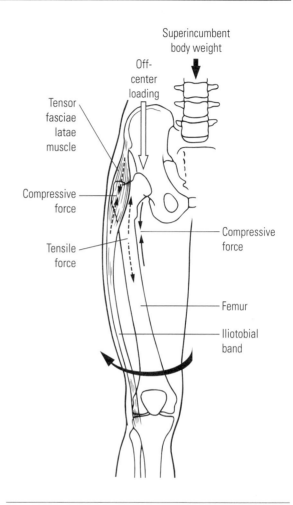

FIG. 48-2 *Bone-sparing role* of the TFL-ITB complex. Eccentric loading of the femur results in compressive forces realized along the medial aspect of the proximal femur and distractive tension along the lateral side. Excessive tension buildup along the convex lateral aspect owing to increased loads may result in a transverse-type fracture at the side under tension. Compressive concentric force generated by TFL provides a counter-tensile force to the lateral (convex) aspect of the proximal femur that cancels the potentially injurious distractive forces. Arrows with dashed lines represent compressive and tensile force vectors that cancel each other.

and gluteus medius at the level of the greater trochanter. The band courses distally down the lateral aspect of the thigh muscles toward the knee where it bifurcates into two functional components. Although the iliopatellar band angulates ventrally to blend with the aponeurosis of the vastus lateralis and lateral patellar border, the iliotibial component continues coursing distally beyond the knee joint. This vertical band, functioning as a long tendinous insertion, is free to glide anteriorly and

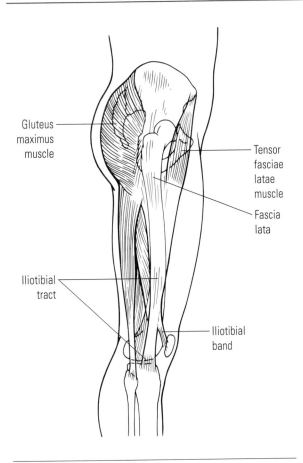

Gluteus maximus muscle

Tensor fasciae latae muscle

Fascia lata

Iliotibial tract

Iliotibial band

FIG. 48-3 Both TFL and gluteus maximus inset on the proximal border of the iliotibial tract and antagonistically work to preserve pelvic balance on the sagittal plane. Shortness or weakness of either will result in pelvic tilt. The iliotibial tract, spanning from the ilium to the tibia, serves as a conjoint tendon to both muscles and endows them with an increased lever arm that enables them to play a role distally in controlling motion at the knee.

posteriorly as it passes over the lateral femoral condyle. Its distal end becomes increasingly thickened as it approaches its insertion and hence becomes endowed with an ability to withstand force to failure comparable with the anterior cruciate ligament. It then terminates at the knee where it reinforces the knee joint capsule before inserting on the lateral tibial prominence on the anterolateral tibial condyle (Gerdy's tubercle).

6. What is the kinesiology of the TFL-ITB complex?

The ITB is a strong lateral band of fascia that serves in a dynamic capacity for the TFL muscle and as part of a functional tendon for the gluteus maximus (Fig. 48-3). Biomechanically, the ITB serves to increase the lever

arm of the muscles that attach to its proximal portion. TFL also plays a role in steadying the trunk on the thigh, as well as counteracting the posterior pull of gluteus maximus on the iliotibial tract.[28] Because the origin of the ITB lies posterior to the level of the hip axis at the level of the greater trochanter, ITB proximally functions to help maintain the hip in extension. Distally, the ITB origin passes anterior to the knee joint axis and thereby creates an extensor moment at the knee. It is this unique reverse alignment with respect to the hip and knee joint axes that endows contraction of the TFL-ITB complex to simultaneously flex the hip and extend the knee joint.

With movement of the lower extremity, such as occurs during walking and running, the ITB translates anteriorly and posteriorly to both the hip and knee joint axes. Swing phase of gait is characterized by shortening of the swing leg via flexion of the hip and knee joints to permit ground clearance. During the swing phase of gait the hip flexor action of the tensor fasciae latae pulls the ITB anterior to the greater trochanter thereby recruiting its leverage to assist with hip flexion. As the knee flexes, the ITB crosses posterior to the knee joint at approximately 30° of knee flexion, and is then positioned to act as a flexor of the knee.[14] This point in the range brings the ITB in contact with the prominence of the lateral femoral condyle.[4,10,19] Thus swing phase is characterized by simultaneous tensing of the ITB across the hip and knee joints. The ITB undergoes maximal tension as it proximally lies anterior to the hip joint and distally lies posterior to the knee joint.

This position of the ITB to both the hip and knee joints is maintained until midstance phase of stance during which the knee undergoes near extension and the hip begins to extend. At midstance, ITB undergoes a reversal in the direction of translation at both the hip and knee as it once again assumes its original position as an extensor of both the hip and knee.[15] As the now taut ITB returns to its original position, it rubs across both the body prominences of the greater trochanter and lateral femoral condyle (Fig. 48-4). This is the basis for repetitive friction that may culminate in snapping hip syndrome or runner's knee.

Distally, ITB serves the knee by augmenting anterolateral stability of the tibia.[14] The deeper fibers of the tibial end of the band may act as a sling behind the lateral femoral condyle that prevents posterior subluxation of the femur on a flexed tibia.[4,8] Thus the ITB shares a similar distal oblique orientation of span with the anterior cruciate ligament and may play a role in re-

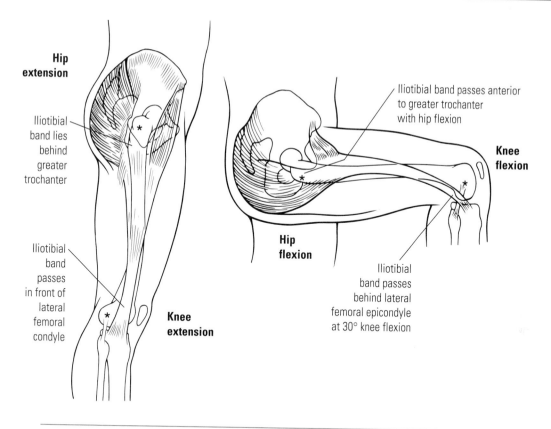

FIG. 48-4 During swing and stance phases of gait, the iliotibial tract translates anterior and posterior with respect to both the hip and knee joint axes. As the hip moves from extension to flexion, the proximal iliotibial tract passes from behind the greater trochanter to in front of it. During knee extension the distal iliotibial band passes from behind to in front of the lateral femoral epicondyle. The repetitive friction caused by a tight iliotibial tract rubbing over the bone prominence of the greater trochanter or lateral epicondyle may result in irritation and inflammation as snapping hip syndrome or runner's knee, respectively.

straining anterior tibial translation and posterior femoral translation. Moreover, the distal ITB may work in concert with the lateral collateral ligament and popliteus to prevent varus opening at the knee joint and may play a role in minimizing excessive external rotation of the tibia on the femur.

7. What patterns of muscle weakness may contribute to ITB tendinitis?

Weakness or tightness of hip musculature is a common sign in patients with ITB tendinitis. Lower extremity disuse as in the case of a relatively sedentary individual who begins intense sudden exercise may incur this disorder. This is because muscle disuse may result in contracture as muscle is denied being worked through its full potential range.

There are essentially 3 key structures that relate to ITB tendinitis. Understanding their interrelationship is essential to understanding the dynamic role of muscles in this disorder. The *iliotibial tract* comprises a lateral reinforcement of the fascia latae from the ilium to the tibia and thus impacts on knee function. En route to its downward descent, the fascia latae encounters the borders of both the *gluteus maximus muscle* and the *tensor fasciae lata muscle*. (Note that *fascia latae* refers to the fascia investing the thigh, which elongates to become the iliotibial tract, whereas the *fasciae lata* is a muscular structure.) Upon reaching the borders of these two muscles the fascia latae divides and invests both the superficial and deep surfaces of these muscles. Finally, both the tensor fasciae lata muscle and the gluteus maximus muscle insert into the iliotibial tract[8] so that its distal extent serves as a conjoint tendon for these muscles.

Gluteus maximus, a powerful hip and trunk extensor that plays its greatest role in stair climbing and running, also functions to stabilize the distal knee joint by virtue of its insertion into the iliotibial tract. The tensor fasciae lata muscle inserts on the other (i.e., anterior) end of the iliotibial tract and works antagonistically by counteracting the backward pull of gluteus maximus on the iliotibial tract. Thus gluteus maximus and the smaller tensor fasciae latae muscle may be viewed antagonistically in relation to their insertion into the iliotibial tract. This is borne out by the opposite actions of these two muscles, namely thigh extension, adduction, and lateral rotation as compared to thigh flexion, abduction, and medial rotation. Thus the pelvis is dynamically balanced by the opposing forces of these two muscles in the sagittal plane. Although tensor fasciae latae generates a moment to tilt the pelvis anteriorly, gluteus maximus works to posteriorly tilt the pelvis. The harmonious interactive dynamic balance among these muscles maintains neutral pelvic obliquity.

The functional significance of the ITB serving as a *conjoint tendon* for both the gluteus maximus and tensor fasciae latae muscles is that both of these proximal thigh muscles have far reaching distal impact on the knee joint. Although both muscles tense the ITB, shortness or weakness of either muscle will upset the balance of the pelvis. If tensor fasciae latae is shortened unilaterally, or unopposed because of a weakened gluteus maximus, loss of dynamic balance may manifest as lateral pelvic tilt to *the side of tightness.* In addition, a shortened tensor fasciae latae would result in tightness of the anterior portion of the iliotibial band. The knee on that side will tend toward a valgus angulation due to bowstringing across the lateral side of the knee. Also, because the distal iliotibial tract sends fibers to the lateral aspect of the patella as well as the lateral intramuscular septum, tightness of the ITB may contribute to lateral patellar displacement, and laterally deflecting the pull of the quadriceps mechanism.

If tensor fasciae latae and other hip flexor muscles are tight, there may be an anterior pelvis tilt and medial femoral rotation. Bilateral shortness of tensor fasciae latae in standing may cause an anterior pelvic tilt, or even bilateral knock-knee. On the other hand, unopposed action of the gluteus maximus muscle due to a weakened TFL muscle may upset the dynamic balance such that unilateral posterior pelvic tilt and varus stress are generated at the level of the knee joint.

8. When does distal ITB anteroposterior excursion across the lateral femoral condyle occur in the gait cycle?

When the knee joint is in the terminal portion of extension, the ITB lies anterior to the axis of the knee joint, but at 30° of flexion it passes posterior to the knee joint axis.[21] Because the distal band is free of attachment along its span between the lateral femoral condyle and the tibial tuberosity, the band undergoes anterior and posterior excursion with extension and flexion of the knee joint, respectively. Repetitive flexion and extension motions of the knee joint that accompany the gait cycle may subject the ITB to increased stress. The excessive friction build-up between the ITB and the femoral condyle may cause irritation and inflammation within the iliotibial band, the bursa underneath, or the periosteum of the lateral femoral epicondyle.[13,23]

Distally, ITB passes to and fro over the lateral femoral epicondyle with each step. At mid-swing phase of gait knee flexion has reduced to 30° and continues to decrease up until terminal swing.[13] During this interim between mid and late swing phase, the distal ITB passes from behind the lateral femoral condyle to a position anterior to the condyle. This movement of the ITB will reverse when flexion beyond 30° occurs, as it does during early swing when the entire limb shortens to allow for ground clearance. Similarly, stance phase is also accompanied by the distal ITB passing anterior to the femoral condyle in the interim between heel strike and midphase of stance. Posterior excursion of the distal band then occurs during the interim between midstance and heel-off phase of gait as the knee flexes, as the distal band returns to a position on or behind the lateral femoral condyle.

9. Which site along the course of ITB-TFL is more commonly irritated in females?

Anatomic differences may account for the increased likelihood of the development of many lower extremity dysfunctions, particularly in unconditioned females. Women have wider pelvises (gynecoid) compared with men (android), and hence a greater varus angulation of the hip and valgus of the knees (Fig. 48-5). The ITB tendon may sustain additional stretch over its length in females due to the greater prominence of the greater trochanter as a direct function of the wider female pelvis. An increase in the Q angle in females is present as a direct function of the greater varus angulation of the hip present in females. As

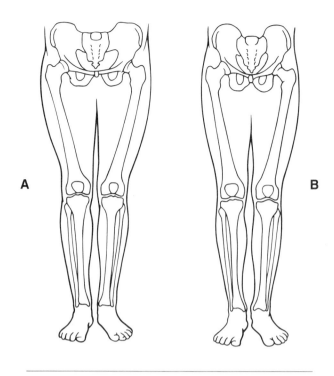

FIG. 48-5 Skeletal differences between the genders. **A,** Women have wider pelvises (gynecoid) compared with **(B)** men (android), and hence a greater varus angulation of the hip and valgus of the knees (genu valgus). An increase in the Q angle in females is present as a direct function of the greater varus angulation of the hip. Subsequently, the ITB tendon may sustain additional stretch over its length in females owing to the greater prominence of the greater trochanter as a direct function of the wider female pelvis.

such, ITB pathology may be more common proximally than distally over the lateral femoral condyle. This tensing effect of the ITB may be highlighted by the presence of femoral anteversion, which serves to increase the Q angle. The presence of femoral anteversion is greater in females than males.[20]

The presentation of ITB tendinitis is rare in endomorphs and may stem from the fact that these individuals do not run as far and also because extra fatty tissue around the knee joint may serve as a lubricant to the taut ITB.[25] Women are less affected by iliotibial band friction syndrome because of the tendency toward valgus at the knee, and because of the presence of more subcutaneous fat as compared to men.[26] The more typical patient will have an ectomorphic habitus and will be an adolescent female who presents with vague knee pain and subluxating patella, both of which could have a tight ITB as a causative factor.[16]

10. What foot deformities are associated with the development of ITB tendinitis?

Prolonged internal tibial rotation associated with abnormal *foot pronation* results in anteromedial traction of the ITB insertion so that its distal span undergoes excessive friction as it is repetitively rubbed across the lateral femoral condyle[14] during stance phase of gait. Foot-fault related dysfunction is extremely common as the foot is the *link* between the ground reaction force and the superincumbent body mass. Forces transmitted to the nonideal foot or even excessive forces imparted to the ideal foot manifest as disruptive force transmitted up the linkage system known as the kinetic chain.

The ITB is stress loaded by TFL during early and midstance phases of gait. This phase of gait is characterized by external rotation of the femur-tibia complex and pronation of the subtalar and midtarsal joints. The impact of this normal sequence of biomechanical events during the phases of stance exerts tension along the length of TFL-ITB in a tug-of-war manner that approaches the limits of its tensile capacity. It is during this period of peak tensile ITB tension that it undergoes anterior excursion across the lateral femoral condyle.

Rather than initiating supination, the *overly pronated foot* tarries into pronation beyond midstance. Excessive pronation is consistent with obligatory internal tibial torsion during stance phase. This excessive tibial torsion migrates proximally and imparts a valgus force at the tibiofemoral joint. The excessive medial tibial torsion associated with excessive and/or late pronation of the subtalar joint has the proximal effect of increasing the linear distance between Gerdy's tubercle at the anterolaterally located tibia (ITB insertion) and the anterior ridge of the iliac crest (TFL origin). Consequently, the TFL-ITB complex undergoes excessive distractive tension (Fig. 48-6). This occurs as the TFL complex contracts during late stance with the other lateral compartment muscles of the hip to provide horizontal stability to the pelvis. Thus additional tension is applied to the ITB secondary to contraction of the TFL. The net effect of both sources of tension upon the ITB, coupled with excursion of the ITB anterior to the femoral condyle may result in rubbing of distal band across the condyle. This represents a *repetitive stress injury* which, if unabated, may lead to eventual fraying or rupture of the band.

In contrast, the foot that demonstrates restricted pronation due to a cavus type foot will cause excessive external rotation proximally along the tibial shaft. This excessive rotation causes genu varum at the knee and

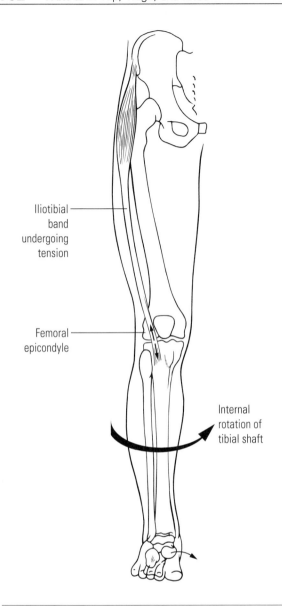

Iliotibial band undergoing tension

Femoral epicondyle

Internal rotation of tibial shaft

FIG. 48-6 The *over-pronated foot type* is implicated as cause of ITB stress syndrome. *Over-pronation of the subtalar joint* results in obligatory and excessive medial tibial rotation. This in turn manifests as a valgus force at the tibiofemoral joint, which has the effect of increasing the linear distance between Gerdy's tubercle at the proximal tibia and the iliac crest. This results in excessive tension along the TFL-ITB complex that may result in excessive rubbing across the greater trochanter or lateral femoral epicondyle.

results in distraction of the lateral tibiofemoral hemi-joint. Consequently, any structure spanning the lateral knee joint, such as the lateral collateral ligament and ITB will undergo distractive tension along its longitudinal axis. The distal ITB is thereby pulled across the

prominence of the lateral femoral condyle and is likely to sustain injury with friction buildup following anteroposterior translation that accompanies the gait cycle (Fig. 48-7). Thus both pes planus and pes cavus represent two extremes along the spectrum of intrinsic foot deformities that cause deviations from subtalar neutral. Both, by way of differing mechanisms, alter the kinesiology at the knee joint such that the ITB undergoes excessive tension before its distal insertion.

11. How does running along a crested surface lead to development of ITB tendinitis?

Iliotibial band tendinitis is frequent in people who jog or run along the beach or other banked surfaces. Pathology may effect the iliotibial band in the upside leg of the drainage pitch or on the low side of the road crown. Both the pronated or supinated subtalar joint (intrinsic) mechanisms may be (extrinsically) mimicked by running along a banked surface. This occurs because a nonlevel surface topography causes diminished medial sole contact of the lower foot, and excessive medial sole contact of the higher foot. The cavus (or supinated) foot is characterized by decreased weight bearing area, whereas the planus (or pronated) foot is characterized by increased surface contact.[27] The foot along the elevated surface undergoes excessive pronation, while the foot along the lower ground undergoes diminished pronation. Thus the topography of the terrain may mechanically force the foot into postures that deviate from subtalar joint neutral and thereby magnify or restrict pronation (Fig. 48-8).

The foot negotiating the uphill side of a pitched road relates to the road surface such that the temporal sequencing of the subtalar and midtarsal joints are altered, so as to maintain pronation beyond midstance. This overpronation imparts an internally rotated moment to the tibial shaft, which manifests as a valgus knee stress and serves to tauten the length of the TFL-ITB complex. In contrast, the foot on the low side of the road crown undergoes restricted pronation. At the tibial shaft this manifests as a diminishment of internal rotation. This excessive external rotation imparts a varus force at the knee joint. A varus angulation at the knee has the effect of distracting the lateral tibiofemoral hemi-joint. Because the ITB crosses the lateral tibiofemoral joint it will undergo distractive tension as it rubs against the lateral femoral condyle.

In contrast, the individual running along a crested road surface subjects their downhill leg[22] and knee into tibia vara and/or genu vara.[5] This posture causes distraction of the iliotibial band that stretches it over the lateral femoral condyle and subjecting it to increased friction. This same varus effect of the leg and knee may stem from running in worn shoes (especially on the lateral side)[4,10] as well as using inflexible (new) running shoes, which restrict subtalar joint pronation.[4]

12. What is the relationship between leg length discrepancy and ITB tendinitis?

The analogy of running along a pitched surface with both feet along different portions of the road is a paradigm for understanding subtalar joint compensation for a leg length discrepancy. The individual with a leg length discrepancy running on a flat surface may sustain stress to the shorter side via over-pronating, while the longer limb maintains weight bearing along the lateral border of the foot, similar to the cavus foot posture. The individual with a limb length inequality running along a horizontal surface is biomechanically equivalent to an individual with limbs of equal length running along a banked surface. In the latter, the foot on the upper portion of the road crown undergoes excessive pronation whereas the foot on the lower portion of the road crown may be analogous to a cavus foot posture. In the individual with a lower limb discrepancy, the longer limb attempts to shorten by undergoing subtalar joint pronation while the shorter limb attempts to lengthen by undergoing diminished subtalar joint pronation. This manifests as increased medial sole surface contact of the longer limb, while the shorter limb effectively lengthens by minimizing surface contact to the outer lateral border of the sole (see Fig. 48-8). The net effect of these compensations allows for more energy efficiency by minimizing the magnitude of vertical pelvic displacement. Although a compensated leg length discrepancy demonstrates normalization of gait, it does so at the price of exposing the longer limb[22] as well as the shorter limb to tendinitis of the ITB.

13. How is hill running contributory to development of ITB tendinitis?

These subtalar joint deviations may also occur from downhill or uphill running. ITB tendinitis is common to downhill runners. Downhill running is characterized by pronation beyond midstance phase of gait, whereas uphill running is characterized by a diminishment of pronation such that supination begins before midstance. The combination of downhill running on a banked surface represents a compounding pronatory effect upon

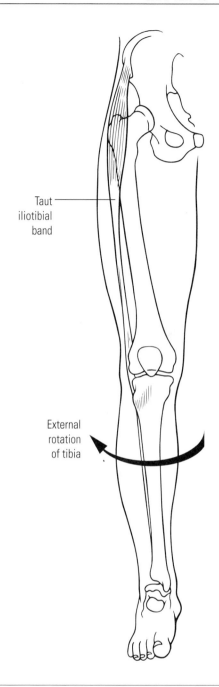

Taut iliotibial band

External rotation of tibia

FIG. 48-7 The *cavus foot type* may be implicated as causative to ITB friction syndrome. *Diminished pronation of the subtalar joint* causes obligatory excessive external rotation of the tibial shaft that manifests as a genu varus. This in turn causes distraction of the lateral tibiofemoral hemi-joint and thereby tautens the iliotibial band spanning across that articulation. Increased distraction along the length of the ITB may cause friction and inflammation as excessive rubbing occurs across the protuberances of the greater trochanter proximally and the lateral femoral epicondyle distally.

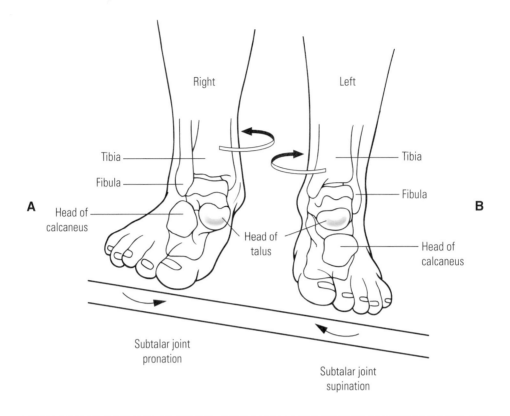

FIG. 48-8 Both an *over-pronated* and *under-pronated* foot may be imposed upon the foot running along a banked surface as body weight and surface topography result in increased or diminished sole contact, respectively. **A,** The elevated foot negotiates the higher slope by increasing sole contact, which is accomplished by subtalar joint pronation. **B,** In contrast, the lower foot undergoes diminished sole contact via subtalar joint supination.

the lower subtalar joint, whereas uphill running compounds the supinatory effect upon the subtalar joint of the higher foot. Both legs are equally susceptible toward developing ITB tendinitis.

14. How does ITB tendinitis occur in cyclists?

Iliotibial band tendinitis is a common lateral overuse disorder plaguing cyclists. This is because with each pedaling stroke, the ITB is pulled anteriorly on the downstroke and posteriorly on the upstroke. Irritation may result from intrinsic causes such as anatomic prominence of the lateral femoral condyle or an inherently tight ITB. Extrinsic factors include excessive saddle height or cleat position of the pedal. If cleats are excessively internally rotated, the tibia will also excessively internally rotate. This results in a valgus force at the knee that acts to distance the lateral femoral condyle from the lateral tibial prominence and thereby tensing that portion of ITB spanning these two bones. Similarly, external foot placement on the bike pedal manifests as sagging of the arches of the foot during the downstroke. This corresponds to foot pronation that is accentuated by deviation of foot placement from neutral to an externally rotated position. Like the internally rotated cleats, the tibia will undergo excessive internal rotation and stress the ITB.[27]

15. What is the classification of ITB tendinitis?

Iliotibial band tendinitis may be classified by four grades based on pain and activity limitation:[7]
* I—Pain beginning after activity that neither restricts distance or speed of athletic activity.

- II—Pain beginning during activity that neither restricts distance or speed.
- III—Pain beginning during activity that may restrict either distance or speed.
- IV—Pain so severe as to preclude athletic participation.

16. What provocative stress tests best reproduce the patients' symptoms?

OBER TEST

This test is diagnostic of tightness of the TFL and the ITB (Fig. 48-9). This provocative maneuver is based on the ideas that tightness of soft-tissue structures occur by passively distracting the attachments of that structure. The clinician first determines the primary, secondary, and tertiary functions of the TFL muscle, namely abduction, flexion, and medial rotation. TFL-ITB is then optimally stressed along its length by serially moving the hip in a reverse passive order.

The patient side lies on the unaffected leg with the hip and knee of the unaffected leg in flexion so as to stabilize the pelvis, flatten the lumbosacral spine, and prevent compensations that may occur from the thorax rolling in either direction during the test. The upper hip is passively lifted by the examiner and the knee is flexed to 90°. The examiner passively moves the hip serially into lateral rotation, hip hyperextension, and maximally adduction. This position places the extensor fascia latae and iliotibial tract posterior to the greater trochanter. Normally, a patient's leg should be capable of descend-

ing to a plane parallel to the examining table owing to the weight of gravity pulling the limb into adduction; this is facilitated by the examiner's gently supporting the descending limb at the ankle. If the test is positive, the patient will complain of pain upon attempted adduction and the limb will remain abducted above the horizontal place.[5] Performing this test may not be possible secondary to a hip flexion contracture (positive Thomas test).

MODIFIED OBER TEST

The patient lies prone and the involved lower extremity is grasped at the ankle. The examiner then abducts the hip, extends the hip, and flexes the ipsilateral knee and then observes how close to midline the knee returns as the hip adducts to swing the limb toward midline.

NOBLE COMPRESSION TEST

This test specifically identifies the presence of distal ITB friction syndrome at the knee. This test results in pain over the lateral epicondyle when pressure is applied to the lateral knee during extension of the knee from 90°. The patient lies in a supine position and the hip and knee of the involved extremity are flexed to 90°. Pressure is applied to or immediately 1 to 2 cm proximal to the lateral femoral condyle during knee extension from 90° of knee flexion. The patient will report a painful arc of movement emanating from the lateral femoral condylar area at 30° of flexion.[18] A variation on this test to further increase tension on the

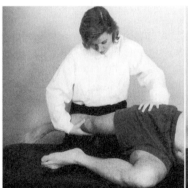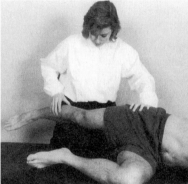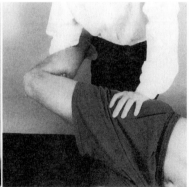

FIG. 48-9 *Ober test* for iliotibial band and tensor fasciae latae tightness. (From Magee DJ: *Orthopedic physical assessment,* Philadelphia, 1997, WB Saunders.)

ITB can be performed with the tibia in forced internal rotation.[29]

CREAK TEST

This test is performed by having the patient support all his or her weight on the affected leg and squat down into knee flexion. During a positive test, the patient will notice a "creak" over the lateral femoral epicondyle at approximately 30° of knee flexion.[14]

17. Rotations of the lower limb result in a snapping sensation of which proximal structures?

The complaint of *painful snapping hip* is a common complaint of ballet dancers, and may either present laterally or inferomedially. Anteroposterior movement of the iliotibial band over the greater trochanter causes a snapping or clicking sensation over the lateral hip that is often incurred during rotational movements of the supported lower extremity. Factors contributing to this snapping include a tight iliotibial band, narrow bi-iliac width, muscular imbalance, and decreased soft-tissue flexibility. In contrast, a painful click or snap that is experienced medially may result from motion of the iliofemoral ligament over the femoral head, or the iliopsoas tendon over the anterior inferior iliac spine, iliopectineal eminence, or the lesser trochanter. The medial clicking phenomenon occurs equally in weight bearing and nonweight bearing when attempting rotational movement.[23]

18. What is the clinical presentation of ITB tendinitis?

Pain is typically diffuse with ITB tendinitis, and presents over the lateral aspect of the knee that may extend just above the lateral joint line.[12] The patient who is a distance runner may complain of pain over the lateral femoral condyle at approximately the same distance each time. In some cases the patient may ambulate with a stiff-legged gait to avoid knee joint flexion if pain is more severe. Symptoms are usually provoked with running activities, and typically appear early in the run and decrease as the runner warms up. Pain is often worse on downhill running or while running along a drainage pitch on a banked surface. Pain may also be aggravated by ascending or descending stairs. Occasionally, swelling may be seen over the lateral femoral epicondyle. Point tenderness may be palpated over the lateral epicondyle, but not over the posterolateral knee capsule, lateral collateral ligament, popliteal tendon, or

anterior lateral fat pad. Generally, patients presenting with ITB tendinitis do not present with any antecedent history of trauma or twisting to the knee before the onset of symptoms. Moreover, patients do not complain of pain during sprinting, walking or squatting, or during such stop-and-go activities as tennis, racquetball, or squash.[16]

19. What is the differential diagnosis?

With iliotibial band disorders, the symptoms of internal knee derangement such as instability (i.e., locking, buckling,) and joint swelling, or joint line tenderness are typically not noted.[10,19] In addition, pain on sitting, or descending stairs and inclines, characteristic of chondromalacia is not evident.

- *Hip pointer injury.* This injury is a localized contusion to the iliac crest due to an unprotected blow (Fig. 48-10). Aside from point tenderness at the injury site that extends to the internal and external oblique musculature, swelling and ecchymosis are often present. Side bending of the trunk away from the injured side increases pain. Often the T12 to L3 lateral cutaneous nerves may be injured, causing numbness and diminished sensation in the lateral buttock and hip region. Radiographs are necessary to rule out iliac fracture. Myositis ossificans may follow. Treatment is with intermittent icing and taping to limit trunk motion. Once the condition is subacute, moist heat followed by ice packs are appropriate.[2] Abdominal strengthening and stretching are gently initiated, and the athlete may return to contact sports when demonstrating pain free trunk range of motion.

- *Iliac crest apophysitis.* This injury occurs in adolescents, and presents as complaints of pain at the TFL muscle origin arises from the growing iliac apophysis. This muscle originates on the ridge of iliac crest immediately superior to the anterior superior iliac spine. This apophysis closes at 13 to 15 years of age and fuses to the ilium by 21 to 25 years of age. Injury most commonly presents subacutely in runners as an overuse syndrome. There is usually no history of trauma. The pelvis is normally subjected to multiplanar motion during running (Fig. 48-11), resulting in repetitive stresses across the iliac crest by two sets of opposing muscles: (1) tensor fasciae latae, abdominal obliquus, and gluteus medius muscles attaching on the anterior portion; and (2) latissimus dorsi, gluteus maximus, quadratus lumborum, or the erector spinae muscles, which attach

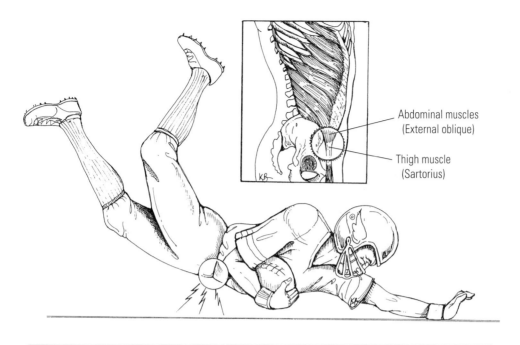

Abdominal muscles
(External oblique)

Thigh muscle
(Sartorius)

FIG. 48-10 Mechanism of a *hip pointer injury:* player falls to turf, sustaining a contusion to the iliac crest and its muscle attachments. Inset shows side profile of thorax and trunk and site of contusion. (From Scuderi GR, McCann PD, Bruno PJ: *Sports medicine: principles of primary care,* St Louis, 1997, Mosby.)

posteriorly (Fig. 48-12). Uphill running accentuates anterior pelvic tilt while downhill running increases posterior pelvic tilt and hyperextends the spine into lordosis. Reciprocal arm swing across the trunk accentuates strain of pelvic rotation. The cumulative effect is a traction force resulting in an avulsion of the apophysis from the iliac crest. Tenderness on palpation of the iliac crest, especially with resisted abduction, suggests apophysitis. Apophysitis usually resolves within 2 to 4 weeks of rest. Stretching and strengthening of the involved muscle groups is appropriately begun once symptoms have improved.

Two other less common forms of iliac crest apophysitis may occur. The traumatic form is the adolescent equivalent of a *hip pointer injury* in the adult and results in a compression fracture following a direct blow over the crest. The other acute form occurs from a sudden directional change while running, as in a lateral cutting or forward lunging movement. These would cause sudden severe abdominal contraction to be opposed by the tensor fasciae latae and gluteus medius in a set and planted leg resulting in an avulsion injury.

- *Bursitis.* A bursa may form in response to friction between the distal ITB and the lateral femoral condyle, and may be ruled out by an absence of palpable soft-tissue mass at that locale. Differentiating *greater trochanteric bursitis* (see Chapter 53) from ITB tendinitis at the greater trochanter is often difficult because of the close association of the superficial trochanteric bursa with TFL. Nevertheless, trochanteric bursitis is not accompanied by a snapping sensation, and the pain associated with bursitis is more posterior to the greater trochanter and may even radiate into the buttock. The friction bursa may be palpable at the greater trochanter.[1]

Midthigh or groin pain, especially that which decreases with rest and increases with activity may indicate a stress fracture of the femoral neck. This may be a potentially career-ending injury for the professional athlete if misdiagnosed. The examiner should be highly suspicious of ipsilateral pain during single-leg stance, pain with a Patrick's or quadrant test; there frequently is a painful Trendelenburg gait. If suspected, patients should not bear weight on the involved leg until a stress fracture is ruled out. This

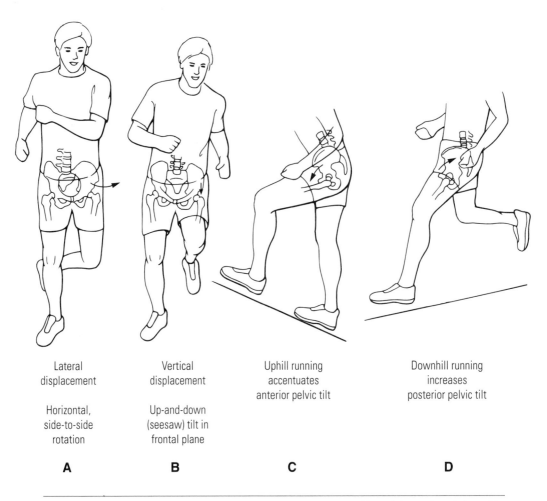

Lateral displacement	Vertical displacement	Uphill running accentuates anterior pelvic tilt	Downhill running increases posterior pelvic tilt
Horizontal, side-to-side rotation	Up-and-down (seesaw) tilt in frontal plane		
A	**B**	**C**	**D**

FIG. 48-11 A, Lateral pelvic displacement occurs by way of horizontal, side-to-side rotation of the pelvis. Swinging arms across the body accentuates the strain of pelvic rotation. **B,** Vertical pelvic displacement occurs by up-and-down tilt in the frontal plane. During midstance, the unsupported side of the pelvis drops or laterally dips. Anterior-posterior pelvic tilting. **C,** Uphill running accentuates anterior pelvic tilt and flexes the spine, whereas **(D)** downhill running increases posterior pelvic tilt and hyperextends the spine into lordosis.

injury is appropriately managed by an orthopaedic surgeon.[9]

- *Iliacus tendinitis.* This condition occurs in the iliacus portion of the iliopsoas muscle of young dancers (Fig. 48-13). The iliacus muscle narrows as it passes through the floor of the femoral triangle. During the développé dance step, the hip is brought into flexion, abduction, and external rotation. This causes the iliopsoas tendon to turn outward at an acute angle as it exits the pelvis. Acute tendinitis may occur in young female dancers following intense activity. Although this condition may be asymptomatic, it may manifest as groin pain and crepitus on palpation over the muscle. Although this condition is self-limiting and does not interfere with continued dancing, the patient must be instructed in slow stretching of the iliopsoas muscle. The patient may use nonsteroidal antiinflammatory medications and ought to decrease her rehearsal regimen.

- *Snapping of the iliopsoas muscle.* This condition occurs mostly in young highly motivated female dancers. Although often asymptomatic, this disorder may present as a deep anterior snapping and pain in the groin that may be disabling enough to require cessation of activity until symptoms subside. The movement that produces snapping is extension of the hip from a flexed, adducted, and externally rotated position. This causes snapping of the iliopsoas tendon over the anterior femoral head and capsule as the tendon moves from lateral to medial with hip exten-

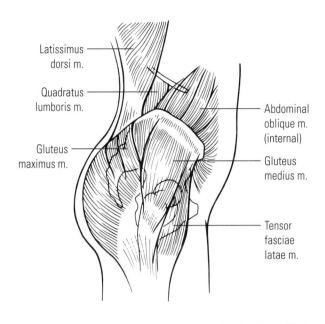

FIG. 48-12 *Iliac crest apophysitis* is an overuse injury due to repetitive stresses across the iliac crest by two opposing sets of muscles. Traction to the apophysis may result in avulsion off the iliac crest.

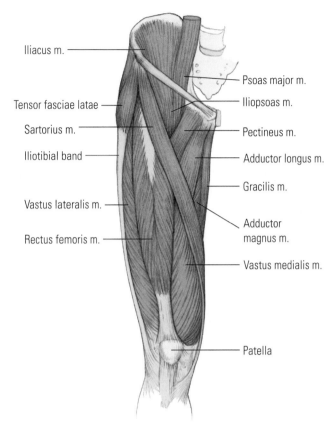

FIG. 48-13 Musculature of the hip showing the position of the iliopsoas muscle. The iliopsoas tendon turns outward at an acute angle as it exits the pelvis during the développé ballet step, resulting in iliacus tendinitis. Crepitus may be palpable inferior and medial to the anterior superior iliac spine. (From Mathers LH et al: *Clinical anatomy principles*, St Louis, 1996, Mosby.)

sion. Over time, the bursa between the tendon and hip capsule becomes inflamed due to friction from the snapping tendon. Management consists of performing slow and gentle stretching exercises for the hip flexor muscle group, reducing the rehearsal regimen, and taking oral nonsteroidal antiinflammatory medications.

• *Abductor snap.* As a jumper or dancer lands from a high leap the pelvis slips into lordosis. As the dancer recovers and rises after landing the iliotibial band may snap forward and it flicks across the greater trochanter. The condition is painful to the jumper and unaesthetic to the audience. Management includes strengthening the ipsilateral abductors and gluteal muscles, as well as prolonged warm-up periods in which the dancer lies on the contralateral side while the affected hip is elevated in abduction; the involved hip is then flexed and extended in its elevated position at about 2 feet off the floor.

20. What therapeutic management is appropriate for the treatment of ITB tendinitis?

Physical therapy strategy is directed at correcting the underlying biomechanical factors contributing to this disorder as well as appropriate modalities to treat symptomology. The therapist should explain to the patient that resolution of symptoms from this overuse injury is not absolutely predictable and the often slow response to treatment may be frustrating. Nevertheless, 4 to 6 weeks of conservative treatment is typically required to adequately manage iliotibial band syndrome as most patients are cured by conservative measures. When local tenderness over the greater trochanter or lateral epicondyle has subsided, the patient may resume running but should avoid prolonged workout. Severe cases require 6 to 8 weeks of rest before athletic activity is permitted. Surgery for this condition is rare and involves release of the posterior band fibers where they overlie the femoral condyle. Operative management is reserved for recalcitrant cases that have responded poorly to physical therapy. Operative management involves surgical release of the posterior fibers of the iliotibial band where they overlie the femoral condyle.

- *Stretching.* Stretch of the ITB-TFL complex using the *Ober test position* and statically holding the lower extremity in the final test position is an effective stretching procedure. This is more effectively performed by two persons. However, those patients with hip flexion contractures will additionally require stretching of the iliopsoas as well as the anterior hip capsule. Repeating this maneuver twice daily while applying gentle pressure on the thigh in the adducted position helps to effectively stretch those muscles. Alternately, an *ITB stretch* is performed by the therapist positioning the patient on the affected side and pulling the lower leg up off the table. The patient may also benefit from stretching of the gluteus maximus, hamstrings, quadriceps, abductor, and adductor muscles as well as those in the low back, by performing exercises such as the Ober self-stretch, the standing fascial stretch or the standing lateral wall lean. Strengthening is an important component of rehabilitation. Any strength deficits should be addressed by beginning with multiple angle isometrics and short arc exercises in a nonpainful range. Although full range isotonic and isokinetic exercises may be helpful in the later stages of rehabilitation, they should preferably not be performed by patients with symptomatic ITB tendinitis.[17]

In the event of a shortened ITB, bowstringing of the lateral tibia and concomitant valgus at the knee is thwarted by working the medial thigh musculature, that is, the adductors, while pelvic obliquity (presence of unilateral tilt) is restored by working the contralateral hip abductors (gluteus medius, minimus, and tensor fasciae latae). A weakened tensor fasciae latae muscle may be strengthened by raising the extended leg diagonally in the direction of hip abduction, flexion, and medial rotation, as well as performing anterior pelvic tilting. In the event of a weakened gluteus maximus, tensor fasciae latae may overpull upset the dynamic balance in its favor. This will result in medial femoral rotation and anterior pelvic tilt. Strengthening to counter this dynamic loss of balance would include working the adductor muscle group (lateral rotators) as well as the hamstring and abdominal muscle groups to facilitate increased posterior pelvic tilt.

A home exercise program must include teaching the patient to stretch the ITB in both the standing and lateral positions as these, although less effective, can be performed without the assistance of a therapist. Such maneuvers include the modified Ober, crossover toe touch, standing lateral fascial stretch, and the lateral hip drop stretches. A complete home program also includes strengthening as well as supplemental exercises.

- *Deep tissue massage proximal to the femoral condyle.* Because the dense fibrous distal portion of the iliotibial tract cannot be stretched effectively longitudinally, the therapist must address the more pliable proximal fascia lata adjacent to the tensor fasciae latae and gluteus maximus muscles.[10,19]
- *Modality.* Management of symptomatic pain and inflammation include the use of *phonophoresis* (10/watts cm) with salicylate cream or 10% hydrocortisone for 10 minutes over the greater trochanter, femoral condyle, or Gerdy's tubercle (6 sessions), and may afford relief.[3] *Icing* the area before and following exercise is helpful during the acute stage, whereas heat may afford relief during the subacute stage. Cryotherapy may be applied for up to 5 minutes or until the area is numb. Although the use of modalities is important, it only treats the symptoms. The use of moist superficial or deep heat may be used before stretching to increase tissue extensibility.[4,10,14,16,19,25]
- *Activity modification.* This includes avoidance of downhill running, decreasing mileage as well as running along a level instead of the drainage pitch of roads; alternatively, the patient may run along alternate sides of the road. A *steroid injection* may be administered by a physician anterior, posterior, and deep to the iliotibial tract at the lateral femoral epicondyle. Nonsteroidal antiinflammatory *medications* may be taken orally for a 14-day period. Patients should be encouraged to partially replace running with activities such as swimming with a minimal kick, or simply reduce their running stride length, overall running distance,[4,10,14,16,19,25] and frequency of run.
- *Orthotic correction of biomechanical discrepancy.* This is an important aspect of management strategy. For the individual with the over-pronated (flat) foot profile, the tibia excessively internally rotates resulting in an increased distance the band must span en route its insertion on the proximal tibia. For this type of patient a 5° or 9° medial heel wedge will help minimize the valgus effect to the knee, and is accompanied by a 1-mm heel height. Other patients may exhibit a varus knee alignment due to a genu varum or

tibia deformity from either a weakened tensor fasciae latae muscle or secondary to excessive foot supination during stance. In the latter, the patient has a cavus foot or a varus heel. Stretch along the ITB is minimized with a 5° or 9° lateral hindfoot wedge, accompanied by a 1-mm heel height.[27] Heel and sole wedges should be used cautiously and closely monitored as they may adversely alter patella tracking.

- *Switching shoe ware from hard shoes to softer running shoes is appropriate.* Switching to new running shoes may alleviate the cause of biomechanical dysfunction as *a shoe with an extremely worn outer heel acts to increase varus loading along the lateral outer aspect of the knee.* Building in a correction in the shoe of the shortened side in the event of a leg-length discrepancy.

- For bikers, cleat position should be corrected to reflect the cyclist's neutral anatomic alignment or a slight degree of external rotation. For those cyclists who use fixed pedal systems, switching to floating pedals may afford relief. Adjusting the stance width via using spacers placed between the pedal and the crank arm may reduce ITB stress by widening the cyclist's stance and thus improve hip-to-foot alignment.

REFERENCES

1. Beal MC: The sacroiliac problem: review of anatomy, mechanics, and diagnosis, *J Am Osteopath Assoc* 81:667-674, 1982.
2. Boland AL, Hulstyn MJ: Soft-tissue injuries of the knee. In Nicholas JA, Hershman EB editors: *The lower extremity and spine,* ed 2, vol 1, St Louis, 1995, Mosby.
3. Donatelli RA: *The biomechanics of the foot and ankle,* ed 2, Philadelphia, 1990, FA Davis.
4. Gose JC, Schweizer P: Iliotibial band tightness, *J Occupational Sports Phys Ther* 11:399-407, 1989.
5. Lindenberg G, et al: Iliotibial band friction syndrome in runners, *Phys Sports Med* 12(5):118, 1984.
6. Grana WA, Coniglione TC: Knee disorders in runners, *Phys Sports Med* 13:127, 1985.
7. Holmes JC, Pruitt AL, Whalen NJ: Cycling injuries. In Nicholas JA, Hershman EB editors: *The lower extremity and spine,* ed 2, vol 2, St Louis, 1995, Mosby.
8. Jones DC, James SL: Overuse injuries of the lower extremity. Shin splints, iliotibial band friction syndrome, and exertional compartment syndromes, *Clin Sports Med* 6:273, 1987.
9. Lilegard WA, Rucker KS: *Handbook of sports medicine,* Boston, 1993, Andover Medical Publishers.
10. McNicol K: Iliotibial tract friction syndrome in athletes, *Canadian J Appl Sports Sci* 6:76-80, 1981.
11. Messier SP, Pittala KA: Etiologic factors associated with selected running injuries, *Med Sci Sports Exerc* 20:501, 1988.
12. Milan KR: Injury in ballet: a review of relevant topics for the physical therapist, *JOSPT,* 19(2):121, 1994.
13. Moore KL: *Clinically oriented anatomy,* ed 2, Baltimore, 1985, Williams & Wilkins.
14. Netter FH: *The Ciba collection of medical illustrations,* vol 8, Part I, Summit, NJ, 1990, CIBA-GEIGY.
15. Noble HB, Hajek MR, Porter M: Diagnosis and treatment of iliotibial band tightness in runners, *Phys Sports Med* 10(4):67-74, 1982.
16. Noble CA: Iliotibial band friction syndrome in runners, *Am J Sports Med* 8:232, 1980.
17. Noble CA: The treatment of iliotibial band friction syndrome, *Br J Sports Med* 13:51, 1979.
18. Ober FR: The role of the iliotibial band and fascia lata as a factor in the causation of low back disabilities and sciatica, *J Bone Joint Surg* 18(1):105-110, 1936.
19. Olson DW: Iliotibial band friction syndrome, *Athletic Training Spring* 32-35, 1986.
20. Perry J: *Gait analysis: normal pathological function,* Thorofare, NJ, 1992, Slack.
21. Pick TP, Howden R editors: *Gray's anatomy,* New York, 1977, Bounty Books.
22. Reilly MA: *Guidelines for prescribing foot orthotics,* Thorofare, NJ, Slack.
23. Renne JW: The iliotibial band friction syndrome, *J Bone Joint Surg* 57A:1110, 1975.
24. Smith WB: Environmental factors in running. In Clancy WG editor: *Runner's injuries, Am J Sports Med* 8:138, 1980.
25. Staheli LT: Rotational problems of the lower extremities, *Orthop Clin North Am* 18(4), 1987.
26. Sutker AN, Jackson DW, Pagliano JW: Iliotibial band syndrome in distance runners, *Phys Sports Med* 9(10):69-73, 1981.
27. Taunton JE, Clement DB: Iliotibial tract friction syndrome in athletes, *Can J Sports Sci* 6:76, 1981.
28. Terry GC, Houghston JC, Norwood LA: The anatomy of the iliopatellar band and iliotibial tract, *Am J Sports Med* 14:39-45, 1986.
29. Tracy JE: Iliotibial band friction syndrome seen often in athletes: A literature review, *Adv Phys Ther* 9, 1991.
30. Xethalis JL, Lorei MP: Soccer injuries. In Nicholas JA, Hershman EB editors: *The lower extremity and spine,* ed 2, vol 2, St Louis, 1995, Mosby.

RECOMMENDED READING

Gose J: Iliotibial band tightness, *J Orthop Sports Phys Ther* 10:399, 1989.

Lindenberg G et al: Iliotibial band friction syndrome in runners, *Phys Sports Med* 12(5):118, 1984.

Noble CA: The treatment of iliotibial band friction syndrome, *Br J Sports Med* 13:51, 1979.

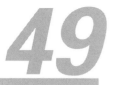

49

Progressive, Aching, Insidious Onset of Pain and Morning Stiffness in the Large Weight-Bearing, Lower-Extremity Joints that is Exacerbated by Inclement Weather Causing Diminished Function

CASE 1: A 58-year-old obese black male anthropologist complains of aching pain in the right groin that is occasionally severe and extends down the anterior thigh to the knee. Symptoms began insidiously 4 months ago when he began golfing several days a week as a post-retirement avocation. Initially, he felt stiffness and aching many hours or the next day following his game. Over time, stiffness would occur whenever he would sit for more than 1 hour, and was especially pronounced after a night's sleep. As his symptoms rapidly progressed, walking became painful and he gradually began to limp. His pain persisted, although in lesser intensity, during his sleep so that he would take a nightly analgesic before going to bed to help him sleep through the night. The patient offers that he cannot walk for as long a distance as he usually could, and that he becomes slightly short of breath if he pushes himself through the pain. Stair climbing is difficult, and must be done one step at a time. Symptoms are unilateral and are not accompanied by similar involvement at any other articulation. The patient offers that he has osteoarthritis of the spine since age 40 that is not nearly as painful as it once was, especially after he lost 45 pounds. While watching him rise out of his chair you note that he does so slowly, using his arms to push up off the arm rests. When asked, he admits to pain and creaking in his left kneecap, especially during standing up and climbing stairs. The patient reports a history of right trochanteric bursitis and left-sided sciatica that have since resolved. The patient is left-handed. He offers that he had congenital right hip dysplasia, which he believed was caused by the way he was carried in a headboard as an infant in his native Africa. He presents a prescription from his orthopaedic surgeon for physical therapy.

OBSERVATION In the standing posture, a pelvic obliquity (with a higher right pelvis) is noted with the right limb in relative adduction and the left hip in relative abduction. The right posterior inferior iliac spine is higher than the left. The levels of the gluteal folds, anal cleft, and posterior knee creases appeared symmetrical. During quiet standing the right knee is slightly flexed and the left ankle is held in slight equinus. Excessive hyperextension of the left knee is noted during stance, and especially during push off phase as the patient ambulates by circumducting the right lower extremity slightly. A shorter stride length and decreased heel strike is noted on the right in an attempt to diminish weight bearing. While the right foot appears postured in decided pronation, the left foot assumes a cavus foot posture.

PALPATION   Normal to the right hip. The left patella emits a creaking noise during patellar compression.

RANGE OF MOTION   Extension, abduction, and internal rotation of the right hip joint are markedly diminished. Rather, the hip is postured in a capsular pattern of right hip flexion, adduction, and external rotation. An abnormal capsular end-feel is imparted to the examiner's hand at the extreme of passive range of motion of the right hip. An 8° right knee flexion contracture and a 5° left plantar flexion contracture are present.

STRENGTH   Strength of the right thigh musculature is assessed to be markedly diminished to approximately one-half compared with the contralateral extremity. Weakness appears most pronounced in the right gluteus medius, maximus, and hamstring muscles. Exact values not possible secondary to pain; however, the following pattern emerges: diminished adductor strength and abductor tightness on the shorter left side and abductor weakness and adductor tightness on the longer right side.

FLEXIBILITY   Significant decrease of right hip extension, abduction, and internal rotation. Sixty degrees of straight leg raising is available on the left leg, whereas 55° is available on the right. Both tensor fasciae latae show significant tightness.

POSTURE   When viewed from behind, scoliotic curves of the low back and cervical spine are pronounced and are corrected during seating, and when placing a 3-cm high block of wood under the shorter left leg during quiet standing.

SPECIAL TESTS   Negative compression and distraction of the sacroiliac joints. Comparative lengths between both lower extremities in supine position show a right leg that is apparently 3 cm longer. When the patient assumed the long-leg sitting posture with the knees extended, the leg length appeared to reduce to only 1.5 cm long, indicating a posterior ilial rotation.

RADIOGRAPHS   Radiographs of the right hip joint show narrowing of the joint space, subchondral sclerosis and cysts, and osteophytic overgrowth. In addition, radiographs of the left knee indicate mild narrowing and sclerosis of the lateral tibiofemoral joint. There is also wedging of the lumbosacral vertebrae.

> *CASE 2:* A slim, white 68-year-old female limps painfully into your office assisted by a cane and her daughter. The patient complains of a poorly defined dull ache that worsens with activity, and stiffness following immobility that is of mild intensity and short duration after a night's rest. Occasionally, the knee joint feels tight. Lately, she reports pain even during rest. She is particularly distraught over the knobby cosmetic deformity developing in the fingers of both hands that "makes her beautiful hands look terrible and ugly" and are painful. Loss of function such as walking and stair climbing are particularly disturbing and make her feel depressed.

OBSERVATION   The patient ambulates with an antalgic gait characterized by diminished left stance time, and decreased knee flexion during swing. Genu varum of the left knee is present. Minimal left knee swelling, particularly of the medial aspect of the joint is readily observable when referenced with the contralateral knee.

PALPATION   This yields point tenderness at the anteromedial aspect of the left knee joint. Joint crepitus during movement occurs, and periarticular bony hypertrophy noted along the medial joint line that is accompanied by increased joint warmth. Polyarticular involvement of the distal interphalangeal joints of both hands shows bony nodules growing from the dorsomedial and lateral aspect of the base of the distal phalanges that are painful and tender, and cause a flexion deformity of the distal the fingers.

RANGE OF MOTION   The last 10° of range of motion of the left knee are lost in both flexion and extension.

STRENGTH   Left quadriceps strength is good minus, whereas left terminal knee extension is fair plus. The left hamstring muscle demonstrates good plus muscle strength. Manual muscle testing does not produce pain.

FLEXIBILITY   Less than 60° of straight leg raising is available. The tensor fasciae latae was mildly tight.

SPECIAL TESTS   Valgus stress testing to the left knee open up the medial side.

GIRTH MEASUREMENTS   These are taken by palpating for the joint line medially and laterally, placing the tape measure at this level. Compared with the contralateral knee, circumferential measurement shows an increase of 3 cm of the left knee.

RADIOGRAPHS   These show localized narrowing of the medial tibiofemoral joint space, subchondral sclerosis and cysts of the medial tibial plateau, and hypertrophic bone formation at the tibiofemoral joint margins.

? Questions

1. What is the cause of pain and disability in these patients?
2. What is cartilage and which elements of its composition endow it with its unique mechanical properties?
3. What is the function of the synovial membrane?
4. What is the role of fatty tissue comprising the subintima layer of synovial membrane at the hip and knee joint, and how may it be injured in the latter?
5. What is the composition of synovial fluid?
6. What is the primary function of hyaluronic acid component of synovial fluid?
7. What is the role of synovial fluid with regard to joint stability?
8. How does nutrition reach the avascular articular cartilage?
9. What is the collagen component of articular cartilage?
10. What are the functions of articular cartilage?
11. What are the stages of articular cartilage deformation during applied stress?
12. What is the morphological structure and organization of articular cartilage?
13. What component within the matrix of articular cartilage retains and regulates the flow of water within the matrix?
14. How do the proteoglycan molecules within the articular cartilage matrix regulate the flow of water within the matrix when the joint is nonweight bearing?
15. What determines the movement of fluid out of the articular cartilage matrix and into synovial fluid?
16. What are the possible etiologic factors in degenerative joint disease?
17. How may angular malalignment in the frontal plane predispose for degenerative joint disease at the hip and knee?
18. How do the normal biomechanical changes that occur with aging of articular cartilage upset its load carriage function?
19. How does wear of the tangential layer of articular cartilage result in diminished chondrocyte nutrition?
20. What is the classification of osteoarthritis?
21. What is the sequential progression of tissue destruction during the evolution of the osteoarthritic joint?
22. How may leg length disparity predispose for unilateral degenerative articular disease at the ipsilateral hip and contralateral patellofemoral joint?
23. What is the clinical presentation of degenerative joint disease at the hip and knee?

24. **Why does pain associated with degenerative joint disease appear to be related to change of barometric pressure?**

25. **What are the clinical manifestations of osteoarthritis distal to the wrist?**

26. **What are the radiographic features of degenerative joint disease at the hip and knee?**

27. **What changes in hip joint mechanics occur due to leg length discrepancy?**

28. **What are the different forms of leg length discrepancy?**

29. **What is the pathogenesis of leg length discrepancy?**

30. **What pathologic conditions may develop secondary to leg length discrepancy?**

31. **What gait deviations may occur secondary to leg length discrepancy?**

32. **What changes in alignment of the spinal column may occur secondary to leg length disparity?**

33. **What postural examination is appropriate in the assessment of leg length discrepancy?**

34. **What are the direct and indirect methods for measurement of total leg length discrepancy?**

35. **What are the two methods for determining which of the long bones of the lower extremity is the source of the total leg length discrepancy?**

36. **When is radiographic measurement for leg length discrepancy appropriate?**

37. **How does rheumatoid arthritis differ from osteoarthritis?**

38. **What conservative management strategy best services these patients?**

---

1. What is the cause of pain and disability in these patients?

Degenerative joint disease of the right hip in Case 1, and the left knee in Case 2. Interestingly, in Case 1, degenerative joint disease of the spine, which may affect the disk, facet joint, or both, is much less common in the elderly than in middle age. This is because the arthritic spine becomes more stable and stiff and subsequently less likely to provoke pain owing to osteophytic bone growth. Moreover, the degenerative process in Case 1 is classified as secondary osteoarthrosis due to apparent leg length discrepancy and congenital hip dysplasia. Swaddling infants or carrying them in headboards is accomplished by maintaining the lower extremities in extension. This position subluxes or dislocates the hip joint. In Case 2, the cause of arthritis was primary. For both patients, pain at rest indicates that an acute phase of an advanced stage of the disease process is predominant.

Alternately known as osteoarthritis in the United States, osteoarthrosis in the United Kingdom,[7] senescent arthritis, hypertrophic arthritis, arthrosis deformans, or simply wear-and-tear disease, *osteoarthritis* is the most common articular disease, and is characterized by progressive degeneration of articular cartilage and secondary inflammation of the synovial membrane. Thus degenerative joint disease or osteoarthrosis are the more accurate descriptions of this joint disorder as they imply degeneration as the fundamental pathologic change deriving from mechanical factors. In contrast, the popular, yet persisting but incorrect term "osteoarthritis" is a misnomer insofar as its suffix implies that the joint deterioration results from inherently inflammatory causes. This condition is a localized one without systemic manifestations. Arthritis of the hip or knee may fall into 5 major categories: osteoarthritis, inflammatory arthritis, metabolic arthritis, infectious arthritis, and the neuropathic joint.* Differentiation among these categories is based upon patient history, physical examination, and radiographic imaging and laboratory testing.[110] Degenerative joint disease occurs as a function of accelerated aging of articular cartilage that may be predisposed by trauma, obesity, or previous infection. A genetic component may also be causative. Degenerative joint disease is much less common in Asiatic

---

*Joints with deficient sensory innervation, as from diabetic neuropathy, may develop a rapidly progressive destructive arthropathy known as *neuropathic arthropathy*. The reason why this occurs is because denervation allows the patient to apply enormous loads to the joint without the normal aches and pains that signal one to stop and rest. The condition was first described by Charcot in patients with tabes dorsalis. The most common causes of neuropathic arthropathy include diabetes mellitus, syringomyelia, late-stage syphilis, pernicious anemia, spinal cord tumors, alcoholism, denervated limbs, idiopathic causes, and patients who are taking large doses of analgesic drugs. Clinical presentation is atypical. The joint is typically inflamed, swollen, grossly unstable, but painless.

persons.[20] Much more than a passive "wear and tear phenomenon," the pathogenesis of osteoarthritis involves a cascade of biochemical, cellular, and metabolic activity within articular cartilage.[66]

A review of diarthrodial joint function will encompass discussion of the interrelationships among the synovial membrane, synovial fluid, and articular cartilage. Before discussing the evaluation and management of patients with this condition it is appropriate to adequately discuss a variety of topics including the structure and function of synovium, cartilage, synovial fluid, malalignment, and leg length discrepancy before fully appreciating both the scope and treatment of degenerative joint disease.

2. What is cartilage and which elements of its composition endow it with its unique mechanical properties?

Articular cartilage is a type of connective tissue that caps the proximal and distal articulating ends of long bones. Also known as *hyaline cartilage* because of its pearly white nature that is translucent to light and endows it with the appearance of frosted glass (Gr: *hyalos,* glass), it is divisible into a central articulating portion and a smaller marginal portion covered by synovial membrane. Hyaline cartilage is composed of cartilage cells (chondrocytes), which produce the two extracellular components known as proteoglycan matrix (ground substance) and type II collagen. The unique mechanical properties of articular cartilage are derived from these two components.

3. What is the function of the synovial membrane?

The inner layer of the articular bursal wall is a connective tissue sac called the *synovial membrane or synovium* because it is in contact with the synovial fluid. The synovial membrane is a joint lining, which encloses the diarthrodial joint as a *synovial cavity*. The synovium is composed of an inner and outer layer: (1) the *intima;* and (2) the *subintima.* The cells of the inner layer of synovial membrane, called synoviocytes, come in two varieties. *Type A synoviocytes* are more numerous and have many features of macrophages as they actively phagocytose. The primary function of the synovial membrane is the production of hyaluronic acid, which is the mucin component of synovial fluid synthesized by *type B synoviocytes* in the intima layer.[11] Because of the countless villi in the synovial membrane its enormous surface area approaches 100 square meters in the human knee.[98,99]

The synovial membrane also acts as a semipermeable membrane that selectively filters blood plasma so as to permit ultrafiltrate into the synovial cavity, and transports needed nutrients into the joint space while removing metabolic wastes through its capillary and lymphatic systems.[40] Moreover, synovium must be elastic enough to be able to adapt to the full range of positions assumed by the articulation. Thus when a joint flexes and extends, the synovium must correspondingly expand and contract over unopposed surfaces of articular cartilage.

For any articulation to function as more than a simple pivot joint, there must, of necessity, be a disparity in the configuration of the surface areas of opposing cartilage, so that when the joint moves, the smaller areas glide across or around the larger one. Cartilage not in contact with opposing cartilage will be temporarily covered by synovium. The moist synovial membrane covering the periphery of cartilage is elastic and stretches when bone either spins or swings near the periphery of its articulating surface only to return to its original size and position when the movement of the bone is reversed. As the cartilaginous surfaces return to their original positions, the synovial fluid secreted by the synovial membrane lubricates the synovium so as to allow it to easily slide out of harm's way and not become pinched. Were this system to fail, repeated hemarthroses of the highly vascular synovial tissue would rapidly incapacitate the affected joint.[103] Thus the synovial membrane and other structures such as menisci and fat pads assist in joint lubrication by evenly spreading synovial fluid throughout the joint and taking up dead space, thereby economizing on the amount of joint fluid necessary.[108] *Synovitis* refers to inflammation of the synovial membrane. Rheumatoid arthritis is primarily a disease of the synovium, whereas the inflammation of the synovium is secondary in osteoarthritis.

4. What is the role of fatty tissue comprising the subintima layer of synovial membrane at the hip and knee joint, and how may it be injured in the latter?

The subintima layer of the synovial membrane is the connective tissue base on which the intima rests and may be fibrous, aerial (loose), or fatty. These fatty portions of intima are thin except in places where they project into the joint cavity as fatty pads. These fat pads serve as joint packing—filling dead space within joint cavities and thereby serving as cushions to the impact of bony processes during movement. Fat pads are known as *plicae adiposae* when wedged shaped in section, and like a meniscus, the base of the wedge rests against a fibrous capsule. These pads are large in the ankle, knee, and elbow joints. In the hip joint a fatty pad is found as the *ligamentum teres,* a triangular band surrounded by a tubular sheath of synovial membrane that, in some persons, connects the acetabulum to the head of the femur. The newborn hip, in contrast to the adult joint, is underdeveloped and prone to dislocation as the acetabulum is small compared with the size of the femoral head. When the lower limbs are in the fetal position, the ligamentum teres prevents the femoral head from becoming dislocated posterosuperiorly. However, if the ligament is abnormally long or absent, dislocation may occur.[82] The ligamentum teres becomes taut when the hip is semi-flexed and the thigh is adducted and externally rotated; in contrast, it is relaxed on hip abduction.[41] Hence, the basis for provocative testing for hip dysplasia in the neonate. The orangutan lacks a ligamentum teres, and consequently has nearly complete rotary action of the hip joint, and relatively diminished stability of that articulation.[31]

At the knee joint, the fat pad is attached superiorly to the suprapatellar and infrapatellar plicae[51] which retract the fat pad within the knee joint[46] so as to avoid pressure upon the pad from bony surfaces within the moving knee. The function of fatty pads at the knee joint is related to fat behaving as a *liquid* fluid when subjected to pressure. Because of their elastic nature, fatty pads are easily deformable and are thus ideal in their ability to tolerate constant joint motion between two, irregular joint surfaces. These pads project into those portions of the synovial-covered joint space in which there would be a likelihood of an eddying (vortical) motion of fluid if that space were occupied by liquid. Thus fat pads contribute to the "internal streamlining" of the joint cavity[31] that facilitates ease of movement by dampening the momentum of the articular joint components and thereby preventing injury to the internal soft-tissue structures surrounding the joint. Of equal importance, the fat pads, by virtue of their presence, maintain lubrication of the joint as they spread synovial fluid throughout the joint cavity during their to-and-fro movement.

The fat pad at the knee receives branches from the femoral, tibial, recurrent, common peroneal, and obturator nerves.[46] Fat pads are thus highly innervated structures that may provoke pain if they become squeezed between two articular surfaces. *Fat pad syndrome* or *Hoffa's disease* refers to thickening and fibro-

sis of the fat pad due to repetitive abrasion from impingement between bony surfaces. Fat pad syndrome is associated with patellar tendinitis[49,54] and tenderness on patellar compression during terminal knee extension.[63] Fat pads may also be impinged upon by internal hemorrhage or increased effusion following trauma to a joint.

5. What is the composition of synovial fluid?

Synovial fluid is normally a viscous, pale yellow, and clear fluid resembling raw egg (Latin *ovum,* meaning egg) white in both appearance and consistency. Like all lubrication mediums, synovial fluid reduces friction and hence wear between the two moving articulating bones by separating the two points of bony contact. Synovial fluid (or synovia) is an *ultrafiltrate** of blood plasma—meaning that it is the portion of blood plasma that has "filtered" through a membrane, except that the mucin lubricant hyaluronic acid,[123] which is produced by the intima layer of the synovial membrane,[18] has been added. It is the synovial membrane that acts as a semipermeable membrane selecting what portions of blood plasma may enter and which may not. The other constituents of synovial fluid such as water, sodium, potassium, and glucose are small enough to enter the small (6-nanometer diameter) pores comprising the surface collagen fibrils of articular cartilage. In contrast, hyaluronic acid molecules are too large to enter into articular cartilage.

Synovial fluid, sparse in normal joints, does not clot as it lacks fibrinogen and prothrombin and contains only a few white blood cells derived from the synovial membrane. The presence of infection in a joint will result in an increase of leukocytes and is diagnosed by joint aspiration. Septic arthritis, which typically results from pathogenic agents such as staphylococcus, streptococcus, and clostridium produce an enzyme, hyaluronidase,[24] which degrades hyaluronic acid. This will result in arthritis of that joint secondary to loss of hyaluronic acid as a lubricant of that articulation.

6. What is the primary function of the hyaluronic acid component of synovial fluid?

Essential to understanding the role of synovial fluid in the diarthrodial joint is an appreciation of the primary component of this liquid medium: hyaluronic acid. *Hyaluronic acid* is a large complex of protein and carbohydrate biochemically categorized as an acid muco-

---

*Also known as *dialysate.*

polysaccharide (*muco,* denoting their slippery mucus-like nature, and *acid,* indicating a preponderance of acidic carbohydrate groups in their polysaccharide chains) that are more recently termed *glycosaminoglycans* (designating the composition of their polysaccharide chains).[18] Hyaluronic acid is alternately known as *mucin,*[98,99] which is the chief constituent of mucus,[24] and endows this substance with viscous and gel-like characteristics.[3]

Before discussing the unique role of hyaluronic acid within the synovial fluid of the diarthrodial joint, it is essential to define the problem encountered between movement of two articulating surfaces. The interaction of sliding surfaces, termed *tribology,* includes an interaction among three phenomenon known as *friction, wear,* and *lubrication.** Kinetic friction* refers to the resistive force encountered when one surface moves against another,[125] as for example, when dragging a concrete slab over a wooden block. High friction is desired for the satisfactory functioning of nuts and bolts or stacking piles of fruit in the supermarket. Constant friction is required in automobile brakes or clutches so as to avoid jerky movement. Low friction is desired in objects that move continuously such as engines, the internal mechanism in watches, and the diarthrodial joint. Wear refers to the removal of material from a solid surface owing to mechanical rubbing by another solid as occurs when lead pencils become worn in the process of writing on paper. Practically everything inanimate wears out over time. Even teeth in humans may wear out eventually. The exception to this almost universal wear phenomenon is the diarthrodial articulation as it is endowed with the property of healing through anabolic regrowth. In addition to its ability to heal, the diarthrodial joint has a unique lubrication medium—synovial fluid.

The unique lubricating quality endowed to synovial fluid is primarily from the thixotropic behavior of hyaluronic acid.[31] *Thixotropy* refers to the reversible behavior of certain gels, such as paint, that liquefy when shaken, stirred, or otherwise disturbed only to revert to a gel-like state when undisturbed. Demonstrating both viscous and elastic behavior, synovial fluid becomes highly viscous when the shear rate is low (corresponding to the slowly moving joint) only to as-

sume the properties of low viscosity—to the point of behaving as an elastic material—as shear increases (corresponding to rapidly moving joint); thus the viscosity of synovial fluid varies in a non-Newtonian manner.[25,87] Hyaluronic acid is endowed with thixotropic properties because of its high molecular weight and its random chain structure, and is especially suitable for lubricating joints that are required to carry load at varying rates of movement.

The elastohydrodynamic property of synovial fluid makes it an ideal *lubricating medium* that is approximately ten times superior to the best mechanical lubrication systems known to modern engineering.[26] The coefficient of friction between the two articulating surfaces of a normal diarthrodial joint is less than that of two pieces of wet ice (0.02) rubbing against one another! There is no one model available to describe lubrication at each point of the articulating cycle as at times the attenuated load may be light whereas at other times it may be heavy. *Boundary lubrication* means that each articular surface is coated with a thin layer of hyaluronate molecules that slide on each other. Graphite dust particles are an example of this type of lubricant. Thus motion occurs between the two thin layers rather than directly between the two surfaces of articular cartilage, so that the respective layers overlying each articular surface slide on one another. This mechanism primarily functions when joints operate under conditions of diminished load, or slow movements[20] typically associated with the starting and stopping of motion,[31] but which ceases to function when loads are excessive[112] or motion commences.

When weight-bearing load is increased, synovial fluid acts as a surface lubricant that tends to be squeezed out from between contacting surfaces of opposing articular ends of bone. This is resisted by a second mechanism, *fluid lubrication,* which involves contact of the articular surface at a limited but changing number of regions as the joint moves through its range of motion. The point(s) of articular contact create a depression within hyaline cartilage that is immediately filled with synovial fluid, which serves to dampen the pressure point of contact and thereby diminish the site of articular wear to minimal attrition.[93,101] The fluid that fills the depression assumes a "wedge-shape." This is because the joint surfaces are not a perfect fit, and the irregularities create a wedge of fluid at the point of contact. This occurs in series throughout the range of motion of the joint, similar to an automobile tire that hydroplanes on the wet road, in which fluid flows between

---

Tribology is an interdisciplinary subject as *friction* is typically categorized under the study of mechanical engineering, whereas *wear* derives from the material science of metallurgy, and *lubrication* falls under the aegis of chemistry.

the rubber tire and asphalt road.[20] Similarly in the diarthrodial joint, synovial fluid is interposed between articulating surfaces and acts to separate them.

7. What is the role of synovial fluid with regard to joint stability?

Normally, only about 0.5 to 4.0 ml of synovial fluid is present within the knee joint[108] so that only a thin film separates the femoral and tibial articular surfaces. Thus the intraarticular cavity is virtually a potential space with an average subatmospheric intracavity knee pressure of −4.0 mmHg. This pressure differential manifests as a suction that draws articulating surfaces into the best possible fit and thereby stabilizes the congruent articulation of large joints, as well as helping to guide the points of surface contact as the joint moves through its range of motion.[103]

8. How does nutrition reach the avascular articular cartilage?

Articular cartilage is particularly susceptible to injury from concussive *impact loading*. The role of shock absorption during impact loading is assumed by the cancellous bone subjacent to the subchondral plate[91] and active muscle contraction,[93] and the elastic nature of periarticular soft tissues,[88] and menisci, all of which act as a soft cushion to protect cartilage.[86] Nevertheless, cartilage must be readily deformable so as to absorb the brunt of concussive weight-bearing forces. However, cartilage is also elastic and therefore capable of recovering its shape quickly when a deforming stress is removed. In contrast, unlike bone, articular cartilage is soft and may be cut by a knife or sustain surface craters from torn menisci or particles of free bone (osteochondritis dissecans). Blood and lymphatic vessels could not tolerate being housed in such a readily deformable material as articular cartilage. Under normal physiologic conditions, articular cartilage may be compressed to as much as 40% of its original height. If vessels or nerves traversed articular cartilage, they would undergo severe trauma and be rendered useless.[65] Because its deeper layers are calcified, nourishment cannot reach cartilagenous cells from underlying bone. It is because of this that hyaline cartilage does not possess the ability to regenerate. That layer of bone serving as the watershed between bone and cartilage is impregnated with calcium salts, and acts as an effective barrier to diffusion. Instead, cartilage cells must obtain their nutrients and oxygen by long-range diffusion from outside the cartilage. The medium for nutrients is the synovial fluid that bathes the free surface of articular cartilage, which derives from capillaries within the synovial membrane.[18] Indeed, the virtual immunologic isolation of chondrocytes is afforded by the articular cartilage being devoid of blood vessels, which accounts for the success of cartilage allografts.[99]

9. What is the collagen component of articular cartilage?

Collagen is the key protein in the musculoskeletal system as it is the most abundant fiber type comprising connective tissue, cartilage, and bone. At present, 11 different types of collagen, designated at types I through XI, have been positively identified. All collagen types are composed of three different amino acids, proline, hydroxyproline, and hydroxine, the relative proportions of which determine the type of collagen. Collagen synthesis occurs within fibroblasts in a series of ten steps followed by two additional extracellular steps in which collagen is assembled.* The fibril making up collagen is first constructed as a precursor known as *procollagen,* which is composed of three helical polypeptide chains having a tropocollagen core. Procollagen then undergoes extracellular assembly to become protein collagen. Generally, collagen has the tensile strength of steel. The source of the tensile force-resisting properties of cartilage derives from the molecular configuration of type II collagen molecules.

---

*A defect in collagen chemistry causes a defect in synthesis of one of the three helical chains comprising collagen, so that, for example, a person with a collagen disorder affecting the composition of collagen in the basement membrane of his kidney tubules will have poor kidney function. In the musculoskeletal system, disorders of connective tissue result in a variety of uncommon, yet clinically significant diseases. *Ehlers-Danlos syndrome* is an inherited connective tissue disorders deriving from defective cross-linking of collagen fibrils. Although patients usually have a normal lifespan, minor trauma (as from a minor bang against a surface) may cause wide gaping wounds with little bleeding. Patients have extremely hypermobile joints and flexible ligaments and may thus contort themselves into bizarre postures typical of "India rubber men" in circus sideshows. *Marfan's syndrome* is autosomal dominant in transmission and is characterized by considerable height, and arm span, as well as long and thin digits, and heart valve defects. *Osteogenesis imperfecta* or *brittle-bone disease* is a condition of newborns affecting approximately 1 out of 25,000 births in which the neonate is born with multiple fractures due to delivery trauma, which results in shortening of the extremities. Some children may exhibit a less severe form of the condition in which they commonly break bones. In addition to bone fragility, the sclera of their eyes is blue instead of a normal white because a deficiency in connective tissue allows the color of the underlying vessels to show through. Mental development is normal unless head trauma with brain injury occurs.

Type II collagen is found in the cornea and vitreous body of the eye, the nucleus pulposus of the interverte-bral disk, and in articular cartilage.[18] In articular carti-lage, collagen functions to bind the cartilage together, protect chondrocytes within their lacunae, facilitate at-tachment of articular cartilage to subchondral bone, and help resist load.[34] Present in hyaline cartilage as both large and small diameter collagen fibrils, type II colla-gen demonstrates a high electrostatic attraction for chondroitin sulfate glycosaminoglycans,[112] and thus helps to stabilize the many proteoglycan aggregate mol-ecules throughout the extracellular matrix of articular cartilage.

10. What are the functions of articular cartilage?

As articulating surfaces are for the most part incongru-ent, the articulating surfaces fit imperfectly. The geo-metrical asymmetry between the two articulating ends of a diarthrodial joint may result in wear and tear of adjacent bone surfaces due to occasional if not con-stant collision. Several strategies have evolved to pre-vent joint incongruity, one of which is the meniscus, which provides improves articular fitting between the two ends of bone. The deformable but elastic nature of articular cartilage represents another such strategy in which hyaline cartilage compensates for bony incon-gruity by increasing the area of contact within a joint, thereby reducing the contact pressures on the bone.[86] In compression, cartilage is twice as stiff as the menis-cus, whereas in tension, the meniscus is 10 times as stiff as cartilage.[31] Similarly, a fluid filled capsule be-tween the bone surfaces permits the disparate architec-ture of the articulating surfaces to accommodate each other by fluid flow, so that contact between bony sur-faces is kept to a minimum, wear is minimized, and du-rable function is ensured. When the two articulating surfaces rub against each other, as does occur, the coef-ficient of friction (0.02 or less[3]) is superior to that of ice skates on ice.[4] Thus the design features and efficiency of articular cartilage, such as the knee and other diarth-rodial joints, is endowed with a lubrication system that is truly an engineering marvel. In summation, articular cartilage functions primarily as a bearing surface that primarily distributes load rather than acting as a shock absorber.[79] Thus although the adjacent subchondral bone serves to absorb the concussive effect of impact loading, articular cartilage serves in an energy-absorbing role by way of load attenuation in which car-tilage deforms and thereby increases the contact area of articulation.

11. What are the stages of articular cartilage deformation during applied stress?

Cartilage negotiates stress in a viscoelastic manner be-cause it is a *two-phase composite* consisting of a solid matrix anchored to bone and a free-flowing fluid phase.[86] The biphasic properties of articular cartilage are directly attributable to two extracellular compo-nents: collagen and proteoglycans. This two-phase composition of articular cartilage further endows it with an energy-absorbing role because fluid dissipates en-ergy by friction of water molecules against the solid in-terstices.[98,99] Because of its two-phase composition, ar-ticular cartilage is a *viscoelastic tissue* composed of a mixture of elastic solid and viscous liquid,[48] and conse-quently, demonstrates a two-stage compression defor-mation phenomenon.[10] A material that yields continu-ally under stress only to return to its original shape when the stress is relieved is said to be viscoelastic. When load is applied to articular cartilage, for example as may occur in the closed packed position when the knee is extended during weight bearing, an *instanta-neous deformation* occurs that results in an indentation over the point of contact that deepens continuously over time despite maintenance of a constant load. Initially, in the first stage, a change of contour in the articular sur-face occurs as an indentation without a simultaneous change in volume. This means that, like a compressed balloon filled with water, articular cartilage under stress will undergo a *bulk movement of both matrix and water* to accommodate to its new shape. This initial phenom-enon is known as *creep*. In mechanical terms, creep re-fers to the phenomenon demonstrated by certain mate-rials, most commonly metals, in which slow change in the dimensions of a material occur with prolonged stress, and in the case of the knee joint for example, with continued application of fixed stress. Thus creep allows the contact area to increase with time, thereby spreading the load over a larger contact area. If load is prolonged, cartilage, which is pliable (viscoelastic) in nature, will continue to deform, although it does so via a flow of water from its matrix and into the synovial fluid in a secondary process known as *stress-relaxation*. Because external pressure is maintained, articular carti-lage acts to relieve stress by reducing its volume such that persistent stress from load is decreased with time. Stress-relaxation, in contrast to creep, is a *gradual deformation*.

In a similar fashion, when the applied load is re-moved, articular cartilage recovers in a two-step man-ner. Initially, instantaneous elastic recovery occurs that

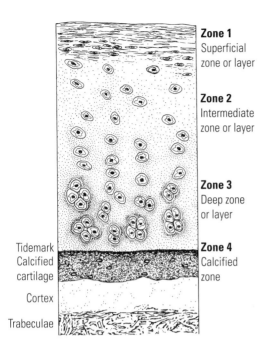

Zone 1
Superficial
zone or layer

Zone 2
Intermediate
zone or layer

Zone 3
Deep zone
or layer

Tidemark
Calcified
cartilage

Zone 4
Calcified
zone

Cortex

Trabeculae

FIG. 49-1 The zones of adult articular cartilage. Collagen fibrils anchor into subchondral bone, which is demarcated by a changed of staining properties termed *the "tidemark line."* (From Turek SL: *Orthopaedics: principles and their application,* Philadelphia, 1977, JB Lippincott.)

is followed by reimbibing water over time. Most weight-bearing joints are subjected to rapidly applied high loads of short duration as a function of the gait cycle. Articular cartilage acts as a shock absorber that protects bone by dampening and attenuating dynamic loads in a viscoelastic fashion.

12. What is the morphologic structure and organization of articular cartilage?

Hyaline cartilage is characterized by sparsely spaced chondrocytes in a matrix of intercellular substance that is histologically organized into three zones (Fig. 49-1). A change in collagen orientation from their rising vertically in the deep layers at the subchondral bone to gradually become horizontal as they reach the joint surface resembles an arcade pattern[5] akin to the curved ribs of an umbrella. The collagen pattern of the surface fibers of articular cartilage are different such that collagen fibers are smaller, packed more tightly together[40] in an orientation tangential (parallel) to the surface. Alternately known as the *tangential* or *sliding zone,* or the *lamina splendans,* this rather thin layer is referred to

as the "armor plate" layer because the tight packing represents a barrier preventing large macromolecules from diffusing in or out of the synovial fluid. Wearing-out of this layer (zone I) is clinically significant to joint nutrition and to understanding the pathohistology of osteoarthritis.

The collagen orientation of the *intermediate* or *transitional zone* are no longer parallel with the surface but are obliquely oriented, whereas in the deep or radial zone, the collagen fiber orientation is vertically arranged with respect to the subcortical bone and thus serves to anchor cartilage to the underlying bone. The fibers in the midzone, although obliquely oriented, appear in a random arrangement. However, when cartilage is subjected to axial compression, these oblique fibers tend to line up perpendicular to the compressive force, the most advantageous arrangement in resisting compressive load.[6] Taken together, the morphologic structure of the zones comprising articular cartilage represent an arcade—a series of arches that represent a strategy for rapid and uniform dissipation of stress[11] from tensile, compressive, and shearing forces (Fig. 49-2).

13. What component within the matrix of articular cartilage retains and regulates the flow of water within the matrix?

The key to understanding the unique properties of articular cartilage, including its resiliency, nutrition, and lubrication under compressive loads[98,99] lies in the chemical structure of the *proteoglycan molecules* comprising a substantial fraction of the articular extracellular matrix. The functional role of articular cartilage is directly related to the chemical structure of these protein-polysaccharide complexes, which have a highly viscous, strongly hydrophilic, and electronegative nature.

Cartilage proteoglycans are protein-sugar macromolecules with a molecular weight in the millions that are synthesized within the endoplasmic reticulum of chondroblasts and chondrocytes and then transported via the Golgi apparatus for extracellular assembly. The core protein of the proteoglycan monomer is divided into 3 regions composed of three carbohydrates classified as glycosaminoglycans that include: (1) hyaluronic acid serving as a core to which sulfated groups bind; (2) chondroitin sulfate; and (3) keratan sulfate. The latter two sulfated groups extend side chains outwardly, like the legs of a centipede, and are simply sulfonated groups attached to a filamentous hyaluronic acid backbone. Chondroitin sulfate extends out relatively farther

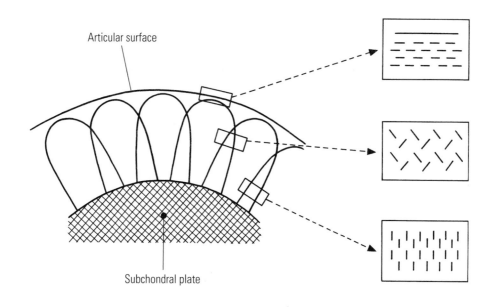

Articular surface

Subchondral plate

FIG. 49-2 Schematic diagram of collagen fiber orientation in articular cartilage. Fibrils are tightly packed near the surface in a tangential layer termed the "armor plate layer." The change in fibril orientation from tangential to perpendicular in deeper layers during joint pressure orients the zones of articular cartilage into an arch-like configuration known as an arcade that resists stress. (From Sledge CB: Structure, development, and function of joints, *Orthop Clin North Am* 6[3]:619, 1975.)

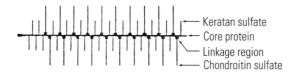

Keratan sulfate
Core protein
Linkage region
Chondroitin sulfate

FIG. 49-3 Proteoglycan monomer. (From Rosenberg L: Structure of cartilage proteoglycan. In Simon WH editor: The *human joint in health and disease,* Philadelphia, 1978, University of Pennsylvania Press.)

as its molecular chain is more complex (Fig. 49-3). The sulfated groups are present in varying proportions in accordance with the age of the individual. After the second decade of life, the proportion of chondroitin sulfate falls and that of keratosulfate rises, corresponding to the diminution of metabolic activity of chondrocytes.

To make the situation more complex, these linear *proteoglycan monomer* subunits aggregate with two other matrix components known as hyaluronic acid and core proteins to form a *giant aggregated proteoglycan* (i.e., protein-polysaccharide) *macromolecule* with a molecular weight approaching 100 million. This aggregate, having the appearance of a baby-bottle brush, is

composed of hyaluronic acid acting as a backbone, a link or core protein attaching the backbone to the sulfated subunit, which correspond to the bristles of the brush (Fig. 49-4).[29] These huge macromolecules are then exported and properly located and secured within the extracellular matrix between the interstices of collagen (Fig. 49-5).

14. How do the proteoglycan molecules within the articular cartilage matrix regulate the flow of water within the matrix when the joint is nonweight bearing?

The matrix of articular cartilage may be described as being *hyperhydrated,* with a water content varying between 60% and 80% of cartilage's total weight.[67] The solid components of the matrix consists of type II collagen, a macromolecule that endows articular cartilage with remarkable elasticity, and the huge proteoglycan aggregates that serve to imbibe water within the matrix. Both collagen and proteoglycans are synthesized by chondrocytes.

The proteoglycan macromolecules have chemical and electrical properties that endow them with the ability to sequester water. These macromolecules are much

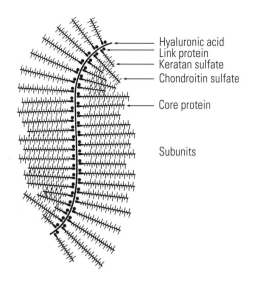

Hyaluronic acid
Link protein
Keratan sulfate
Chondroitin sulfate

Core protein

Subunits

FIG. 49-4 Giant aggregated proteoglycan macromolecule. (From Rosenberg L: Structure of cartilage proteoglycan. In Simon WH editor: *The human joint in health and disease*, Philadelphia, 1978, University of Pennsylvania Press.)

too large to move between the fibrils of collagen, or exit the armor plate layer comprising the surface of articular cartilage as the 6 nm diameter of those surface pores are too small.[104] Because of the high degree of entanglement of proteoglycans, the tight packing of surface collagen acts as a molecular sieve to keep proteoglycans in while keeping hyaluronidase out.[82,83]

The side chains of the proteoglycan aggregate, composed of proteoglycan monomers, contain many electronegative surface charges (on the sulfated sugars and carboxyl groups) that repel each other, causing the molecules to attempt to unwind and enlarge their domain within the cartilagenous extracellular matrix. The water molecules in the extracellular fluid act as dipoles: the positively charge hydrogen atoms are to the negatively charged sulfate domains, whereas the negatively charged oxygen atoms comprising the water molecules repel one another.[1,80] The net effect of these reactions is the attraction of water molecules in between the monomers, which serve as a molecular sponge. Moreover, because the proteoglycan aggregates within the extracellular matrix are larger than the hyaluronidase molecules within synovial fluid, a *concentration gradient* is created in the direction of the extracellular matrix so that water tends to flow from the synovial fluid into cartilage across the surface layer of articular cartilage as a

function of *simple passive diffusion.* Thus both the size and the electrochemical properties of the proteoglycan molecule aggregates act like a hydrophilic "pump." This tendency to *imbibe water* creates a swelling pressure within cartilage, which acts as an enormous hydration sphere surrounding the proteoglycan aggregates within the extracellular matrix. Articular cartilage is thus pressurized by the presence of water, and uses its incompressibility to protect against the deleterious effects of concussive force during weight bearing and joint loading. This is referred to the *load carriage role* of articular cartilage.

15. What determines the movement of fluid out of the articular cartilage matrix and into synovial fluid?

Movement of fluid (liquid water) is the mechanism by which load bearing, nutrition, and lubrication occur. Normally, net flow of fluid into and out of cartilage is induced by the normal weight-bearing function of synovial joints. During weight bearing, the external pressures of superincumbent body weight and ground reaction force collide at the articulating surfaces of the joint. If the external pressure exceeds the internal swelling pressure of the fluid contained within the extraarticular matrix, fluid will flow outward. Thus water is forced out of the extracellular matrix against the concentration gradient, across the surface layer of articular cartilage, and into synovial fluid when joint compression occurs during weight bearing. This *dissociation of fluid* increases the volume of synovial fluid and is expressed out of cartilage in front of the advancing contact surfaces of cartilage so as to minimize cartilage-to-cartilage contact.[98,99] This causes a wedge of fluid to become interposed between the points of contact (fluid lubrication) and thus minimizes articular wear. The direction of fluid flow is reversed and equilibrium is reestablished once weight bearing ceases. Thus for example, during unloading of the knee joint during swing phase, water is reimbibed back into the proteoglycan macromolecules within the extracellular matrix.

Fluid movement has the triple function of lubricating the joint, providing nutrients for chondrocytes, and load carriage. Loading cartilage for long periods without allowing for intermittent relaxation will lead to decreased diffusion, resulting in diminished nutrition to articular cartilage. By contrast, prolonged immobilization of a synovial joint leads to stasis of synovial fluid, diminished nutrition, and disuse atrophy of articular cartilage.[98]

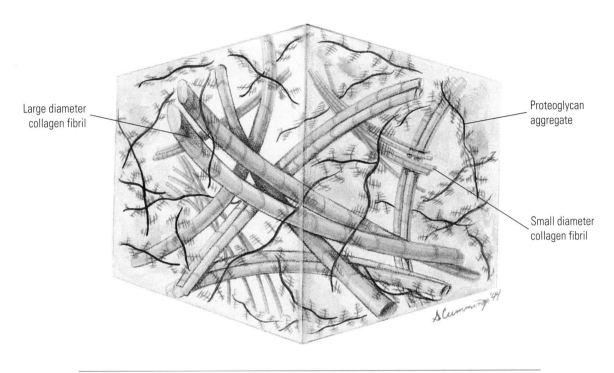

Large diameter
collagen fibril

Proteoglycan
aggregate

Small diameter
collagen fibril

FIG. 49-5 The extracellular matrix of articular cartilage showing the proteoglycan aggregates and their monomer side chains secured within the interstices of collagen fibrils. (From Cramer GD, Darby SA: *Basic and clinical anatomy of the spine, spinal cord, and ANS*, St Louis, 1995, Mosby.)

16. What are the possible etiologic factors in degenerative joint disease?

Several etiologic factors have been postulated to precede the development of degenerative joint disease. These include:

- *Articular cartilage defects.* Articular cartilage defects may occur secondary to a history of meniscus derangement or an osteochondritic lesion. Indeed, weight bearing upon a knee that has become locked because of meniscal impingement or a flit of osteochondritic bone may cause a partial-thickness crater-like defect in the surface of articular cartilage. Although small defects undergo spontaneous healing, particularly from continuous passive motion (CPM),[3] defects greater than ⅛ inch are beyond the capacity of effective response by the cells of subchondral bone. These larger size defects become filled with fibrocartilage that never reaches the normal joint surface and therefore does not articulate with the opposing cartilage. Thus the typical defect derived from osteochondritis dissecans will not fill in to the extent required for a stable joint interface,[90] resulting in degenerative arthrosis of the medial tibiofemoral articulation.

- *Subchondral bone fatigue.* Subchondral bone and the menisci function primarily as shock absorbers to dampen the caudally migrating ground-reaction forces generated at heel strike.[89] Articular cartilage, by virtue of its elastic properties also serves to attenuate these forces by undergoing instantaneous deformation during contact. However if weight bearing is prolonged, repetitive,[91] or forceful it may result in extensive wear of the articular surface and eventual degenerative arthrosis.[23]

- *Joint contracture.* Mathematical analysis of the force acting on the knee in the sagittal plane shows that weight bearing on a knee flexion contracture brings extensive forces to bear on both the tibiofemoral and patellofemoral joint surfaces, thus predisposing for degenerative change.[120] Moreover, in the presence of flexion contracture, infiltration of pannus, erosion, and osteophyte formation occur in a triangular area on the medial femoral condyle and along the strip on the lateral femoral condyle corresponding to the areas normally in contact with the anterior meniscal horns when the knee is fully extended.[23]

- *Obesity.* Obesity represents a significant risk factor in the development of degenerative joint disease at the hip and knee joints. As opposed to quiet standing, during stance phase the forces acting on the single stance leg are represented by twice the magnitude of force, so that the forces acting through the joints are multiple of body weight. This is magnified in the case of obesity, which causes an increase in peak dynamic loads and focal overloading of the articular cartilage and subchondral bone.[115]

- *Occupation and recreation.* These represent factors in the development of degenerative joint disease. This is borne out by the many incidences of premature degenerative joint disease in retired Olympic gymnasts who, having pushed their bodies beyond the physical limit during their teenage years, experience premature signs and symptoms of osteoarthritis in their late twenties. Heavy physical workloads have been found to contribute to the development of osteoarthrosis at the knee in farmers, firefighters, and construction workers.[58]

17. How may angular malalignment in the frontal plane predispose for degenerative joint disease at the hip and knee?

Before a discussion of the effects of malalignment of the hip and knee joints, it is essential to establish the importance of normal anatomic alignment of the lower extremity. The load transmitted across a joint is expressed as a direct function of the alignment of the bones relative to that articulation.[107] Normal orientation of the hip and knee joints in the coronal, sagittal, and transverse planes is imperative to adequate distribution of forces. These forces include both ground reaction force and superincumbent body weight across the weight bearing joints of the lower extremity.* The horizontal orientation of joint lines at the hip, knee, and ankle is an essential anatomic determinant for all weight-bearing functions.[45] The lack of a normal hori-

---

*During walking a force is created against the ground in concurrence with Newton's third law, which states that for every action there is an equal and opposite reaction. Thus the downward force of superincumbent body weight generates an upward ground reaction that is equal in magnitude but opposite in direction. As force is directly proportional to both mass and acceleration, as the speed of gait increases, so does the force involved. Consequently, greater wear occurs as the speed of gait increases. Running creates forces across the hip joint of four to five times the body weight.

zontal joint-line orientation because of joint tilting secondary to axial malalignment generates translation or shear forces across the joint.[35] This obliquity of the joint line, secondary to angular deformity, may alter the biomechanical distribution of forces, hasten the normal aging of articular cartilage, and result in osteoarthritis.[55]

The femoral head, described by some as spherical[97] and by others as ellipsoid and compressed in an anteroposterior direction,[40] has a smooth surface that snugly fits into the half-moon shaped acetabular (*acetabulum* means "cup" in Latin) socket. The function of the human hip is to sustain and distribute load, and to allow for motion between the thigh and trunk. Because the hip joint is part of a closed kinetic chain, any abnormal stress on this joint due to less-than-ideal joint line orientation will predispose for premature wearing of the articular surface. Diminished horizontal joint orientation may follow infection or trauma to the hip joint as the articulating surface becomes irregular, and may result in premature arthritis. Normally, a dynamic balance between the agonist and antagonist muscle couples surrounding the hip joint provides equal tension to the hip that contributes to joint stability. Any disturbance in this equal tension owing to muscle weakness or spasticity will shift the pelvis to one side, with the net result of disproportionate distribution of forces and eventual wear of that portion of the femoral head in excessive contact with the acetabulum. In contrast, axial malalignment secondary to leg length discrepancy, either due to osseous malformations of the hip or from shortening or lengthening of one lower limb, may cause excessive weight bearing of one aspect of the joint, and predispose for degenerative arthrosis. These three mechanisms are some of the more common pathways for articular wear of the hip joint. Moreover, abnormal distribution of stress at the hip will have biomechanical repercussions as asymmetries are expressed superiorly to the trunk and neck and inferiorly to the knee, ankle, and foot.[20]

The medial tibiofemoral compartment of the knee is more often affected by osteoarthritis than the lateral compartment.[109] This derives from the geometric asymmetry between the medial and lateral portions of the joint. The medial femoral condyle is larger and longer than the lateral femoral condyle (see Fig. 41-4). This results in slight valgus of the normal knee as a direct function of the greater anteroposterior projection of the medial femoral condyle.[109] If a line showing the mechanical axis of the lower limb is drawn from the center of the femoral head to the center of the ankle joint, it will pass medial to the center of the knee.[71] Thus normal human anatomy represents a medial deviation of the axial alignment of the load-bearing axis. This creates a moment arm acting to increase force transmission across the medial tibiofemoral compartment.[122] Thus human anatomy, characterized by uneven load distribution at the knee, is itself a risk factor for degenerative changes at the tibiofemoral joint. The consequence of tilting of the tibial plateau results in relatively excessive weight bearing at the medial tibiofemoral joint. As the medial compartment becomes progressively worn, varus will increase, more load is assumed by the medial compartment, the wear increases, and the deformity worsens in a characteristic vicious cycle.

18. How do the normal biomechanical changes that occur with aging of articular cartilage upset its load carriage function?

Age-related changes in articular cartilage, beginning in early adult life, involve biochemical changes that parallel the metabolic slow-down occurring throughout the body. The overall effect of these changes is the loss of water content from cartilage. This is important because, as water is an incompressible fluid, healthy articular cartilage makes use of this incompressibility to withstand the continual concussive brunt of weight bearing, and thereby protect articular cartilage from wear and tear. It is the fluid component that accounts for the viscous nature of cartilage. Without the benefit of fluid kept within the matrix of articular cartilage, the loss of resiliency subjects cartilage to excessive tension, compression, shear, and torsional forces.

Specifically, the molecular changes within the matrix of articular cartilage occur as a gradual loss of proteoglycan content, and a significant change within the remaining proteoglycan molecules. The latter refers to what normally occurs after the second decade of life, in which the proportion of chondroitin sulfate falls and that of keratosulfate rises, corresponding to the diminution of metabolic activity of chondrocytes. Chondroitin sulfate is a longer molecule then keratosulfate, and therefore has greater hydrophilic characteristics. Moreover, as we age, chondroitin 4 sulfates, which are relatively less electronegative and subsequently less hydrophilic, replace the existing chondroitin 6 sulfate molecules.

The cumulative effects of these biochemical changes have a profound effect on the load-carriage function articular cartilage. It is because of the many proteoglycan aggregates, and the longer-chain chondroitin 6 sulfate molecules that endow the extracellular matrix of cartilage with its ability to sequester fluid during nonweight bearing and reimbibe fluid following weight bearing. Under normal circumstances, articular cartilage acts as a shock absorber that protects bone by dampening and attenuating dynamic loads in a viscoelastic fashion. Diminishment and alteration of proteoglycans with the passage of time results in the loss of the biphasic properties of articular cartilage with a net result of cartilage gradually losing its shock absorbing capacity. As a result, the surface of articular cartilage is exposed to relatively more friction and eventually succumbs to wearing of the tangential layer of cartilage.

19. How does wear of the tangential layer of articular cartilage result in diminished chondrocyte nutrition?

In addition, the cumulative effect of friction wears down the surface layer of articular cartilage. The thin tangential surface layer, only 1 to 7 mm thick in healthy joints,[67] is referred to as the "armor plate" layer because its tight packing represents a barrier preventing large macromolecules from diffusing in or out of the synovial fluid. Normally the proteoglycan aggregates cannot exit the armor plate layer comprising the surface layer of articular cartilage as the 6 nm diameter of those surface pores are too small.[104] Thus the tight packing of surface collagen acts as a molecular sieve to keep proteoglycans in while keeping hyaluronidase out.[66] Wearing-out of this layer (zone I) is critically significant to understanding the histopathology of osteoarthritis as it causes proteoglycans to escape across the tangential layer into synovial fluid thus endowing it with greater viscosity. Moreover, the concentration gradient is reversed so that the larger proteoglycan molecules act as a reverse pump to pull water out of the extracellular matrix and into synovial fluid. Loss of the tangential layer upsets the normal concentration gradient maintained between the extracellular matrix and synovial fluid, and results in diminished chondrocyte nutrition. Thus wear of the tangential layer initiates the degenerative sequence of pathologic degeneration of diarthrodial joints. These changes described in the pathogenesis of osteoarthritis demonstrate that degenerative joint disease is much more than a passive "wear and tear phenomenon," but rather a disease characterized by much cellular and metabolic activity within articular cartilage.[98,99]

20. What is the classification of osteoarthritis?

Primary degenerative joint disease develops spontaneously during or past middle age and, similar to premature graying hair, represents an acceleration of the normal aging process of joints.[98,99] Exactly why certain individuals are prone to accelerated articular wear may be because of unknown constitutional factors or have a genetic basis. Thus primary osteoarthritis is considered idiopathic involving many joints without any know preexisting abnormality, and is more common in females[20] during their fifth and sixth decades as polyarticular involvement of many joints. The onset may be relatively sudden with hot, inflamed distal interphalangeal joints. Primary arthritis in males typically involves the hip joint unilaterally, with no obvious precipitating cause and no other joint involvment.[31]

Secondary degenerative joint disease occurs in the presence of predisposing factors or preexisting conditions that produce the initial lesion in articular cartilage. Here, secondary osteoarthritis occurs as a sequel to infection, internal derangement, extraarticular malalignment, lax or sprained ligaments, microtrauma from occupational stress, hemarthrosis from hemophilia, metabolic forms of arthritis such as gout, and inflammatory joint disorders such as rheumatoid arthritis or ankylosing spondylitis. Other predisposing factors include congenital joint abnormalities such as hip dysplasia, pelvic obliquity secondary to leg length discrepancy, trauma from fracture through the joint line, slipped capital femoral epiphyses, injury to the epiphyseal plate, osteochondroses such as Legg-Calve-Perthes disease or osteochondrosis dissecans, neuropathies that cause joint denervation, Charcot joint, immobilization, or iatrogenic damage. These or other insults to the joint may initiate wearing of the tangential layer of articular cartilage and degeneration, which with continued use and abuse will rapidly evolve into the progressive cycle characterizing arthrosis of that joint. The joints typically involved are the weight bearing synovial joints such as the hip, knee, and the intervertebral joints of the lower spine. Secondary degenerative disease usually involves a single joint and commonly develops in younger males.

Traumatic injuries do not typically result in degenerative joint disease unless the joint is permanently injured from the initial trauma. With occupational injuries, the cumulative microtrauma generated by vibrations, for example, from heavy pneumatic drills, is particularly damaging to joints. For those children not born with dysplasia of the hip joint, it is believed that subluxation or dislocation may result after birth by swaddling infants or carrying them in headboards, both of which maintain the thigh in an extended posture, thus forcing the femoral head out of its normal relationship with the acetabulum.[104]

21. What is the sequential progression of tissue destruction during the evolution of the osteoarthritic joint?

The pathogenesis of degenerative arthrosis refers to the sequential degenerative changes characteristic of osteoarthritis that may be provoked by any number of factors. Whether degenerative joint disease is primary, secondary, or a combination of both, the pathologic sequence causing joint destruction is the same once the pore size of the surface layer of articular cartilage is altered through wear causing proteoglycans to leak out into the synovial fluid resulting in impaired chondrocyte nutrition. With loss of proteoglycan content from the matrix, the collagen fibers become more susceptible to mechanical damage secondary to wear.[93] As a result, the elastic resilience of cartilage becomes impaired so that the articular surface becomes increasingly less able to withstand even minor stress. Moreover, the poorly nourished chondrocytes must bear the brunt of direct frictional stress while protease, a lysosomal enzyme normally intracellular, is released owing to chondrocyte damage. The chondrocytes, in turn, respond defensively by increasing the rate of proteoglycan synthesis in an effort to ward off the damage. However, the rate of mechanical wear outstrips any attempted repair in those sites subject to the greatest load bearing or shearing stress. Enzymatic degradation due to marked lysosomal activity[17] results in thwarting proteoglycan synthesis, and the creation of cartilage debris, which consists of small fragments of abraded dead cartilage that is released into the joint and swept about because of joint motion producing a reactionary synovitis,[98,99] so that what began as a purely degenerative process progresses to focal areas of secondary inflammatory synovitis. This results in a villous hypertrophy and fibrosis of the synovium with subsequent moderate synovial effusion, increased mucin content, and greater viscosity.[105] Changes in the synovial membrane are often accompanied by fraying and instability of the cruciate ligaments and menisci at the knee.[23] Moreover, as bone is lost and the joint surfaces approximate, the ligaments become more lax. In addition, fibrosis and thickening spreads to the adjacent fibrous joint capsule, which further limits joint motion so that the endstage may be a fibrous ankylosis of the joint. The muscles adjacent to the affected joint demonstrate spasm in response to pain, and the flexors, typically the hamstrings, undergo contracture and cause joint deformity and further restriction of motion. Thus osteoarthritis represents a failure in repair that occurs when chondrocyte proliferation and proteoglycan production cannot keep pace with the destruction.[20] This sets into motion a cascade of degeneration of the articular cartilage and surrounding soft tissue.

Once the tangential layer of the central, weight-bearing aspect of articular cartilage undergoes shredding, fraying, and fibrillation of the weakened area minor stress renders the cartilage matrix more susceptible to friction. *Fibrillation* refers to vertical splitting of the superficial portion of articular cartilage causing softening (malacia) as the surface become rough, resembling a shaggy carpet.[113] The articular surface, which is normally a bluish-white, smooth and glistening, becomes yellow, granular, and dull with fibrillation. It is at this point that conservative intervention is most helpful in the form of nonsteroidal antiinflammatory medications, which inhibit prostaglandin synthesis by fibroblasts, as prostaglandin is an intermediary in releasing catabolic enzymes.[92] In addition, the short-term benefits of steroid injection serve to stabilize the lysosomal membranes containing these enzymes within cartilage cells, while rendering white cells less sticky and thereby minimizing their ability to generate an inflammatory response. An assistive device during weight bearing is especially helpful at this time.

If the degenerative process is not interrupted, fibrillation gives way to deep *fissures* or cracks representing partial-thickness defects within the articular surface. Clusters of chondrocytes proliferate clusters called *clones* around the fissures in an attempt to ward off impending disaster by metabolizing collagen and proteoglycan at a more rapid rate than usual. Despite these efforts, fissuring represents a point of no return in the degenerative process. Eventually, all four layers of articular cartilage are worn away and the joint is *denuded.* Once the fissures have grown deep enough to penetrate subcortical bone, an influx of marrow cells allows fibrocartilage to grow upward at an attempt at repair. Healing of the surface defect at best occurs as the form of a scar composed of fibrocartilage, which is made up of randomly oriented fibrils unsuited for load bearing. In addition, because fibrocartilage is unlike hyaline cartilage, which is a vascularized tissue, continued wearing over these defects causes bleeding into the joint, which further contributes to degradation of any remaining or adjacent articular cartilage. As weight bearing continues over this defect and fibrocartilage is progressively worn away, the subchondral bone serves at the joint surface causing raw bone to rub against raw bone. In response, the subchondral bone undergoes *eburnation* in which it becomes as smooth as polished ivory, and hypertrophies to the point of becoming *sclerotic* (having increased radiographic density) on a radiograph. Sclerosis represents a healing process, similar to callus formation, of microfractures in subchondral bone.[105] In contrast, in the peripheral areas, which are characterized by minimal stress, the subchondral bone atrophies and becomes radiographically *rarefied* (less dense). The trabeculae in these central areas of maximum stress and friction suffer fracture and heal with callus, which increases the rigidity of bone so that the bone becomes denser and less resilient. As the normal architecture of bone is lost, the trabeculae undergo mucoid and fibrous degeneration and are replaced by cystic areas of rarefaction of bone radiographically apparent just beneath the eburnated surface and may be filled with pockets of synovial fluid[98,99] that leak in from the joint surface via defects in the subchondral bone.[73] Eventually, continued wear through to these cysts appears as multiple pits on the eburnated surface.

Although the proportion of bone increases centrally, cartilage behaves differently in that it decreases centrally and increases peripherally. At the peripheral border of the joint cartilage undergoes hypertrophy and hyperplasia to form a thickened rim of cartilage around the joint margin. This cartilaginous outgrowth is called a *chondrophyte* and undergoes endochondral ossification to become a peripheral bony outgrowth known as a bone spur or *osteophyte* as an attempt to minimize joint motion and more broadly distribute loading forces. This topologic change in the shape of bone at the joint margins involves stretching of the highly innervated periosteum that is painful. This new bone may even grow inwardly into the joint space. This loss of cartilage centrally and simultaneously growth peripherally represents a protective strategy to minimize joint motion. In the process, however, incongruity of the joint surfaces increases so that an alteration of the distribution and magnitude of the biomechanical stresses on the joint occurs. In this way, this form of remodeling may have the short term benefit of minimizing pain by way of restricting motion, but does so at the expense of worsening joint congruity, which leads to progressive arthrosis of that joint. Thus the body's various attempts to ward off the effects of degeneration throughout the evolution of osteoarthrosis are met with increasing failure that only, in the long run, contributes to the ultimate demise of the joint, characteristic of a vicious cycle of degeneration.

22. How may leg length disparity predispose for unilateral degenerative articular disease at the ipsilateral hip and contralateral patellofemoral joint?

Leg length discrepancy has been cited[36,37] as a factor predisposing unilateral degenerative arthritis of the hip on the side of the longer leg.[117] In the standing posture, the pelvic obliquity resulting from a disparity in leg lengths would cause the longer lower limb to assume a position of relative adduction. The relative tilting of the acetabulum results in reduced coverage of the femoral head, and increased joint congruence that focuses proportionally greater compressive force along the lateral acetabular roof. The resultant increased loading on the lateral acetabular edge may act to increase the vertical compressive forces on the medial and middle aspects of the femoral head, which, over time, may result in degenerative changes of the femoral head. In contrast, chondromalacia patellae may develop at the knee of the shorter leg in patients with leg length discrepancy possibly due to excessive knee hyperextension throughout stance and particularly during push-off phase of gait.[14]

23. What is the clinical presentation of degenerative joint disease at the hip and knee?

Degenerative joint disease of the hip joint is the most common painful condition of the hip joint[57] that is estimated to affect as much as 20% of all persons over the age of 55 years,[56] and in a female to male ratio of 3:2.[118] The three principal features of the clinical presentation are pain, loss of movement, and altered function. Early on, pain is absent with movement, but later becomes painful on the next day because of wear particles that cause a reactionary synovitis after exercise has ceased. Pain during rest is an indication that joint degeneration has significantly progressed to the acute phase of the disease process. Loss of movement secondary to remodeling occurs from change in the shape of the articular surface due to central and peripheral changes. This occurs so slowly that few patient notice any sudden change. Similarly, alterations in joint function occur imperceptibly so that the patients may not choose to work as long or as hard as they once did, or

walk as far as they used to ambulate. These limitations gradually increase and diminish patient stamina.

The initial degenerative pathology at the hip begins as fibrillation of one or both articular surfaces and the formation of wear particles, which are swept to the side of the joint where they irritate the synovium. This synovial irritation corresponds to the initial ache felt by the patient. As synovial irritation continues, the synovial membrane and adjacent capsule undergoes fibrosis, which in turn interferes with the normal function of the hip joint capsule. The thick articular joint capsule contributes to hip joint stability during weight bearing by holding the femoral head snugly into the acetabulum. Stability of the hip joint during weight bearing is best afforded by a taut hip capsule, which occurs when the hip is in extension, abduction, and internal rotation.[20] Fibrosis of the capsule causes shortening resulting in instability and muscle spasm setting in to prevent those positions that stretch the hip capsule; the opposite posture of hip flexion, adduction, and external rotation results and may become fixed and contractured.

The most prominent symptom of the osteoarthritic hip is aching pain, which may be severe, during weight bearing and radiates to the groin, the medial aspect of the thigh, and distally to the knee. In some persons, pain manifests primarily in the distal thigh. This is because the hip and distal femur both derive from the same sclerotome, so that the perceived pain is referred distally. As the disease progresses, pain becomes sharper, and may occur at rest so as to disturb sleep. Once articular cartilage is lost, subchondral bone is exposed, and grooves form in the eburnated joint surface so that the hip is gradually converted from a ball and socket into a *roller bearing*.[19] As cysts form in the femoral head and acetabulum, the bone softens and crumbles, the femoral head collapses and flattens, and osteophytes grow around the acetabular rim. Subsequently, joint motion becomes even more limited. In addition to loss of motion, morning stiffness occurs, and diminished function, and antalgic gait. Because the inflammation of the joint spreads to the greater and lesser trochanters, the hip abductors will be affected, resulting in a Trendelenburg lurch over the unilateral arthritic hip. In bilateral osteoarthritis of the hip joints, the patient will exhibit a *waddling gait* as their trunk lurches from side to side. An *abnormal capsular end-feel* imparted to the therapist's hand suggests a nonacute arthritis. End-feel refers to the sensation imparted to the examiner's hand at the extreme of the possible passive range of motion of the joint.[83]

Of the large joints, the knee is the most often affected by degenerative arthrosis.[42] The most common symptom is poorly defined pain that is variable in location, but most typically located over the *anteromedial aspect of the joint,* with point tenderness at that location. Patients describe an omnipresent dull *ache* that worsens with activity, diminishes with rest although not sufficiently to allow for painless relief during sleep. Complaints of *stiffness* following immobility known as a *gelling phenomenon* derives from the joint remaining in a fixed position for any length of time only to abate with activity resumption. The tendency toward gelling derives from a higher than normal viscosity of synovial fluid because of the synovial reaction to inflammation. In contrast to rheumatoid arthritis, morning stiffness is usually of mild intensity and short duration. A sense of *joint tightness* may wax and wane in accordance with episodes of *joint effusion,* which does not increase patient perception of pain. *Diminished muscle strength* of the quadriceps muscles, particularly during terminal knee extension may be evident in the knee that experiences effusion. Quadriceps *atrophy,* particularly involving the vastus medialis oblique muscle may be evident. *Function* is compromised as diminished tolerance to standing, walking, and stair climbing. An antalgic gait may be present. The gluteus maximus muscle can become significantly weak from inactivity. A shortening of single leg stance time of the affected limb may create disuse weakness in the ipsilateral gastrocnemius-soleus and gluteus medius muscles.[110] *Angular malalignment,* typically genu varum, is observed to advance with progression of the disease, although neutral alignment is also common.[20] A valgus strain will open up the medial side as the tibia returns to its normal neutral position.[23] Angular deformity is accompanied by *rotatory deformity* so that varus of the knee is accompanied by internal tibial rotation, while valgus of the knee is accompanied by slight external tibial rotation.[20] Joint line *crepitus* may be present as creaking, squeaking, or grating during movement and assessed by palpation along the joint lines. Crepitus may be audible. The therapist may also palpate for *periarticular bony hypertrophy* and tenderness along the medial joint line, accompanied by increased *warmth.* Some *loss of range of motion,* particularly the extremes of flexion and extension may occur. Laboratory data, in contrast to inflammatory, metabolic, infectious, and neuropathic forms of arthritis, are often within normal limits. Valgus testing of the knee joint will open up the medial site due to wear of the medial compartment and not because

the medial ligament has become lax.[23] When arthritis is advanced, the knee may exhibit a flexion contracture, and diminished size and tone of the quadriceps musculature.[110]

24. Why does pain associated with degenerative joint disease appear to be related to change of barometric pressure?

For many patients, the pain associated with osteoarthritis is often worsened before or just following a bout of inclement weather. Weather sensitivity may result from changes of trabecular subchondral bone beneath the surface of the joint. Cancellous bone normally contains fluid and blood within chambers known as *lacunae* that communicate by way of minute channels known as canaliculi. Hypertrophic bone formation in the central, weight-bearing portion of bone appears as sclerosis of bone, and represents bone remodeling walling off lacunae from each other. These sealed chambers and cysts contain fluid and resemble barometers. When barometric pressure drops suddenly, the encased fluid expands but cannot escape. This is experienced as pain by the patient before or just following periods of inclement weather and resultant barometric pressure changes.

25. What are the clinical manifestations of osteoarthritis distal to the wrist?

Many patients with arthrosis of the weight bearing joints demonstrate concomitant degenerative and nodular changes despite osteoarthritis not being a systemic disease. A single gene, dominant in females and recessive in males is believed to be instrumental in genetic expression of hand nodules. Osteoarthritic changes of the hand and wrist more commonly affect females. The joints of the digits most commonly involved include the distal and proximal interphalangeal joints in that order. In the hand, the carpometacarpal joints of the wrist, particularly that of the first digit and thumb, are more often involved in women. Arthrosis of the first carpometacarpl articulation presents as severe local pain and tenderness that is exacerbated by firm grasping and by moving the wrist. Finger nodules known as Heberden's nodes, considered a hallmark of osteoarthritis, develop at the terminal joints of the fingers. *Heberden's nodes* are extraarticular osteophytic spurs that initially occur at the *distal interphalangeal joints.* As the cartilage of the distal interphalangeal joint degenerates, osteophytes, which represent reactive outgrowths of articular cartilage away from the joint margins, grow from the dorsomedial and lateral aspects of the base of the distal phalanx to form painful and tender nodular protuberances. A permanent flexion or angular deformity may set in when degeneration is severe. When nodules less commonly develop at the *proximal interphalangeal joints,* they are called *Bouchard's nodes.* These hard, bony outgrowths are not to be confused with rheumatoid nodules that also occur at the proximal joints.

26. What are the radiographic features of degenerative joint disease at the hip and knee?

Plain radiographs of degenerative joint disease of the hip and knee joints are one of the primary determinants for arthritis, as radiographic changes often mirror clinical changes. There is loss of articular space, which is viewed as a narrowing of the cartilage space on radiograph. Bone may be sclerotic in those areas of maximal weight bearing or osteoporotic in adjacent areas of diminished weight bearing, and may include osteophyte formation or subchondral cysts, which may be central or peripheral. During the early stages of arthritis, radiographic changes are clear and easily identified, whereas once joint pathology progresses the joint destruction becomes more diffuse and radiographs become similar in appearance regardless of the specific angle the radiograph was taken. The roentgenographic changes in different forms of arthritis vary and may be summarized in Box 49-1.[6] Although these criteria are not diagnostic by themselves, when combined with patient history, physical examination, and laboratory tests, they may be used to point to a specific disease entity.[98,99] Paradoxically, the severity of perceived pain is not necessarily related to the severity of arthrosis as evidenced by radiographic changes.[23] Scintigraphy as a diagnostic tool is not helpful in the early stages of osteoarthrosis. Magnetic resonance imaging is a time-consuming and costly imaging tool that is not indicated in the evaluation of routine cases of osteoarthrosis.[20]

The radiologic changes associated with osteoarthritis of the hip joint include narrowing of the joint space, cyst formation in the femoral head and the acetabulum, sclerosis of subchondral bone, osteophyte formation, and periosteal thickening of the medial side of the femoral neck. If there is bone destruction as well, Shenton's line will be disturbed, indicating true limb shortening[62] (Fig. 49-6). In additional, over time, flattening of the femoral head and acetabulum will become evident,[56] and narrowing of the joint space.[69]

An anteroposterior radiograph of a healthy knee demonstrates subchondral sclerosis of an even width and pattern under both tibial plateaus, indicating even

BOX 49-1 Roentgenographic Changes in Arthritis

Osteoarthritis
Joint space narrowing (often localized)
Subchondral sclerosis
Osteophytes
Subchondral cysts

Inflammatory arthritis
Diffuse joint space narrowing
Absent subchondral sclerosis
Absent osteophytes
Subchondral cysts
Periarticular soft tissue swelling (symmetric)

Metabolic arthritis
Localized joint space narrowing
Marginal erosions
Asymmetric soft tissue swelling
Limited subchondral sclerosis
Chondrocalcinosis

Infectious arthritis
Joint space destroyed
Joint effusion
Symmetric soft tissue swelling
Osteoporosis

Neuropathic arthritis
Joint space destroyed
Periarticular debris
Joint instability
Joint effusion

From Tria AF, Klein KS: *An illustrated guide to the knee,* New York, 1992, Churchill Livingstone, p. 126. Table 9-2.

distribution of joint surfaces. Uneven distribution of weight bearing forces on the articular surfaces is radiographically revealed by a change in the shape of the subchondral sclerosis under the overstressed portion of cartilage in conjunction with a regression of sclerosis under the unloaded joint compartment.[2] Osteoarthrosis of the medial tibiofemoral joint usually begins on the tibial side rather than the femoral side.[94] Other radiographic changes include subchondral cyst formation and hypertrophic osteophytic lipping at the periarticular margins of the femur and tibia, and the intercondylar eminences of the tibia. Narrowing of the joint space should preferably be evaluated on the basis of weight-bearing films taken at both 0° and 45° of flexion. This

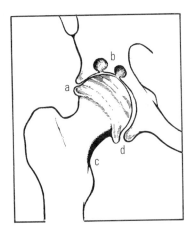

FIG. 49-6 Radiological appearance of osteoarthritis of the hip: *(a)* narrowing of the joint space; *(b)* subchondral bone cysts; *(c)* sclerosis; *(d)* osteophyte formation at the margin of the acetabulum. (From Dandy DJ: *Essential orthopaedics and trauma,* ed 2, Edinburgh, 1993, Churchill Livingstone.)

is because articular cartilage loss usually affects the portion of the femoral condyle that contacts the tibia between 30° and 60° of flexion, and joint space compromise may not be evident on weight-bearing films with the knee in full extension.[47]

27. What changes in hip joint mechanics occur due to leg length discrepancy?

Mathematical analysis of weight-bearing distribution across the hip joint in leg length discrepancy shows that the shorter leg undergoes *diminished load* as lesser force is transmitted across the hip. Because the pelvis on the shorter side drops, the lever arm between the center of gravity and the hip joint axis becomes *shorter,* and the abductor muscles' line of pull is changed, thus diminishing the total forces about the hip. Bilateral comparison of adductor strength will show weakness on the shorter side. The approximation of the greater trochanter to the iliac crest favors tightness and even contracture of the hip abductors. Leg length discrepancy acts on the shorter leg like a coxa vara deformity. In contrast, the longer leg undergoes increased load bearing at the hip joint, that is accompanied by upward pelvic obliquity and adductor tightness or contracture on that side.

A bilateral comparison of abductor strength will show weakness on the longer side. Vertical compressive forces are increased on the hip of the longer side

because the abductors must contract ever more forcefully to prevent the pelvis from dipping to the short side during stance phase of the longer limb.[52] Thus leg length discrepancies act on the longer leg like a coxa valga* deformity.[96]

28. What are the different forms of leg length discrepancy?

Leg length discrepancy, referred to as *anisomelia* or *pelvic tilt syndrome,* includes any inequality in length spanning proximally from the pelvis to the foot, distally. Most leg length discrepancies are less than 2 cm in magnitude,[106] although discrepancies of 1 cm or more are considered clinically significant.[53] Shortening of the right leg is more common in the general population.[72] The increase in length of the left leg seems to be related to the higher incidence of right handedness. Patients whose dominant hand is the right are more prone to use the left leg as their supporting extremity during quiet standing.[52] Discovery of pelvic tilt and associated limb length inequality is often made by a tailor fitting his clientle.[77]

True leg length discrepancy means that disparity between length of the lower limb derives from a dif-

---

*Coxa vara and valga represent focal osseous abnormalities of the proximal femur in which the angle of inclination causes a relative shortening or lengthening, respectively, of the limb on the involved side. During embryonic development, the neck (and head) and the femoral shafts become angulated in two planes. In addition to the *angle of torsion* between the femoral neck and shaft in the transverse plane, another angle known as the *angle of inclination* measures the relative medial or lateral deviation of the femur in the frontal plane, and is alternately known as the *neck-shaft angle*. The range of the angle of inclination is between 90° and 135° with an average of 125°. An angle of inclination in excess of 125° results in a *coxa valga* deformity in which the femoral shaft deviates laterally. An angle of inclination less than 125° will produce a *coxa vara* deformity in which the femoral shaft deviates medially. Because of the linkage between the hip and knee joints, coxa valga is often accompanied by compensatory genu varum (bowleg) whereas coxa vara is often accompanied by compensatory genu valgum (knock knees). In the newborn, the angle of inclination is approximately 150° and diminishes with normal growth and the effect of weight bearing to approximately 125° by skeletal maturity. Coxa valga is an abnormality of the proximal femur that represents undergrowth of the neck-diaphysis angle. Coxa valga may occur from multiple causes such as congenitally short femur in which dysplasia, which is most often bilateral, results in diminished medial-ward development of the shaft of the femur in relation to the head and neck of the femur. This condition may also present unilaterally following a traumatic incident, from spastic paralysis of the lower limb, or may derive from the elimination of weight bearing in early childhood.

ference in the length of the long bones of the lower extremity in which either the femur or tibia are shorter or longer. Here, the discrepancy is known as *structural* or *anatomical anisomelia*. In contrast, the state of *apparent leg length discrepancy* means that there is no true bony inequality. Apparent shortening occurs because of a right or left asymmetry in joint position resulting in pelvic obliquity, contracture of the hip adductors or knee flexors, abnormal positioning of the hip or knee with muscle spasm, or from unilateral excessive pronation (resulting in shortening) or a cavus posture (causing lengthening) of that leg. This form of disparity is known as a *functional anisomelia*. It is essential for the clinician to determine whether the discrepancies are structural or functional because corrections are specific for the type of length discrepancy.

29. What is the pathogenesis of leg length discrepancy?

Lower limb-length discrepancy has numerous congenital and acquired causes. Until the advent of effective vaccination poliomyelitis was the most common cause of leg length discrepancy causing shortening of the affected lower limb. Today, most significant leg length discrepancies are caused by congenital abnormalities, epiphyseal plate injuries secondary to trauma with subsequent growth disturbance, infection, which leads to damage of the growth plate, Legg-Calvé-Perthes disease, slipped capital femoral epiphysis, radiation therapy,[95] juvenile rheumatoid arthritis, arthrodesis of the knee, arthroplasty of the hip,[78] or following a stone-girdle hip procedure.

It is essential for the clinician to consider both the length parameter in a patient with limb length disparity and the difference in growth rate, particularly in the adolescent, to implement effective management. The causes of leg length discrepancy may be classified into three pathologic categories. One category includes a difference in length but not in growth rate, as in fractures that heal with overlapped fragments and cause an immediate discrepancy, but not a long-term difference the rate of long limb growth. Another category of disparity may arise from a difference in growth rate, but not initially in longitudinal length of the limb. For example, radiation may affect the growth plate with a change in the growth rate of the leg but no immediate shortening. Finally, the congenitally short femur may manifest as a difference in both length and growth with significant growth inhibition.

30. What pathologic conditions may develop secondary to leg length discrepancy?

Pelvic obliquity secondary to leg length discrepancy may place many of the soft and osseous tissue structures spanning between the pelvis and foot at potential risk for injury due to biomechanical imbalance. Every leg length discrepancy presents with both a shorter and longer leg. Consequently, pathologic changes and stress rise will consistently occur at sites specific to both the shorter and longer leg. The longer leg, usually on the left side,[52] is characterized by a higher pelvis and a hip joint that is held in adduction. This results in an increase in the distance between the origin and insertion of the hip abductors of the longer leg, which tends to increase their tension while decreasing their mechanical efficiency.[9] Moreover, the greater trochanter will protrude more laterally than in the normal hip. This may lead to trochanteric bursitis or iliotibial tract tendinitis[12] as the iliotibial tract is pressed ever more tightly over the greater trochanter. Other forms of tendinopathy reported at the longer side include the insertion and origin of iliopsoas at the lesser trochanter, at the transverse processes of the lumbar vertebrae, and at the origin of the hip adductors at the pubis. Pyriformis tightness with sciatic impingement may also occur.[13] Furthermore, arthritis of the hip joint is likely to develop because weight bearing from the acetabulum is focused at the center of the femoral head instead of uniformly. This subtle shift in weight-bearing distribution proximally at the hip results in excessive weight bearing distally at the medial compartment of the knee, and may result in eventual degenerative changes at the medial knee. Both proximal and distal joints attempt self-correction of the longer leg and include the ipsilateral sacroiliac and subtalar joints. In an attempt to equalize the longer limb, the sacroiliac joint posteriorly rotates the innominate bone and corrects for a difference of as much as 6 mm while the subtalar joint may posture in pronation so that the foot is characterized by a pes planus type deformity.[9]

In contrast, the shorter leg, usually on the right side, is characterized by a lower pelvis and a hip joint postured in decided hip abduction. The diminished distance between the origin and insertion of the hip abductor muscle results in minimized tension production. The greater trochanter assumes a more highly placed position closer to the ipsilateral iliac crest. The resultant change of location of this osseous landmark may result in tightness of the tensor fasciae latae leading to iliotibial tract tendinitis and trochanteric bursitis. Furthermore, because the superolateral portion of the hip joint undergoes higher stress per square centimeter of weight-bearing pressure, arthritis of the hip joint is likely to develop. This subtle shift in weight-bearing distribution proximally results in excessive weight bearing distally of the lateral compartment of the knee, and may result in eventual degenerative changes at the lateral knee. Finally, in an attempt to equalize the shorter limb, the sacroiliac joint attempts self-correction by undergoing anterior innominate torsion to lengthen the short side while the subtalar joint may posture in supination so that the foot is characterized by a pes cavus type deformity.[52]

31. What gait deviations may occur secondary to leg length discrepancy?

During quiet standing, compensation for leg length discrepancy is accomplished by flexing the knee on the long side, or by standing with the shorter limb in equinus. Both strategies accomplish the goal of leveling the pelvis. During gait, discrepancy results in stooping down onto the short leg and vaulting over the longer leg. However, gait is ideally characterized by a vertical displacement of the center of gravity via a shallow sinusoidal curve when both legs are of equal length.[27] The apex of this curve occurs when the supporting limb is at midstance, whereas the lowest point occurs at the time of double support when both feet are on the ground. The center of gravity, located at the first or second sacral level, lies within the pelvis, and its vertical path is kept at a minimum of 5 cm in the adult male.[78] Abrupt deviation from this smooth path represents inefficiency that requires more energy expenditure. A shorter or longer leg causes marked distortion of this curve, as the center of gravity is forced to change its position in the vertical plane, resulting in increased energy consumption[78] and poor cosmetic appearance. Younger patients often prefer to compensate by walking on the toes of the shorter leg. This diminishes the stimulus for growth of the calf muscles and may result in a progressive contracture in the shorter limb. Older patients often prefer to compensate for inequality by flexing the long leg.[32] Alternately, *circumduction* allows the longer limb to advance forward during swing phase, whereas *vaulting* results in an energy consuming rise and fall of the body.

32. What changes in alignment of the spinal column may occur secondary to leg length disparity?

A strong association is recognized between leg length discrepancy and the occurrence of low back pain.[38,43] Asymmetric tensions generated by pelvic obliquity result in compensatory scoliotic curves primarily in the low back and cervical spine.[13] In the lower back, standing with the knees straight and both soles flat against the floor tilts the lumbosacral junction in a person with a leg length discrepancy. The resultant scoliosis is not a fixed deformity, especially in a young person, as it is completely corrected when seated or when the discrepancy is corrected for by placing a board of appropriate height under the shorter leg. Over time, this *postural scoliosis* may eventually develop into a structural curve secondary to adaptive changes in soft and osseous tissue. There is no consistent correlation between pelvic tilt and the convexity of lumbar scoliosis,[53] although the convexity is often reported to be associated from a pelvic droop stemming from a shorter lower limb.[77] Wedging of the vertebral bodies may occur secondary to pelvic obliquity in those cases in which lateral deviation of the spine originated during a period of skeletal growth.[77] The uncorrected state of leg length discrepancy may predispose for degenerative disk disease in the lumbosacral spine later in life[53] owing to the reduced facet angle on the shorter side.

33. What postural examination is appropriate in the assessment of leg length discrepancy?

Before measurement of any potential discrepancy it is important to visually assess the patient from behind and in front, observing for any subtle differences in skin folds or postural asymmetries. During a standing *posture examination* the clinician both *visually inspects* and *palpates* a series of bone and soft-tissue landmarks in the effort to assess asymmetries secondary to leg length disparity. A marking pencil may be used to mark key anatomic landmarks such as the spinous processes, scapular borders, anterior superior iliac spines, iliac crests, posterior superior iliac spine, greater trochanters, patellae, the medial malleoli and the navicular of both feet. When comparing the heights of the pelvic crests it is also necessary to observe the gluteal cleft, which should ideally be in true vertical alignment in the absence of pelvic obliquity.[30] Following observation, a manual examination ensues. The patient stands with equal weight on each leg and with feet shoulder-width apart. The therapist places his or her hands on the iliac crests to assess for differences in pelvic obliquity, comparing the right with the left side. This may be repeated with the examiner's hands on the anterior superior iliac spines and on the superior aspect of each greater trochanter.[61] It is especially important to note the relative levels of the knees and iliac crests, the verticality of the lumbar spine, any differences in the size of the feet, and the configuration of the trunk. An asymmetry suggests a leg length discrepancy. Only clinical measurement will determine if the disparity is apparent, for example, stemming from a right-left joint asymmetry, or true and deriving from an actual right-left discrepancy of longitudinal bone length.

34. What are the direct and indirect methods for measurement of total leg length discrepancy?

Several methods of clinical measures of discrepancy are available. Both the indirect and direct methods may be used to complement each other. The *indirect method* uses blocks of wood or rubber of known thickness while the patient stands against a wall with the feet slightly apart and parallel, knees straight ahead, and arms hanging naturally to the sides. The therapist places calibrated blocks of 2-mm thickness under the short side until symmetry, defined by elimination of pelvic obliquity or leveling an anatomic landmark, is achieved. Compensation of disparity is ascertained by building up the plantar surface of the foot of the short leg side, using different thickness of blocks, until the greater trochanters and iliac spines are level, and obliteration of the postural lumbar scoliosis occurs. The patient will often sense when leveling is established. The indirect method of assessment does not differentiate between length disparities deriving from joint contractures (apparent discrepancies) or discrepancies in long bone length (true disparities).

The *direct method* for measurement of leg length is to perform a linear measurement of the distance between two anatomic landmarks and, using the same method, measure the contralateral extremity for comparison. The distance measured corresponds to the long axis of the long bone to be measured. The accuracy of measurement depends upon the precise determination of well-defined landmarks serving as anatomic reference points. The choice of these starting and ending points should correspond to the ends of long bones. However, because the proximal femur is difficult to palpate owing to the thick and deep surrounding layer of soft tissue, the greater trochanter is often used as the reference point. In obese patients who present difficulty in readily palpable greater trochanters, the anterior superior iliac spine may substitute. If the patient is morbidly obese, and difficulty is encountered in correctly identifying the anterior superior iliac spines, then the iliac crest, umbilicus or xiphisternal juncture may be substituted, in that order, as a proximal site. The prob-

lem with the latter three sites is that a positive finding is less specific for the true length of the femur, and may indicate the etiology of disparity to come from the hip or sacroiliac joint. A positive finding using either the anterior superior iliac spine or the umbilicus only confirms an apparent leg length discrepancy, but does not necessarily rule out true leg length inequality. The latter two sites are least preferred, as their position is inconstant.[30]

The patient lies in the supine position with the legs parallel to each other and 15 to 20 cm apart.[64] The placement of the proximal end of the tape measure is pressed at the protuberance of the greater trochanter. The greater trochanter is palpated as a prominence at the broadest part of the hips. In the female, this may be a little lower because of the greater proportion of fat infesting this region of the thigh.[8] Although the anterior and lateral portions of the greater trochanter are less accessible as they are covered by the tensor fasciae latae and gluteus medius muscles, the posterior edge of the trochanter is readily palpable. The tape measure is then extended distally to the tip of the lateral malleolus and a numerical measure from one bony landmark to another on the same extremity is recorded. The lateral malleolus is chosen over the medial malleolus because crossing the thigh may confound the measurement due to a potential difference in thigh circumference thereby introducing error into the measurement. This is because passing the tape obliquely across the thigh will cause the measuring tape to be displaced more anteriorly by an ipsilaterally hypertrophied quadriceps. Cloth or plastic tape measures are preferred to metal ones as the latter are smaller in width, have sharper edges, do not as easily conform to the contour of the lower limb, and feel cold to touch.[30] The tape measure should be stretched firmly between both end points, should be placed in as straight a line as possible,[16] and measurements should be rounded off to the nearest 0.5 cm. This measurement is then repeated on the contralateral extremity. When comparing the two sides, unequal values between the right and left extremities indicates that one leg is shorter and one leg is longer (Fig. 49-7).

In addition, using the lateral malleolus instead of the medial malleolus as a reference point translates into a slightly shorter distance in the presence of a genu valgum deformity and a slightly longer distance in the presence of a genu varum deformity. This is because a genu valgus deformity results in a measurement that is actually shorter than the real length of the leg, which is caused by the straight course of the tape measure. In

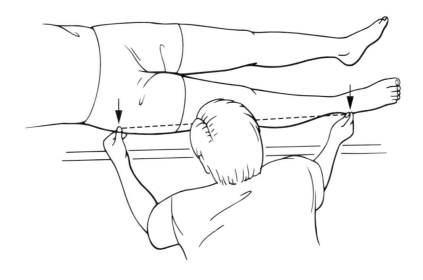

FIG. 49-7 *Direct method* for detecting *true leg length discrepancy* is assessed by measuring from one fixed bony point (greater trochanter) to another (lateral malleolus.

contrast, a genu varum deformity necessitates measuring an arc resulting in a measurement that is longer than the real leg length.[30]

35. What are the two methods for determining which of the long bones of the lower extremity are the source of the total leg length discrepancy?

After establishing a difference in *total leg length,* one must then determine whether the discrepancy derives from the femur or the tibia. This may be accomplished in one of two ways. The direct method measures the thigh (i.e., femoral) length and lower leg (i.e., tibial) length, and compares it to the opposite side. The proximal anatomic landmark, as with measurement of total discrepancy, is the ipsilateral greater trochanter. The distal end of the femur is best palpated as the interarticular space between the distal femur and proximal tibia at the lateral tibial plateau.

Alternately, determination of whether the discrepancy lies in the tibia or femur may be accomplished by observing the patient from the front and laterally. The patient is asked to lie supine with the knees flexed to 90° and the feet flat on the table. The therapist then stands at the feet of the patient and looks at the peaks created by the flexed knees. If one knee projects higher than the other does, then the tibia of that extremity is longer. If no change in height is noted during this comparison, one then views the tops of both knees laterally.

If one knee projects further anteriorly than the other, the femur of that extremity is longer (Fig. 49-8).[50]

36. When is radiographic measurement for leg length discrepancy appropriate?

Because as much as 30%[95] of clinical measurements of leg length discrepancy differ from radiographic measurements, clinical assessment of inequality is considered less reliable as it may be influenced by landmark palpation difficulties in patients with hypoplastic iliac crests, pronation of the feet, concomitant sacroiliac torsion, or obesity. Moreover, methodologic error owing to intertester and intertester assessment may lead to errors of as much as 1.5 cm.[30] The gold standard of accuracy in measurement for leg length discrepancy and pelvic obliquity is the standing anteroposterior radiograph of the pelvis.

37. How does rheumatoid arthritis differ from osteoarthritis?

Rheumatoid arthritis belongs to the group of autoimmune inflammatory arthritides that includes psoriatic arthritis, Reiter's syndrome, ankylosing spondylitis, sarcoidosis, and the crystal arthropathies such as gout and pseudogout. Both rheumatoid and osteoarthritis share in common their principal affectation of connective tissue comprising articular cartilage and the synovium. However, whereas rheumatoid arthritis is primarily an inflammatory process of the synovium,

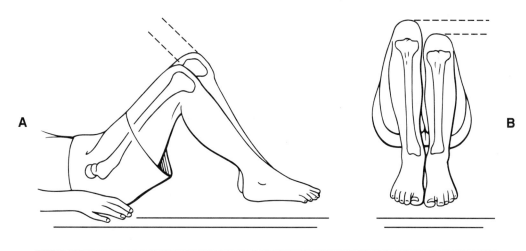

FIG. 49-8 Indirect method for determining if a positive leg length discrepancy derives from the femur or tibia. **A,** Femoral length discrepancy. **B,** Tibial length discrepancy.

osteoarthritis is principally a degenerative process of the articular cartilage. The division between these two disease processes is arbitrary because an inflammatory reaction occurs in osteoarthritis as well, although is occurs secondary to degeneration. With rheumatoid arthritis, the affected synovium contains plasma cells and lymphocytes, suggesting an autoimmune mechanism as the origin of the disease. Eventually, the rheumatoid inflammation that began in the synovium spreads to adjacent structures such as the articular cartilage.

The clinical features of osteoarthritis and rheumatoid arthritis differ considerably. Rheumatoid arthritis is characterized by symmetrical swelling in the small joints of the hands and feet of young adults, particularly females, between the ages of 15 and 35. Rheumatoid arthritis is a systemic disease that may affect any body organ and may present as one of two types: the juvenile or adult form. In contrast, osteoarthritis is a nonsystemic, localized disease usually affecting the large weight-bearing joints of older persons.

38. What conservative management strategy best services these patients?

The role of physical therapists in the prophylactic treatment of patients with a diagnosis of osteoarthritis of the hip and knee is to assist in achieving the highest functional outcome possible. Degenerative joint disease has a relatively poor prognosis in the lower extremities because of the continuing demands placed upon the affected joint with ordinary walking. There is, as yet, no cure for degenerative joint disease. The long-term re-

sults of uncemented total joint arthroplasty in young patients (less than 60 years of age) remain unknown. Patients in their fourth and fifth decades undergoing total joint arthroplasty present with the problem of possible mechanical failure and the need for revision in subsequent years.[28] Physical therapy intervention helps extend the time until total hip or knee replacement while assisting the patient in maintaining their optimal functional level.[59] The goals of physical therapy management of patients with osteoarthritis include pain control, prevention of strain or further damage to the affected joints, improved range of motion and muscle strength, and maintenance of or improvement in functional independence.[119]

- *Increased muscle strength.* Patients with osteoarthritis typically exhibit Type II fiber atrophy in muscles supporting the joints.[102] Strengthening exercises are used to gain increased muscle strength to provide better shock-absorbing capabilities to the joint and thereby diminish the magnitude of concussive force to the joint. In the case of knee involvement, exercises should include strengthening of the quadriceps, hamstring, and gastrocnemius-soleus muscle group. For the hip joint, strengthening exercises for all hip musculature is essential, particular the abductors. Biking and swimming are important because they avoid excessive stress on the hip joint while maintaining fitness and range of motion.

In the acute phase, isometric exercise produces a greater amount of muscle tension compared with concentric contractions[114] while creating the least amount of joint stress. Isometric exercise is thus the ideal starting point for strengthening of the periarticular musculature as it eliminates the rolling and sliding forces present during isotonic exercises. However, muscle strengthening should be progressed to include isotonic contractions as soon as possible to incorporate functional movement into the exercise program.[22] Concentric and eccentric exercises, in both the open and closed kinetic modes, should be performed. Incorporating eccentric exercises into the strengthening program is especially important because much of functional lower extremity muscle activity is eccentric and occurs in the first 45° of knee flexion.[76] The patient should be progressed carefully, and if increased pain lasts for more than 2 hours after exercise, exercise intensity should be decreased.[121] Although the lower extremity primarily functions in a closed kinetic chain, the full brunt of weight bearing creates forces in the knee that are equal to approximately three times body weight. Because of this, full weight-bearing strengthening exercises should be reserved for the subacute and chronic forms of the disease, and avoided in the acute phase of arthritis unless performed in water.

- *Assistive device.* A cane used on the unaffected side can reduce the forces on the affected side to just slightly more than body weight.[97] This form of external unloading diminishes the moment of force eccentrically exerted by the mass of the body on the loaded knee by transmitting a part of this force directly to the ground. Thus the magnitude of the resultant force acting on the joint is decreased.[70]

- *Orthotic correction.* The use of a viscoelastic arch support provides considerable reduction in the amplitude of concussive forces induced during stance.[116] Using a lateral-wedge insole for patients with medial joint osteoarthritis aligns the femur and tibia to a more upright position by reducing the mechanical axis without any change in the tibiofemoral angle, and shifts the calcaneus to a more upright position with respect to the tibia.[124] This relieves pain by unloading the medial knee compartment and reducing the tensile forces in the lateral ligamentous structures, and is effective in the treatment of mild medial joint osteoarthrosis.[100]

- *Lift therapy.* This refers to applying lifts to shoes so as to increase the length of the short limb and may be useful in discrepancies greater than 2 to 3 cm. Lifts may be flat, tapered, or rounded, and may be applied inside the shoe or on the heel. Although lifts are usu-

ally of a solid design, a slotted lift increases flexibility of the sole. It is important for the patient's self image to attempt to make the lift as inconspicuous as possible.[106] Lifts are ideally made of lightweight, high-density materials such as rubber or cork. A lift may extend the entire length of the sole or may only underlie the heel.

- *Correction of flexion contracture.* Prolonged weight bearing on a flexed knee can accelerate the degenerative process due to focal overloading. Restoration of the knee to full extension enlarges the tibiofemoral weight-bearing surfaces, and thereby diminishes the focal articular compressive stress. A light and durable knee extension long-leg brace with a knee extension spring may be helpful if worn constantly. Otherwise, serial splinting is used to gradually increase knee joint extension. This is helpful if the flexion contracture is between 5° to 10°. Active assistance and heat modalities may be helpful in gaining soft-tissue extensibility.

- *Soft-tissue flexibility.* Stretches of the iliopsoas, hamstring, quadriceps, pyriformis, and triceps surae muscle groups are important in maintaining tissue extensibility. Hold-relax techniques may be helpful. When patients spend excessive time in the sitting posture, the hip flexor and hamstring muscles are placed in an adaptively shortened position. Muscle tightness in these muscle groups will contribute lack of hip and knee extension, and ankle plantar flexion at the end of single limb stance, and thereby increase the force generated within these joints during walking.[75] The hamstring muscles, in particular, become tight and inflexible owing to secondary reflex muscle spasm derived from a joint capsule distended by joint effusion.[21] Thus stretching plays an important role in the management of the osteoarthritic hip or knee.

- *Patient education.* Joint protection plays an important role in daily activities. Patients are instructed to avoid low chairs and sustained weight bearing. Deep knee bends are to be avoided, and the patient is advised to sit in a high chair and elevated toilet seat. The importance of a daily home exercise program is explained to the patient, with emphasis on range-of-motion activities in the early morning to diminish the effects of stiffness. The use of a neoprene *knee brace* may be helpful as it gives the patient subjective support while the knee is weight bearing. It is helpful to reassure patients that their disease, while progressive, is only an exaggeration of the normal wear-and-tear process of the weight bearing joints and not a generalized disease process like rheumatoid arthritis. Getting patients to understand those factors such as excess weight bearing on the affected joint may help retard the arthritic process as they assume a proactive role in their own management.

- *Weight reduction.* Loss of excess weight may reduce the load assumed by the weight-bearing joints, and may be accomplished by a combination of both dieting and exercise.[14]
- *Endurance.* Poor cardiovascular status and deconditioning are significant problems in patients with arthritis owing to decreased activity levels.[85] A cardiopulmonary exercise program may be initiated once the arthritic joint is less acute. Because jogging and running cause repetitive stress in the knee joint,[85] walking, stationary biking, and swimming are three forms of fitness training often recommended because of the low-impact nature of these activities.[15] Both raising the seat height and decreasing the workload will decrease the amount of compressive force across the knee.[81] Walking through water further reduces the weight-bearing forces across the knee joint and is an excellent way to increase heart rate while allowing the buoyancy of the water to decrease the force of gravity affecting the weight-bearing joints.[39] A water temperature of 86°F is recommended.[33]
- *Modality application.* Modalities such as cold, heat, transcutaneous electrical neuromuscular stimulation (TENS), and hydrotherapy to minimize swelling and decrease pain are important components in the treatment of arthritic patients.[44,74] Cold is most effective in the acute stage of the disease, whereas heat is more effective in the subacute or chronic stages.[112] When applying cold in the acute state, it is best not to apply cooling for greater than 15 minutes to avoid a rebound vasodilation of the blood vessels within the cooled tissue.[74] Heat therapy may be used to decrease pain, joint stiffness, and muscle spasm, and increase the extensibility of contracted connective tissues. TENS electrode placement may ideally reduce pain when placed directly over area of pain.[68]
- *Medications.* Medications that have an analgesic and/or antiinflammatory effect are useful in diminishing symptoms associated with osteoarthritis. These medications share the ability to inhibit biosynthesis of prostaglandin[60] by blocking the production of the cyclooxygenase enzyme.[84] However, nonsteroidal antiinflammatory medications also suppress prostaglandin production in the stomach, which normally protects the stomach from its own acids. The long-

term hazard associated with aspirin usage is gastritis secondary to asymptomatic gastric erosions because the effect of even a small amount of daily salicylate intake (300 mg) increases bleeding time by inhibiting platelet aggregation. The earliest toxic symptoms in adults are usually tinnitus or deafness.[23] Because of this, aspirin has been largely replaced by other nonsteroidal antiinflammatory agents, which despite their greater expense, are safer to use. The intraarticular injection of steroids should be used sparingly. Multiple injections should be avoided as they may cause steroid arthropathy.

REFERENCES

1. Advances in bioengineering: transactions of the American society of mechanical engineers, *Am Soc Mech Eng* 177, 1974.
2. Ahlback S: Osteoarthrosis of the knee: a radiographic investigation, *Acta Radiol Suppl(Stockh)* 277:7, 1968.
3. Akeson WH, Amiel D, Lee J et al: Cartilage and ligament: physiology and repair processes. In Nicholas JA, Hershman EB editors: *The lower extremity and spine in sports medicine,* St Louis, 1995, Mosby.
4. American Academy of Orthopaedic Surgeons: *Symposium on osteoarthritis,* St Louis, 1976, Mosby.
5. Amiel D, Akeson D, Harwood FL et al: The effect of immobilization on the types of collagen synthesized in periarticular connective tissue, *Connect Tissue Res* 8:27, 1980.
6. Anderson CE: The structure and function of cartilage, *J Bone Joint Surg* 44A:777, 1962.
7. Arondheim JC: *Case studies in geriatrics for the house officer,* Baltimore, 1990, Williams & Wilkins.
8. Backhouse KM, Hutchins RT: *Color atlas of surface anatomy: clinical and applied,* Baltimore, 1986, Williams & Wilkins.
9. Baxter DE: The foot in running. In Mann RA, editor: *Surgery of the foot,* St Louis, 1986, Mosby.
10. Benninghoff A: Form and Bau der Gelenkknorpel in ihren Beziehungen zur Funktion, *Z Anat Entwicklungsgesh* 76:43, 1925.
11. Biology of connective tissue and the joints, *JAMA* 224(supl 5):669, 1973.
12. Bopp HM: *Orthop Praxis* 10:261, 1971.
13. Botte RR: An interpretation of the pronation syndrome and foot types of patient with low back pain, *J Am Podiatry Assoc* 71:243-253, 1981.
14. Calliet R: *Soft tissue pain and disability,* Philadelphia, 1977, FA Davis.
15. Cavanagh PR, Lafortune MA: Ground reaction forces in distance running, *J Biomechanics,* 13:397, 1980.
16. Chapchal G: *Untersuchung des Bewegungssystems Handbuch der Orthopadie,* vol I, Stuttgart, 1957, Thieme.
17. Chrisman OD: Biochemical aspect of degenerative joint disease, *Clin Orthop* 64:77, 1969.
18. Cormack DH: *Introduction to histology,* Philadelphia, 1984, JB Lippincott.

19. Cyriax J: Diagnosis of soft tissue lesions. In Cyriax J, editor: *Textbook of orthopaedic medicine,* vol 1, London, 1978, Balliere Tindall.

20. Dandy DJ: *Essential orthopaedics and trauma,* Edinburgh, 1989, Churchill Livingstone.

21. deAndrae JR, et al: Joint distension and reflex muscle inhibition in the knee, *J Bone Joint Surg* 47A:313, 1965.

22. Delateur BJ, Lehmann J, Stonebridge J: Isotonic versus isometric exercise: a double shift transfer of training study, *Arch Phys Med Rehabil* 53:212, 1973.

23. DiStefano VJ: Skeletal injuries of the knee. In Nicholas JA, Hershmann EB editors: *The lower extremity and spine in sports medicine,* St Louis, 1995, Mosby.

24. *Dorland's Illustrated Medical Dictionary,* ed 27, Philadelphia, 1988, WB Saunders.

25. Dowson D: Lubrication and wear of joints, *Physiotherapy* 59(4):104, 1973.

26. Dowson D, Wright V, Longfield MD: Human joint lubrication, *Bio-Medical Engineering* 4:160, 1969.

27. Edelstein JE: *Lower-Limb orthotics* New York University Medical Center, 1986.

28. Eftekhar NS: *Total hip arthroplasty,* St Louis, 1993, Mosby.

29. Eichelberger L, Akeson WH, Roma M: Biochemical studies of articular cartilage. I. Normal values, *J Bone Joint Surg* 40A:142, 1958.

30. Eichler J: Methodological efforts in documenting leg length and leg length discrepancies. In Hungerford DS editor: *Leg length discrepancy: the injured knee,* Berlin, 1977, Springer Verlag.

31. Encyclopaedia Britannica ultimate CD 99 edition.

32. Friberg O: Clinical symptoms and biomechanics of lumbar spine and hip joint in leg length inequality, *Spine* 8:643-651, 1983.

33. Gerber LH, Hicks JE: Exercise in the rheumatic diseases. In Basmajian JV, Wolf SL editors: *Therapeutic exercise,* Baltimore, 1990, Williams & Wilkins.

34. Giles LG: The pathophysiology of the zygapophyseal joints. In Haldeman S, editor: *Principles and practice of chiropractic,* ed 2, East Norwalk, Conn., 1992, Appleton & Lange.

35. Gilmet T, Masse JP, Ryckewaert A: Etude radiologique des genoux indolores de 50 femmes de plus de 65 ans, *Revue du Rhumatisme* 46:589-592, 1979.

36. Gofton JP, Trueman GE: Studies in osteoarthritis of the hip: II osteoarthritis of the hip and leg length disparity, *Can Med Assoc J* 104:791-799, 1971.

37. Gofton JP, Trueman GE: Studies in osteoarthritis of the hip: IV. Biomechanics and clinical considerations, *Can Med Assoc J* 104:1007-1011, 1971.

38. Gofton JP: Persistent low back pain and leg length disparity, *J Rheumatol* 12:747-750, 1985.

39. Golland A: Basic hydrotherapy, *Physiotherapy* 67:258, 1981.

40. Gould JA: *Orthopaedic and sports physical therapy,* ed 2, St Louis, 1990, Mosby.

41. Gray H: *Anatomy: descriptive and surgical,* ed 15, New York, 1977, Bounty Books.

42. Greenfield BH: *Rehabilitation of the knee: a problem-solving approach,* Philadelphia, 1993, FA Davis.

43. Greenman PE: *Principles of manual medicine,* Baltimore, 1989, Williams & Wilkins.

44. Haralson K: Physical modalities. In Banwell BF, Gall V editors: *Physical therapy management of arthritis,* New York, 1987, Churchill Livingstone.

45. Harding ML: A fresh appraisal of tibial osteotomy for osteoarthritis of the knee, *Clin Orthop* 114:223, 1976.

46. Henry JH: The patellofemoral joint. In Nicholas JA, Hershman EB editors: *The lower extremity and spine in sports medicine,* St Louis, 1995, Mosby.

47. Hertling D, Kessler RM: *Management of common musculoskeletal disorders,* ed 2, Philadelphia, 1990, JB Lippincott.

48. Hirsch C: The pathogenesis of chondromalacia of the patella, *Acta Chir Scand* 90(suppl 83):9, 1944.

49. Hoffa A: The influence of the adipose tissue with regard to the pathology of the knee joint, *JAMA* 43:795, 1904.

50. Hoppenfeld S: *Physical examination of the spine and extremities,* Norwalk, Conn., 1976, Appleton-Century-Crofts.

51. Hughston JC, Walsh WM, Puddu G: *Patellar subluxation and dislocation: Saunders monographs in clinical orthopaedics,* Philadelphia, 1984, WB Saunders.

52. Hungerford DS: *Leg length discrepancy: the injured knee,* Berlin, 1977, Springer-Verlag.

53. Inglemark BE, Lindstrom J: *Acta Morph Scand* 5:221, 1963.

54. James SL, Bates BT, Osterling RL: Injuries to runners, *Am J Sports Med* 6:40, 1978.

55. Johnston R: Mechanical consideration of the hip joint, *Arch Surg* 107:411, 1973.

56. Jorring K: Osteoarthritis of the hip, *Acta Orthop Scand* 51:523, 1980.

57. Kellegren J: Osteoarthritis in patients and populations, *Br Med J* 2:1, 1961.

58. Kettelkamp DB, Hillberry BM, Murrish DE et al: Degenerative arthritis of the knee secondary to fracture malunion, *Clin Orthop* 234:159, 1988.

59. King L: Case study: physical therapy management of hip osteoarthritis prior to total hip arthroplasty, *J Orthop Sports Phys Ther* 26(1):35-38, 1997.

60. Kulund DN: The injured athlete's pain, *Curr Concepts Pain* 1:3, 1983.

61. Lillegard WA, Rucker H: *Handbook of sports medicine: a symptom-oriented approach,* Boston, 1993, Andover Medical Publishers.

62. Lloyd-Roberts G: Osteoarthritis of the hip, *J Bone Joint Surg* 37B:8, 1955.

63. Lynch MA, Henning CE: Physical examination of the knee joint. In Nicholas JA, Hershman EB editors: *The lower extremity and spine in sports medicine,* St Louis, 1995, Mosby.

64. Magee DJ: *Orthopedic physical assessment,* Philadelphia, 1987, WB Saunders.

65. Mankin HJ, Radin E: Structure and function of joints. In McCarty DJ editor: *Arthritis and allied conditions,* Philadelphia, 1979, Lea & Febiger.

66. Mankin HJ: The reaction of articular cartilage or injury and to osteoarthritis, Part I. *N Engl J Med* 291:1285, 1974.

67. Mankin HJ, Thrasher AZ: Water content and binding in normal and osteoarthritic human cartilage, *J Bone Joint Surg* 57A:76, 1975.

68. Mannheimer C, Lund S, Carlsson CA: The effect of transcutaneous electrical nerve stimulation of joint pain in patients with rheumatoid arthritis, *Scand J Rheumatol* 7:13, 1978.

69. Maquet P: Biomechanics and osteoarthritis of the knee, *J Bone Joint Surg* 61B:252, 1979.

70. Maquet P: *Biomechanics of the knee with application to the pathogenesis and the surgical treatment of osteoarthritis,* Berlin, 1976, Springer-Verlag.

71. Maquet PGJ: *Biomechanics of the knee: with application to the pathogenesis and the surgical treatment of osteoarthritis,* ed 2, New York, 1984, Springer-Verlag.

72. Marsk A: *Acta Orthop Scand* suppl 31, 1958.

73. Merchant AC: Hip abductor muscle force, *J Bone Joint Surg* 47A:462, 1965.

74. Michlovitz SL: The use of heat and cold in the management of rheumatic diseases. In Michlovitz SL editor: *Thermal agents in rehabilitation,* Philadelphia, 1990, FA Davis.

75. Morrison JB: Bioengineering analysis of force actions transmitted by the knee joint, *Biomedical Engineering* 3:164, 1960.

76. Morrissey MC: Reflex inhibition of thigh muscles in knee injury: causes and treatment, *Sports Med* 7:263, 1989.

77. Morscher E: Etiology and pathophysiology of leg length discrepancies, *Prog Orthop Surg* 1:9-19, 1977.

78. Moseley CF: Leg length discrepancy, *Orthop Clin North Am* 18(4), 1987.

79. Mow VC, Fithian DC, Kelly MA: Fundamentals of articular cartilage in meniscus biomechanics. In Ewing JW editor: *Articular cartilage and knee joint function: basic science and arthroscopy,* New York, 1990, Raven Press.

80. Mow VC, Mansour JM, Redler I: The movement of interstitial fluid through normal and pathological cartilage during articulation. In Brighton JA, Goldman S editors:

81. Namey TC: Adaptive bicycling, *Rheum Dis Clin North Am* 16:4, 1990.

82. Netter FH: *The Ciba collection of medical illustrations,* vol 8, Part 1, Musculoskeletal system: anatomy, physiology, and metabolic disorders, Summit, N.J., 1991, CIBA-GEIGY.

83. Netter FH: *The Ciba collection of medical illustrations,* vol 8, Part II, Musculoskeletal system: developmental disorders, tumors, rheumatic diseases, and joint replacement, Summit, N.J., 1990, CIBA-GEIGY.

84. Outfoxing pathways of pain, *US News and World Report* Dec. 14, 1998.

85. Panush RS, Brown DG: Exercise in arthritis, *Sports Med* 4:54, 1987.

86. Pitman MI, Frankel VH: Biomechanics of the knee in athletes. In Nicholas JA, Hershman EB editors: *The lower extremity and spine in sports medicine,* St Louis, 1995, Mosby.

87. Pond MJ: Normal joint tissues and their reaction to injury, *Bet Clin North Am I* 3:523, 1971.

88. Radin EL, Paul IL: Does cartilage compliance reduce skeletal impact loads? The relative force-attenuating properties of articular cartilage, synovial fluid, periarticular soft tissues and bone, *Semin Arthritis Rheum* 13(2):139, 1970.

89. Radin EL, Orr RB, Kelman JL et al: Effect of prolonged walking on concrete on the joints of sheep: ARA abstracts, *Arthritis Rheum* 22:649, 1980.

90. Radin EL, Paul IL, Lowry M: A comparison of the dynamic force-transmitting properties of subchondral bone and articular cartilage, *J Bone Joint Surg* 52A:444, 1970.

91. Radin EL, Paul IL: Response of joints to impact loading, *Arthritis Rheum* 14:356, 1971.

92. Radin EL, Rose RM: Role of subchondral bone in initiation and progress of cartilage damage, *Clin Orthop* 213:34, 1986.

93. Radin EL: The physiology and degeneration of joints, *Semin Arthritis Rheum* 2(3):245, 1972-1973.

94. Rosenberg TD, Paulos LE, Parker RD et al: The forth-five degree posteroanterior flexion weight-bearing radiograph of the knee, *J Bone Joint Surg* 70A:1479, 1988.

95. Rothernberg RJ: Rheumatic disease aspects of leg length inequality, *Semin Arthritis Rheum,* 17:196-205, 1988.

96. Rush WA, Steiner HA: *AJR* 56:616, 1946.

97. Rydell N: Biomechanics of the hip joint, *Clin Orthop* 92:6, 1973.

98. Salter RB, Simmonds DF, Malcolm BW et al: The biological effect of continuous passive motion on the healing of full-thickness defects in articular cartilage, *J Bone Joint Surg* 62A:1232, 1980.

99. Salter RB: *Textbook of disorders and injuries of the musculoskeletal system,* ed 2, Baltimore, 1983, Williams & Wilkins.

100. Sasaki T, Yasuda K: Clinical evaluation of the treatment of osteoarthritic knees using a newly designed wedged insole, *Clin Orthop* 221:181, 1987.

101. Schmid FR, Ogata RA: The composition and examination of synovial fluid, *J Prosthet Dent* 18(5):449, 1967.

102. Semble EL, Loeser RF, Wise CM: Therapeutic exercise for rheumatoid arthritis and osteoarthritis, *Semin Arthritis Rheum* 20:32-40, 1990.

103. Simkin PA: Synovial physiology. In McCarty DJ editor: *Arthritis and allied conditions,* Philadelphia, 1979, Lea & Febiger.

104. Sledge CB: Structure, development and function of joints, *Orthop Clin North Am* 6(3):619, 1975.

105. Sokoloff L: Pathology and pathogenesis of osteoarthritis. In McCarty DJ editor: *Arthritis and allied conditions,* Philadelphia, 1979, Lea & Febiger.

106. Staheli LT: *Fundamental of pediatric orthopedics,* New York, 1992, Raven Press.

107. Steindler A: Biology of functional restoration, *Clin Orthop* 177:4, 1983.

108. Stravino VD: The synovial system, *Am J Phys Med* 51(6):312, 1972.

109. Tetsworth K, Paley D: Malalignment and degenerative arthropathy, *Orthop Clin North Am* 25(3), 1994.

110. Tria AJ, Klein KS: *An illustrated guide to the knee,* New York, 1992, Churchill Livingstone.

111. Turek SL: *Orthopaedics: principles and their application,* Philadelphia, 1977, JB Lippincott.

112. Utsinger PD, Bonner F, Hogan N: Efficacy of cryotherapy and thermotherapy in the management of rheumatoid arthritis pain: evidence for endorphin effect (abstr), *Arthritis Rheum* 25(suppl):113, 1982.

113. Vane J: Inhibition of prostaglandin synthesis as a mechanism of action of aspirin-like drugs, *Nature New Biol* 231:232, 1971.

114. Van Eijden TMGJ, de Borr W, Verburg J: A dynamometer for the measurement of the extension torque of the lower leg during static and dynamic contractions of the quadriceps femoris muscle, *J Biomech* 16:1019, 1983.

115. Vingard E, Alfredsson L, Goldie I et al: Occupation and osteoarthrosis of the hip and knee: a register-based cohort study, *Int J Epidemiol* 20(4):1025, 1991.

116. Voloshin A, Wosk J: Influence of artificial shock absorbers of human gait, *Clin Orthop* 160:52, 1981.

117. Walker H, Schreck R: Relationship of hyperextended gait pattern to chondromalacia patellae, *Phys Ther* 55:259-262, 1975.

118. Walmsley T: The articular mechanism of the diarthroses, *J Bone Joint Surg* 10A:40, 1928.

119. Ward DJ, Tidswell ME: Osteoarthritis. In Downie PA editor: *Cash's textbook of orthopaedics and rheumatology for physiotherapists,* London, 1984, Faber & Faber.

120. Waugh W, Newton G: Articular changes associated with flexion deformity in rheumatoid and osteoarthritic knees, *J Bone Joint Surg* 62B:180, 1980.

121. Wickersham BA: The exercise program. In Riggs GK, Gall EP editors: *Rheumatic diseases: rehabilitation and management,* Boston, 1984, Butterworth.

122. Wright V, Dowson D, Kerr J: The structure of joints, *Int Rev Connect Tissue Res* 61:105, 1973.

123. Wright V, Dowson D, Seller PC: Bio-engineering aspect of synovial fluid and cartilage, *Mod Trends Rheumatol* 2:21, 1971.

124. Yasuda K, Sasaki T: The mechanics of treatment of the osteoarthritic knee with a wedged insole, *Clin Orthop* 215:162, 1987.

125. Zebrowski E: *Physics for technicians,* New York, 1974, McGraw-Hill.

RECOMMENDED READING

Mankin HJ, Radin E: Structure and function of joints. In McCarty DJ editor: *Arthritis and allied conditions,* Philadelphia, 1979, Lea & Febiger.

Moseley CF: Leg length discrepancy, *Orthop Clin North Am* 18(4), 1987.

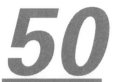

50

Quadriceps Contusion After a Swimming Pool Diving Injury Resulting in Palpable Lump, Restricted Knee Range, Progressively Increasing Daytime Pain Upon Activity

A 16-year-old male lifeguard is referred to your clinic by his physician for treatment of a "right deep quadriceps contusion." The patient reports diving off the side of a swimming pool 3 weeks ago during a successful lifesaving attempt. As he entered the water he accidentally struck his anterior right thigh against a swimmer beneath him. He subsequently developed a small contusion over his mid anterior right thigh but nevertheless continued his work and even swam during the remainder of that afternoon. He admits to passing off the injury "as nothing" and continued to adhere to his work routine, although he initially had some difficulty bending his knee and walked with a slight limp. Approximately 6 or 7 days later, instead of resolving, the pain and swelling increased, particularly during activity. During the second week postinjury his pain was increasingly present during stair descent. Although walking was painless, running provoked a sharp pain in the right anterior thigh. The patient does not report pain at night. There is no history of any previous related injury, nor could the patient remember any history of joint pain, muscular ache, sickness, or fatigue. He takes no medications.

OBSERVATION   There are no signs of redness or streaking around the mass. The ipsilateral midquadriceps region appears approximately one-quarter larger in girth than the uninvolved thigh. Effusion appears to extend distally to include the right knee joint.

PALPATION   This demonstrates a well circumscribed fixed mass approximately 5 × 10 cm in the right mid quadriceps that elicits pain upon direct palpation.

RANGE OF MOTION   The right hip was decreased by one-quarter hip flexion and extension, and one-third right knee flexion and extension.

STRENGTH   Testing yields a grade of a least good minus to the right quadriceps muscle group; note that grading may have been obscured by patient pain during manual muscle testing.

SELECTIVE TENSION   Pain with isometric and resistive left knee extension; symptoms are reproduced with resistive right knee flexion. Resistive right hip flexion and extension are mildly painful at the extremes of range.

FLEXIBILITY TESTING   Bilateral straight leg raise measures at 70°; otherwise normal.

SPECIAL TESTS   Positive right femoral nerve stretch maneuver.

SENSORY TESTING   Intact to light touch and pinprick throughout bilateral lower extremities.

CLUE

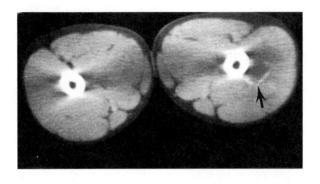

(From Nicholas JA, Hershman EB editors: *The lower extremity and spine in sports medicine,* ed 2, St Louis, 1995, Mosby.)

? Questions

1. The therapist should communicate with the referring physician and suggest the possibility of investigating any possible pathology?
2. What is myositis ossificans?
3. What anatomic sites are most likely candidates for the development of this condition?
4. What two traumatic injuries to the cubital area predispose for the development of myositis ossificans?
5. What is the clinical presentation?
6. What is the classification of quadriceps contusion?
7. How may acute treatment of soft-tissue injury minimize magnitude of reactive calcification?
8. What management regimen is appropriate during the acute and subacute stage of muscle injury?
9. What are the radiographic features of myositis ossificans?
10. What is the differential diagnosis for this condition?
11. What is the prognosis of this condition?
12. What is the rationale for use of acetic acid iontophoresis as a treatment strategy in the reduction of the developing calcific mass?
13. Why is direct injection not an appropriate vehicle for introduction of acetic acid?
14. What therapeutic strategy may result in a quicker, safer return to activity while precluding surgery?

1. The therapist should communicate with the referring physician and suggest the possibility of investigating any possible pathology?

Myositis ossificans of the right anterolateral thigh following traumatic contusion to the quadriceps muscle group. The Clue shows a computed tomography scan of myositis ossificans developing in the right quadriceps.

An area of higher density signifies calcification is present deep with the quadriceps muscle *(arrow).*

2. What is myositis ossificans?

Posttraumatic *myositis ossificans* or *myositis ossificans traumatica* is a nonneoplastic reactive calcification with subsequent ossification of soft tissue following recurrent injuries or blunt trauma such as direct trauma resulting in massive contusion; it is not seen with a strain injury.[39] The incidence of myositis ossificans following a contusion ranges between 9% to 20%.[13,27,30,32] Inadequate management following a deep intramuscular hematoma may be contributory to this disorder. The disorder commonly occurs in muscles in the region of the thigh[28] and elbow of children and young adults. A rapidly enlarging painful and tender mass, which is part hematoma and usually connected to the underlying femur,[13,27,30,32] undergoes heterotopic bone formation (calcification and ossification). Calcification appears some 2 to 3 weeks postinjury whereas ossification develops approximately 4 to 8 weeks following trauma, and is often, but not always, related to disrupted healing owing to repeated impact or contraction in the absence of rest. As the acute symptoms subside, a painless mass remains, and corresponding adjacent hip motion may be lost as a result of restricted muscle function. The resultant mass may enlarge or become symptomatic for several months before stabilizing. Myositis ossificans appears to be a self-limiting disease as spontaneous resolution after maturation occurs in many cases.[38]

Myositis ossificans may also occur following joint dislocation, or as exuberant callus following fracture. Involvement of small joints is uncommon.[21] A significant number of patients undergoing acetabular open reduction and internal fixation (ORIF)[20] and total hip arthroplasty[4,6,29] develop heterotopic ossification. Neurogenic causes of heterotopic bone formation include spinal cord injury (in which the lesion develops below the level of lesion)[28] and closed head injury.[33]

A high index of suspicion is applied to any injury that may develop into heterotopic bone deposition. This unfortunate possibility is staved off by the immediate protection of the injured area from further movement, followed by ice, elevation, compression, and graduated exercises to rapidly regain continuous function and motion.

3. What anatomic sites are most likely candidates for the development of this condition?

Heterotopia refers to tissue formation in a place where its presence is abnormal. Heterotopic ossification associated with myositis ossificans develops between rather than within strained muscle fibers. The most common sites of incidence include the anterior thigh, the anterior arm, and buttocks. Drug abuser's elbow refers to myositis ossificans following injury to the bra-

chialis muscle[12] following inept needle manipulation by the addict. In the lower extremity, the most commonly affected site is the quadriceps muscle[12,14]; in soccer, the lateral hamstring is often involved. This is because these two muscle groups are the most frequently contused.

4. What two traumatic injuries to the cubital area predispose for the development of myositis ossificans?

Two forms of elbow injury that result in displacement of bony parts and concomitant contusion to the distal brachialis muscle belly include supracondylar elbow fractures and posterior dislocation of the ulna on the humerus. Fractures and dislocation of the elbow occur most commonly in children; they result in contusion of the adjacent distal brachialis muscle as the belly of that muscle overlies and is in close contact with the distal end of the humerus. Myositis ossificans may be the eventual consequence of *brachialis contusion,* and usually results in permanent restriction of elbow motion; extension is restricted more than flexion.[11]

5. What is the clinical presentation?

A history of severe thigh contusion should alert the clinician to the possibility of myositis development. Diagnosis is pronounced based on clinical presentation and confirmed by radiologic films and sometimes laboratory studies. Laboratory studies include a transient depression in serum calcium that may occur before an acute rise in the serum alkaline phosphatase level, which occurs at approximately 2 weeks postinjury.[3,26] This relates to why development of heterotopic bone formation begins approximately 2 weeks after insult.[28] Signs and symptoms include pain and swelling that subside following the acute stage and a focal site of acute inflammation sets in. Palpation yields a tender, firm, and hot mass within the involved muscle accompanied by considerable loss of range of motion of the related joint(s). Following the acute stage, the mass is still palpable but painless, although adjacent hip and knee motion may be lost as a result of restricted muscle function.[39] Fortunately for the diver, this condition becomes suspect before significant loss of range of motion. As time progresses, inhibition of quadriceps mobility with continued loss of leg function may result. Identified risk factors for the development of myositis ossificans following a quadriceps contusion include a decrease in knee joint motion by

120°, a history of traumatic injury following a football tackle or other kind of injury, a history of previous quadriceps injury, delayed initial treatment for more than 3 days, and development of ipsilateral knee joint effusion.[32]

6. What is the classification of quadriceps contusion?

A contusion is a common athletic injury[8] and is most frequently caused in American football by a direct blow by a knee to the thigh muscles.[30,31] (See the discussion of compression ruptures ["charley horse"] on page 284 in Chapter 25.) Quadriceps contusions are classified according to the amount of available knee range of motion between 12 and 24 hours following injury.[32] Mild *contusions* have greater than 90° of available range of knee motion, *moderate contusions* have 45° to 90° of knee range of motion, whereas *severe contusions* demonstrate less than 45° of knee range of motion.[19]

7. How may acute treatment of soft-tissue injury minimize magnitude of reactive calcification?

Acute injury of soft tissue such as muscle may quickly escalate into a deleterious cycle in which the healing process is adversely effected. Following soft-tissue injury, resultant bleeding occurs and rapidly spreads into adjacent soft tissue, which becomes tense and tender owing to increased pressure. This increased pressure causes pain in sensitive tissue and causes impaired healing owing to vascular congestion that prevents removal of debris and anabolic healing. Because of this, the initial acute management of a muscular or soft-tissue injury can be the most importing factor influencing recovery. Because of this, treatment should be *immediately* initiated. After bleeding has been controlled, the remaining extravascular blood collected at the injury site is gradually removed mainly by the lymphatics. Scar tissue then forms in that area and constitutes a potentially weak point in the injured muscle, tendon, or ligament. The application of heat, continuous ultrasound, massage, stretching, and exercise should be avoided initially so as not to induce further bleeding in this area.[23] If too early or too heavy a load is applied to this scarred tissue, injury is liable to occur, or, as in the case of muscle, ossification may manifest or expand its perimeter. Sometimes, however, despite the best and earliest intervention, calcification may still occur, albeit to a smaller magnitude than had early intervention not occurred.

8. What management regimen is appropriate during the acute and subacute stage of muscle injury?

Generally, the lighter the bleeding, the faster the effusion of blood disappears and the less scar tissue forming in the injured tissue. Thus immediate treatment at the scene of injury mandates reduction in the magnitude of bleeding by way of application of rapid cooling, compression bandaging, elevation of the injured limb, and rest. However, patients with extensive injury, particularly to the quadriceps mechanism, may need to be admitted to the hospital to rule out the possibility of compartment syndrome.

Management of quadriceps contusion follows a three-phase rehabilitation protocol.[32] Phase I is characterized by the acute stage in which the primary goal of management is to reduce hemorrhage.

PHASE I—ACUTE STAGE

Cryotherapy provides a local pain-relieving effect that causes contraction of blood vessels thereby reducing blood flow and minimizing hypoxic injury from edematous swelling[18] to the injured area and allowing healing to proceed more rapidly. For cooling to be effective, it must be applied long enough to penetrate deep into the injured tissue. Generally, the larger the injured muscle or joint, the longer should cooling continue. A cold modality should not be used directly on an open wound, nor should it be placed directly on the skin. Cryotherapy may be applied to a thigh muscle for up to 45 minutes.

During or in conjunction with cooling, a compression bandage should be applied to the injured area. Cooling and compression may be achieved simultaneously by positioning an ice pack with the help of an elastic bandage. A compression bandage often consists of an elastic bandage applied with some degree of tension. Compression provides counter pressure to bleeding that allows the body's hemostatic function to take effect. Compression bandaging is replaced by support bandaging after a few hours when the desired outcome has been achieved. (Although cryotherapy has a delayed response in decreasing blood flow and is therefore less effective at reducing hemorrhage,[37] compression has the advantage of instantaneously reducing blood flow and minimizing hemorrhage and should be applied immediately.[36])

Elevation of the injured limb reduces swelling by reducing blood flow and allowing for expelled blood to be transported away more easily. With the patient lying supine, the injured thigh should be elevated at an angle of at least 45° to the horizontal, and as long as 24 to 48 hours in the case of extensive bleeding. The injured thigh should not be subject to loading and the athlete must obey a mandatory rest period for 24 to 48 hours. Crutches may be used if walking is necessary so as to unload the injured lower limb as per patient tolerance.[19]

The use of heat therapy or massage is contraindicated during the acute stage on injury as this modality facilitates expansion of the blood vessels and potential interference of blood clotting. In addition, the amount of fluid in the tissue increases and leads to swelling and higher pressure in the surrounding tissues. This may result in increased pain and slowed healing. Thus the use of heat or massage should not be started until 48 hours, at the very earliest, following injury.

PHASE II—SUBACUTE STAGE

Phase II management may begin when pain has subsided with rest. The purpose of this second phase of management is to restore pain-free range of motion. The importance of preserving knee range of motion early on following injury cannot be overemphasized; this may be facilitated by the use of a knee flexion brace.[2]

Stretching exercises are initiated as soon as possible to prevent contracture in the involved muscle group.[40] For example, an anterolateral hematoma is managed by stretching of the quadriceps and the iliotibial band. Careful static (isometric) quadriceps muscle contractions and active contractions by way of active knee flexion exercises, and low-resistance stationary cycling may be initiated. This may be accompanied by contrast baths and gentle massage to the surrounding muscle. Progressive resistance exercises are begun for the involved muscle group as soon as symptoms permit and include rehabilitation of the entire extremity. Athletic involvement before resolution may maximize intermittent problems such as decreased range of motion, muscle spasm, or disuse atrophy.

PHASE III

The purpose of the last phase of management is sport-specific rehabilitation with exercises to restore strength and function. Return to athletic activities may be permitted only after full strength, motion, and coordination have returned. The criteria for full strength at this stage refer to pain-free resisted motion throughout the quadriceps range of motion. When contact is anticipated in sport, the athlete must wear protective padding in the area of the previous contusion to minimize further insult.[35]

9. What are the radiographic features of myositis ossificans?

It is essential to take radiographs early so as to avoid confusion with a juxtacortical osteogenic sarcoma. At a later date the athlete may not recollect a specific traumatic event several weeks earlier and may cause increasing concern to caregivers had radiographic documentation been done initially following injury. Radiographic changes associated with myositis ossificans parallel a definable histopathologic evolution (Fig. 50-1).[25] Shortly after injury, a soft-tissue mass may be visibly detected whereas faint calcification may be seen as early as the third or fourth week. At 6 to 8 weeks following injury, a sharply circumscribed cortical periphery forms around a central lacy pattern of new bone. This pattern of subtle circumferential ossification in the relatively early stages of this condition can be diagnostic. A radiolucent thin cleft separates the juxtacortical lesion from the adjacent bone. It may not be visible on plain films although special tangential views may show the lesion; because of this, computed tomography is advocated.[22] The ossified lesion may develop cysts that may enlarge and coalesce into an eggshell cyst.[25] Maturity is reached anywhere between 6 to 18 months, and the ossified mass may regress in size as remodeling commences. The mature lesion is characterized by a mature contoured appearance of the outer surface of bone commensurate with surrounding muscle activity and a mature trabecular pattern of bone within the lesion. The mass typically disappears within a year, although a residual exostosis with an attachment to bone may remain.[7]

10. What is the differential diagnosis for this condition?

The differential diagnosis of myositis ossificans includes infection, deep venous thrombosis, and tumor[10] as well as:

- *Periosteal osteogenic sarcoma.* This is a malignant bone tumor and has a predilection for patients above thirty years of age. Myositis ossificans may be confused with malignant bone tumor if one is not aware

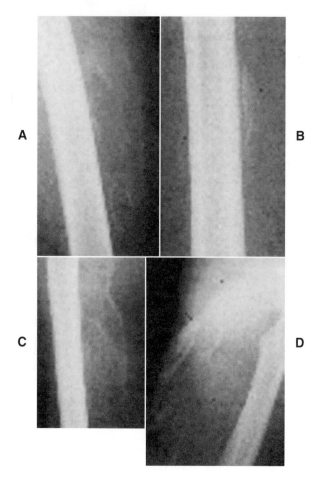

FIG. 50-1 Examples of myositis ossificans. **A,** The typical early (2½ weeks) roentgenographic appearance. **B,** A more broad-based variety. **C,** Massive involvement of the hamstring area. **D,** The same case as C after maturity. These injuries can occasionally be confused with malignant bone lesions, but in contrast to tumors, there is no involvement of the adjacent bone. (From Mercier LR: *Practical orthopedics*, ed 5, St Louis, 2000, Mosby.)

sents the reverse radiologic appearance. In addition, histopathologic tissue examination may also differentiate these two conditions. Although alkaline phosphatase levels are elevated with sarcoma, histologic examination may be required for differentiation. Although myositis ossificans contains abnormal cells within the depth of the lesion and mature, well developed cells at the periphery of the lesion, osteogenic sarcoma demonstrates abnormal cells on the periphery of the mass. Careful attention to these findings underscores the need for initial radiographs in the suspected myositis ossificans and prevents unnecessary initiation of cancer therapies or amputation.[15]

- *Soft tissue sarcoma.* Myositis ossificans is classified as extraosseous pseudomalignant metaplasia of muscle, and may very easily be mistaken during its active stage for a *soft tissue sarcoma* (extraosseous sarcoma), which is a malignant neoplasm. The incidence of soft tissue sarcoma equals that of malignant bone tumor, although diagnosis is more difficult as they are not well visualized on radiographs. Because of this, a presentation of a firm, and deeply palpable tumor on the anterior proximal thigh may be passed off and managed as a hematoma, thrombophlebitis, cyst, or abscess. However, the tumor may be viewed with computerized tomography and confirmed following biopsy by histologic examination.[24]

11. What is the prognosis of this condition?

Full maturity of the osseous lesion is reached by 5 to 6 months, but may take up to 2 years to resolve. Early surgical removal of the ossified mass is often a debilitating option as it compromises the integrity of the muscle as a working unit, serves to tear more muscle fibers, may aggravate the entire process, and stimulate an even more voluminous reaction. Thus early surgery is best avoided because it may exacerbate heterotopic bone formation and prolong disability.

The natural history of myositis ossificans is related to lesion location. Typically, if myositis ossificans is located within a large muscle mass, such as the quadriceps muscle, it becomes progressively resorbed and shrinks. However, when the lesion occurs in an area of the body that has limited muscle mass, resorption becomes less likely, in which case the ossified mass may cause continued sensitivity and motion restriction. Regardless of location of the mass, surgical removal ought to be delayed for at least 12 to 18 months so as to allow for maturation of the lesion and resultant disability such as loss of range and muscle contracture is manifest.[15]

of the preceding traumatic injury to the quadriceps muscle. The histologic features of both conditions may be similar, especially if a biopsy is performed early in the course of myositis ossificans.[9] Pain is typically of a constant nature, whereas pain associated with myositis ossificans is related to activity. Clarification of diagnosis is facilitated by radiographs. Myositis ossificans is radiologically characterized by peripheral maturation with distinct margins and a radiolucent center, whereas osteosarcoma pre-

12. What is the rationale for use of acetic acid iontophoresis as a treatment strategy in the reduction of the developing calcific mass?

Iontophoresis is the introduction of topically applied, physiologically active ions through the epidermis using continuous direct current,[38] and is based on the principle that an electrical charge will repel a similarly charged ion.[5] Before complete ossification, myositis ossificans consists of precipitates of calcium carbonate that are not soluble in normal blood pH levels.[16] Presumably, the acetate radical binds with calcium carbonate by displacing the carbonate radical and, in so doing, allows the newly formed calcium acetate to be more soluble and therefore removable.[17]

$$CaCO_3 + 2H(C_2H_3O_2) = Ca(C_2H_3O_2)\,2 + H_2O + CO_2$$

13. Why is direct injection not an appropriate vehicle for introduction of acetic acid?

Because recurrent injury resulting in additional bleeding is often a precursor to formation of myositis ossificans, additional tissue damage with concomitant bleeding may occur by the invasive injection of a syringe and needle.[1]

14. What therapeutic strategy may result in a quicker, safer return to activity while precluding surgery?

Ossification and resolution is typically a lengthy process for which many authorities are reluctant to recommend active treatment for a long period of time in fear of aggravating the process. Nevertheless, therapeutic intervention supplementing a prescription of rest and inactivity includes the following regimen performed prior to complete ossification:

- The use of 3 ml of a 2% acetic acid *iontophoresis* with the negative electrode placed over the site of ossification at a 4 mA direct current for 20 minutes, for a total of 80 mA/minute.
- The above is then followed by 8 minutes of 1.5 W/cm^2 pulsed *ultrasound* at 50% duty cycle to facilitate dispersal of the acetic acid throughout the injury site, and for the purpose of decreasing skin irritation. This is followed by mild passive range of motion within pain-free range for 5 minutes. Avoidance of any painful activity such as stair climbing, squatting, and participation in sports is essential.

Sharp's protocol[34] of iontophoresis, ultrasound, and passive stretching should be administered on alternate days, 3 times per week for 3 weeks. After several treatments the mass may become increasingly compressible. An increase in the painless range of motion may be observed and also radiographic evidence for the decrease in the size of the mass.

RECOMMENDED READING

Antao NA: Myositis of the hip in a professional soccer player, *Am J Sports Med* 16:82-83, 1988

Pittenger DE: Heterotopic ossification, *Orthop Rev* xx(1), January 1991.

Wieder DL: Treatment of traumatic myositis ossificans with acetic acid iontophoresis, *Phys Ther* 72(2), February 1992.

REFERENCES

1. Antao NA: Myositis of the hip in a professional soccer player, *Am J Sports Med* 16:82-83, 1988.
2. Aronen JG, Ove NP, McDevitt ER: Thigh contusions: minimizing the length of time before return to full athletic activities with early immobilization in 120 degrees of knee flexion, *Am J Sports Med* 18:547, 1990.
3. Bolger J: Heterotopic bone formation and alkaline phosphatase, *Arch Phys Med Rehabil* 56:36-39, 1975.
4. Brooker A, Bowerman J, Robinson R et al: Ectopic ossification following total hip replacement: incidence and a method of classification, *J Bone Joint Surg* 55A(8):1629-1632, 1973.
5. Cummings J: Iontophoresis. In Nelson RM, Currier DP editors: *Clinical electrotherapy*, East Norwalk, Conn., 1987, Appleton & Lange.
6. DeLee J, Ferrari A, Charnley J: Ectopic bone formation following low friction arthroplasty of the hip, *Clin Orthop Rel Res* 121:53-59, 1976.
7. Edeiken J: *Roentgen diagnosis of diseases of bone*, ed 3, Baltimore, 1981, Williams & Wilkins.
8. Ekstrand J, Gillquist J: The avoidability of soccer injuries, *Int J Sports Med* 4:124, 1983.
9. Garrett WE Jr: Basic science of musculotendinous injuries. In Nicholas JA, Hershman EB editors: *The lower extremity and spine*, ed 2, vol 1, St Louis, 1995, Mosby.
10. Goldberg M, Schumacher H: Heterotopic ossification mimicking acute arthritis after neurologic catastrophes, *Arch Intern Med* 137:619-621, 1977.
11. Hertling D, Kessler RM: *Management of common musculoskeletal disorders: physical therapy principles and methods*, ed 2, Philadelphia, 1990, JB Lippincott.
12. Huss CD: Myositis ossificans of the upper arm, *Am J Sports Med* 8:419-424, 1980.
13. Jackson DW, Feagin JA: Quadriceps contusion in young athletes, *J Bone Joint Surg* 55A:95, 1973.
14. Jackson DW: Managing myositis ossificans in the young athlete, *Phys Sports Med* 3(10):56, 1975.
15. Jaivin JS, Fox JM: Thigh injuries. In Nicholas JA, Hershman EB editors: *The lower extremity and spine*, ed 2, vol 2, St Louis, 1995, Mosby.
16. Kahn J: Acetic acid iontophoresis for calcium deposits: suggestion from the field, *Phys Ther* 57:658-659, 1977.
17. Kahn J: *Principles and practice of electrotherapy*, New York, 1987, Churchill Livingstone.

18. Knight KL: Cold as a modifier of sports-induced inflammation. In Leadbetter WB, Buckwalter JA, Gordon SL editors: *Sports-induced inflammation,* Park Ridge, Ill., 1990, American Academy of Orthopaedic Surgeons.

19. Magnusson SP, McHugh MP: Current concepts on rehabilitation in sports medicine. In Nicholas JA, Hershman EB editors: *The lower extremity and spine* ed 2, vol 1, St Louis, 1995, Mosby.

20. Mears D, Rubash H: *Ectopic bone formation, in pelvis and acetabular fractures,* Thorofare, N.J., 1986, Slack.

21. Mital J, Garber J, Stinson J: Ectopic bone formation in children and adolescents with head injuries: its management, *J Ped Orthop* 7(1):83-90, 1987.

22. Moss AA, Gamsu G, Gannant HK: *Computed tomography of the body,* Philadelphia, 1983, WB Saunders.

23. Nalley J, Susan Jay M, Durant RH: Myositis ossificans in an adolescent following a sports injury, *J Adolesc Health Care* 6:460-462, 1985.

24. Netter FH: *Developmental disorders, tumours, rheumatic diseases and joint replacement,* vol 8, Part II, 1990, CIBA-GEIGY.

25. Norman A, Dorfman HD: Juxtacortical circumscribed myositis ossificans: evolution and radiographic feature, *Radiology* 96:301, 1970.

26. Orzel J, Rudd T: Heterotopic bone formation: clinical, laboratory and imaging correlation, *J Nucl Med* 26(2):125-132, 1985.

27. Peterson L, Renstrom P: *Sport injuries—their prevention and treatment,* Chicago, 1986, Yearbook Medical Publishing.

28. Pittenger DE: Heterotopic ossification, *Orthop Rev* 20(1):34, 1991.

29. Riegler H, Harris C: Heterotopic bone formation after total hip arthroplasty, *Clin Orthop Rel Res* 117:209-216, 1976.

30. Rothwell A: Quadriceps hematoma: a prospective clinical study, *Clin Orthop* 171:97, 1982.

31. Ryan AJ: Quadriceps strain, rupture, and charlie horse, *Med Sci Sports Exerc* 1:106, 1969.

32. Ryan JB, Wheeler JH, Hopkinson WJ et al: Quadriceps contusions: West Point update, *Am J Sports Med* 19:299, 1991.

33. Sazbon L, Najenson T, Tartakovsky M et al: Widespread periarticular new-bone formation in long-term comatose patients, *J Bone Joint Surg* 63B(1):120-125, 1981.

34. Sharp N: Acetic acid: a solution for some frozen shoulders, *Phoresor Forum* 7(5):1, 1988.

35. Sim FH, Rock MG, Scott SG: Pelvis and hip injuries in athletes: anatomy and function. In Nicholas JA, Hershman EB editors: *The lower extremity and spine,* ed 2, vol 2, St Louis, 1995, Mosby.

36. Thorsson O, Hemdal B, Lilja B et al: The effect of external pressure on intramusculature blood flow at rest and after running, *Med Sci Sports Exerc* 19:469, 1987.

37. Thorsson O: Symposiet: behandling vid akut mjukdelsskadatro och vetenskap, *Lakarsallskapets Riksstamma* 5, 1990.

38. Wieder DL: *Treatment of traumatic myositis ossificans with acetic acid iontophoresis,* vol 72, no. 2, Cleveland, OH, 1992, Ohio Physical Therapy and Sports Medicine.

39. Xethalis JL, Lorei MP: Soccer injuries. In Nicholas JA, Hershman EB editors: *The lower extremity and spine,* ed 2, vol 2, St Louis, 1995, Mosby.

40. Yost JG Jr, Schmoll DW: Basketball injuries. In Nicholas JA, Hershman EB editors: *The lower extremity and spine,* ed 2, vol 2, St Louis, 1995, Mosby.

51

Anterolateral Thigh Paresthesia without Muscle Weakness

A 52-year-old truant officer just spent his summer vacation learning to prepare new culinary dishes of steak and spare rib on the barbecue grill his wife bought him for Father's Day. Following a weight gain of some 10 pounds over the past month he has begun a strengthening and stretching regimen that involves, among others, sit-up exercises. Lately, he reports an annoying and increasingly more obvious tingling of his front thigh corresponding to the area of his front left pants pocket. The sensation is occasionally itchy or even burning in nature. When asked, he admits that the area feels a peculiar numbness at times. There is no history of any precipitating injury although the patient suffered an L5 to S1 disk herniation 7 years ago. This back injury had spontaneously resolved although he occasionally experiences a backache after "overdoing it." He reports that he is a non–insulin-dependent diabetic. The patient offers that he has no trouble with urination. When asked to demonstrate the stretch exercises performed daily, he performs a quadriceps stretch in the supine position with both feet tucked under his buttocks. This position, he claims, exacerbated his symptoms, which are relieved by assuming the sitting position.

HISTORY   The patient underwent a right total hip replacement 5 months ago.

OBSERVATION   There is no postural deviation although the patient appears to exhibit a slight lateral tilting of the right pelvis, some adduction of the left leg during swing, and slightly decreased stance time of the right foot.

PALPATION   Palpation of the paraspinal muscles yields no evidence of muscle spasm, but imparts a sensation of moderate tightness.

RANGE OF MOTION   Range of motion within functional limits and pain free throughout trunk and extremities.

STRENGTH   This is graded good throughout trunk and bilateral upper and lower extremities.

SELECTIVE TENSION   This yields negative results for a resistive testing throughout.

SENSATION   This is decreased to light touch and pinprick over anterolateral skin of left thigh.

DEEP TENDON REFLEXES   This yields a normal (2+) response for the patellar tendon reflex.

SPECIAL TESTS Negative straight and crossed leg raising, and negative Lasègue's test. Positive inverse Lasègue sign. A positive 1-inch left leg length discrepancy is discovered. A rectus femoris stretch in the prone positive acutely provokes symptoms.

CLUE:

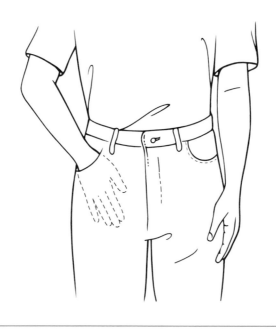

? Questions

1. What is most likely causing this man's symptoms?
2. What is the etiology of meralgia paresthetica (MP)?
3. What cutaneous area does this nerve supply?
4. What is the anatomic course of the lateral cutaneous femoral nerve?

5. What is the clinical presentation?
6. What is the differential diagnosis?
7. What is the course and treatment of this condition?

1. What is most likely causing this man's symptoms?

Meralgia paresthetica (MP) is derived from the terms *meros,* meaning "thigh" and *algo,* meaning "pain."[1] MP refers to lateral femoral cutaneous nerve to the thigh (LCNT) entrapment beneath the inguinal ligament[2] and is identified as the illness afflicting Sigmund Freud who initially ascribed his symptoms to a psychological origin, although his view changed in later years.[4]

2. What is the etiology of meralgia paresthetica (MP)?

The mechanical causes of MP include blunt trauma or penetrating (knife or bullet) wounds to the anterior thigh, or sudden weight loss or gain. Injury to this superficial nerve may occur from seat belt trauma.[2] An example of local trauma in a young male may be a young lady sitting on his lap.[7] MP due to compression or traction of the LCNT may occur, as people of either gender grow older and more obese,[8] especially as the abdomen bulges over the inguinal ligament. Similarly, MP may occur during late pregnancy when the abdomen protrudes or immediately or several weeks after pregnancy when the abdomen suddenly flattens.[7] It may be that the sagging anterior abdominal wall pulls on the nerve. However, patients often cannot offer any predisposing factor. MP may also occur to individuals wearing tight-fitting clothes or corsets. MP may also be a complication of abdominal surgery in which the nerve gets caught up in scar tissue. Diabetes is a risk factor for MP and positive findings in a supposedly nondiabetic indicate the need for blood-sugar analysis.

3. What cutaneous area does this nerve supply?

The entire area supplied by the LCNT is quite large and includes a wrap-around distribution of the anterolateral, and some of the posterolateral skin of the thigh (Fig. 51-1). However, in most instances, the area of sensory loss due to MP is much smaller than this topographic distribution and corresponds to a patch of skin more or less the size and location of the front pocket of a pair of pants[8] (see Clue).

4. What is the anatomic course of the lateral cutaneous femoral nerve?

The LCNT to the thigh derives from L2 and L3 nerve roots in the lumbosacral plexus and emerges from under the lateral margin of psoas major to travel through

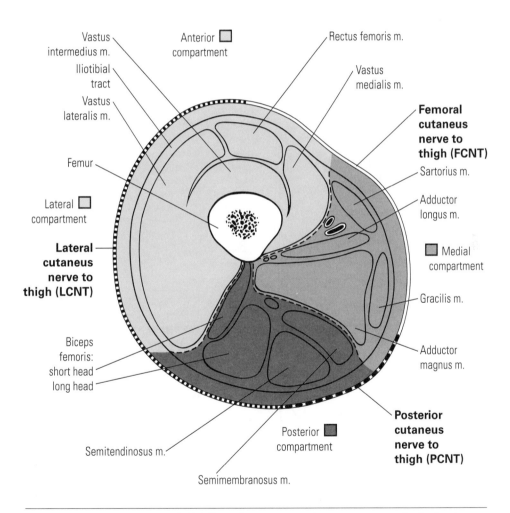

FIG. 51-1 Cross-section of proximal thigh illustrating a wraparound cutaneous sensory distribution. Innervation derives from the lumbar plexus for the lateral and femoral cutaneous nerves, and the cutaneous branch of the obturator nerve all derive from the lumbar plexus. The posterior cutaneous nerve to the thigh, however, derives from the sacral plexus.

the lower pelvic cavity coursing through iliacus fascia. The nerve then takes leave of the pelvis to enter the thigh lateral to the femoral triangle beneath the upper lateral end of the inguinal ligament at an angle of 70° to 90°.[8] The nerve enters the thigh medial to the anterosuperior iliac spine (ASIS) by way of a small hiatus, where it then enters the fascia lata tissue and branches

into anterior and posterior branches 5 inches below the anterior superior spine[5] (Fig. 51-2). The thinner posterior branch runs deep under tensor fasciae latae to innervate the lateral and posterior portions of the thigh from the trochanteric region to the middle thigh. Anomalous passages of this nerve from the pelvis into the thigh do occur and may contribute to the incidence of entrap-

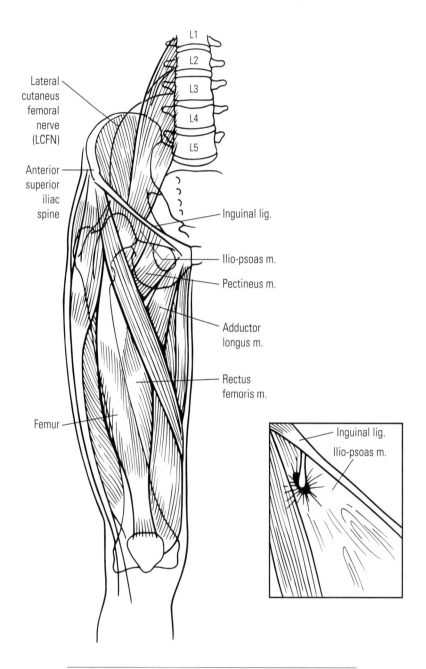

FIG. 51-2 Anatomic course of the lateral cutaneous femoral nerve.

ment. Entrapment of the anterior branch of the LCNT occurs at its binding point, beneath the lateral end of the inguinal ligament, just medial to the ASIS. Beyond this point, the nerve is distally bound by the *fascia lata*, the deep fascia investing the thigh.

5. What is the clinical presentation?

Patients often cannot identify a predisposing factor before onset of symptoms. Symptoms are mild and consist of well-delineated unpleasant and peculiar paresthesias, itching, aches, burning, or numbness over the anterior and anterolateral thigh. The patient may be aggravated by the touch of clothing, leg extension while sleeping, or the avoidance of placing keys in the pocket over the affected thigh.[8] Symptoms may be aggravated by hip extension or walking and are often relieved by the sitting position. Tapping the nerve over the inguinal ligament[3] may reproduce complaints of tenderness compared to the contralateral side, or reproduce symptoms. There may be trophic skin changes and hair loss with long-standing neuropathy. Because the LCNT is entirely sensory, there are no motor symptoms or signs.[3]

Symptoms may be reproduced by placing the LCNT on stretch. Given the knowledge of the nerve's course through the lower trunk and thigh we may modify the prone knee bend to tension test the nerve.[2] If this test is performed in hip extension *(inverse Lasègue's sign)*, more tension is placed along the LCNT because the nerve is anterior to the hip axis of flexion and extension and to the main femoral nerve trunk. This is best accomplished by superimposing hip extension and some measure of hip adduction on the prone knee bend test so as to tether the nerve and stretch it across the inguinal ligament[2] (Fig. 51-3).

Arguably, the location of the nerve's course may subject it to tension by way of truncal shifts. Whereas a posterior pelvic tilt may tauten the nerve along its length, anterior tilting may cause nerve compression as this posture permits the belly to protrude more obviously over the waistline. A lateral pelvic tilt due to leg length discrepancy in which the contralateral leg is shorter may result in adduction of the longer involved leg.[5]

6. What is the differential diagnosis?

Because the LCNT is purely sensory, radiculopathy involving the second, third,[8] and half of the fourth lumbar roots are excluded. Femoral neuropathy is similarly excluded. In addition, the latter two conditions may ex-

press as a weakened knee reflex (L4) and possible quadriceps muscle wasting. High-herniated lumbar disks may produce radiating pain to the upper thigh. However, it is unlikely that disk pathology manifests only along the sensory portion of these nerve roots, thus masquerading as MP. Also, with radiculopathy, provocative signs may prove positive, as may various lumbar movements. Thus if strict anatomic criteria are applied it is not possible to link MP to lumbar radicular lesions. However, an indirect link may be drawn between these two pathologies if we consider that a lumbar spine derangement may result in tightness of the fascia lata, with consequent tethering of the LCNT.

- *Diabetic amyotrophy of Garland.* This affects either the femoral nerve or the three lumbosacral roots (L2, L3, L4) contributing to it. This condition typically occurs in the non–insulin-dependent diabetes mellitus and is more common in males. Symptomatology is characterized by excruciating pain down the front of the thigh that may even radiate down the

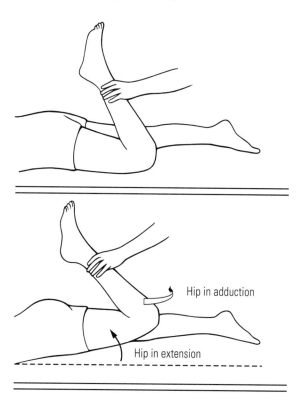

FIG. 51-3 Tension biasing of the LCNT is accomplished by superimposing hip extension and hip adduction on the prone knee bend test. This may provide clinical confirmation of meralgia paresthetica by reproducing symptoms.

medial border of the leg to the medial malleolus. There is often a history of rapid weight loss and general ill-health several weeks before onset. The pain may require narcotic management and abates within several days of initial onset. The disease then results in rapid wasting and weakness of the quadriceps muscle, which makes normal walking impossible. This condition usually self-improves to the point of full recovery over a time period of 18 to 24 months although 6 months may elapse before any recovery begins. Insulin therapy will guarantee that the patient recovers from this disabling condition.[7]

- *Cancer of the prostate. Prostatic adenocarcinoma* is the second most common cancer in men. Occurring in males over 50 years of age, the etiology is unknown but appears to be hormone related. This condition is slowly progressive and may cause no symptoms. Later in the course of the disease the condition is often diagnosed when the man seeks medical attention because of symptoms of urinary obstruction or low back pain. Low back pain or sciatica is caused by metastasis of the cancer to the bones of the pelvis, lumbar spine, or femur.[6]

7. What is the course and treatment of this condition?

MP is not a serious condition and as most patients have mild symptoms, conservative management ought to be followed. A period of paresthesia and pain is often followed by gradual remission of symptoms, and replacement by relatively minor and asymptomatic sensory loss in the nerve's distribution. Sensory loss may persist. Surgical decompression should be avoided because of the subsequent and permanent entrapment of the nerve in scar tissue that may cause the pain to assume a more severe, causalgic quality. Occasionally, nerve blocks or local steroid injections may be of help. Management includes:

- Weight reduction
- Removal of constricting corsets and loosening of tight belts
- Insertion of heel lifts serves to relieve pressure on the nerve by approximating the pelvis to the lower extremity. By way of biomechanical linkage, this serves to ease tension in soft-tissue structures such as the psoas muscle and fascia lata, thus preventing ischemic straddling of the LCNT across the inguinal ligament. The philosophical problem with this management approach is that it does not seek to redress the source of the patient's pathology. Rather, it is intended to supply relief by providing a short-term

solution. Although initially offering relief, the soft tissue supporting the nerve may adaptively foreshorten. Thus the long-term effect may place the LCNT at potentially greater risk for injury across the inguinal ligament.

- By identifying those tightened soft-tissue structures implicated in reproduction of symptoms, the position of detection may now be used as a treatment position to facilitate improved nerve mobility. The premise here is that nerves are not static structures but are rather dynamic and normally move relative to their surrounding tissue during normal kinesiology. Nerve mobilization should occur with gradual introduction of relevant hip and knee movements.[2]
- Stretching of tightened ventral soft tissue such as iliopsoas, the fascia lata, and the abdominal musculature. The tension bias position for the LCNT may be used.
- When a lateral pelvic tilt is present, a heel lift for the contralateral shoe should be tried. This may decrease excessive adduction at the affected hip, which will in turn slacken tension off the nerve and fascia.[5]
- Massage and soft-tissue techniques to gain improved muscle and soft-tissue extensibility.

If conservative management yields no relief, then neurolysis or nerve resection may be performed, as patients prefer hypesthesia to burning pain.[8]

RECOMMENDED READING

Kopell HP: *Peripheral entrapment neuropathies,* Huntington, N.Y., 1976, Robert E Krieger.

Pecina MM, Krmpotic-Nemanic J, Markiewitz AD: *Tunnel syndromes,* Boca Raton, Fla., 1991, CRC Press.

REFERENCES

1. Bernhardt M: Uber isoliert in gebiete des nervus cutaneus femoris externe vorkommende, *Paresthesiea Neurol Centralbl* 14:242, 1895.
2. Butler DS: *Mobilisation of the nervous system,* United Kingdom, 1991, Churchill Livingstone.
3. Dawson DM, Hallett M, Millender LH: *Entrapment neuropathies,* ed 2, Boston/Toronto, 1990, Little, Brown and Company.
4. Freud S: Uber die bernhardt sche sensibilitats-storungam oberschenkel, *Neurol Centralbl* 14:491, 1895.
5. Koppel HP: *Peripheral entrapment neuropathies,* Huntington, N.Y., 1976, Robert E Krieger.
6. *Merck Manual,* ed 15, Rahway, N.J., 1987, Merck, Sharp, and Dohme Research Laboratories.
7. Patten J: *Neurological differential diagnosis,* ed 2, London, 1995, Springer.
8. Pecina MM, Krmpotic-Nemanic J, Markiewitz AD: *Tunnel syndromes,* Boca Raton, Fla., 1991, CRC Press.

52

Miserable Malalignment Syndrome in an Aspiring Ballerina

During the last several months a number of dancers from the local ballet repertory have sought physical therapy for a variety of lower extremity disorders including the hip, knee, and ankle. The director of the ballet company, concerned with the ever increasing rate of injury, sponsored a physical therapy presentation regarding prevention of overuse pathology, with an emphasis on ballet. The board of directors of the company included a pediatrician, orthopaedic surgeon, and school nurse as well as other health professionals. A key focus of the discourse centered on a 15-year-old female student with biomechanical malalignment including femoral anteversion, genu valgum, and pronation of the feet. The discussion concerned the importance of selection of adult dancers with good axial alignment during the auditioning process. Because the company also offered ballet school to young children, the discussion following the presentation debated the benefits of accepting children into ballet school who had less-than-ideal axial alignment due to rotational and angular deformities of the lower extremities. A physical therapist presided over the discussion and presented the lecture with a question-and-answer session. A compilation of various comments as well as specific questions and discussion follow the case presentation.

A 15-year-old female ballet student with a history of reversed tailor sitting as a child complains of knee pain. Frontal observation during quiet standing shows kissing patellae and foot pronation. In addition, she appears to demonstrate a mild knock knee angular deformity with a slightly increased distance between the feet when the medial aspects of both knees approximate. During gait she exhibits an adducted gait pattern that is most pronounced during running. During swing phase of gait, both her legs move out laterally. Her Q angle measures 18°. A minus 10° foot-progression angle is noted, as well as a positive Craig's test. Radiographs of both lower extremities were normal.

? Questions

1. What is ballet?
2. What are the physical rigors involving ballet?
3. What types of injury are ballet dancers exposed to?
4. What is the significance of floor type and footwear in ballet?
5. What foot-type is ideal for participants in ballet?
6. Which positions are the basis for all beginning or ending movements in ballet?
7. What common forms of axial misalignment of the lower extremity signify an increased likelihood for injury in ballet?
8. What are the physiologic and pathologic angular deformities of the knees and legs in the frontal plane?
9. What types of rotational deformities of the hip, knee, leg, and foot may typically occur in the general population?
10. What is meant by "version" of the lower extremity?
11. What is femoral antetorsion?
12. Which osseous or soft-tissue structures may be identified as causative in excessive femoral torsion?

13. What causative factors contribute to excessive torsion of the lower extremity?
14. What is the relationship between excessive femoral anteversion and early arthritis of the hip joint?
15. How is excessive femoral anteversion detected?
16. How is femoral neck anteversion assessed?
17. What are the clinical manifestations of excessive femoral anteversion?
18. What are the components of a torsional profile of the lower extremity?
19. What is metatarsus adductus?
20. What is the origin of internal tibial torsion?
21. What is the origin of external tibial torsion?
22. What is the origin of miserable malalignment syndrome?
23. How would the biomechanical interdependency of the lower extremity articulations reinforce femoral anteversion in an individual with femoral antetorsion?
24. What is meant by the ballet term "hip turnout?"
25. What treatment is appropriate in management of femoral anteversion?
26. What is the role of physical therapy in the management of ballet-related injury?

1. What is ballet?

Classical ballet is an exacting art form that has its roots in the triumphal pageantry, religious rites, and royal banquets of the Italian Renaissance. The ballet, when combined with music, attempts to creatively express human emotion through bodily movement and facial gesture. It was imported to France by Louis the "Sun King," who founded the first ballet school in the midseventeenth century so that dancers could train for elaborate court presentations. The ease and grace of ballet performance and the seemingly effortless movement that appear, at times, to defy gravity mask the extraordinary physical demands placed on dancers. Today's classical ballet dancer has the "Balanchine" shape consisting of a small head, long neck, slightly shortened torso, small waist, and long thin legs as these traits are considered by some to be the ideal of the classic stage silhouette.[21]

2. What are the physical rigors involving ballet?

As an artistic endeavor, ballet demands a highly skilled and trained athlete. Few professional sports require the duration, intensity, and time that are demanded of the ballet. Ballet class prepares the dancer to meet the physical demands of this most vigorous art form. Class lasts for approximately 90 minutes and begins with warm-up exercises at the barre—a wooden rail along the wall that provides external support. Barre exercises include a variety of stretching and bending movements for the legs, which gradually increase in speed and scope as the leg is lifted from the floor (Fig. 52-1). Barre, lasting between 25 to 45 minutes, involves a progression of exercises beginning with pliés (knee bends) and battements (beating foot movements performed with the leg elevated or close to the floor), ronds de jambe (circular movements of the leg across the floor

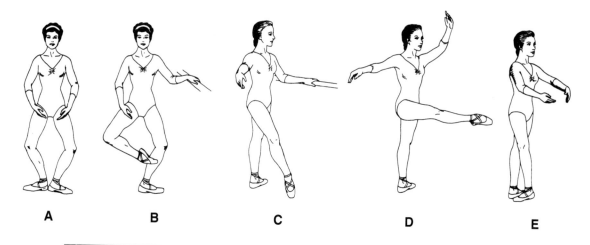

A   **B**   **C**   **D**   **E**

FIG. 52-1 Sequential exercises performed during barre. **A,** Pliés are knee-bending movements that are practiced in all classical positions of the feet. **B,** Battements are beating movements performed with the foot close to the floor or with the leg elevated. **C,** Rond de jambe involves movements of the leg across the floor and in the air. **D,** In développé, the leg is smoothly unfolded in space. **E,** Port de bras refers to leg movements that are coordinated with graceful movement of the arms. (From Malone TR, Hardaker WT: Rehabilitation of foot and ankle injuries in ballet dancers, *JOSPT* 11:8, February, 1990.)

and in the air), and développés (unfolding of the leg in space). Leg movements are coordinated with graceful movements of the arm known as port de bras.[19]

Following barre, class moves to the central floor exercise where dancers perform more complicated movements that are at first slow and progress in speed all the while concentrating on balance, strength, and aesthetic line. Class culminates with grand allegro comprised of multiple sequences of footwork combinations, turns, jumps, leaps, and turns as dancers migrate across large areas of the dance floor. Dancers often participate in 2 or 3 such classes per day, and in addition, may engage in cross training such as modern dance, jazz, folk dancing, ethnic dancing, or variety dance as in Broadway shows. Afternoons are usually spent in long rehearsals that may last as long as 4 to 5 hours per day, and may be followed by an evening performance.[19] The convention of dancing on the point of one's toes is almost exclusively reserved for female dancers and it attempts to express a floating ethereal airiness, a quality endeared in many Romantic ballets of the 19th century. It is no wonder then that ballet dancers are liable to a variety of lower extremity musculoskeletal pathologies, the majority of which involve the foot and ankle.

Advancing a dancer beyond his or her ability and training can lead to both acute and chronic injury.[26] It

is for this reason that ballet training begins before a child is 5 years old. The beginning student is at least 11 years old and has undergone a minimum of 3 years uninterrupted training before having mastered basic dance steps and developing physical strength.[1] In classical ballet, girls are not permitted to attempt "pointe dancing" before having developed the proper balance, coordination, and mental maturity required to concentrate continuously for periods up to 1 hour.[29] The dancer's advancement is predicated upon these prerequisites so as to prevent future injury. "Taking on too much too soon" is a problem commonly associated with dancers. In contrast, dancers returning from a furlough push themselves to the limit to make up for lost practice time.

3. What types of injury are ballet dancers exposed to?

Common injuries include lateral ankle sprain, stress fractures of the second or fifth metatarsal, plantar fasciitis, flexor hallucis longus tendinitis, trigger toe, shin splints, anterior and posterior compression syndrome, Achilles tendinitis, anterior and posterior impingement syndrome, hallux rigidus, cuboid subluxation, bunions, blisters, and corns. Other injuries, which ballet dancers are prone to, include periostitis of the dorsal spine from repetitive lying with the back on the floor; stress fracture of the pars interarticularis from excessive strain to the male lumbar; pars interarticularis during partnering; herniated disk from continuous bending and twisting; back strain or sprain resulting from poor technique; and sacroiliac joint dysfunction due to diminished flexibility. Proximal pathologies of the lower extremity include anterior hip click from the iliopsoas tendon snapping across the anterior hip capsule as the abducted lower extremity is brought back into the first position; abductor snap as the dancer lands from a leap; iliacus tendinitis during the *développé* dance step; femoral nerve neurapraxia due to *hinging**; meniscal derangement from "screwing the knees" to achieve the fifth classical dance position; and quadriceps avulsion at the superior patellar pole from performing *grande tours jete*.[29] In addition to falling prey to a myriad of lower extremity injuries, dancers are targets of the female athlete triad: a syndrome that combines disordered eating, amenorrhea, and osteoporosis. The latter results in reduced bone density and may culminate in repetitive fractures,[34] especially as dancers perform great leaps and turns in the air.

4. What is the significance of floor type and footwear in ballet?

Although injury may be caused acutely by a single impact, the majority are chronic in nature and due to overuse in which the lower extremity undergoes repetitive impact on a relatively hard, unyielding surface—the dance floor.[9,10,32] The ideal dance surface is made of hardwood with springs beneath and provides an optimal dampening mechanism to cushion the repetitive impact characterizing the dance routine.[33] The most important properties of dance surface are resiliency, shock absorption, and appropriate surface friction.[33] Unlike other athletic footwear designed to absorb shock and stabilize the foot, ballet slippers are neither designed to provide the foot with stability nor absorb shock.[23] Ballet footwear includes either slippers or toeshoes constructed of canvas or leather, and covered by satin.

5. What foot-type is ideal for participants in ballet?

The burden of bearing shock absorption in ballet is relegated, in large part, to the lower extremity. In modern dance, performers may not wear shoes at all. The best foot to accommodate dancing in pointe shoes is the squared foot type, occurring in approximately 9%[18] of the population and is one in which the first, second, and

third toes are the same length across. Second best is the Grecian (or Morton's) type foot, occurring in approximately 22% of the population and characterized by a middle toe that is slightly longer than the others. A ballet dancer having a foot in which the big toe is the longest (known as an Egyptian foot type) may encounter the most difficulty because the foot will have the greatest tendency to develop a bunion.[34] The latter is the most common foot type (69%).[18] It is the failure of the lower extremity to sufficiently absorb ground reaction that leads to injury.

Neither extreme of foot types is useful to aspiring ballet dancers. A cavus foot, with its rigid transverse tarsal joint absorbs energy poorly and transmits the brunt of ground reaction force to adjacent structures unaccustomed to absorbing stress. In contrast, a flatfoot may lead to breakdown of the intertarsal ligaments.[34]

6. Which positions are the basis for all beginning or ending movements in ballet?

The choreographer of Louis XIV codified the five basic positions of the lower extremities, postures that are characterized by the way a dancer's feet point outward. Indeed, all ballet movements begin or end with one of these positions (Fig. 52-2). The common denominator for these positions is that all are characterized by maximum external rotation of the lower extremity known as

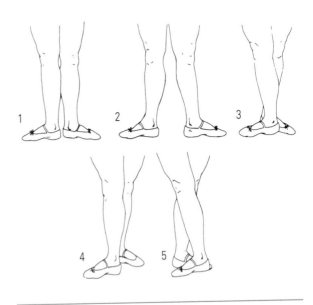

FIG. 52-2 The five classical ballet positions. All of these are characterized by maximum external rotation of the lower extremity. (From Malone TR, Hardaker WT: Rehabilitation of foot and ankle injuries in ballet dancers, *JOSPT* 11:8, February 1990.)

---

*Hinging refers to backward bending while sitting on the floor with the knees bent beneath the body.

turnout. Turnout is imperative to classical ballet as it enables the dancer to face the audience instead of profile in silhouette while simultaneously allowing the dancer to leap and pivot as quickly as possible. Turnout is primarily accomplished by maximum external rotation of the hip, with smaller contributions from the knee, ankle, and joints of the foot.[4] Factors contributing to external hip rotation include the amount of diminished anteversion angle at the hip, acetabular orientation, elasticity of the anterior hip capsule, particularly, the iliofemoral ligament, and the flexibility of the muscles crossing the hip joint. After the age of 11 in females, the femoral neck can no longer be anatomically altered into a position of relative retroversion.[29] Dance students may demonstrate poor turnout because of osseous factors such as femoral anteversion. In such instances, the dancer may improve turnout by stretching the hip capsule over the head of the femur anteriorly.[7,27] Dancers who exhibit tightness at the hip may compensate by imposing external rotation at the knee and ankle joints.[8,31] Some dancers may resort to a maladaptive technique known as rolling in that is characterized by extreme forced pronation of the midfoot and forefoot as well as hindfoot eversion in an attempt to compensate for inadequate external rotation at the hip.[3] This places additional strain on tibialis anterior and posterior and may precipitate shin splint syndrome.[23]

7. What common forms of axial misalignment of the lower extremity signify an increased likelihood for injury in ballet?

Axial malalignment of the lower extremities includes both *rotational* and *angular* deformities. Both transverse and frontal plane deformities are normal and quite common, especially during the child's first 2 years of life. When axial misalignment is excessive and persists beyond childhood, the likelihood for a diminished aesthetic and an increased likelihood of pathologic breakdown are highly significant for the potential ballet dancer. A dancer who has an inherent anatomic deviance diminishes the proper aesthetic line so essential for dance.

8. What are the physiologic and pathologic angular deformities of the knees and legs in the frontal plane?

The most common forms of lower extremity angular deformity in the frontal plane include *genu varum* (bow leg) and *genu valgum* (knock knees). These malalignments are termed physiologic to represent the normal developmental profile of the lower extremities in

infants and young children. The normal *tibiofemoral angle* changes with age. Both types of frontal plane deformities are often accompanied by foot pronation. Because of the linkage of the leg to the foot, overpronation of subtalar joint (compensation) is necessary to allow the calcaneus to maintain a normal vertical position relative to the supporting surface.

In the newborn the tibiofemoral angle is 15° and is characterized by lateral bowing of the tibiae. Varus positioning of the heel with pronation of the feet may be noted during standing, and while the child may ambulate with a waddling gait,[43] no lateral thrusting occurs.[25] Internal tibial torsion often accompanies physiologic bowleg, and serves to accentuate genu varum when the child stands or walks. Moreover, tibial varum is often associated with genu varum and ranges between 5° and 10° at birth to a gradual reduction of 2° to 3° between the ages of 2 and 4 years where it remains constant into adulthood.

The limbs appear to straighten at approximately 18 months of age, whereas between 2 and 4 years of age, the tibiofemoral angle reverses to 12° of valgus[28] as a consequence of normal osseous remodeling. Pronounced physiologic knock knees are more frequently seen in females. During quiet standing, the child is observed to have an increased distance between the feet when the medial aspects of both knees approximate. In addition, the child may place one knee behind the other in an attempt to place the feet together. Occasionally, a valgus alignment of the feet and pes planus deformity may present concomitantly.[43] This is because increased angles of genu valgum shift overall body weight to the medial aspect of the developing foot, and thereby increase the tendency for excessive pronation.[42] External tibial torsion may accompany a knock knee deformity and accentuate the genu valgum during standing and walking.[25] As the child undergoes skeletal maturation, this valgus angulation slightly persists as a function of the more distally projecting medial femoral condyle (see Fig. 41-4).[39] Proportionally greater distal overgrowth of the medial femoral condyle occurs when compared to the lateral femoral condyle as a function of normal development and weight bearing.[42] Treatment is not indicated in physiologic angular deformities as the malalignment gradually self-corrects over time. Reassurance and observation are the only form of management, whereas the application of splints, corrective shoes, or exercise does not change the outcome.

The clinical challenge is to differentiate between physiologic and pathologic types of angular deformity. It is important to remember that when screening a child for possible pathologic angular deformity a lateral and medial thrust during ambulation are characteristic of the pathologic and not physiologic forms of bow leg and knock-knee deformities, respectively.[25] The degree of genu varum or valgum may be assessed clinically or radiologically with the child either supine or standing. Any measured value greater than 30°, or persistence of angular deviation beyond what is normally expected given the patient's age warrants additional evaluation.[42]

Pathologic bowleg most commonly occurs from either *Blount disease,* also known as *tibia vara* or *tibial osteochondrosis* and is classified as a *focal* pathologic cause of bowleg. Less commonly, when pathologic bowleg occurs from *rickets,* the resultant angular deformity is considered generalized. Pathologic bowleg may occur from either a vitamin D dependent or resistant type rickets.

Blount disease is an isolated growth disturbance of the medial aspect of the proximal tibial growth plate (medial tibial epiphyses). Although the etiology of Blount disease is uncertain, the condition is thought to derive secondary to mechanical stress of weight bearing on the medial tibiofemoral compartment. Normally, the overall valgus of the knee is derived from the larger and longer medial femoral condyle extending distal to the lateral condyle.[39] This may concentrate uneven weight bearing across the tibiofemoral articulation, focusing undue pressure through the medial tibiofemoral joint. Because the growth plate is vulnerable, the epiphyses may suffer damage and thus a process of progressive medial angulation (genu varum) of the metaphysis of the tibia is initiated. The incidence of occurrence is higher if the child is black, obese, has an affected family member,[37] or typically initiated ambulation at an early age. Two clinical patterns of Blount disease occur. The early *infantile form,* which is commonly bilateral and progressive, is associated with significant tibial torsion and is often difficult to distinguish clinically from severe physiologic bowing without the benefit of radiographs or a bone scan. Progression of the disease is often rapid during the first 4 years, and slows for the remainder of the growth period. The *juvenile form* of tibia vara is typically unilateral, less severe, lacks an internal tibial torsion component, and becomes apparent between 6 to 14 years of age. This less common form of Blount disease often occurs following trauma and is associated with arrest of the physes.[42] Satisfactory management is based upon the age of the child and the stage of the disease process. The disease is reversible during stages I and II provided early recognition has occurred. In the infantile form, observation is often sufficient until the child is 18 months of age, after which, treatment takes the form of a long leg brace such as an A-frame or Blount brace until the age of 3 and worn at night and during active play. Bracing helps leg realignment and prevents further progression. Osteotomy is indicated if the disease progresses to stage III or IV, and should preferably be performed before age 4.[37]

Pathologic knock knee may result from rickets secondary to renal insufficiency known as renal osteodystrophy. The child with rickets presents with a number of coexistent physical findings including musculoskeletal abnormalities such as short stature, thoracic kyphosis, symmetric enlargement of the ends of long bones (such as the wrist and elbows), frontal bone prominence, skull deformity, knock knees, or less frequently, bow legs, as well as rib flaring and funnel chest deformity. Children are often apathetic or irritable and frequently remain immobile, which with their potbelly, gives them a Buddha-like appearance. Respiratory infections and a chronic cough are common.[25] Radiographs confirm the diagnosis. The value of bracing these children remains controversial. Osteotomy is best reserved until after skeletal growth is complete.[37]

9. What types of rotational deformities of the hip, knee, leg, and foot may typically occur in the general population?

Because the position of the foot is the most obvious clinical manifestation, rotational problems of the lower extremities are typically referred to as toe-in and toe-out. However, the causes of in-toeing, for example, may stem from femoral anteversion, medial tibial torsion, or metatarsus adductus. Identifying the correct source of in-toeing is the challenge presented to the therapist examining the patient. Early identification of these malalignments may be significant in the selection process of young students because these malalignments result in inefficient motion, require more energy to move, and may be indirectly responsible for injury. Because of this, a proper aesthetic line in the axial alignment of the lower extremities is essential in selection of the aspiring ballerina.

10. What is meant by "version" of the lower extremity?

Version refers to limb rotation and may be defined as the angular difference between the transverse axis of each end of a long bone. The lower limb bud appears during the third week of embryonic life, and undergoes rotation about their long axes during the seventh fetal week so as to situate the great toe at the medial side of the foot. A second rotation involving both the tibia and femur occurs later at both the femoral and tibial levels.[38] Because of the position of the infant in utero, internal rotation and flexion of the hip occurs during the final months of pregnancy due to a variety of factors including uterine pressure.[42] This internal rotation is referred to as femoral neck anteversion, and represents the angle between the neck and shaft of the femur.[39] This is most easily visualized by considering an isolated femur lying in the anatomical position on a plinth. Viewing the femur distal-to-proximal along its longitudinal axis demonstrates a 30° internal angulation of the distal femoral condyles relative to the head and neck of the femur. Just after birth, anteversion is typically 30° to 40°, while the magnitude of femoral anteversion progressively declines as the child develops into an adult. Until the child is 2 years of age, the total range of hip rotation is approximately 120°. A gradual unwinding of this angular relationship between the shaft and neck occurs as maturity commences. This is facilitated by assuming the standing posture as the hip is postured in extension after the child begins walking. The anterior hip capsule tightens when the hip is extended and results in an external torsional strain along the malleable femoral neck. Thus normal tensing of the ligaments comprising the anterior hip capsule acts to reduce the magnitude of femoral neck anteversion.[35,36] If these ligaments are lax, as may occur in a child with Down syndrome, the forces necessary to assist in reduction of femoral torsion may be absent. Thus derotation occurs rapidly during the first 2 years of life, after which derotation occurs more slowly and reaches a plateau at about 8 to 9 years of age to approximately 16° in adulthood. Thus the total range of hip rotation in the mature individual varies between 90° and 110°, with internal and external rotation being approximately equal (45° to 50°).[25]

Anteversion decreases to approximately 8° in the male and 14° in the female at skeletal maturity. The normal pediatric and adult femur is anteverted. When excessive femoral anteversion exists, it is usually most severe between the ages of 4 and 6 years before resolving beyond that time.[37] Resolution results from a combination of spontaneous femoral derotation and lateral tibial rotation. Excessive femoral anteversion during childhood undergoes *spontaneous derotation* by the time adolescence occurs in the majority of children. Torsional growth may be slower than usual and, in some children, the angle may not reduce to normal until several years later. In others, the common rotational patterns of infancy may persist if the normal lateral rotational process is altered by either genetic or environmental factors.

11. What is femoral antetorsion?

Where version describes normal limb rotations, *antetorsion* is reserved for excessive, medial femoral rotation; that is, excessive *femoral anteversion*. In contrast, the lower limb may be excessively laterally rotated, also referred to as *femoral retroversion* or retrotorsion. Excessive femoral anteversion, or antetorsion, refers to an abnormal relationship of the femoral diaphysis and condyles to the neck and femur. Defined another way, the neck of the femur points more directly forward than normal[22] so that the femur is excessively internally rotated. Excessive anteversion is twice as common in females compared with males,[18] and if present unilaterally, causes an apparent leg-length discrepancy and predisposes the adult to lower back pain or sacroiliac joint dysfunction.[5] In contrast, some children may have overgrowth in the transverse plane with excessive external rotation known as *retrotorsion* (Fig. 52-3).

12. Which osseous or soft-tissue structures may be identified as causative in excessive femoral torsion?

Acetabular position appears to influence the rotational status of the femur. An internally rotated acetabulum will contribute to an internally positioned limb. More commonly, the acetabulum is more externally rotated.[15,40] Persistent femoral anteversion may result from contracture of the iliofemoral and pubofemoral ligaments, as well as the iliopsoas, tensor fasciae latae, gluteus medius, and gluteus minimus muscles. In contrast, retrotorsion may result from contracture of the ischiofemoral ligament, as well as the gluteus maximus, obturator externus and internus, gemelli, quadratus femoris, piriformis, sartorius, and the adductors magnus, brevis, and longus muscles.[41]

13. What causative factors contribute to excessive torsion of the lower extremity?

The etiology of excessive rotation includes genetic, positional, iatrogenic, or compensating mechanisms. Rotational variations tend to run in families. However, the most common cause of torsional deformity, particularly tibial torsion and metatarsus adductus, derives from intrauterine position. Certain common habitual positions

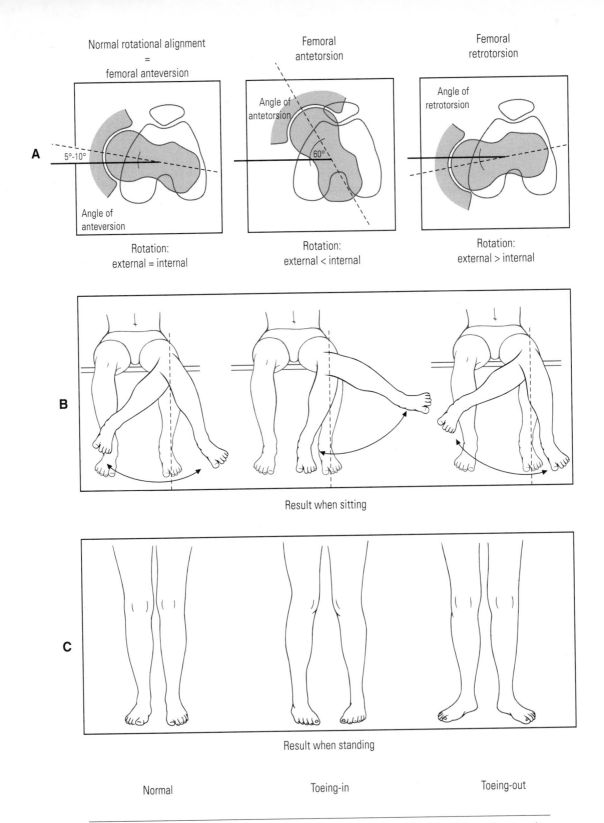

FIG.52-3 A, The normal rotational alignment of the femoral shaft and neck is one of femoral anteversion, which manifests as roughly equivalent range of external and internal rotation; the toes point slightly outward in the anatomical position. **B,** Femoral antetorsion refers to excessive anteversion that manifests as excessive medial hip rotation and toeing-in. **C,** Femoral retrotorsion refers to relative external rotation of the femoral shaft in relation to the femoral neck, resulting in proportionately more external rotation of the hip, and outtoeing.

of sleeping and sitting may contribute to molding the femur into an excessively anteverted relationship between the neck and shaft of the femur. Sleeping with the feet turned in under the buttocks exerts a medial rotational strain along the length of the femur. In contrast, sleeping prone with the hips in external rotation in the "frog sleeping posture" may predispose excessive external rotation. Both positions most certainly cause soft-tissue contractures of the hip that reinforces osseous torsional change (Fig. 52-4).

Similarly, *reverse "W" sitting,* also known as the *tailor's posture,* for long periods, as may occur when children sit on the floor in front of a television, acts to exert a medial torsional force upon the femoral neck and simultaneous external torsion upon the tibial shaft. The latter is particularly offensive as it promotes a compensating torsional deformity in which pronation of the foot compensates for external tibial torsion, which in turn compensates for excessive femoral anteversion. Moreover, this posture promotes contracture of the il-

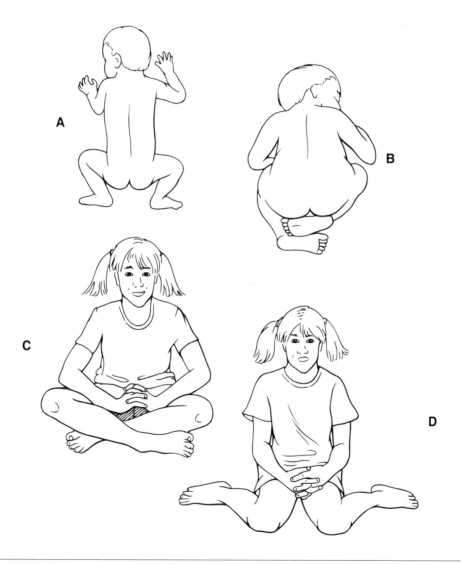

FIG. 52-4 Infantile sleeping postures causing excessive torsion. **A,** The spread-eagle or frog sleeping position may contribute to external rotation of the hips, manifesting as femoral retrotorsion. **B,** Sleeping with the feet turned in under the buttocks exerts a medial rotational strain manifesting as femoral antetorsion. **C,** Sitting cross-legged (tailor or indian position) applies external torsion of the femurs and internal torsion to the tibiae. **D,** Reversed tailor position places internal torsional stress on the femurs and external torsion on the tibiae.

iofemoral and pubofemoral ligaments by approximating their attachments while causing stretching of the ischiofemoral ligament. Consequently, the most comfortable way of standing and ambulating is to rotate the femur inward thereby avoiding the painful discomfort of stretching the capsule. Because of the linkage between the joints of the lower extremity, the knees and toes undergo simultaneous obligatory pointing inward as well. Iatrogenic causes of torsional deformity by the use of long leg cases or Denis Browne splints that attempt to correct for excessive internal tibial torsion, or "horizontal breach" clubfoot management, may result in external tibial torsion.

14. What is the relationship between excessive femoral anteversion and early arthritis of the hip joint?

The internally rotated position of the femoral shaft associated with excessive anteversion impacts on the femoral neck angle and hence the relationship of the femoral head with the acetabular socket. An excessively anteverted femur allows the head to exert increased pressure against the superior and anterior parts of the acetabulum.[5] This causes weight-bearing forces to be transmitted over a smaller area of contact over the articular surface of the hip joint. Thus ambulation with hip incongruity may accelerate wear of the hip articular surface and lead to degenerative hip disease. Persistent infantile femoral anteversion is thought to contribute to osteoarthritis at a later age although this has not been proven.[6]

15. How is excessive femoral anteversion detected?

Excessive femoral anteversion is typically detected during gait analysis. Ambulation, especially running, may be characterized as an internal rotation of the lower extremities during swing phase of gait, which may appear ungainly and a potential source of embarrassment to the self-conscious child. This awkward pattern of ambulation has been described as an "eggbeater" type gait. In addition, the foot posture may be characterized as pigeon-toed, while an adducted gait pattern may describe the proximal lower extremity. An adducted pattern of gait may result from an anteriorly located acetabulum, a tight hip capsule, a tight iliotibial band, or short or tightened anterior hip muscles.[16] A child with femoral antetorsion may exhibit an eggbeater running pattern with the legs flipping laterally during swing phase.[37] In contrast, femoral retrotorsion may be char-

acterized by toeing-out. A larger than normal value for Q angle will be present.

16. How is femoral neck anteversion assessed?

The internal rotation characterizing femoral neck anteversion indicates a value measuring the angle between the neck and shaft of the femur. The shaft of the femur is defined by the coronal plane of the femoral condyles. Femoral anteversion refers to the degree of forward projection of the femoral neck from the coronal plane. This value may be assessed with Craig's (also known as Ryder's) test which considers comparative ranges of internal and external hip rotation suggesting antetorsion or retroversion, respectively. This is performed with the patient lying prone with the knee flexed to 90°. The therapist palpates the posterior aspect of the greater femoral trochanter. The hip is passively internally and externally rotated until the greater trochanter is parallel with the examining surface or until it reaches its most lateral position. The degree of femoral anteversion may then be estimated, based on the angle of the lower leg with the vertical.[18]

17. What are the clinical manifestations of excessive femoral anteversion?

Before performing a physical examination it is essential to inquire whether a family history of rotational problems exists, and whether a delay in walking, suggesting a neuromuscular disorder, was present during infancy. There may be a history of sitting on the floor with the legs in the *reverse tailor position*.[43] The onset, severity, disability, and previous management of a rotational problem should be established.[37] This is followed by ruling out other conditions, such as congenital hip dysplasia or cerebral palsy,[38] or subtle onset of peroneal muscle atrophy. On examination the child is observed to stand with the knees and feet turned inwards. Radiographic examination is usually normal.[43]

18. What are the components of a torsional profile of the lower extremity?

A proper evaluation is predicated on a cooperative child so that the lower limb is examined in a sequential manner, so that the foot, tibia, femur, and the joints between may be isolated in turn. Patients may have a combination of deformities such as medial femoral and tibial torsion or medial tibial torsion and metatarsus adductus. The clinical examination should include a torsional profile, which provides the information necessary to establish the current level and severity of torsional pathology. This evaluation occurs in four steps that include: the foot-progression angle, hip rotation assessment, tibial rotational assessment, and forefoot adduction.

FOOT-PROGRESSION ANGLE

This is assessed by having the patient walk and run without shoes. The foot-progression angle (FPA) is defined as the angle between the axis of the foot and the line of forward progression; an average negative value is assigned to an in-toeing gait, and a positive value is assigned to an out-toeing gait. These gait deviations may be accentuated when the patient is fatigued. A value of 5° to 10° is considered mild, 10° to 15° moderate, and a value greater than 15° is severe.[37]

FEMORAL ROTATION

Femoral version is best assessed with the patient recumbent in either the prone or supine position. The examination should not be performed with the patient sitting, as a flexed hip relaxes the anterior capsule, and leads to an inaccurate evaluation by permitting a greater range of external rotation. Medial rotation is slightly greater in girls. Both hips are tested simultaneously. The patient has a positive score for a medial femoral torsional deformity if medial rotation is greater than 70°. A value of 70° to 80° is considered mild, 80° to 90° is considered moderate, and a value greater than 90° is considered severe.[38]

Prone testing keeps the pelvis level as the knees are flexed. Internal rotation of the hip is assessed by allowing the weight of the lower limb to fall outward by gravity alone, whereas external hip rotation is assessed by allowing both legs to cross. A substantial increase in internal versus external rotation becomes apparent in individuals with excessive femoral anteversion. The converse is true with femoral antetorsion.

Supine testing is performed by having the patient lie with both knees extended on the examination table in a relaxed manner. The person with normal femoral anteversion will demonstrate toe-out of approximately 45° when lying in the anatomic position, whereas the patient with excessive femoral anteversion will show a neutral rotational position of the lower limb and lack of toe-out with toes are pointing upward (Fig. 52-5). The therapist then attempts to maximally rotate the feet inward and then outward. Excessive femoral anteversion is suggested by the knees facing each other with medial

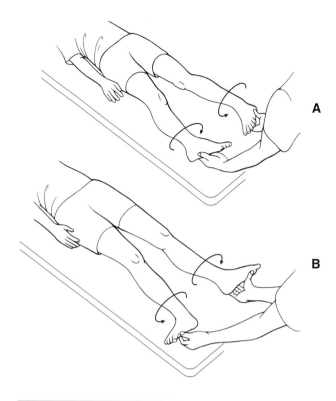

FIG. 52-5 Supine testing for femoral antetorsion. **A,** With the feet turned maximally inward, the knees point directly medially so that they face each other. **B,** With the feet turned maximally outward, the knees rotate only slightly beyond the neutral position.

foot rotation. However, when these same feet are manually externally rotated, the examiner meets with resistance as the knees rotate only slightly beyond the neutral position.[25]

TIBIAL ROTATIONAL ASSESSMENT

This may be assessed by determining the *thigh-foot angle* (TFA) defined as the angular difference between the axis of the thigh and foot. This is determined by having the patient lie prone with the knees flexed to 90°, as the examiner views the foot and thigh directly from above. The axis of the foot is then compared with the axis of the thigh and a value is estimated. Alternately, tibial version may be assessed by determining the transmalleolar axis (TMA). This is accomplished by comparing the bimalleolar axis, described as the oblique line drawn between the medial and lateral malleoli, and noting the angle it makes when comparing it with the axis of the thigh. This value is then the trans-malleolar axis. Manipulating the foot may result in assessment errors.

FOREFOOT ADDUCTION

The forefoot adduction and convexity of the lateral border is evidence of metatarsus adductus, as the lateral border of the foot is normally straight. An everted foot may contribute to toe-out.

19. What is metatarsus adductus?

Metatarsus adductus, also known as *metatarsus varus,* is the most common foot deformity in children and is characterized by medially deviating metatarsals. Other than metatarsal deviation, there are no pathologic changes in foot structure. Radiographs will confirm abnormal metatarsal deviation without osseous abnormalities. This forefoot deformity is usually bilateral and is due to intrauterine positioning. Some patients may have a concurrent internal tibial torsion deformity, although the calf is of normal size. Metatarsus adductus represents just one component of congenital clubfoot deformity.[22] It carries a benign prognosis compared with the former complex deformity. Indeed, patients with metatarsus adductus are asymptomatic, although the spectrum of severity and magnitude of in-toeing may be classified as mild, moderate, or severe. Tests for stiffness or suppleness of the foot are done by holding the heel firmly and attempting to position the forefoot laterally into an overcorrected posture. A positive examination yields a forefoot that reassumes its medially deviated or varus position. When observing the plantar surface of the foot, a convexity is present along the lateral border of the foot, a concavity medially, as well as widening between the great and second toes. A plantar skin crease may be seen and palpated over the medial aspect of the longitudinal arch.

A mild metatarsus adductus deformity is one that is either actively correctable by the patient or passively corrected by the clinician. Active correction may be elicited by gentle stroking over the lateral leg and foot, stimulating the peroneal muscles to contract.[43] In more involved cases, deviation may only be partially correctable by active or passive stretching. Rigidity and heel valgus should alert the therapist to the possibility of a more complex problem. Management depends upon the severity of the condition. Mild cases may be addressed by teaching the mother passive forefoot stretching exercises approximately ten times with each diaper change. With moderate deformity, a combination of manipulative stretching with straight or out-flare shoes are appropriate between exercises to keep the foot in an overcorrected posture. If improvement does not occur after a few months, or in more severe cases if the forefoot is more rigid or resistant to passive stretch, and exhibits a prominent deformity and skin crease, then serial casting over a period of 6 to 8 weeks should proceed. Casts should be changed every 1 to 2 weeks. Casting as a treatment approach is feasible up to the ages of 4 to 5 years.[37] When treatment is initiated before a child turns 8 to 10 months old, a satisfactory result usually occurs. However, if management is delayed beyond 1 to 5 years of age, bone and soft-tissue changes may not be reversible, as the foot assumes an unusual appearance characterized by an adducted forefoot and prominent base of the fifth metatarsal. This necessitates a wider than normal shoe. Improved cosmesis may be accomplished in the older child by a metatarsal osteotomy.[25]

20. What is the origin of internal tibial torsion?

Internal tibial torsion, the most common cause of in-toeing, is characterized by a tibia that is internally rotated on its long axis, causing the foot to point inward. This deformity, attributed to internal molding of the foot and leg in utero, is often symmetric, but if unilateral it most commonly presents with the left side being more severely involved.[38] This left-sided propensity may be attributable to the fact that most babies are carried with their backs to the left side of the mother, thereby causing the child's left leg to abduct and cross the right leg.[41] Internal tibial torsion may therefore be considered normal in the infant and is most commonly noticed during the second year of life when the infant begins to walk although it gradually disappears with growth and further weight bearing. Thus internal tibial torsion is a nonpathologic variation of normal in the lower extremity of the child under 5 years of age. The parent may be concerned because of prominent in-toeing during gait and frequent tripping. Examination is best performed with the child seated showing hips and knees that are normally aligned and anteriorly facing patellae, whereas the lower legs and feet are internally rotated. The lateral malleolus is normally positioned slightly posterior to the medial malleolus resulting in an oblique transmalleolar axis. With internal tibial torsion the two malleoli may be in alignment with each other or the lateral malleolus may be anteriorly displaced, causing the ankle mortise to shift to a medially directed orientation, which accounts for the in-toeing.[43] An alternative method of measurement is to use the thigh-foot angle (see earlier discussion). Radiographs are normal. Observational management is best as internal tibial torsion improves spontaneously as bone remodeling gradually corrects this condition as the child grows. The use of bracing and night splinting is discouraged as they are of no proven benefit. The former may slow the child's running and be deleterious to the child's self-image.[37] Children who are in the habit of sitting or sleeping with their feet tucked under the buttocks are discourage from doing so as this posture may inhibit the normal remodeling process. Instead, children are encouraged to sit cross-legged (tailor or Indian positions).[25]

21. What is the origin of external tibial torsion?

External tibial torsion is more common in the older child and represents excessive derotational growth out of the internally rotated position of the tibia. Thus unlike medial tibial torsion, external tibial torsion becomes worse over time, and may result in patellofemoral pain. This occurs because optimal patellofemoral joint congruity depends upon, among other factors, neutral alignment of the tibia. As the knee is the central link in the lower extremity, compensation above the knee in the form of femoral anteversion may facilitate restoration of balance to patellofemoral biomechanics. In addition to proximal compensation, additional compensation occurs distally at the subtalar joint in the form of foot pronation. The summation of external tibial torsion with its proximal and distally generated compensatory malalignments results in miserable malalignment syndrome (see the following discussions), a condition that produces an inefficient and therefore more energy expending gait, as well as patellofemoral joint pain. On observation, the feet are turned outward while the knees point directly forward, indicating that toeing out is due to tibial, and not femoral, external torsion.* Conservative management of external tibial torsion is controversial. Tibial rotational osteotomy is only indicated in the older child over 8 to 10 years of age who has a significant cosmetic and functional deformity.[37]

22. What is the origin of miserable malalignment syndrome?

Although torsional deformity may be simple, involving one level, complex torsion involves multiple lower extremity segments. Complex deformity is characterized

by being either additive or compensating. Although medial tibial and femoral torsion are additive,[37] medial femoral torsion and lateral tibial torsion are compensating. Standing and ambulation may cause compensations to occur distally along the lower extremity, which is characterized by femoral anteversion. The most common pattern of compensation is secondary external rotation of the tibiae and tertiary compensation of the feet into excessive pronation. The patellae, comprising the central component of malalignment, face toward each other during quiet standing, and almost face each other ("kissing patella") at termination of stance phase. This pattern of deviation is known as *miserable malalignment syndrome*[14] as it signifies considerable deviation from ideal anatomic axial alignment of the lower extremities. Because of the linkage between the joints of the lower extremity, the knees and toes undergo simultaneous obligatory pointing inward as well. This malalignment increases joint forces across the knee and ankle, wreaks havoc at the patellofemoral joint, and may be indirectly responsible for injury.[9] The excessive pronation at the subtalar joints is thought to be primarily responsible for chondromalacia patellae.[2] It is for this reason that near normal or normal axial alignment of the lower extremities is selected for ballet, for both aesthetic and physical reasons.[10] Thus axial malalignment such as significant femoral neck anteversion or retroversion, genu valgus or varum, or internal or external tibial torsion breaks the aesthetic line. These body types are not preferable for participation in ballet as these persons may be more susceptible to injury and poorly tolerate the physical rigors of ballet. The presence or absence of axial malalignment noted during auditioning is thus of considerable importance to the artistic director of a dance company.

23. How would the biomechanical interdependency of the lower extremity articulations reinforce femoral anteversion in an individual with femoral antetorsion?

During ambulation, rotation of the pelvis causes the femur, fibula, and tibia to rotate about the long axis of the limb.[13] The lower extremity rotates laterally beyond midstance and until toe off has occurred during late stance. In contrast, the lower limb rotates medially during swing phase and early stance.[20]

Excessive femoral anteversion results in decreased congruity of the hip joint surfaces. During late stance phase, as the femur externally rotates on the pelvis, the individual with excessive femoral anteversion will not undergo enough external rotation compared with the

---

*In contrast, where the origin of external rotation is at the hips, the knees are in neutral or slight internal rotation when the feet are positioned maximally inward.

normal hip. Consequently, the tibia and fibula undergo a corresponding internal rotation as a result of the biomechanical interdependency linking the articulations spanning these long bones. This internal tibial rotation is primarily transmitted to the subtalar joint, which is best suited to negotiate transverse rotations at the foot. Subsequently, this causes pronation of the hindfoot as the foot untwists and the arch flattens. Delayed or absent resupination of the subtalar joint during late stance causes delayed external tibial torsion, which, in turn delays external femoral rotation. In this manner, the subtalar joint may reinforce excessive femoral anteversion by stressing the soft-tissue structures surrounding the proximal femur by prolonging the internal rotary moment of the lower limb.

24. What is meant by the ballet term "hip turnout?"

The singularly most essential component of classical ballet is for the dancer to be able to achieve proper turnout, referring to maximal external rotation of the hip common to each of the five basic dance positions. Also, turnout positions the lower limb in profile with the dancer facing the audience so that position, intent, and movement may be implied without the dancer moving.[30] Several factors contribute to external rotation of the hip during turnout, and include the amount of relative femoral antetorsion or retrotorsion, acetabular orientation, the elasticity of the anterior hip capsule (particularly the iliofemoral ligament), and the flexibility of the musculotendinous units crossing the hip.[10] Until age 11, osseous molding of the acetabulum and the angle of orientation of the femoral neck may be molded into a relatively retroverted femur. Beyond this time, however, passive stretching of the hip in external rotation and active muscle contraction will not change osseous relationships of the acetabulum or femoral neck angle as bone is considerably less deformable beyond puberty. To maintain proper turnout in a dancer who has not had the good fortune of beginning dance before age 11, the above mentioned muscle exercises must be continuously performed so as to stretch the hip capsule over the femoral head anteriorly.[7,27] Ideally, turnout is primarily achieved at the hip joint, with smaller contributions deriving from the knee, ankle, and joints of the foot.[4] Some dancers may be predisposed toward better turnout by having the good fortune of being more flexible, whereas others who are less flexible may compensate for poor turnout by maladaptive techniques at the knee or foot-ankle complex that stress these joints beyond their anatomic limit.[30]

Dancers with poor turnout have difficulty in achieving the fifth position and may compensate by a maneuver known as "screwing the knees."[12] This may cause rotational stress and resultant tear of the meniscus. Another maladaptive technique that compensates for poor turnout at the hip is rolling-in, which involves forced pronation of the midfoot and hindfoot secondary to extreme eversion of the hindfoot. This maneuver places excessive strain on the medial structures of the foot and ankle and may lead to chronic injuries in this region.[10]

25. What treatment is appropriate in management of femoral anteversion?

Treatment for femoral anteversion is controversial.[25] Bracing is not appropriate as it may simply generate adjacent angular and/or torsional deformities. Similarly, the use of shoe wedges and inserts has been proven ineffective in changing the foot-progression angle.[17] The use of twister cables during the day is poorly tolerated as they limit the child's mobility. Night splints, which externally rotate the feet, are better tolerated, but have not been proven to be of long-term benefit. Because ballet is predicated upon vigilant maintenance of the lower extremity in the externally rotated posture, ballet has been recommended as a therapeutic activity for individuals with excessive internal rotation.[24] Although practicing turnout during an early age may indeed alter the bony relationship of the femoral neck and shaft, any gain in external rotation beyond the age of osseous maturity is caused by soft-tissue adaptation.

Observational management is best when dealing with rotational problems in children, unless pathology is suspected. Parents of children must be educated that only rarely (less than 1%) do torsional problems fail to resolve. Attempting to control the child's walking, sitting, or sleeping postures is virtually impossible and likely to engender frustration and conflict between the parent and child. Instead, education, reassurance, and follow up are often all that is necessary in management.

In the adult, facilitating increased external rotation is a worthwhile therapeutic endeavor because excessive femoral anteversion may generate pathomechanics at the spine, knee, and foot. Early detection may stave off stress-related symptoms if therapeutic soft-tissue intervention is initiated early. Joint mobilization to facilitate improved capsular extensibility is an important soft-tissue technique, especially in stretching the iliofemoral and pubofemoral ligaments. Relative imbalance between opposing muscle groups should be corrected by a program of strengthening of the external rotators and stretching of the internal hip rotators.

26. What is the role of physical therapy in the management of ballet-related injury?

It is essential for the therapist to appreciate the enormous pressure dancers are under to maintain their strength and flexibility. Asking a dancer to stop dancing is unrealistic and may prevent the patient from returning. Instead, the treatment focus must revolve around relative rest. Moreover, many dancers wait too long before coming for treatment as they may feel their career may be jeopardized if they are labeled as "high risk" in terms of their injury.[34]

Muscle imbalance due to diminished flexibility in the pelvis and hip may result in neuromusculoskeletal pathology. The therapist's goals include restoration of motion, strength, flexibility, endurance, and proprioception. Of equal importance is a thorough musculoskeletal evaluation to ascertain potential risk factors for injury, including anatomic malalignment, muscle imbalance, poor technique, and training errors. Prevention is an essential component of management. Following injury, the dancers should perform many warm up exercises and "take it slowly." Dancers must be reminded not to take on "too much too soon." Performing the barre in a pool with ankle weights is very helpful. The Pilates-based system of exercises is performed on floor mats and use apparatus that employ springs as resistance. This method of rehabilitation is gentle and employs both body and mind in maintaining flexibility, strength, and range of motion while resting and rehabilitating from injury.

RECOMMENDED READING

Milan KR: Injury in ballet: a review of relevant topics for the physical therapist, *JOSPT* 19(2), February 1994.

Sammacro GJ: Dance injuries. In Nicholas JA, Hershman EB editors: *The lower extremity and spine in sports medicine*, St Louis, 1995, Mosby.

Staheli LT: Rotational problems of the lower extremities, *Orthop Clin North Am* 18(4), October, 1987.

REFERENCES

1. Beaumont CW, Idzikowski S: *A manual of the theory and practice of classical theatrical dancing*, New York, 1970, Dover Publications.
2. Buchbinder MR, Napora NJ, Biggs ES: The relationship of abnormal pronation to chondromalacia of the patella in distance runners, *Pod Sports Med* 69:159, 1979.
3. Dunn B: Physiotherapy and the ballet, *Physiother* 51:125-128.
4. Gelabert R: Turning out, *Dance Magazine*, 86, February 1977.
5. Gould JA: *Orthopaedic and sports physical therapy*, ed 2, St Louis, 1990, Mosby.
6. Halpern A, Tanner J, Rinsky L: Does persistent femoral anteversion contribute to osteoarthritis? *Clin Orthop* 145:213, 1979.
7. Hamilton WG, Hamilton LH, Marshall P et al: A profile of the musculoskeletal characteristics of elite professional ballet dancers, *Am J Sports Med* 20:267, 1992.
8. Hamilton WG: Tendinitis about the ankle joint in classical ballet dancers, *Am J Sports Med* 5:84, 1977.
9. Hardaker WT Jr, Erickson L, Myers M: The pathogenesis of dance injury. In Shell CG editor: *The dancer as athlete*, Olympic Scientific Conference Proceedings, Champaign, Ill., 1984, Human Kinetic Press.
10. Hardaker WT Jr, Margello S, Goldner JL: Foot and ankle injuries in theatrical dancers, *Foot Ankle* 6:59-69, 1985.
11. Reference deleted.
12. Howse AJG: Orthopaedists aid ballet, *Clin Orthop* 89:52, 1972.
13. Inman VT, Ralston HJ, Todd F: *Human walking*, Baltimore, 1981, Williams & Wilkins.
14. James SL, Bates BT, Osterning LR: Injuries to runners, *Am J Sports Med* 6:40, 1978.
15. Khermosh O, Lior G, Weissman SL: Tibial torsion in children, *Clin Orthop* 25:679, 1971.
16. Kleiger B: The anteversion syndrome, *Bull Hosp Joint Dis* 29:22, 1968.
17. Knittel G, Staheli LT: The effectiveness of shoe modifications for intoeing, *Orthop Clin North Am* 7:1019-1025, 1976.
18. Magee DJ: *Orthopedic physical assessment*, ed 3, Philadelphia, 1997, WB Saunders.
19. Malone TR, Hardaker WT Jr: Rehabilitation of foot and ankle injuries in ballet dancers, *JOSPT* 11:8, February, 1990.
20. Manley MT: Biomechanics of the foot. In Helfet AJ, Gruebel Lee DM editors: *Disorders of the foot*, Philadelphia, 1980, JB Lippincott.
21. McLain D: Artistic development of the dancer, *Clin Sport Med* 2:563, 1983.
22. Meals RA: *One hundred orthopaedic conditions every doctor should understand*, St Louis, 1992, Quality Medical Publishing.
23. Milan KR: Injury in ballet: a review of relevant topics for the physical therapist, *JOSPT* 19(2), February 1994.
24. Miller EH, Schneider HJ, Bronson JL et al: A new consideration in athletic injuries. The classical ballet dancer, *Clin Orthop* 111:181, 1975.
25. Netter FH: The Ciba collection of medical illustrations, vol 8, *Musculoskeletal system, part II: developmental disorders, tumors, rheumatic diseases, and joint replacement*, Summit, NJ, 1990, CIBA-GEIGY.
26. Nixon JE: Injuries to the neck and upper extremities of dancers, *Clin Sports Med* 2:459, 1983.
27. Reid DC, Burnham RS, Saboe LA et al: Lower extremity flexibility patterns in classical ballet dancers and their correlation to lateral hip and knee injuries, *Am J Sports Med* 15:347, 1987.
28. Salenius P, Vankka E: The development of the tibiofemoral angle in children, *J Bone Joint Surg* 57A:259-261, 1975.

29. Sammacro GJ: Dance injuries. In Nicholas JA, Hershman EB editors: *The lower extremity and spine in sports medicine,* St Louis, 1995, Mosby.

30. Sammarco GJ: The dancer's hip, *Clin Sports Med* 2:485, 1983.

31. Sammarco GJ: The foot and ankle in classical ballet and modern dance. In Jahss MH editor: *Disorders of the foot,* Philadelphia, 1982, WB Saunders.

32. Seals JG: A study of dance surfaces. In Sammarco GJ editor: Symposium on injuries to dancers, *Clin Sports Med* 2:557-561, 1983.

33. Seals JG: Dance floors, *Med Prob Perf Art* 1(3):81, 1986.

34. Sephton S: Foot injuries in dancers. Advance directors rehabilitation, September, 1998.

35. Somerville EW: Development of congenital dislocation of the hip, *J Bone Joint Surg* 39B:106-113, 1957.

36. Somerville, EW: Development of congenital dislocation of the hip, *J Bone Joint Surg* 35B:568, 1953.

37. Staheli LT: *Fundamentals of pediatric orthopedics,* New York, 1992, Raven Press.

38. Staheli LT: Rotational problems of the lower extremities, *Orthop Clin North Am* 18(4), October, 1987.

39. Tria AJ, Klein KS: *An illustrated guide to the knee,* New York, 1992, Churchill Livingstone.

40. Valmassy RL, DeValentine SJ: Torsional and frontal plane conditions of the leg and idiopathic toe walking. In DeValentine S, editor: *Foot and ankle disorders in children,* New York, 1992, Churchill Livingstone.

41. Valmassy RL: Torsional and frontal plane conditions of the lower extremity. In Thomson P, editor: *Introduction to podopaediatrics,* London, 1993, WB Saunders.

42. Valmassy RL: *Clinical biomechanics of the lower extremities,* St Louis, 1996, Mosby.

43. Ziteli BJ, David HW: *Atlas of pediatric physical diagnosis,* St Louis, 1987, Mosby.

53

Pain Over Lateral Aspect of Hip and Proximal Thigh with Site of Maximal Tenderness Posterior to the Greater Trochanter

A 26-year-old graduate student plays college soccer and prefers the inside kick technique on the playing field. Before practice he maintains his level of stamina by running 3 miles along a banked road surface. Following a vigorous game last week he complains of aching pain that is deep and diffuse, although occasionally sharp over the lateral aspect of the right hip and thigh that radiates into the buttock and down toward the knee. Pain is reproduced when attempting to cross his right leg over his left leg while sitting, when lying on either side, and when ascending the stairs. He offers that he often falls upon, and receives blows to his right lateral side during athletic competition. When asked whether he stretches adequately before and after playing, he claims that he is very careful about stretching his hamstrings, quadriceps, and calf muscles. He offers that he is now taking nonsteroidal antiinflammatory medications to relieve his pain in conjunction with cold packs to the painful site.

OBSERVATION   This shows normal pelvic obliquity. Excessive pronation of the left foot is observed. No edema or ecchymosis is observed over the lateral right hip. No swelling noted over the right greater or lesser trochanters. A mild antalgic limp is noted with increased stance time on the left lower extremity.

PALPATION   Palpation over the posterolateral aspect of the greater trochanter reveals mild warmth and pain and maximal tenderness. Minimal crepitus is palpated over the greater trochanter with flexion and extension of the right hip joint. No point tenderness noted over the ischial tuberosities.

PASSIVE RANGE OF MOTION   Extreme internal rotation is painful.

ACTIVE RANGE OF MOTION   External rotation, adduction, as well as flexion and extension of the right hip are painful.

STRENGTH   This is normal; resisted abduction increases patient symptoms.

FLEXIBILITY   This shows tightness to bilateral iliotibial bands, and the right hamstring muscle.

SELECTIVE TENSION   Resistive right hip adduction reproduces pain whereas hip abduction does not.

JOINT PLAY   This is normal.

SPECIAL TESTS   Positive Patrick-Faber test. Normal leg lengths noted. Negative hop test, straight leg raising, and femoral nerve stretch tests.

? Questions

1. What is most likely causing this patient's symptoms?
2. What anatomy is relevant to understanding this pathology?
3. What is the anatomy of that longitudinal thickening of fascia lata known as the iliotibial band?
4. Why does the iliotibial band translate anteriorly with flexion and posteriorly with extension of the hip joint?
5. What is the traumatic mechanism of injury to the trochanteric bursa?
6. What biomechanical imbalance is implicated in the etiology of greater trochanteric bursitis?
7. Why are females more likely at risk in developing greater trochanteric bursitis?
8. What is the clinical presentation?
9. What is the "Faber" test and how does it detect for inflammation of the trochanteric bursa?
10. What is the differential diagnosis?
11. What other forms of bursitis may occur at the hip or pelvis?
12. What therapeutic intervention is appropriate in management of this condition?

1. What is most likely causing this patient's symptoms?

Greater trochanteric bursitis is the most common form of bursitis in the vicinity of the hip[27] and is frequently seen in soccer players.[51] This pathology is the second most frequent cause of lateral hip pain, after osteoarthritis.[36] Trochanteric bursitis has been reported in all age groups, although peak incidence occurs between the fourth and fifth decades of life,[39] except when occurring from external trauma, as in young soccer players. The male-to-female ratio for this condition is 2 to 4.[46] The pathogenesis of trochanteric bursitis is varied and stems from a variety of extrinsic and intrinsic factors. Understanding this overuse syndrome necessitates an appreciation of the anatomy of the region and the dynamic relationship of the iliotibial band to the greater trochanter during gait.

2. What anatomy is relevant to understanding this pathology?

Approximately 14 to 21 bursae have been described in the hip region.[8,41,50] Three bursae—2 major and 1 minor—are present in the vicinity of the greater trochanter (Fig. 53-1). The superficial trochanteric bursa, also known as the gluteus minimus bursa is a minor bursa that lies above and slightly anterior to the proximal superior surface of the greater trochanter.[39] The deep trochanteric bursa, otherwise known as the subgluteus medius bursa is a major bursa located beneath the gluteus medius muscle, situated posterior and superior to the proximal edge of the greater trochanter. The subgluteus maximus bursa is the other major peritrochanteric bursa that is consistently found, and is lateral to the greater trochanter. Functioning to facilitate gliding of the anterior portion of the gluteus maximus tendon as it passes over the greater trochanter to insert into the iliotibial band, this bursa lies beneath the converging fibers of the tensor fasciae latae and gluteus maximus muscles onto the fascia lata as they join to form the iliotibial tract. The subgluteus maximus bursa, representing a third bursa that may be implicated in trochanteric bursitis, is separated from the trochanter by the gluteus medius muscle.[39]

3. What is the anatomy of that longitudinal thickening of fascia lata known as the iliotibial band?

The *iliotibial band* (ITB) is a nonelastic, dense, collagenous, longitudinal thickening of the fascia lata that connects the ilium to the tibia[19] by extending from the pelvis across the lateral aspect of the knee. The fascia lata is a complete stockinglike investment of the thigh. En route in its downward descent, the fascia latae encounters the borders of both the *tensor fasciae lata femoris muscle,** and the *gluteus maximus muscle,* a powerful hip and trunk extensor that plays its greatest role in stair climbing and running.

---

*Note that *fascia latae* refers to the fascia investing the thigh, which elongates to become the iliotibial band, whereas the *fasciae lata* is a muscular structure.

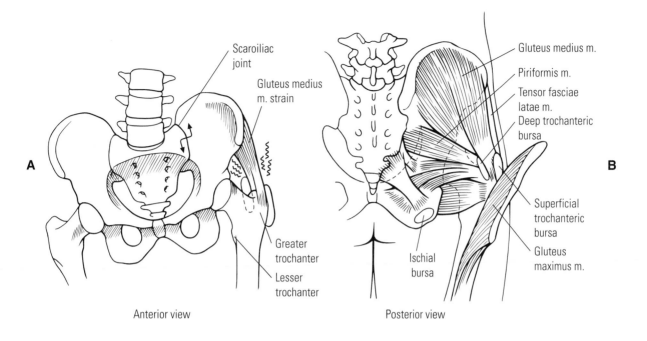

FIG. 53-1 Anatomic relationships between the trochanteric bursae and adjacent osseous and soft tissue. **A,** Anterior view. **B,** Posterior view.

Function of the gluteus maximus and the smaller tensor fasciae latae muscles may be viewed antagonistically in relation to their insertion into the iliotibial band. The proximal aspect of the ITB is held posterior to the hip axis at the level of the greater trochanter by the combined pull of the gluteus maximus posteriorly, the tensor fasciae latae muscle anteriorly, and maximus's deep attachment into the gluteal tuberosity of the femur. Both the tensor fasciae latae muscle and the gluteus maximus muscles insert into the ITB[33] so that their distal extent serves as a conjoint tendon for these muscles. The tensor fasciae latae muscle inserts on the anterior side of the ITB and works antagonistically by counteracting the backward pull of gluteus maximus. The antagonistic function of these two muscles is borne out by their opposite actions, namely thigh extension, adduction, and lateral rotation as compared to thigh flexion, abduction, and medial rotation. Thus the pelvis is dynamically balanced by the opposing forces of these two muscles in the sagittal plane. Although the tensor fasciae latae generates a moment to tilt the pelvis anteriorly, the gluteus maximus works to posteriorly tilt the pelvis. The dynamic balance between these muscles maintains neutral pelvic obliquity.

4. Why does the iliotibial band translate anteriorly with flexion and posteriorly with extension of the hip joint?

Because the origin of the of the ITB lies posterior to the level of the hip axis at the level of the greater trochanter, ITB proximally functions to help maintain the hip in extension. With movement of the lower extremity, during walking and running, the ITB translates anteriorly and posteriorly relative to the hip joint axis. Swing phase of gait is characterized by shortening of the swing leg via flexion of the hip and knee joints to permit ground clearance. During the swing phase of gait the hip flexor action of the tensor fasciae latae pulls the ITB anterior to the greater trochanter, and thereby improving its leverage to assist with hip flexion. The ITB generates maximal tension anterior to the hip joint between swing and midstance phases of gait.

Just after heel strike the tibia rotates medially as a function of subtalar joint pronation and knee flexion due to unlocking of the screw-home mechanism. This has the effect of tensing the distal aspect of ITB (at Gerdy's tubercle) pulling it away from its proximal origin. At the same time, the tensor fasciae latae muscle contracts in an effort to stabilize the pelvis. This represents a proximal source of tension to the ITB, and may be thought of as a tug-of-war along the length of ITB causing it to rub over the greater trochanter during midstance. At midstance, ITB undergoes a reversal in the direction of translation at both the hip and knee as it once again assumes its original position as an extensor of both the hip and knee.[31] As the now tense ITB returns to its original position, it rubs across the bony prominence of the greater trochanter (see Fig. 48-1). This is the basis for repetitive friction and subsequent microtrauma that may culminate in snapping hip syndrome or greater trochanteric bursitis.

5. What is the traumatic mechanism of injury to the trochanteric bursa?

The two inciting factors implicated in injury to the greater trochanteric bursa in soccer players include repetitive inside kicks and recurrent blows and falls sustained to the bony prominence of the greater trochanter causing contusion to the underlying bursa.[51] In the former, repetitive and forceful adduction associated with inside kicking maximally tenses the iliotibial band and compresses the bursa against the greater trochanter.

In the event of a fall or blow, the superficial bursa may become the site for bleeding (haemobursa). Although minor bleeding spontaneously resolves, a major bleed may result in clot formation that may cause adhesions or undergo calcification and contribute to chronic inflammation and fluid effusion. These may be palpated as crepitus over the greater trochanter.[32] Calcification in the region of the greater trochanter in association with bursitis is common,[24] and may be found in either the tendons of the gluteal muscle or the surrounding bursae.[14] When calcification occurs within the tendon it is referred to as enthesopathy of the gluteus medius tendon insertion. Enthesopathy is a rheumatologic term referring to a locus of inflammation at the site of ligament, tendon, or joint capsule attachment to bone in which microtears at the soft-tissue–bone junction give rise to bone spurring and are accompanied by joint stiffness and pain. Calcification varies in shape and size, from a few millimeters to 3 to 4 cm in diameter, appearing as linear or small rounded masses that are either separated or grouped together.[39]

6. What biomechanical imbalance is implicated in the etiology of greater trochanteric bursitis?

Trochanteric bursitis may occur from alteration in the biomechanics of the lower extremity. A common cause of bursitis relates to the iliotibial band, a dynamic structure over the bursa, which moves anteriorly with flexion and posteriorly with extension. If flexibility of the iliotibial band is compromised, it may rub across the greater trochanteric bursa with excessive force, resulting in inflammation of the bursa. This may occur from a variety of intrinsic or extrinsic factors, or both. Intrinsic factors contributing toward bursal irritation may include running with asymmetric pelvic height (pelvic obliquity), which causes an imbalance in normal length between the adductors and abductor muscles. Similarly, an imbalance in muscle strength between the adductors and abductors caused, for example, by a previous injury with residual weakness, or a contracture of the gluteus medius may concentrate stress at the greater trochanter.[40] Moreover, excessive stress in the various muscle attachments to the greater trochanter may also initiate bursal inflammation. The terrain may also be a contributing factor toward developing bursitis.[23] Running with one foot lower than the other, such as on a banked surface, may simulate a leg-length discrepancy, as would running with one foot excessively pronated. Here the pronated foot corresponds to the shorter extremity, whereas a supinated foot is relatively higher owing to the stacking of the talus atop the calcaneus. This mechanism may also occur from running on or off curbs, or with a poor running gait such as crossing feet over midline.[7] In the latter, abnormal running mechanics increase the adduction angle causing a rise in friction between the trochanter and the overlying ITB. The final common etiologic pathway resulting in pathology is one in which the longer lower limb is postured in obligatory adduction in relation to the hip joint, causing trochanteric bursitis to occur in the longer of two legs.[2] Adduction of the longer leg results in tension of the ipsilateral ITB, which in turn compresses the bursa against the greater trochanter. When this happens as the ITB moves to and fro over the greater trochanter during gait, the underlying bursa is subject to excessive friction and may develop inflammation. Prolonged sitting approximates the origin and insertion of ITB, and in the typical armchair executive results in tightness of the ITB and excessive stress concentration over the greater trochanter during ambulation.

7. Why are females more likely at risk in developing greater trochanteric bursitis?

Inflammation of the greater trochanteric bursa is common in the female runner because of the broad configuration of the female pelvis.[40] Women have wider pelvises (gynecoid) compared with men (android), and hence a greater varus angulation of the hip and valgus of the knees. There is greater prominence of the greater trochanter as a direct function of the wider female pelvis. This causes additional longitudinal stretch of the ITB along its length in females. An increase in the Q angle in females is present as a direct function of the greater varus angulation of the hip present in females. As such, ITB pathology may be more common proximally than distally over the lateral femoral condyle. This tautening effect of the ITB may be highlighted by the presence of femoral anteversion, which serves to increase the Q angle. The presence of femoral anteversion is greater in females than males.[44]

8. What is the clinical presentation?

Patients may or may not present a history of antecedent trauma. Pain is deep, aching, intermittent, and diffuse[30] at the greater trochanter and may radiate to the distal lateral thigh (pseudoradiculopathy), groin, and gluteal areas[48] with maximal tenderness laterally over the greater trochanter. The quality of the pain may be sharp and intense, and extends into the thigh in less than half of all cases.[15] Pain may increase with certain hip motions such as external rotation and abduction, as the insertions of these muscles attach upon the greater trochanter and causes rubbing of the adjacent sensitive bursae. Internal hip rotation is not painful.[48] Because a bursa is an inert and noncontractile structure, resistive abduction is painless whereas resistive adduction would elicit pain.[9] The patient may exhibit an antalgic limp[32] with asymmetrical stance time. Pain may be provoked by standing up out of a deep chair, stair climbing, running, or lying on the affected side. Rolling over in bed onto the affected trochanter may cause nocturnal pain. Lying on the unaffected side may cause pain because the hip with the inflamed trochanteric bursa may fall into adduction, thus stretching the fascia lata over the prominence of the greater trochanter. For similar reasons, there is usually a positive Ober test (see Fig. 48-9), while sitting cross-legged is also uncomfortable. Obvious swelling, redness, and heat so common in others forms of bursitis, is unusual because the trochanteric bursae are relatively deeply placed structures to a substantial number of muscular insertions.[39] Crepitus may be present. No specific radiographic findings are diagnostic of trochanteric bursitis. Bursal aspiration may yield serous, blood-tinged, or entirely clear fluid.[51]

9. What is the "Faber" test and how does it detect for inflammation of the trochanteric bursa?

The Patrick test is also known as the Faber test (flexion, abduction, and external rotation), which is the position of the hip when the patient begins the test. This test, which postures the lower limb into the "number four," stretches the anterior hip capsule, and is used to detect an inflammatory disease of the hip,[49] sacroiliac joint dysfunction, and spasm of iliopsoas.[26] Incidentally, these same motions will provoke pain in an already inflamed trochanteric bursa by way of applying pressure to it via stretching or compression of adjacent soft-tissue structures. More that half of all patients with trochanteric bursitis exhibit pain on Patrick-Faber testing.[15] This test is performed with the patient lying supine, with the test leg so positioned that the foot of that leg lays atop the opposite knee. The clinician then slowly lowers the knee of the test leg toward the examining table, forcing the involved hip into maximal abduction and external rotation. Although a negative test is indicated by the test leg failing to lie in a plane parallel with the opposite leg, a positive test is indicated by a test leg that remains above the contralateral leg in which the knee points upward. A positive score affirms the restriction of hip joint range of motion.

10. What is the differential diagnosis?

The diagnosis of trochanteric bursitis is clinically determined and often confirmed by resolution of symptoms after glucocorticoid intrabursal injection.[39] The absence of painful movement on hip flexion and extension helps distinguish trochanteric bursitis from intraarticular hip disease.[39] The differential diagnoses should encompass other conditions that may cause hip or low back pain and include:

- *Snapping hip syndrome.* This refers to painful irritation of the proximal iliotibial band over the greater trochanter. The complaint of painful snapping hip is commonly encountered in ballet dancers, and may either present laterally or inferomedially. Anteroposterior movement of the iliotibial band over the greater trochanter causes a snapping or clicking sensation over the lateral hip that is often incurred during rotational movements of the supported lower extremity. Factors contributing to this snapping include a tight iliotibial band, narrow bi-iliac width, muscular imbalance, and decreased soft-tissue flexibility. Because of the close association between the superficial trochanteric bursa and the tensor fasciae latae, differentiating snapping hip syndrome (see p. 745) from greater trochanteric bursitis is difficult. Nevertheless, greater trochanteric bursitis manifests as pain that is more posterior to the greater trochanter, and that can often radiate into the buttock.[25] However, trochanteric bursitis may develop secondary to snapping hip syndrome.[40]

- *Gluteus medius muscle strain.* This may occur in association with chronic tendinitis of its attachment to the greater trochanter, and is seen in football, swimming, or ice hockey. An association between gluteus medius strain and pronated feet may exist.[6] Although passive range of motion is painless, resisted abduction provokes symptoms. Pinpoint tenderness occurs over the greater trochanter. If an acute strain of gluteus medius occurs, prompt attention is essential as the gluteus medius is the primary lateral hip stabilizer. Mild weakness resulting from an unattended strain may have negative repercussions on the biomechanics of the entire hip and pelvis region. The gluteus medius is a hip abductor in the open kinetic chain, which, in the closed kinetic chain stabilizes the pelvis when weight is put on one leg. Slight weakness of the gluteus medius causes adduction of the hip in relation to the pelvis with an ipsilateral high pelvis and lumbar curvature toward the opposite side. Similarly, gluteus medius strain may occur in persons with leg length discrepancy.[34] With pronounced weakness, the abductors cannot keep the pelvis horizontal when weight is placed upon a single leg (gluteus medius limp).[40] Contracture of this muscle may result from a coxa vara deformity[27] and results in an abduction deformity.[40] Management is by daily stretching and strengthening of the hip abductors, and a 5° or 9° medial hindfoot wedge.[34]

- *Bone contusion.* The greater trochanter is the most frequently contused area of the hip[20] and is often injured from a fall or collision. A bone contusion represents the mildest level of bone injury and causes bleeding into the surrounding deep tissue. The greater trochanter is particularly vulnerable because of its superficial location. Greater trochanteric contusion may give rise to greater trochanteric bursitis.[40]

- *Stress fractures of the femoral neck.* Femoral neck fractures are potentially career ending injuries if misdiagnosed.[25] If undetected, a femoral neck stress fracture can lead to disastrous results with displacement and the possibility of inducing avascular necrosis.[18,28] Displaced femoral neck fractures represent surgical emergencies.[12] Stress fractures (see pp. 504-505) are a severe form of overuse injury, which occur

when bone is subjected to a magnitude of stress that outpaces the ability of osseous tissue to adapt by the normal process of work hypertrophy.[37] Although femoral stress fractures typically occur in the older athlete, the younger athlete more likely experiences tibial stress fractures. Risk factors include biomechanical malalignments of the lower extremity including excessive genu varum, tibial varum, subtalar joint varus, and forefoot varus.[40] These malalignments may cause suboptimal loading of the femoral neck and thereby contribute to stress fracture.

Stress fractures are characterized by a sudden onset of pain and a recent change in activity level.[45] There may be an antalgic gait, deep tenderness in the anterior aspect of the hip, and slight limitation of flexion and internal rotation with discomfort at the extremes of these movements. In the early stages, localized pain is present that worsen with activity and improves with rest.[45] As with trochanteric bursitis, localized tenderness may occur at the greater trochanter, although injection with a local anesthetic will not obliterate pain as it does with trochanteric bursitis.[48] Pain may be present on single leg stance, and a painful Trendelenburg gait may be present.[25] Radiographs of femoral neck stress fractures are often negative[5] for as long as 4 to 6 weeks.[21] When a stress fracture is suspected, a bone scan (scintigraphy) allows for early detection.[13] Clinical determination of the presence of a stress fracture is the hop test in which the patient attempts to hop on the injured leg, invariably reproducing the pain.[40] Although medial rotation may be painful in a femoral neck stress fracture, this is not the case in trochanteric bursitis.[48]

Management of stress fractures is determined by the type of fracture. A tension-side cortical bone fracture manifests as a transverse break across the femoral neck. If undisplaced, complete bed rest is required.[12] If displacement has occurred, then internal fixation by way of percutaneous pinning is mandatory to halt progressive displacement that may lead to avascular necrosis, varus deformity, or nonunion. In contrast, compression-side fractures are less likely to undergo displacement, and conservative treatment with gradual protected weight bearing with crutches may be indicated.

- *High lumbar radiculopathy.* This is characterized by pain, paresthesia, and weakness in the dermatomal and myotomal distribution of the upper lumbar levels. The L2 nerve root is predominantly responsible for hip flexion via the iliopsoas muscle, and makes a major contribution to hip adduction. The L2 root contributes to the cremasteric reflex. The L3 nerve root contributes significantly to knee extension (quadriceps) and the hip adductors. The adductor jerk is an L3 reflex conveyed through the obturator nerve. The patient with greater trochanteric bursitis does not demonstrate weakness or sensory loss consistent with nerve root pathology. Moreover, a femoral nerve stretch will be positive with lumbar radiculopathy.

- *Slipped capital femoral epiphysis.* This is an uncommon condition referring to displacement of the epiphysis of the femoral head (capitus) that differs from traumatic epiphyseal fractures because the displacement occurs through a different area of the growth plate. This childhood condition is the anatomic equivalent of an intracapsular fracture of the adult femoral neck, which cuts off the blood supply to the femoral head.[10] This condition, occurring during the adolescent growth spurt before epiphyseal plate closure, is twice as frequent in boys than girls;[17] occurs more often in blacks; bilaterally in approximately one quarter of all patients; and most commonly occurs between 10 and 17 years of age with an average age of onset of 12 years.[31] There is a strong familial pattern with incidence among family members higher than the general population.[35] Multiple etiologies have been linked to mechanical failure of the growth plate. In particular, this condition has been linked to subtle endocrine imbalance and is reflected by the occurrence of disease in children of two somatic body types: those who are tall and thin and those who are large and obese and exhibit delayed sexual maturation. It may be that hormonal changes at the time of puberty contribute to loss of mechanical integrity of the growth plate. These children may be predisposed to this condition so that mechanical injury may precipitate slippage of the femoral head.

The adolescent hip is biomechanically vulnerable because the position of the proximal femoral growth plate normally changes from horizontal to oblique during puberty, thus subjecting the epiphyseal plate to shear forces.[31] An associated growth spurt and accompanying rapid weight gain during preadolescence and adolescence amplify the shear stress such that loading across the joint is approximately four times body weight.[46] The growth plate at the femoral head is relatively weaker than other skeletal components during puberty. Overloading of the growth plate results in failure due to excessive mechanical stresses that exceed the strength of the plate.

Softening of the physeal junction between the femoral head and neck weakens. As a result of weight-bearing forces and muscular pull, the femoral head, gradually or suddenly, slips downward and backward within the acetabulum giving the radiological appearance of a scoop of ice cream sliding off a cone.[29] The femoral neck, in turn, migrates superiorly and rotates externally. Classification of slippage may be described either on the duration (in weeks) of the pathologic process, the amount of slippage measured according to the diameter of the femoral head, or the amount of angulation of the head relative to the neck.

Detection of slipped upper femoral epiphysis is difficult because symptoms are insidious while pain is often referred to the knee. The typical presentation is groin pain that is referred to the anteromedial thigh, and often confined to the area of the vastus medialis. There may be a history of injury if the presentation is acute. Chronic, or graduate slipping is the most common variety in which an antalgic limb accompanies mild aching pain and loss of hip motion, especially medial rotation. When long-standing, the slipping progresses, manifesting as an abductor lurch and out-toeing gait[46] as well as a hip flexion contracture. Because the femoral head is slipping down and behind its normal location, external rotation and adduction of the hip will be accentuated as these motions bring the femoral head into its normal relationship with the acetabulum.[29] Consequently, a limitation in range of motion of flexion, abduction, and internal rotation will occur. When suspected, the best screening for chronic slipped upper femoral epiphysis is to position the patient in the prone posture and assess for symmetry of medial hip rotation.[46] Alternately, flexing the suspected hip causes the hip to roll into external rotation and abduction. The acute presentation of a slipped epiphyses is very much like that of a femoral neck fracture, with the involved leg slightly shorter and externally rotated.[10] The sudden onset of pain is so severe as to preclude weight bearing. Radiographic confirmation is best performed with lateral views, which provide the best assessment without the possibility of further slip from a frog lateral view.[20]

The goal of management is stabilization of the growth plate to prevent further slippage. Without intervention, the femoral head heals to the neck in a grossly abnormal position, resulting in joint incongruity and accompanying arthritis. Forceful manipulation to achieve reduction is contraindicated as damage to the blood supply to the femoral head may occur and lead to avascular necrosis. Whether or not any reduction can be achieved by gentle repositioning, the physeal plate is stabilized with pins or screw fixation. Correct pin placement is essential to avoid damage to the blood supply of the femoral head.

- *Osteomyelitis.* This refers to infection of the bone marrow by bacteria,* fungi, or mycobacteria and takes two forms, depending on the source of contamination. Exogenous osteomyelitis involves direct contamination caused by the spread of nearby infection,† open fractures, surgical procedures, pressure ulcers, and third-degree burns causing bone penetration and contamination. Hematogenous osteomyelitis results from infection carried in the bloodstream. Hematogenous osteomyelitis may arise from a clinically evident infection elsewhere in the body including the throat, teeth, skin, urinary tract, gastrointestinal tract, and lungs.[31] Osteomyelitis of the skull typically arises from dental or sinus infections. In diabetic patients, or those with atherosclerotic arterial insufficiency of the lower extremities, pathogens usually reach bone by entering the soft tissues through a cutaneous foot ulcer. Diabetic feet are particularly susceptible to bone infection, secondary to chronic skin ulceration, due to a combination of immunocompromise and vascular insufficiency. These distant infections produce showers of bacteria into the bloodstream that are usually cleared by the reticuloendothelial system, although some escape this filtration, and settle in bones with a good blood supply and rich marrow.

Children, having an immature immune system, are particularly susceptible to bacterial infections. In children, the most common sites of seeding are the ends of long bones, particularly in metaphyseal bone near the epiphyseal plate at the end of the shaft and just beneath the growth plate. Here, the large terminal branches of the metaphyseal arteries form loops as they meet the relatively smaller caliber venous sinusoids. This causes an abrupt change in the dynamics of blood flow at this region causing turbulence as the speed of blood flow is suddenly slowed. This allows bacteria to congregate and proliferate as a focus of infection, especially because little phagocytic activity occurs in the region of the venous sinusoids. Thus the region beneath the growth plate represents an ideal environment for bacterial growth. Alternately, disease may be initiated following relatively minor trauma, possibly because the trauma causes a small hematoma from rupture of very profuse vessels near the epiphyseal plate of the proximal femur. This provides an ideal breeding ground for bacteria reaching this site from the bloodstream.[10] Because fat replaces marrow in these sites during adolescence, causing a substantial reduction in vasculature, hematogenous osteomyelitis in the long bones of adults is rare.

In adults, the vertebrae are the most common location for the development of hematogenous osteomyelitis. Hemodialysis patients and drug abusers are particularly prone to hematogenous osteomyelitis in the clavicle or pubic bone. In addition to trauma, osteomyelitis may occur in areas of bone damaged by radiation therapy or malignancy. Radiation destroys adjacent soft tissue and damages periosteum causing bone and surrounding soft tissue to become more vulnerable to infection.

Once bone is seeded, rapid pathogen duplication creates a localized abscess just beneath the growth plate and extends along Volkmann's canals along the shaft of the bone. At this point the disease is in its acute state. Once this occurs, the infection assumes control of a portion of blood supply to the shaft and is directly nourished. What follows is that the devitalized portion of cortical bone, known as a sequestrum, acts as a nidus for persistent infection as it now lacks a blood supply to deliver antibiotics or inflammatory cells to fight infection. Infection erodes the surrounding bone and pus elevates the periosteum. The infection works inside out, as pus ruptures through the periosteum, extends to the subcutaneous tissue, and eventually discharges through the skin creating a draining sinus releasing a foul odor. At this stage the patient has *chronic osteomyelitis.*[10] If discharge occurs into a joint space, septic arthritis will ensue.‡ Chronic osteomyelitis has disastrous complications including nonunion, deformity following growth arrest, and skin cancer at the margin of the sinus, which may even require amputation.

---

*Similar to infectious arthritis, *Staphylococcus aureus* is the most common pathogen.

†Soft tissue infection as apparently insignificant as a felon. An infection of the pulp of the fingertip may cause infection of the distal phalanx.

‡The course of osteomyelitis does not always occur in this manner. The infection may be entirely overcome by natural defenses or partly overcome and remain confined in an abscess lined by cortical bone known as Brodie's abscess. Brodie's abscess acts to quarantine quiescent pathogens within a small cavity, out of harm's way to the body.

Clinical manifestations include pain in the infected bone and fever that is accompanied by malaise, decreased appetite, and generalized weakness. The latter may precede pain several days. Pain may be excruciating owing to rising tissue tension within bone.[10] Point tenderness and warmth are present at the hip, and pain is provoked when the hip is moved. Active range of hip motion is diminished, and the child is reluctant to stand or walk. Elevated sedimentation and white blood cell counts are typical. Radiographs show bone destruction as radiopaque sequestra, which usually take 3 or more weeks to become visible. Medical management includes administration of bacteria-specific antibiotics. If the patient has not shown signs of clinical improvement in 2 days, the affected area of bone is exposed and drilled to release pus. Exogenous osteomyelitis is prevented following open fracture with thorough debridement of contaminated bone and administration of broad-spectrum antibiotics.

• *Transient synovitis of the hip joint.* This is also known as toxic synovitis, it is a self-limiting nonbacterial inflammatory condition of unknown etiology that causes unilateral hip pain in children less than 10 years of age.[47] In more than half of all patients, an upper respiratory infection preceded the onset of synovitis.[43] The pathogenesis remains obscure but has been postulated to be related to trauma, infection, or allergy. The child may report a gradual or acute onset of pain in the inguinal region, thigh, or knee, an antalgic limp, and restriction in range of motion. Synovial effusion within the hip joint capsule causes the hip to assume the open packed position of flexion, abduction, and external rotation.[37] Other conditions that mimic transient synovitis include Legg-Calvé-Perthes disease,[42] rheumatoid arthritis, and septic arthritis. Joint aspiration and blood tests are of value when septic arthritis is suspect. As much as 10% of all cases of transient synovitis progress to Perthes disease, which is suspected if mild synovitis persists or if synovitis recurs. Because of this, following resolution of synovitis, children should have radiographs of their hip joint taken to detect the earliest evidence of Perthes' disease, should it occur.[37] Transient synovitis has a benign course with resolution occurring over several days to 1 week. Treatment consists of bed rest with the hip postured in the position that is most comfortable for the patient. Traction is contraindicated as it increases intraarticular pressure. Activity is allowed to increase if the hip can be rotated smoothly without guarding or limitation in the arc of motion.[43]

• *Infectious arthritis.* This refers to arthritis resulting from infection of the synovial tissues lining an articular joint due to an infectious agent such as bacteria, virus, fungi, and yeast. Bacteria (causing septic arthritis) are the most common pathogenic organism, typically *Staphylococcus aureus* and gonococci in adults and *Haemophilus influenzae* in toddlers and infants. Viral infections such as rubella, mumps, or hepatitis B may also be implicated.[3] Pathogenic agents may be blood borne (hematogenous) or introduced directly from an external source such as a penetrating wound, surgery, or intraarticular injection. Diabetic patients are particularly susceptible to infection. Hematogenous infectious arthritis is particularly common in children, especially at the hip as the femoral head has a precariously vulnerable blood supply. The blood vessels supplying the femoral head course through the femoral neck inside the joint capsule. The pathogen reaches the joint from the bloodstream via direct seeding or indirectly settling in the metaphyseal bone and breaking through into the joint. Microorganisms first invade the synovial membrane surrounding the joint where they compete with chondrocytes for synovial fluid nourishment and proliferate. This incites an acute inflammatory process that ushers in leukocytes. Accumulating pus distends the capsule and increases pressure and may compress the nutrient vessels and diminish blood supply to the vulnerable femoral head. This alone may cause osteonecrosis if the pressure persists for more than a few hours, with ensuing epiphyseal growth arrest, and eventual arthritis. Moreover, degradative enzymes released from the bacteria and leukocytes rapidly erode articular cartilage, resulting in severe irreversible structural damage to the articular surface, permanent deformity, limb-length discrepancy, and early arthritis.

Detection of infectious arthritis requires a high index of suspicion in adults and children presenting with chills, fever, and monoarticular arthritis. Infectious arthritis represents a medical emergency, which, if not identified, has the devastating consequences of joint destruction and bony ankylosis. Clinical manifestations include fever and acute pain, tenderness, and holding of the involved joint in the open packed position. The systemic response in infants may be deceiving as it may present with a normal temperature and white blood cell count. Elevated sedimentation will, however, be present. In the case of gonococcal arthritis, commonly occurring in the adult, this condition may follow a more generalized arthritis and feverish state that evolves into monoarticular arthritis. Following acute and incapacitating pain of a single joint, cutaneous lesions frequently appear on the limbs and trunk.[31] Management is by (diagnostic) joint aspiration, antibiotics, surgical drainage, and irrigation. Rehabilitation may be required to address any residual dysfunction of the joint.

- *Avascular necrosis.* This is also known as *aseptic necrosis* and *osteonecrosis* and refers to bone death in the absence of infection. Avascular necrosis commonly occurs in bones such as the femoral head, the scaphoid, and talar head, which derive the majority of their blood supply from the medullary cavity rather than the periosteum or surrounding soft tissue.[10] This may occur to the femoral head following a femoral neck fracture or femoral head dislocation, or idiopathically. The femoral head is especially susceptible to avascular necrosis as virtually all the vessels to the femoral head traverse the femoral neck. A high femoral neck fracture, known as an intracapsular fracture involves a fracture line inside the capsule. Because of this, blood is contained within the capsule thereby raising intracapsular pressure and causing tamponade of the blood vessels to the femoral head. Avascular necrosis may occur at any time postoperatively, even up to 20 years later[16] and may occur in part or all of the head. Alcoholism may be related to incidence of avascular necrosis of the femoral head.[10] An athlete with a history of high-dose steroid usage is also at increased risk.[25] The prognosis is worse for adults as regrowth is no longer possible. Clinical findings include unexplained aching at the hip joint and complaints of being unable to sit for prolonged periods because of stiffness. The patient may exhibit a limp. During the early stages of avascular necrosis, the avascular segment of dead bone is characterized by a very dense appearance on radiograph. This is because the surrounding living bone, undergoes disuse osteoporosis, a normal phenomenon seen in the early stages of fracture healing. The necrotic fragment however, does not undergo osteoporosis and appears relatively dense.[31] A bone scan and magnetic resonance imaging are indicated if avascular necrosis is suspected. If complete head collapse has occurred in the adult, then a prosthetic replacement is performed. If the condition is not severe, physical therapy maintains strength and mobility of the joint. Assistive devices, and a home exercise program are also prescribed.

11. What other forms of bursitis may occur at the hip or pelvis?

ISCHIAL BURSITIS

This is also known as ischiogluteal bursitis, or *tailor* or *weaver's bottom,*[22] or *bench warmer's bursitis*[40] occurs much less frequently than trochanteric bursitis and is much easier to treat.[27] This bursa lies between the ischial tuberosity and the gluteus maximus muscle, and is most often inflamed in individuals whose occupations require prolonged sitting on a hard surface, particularly with the legs crossed as this focuses both body weight and the weight of the crossed leg upon a single ischial tuberosity. Weavers extend first one leg, and then the other during their work, causing excessive friction to the bursa. This leads to inflammation of the bursal walls, which causes painful swelling.[30] Bursitis may also occur from a direct blow to the ischial bursa following a fall onto the buttocks. In soccer players, the mechanism is often from repeated falls onto the buttocks, or following drills that emphasize speed work.[51] Clinical findings include tenderness upon palpation around the ischial tuberosities during stair climbing, or even walking as both require gluteus maximus contraction. Consequently, jumping or stair climbing may provoke symptoms. Tight hamstrings may occur secondary to pain. Subsequently, hip or trunk flexion compresses the painful bursa and reproduces pain. Sitting provokes symptoms as soon as the ischium touches the chair, especially if the chair is hard, but eases the moment the patient stands up.[9] The common practice of carrying one's wallet in the back pocket may aggravate symptoms. If the adjacent sciatic nerve becomes irritated from bursal swelling, symptoms of sciatica may manifest[22] as pain radiating to the hamstrings. Treatment involves having the patient sit with chair padding or use of a donut pad. Acute pain is eased by using ice whereas the subacute state is managed by heat. Phonophoresis with analgesic, and hamstring stretching are often helpful, as are nonsteroidal antiinflammatory medications.

ILIOPECTINEAL BURSITIS

This is also known as psoas bursitis. The iliopectineal bursa lies deep to the tendon of the iliopsoas over the front of the hip joint. A common cause of bursitis is osteoarthritis of the hip articulation, which causes incongruity of the joint surfaces, shortening of the limb, and consequently altered biomechanics immediate to, and distal to the hip. Bursitis may also be caused by a tight iliopsoas muscle, as may occur in prolonged sitting. Clinical signs include pain upon passive stretch of the iliopsoas during hip extension in the prone posture, active hip extension, and isometric tensing of the iliopsoas muscle during resisted flexion.[27] The patient typically complains of disabling pain in the groin and anterior thigh that causes an antalgic gait. The person may assume a position of flexion and external rotation of the hip.[40]Adduction during hip flexion is the most painful movement as this squeezes the bursa. Although passive lateral rotation is painful, medial rotation is not.[9] Maximal point tenderness is found over the inguinal area. Pain in the anterior knee may occur from irritation or compression of the adjacent femoral nerve (neuritis), especially if the bursitis is large. The bursa may grow so large as to be misinterpreted as a primary bone or soft-tissue malignancy.[4] Patients with iliopectineal bursitis may display hip flexor tightness, because flexion of the anterior thigh musculature may relieve painful tension over the bursa. A hip flexion contracture may be present,[27] particularly in persons who must sit a great deal. The iliopectineal bursa may communicate with the hip joint. Differential diagnoses for this condition includes: ganglion cysts, glenoid labrum tears, or primary degenerative arthritis of the hip, and a femoral hernia.[40] Decompressive surgery is recommended for patients who feel embarrassed by the large proportions the bursa may grow.[40] Treatment includes addressing osteoarthritis if present, stretching of the iliopsoas muscle if muscle tightness is found, nonsteroidal antiinflammatory medications, and ultrasound application.

12. What therapeutic intervention is appropriate in management of this condition?

With prompt and appropriate symptomatic management, most patients with trochanteric bursitis recover satisfactorily. The disadvantages of resolving trochanteric bursitis with a peritrochanteric intrabursal corticosteroid injection includes adverse effects including sterile abscess, granulomatous reaction, soft tissue and nerve injury, and skin atrophy, especially with repeated injections.[39] Although this approach alone may offer temporary relief, it does not consider the biomechanical pathogenesis of trochanteric bursitis and may only provide a short-term solution to a condition that may return. Identification of the specific pathokinesiology

causing the lower extremity malalignment and addressing its resolution is the surest approach toward preventing recurrence. Only rarely is surgical release of the tight fascia over the trochanter and excision of the bursal sac with removal of any calcified tissue performed, and is reserved for refractory and recalcitrant cases.

Bursitis may be acutely managed with cryotherapy and iontophoresis with an analgesic, and possibly nonsteroidal antiinflammatory medications. Rest from athletic activity is essential. Phonophoresis with ultrasound may be used.[25] Using a unilateral assistive device in the contralateral upper extremity may alleviate some pain. Identification of any lower extremity malalignment is imperative. Although a medial hindfoot wedge is prescribed for the over-pronated foot, a lateral hindfoot wedge is applied to the cavovarus foot type.[34] Leg length discrepancies must be balanced by a lift placed in the shoe on the short side. Stretching of the iliotibial band[11] should begin immediately. Because the dense fibrous distal portion of the iliotibial tract cannot be stretched effectively, the therapist should address the more pliable proximal fascia lata adjacent to the tensor fasciae latae and gluteus maximus muscles.

Passive stretching of the iliotibial band-tensor fascia lata complex using the Ober test position and statically holding the lower extremity in the final test position is an effective stretching procedure. This is more effectively performed by two persons. However, those patients with hip flexion contractures will additionally require stretching of the iliopsoas and the anterior hip capsule. Repeating this maneuver twice daily while applying gentle pressure on the thigh in the adducted position helps to effectively stretch those muscles. Alternately, an ITB stretch is performed by the therapist positioning the patient on the affected side and pulling the lower leg up off the table. The patient may also benefit from stretching of the gluteus maximus, hamstrings, quadriceps, abductor, and adductor muscles and those in the low back. Stretching may more easily be performed by applying moist heat to facilitate improved extensibility of soft tissue. Stretching may also be facilitated by contract-relax techniques or other forms of proprioceptive neuromuscular facilitation. Strengthening is an important component of rehabilitation. Any strength deficits should be addressed by beginning with multiple angle isometrics and short arc exercises in a nonpainful range. Although full range isotonic and isokinetic exercises may be helpful in the later stages of rehabilitation, they should preferably not be performed by patients with symptomatic ITB tendinitis.

A home exercise program must include teaching the patient to stretch the ITB in both the standing and lateral positions as these, although less effective, can be performed without the assistance of a therapist. Such maneuvers include the modified Ober, crossover toe touch, standing lateral fascial stretch, and the lateral hip drop stretches. A complete home program also includes strengthening and supplemental exercises. Deep tissue massage distal to the greater trochanter also facilitates improved tissue extensibility.

RECOMMENDED READING

Jones DL, Erhard RE: Diagnosis of trochanteric bursitis versus femoral neck stress fracture, *Phys Ther* 77(1):58-67, January, 1997.

Shbeeb MI, Matteson EL: Trochanteric bursitis (greater trochanteric pain syndrome), *Mayo Clin Proc* 71(6):565-569, 1996.

REFERENCES

1. Arendt EA, Clohisy DR: Stress injuries of bone. In Nicholas JA, Hershman EB editors: *The lower extremity and spine in sports medicine,* ed 2, St Louis, 1995, Mosby.
2. Baxter DE: The foot in running. In Mann RA, editor: *Surgery of the foot,* St Louis, 1986, Mosby.
3. Berkow R: *The Merck manual of diagnosis and therapy,* ed 15, Rahway, N.J., 1987, Merck Sharp & Dohme Research Laboratories.
4. Blinck R, Levinsohn EM: Enlarged iliopsoas bursa: an unusual pain, *Clin Orthop* 224:158, 1987.
5. Brake D: Imaging of femoral neck stress fracture, *Kan Med* 95:49, 1994.
6. Brody D: Rehabilitation of the injured runner. In *American Academy of Orthopedic Surgeons' instructional course lecture,* St Louis, 1984, Mosby.
7. Brody DM: *Running injuries,* Clinical Symposia, Summit, N.J., 1987, CIBA-GEIGY.
8. Bywaters EGL: The bursae of the body (editorial), *Ann Rheum Dis* 24:215-218, 1965.
9. Cyriax J: Diagnosis of soft tissue lesions. In Cyriax J, Coldham M: *Textbook of orthopaedic medicine,* vol 1, London, 1982, Bailliere Tindall.
10. Dandy DJ: *Essential orthopaedics and trauma,* ed 2, Edinburgh, 1993, Churchill Livingstone.
11. Dugas R, D'Ambrosia RD: Causes and treatment of common overuse injuries in runners. *J Musculoskeletal Med* 68, May 1991.
12. Fullerton LR, Snowdy HA: Femoral neck stress fractures, *Am J Sports Med* 1988:16:365-377.
13. Geslien GE, Thrall JH, Espinosa JL et al: Early detection of stress fractures using 99m Tc-polyphosphate, *Radiology* 121:683, 1976.
14. Reference deleted.
15. Gordon EJ: Trochanteric bursitis and tendinitis, *Clin Orthop* 20:193-202, 1961.
16. Iverson L, Clawson D: *Manual of acute orthopaedic therapeutics,* Boston, 1982, Little, Brown, and Company.

17. Jacobs B: Diagnosis and history of slipped capital femoral epiphysis. In *American Academy of Orthopaedic Surgeons: instructional course lectures,* vol 21, St Louis, 1972, Mosby.
18. Johansson C, Ekenman I, Tornkvist H et al: Stress fractures of the femoral neck in athletes: the consequence of a delay in diagnosis, *Am J Sports Med* 18(5):524, 1990.
19. Jones DC, James SL: Overuse injuries of the lower extremity. Shin splints, iliotibial band friction syndrome, and exertional compartment syndromes, *Clin Sports Med* 6:273, 1987.
20. Karlin LI: Injuries to the hip and pelvis. In Nicholas JA, Hershman EB editors: *The lower extremity and spine in sports medicine,* ed 2, St Louis, 1995, Mosby.
21. Kelley WN, Harris ED, Ruddy S et al: *Kelley's textbook of rheumatology,* ed 4, vol 2, Philadelphia, 1993, WB Saunders.
22. Kisner C, Colby LA: *Therapeutic exercise: foundations and techniques,* ed 2, Philadelphia, 1990, FA Davis.
23. Kulund DN: *The injured athlete,* Philadelphia, 1982, JB Lippincott.
24. Lecocq E: Peritrochanteric bursitis, *J Bone Joint Surg* 13:872-873, 1931.
25. Lillgard WA, Rucker KS: *Handbook of sports medicine: a symptom-oriented approach,* Boston, 1993, Andover Medical Publishers.
26. Magee DJ: *Orthopedic physical assessment,* ed 3, Philadelphia, 1997, WB Saunders.
27. Malone TR, McPoil T, Nitz AJ: *Orthopedic and sports physical therapy,* ed 3, St Louis, 1997, Mosby.
28. Matheson GO, Clement DB, McKenzie DC et al: Stress fractures in athletes: a study of 320 cases, *Am J Sports Med* 15(1):46, 1987.
29. Meals RA: *One hundred orthopaedic conditions every doctor should understand,* St Louis, 1992, Quality Medical Publishing.
30. Moore KL: *Clinically oriented anatomy,* ed 2, Baltimore, 1995, Williams & Wilkins.
31. Netter FH: *The Ciba collection of medical illustrations,* Summit, NJ, 1991, CIBA-GEIGY.
32. Peterson L, Renstrom P: *Sports injuries—their prevention and treatment,* Chicago, 1986, YearBook Medical Publishers.
33. Pick TP, Howden R editors: *Gray's anatomy,* New York, 1977, Bounty Books.
34. Reiley MA: *Guidelines for prescribing foot orthotics,* Thorofare, N.J., Slack.
35. Rennie AM: The inheritance of slipped capital femoral epiphysis, *J Bone Joint Surg* 64(B):180, 1982.
36. Roberts WN, Williams RB: Hip pain, *Primary Care* 15:783-793, 1988.
37. Salter RB: *Textbook of disorders and injuries of the musculoskeletal system,* ed 2, Baltimore, 1983, Williams & Wilkins.
38. Reference deleted.
39. Shbeeb MI, Matteson EL: Trochanteric bursitis (greater trochanteric pain syndrome), *Mayo Clin Proc* 71(6):565-569, 1996.
40. Sim FH, Rock MG, Scott SG: Pelvis and hip injuries in athletes: anatomy and function. In Nicholas JA, Hershman EB editors: *The lower extremity and spine in sports medicine,* ed 2, St Louis, 1995, Mosby.

41. Spear IM, Lipscomb PR: Noninfectious trochanteric bursitis and peritendinitis, *Surg Clin North Am* 32:1217-1224, 1952.

42. Spock A: Transient synovitis of the hip joint in children, *Pediatrics* 24:1042, 1959.

43. Staheli LT: *Fundamental of pediatric orthopedics,* New York, 1992, Raven.

44. Staheli LT: Rotational problems of the lower extremities, *Orthop Clin North Am* 18(4):506, 1987.

45. Sterling JO, Edelstein DS, Calvo D et al: Stress fractures in the athlete: diagnosis and management, *Sports Med* 14:336-346, 1992.

46. Swezey RL: Pseudo-radiculopathy in subacute trochanteric bursitis of the subgluteus maximus bursa, *Arch Phys Med Rehabil* 57:387-390, 1976.

47. Tachdjian MO: *Pediatric orthopedics,* vol 1, Philadelphia, 1972, WB Saunders.

48. Traycoff RB: Pseudotrochanteric bursitis: the differential diagnosis of lateral hip pain, *J Rheumatol* 18:1810-1812, 1991.

49. Turek SL: *Orthopedics: principles and their application,* ed 4, Philadelphia, 1984, JB Lippincott.

50. Williams PL, Warwick R, Dyson M et al editors: *Gray's anatomy,* ed 37, Edinburgh, 1989, Churchill Livingstone.

51. Xethalis JL, Lorei MP: Soccer injuries. In Nicholas JA, Hershman EB editors: *The lower extremity and spine in sports medicine,* ed 2, St Louis, 1995, Mosby.

PART XI
PELVIS

54

Unilateral Pubalgia in a Soccer Player that is Aggravated by Performing an Inside Kick

A 27-year-old Olympic soccer team member complains of new onset of right groin pain while performing an inside kick to "shoot" the ball forward. Approximately 6 months ago he experienced a pulled groin injury to the ipsilateral gracilis muscle after which he underwent physical therapy before complete resolution 2 months ago. He also reports a previous history of strain of his rectus abdominis muscle on the side opposite to the present groin pain due to a weight lifting injury. Over the last few months he has maintained his cardiovascular fitness by running along a banked road for 10 miles a day. He describes his symptoms as a gradual onset of mild groin pain that began after several practice sessions in cold weather, the last of which occurred in the rain. When asked whether he played with a leather or synthetic ball, he affirmed the former. There is no history of developmental dysplasia of either hip joint. While observing him perform during a soccer game you note that he kicks the ball directly in front of his body while avoiding inside kicks. When asked to stand on either leg for a prolonged time he complains of discomfort in the groin, as does repeated hopping on either leg. The patient reports no feeling of morning stiffness in his back or hips. Symptoms are not aggravated by forced coughing.

OBSERVATION   A slightly antalgic limp is noted during gait. The athlete is strongly built with prominent musculature in both thighs. When the lower abdominal musculature is observed, there appears to be a mild loss of symmetry between the two sides such that "relaxation" or loss of the normal integrity of the fascia of the anterior abdominal wall at its insertion on the pubis occurs.

PALPATION   This yields point tenderness over the symphysis pubis, the right inguinal canal, the right adductor tendons, and the contralateral rectus abdominis. Tenderness is more prominent at the pubis than the adductor tendons.

PASSIVE AND ACTIVE RANGE OF MOTION   This yields pain on right hip abduction and external rotation. There is normal range of motion in the spine and hips.

STRENGTH   Testing reveals a good grade of the right gluteus medius and tensor fasciae latae muscles as compared to the contralateral side.

SELECTIVE TENSION   Selective tension of right hip abduction or adduction is painful, as is a resistive right straight leg raise. Pain is also elicited upon resistive trunk flexion.

SENSATION   This is intact to light touch throughout both lower extremities.

SPECIAL TESTS   A leg length discrepancy of 2 cm is measured on his right lower extremity. During single leg stance on his right lower limb you note a slightly positive Trendelenburg sign during which the left pelvis dips inferiorly. There is a negative straight leg raise and negative Patrick's test.

RADIOGRAPHS   Flamingo views reveal bilateral sclerosis of the pubic symphysis, presence of traction osteophytes along the superior pubic ligament, as well as an asymmetric height difference greater than 2 mm of the right superior pubic ramus. Bone scan of the femoral neck was negative.

? Questions

1. What disorder is most likely afflicting this patient?
2. What anatomy is relevant to understanding this disorder?
3. Are the secondary movements of muscles across the hip joint less functionally important than the primary motions?
4. What is meant by inversion of muscle action in relation to a joint with universal movement capability?
5. Are the consequences of contraction of those muscles enveloping the hip joint dependent on whether the lower limb function is in the open or closed kinetic mode of function?
6. What are the various displacements of the pelvis during ambulation?
7. When do single and double limb support occur during gait?
8. What are the parameters of medial pelvic inclination in the horizontal plane?
9. What mechanism initiates and perpetuates the gait sequence?
10. What are the parameters of vertical pelvic inclination or tilt in the sagittal plane?
11. What is the relationship between pelvic tilting, lower limb muscle imbalance, and asymmetric loading of the intervertebral disk?
12. What passive structure restrains excessive posterior pelvic tilt?
13. What are the parameters of vertical pelvic displacement in the frontal plane?

14. What are levers and what mechanical advantage do they offer the musculoskeletal system?
15. How many kinds of lever systems are present in the human musculoskeletal system?
16. What bone sparing function do eccentric contractions offer?
17. What is the dual dynamic role of the hip abductors and what gait deviation results from their weakness?
18. How would an alteration in the length-tension of a single contractile component of the pelvic force couple result in excessive shear stress at the pubic symphysis?
19. What is the etiology and observed gait deviation derived from gluteus medius weakness?
20. What other compensating gait deviations may alternately manifest secondary to paresis of the abductor mechanism?
21. How are shear forces imparted to the pubic symphysis during normal gait?
22. What is the classification of the etiologic mechanism of injury in soccer players with biomechanically sound lower limbs?
23. What factors predispose for the development of osteitis pubis?
24. What is the clinical presentation?
25. What three clinical tests confirm the diagnosis of suspected osteitis pubis?
26. What imaging techniques are appropriate following suspected osteitis pubis?
27. What is the differential diagnosis?

28. How is osteitis pubis differentiated from adductor muscle strain?

29. What treatment strategy best manages this condition?

1. What disorder is most likely afflicting this patient?

Traumatic *osteitis pubis* is an inflammatory condition of the pubic symphyseal joint due to excessive biomechanical stress across that articulation. The nomenclature describing this condition includes osteochondritis of the symphysis pubis, gracilis syndrome, osteochondrosis of the pubis, pubalgia, osteitis necroticans pubis, rectus adductor syndrome, traumatic inguinal leg syndrome, anterior pelvic joint syndrome, osteoarthropathy of the symphysis pubis, and Pierson syndrome.[32] The majority of cases typically affect soccer players, owing to repetitive kicking of the ball at high speed while twisting on one leg.[9] This maneuver may exceed the capacity of the adductor muscle fibers originating from the inferior ischial rami, which may be responsible for the transmission of shear force to the pubic symphysis.[14] This disorder may manifest unilaterally or bilaterally, occurs in adults, and is cause for alarm when occurring in the elite athlete as it may have career ending consequences owing to its chronicity and resistance to treatment.

As the symphysis pubis is an important joint of the pelvis, any discussion of its function must be prefaced by its role in relation to the pelvic girdle. Moreover, any analysis of motion of the hip and pelvis must begin with the role of the muscles moving these bones, and how this movement varies in relation to open or closed kinetic chain function. In addition, the mechanical interaction between the osseous and contractile components to perform movement must be defined.

2. What anatomy is relevant to understanding this disorder?

The *pelvis* (or "basin" in Latin) is that ringlike osseous bowl comprised of four bones including the two hip bones, the sacrum, and coccyx. This girdle of bone is united by seven joints including the lumbosacral, sacroiliac (two), symphysis pubis, and the hip (two). The two hip joints are considered in the discussion of the pelvis because body weight is transmitted through the pelvis to the femur, while ground reaction force is imparted to the pelvis through the hip joints.[30] The two hip bones, otherwise known as the ossa coxae,

coxal bones, or *innominate** bones are ossified from three primary centers corresponding to the ilium, ischium, and pubis in the adult. All three hip bones fuse in the deep hemispheric cavity known as the acetabulum. The ilium is a fan or propeller shaped bone whose large surface area holds and protects the abdominal contents and uterus, and provides attachment for abdominal muscles and fasciae. Twenty-eight muscles attach on the pelvis, with the majority located on the ilium.[30] The ischium is the heavy posteroinferior portion of the coxal bone that is colloquially known as the "sit bone."

The pubis is the smallest of the three parts of the coxal bone that, together with the contralateral pubis, articulate anteriorly as the symphysis pubis. The *interpubic joint* is a cartilaginous articulation and is normally a slightly moveable joint that is constrained by three static structures. The superior pubic ligament connects the superior border of the joint, the inferior pubic ligament borders the inferior aspect of the joint, and a fibrocartilaginous interpubic disk (thicker in females)[23] is interposed between the articular pubic surfaces.

The pubis is the proximal site of attachment of the entire medial compartment of the thigh (the adductor group) as well as the deep, short, external rotators located in the deep posterior compartment musculature. Moreover, the hamstring muscles take their origin adjacent to the pubis on the ischium. The presence of tightness, contracture, or flaccidity of one or more components may alter pelvo-femoral mechanics causing a dynamic imbalance. This alteration in kinesiology is hypothesized to generate a rise in shear forces across the symphysis that results in pain and degeneration characteristic of osteitis pubis.[22]

3. Are the secondary movements of muscles across the hip joint less functionally important than the primary motions?

Muscles crossing the hip joint generally span from the pelvis to the femur and produce movement in three planes. The nomenclature describing the types of movements have, for the purpose of simplicity, been defined anatomically in the open kinetic chain mode of

---

*In Latin this means *nameless*. This term is reserved for those anatomic structures better named after their description.

function in which the distal segment moves on a stable proximal segment. Thus sagittal plane movement is provided by the flexors and extensor, frontal plane movements by the abductors and adductors, and transverse plane movements by the hip rotators. These positions, based on the human body in the anatomically neutral position, serve as a reference for understanding muscle function and are called *primary movements.* Most of these muscles are quite long and do not run in a perfectly straight vertical direction and therefore perform more than one movement when they contract. These latter movements are known as the *secondary functions* of muscle. These motions are wrongly relegated to secondary importance, however, as their kinesiologic contribution is indispensable in the understanding of function.

4. What is meant by inversion of muscle action in relation to a joint with universal movement capability?

Because the hip is a ball-and-socket joint, motion of the femoral head in relation to the acetabular cup will change the orientation of the muscles relative to the hip joint axis. Thus the action of particular muscles may vary according to the position of the hip joint and may even diametrically change its action. For example, when the hip is in the neutral position, the piriformis muscle produces lateral rotation, flexion, and abduction; whereas when in a position of exaggerated hip flexion, piriformis becomes a medial rotator, extensor, and abductor![17] This illustrates how an agonist may, by virtue of a change in joint position, suddenly demonstrate motions antagonistic to its primary motion. In addition to understanding the primary and secondary actions of the hip joint in the neutral position, it is important to appreciate the *inversion of muscular action* when the position of the hip is other than anatomically neutral.[18] Without comprehension of the varied repertoire of movement of which the hip joint is subject, the clinician cannot fully understand the kinesiology and pathokinesiology of biomechanical systems.

5. Are the consequences of contraction of those muscles enveloping the hip joint dependent on whether the lower limb function is in the open or closed kinetic mode of function?

Important to the understanding of muscle function at the hip joint is the inversion of anatomic origin and insertion as a function of kinetic mode of action. Although we previously defined motions in the sagittal, frontal, and transverse planes in relation to the thigh

bone moving on a stationary pelvis, we may also reverse our orientation to define hip joint musculature in relation to pelvic movement. Thus if our frame of reference is the closed kinetic chain then muscular action is now defined as movement of the mobile pelvis on a fixed femur. Thus we have anterior and posterior pelvic tilt in the sagittal plane, vertical (i.e., up-and-down) dip or inclination in the frontal plane, and lateral (i.e., side-to-side) displacement or rotation in the transverse plane. As human locomotion involves both the open (swing) and closed (stance) kinetic modes of function, our analysis of muscular function is incomplete without this final analysis.

6. What are the various displacements of the pelvis during ambulation?

If the lower limbs terminated in wheels instead of feet, the imaginary line drawn by forward locomotion would yield a straight line path. Since this is not the case, the body's center of gravity, located at S2 and adjacent to the pelvis, deviates from a straight line as a gentle sinusoidal curve in an attempt to minimize pelvic excursion to as narrow range as possible. Sinusoidal movement insures the least amount of energy is expended when the body moves along as straight-a-line as possible, while the center of gravity deviates neither up and down, nor side to side excessively (Fig. 54-1). Analyzing the various component motions involved in rhythmic pelvic excursion throughout the gait cycle yields displacement in all three dimensions. Medial-lateral pelvic inclination occurs in the horizontal plane, anterior posterior tilt occurs in the sagittal plane, whereas vertical displacement occurs in the frontal plane.

7. When do single and double limb support occur during gait?

We are balanced when standing or ambulating when the vertical projection of the center of gravity (our pelvis) is contained within our base of support. Walking consists of throwing ourselves off balance by leaning forward and then catching ourselves before we fall by moving our foot ahead into a new position. Thus our legs are always kept one step ahead of us as we ambulate forward.[1] Movements of the lower limbs during ambulation follow a particular sequence during the gait cycle. Before discussing specific pelvic displacements, it is necessary to discuss those parameters of gait known as single and double support. *Single limb support* refers to the period in the gait cycle when only one extremity is in contact with the floor; this occurs when the opposite leg is lifted for swing. Single limb support

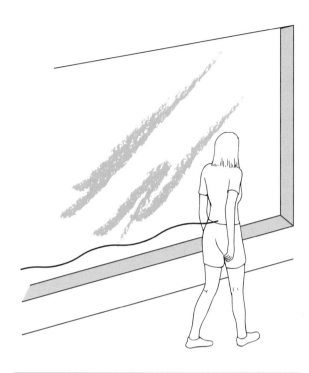

FIG. 54-1 If the lower limbs terminated in wheels instead of feet, the imaginary line drawn by forward locomotion would yield a straight line path. Since this is not the case, the body's center of gravity, located at S2 and adjacent to the pelvis, deviates from a straight line as a gentle sinusoidal curve in an attempt to minimize pelvic excursion to as narrow a range as possible. Sinusoidal movement ensures the least amount of energy is expended when the body moves along as straight a line as possible, while the center of gravity deviates neither up and down, nor side to side excessively. The line drawn on the glass window represents the approximate sinusoidal pathway of the center of gravity.

occurs twice during each gait cycle, as each extremity undergoes the midstance subphase of gait. Right single limb support occurs during the same time interval as left swing, whereas during right swing there is left single limb support (Fig. 54-2). *Double limb support* (occurring 11% of the gait cycle) means that both feet are in contact with the ground simultaneously. This occurs twice during a single gait cycle, both at the start and end of stance in which one limb undergoes toe-off while the other experiences heel strike. Double limb support occurs for a much shorter interval than single leg stance.*

---

*The absence of a period of double support distinguishes running from walking. While running, the period of double support is entirely eliminated. However, single limb support must be maintained so as to propel the body forward.

8. What are the parameters of medial pelvic inclination in the horizontal plane?

Medial pelvic displacement or horizontal, side-to-side rotation on the longitudinal axis of the body occurs in the horizontal (transverse) plane as weight is transferred from one leg to the other. Medial pelvic oscillation, in particular, is integral to the initiating mechanism of gait. Normally, the pelvis rotates medially just before heel strike, so that, for example, a pelvis rotating medially to the left is consistent with right limb stance and left limb swing.

The total amount of side-to-side displacement is approximately 5 cm. The horizontal limits of pelvic, and hence center of gravity deviation, is reached as each supporting limb is at its midstance point.[10] Displacement may be increased by increasing reciprocal arm swing across (rather than alongside) as the body rotates the pelvis and trunk excessively, and may painfully strain the attachment of the thoracolumbar muscles on the iliac crest.[6]

During each stride the pelvis moves through an arc of internal rotation followed by an arc of external rotation that averages at 8°. Maintaining this motion within this margin is accomplished by the cooperative (concentric and eccentric) action of the internal and external rotators. Normally, the external rotators are stronger than the internal rotators. Balance is maintained however by the passive restraint of the iliofemoral and pubofemoral ligaments, which limit external rotation. An imbalance in favor of shortened external rotators may result in toeing-out, whereas tight internal rotators may cause toeing-in.

9. What mechanism initiates and perpetuates the gait sequence?

The fact that mankind can ambulate almost indefinitely for long periods suggests a rhythmicity and near-perpetual quality to human locomotion. How does this occur? Human locomotion is defined as *reciprocal alternating standing bipedalism,* and involves repetitively throwing ourselves off balance by leaning forward and then catching ourselves before we fall by moving our foot ahead into a new position. Throwing ourselves forward occurs by way of lower limb swing due, in part, to *concentric* muscular activity. As our center of mass is forward fall, we catch our falling body weight by planting our forward swing foot forward. Stabilization after ground contact is afforded by *eccentric* muscle activity despite the considerable magnitude of opposing forces in the form of superincumbent body mass, by way of the forward leg contacting and pushing

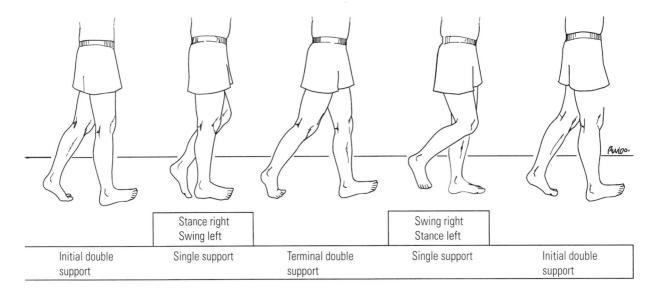

Stance right Swing left		Swing right Stance left	
Initial double support	Single support	Terminal double support	Single support	Initial double support

FIG. 54-2 Subdivisions of stance, swing, and single and double support. (Note: the swing phase of one limb comprises the entire single support period of the opposite limb.) (From Valmassy RL: *Clinical biomechanics of the lower extremities,* St Louis, 1996, Mosby.)

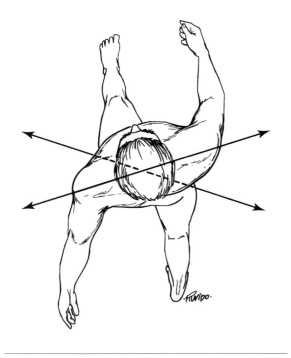

FIG. 54-3 *Adversal truncal rotation* refers to the fact that the upper and lower limbs demonstrate movement (such as swing) that are opposite in nature. (From Valmassy RL: *Clinical biomechanics of the lower extremities,* St Louis, 1996, Mosby.)

down on the ground, and ground reaction force pushing upward on the forward leg (Newton's third law). In such a fashion, the weight-bearing limb serves as a *lever* that effectively thrusts the ground backward while levering the body forward causing the stance side pelvis to rotate medially. This cyclic progression is serially perpetuated by reciprocal action of both lower limbs using one's own body mass as a prime mover.[8] The pelvis is the location of the body's center of mass and is located midway between the upper and lower extremities. Its anatomic location corresponds to the site of movement differential between the upper and lower extremities during ambulation known as *adversal truncal rotation.* This refers to the fact that the upper and lower limbs demonstrate movement (such as swing) that are opposite in nature (Fig. 54-3). For example, if the pelvis medially rotates to the left in at attempt to swing the right lower extremity forward, it is accompanied by lateral trunk rotation and hence, left forward arm swing and right backward arm swing; the latter is referred to an *reciprocal arm swing.* As the pelvis rotates medially, reciprocal alternating arm swing, emanating from the shoulder, causes relative opposite (adversal) truncal rotation, thus helping to narrowly preserve the side-to-side displacement of the center of gravity.

These reverse rotations between the pelvis and trunk are the source of an *energy storage and return mechanism* in which potential energy is stored in the fascia, muscles, and ligaments of the back. Thus the spine serves as a "gait-driving engine," that stores and releases potential energy. Once sufficient tension occurs, active release occurs as reverse rotation between the pelvic and shoulder girdles as stored energy is expressed as elastic recoil. The locus of this recoil occurs at the mid-juncture point of the body located at the pelvis, and is the source of medial pelvic rotation that corresponds to ipsilateral leg acceleration (hip flexion).[13]

10. What are the parameters of vertical pelvic inclination or tilt in the sagittal plane?

During normal walking the pelvis also undergoes a rhythmic upward and downward motion called *pelvic tilt*. Pelvic tilting occurs in the sagittal plane, and may be measured with reference to upward or downward movement of the anterior superior iliac spines (ASIS). Since the pelvis and spine articulate at the lumbosacral joint, a relationship exists between the pelvis and the spine such that the orientation of tilt directly determines the magnitude of spinal curve. When the ASIS is tilted relatively forward, as during hip flexion, the ischium tilts backward and the pelvis undergoes an *anterior pelvic tilt* accentuating the lumbar curve, causing *hyperlordosis*. Conversely, a posterior pelvic tilt is defined by the relative backward rotation of the pelvis in the sagittal plane, in which the ASIS tilts backward (while the ischium rotates forward.) This causes a flattening of the lumbar spine. Thus a definite and direct relationship exists between spinal configuration and pelvic alignment. Chronic postural anterior pelvic tilt is increased and may be due to tightness of the prefemoral muscles whereas posterior pelvic tilt is increased owing to tightness of the postfemoral muscles. Unlike muscle shortness in the hip abductor musculature in relation to lateral displacement in the frontal plane, excessive anterior or posterior pelvic tilt is not obviated during gait. Were excessive tilting be allowed to occur in the sagittal plane, survival would be endangered as forward vision would deviate from the horizontal. As such, compensation effectively skips over the pelvis to manifest as accentuation or minimization of the lumbar lordosis alternately known as "swayback" or "flat-back'" posture, respectively.

11. What is the relationship between pelvic tilting, lower limb muscle imbalance, and asymmetric loading of the intervertebral disk?

The two postural extremes of lordosis or flat back may lead to an asymmetric loading of the intervertebral disks of the spine. The pathologic ramification of asymmetric disk loading is implicated as a mechanism contributing to low back pain. As the lumbar spine moves into excessive lordosis, the posterior spinal joints are approximated, causing excessive posterior disk compression. Concomitantly, the distance anteriorly between the vertebral bodies increases. Thus posterior compression and anterior dysfunction lead to anterior bulging of the nucleus pulposus. In the flattened lumbar spine these events are essentially reversed causing posterior or posterolateral disk displacement.

12. What passive structure restrains excessive posterior pelvic tilt?

The fibrous capsule of the hip joint is a cylindrical sleeve that is strengthened by three distinct capsular thickenings known as the ischiofemoral, pubofemoral, and iliofemoral ligaments. All three ligaments become taut in hip extension and relax in hip flexion. In addition, the ischiofemoral ligament has twisted fibers that span the posterior aspect of the hip joint so as to limit medial rotation.[17] The pubofemoral ligament strengthens the medial aspect of the hip joint and thereby tenses during abduction to prevent excessive abduction;[23] it also tightens during external rotation.[19]

The iliofemoral ligament is known as the "Y" ligament because of its resemblance to an inverted Y as it overlies the superior-anterior aspect of the capsule. Its attachments span from the anterior-inferior iliac spine (AIIS) and acetabular rim to distally insert on the intertrochanteric line located on the femoral neck.[23] The function of this passive restraint is to limits posterior pelvic tilt and hence limit active hip extension to approximately 0° to 10° beyond neutral, and passive hyperextension beyond 40° to 50°. In the sitting posture these ligaments no longer restrict posterior pelvic movement, which may increase to the point of obliteration of the lordotic lumbar curve. Conversely, the lying-prone position places the pelvis in anterior pelvic tilt and accentuates lumbar lordosis.

Function of the Y-ligament is intimately related to quiet standing posture otherwise known as the "stand easy" posture of the armed forces.[23] In symmetric stance the body stands comfortably erect and expends a minimal of energy. In this posture, the vertical projection of the center of gravity of body mass falls just behind the hip joint, just anterior to the knee joint, and anterior to the axis of the upper ankle joint. Why is this significant? Because such a position makes use of the ligamentous restraining mechanism afforded by the Y-ligament at the hip and the bony locking of the knee into extension; in such a manner, standing is passively accomplished (the exception is the ankle joint, which requires tonic contraction of gastroc-soleus.) This posture is accomplished by tipping the pelvis back posteriorly so as to locate the center of gravity just posterior to the common hip axis. Also known as the *model's posture,* this posture is assumed by the paraplegic wearing long leg braces without spinal support. Passively hanging on the taut Y-ligament requires no active energy expenditure at the thigh. Should one suddenly "assume position" of the military posture, active energy is required to stand still as the center of gravity is placed in front of the base of support. In the paraplegic, this would cause loss of balance by way of "jackknifing," in which gravity pitches body weight forward owing to loss of active hip extension.

13. What are the parameters of vertical pelvic displacement in the frontal plane?

During normal walking the pelvis tips on the nonstance side in the coronal (frontal) plane. Why does this occur? To answer this question we must first begin with the introduction of kinesiologic function of the hip abductor muscles. Although gluteus medius, gluteus minimis, and tensor fasciae latae are anatomically classified as performing hip abduction, their major functional role is to maintain pelvic stability during unilateral stance by keeping the pelvis level. Contraction of the hip abductors in the open kinetic chain is defined by movement of the hip with fixation of the proximal iliac attachment yielding hip abduction, whereas contraction of these same muscles with fixation on the trochanteric attachment manifests as horizontal pelvic stability during closed chain function (such as standing on one leg or during gait).* In addition, essential to understanding the weight-bearing function of the pelvis is the biomechanical role of levers. Although the forces on the pelvis while standing on both feet corresponds to a second class lever, unilateral stance forms a first class lever.

14. What are levers and what mechanical advantage do they offer the musculoskeletal system?

The human skeleton is comprised of 206 bones and represents the structural chassis that, together with 650 muscles anchored to the skeleton, power a dynamic system of struts and levers resulting in movement. What is a lever and what does it do?

---

*This example beautifully shows the folly of thinking in purely anatomic terms with regard to the origin and insertion of muscle. Here, anatomic hip abductors are kinesiologically pelvic stabilizers as their origin and insertion are reversed relative to which segment is stable and which is mobile.

To begin with, let us consider a thought experiment in which a prehistoric man or woman encountered a number of rocks barring his way. Over time, he could slowly but surely lift and carry out of his way 20 rocks to another locale some one hundred feet away. In doing so he would "toil" or "labor" by the sweat of his brow to interact with two constants—the force of the rocks and the distance they are carried. He would expend energy by performing *work,* which is defined as force multiplied by distance.

However, if the 20 fifty-pound rocks were united into one half-ton boulder, our man could not accumulate enough energy nor expend it quickly enough to lift the boulder in one stroke. The rate at which energy is expended is called *power.* Man does not possess sufficient power to perform certain activities because there remains a limit to the rate at which any living creature can expend energy. However, if a beam were inserted under the boulder and pivoted over a small rock nearby, this multiplies the force output at the other end of the beam so that a single man could move the boulder that could not previously be moved. This is an example of a simple lever whose parameters were first defined by the Greek mathematician Archimedes (287-212 B.C.), and represents a simple machine. A *machine* is a tool whereby effort (or energy) applied at one point is transmitted, in more useful form, to another point or in another direction.† Thus machines are devices that

---

†The anthropological consequences of simple tools by early man represent an extension of the human hand that irrevocably changed history as it freed him from operating within the confines of his own puny physical capacity. It spawned an agricultural revolution with the introduction of the plow, which is a wedge dividing the soil, and thereby much improved the quality of his life by creating surplus food. The significance of this invention may be compared to the change in man's diet from vegetarian to that of meat eating. Because meat is a higher link in the food chain, it is a more concentrated form of protein compared with plant, and so eating meat cuts down the bulk and time spent in foraging and eating to live by two-thirds. (From Bronowski J: *The ascent of man,* London, 1981, Macdonald Futura Publishers.) The advantages of both these monumentous changes for the evolution of man were far reaching as they provided more free time. At some point man learned that a beast of burden, such as a cow or horse, can multiply the available energy supply 10-fold. And so the domestication of animals ensued in which the power output of animals was marshaled to pull the plow. With time man learned to make use of inanimate sources of energy such as wind and water, although the culmination of this quest ended with the Promethean discovery of fire. Fire is a concentrated source of energy that is virtually limitless if properly marshaled. Man finally discovered a means to free himself from bondage to a limited energy source eked out by the beasts he domesticated. It is for this reason that fire is considered the greatest single human achievement.

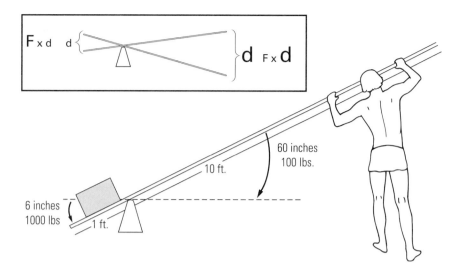

FIG. 54-4 A *lever* is a simple machine that multiplies the magnitude or direction of force, or increases the speed with which a task is performed. The fulcrum can be placed near one end of the lever, which then divides the shaft into a shorter and longer shaft. By applying a *small force* through a *large distance* one focuses a large force across a short distance. A lever is simply a vehicle for manipulating these two variables by way of equal exchange. Based upon the concept of equilibrium, that balance is such that the product of applied force and the shaft length is the same at either end. Thus a lever doesn't increase the work capacity, but merely trades distance for force.

perform tasks that require more strength than our muscles can supply by multiplying the magnitude or direction of force, or by increasing the speed with which a task is performed.*

When we consider the human body as a work-yielding machine, the vehicle used to generate force and power is through a simple machine known as the lever. By applying a *small force* through a *large dis-*

---

*The speed with which any machine performs work is termed *power*, and the efficiency of different machines varies according to the rate at which energy can be expended. No machine is 100% efficient. The human body is only about 24% efficient, that is, only 24% of the energy supplied by the food we eat goes into doing useful work. The other 76% is neither wasted or lost, but is necessary to maintaining the life processes (metabolism) of the body. Moreover, the materials comprising the body machine actually limit power. It has been estimated that if a man could drive his legs as quickly as an ant, we would be capable of running at speeds greater than 100 miles (160 km) per hour. However, due to our design and material limitations, if we could run at this speed, something would give—bones would soon snap and muscles would tear. The significance of using machinery allows man to be more productive than he might otherwise become. The automobile is only 25% efficient but, unlike humans, can run for hours on end. The steam locomotive is 10% efficient, the turbine engine is 40% efficient, the steam engine up to 85%, while the electric motor demonstrates up to 95% efficiency.

tance we can focus a large force across a short distance. A *lever* is simply a vehicle for manipulating these two variables by way of equal exchange; it does not invent more energy (energy conservation law) or work, although it may give the appearance of doing so (Fig. 54-4). The lever performs in so uncomplicated a fashion that it cannot be further simplified, and is therefore considered a *simple machine*.

There are six classes of simple machines that include the inclined plane, the wedge, the screw, the lever, the pulley, and wheel and axle. This expanded classification may be reduced to inclined planes and levers, as the former two machines are special cases of the inclined plane. Similarly, the latter two machines may be derived from the lever.

15. How many kinds of lever systems are present in the human musculoskeletal system?

Every time we nod yes and no, stand on our toes, or perform a biceps curl, we engage a type of lever in our body (Fig. 54-5). The lever where the fulcrum (joint) is positioned between the applied force (muscular effort) and the applied load and the applied force is called a *class I lever.* An example of such a lever system in the body is the atlanto-occipital joint

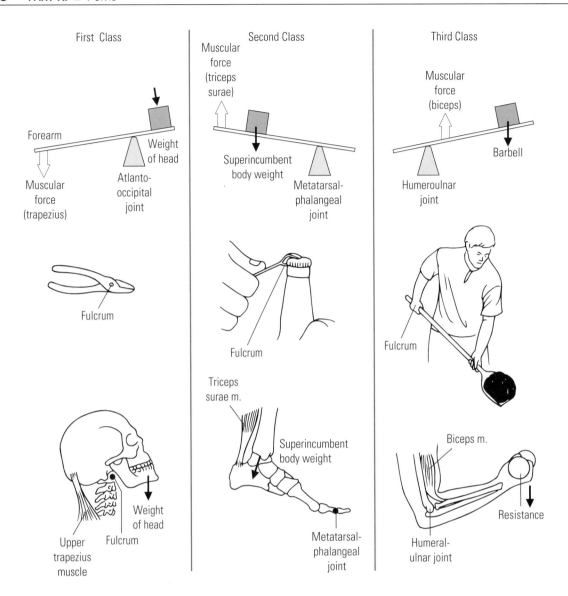

FIG. 54-5 Examples of classes of levers that differ based upon the positions of the *weight* (resistance) and *force* in relation to the *fulcrum* (joint axis). The permutations of these three variables represent three different possibilities as to placement of these parameters. With a ***first class lever,*** the fulcrum (joint) always lies between the effort (muscular force) and the resistance (load). This is the most efficient class of lever. With a ***second class lever,*** the resistance always lies between the fulcrum and the effort. With a ***third class lever,*** muscular effort is placed between the weight and the joint, providing the least efficient mechanical advantage.

located at the summit of the cervical spine. If we fall asleep in the sitting posture, the weight of the head forces it forward because of the relaxed tone in the posterior musculature. When awake, this first class lever engages so that the intrinsic back muscles and paracervical muscles of the neck serve at the counter balance in this see-saw type lever. This is the most efficient type of lever system for overcoming heavy resistive loads. Another example of a first class lever is the intervertebral joints in which the weight of the trunk is balanced by the erector spinae muscles.[20]

A *class II lever* is one in which the load (resistance) is between the fulcrum (joint) and the applied force (muscle). This type of lever is intuitively understood when we appreciate the large load we can transfer by using a wheelbarrow, or a crowbar for prying. A second class lever system is operative when we stand on our toes. Here, the gastrocnemius muscle lifts the body weight onto the metatarsal heads; the metatarsophalangeal joints serve as the fulcrum.

In a *class III lever*, of which the elbow joint is an example, the applied (muscle) force is located between the resistive load (held weight) and the fulcrum (joint). Other examples include the deltoid muscle acting on the glenohumeral joint and the tibialis anterior at the ankle joint. This class of lever is the most common in the musculoskeletal system despite its providing the poorest *mechanical advantage*. Compare the effort required to lift a load using a second and third class lever; it requires considerably more muscular effort to perform lifting a 50-lb weight as compared with a body weight of 150 lbs by standing on one's metatarsal heads. Although less than adequately adapted to negotiate heavy resistive loads, this class of lever is suited to negotiate high-velocity contraction. What benefit would this serve?

16. What bone sparing function do eccentric contractions offer?

It must be remembered that the biceps muscle corresponds to the hamstring muscle in the lower extremity, and was very likely relocated to lie on the dorsal humerus when our species was quadruped. Now, these muscles span across long bones that possess an inherent convexity and concavity, which means that although the concave portion undergoes *compressive loading,* the convex aspect undergoes *tensile loading.* Although bone is quite capable of negotiating compressive loading, it is less able to negotiate tensile forces. Tension is magnified during the high velocity forces that may occur during walking or running. In response, the musculoskeletal system developed a *bone-sparing strategy* to minimize excessive force build-up along the convex aspect of long bones by way of eccentric contraction. *Eccentric contractions* offer a compressive or counter-tensile force so as to neutralize excessive tension accrued during locomotion, and represent a strategy to minimize the poten-

tially injurious forces incurred during high velocity contractions.

17. What is the dual dynamic role of the hip abductors and what gait deviation results from their weakness?

Consider the right single leg during the mid-subphase of stance in the normal individual. The unsupported swing side of the pelvis tilts downward below the horizon as a direct function of gravity no more than 5° to 8° before the stance side abductors activate and contract to prevent further tipping in the coronal plane by offering a counter tilt that keeps the pelvis level. Why does this occur? If we consider the magnitude of force due to super-incumbent load applied to the vulnerable neck and head of the stance side limb, we note that joint compressive forces are magnified to approximately 2.5 times body weight.[11] The proximal femur, particularly the femoral neck, is particularly vulnerable to fracture by virtue of its inherent architectural design. Because of the convex and concave topography of the proximal femur, loading will manifest as compressive forces on the medial concave side and tensile force along the lateral convex aspect. As bone is poorly adapted to negotiate tensile force, excessive tension secondary to increased load from carrying a refrigerator on one's back may exceed bone strength and result in a transverse fracture on its convex aspect. During normal function, force across this potentially weak site increases to 3 times body weight during stair climbing, whereas running may elevate force to as much as 5 times body weight.[29] A considerable safety margin is provided for as the femoral neck will normally tolerate as much as 15 times body weight before sustaining fracture. The body has evolved a dynamic strategy to help circumvent the focus of excessive force to the proximal femur by way of active contraction of three muscle groups accomplished by combined synergy of the stance leg abductors and adductors*, as well as the swing side erector spinae and abdominal musculature by way of a *force couple* mechanism. Working in synergy these compartment muscles provide a counter-tensile compressive force, so that the net tensile force developing along the lateral femur is canceled. Thus the lateral compartment muscle

---

*It is essential not to confine our thinking of muscle groups such as the hip abductors and adductors to agonist-antagonist relationship, as they are clearly functioning simultaneously and mutually toward a singular goal—pelvic stabilization.

serves to unload the lateral side of the femur secondary to eccentroic loading of the femoral head.

Of equal importance is the role of the lateral compartment muscle working as pelvic stabilizers. If we analyze the forces operating here with respect to the femoral head and pelvis we note a first class lever system consisting of two levers of different lengths generating two forces and balanced across the femoral head which serves as the fulcrum.

Torque generated by the lateral compartment hip muscles on the stance side normally balances torque generated by the center of gravity of the body wanting to rotate the pelvis away from the stance-side hip. If the torques are equal than the contralateral pelvis rotates no more than 5° to 8°. Recovery from excessive dip, known as a *Trendelenburg lurch,* is normal and the pelvis is maintained more or less parallel with the horizontal.

Loss of stance side lateral compartment muscles causes a disruption of this balance. The contralateral hip rotates away from the stance side hip and causes the contralateral hip to drop greater than 5° to 8° known as a *positive Trendelenburg sign* (Fig. 54-6).

A compensatory maneuver during gait is a lurching gait or gluteus medius lurch in which the patient moves the center of gravity of the body toward or over the stance-side hip. This reduces the contralateral tipping to approximately zero by reducing the torque to a zero value, and thereby maintaining the pelvis parallel with the horizon which facilitates swing-through of the non-stance side limb. Thus the patient lurches toward the weak side.

18. How would an alteration in the length-tension of a single contractile component of the pelvic force couple result in excessive shear stress at the pubic symphysis?

The co-dependence of function of three muscle groups, namely the hip abductors, adductors, and erector spinae, is illustrated by considering the deleterious effects of muscle imbalance of this force couple. An analogy may be drawn to the scapula of the upper extremity in which imbalance of one or more muscles of the shoulder girdle alters the precisely orchestrated length-tension of the other shoulder elevators, thereby predisposing disorders of the rotator cuff. Here too, tightness or stretching of either of the abdominal or paraspinal muscles (owing to a sway-back or flat-back posture) or of either adductors or abductors of either hip may deleteriously alter length-tension of the adductor muscula-

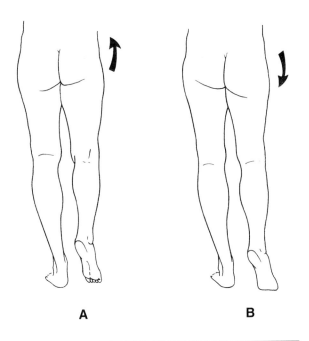

FIG. 54-6 *Trendelenburg's sign.* **A,** Negative test. **B,** Positive test. (From Magee DJ: *Orthopedic physical assessment,* Philadelphia, 1997, WB Saunders.)

ture such that its capacity to negotiate shear* stress is compromised. As a result, the mechanism for limiting lateral dip in the frontal plane remains unchecked, and a vicious cycle is set for the delivery of excessive shear to the pubic symphysis.

It is in this context that we may attempt to understand why osteitis pubis often develops as a sequel to urologic surgery (such as retropubic prostatectomy) or gynecologic procedures (such as cystocele repair).[28] Our frame of reference in understanding how disruption of those muscles involved during surgery causes an alteration in the precisely orchestrated force couple and thereby disturbs muscle balance resulting in excess shear delivery to the symphysis pubis.

19. What is the etiology and observed gait deviation derived from gluteus medius weakness?

One may have gluteal muscle weakness from a variety of reasons such as a herniated spinal disk that compresses the fourth or fifth lumbar roots; from a peripheral nerve injury to the superior gluteal nerve due to a gunshot wound; from a congenitally unilateral dislo-

---

Shear is defined as the confluence of two forces applied to a single object in opposite directions along a single plane.

cated hip joint, or unilateral Legg-Calve-Perthes disease; from altered muscle length due to osteoarthritis, or shortening of the ipsilateral hip. The ipsilateral gluteus medius may be mechanically disadvantaged by becoming lengthened in the event that the contralateral leg is longer. Either an abduction or adduction contracture will cause the pelvis to assume an asymmetrical posture. An adduction contracture raises the pelvis on the affected side and creates as apparently shorter leg, and abduction contracture results in an apparently shorter leg.[12]

Whatever the mechanism of weakness, ipsilateral gluteal muscle weakness manifests as tipping of the contralateral side, that is on the swing side. During one-legged standing this is known as a positive *Trendelenburg sign* and is apparent as the pelvis on the opposite side is displaced inferiorly and is indicative of weakness or paralysis of the stance-side abductors. This asymmetric pelvic posture appears as lateral inferior droop of the pelvis of the unsupported (swing) side until the supported (stance) hip becomes maximally adducted. At this point tension the capsule, ligaments, and iliotibial tract passively prevents further lateral dip.

When observed during walking, this is known as a *Trendelenburg gait,* or *lurching gait,* or *gluteus medius gait.* This gait is actually a compensatory strategy to cope with excessive contralateral pelvic tipping secondary to ipsilateral weakness of the gluteus medius and tensor fasciae latae muscles. A bilateral Trendelenburg gait is known as a *waddling gait,* and is common in neuromotor diseases such as multiple sclerosis with symmetrical involvement, muscular dystrophy, or amyotrophic lateral sclerosis.

20. What other compensating gait deviations may alternately manifest secondary to paresis of the abductor mechanism?

The patient with ipsilateral weakness or paralysis of the hip abductor mechanism has an apparent leg length discrepancy with a longer swing leg. Two alternate deviations of gait would include *circumduction* or *lower limb flexion* of the swing leg. Normal gait involves the precise swing of one leg while the other leg undergoes stance. Weakness of the gluteus medius mechanism does not affect the lower limb's ability to perform stance. However, it does manifest as compromised swing function because that limb is now too long. Circumduction strategy attempts to swing the leg around the body's center of gravity since it does not swing underneath the body; whereas as shortening the limb by way of excessive flexion of the ipsilateral hip, knee, and ankle on the

same side of gluteal dysfunction shortens the limb and allows for it to swing underneath the carriage. A Trendelenburg gait is simply another form of gait deviation compensatory strategy to negotiate an apparently longer leg on the (swing) side of gluteal dysfunction.

An individual with weakness of a unilateral gluteus medius muscle will attempt to compensate for lost pelvic stability by one of several mechanisms. Most simply, compensation may occur by way of walking with a cane on the (contralateral) swing side that provides an upward force at a long distance from the joint axis, thereby counterbalancing the unwanted torque derived from superincumbent body weight that results in excessive swing side dip. A positive Trendelenburg test for a left hip observed from behind shows the right hip dropping, indicating weakness of the left gluteal muscle. A unilateral assistive device, such as a cane, in the right hand functions in lieu of the paretic or paralytic right hip abductor mechanism and serves to minimize or mask right pelvic tip.[3] The patient may alternately carry a weight in the left (stance) hand to counterbalance the weight of unsupported superincumbent body weight that tips the contralateral pelvis.

Another method of compensation for stance side gluteus medius paresis manifesting as swing side pelvic droop is by way of *trunk shifting.* By inclining the trunk laterally toward the stance side so as to shift the center of gravity closer to the base of support, the torque generated by the unbalanced pelvis minus a contralateral hip abductor mechanism is minimized, at the price of altering spinal alignment. Thus long standing gluteal weakness will result in a primary scoliotic curve on the side opposite to compromised gluteal function and a secondary curve on the same side.

21. How are shear forces imparted to the pubic symphysis during normal gait?

The pelvis with articulated hip complex approximate a first class lever system during single leg stance. In this "see-saw analogy" the fulcrum is the femoral head and the pelvis may be compared to a scale that is pulled to the swing side leg by gravity, but is counterbalanced by the abductor mechanism on the stance side. Since the lever arm of body weight is longer than that of the hip abductors, the latter are at mechanical disadvantage. Hence, the stance-side abductors are assisted by the swing side erector spinae as well as the abdominal musculature.[32] In the event that any one or more of the components involved in maintaining vertical hip displacement is compromised, excessive shear (Fig. 54-7)

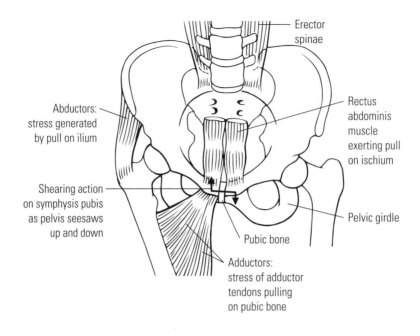

Abductors: stress generated by pull on ilium

Erector spinae

Rectus abdominis muscle exerting pull on ischium

Shearing action on symphysis pubis as pelvis seesaws up and down

Pelvic girdle

Pubic bone

Adductors: stress of adductor tendons pulling on pubic bone

FIG. 54-7 Shearing action of symphysis pubis as the pelvis seesaws up and down.

will occur between the two pelvic bones—the cartilaginous symphysis pubis. Predisposition to osteitis pubis may be attributable to imbalance such as shortness or either the hip abductors or adductors, erector spinae, or abdominal wall musculature. Excessive shear may also occur from a leg length discrepancy, a unilaterally pronated foot (causing an apparently shortened limb) running on a banked surface, or in advanced runners who increase their mileage or add interval training or speed work to their training routine. In the latter, there is no muscle deficit but rather, the athlete subjects his or her body to quick, repetitive, and sudden pelvic drops while quickly and forcefully alternating between midstance phase of either foot. The common etiologic denominator to these varied mechanisms is the application of excessive shear force to the symphysis pubis, which may result in small avulsion fractures at the site of attachment of the adductor muscles to the pubic bones.[5,6]

22. What is the classification of the etiologic mechanism of injury in soccer players with biomechanically sound lower limbs?

The mechanism of acute injury is attributable to repetitive inside kicking, by overextending and externally rotating the hip so as to kick the ball harder thus recruiting the adductors and rotators. Known as "shooting practice," this mechanism is common during preseason training when the player lacks flexibility and kicks a poorly conditioned leg. This causes excessive shear stress at the pubic symphysis and strain of the adductor muscles, particularly adductor longus. Thus injurious force may either involve the pubic joint resulting in osteitis pubis or may be absorbed by the adductor muscle(s) resulting in adductor strain. Another mechanism of injury in soccer is by direct contusion to the pubic area by an opponent's knee or by the ball.[32]

Although osteitis pubis may manifest following acute trauma, evidence favors repeated minor trauma from excessive or repetitive biomechanical stresses transmitted to the symphysis. Osteitis pubis also occurs in race walkers and runners,[31] particularly long distance or elite marathon runners who suddenly increase mileage or add interval training with speed work to their training routine. Running for many years may lead to asymptomatic osteitis pubis (with positive radiographic signs) as well as to osteitis condensans ilii, which involves the sacroiliac joint.[5]

23. What factors predispose for the development of osteitis pubis?

Osteitis pubis typically occurs secondary to one of three predisposing patterns, which are primary characteristics in athletes. The first pattern is in athletes with strong musculature and 'tight' ligaments; the second in patients who are often young. Almost all affected soccer players are between the ages of 20 to 30 years (Imbert JC et al, 1992, personal communication). This may be related to the fact that the symphysis pubis reaches articular maturity in the third decade.[7] The third predisposing pattern is limitation of hip joint motion caused by degenerative hip disease in adolescents.[24] Other factors include hard training, frequent competition, poorly maintained grounds, cold weather, inadequate warm-up and stretching, and a wet soccer ball. It has been estimated that a leather ball can be as much as twenty percent heavier during wet weather, whereas the weight of synthetic balls are not significantly affected by wet weather.[32]

24. What is the clinical presentation?

Osteitis pubis is clinically characterized by gradual onset of dull ache in the groin or mild, deep seated pain localized to the region of the pubis, which may extend to the groin or lower aspect of the abdomen. If attributable to a shooting-type kick injury in soccer, pain increases during the subsequent night and the athlete is unable to kick a ball the next morning. The acute phase lingers over the first few days following injury and is characterized by pain and tenderness over the adductor tendon area, the symphysis pubis (pubalgia), inguinal ligament, as well as the lower abdominal musculature (rectus abdominis).[32] This combined tenderness of the abdominal and adductor muscles is pathognomic for injury to the symphysis pubis.

Symptoms are intensified by passive or active abduction and external rotation of the thigh or on resistive adduction or abduction of the involved thigh; the latter provokes stretching of the involved adductors. In addition, resisted flexion of the trunk may elicit pain, which occurs because the insertion of rectus abdominis inserts just above the pubis. An *antalgic limp* may be exhibited, and if the condition is severe, adductor spasm may set in, which results in a *waddling gait*. In addition, a clicking sensation may be present, indicating instability.[31]

A soccer player may attempt to conceal the injury by kicking the ball directly in front of the body and by avoiding inside kicks. This compensating mode of kicking uses the hip flexors and abductors while bypassing the need for adductor recruitment, thus lessening the shear force across the symphysis. The clinician should be watchful for the seasoned player who exhibits abnormal modes of kicking during the game.[32]

25. What three clinical tests confirm the diagnosis of suspected osteitis pubis?

During the physical examination, the presence of three signs (Imbert et al, 1992, personal communication) confirm diagnosis of osteitis pubis and include: (1) "relaxation" or loss of the normal integrity of the fascia of the anterior abdominal wall at its insertion on the pubis; (2) pain on resisted elevation of the leg in the supine position; and (3) tenderness and "relaxation" of the inguinal canal. Some 80% of patients with these signs also have tenderness of the adductor muscles.

26. What imaging techniques are appropriate following suspected osteitis pubis?

Radiographs should include stress anteroposterior, inlet and outlet views of the pelvis, as well as stress anteroposterior views of the symphysis pubis. Stress is most easily applied by taking the radiograph with the patient in single leg stance known as the "flamingo view"[4] and are obtained while the patient performs single leg support for one view and the other leg for the comparison view. Positive radiographs reveal either unilateral or bilateral sclerosis of the pubic symphysis.[5,6] It is also characterized by erosive lucencies (indicating bone rarefaction secondary to local osteoporosis) at the origins of the adductor and gracilis musculature indicating: periosteal reaction at the muscle attachments (the symphysis); frayed corners and fluffy margins[2] of the symphysis pubis; mottled areas of rarefaction; (primer) symmetric bone resorption at the medial ends of the pubic bones; presence of traction osteophytes at the insertion of the superior pubic ligament; in severely unstable joints that have been subjected to considerable trauma; osteophytic progression represents an attempt to stabilize the joint.[32] Instability is also indicated by widening of the symphysis[5,6] or shifting of the relationships of the pubic bones between flamingo views. A difference in height of the superior pubic ramus on each side of more than 2 mm, or width exceeding 10 mm, may be considered abnormal and positive for osteitis pubis.

It takes approximately 1 month after the initial injury or onset of symptoms for radiographic changes to manifest, although radiographic signs tend to persist even after symptoms have receded following resolution of this disorder.[31] The use of bone scans is more helpful early after the onset of pain, which demonstrates increased bone metabolic activity in the area of the symphysis. Computed tomography provides the earliest detection of traumatic osteitis pubis, and demonstrates hematomas, soft tissue swelling, and small avulsions not discernible on plain radiographs.[32]

27. What is the differential diagnosis?

Osteitis pubis is a localized inflammation of bone in contradistinction to the generalized osteitis (deformans) of Paget's disease. Other causes of osteitis pubis that must be excluded include adductor muscle strain, hernia, infection, ankylosing spondylitis,[16] osteitis secondary to chronic prostatitis in men, traumatic delivery in woman, and femoral neck fracture.[5,6] The latter is a potentially career-ending injury if misdiagnosed, and the examiner should be highly suspicious of any hip or groin pain in the running athlete. Clinical presentation reveals pain during single leg stance on the affected side; pain elicited during Patrick's test; and a frequently painful Trendelenburg test. If a bone scan is positive, then the patient should be immediately referred to an orthopaedic surgeon.[21]

28. How is osteitis pubis differentiated from adductor muscle strain?

Adductor strain, also known as *groin pull,* is easily confused with traumatic osteitis pubis because of the adjacent area of injury and also because of a common mechanism of injury. Similar to osteitis pubis, adductor strain may also result from passing or "shooting" the ball during soccer or from sprinting, or a sudden directional change while running.[21] These latter cases are examples of a traumatic mechanism of injury. In addition, adductor strain may also occur from repetitive abduction of the free leg in skating, cross-country skiing, in which case the mechanism involves repetitive stress. The adductor of the hip joint includes the adductor longus, adductor magnus, adductor brevis, and pectineus muscles. Although the gracilis and the lower fibers of gluteus maximus also manifest an adduction capacity, it is mainly the adductor longus that sustains injury during sport.[25]

A alternate traumatic mechanism implicated in adductor strain during soccer may happen when a player has one foot planted on the ground and brings the kicking leg forward in an abducted, flexed, and externally rotated position to reach the ball. This excessive external rotation and abduction movement at the hip has the effect of momentarily overstretching the adductor muscles. Although adductor strain may occur either by way of momentary overstretching or sudden contraction, osteitis pubis is incurred by way of excessive shear owing to a contractile mechanism of injury.

Although adductor strain involves injury to contractile tissue of the adductor longus muscle or musculotendinous junction[25] osteitis pubis involves injury to osseous tissue, at or adjacent to the locale of the adductor longus insertion. Although clinical presentation of both types of injury are often identical, adductor tendinitis exhibits groin tenderness maximally at the distal muscle insertion; osteitis pubis is maximally tender at the pubic bone. Moreover, complete adductor tear exhibits an inability to contract the adductor longus upon selective manual muscle testing, whereas some degree of adductor contraction may be elicited, despite pain, following traumatic osteitis pubis. The latter manifests severe pain that precludes further participation following traumatic osteitis pubis from direct contusion or an excessively powerful adductor contraction. Pain lingers and the player is unable to stand and may be taken to the hospital for evaluation.[32] Adductor strain typically manifests as a knifelike stabbing pain in the groin at the time of injury only, followed by returning pain only if the patient attempts to restart activity. Swelling associated with adductor strain does not occur until several days following the injury. Treatment for both injuries is similar.

29. What treatment strategy best manages this condition?

Osteitis pubis appears to be a self-limiting disorder, usually lasting several months. Most patients respond to conservative treatment[15] which may shorten the duration of this disorder, and is recommended for at least six months.[32] Immediately following injury, **ice massage** with cold cups may be applied to the groin area. The sine qua non treatment for osteitis pubis is **rest** from physical exertion that may have precipitated pubalgia. Bed rest for up to 2 to 3 weeks may be indicated for patients with severe symptoms. **Moist heat** by way of whirlpool or a bath at a temperature of 38.9°C (102°F) is indicated for symptomatic relief of pain. After pain subsides, **range of motion** exercises may begin with emphasis on gentle abduction of the hip joint and **strengthening** of the abdominal musculature.[27] **Resistive exercises** may begin when range of motion is full and can be performed without pain. Although this condition heals, an alternate substitute upper body exercise program should be instituted, and may include freestyle swimming (Australian crawl) using a flotation device (pull-buoy or life jacket) with the legs tied together so as to avoid stress across the pubis. Using the scissor or "frog kick" during swimming, or performing bicycling activities is contraindicated as these motions may reproduce symptoms. The use of nonsteroidal antiinflammatory drugs and phenylbutazone[15] as well as oral cortisone[26] have been effective in relieving symptoms. Some patients may experience relief of symptoms after steroid injection[27] although this is preferably avoided because of the possibility of infection. In contrast to adductor muscle strain, which is derived from poor flexibility of these muscles and is managed by stretching, adductor stretching may aggravate the patient with osteitis pubis.[14] Instead, patients with osteitis pubis should perform strengthening exercises to their adductor musculature. In addition to performing concentric exercises, **eccentric exercises** are particularly helpful as this form of contraction attenuates high velocity or heavy resistive loads, and thereby helps stave off injury. Training modifications should include mileage reduction, prevention of overstriding, and elimination of downhill running.[21] A heel lift is to be used to correct a leg length discrepancy, while any excessive pronation should be checked with an appropriate orthoses. Following approximately 2 months of conservative treatment, early recalcification is usually noted on the radiograph, and light jogging may be initiated. Running or cutting are not permitted until the eighth week, after which kicking the ball is gradually introduced.[32] Athletes may return to sport approximately 3 months following onset.

RECOMMENDED READING

Hanson PG, Angenine M, Juhl JH: Osteitis pubis in sports activities, *Phys Sports Med* 6:111, 1978.

Pyle LA Jr: Osteitis pubis in an athlete, *J Am Coo Health* 23:238, 1975.

REFERENCES

1. Asimov I: *The human brain: its capacities and functions,* 1965, New American Library.
2. Birrer RB, Robinson T: Pelvic fracture following karate kick, *NY State J Med* 11:503, 1991.
3. Lount W: Don't throw away that cane, Presidential Address, Annual Meeting, Academy of Orthopaedic Surgeons, *J Bone Joint Dis* 38A:695, 1956.
4. Bowerman JW: *Radiology and injury in sport,* New York, 1977, Appleton-Century-Crofts.
5. Brody DM: *Running injuries.* In Clinical symposia, West Caldwell, N.J., 1987, CIBA-GEIGY.
6. Brody DM: Running injuries. In Nicholas JA, Hershman EB editors: *The lower extremity and spine in sports medicine,* St Louis, 1995, Mosby.
7. Burman M, Weinkel IN, Langston MJ: Adolescent osteochondritis of the symphysis pubis with a consideration of normal roentgenographic changes in the symphysis pubis, *J Bone Joint Surg,* 16:649, 1934.
8. Dananberg HC: Functional hallux limitus and its relationship to gait efficiency, *J Am Podiatr Med Assoc* 76:6-18, 1986.
9. Dandy DJ: *Essential orthopaedics and trauma,* Edinburgh, 1989, Churchill Livingstone.
10. Edelstein JE editor: *Lower limb orthotics,* New York, 1986, New York University Post-Graduate Medical School of Prosthetics and Orthotics.
11. Frankel VH, Nordin M: *Basic biomechanics of the skeletal system,* Philadelphia, 1980, Lea & Febiger.
12. Gould JA: *Orthopaedic and sports physical therapy,* ed 2, St Louis, 1990, Mosby.
13. Gracovetsky S: *The spinal engine,* Vienna, 1988, Springer-Verlag.
14. Hanson PG, Angevine M, Juhl JH: Osteitis pubis in sports activities, *Phys Sports Med* 6:111, 1978.
15. Harris WR: The endocrine basis for slipping of the upper femoral epiphysis: an experimental study, *J Bone Joint Surg* 32B:5, 1950.
16. Hollander JL, McCarty DJ Jr: *Arthritis and allied conditions: a textbook of rheumatology,* ed 8, Philadelphia, 1972, Lea & Febiger.
17. Kapandji IA: *The physiology of the joints: lower limb,* ed 2, vol 2, London, 1970, ES Livingstone.
18. Kapandji IA: *Physiology of the joints: lower limb,* vol 2, New York, 1975, Churchill Livingstone
19. Kapandji IA: *The physiology of the joints,* ed 2, New York, 1976, Churchill Livingstone.
20. Lehmkuhl LD, Smith LK: *Brunnstrom's clinical kinesiology,* ed 4, Philadelphia, 1989, FA Davis.
21. Lillegard WA, Rucker KS: *Handbook of sports medicine: a symptom-oriented approach,* Boston, 1993, Andover Medical Publishers.
22. Lockhart RD, Hamilton GF, Fyfe FW et al: *Anatomy of the human body,* Philadelphia, 1969, JB Lippincott.
23. Moore KL: *Clinically oriented anatomy,* ed 2, Baltimore, 1985, Williams & Wilkins.
24. Oka M, Hatanpaa S: Degenerative hip disease in adolescent athletes, *Br J Sports Med* 12:4, 1978.
25. Peterson L, Renstrom P: *Sports injuries: their prevention and treatment,* Chicago, 1986, YearBook Medical Publishers.
26. Pyle LA Jr: Osteitis pubis in an athlete, *J Am Coo Health* 23:238, 1975.
27. Rispoli FP: Sindrome pubica dei calciatori socemiliana romagnola triveneta ortop, *Traumatol Atti* 8:331, 1963.
28. Rodnan GP, Schumacher HR: *Primer on the rheumatic diseases,* ed 8, Atlanta, 1983, The Arthritis Foundation.
29. Rydell N: Biomechanics of the hip joint, *Clin Orthop* 92:6, 1973.
30. Scully RM, Barnes MR: *Physical therapy,* Philadelphia, 1989, JB Lippincott.
31. Sim FH, Rock MG, Scott SG: Pelvis and hip injuries in athletes: anatomy and function. In Nicholas JA, Hershman EB editors: *The lower extremity and spine in sports medicine,* St Louis, 1995, Mosby.
32. Xethalis JL, Lorei MP: Soccer injuries. In Nicholas JA, Hershman EB editors: *The lower extremity and spine in sports medicine,* St Louis, 1995, Mosby.

55

Deep Buttock Pain and Numbness in the Peroneal Distribution

CASE 1: A slim 37-year-old unemployed female spent her newfound leisure time pursuing nirvana at the local yoga retreat. She spends 6 to 7 hours a day in the lotus meditative posture for several weeks and now complains of left numbness, tingling, and deep ache in the left buttock that migrates down the length of the back of her thigh, leg, and shin and is relieved by standing upright. She presents a prescription from her family physician that reads: "Vague low back and sciatic pain—please evaluate." When asked, the patient reports no history of injury. She claims that she has been healthy her entire life, and offers that symptoms are reproduced during sexual intercourse and recently during a constipated bowel movement. Symptoms increase with sitting and walking but decrease when she lies down. The patient runs along a hard concrete surface 3 miles per day, 6 days per week.

OBSERVATION   A bilateral forefoot varus foot deformity is observed, left greater than right. A kyphosis-lordosis type thoracic posture is observed; the pelvis is tilted in excessive anterior pelvic tilt.

PALPATION   This yields deep localized pain elicited in the posterior aspect of the hip near the sciatic notch.

ACTIVE RANGE OF MOTION   Internal rotation of the left hip is decreased by 25%.

PASSIVE RANGE OF MOTION   Extremes of left internal hip rotation yields pain. Passive hip extension is painless.

STRENGTH   There is some weakness indicated in the lateral hamstring muscle G (good), and a G−/G grade to the left ankle evertors and dorsiflexors.

FLEXIBILITY   Excessive tightness noted in the iliopsoas, quadriceps, and paraspinal muscle groups, as well as extensibility of the hamstrings and abdominal muscles.

SELECTIVE TENSION   Resisted external rotation of the femur and medial pelvic rotation are painful. Resistive hip extension is also painful.

GIRTH MEASUREMENT   Left calf muscle shows atrophy by one third compared with the contralateral calf.

SENSATION   Decreased light touch and pressure in the peroneal distribution.

856

DEEP TENDON REFLEXES A 2+ Achilles and medial hamstring jerks; 1+ lateral hamstrings jerk test.

SPECIAL TESTS Positive straight leg raise. The left Q angle measures 18°, compared with 16° on the right.

CLUE Passive left internal hip rotation, flexion, adduction, and knee flexion produce pain. Resistive left external rotation in this posture affords relief.

CASE 2: A 28-year-old female complains of severe left ischial pain with sciatic radiation of 5 months duration. Her ischial pain has not decreased in intensity since the onset of symptoms nor has pain radiation progressed further distally than when symptoms appeared. A history of a fall in which she struck her left buttock along the edge of a carpeted stairway 2 months before onset while carrying a heavy object only after much memory dredging. She describes in detail how she was "black and blue" for 3 weeks on her left buttock. Since the onset of symptoms she has undergone an extensive medical work-up, including magnetic resonance imaging and computerized tomography that scored negative for lumbosacral radiculopathy. The patient reports exacerbation of pain on sitting or standing, and relief when lying. Despite her pain, the patient consistently exercises on a stair-climbing machine for 30 minutes per day.

OBSERVATION A miserable malalignment of the lower extremities is observed in both lower extremities as excessive femoral internal rotation, lateral tibial torsion, and over-pronated feet.

PALPATION This yields extreme tenderness in the buttock area between the ischium and greater trochanter.

ACTIVE RANGE OF MOTION This is within functional limits.

PASSIVE RANGE OF MOTION Painless internal rotation.

STRENGTH Hamstring muscle strength is graded at G−.

FLEXIBILITY There appears to be mild to moderate tightness of the left medial hamstrings.

SELECTIVE TENSION This yields pain on resistive external rotation and hip extension.

GIRTH MEASUREMENT The left calf muscle shows atrophy by one third as compared with the contralateral calf.

SENSATION There is decreased sensation and trophic changes along the entire peripheral sciatic nerve distribution.

DEEP TENDON REFLEXES A 1+ grade for patellar, hamstrings, and calcaneal tendon reflexes.

SPECIAL TESTS There is a positive straight leg raise.

CLUE Resisted contraction of the left hip external rotators reproduces pain when the involved leg is positioned in extremes of left hip internal rotation, flexion, adduction, and knee flexion. Passive internal rotation yields relief.

❓ **Questions**

1. What is the cause of these women's symptoms?
2. What is the anatomy of the sciatic nerve in relation to the piriformis?
3. What are the short rotators of the hip joint and what is their functional anatomy during open and closed kinetic chain function?
4. What is the significance to the course of the sciatic nerve in relation to the short hip rotators?
5. What is the significance of intrapelvic division of the sciatic nerve?
6. How may activities that increase intraabdominal pressure be related to strain of the piriformis muscle?
7. How does femoral anteversion tense the sciatic nerve?
8. How is hyperlordosis of the lumbar spine related to tension applied to the sciatic nerve?

9. What is the traumatic mechanism implicated in the acute form of this disorder?
10. What vascular mechanism has been proposed in the etiology of piriformis syndrome?
11. What is the role of the external and internal rotators in relation to transverse plane motion of the femur?
12. What is the decelerating role of the short rotators in relation to medial pelvic and ipsilateral lower limb rotation beyond midstance phase of gait?
13. How may a forefoot varus postural abnormality of the foot predispose for the development of piriformis syndrome?
14. What is the clinical presentation?
15. What is the differential diagnosis?
16. What therapeutic intervention is appropriate in management of piriformis syndrome?

1. What is the cause of these women's symptoms?

Piriformis syndrome is a *peripheral neuropathy* of the sciatic nerve secondary to compressive entrapment of the nerve as it passes adjacent to the external hip rotators en route to its exit from the gluteal region by way of the greater sciatic foramen. Piriformis syndrome may be thought of, by way of analogy, as the lower extremity correlate of thoracic outlet compression in the upper extremity of the *brachial plexus.* In a similar way, piriformis syndrome may cause a sciatic nerve palsy, or selective entrapment of the common peroneal nerve. There is considerable debate about the etiologic origins of piriformis syndrome, and the matter remains one of some uncertainty. Multiple etiologies have been proposed and include muscle spasm,[16] contracture, compression, trauma, vascular compromise, and increased muscle mass due to hypertrophy.

In Case 1, which most likely involved selective compression of the common peroneal nerve, weakness of the peroneal muscles supplied by that nerve would be a consistent finding. Occasionally, the common peroneal nerve may pass through the piriformis muscle and separate it into two bellies.[1,2,7,10,13,14,26] The common peroneal nerve supplies the short head of the biceps femoris, the anterior compartment

muscles of the leg (foot and ankle dorsiflexors), and the evertors (peronei) in the lateral compartment of the leg. Also, because the lateral hamstring deep tendon reflex is conveyed through the S1 root of the peroneal division of the sciatic nerve, a depressed reflex is suggestive of common peroneal entrapment. Whereas if the medial hamstring reflex was also depressed or absent, compression of both the tibial and common peroneal sciatic components is suggested. Pain is reproduced by simultaneous stretching of the piriformis muscle and the sciatic nerve running through it. Here the mechanism is intrinsic secondary to stretching of the piriformis muscle owing to distancing of the bony attachments of piriformis as a function of over-pronation secondary to a forefoot varus deformity. Relief is afforded to the nerve passing between the two heads of piriformis by contraction of the external rotators, which temporarily decreases tension along the nerve by momentarily restoring the muscle to its normal length. Sexual intercourse with the female in the recumbent position may cause compression of the gluteal muscle mass and those structures deep to it such as the sciatic nerve.

Case 2 is probably involves compression of the entire sciatic trunk, and occurred secondary to an external cause such as trauma. Predisposition toward the development of piriformis syndrome may have contributed to contracture or hypertrophy of the short rotators. Here, resistive contraction would only further aggravate the sciatic nerve, especially if it passes through the substance of piriformis. Pain is momentarily relieved by stretching into internal rotation as this relieves contraction of the muscle on the intervening nerve.

2. What is the anatomy of the sciatic nerve in relation to the piriformis?

One of the principal nerves of the lumbosacral plexus is the *sciatic nerve,* which is comprised of two terminal nerves. Composed of an anteriorly derived tibial and posteriorly derived *common peroneal component,* the sciatic nerve derives from the anterior ventral rami of the fourth lumbar to the second sacral nerve roots and converges as a singular triangular trunk, the apex of which passes through the *greater sciatic foramen* into the buttock, covered by gluteus maximus. These two nerves, usually combined (in approximately 85% of the population)[16] in a single sheath, exit the pelvis to enter the posterior gluteal region by passing *underneath* (and not through) the lower border of that pear-shaped and uppermost of the short rotators of the hip joint: the *piriformis muscle* (L. *Pirum,* pear) (Fig. 55-1). The piriformis, the only *sacroiliac muscle,* connects the anterior surface of the sacrum to the greater trochanter of the femur.[27] The sciatic nerve then traverses over the other short rotators and enters the gateway to the thigh by passing *over* the quadratus femoris muscle through the hollow

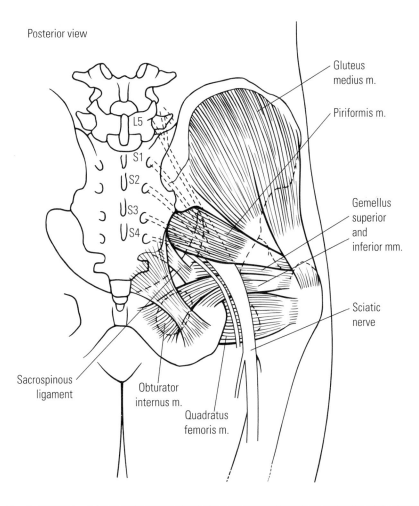

Posterior view

Gluteus medius m.

Piriformis m.

L5

S1

S2

S3

S4

Gemellus superior and inferior mm.

Sciatic nerve

Sacrospinous ligament

Obturator internus m.

Quadratus femoris m.

FIG. 55-1 Anatomy of the *piriformis muscle.* Piriformis divides the greater sciatic foramen into the *suprapiriformis* and *infrapiriformis regions.* The sciatic nerve passes underneath piriformis in most persons.

between two osseous gateposts; that is, the greater tuberosity and the greater trochanter.

3. What are the short rotators of the hip joint and what is their functional anatomy during open and closed kinetic chain function?

The deep layer of the posterior compartment of the hip is composed of 6 *short rotators* of the hip joint. Running under cover of the gluteus maximus muscle, these small muscles originate on the ischial portion of the innominate bone and/or within the pelvis and insert on the posteromedial aspect of the greater trochanter of the femur. Their horizontal orientation of span falls to the posterior side of the transverse axis of the hip joint so that contraction results in *external rotation of the hip* joint in the *open kinetic chain,* in which the femur moves on a fixed pelvis. This occurs in early to mid swing phase of gait. In contradistinction, movement of the pelvis on a fixed femur corresponding to the *closed kinetic chain* during stance phase of gait results in *me-dial pelvic rotation* of the stance leg (Fig. 55-2). The lower short rotators also help extend and adduct the hip joint by virtue of their relation to the hip joint axis.

4. What is the significance to the course of the sciatic nerve in relation to the short hip rotators?

The uppermost of the six short hip rotators is the triangular shaped piriformis muscle, whereas the lowermost muscle border is the rectangular quadratus femoris muscle. The relationship of the sciatic nerve to these two muscles is particularly relevant to understanding piriformis syndrome. Because the sciatic nerve usually runs beneath the upper most short rotators and superior to the lower most of these muscles, shortness, contracture, or even hypertrophy of the short rotators may tense that span of intervening nerve. Thus mechanical compression causing localized ischemia of both components of the sciatic nerve may be implicated in the etiology of this sciatic entrapment neuropathy.

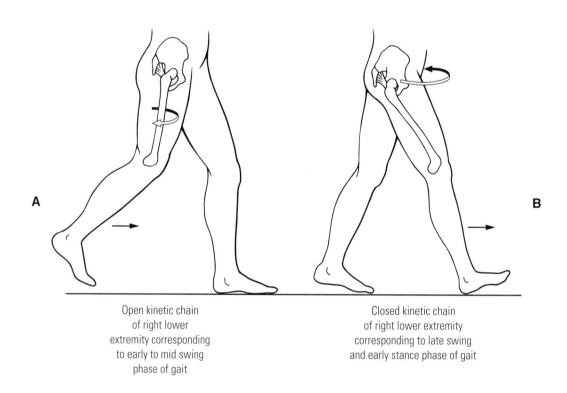

A, Open kinetic chain of right lower extremity corresponding to early to mid swing phase of gait

B, Closed kinetic chain of right lower extremity corresponding to late swing and early stance phase of gait

FIG. 55-2 Open and closed chain function of the short rotators of the hip. **A,** In the open kinetic chain, corresponding to late stance and early to mid swing phase of gait, the femur moves on a fixed pelvis and causes the hip joint to undergo external rotation. **B,** In the closed kinetic chain, corresponding to late swing and into early stance, the pelvis rotates internally on a relatively fixed femur.

5. What is the significance of intrapelvic division of the sciatic nerve?

A variation in the course of the sciatic nerve involves a separation of its constituent nerves by all or part of the piriformis muscle in approximately 15%[6] of the population owing to absence of a common sheath binding these nerves together; in these patients, the sciatic nerve courses through the piriformis muscle. In this case the more posterolateral placed common peroneal nerve may pass through the substance of the piriformis muscle (Fig. 55-3). As a result, shortness or an excessively forceful contraction of the short rotators may entrap the nerve resulting in ischemia. Alternately, the entire sciatic nerve and its sheath pierce the substance of the piriformis. Either variation may separate piriformis into two bellies.

If the sciatic nerve or the common peroneal nerve pass between the two tendinous heads of the piriformis, compression occurs with muscle stretch rather than muscle contraction (Fig. 55-4). Piriformis is maximally stretched by simultaneous hip internal rotation, flexion, adduction, and knee flexion. This posture also maximally tenses the sciatic nerve.[4]

6. How may activities that increase intraabdominal pressure be related to strain of the piriformis muscle?

The muscles of the pelvic floor include, among others, the piriformis, levator ani, and coccygeus, which together form a contiguous muscular sling that closes the posterior part of the pelvic outlet. The latter two muscles form the pelvic diaphragm surrounding the sphincters of the excretory and reproductive systems. The pelvic floor is strong enough to passively support the abdominal contents during running or jumping activities, and yet resilient enough to allow passage of a full term infant. Loss of tone of the pelvic floor musculature may occur in multiparous women and often results in stress incontinence. Repetitive muscular stresses to the pelvis in athletics or in activities involving frequent increases of inner abdominal pressure may result in a tension myalgia of the pelvic muscles known as *pelvic floor myalgia*. This condition also occurs by reflex contraction of these muscles secondary to pain arising anywhere in the lumbosacral spine, sacroiliac joint, coccyx, or hips.[23]

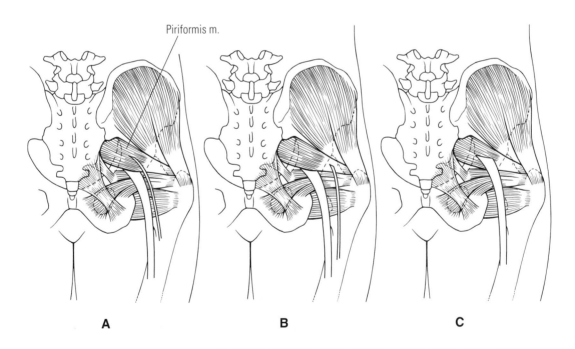

Piriformis m.

A   **B**   **C**

FIG. 55-3 Intrapelvic division of the sciatic nerve owing to the absence of a common neural sheath. **A,** This variation shows the common peroneal nerve passing through the muscular fibers of piriformis. **B,** In another variation, the common peroneal nerve may course between the tendinous portions of piriformis. **C,** Alternately, the entire sciatic nerve and its sheath pierce the substance of the piriformis.

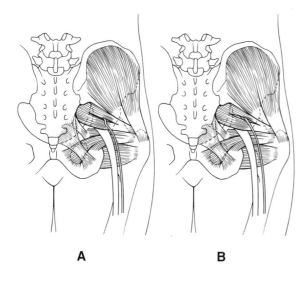

A   **B**

FIG. 55-4 Intrapelvic division of the sciatic nerve may cause compromise of the common peroneal nerve during both passive stretching. **A,** During passive stretching of piriformis by simultaneous hip internal rotation, flexion, adduction, and knee flexion, the tendinous portions of the muscle compress the nerve. **B,** During concentric contraction of piriformis the space between the tendons enlarges and the nerve is free to pass.

Although a loss of tone of the pelvic floor muscles may not adversely affect the sciatic nerve, hypertrophy, or strain of piriformis in athletes of either gender may entrap the sciatic nerve, viselike, at the inferior aspect of that muscle. The resulting nerve distortion with limb motion may result in pain in the ipsilateral buttock, hip, or down the posterior portion of the leg. Although passive tensing and subsequent compression of the sciatic nerve may occur by way of medial femoral rotation and adduction of the hip joint, active contraction of hypertrophied short hip rotators may act to dynamically constrict the sciatic nerve. The latter may be implicated as a possible *dynamic mechanism* of sciatic nerve compression because piriformis functions as a lateral hip rotator and may thereby contribute to excessive tension upon the nerve during repetitive forceful contraction.

7. How does femoral anteversion tense the sciatic nerve?

A *miserable malalignment syndrome* (Chapter 52) involving the triad of *femoral anteversion* (i.e., excessive internal rotation, external tibial torsion, and foot pronation) will tether the sciatic nerve along its length. This tenses the nerve in much the same way that the nerve is

tension biased during a straight leg raise in which hip adduction and medial rotation is superimposed on the provocative maneuver. The sciatic nerve may be passively compromised across its length of span of the short hip rotators due to shortening of those muscles.

8. How is hyperlordosis of the lumbar spine related to tension applied to the sciatic nerve?

A postural etiology may be related to the development of piriformis syndrome. Sagittal plane postural balance is maintained by reciprocal contractions of the extensors and flexors. An individual, such as the perpetual armchair executive, with shortness or contracture of bilateral hip flexors will, to some degree, maintain his or her sitting posture when standing upright. This occurs because the sitting position approximates the origin and insertion of the iliopsoas and rectus femoris muscles. To prevent the eyes from looking downward, righting reactions cause compensatory hyperlordosis of the lumbar spine. This results in an overall approximation and eventual shortening or contracture of the paraspinal muscles. The net effect of these two synergistic muscle groups with reference to the pelvis is an *anterior pelvic tilt*. Lordotic compensation occurs with the lordosis postural pattern, and the kyphosis-lordosis postural pattern. This state of inadequate thoracic stabilization results in increased tension of the pelvifemoral muscles as they contract in the attempt to stabilize the pelvis and spine in the new position. The short rotators, including piriformis, hypertrophy in response. However, this hypertrophy causes narrowing of the infrapiriformis foramen and may lead to sciatic nerve compression.[15,17,18] The clinical relevance of these postural and soft-tissue changes is that the now anteriorly tilted pelvis tautens the sciatic nerve, causing it to rub against the sharp edge of the sciatic notch.[9]

9. What is the traumatic mechanism implicated in the acute form of this disorder?

A sciatic nerve palsy, as a result of direct external trauma[16] at the sciatic notch, is uncommon because of the protection afforded by the overlying gluteal musculature.[9] Protection is also provided by a fat pad that ensheaths the sciatic trunk as it lies against the underside of the short rotator. However, injury may nevertheless occur from an excessively hard fall in the sitting position onto a hard object as in Case 2. Sudden upward pressure may injure the nerve directly or may suddenly compress it against the sciatic notch owing to the close apposition of the sciatic nerve to the sharp edge of the sciatic foramen. Alternately, distortion of the underlying nerve may occur secondary to a muscle contusion or hematoma of the gluteus maximus. Sciatic nerve injury may also occur from a penetrating knife or bullet wound, or from a medially placed intramuscular injection. A prolonged spasm of piriformis may occur following a twisting injury sustained during single leg stance.[11] Palpation of piriformis spasm is assessed by performing a rectal examination,[20,24] or by external palpation over the greater sciatic foramen.

Some people may develop sciatic pain particularly on the right during prolonged driving. This may be attributed to one of several reasons. The seat may be of such construction that its forward edge is at about the middle of the thigh. When the posterior thigh "breaks" over the edge at this point with the knee in near extension external force may result in sciatic nerve distress. In addition to being primed for tension by knee extension, the sciatic nerve is also proximally tautened owing to the spine-seat configuration, which essentially reproduces the straight leg raise posture. The middle of the posterior thigh is particularly vulnerable to sciatic nerve distress when the knee is almost extended as may occur when the seat is adjusted backwardly. At the mid-posterior thigh, the long head of biceps femoris diverges from the semitendinosus so that the nerve does not have the benefit of much flesh intervening between it and the skin. The sciatic nerve therefore lies in the invagination between the short biceps head and the adductor magnus muscles. The nerve may be compromised by the forward seat edge pressing it against the sharp posterior edge of the femoral crest resembling the apex of a triangle known as the *crista femoris* (Fig. 55-5). The remedy is to either increase knee flexion or alter the seat position. This serves to slacken the sciatic nerve as well as the adductor magnus and the short head of the biceps; the nerve is no longer pulled across the sharp edge of the crista, which bears down upon it with thigh weight. Also, the two muscles may actually provide a cushioning effect to the nerve trunk.[9]

10. What vascular mechanism has been proposed in the etiology of piriformis syndrome?

A branch of the inferior gluteal artery known as *commitans nervi ischiadici* accompanies the sciatic nerve for a short distance as it crosses the inferior margin of the piriformis. This vessel nurtures the sciatic nerve by way of feeding into the sheath enfolding the nerve. Constant or repeated muscle spasm may compress this vessel and result in sciatic nerve ischemia.[16]

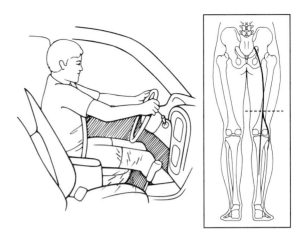

FIG. 55-5 Mechanical mid-thigh compression of the sciatic nerve. The nerve may be compromised by the forward seat edge pressing it against the sharp posterior edge of the femoral crest.

11. What is the role of the external and internal rotators in relation to transverse plane motion of the femur?

As piriformis is a muscle involved in rotation, any analysis of piriformis dysfunction must of necessity take into account rotary movement of the lower limb. *Transverse motion* refers to rotational movements that occur in direct response to alignment changes during stride as the body (hence, center of gravity) swings from behind the supporting limb to the contralateral advancing leg. Rotations function to smooth out the path of center of gravity so that gyrations are at a minimum and thus reduce the energy expenditure incurred during gait. With each stride the lower limb accommodates changes in alignment by moving through an arc of internal and external rotation. During stance phase the femur and tibia rotate in unison, except momentarily during midstance, whereas in swing phase they rotate in opposing directions. Moreover, during swing and early stance phases of gait the lower limbs rotate medially and then laterally beyond midstance phase of stance until toe off.[21] The purpose of dynamic internal rotation of the pelvis, and hence the femur, which occurs during swing just before heel strike, is to render the posture of the knee and ankle joints optimal in preparation for heel strike.

During walking, rotation of the pelvis causes the femur, tibia, and fibula to rotate about the long axis of the lower limb.[8] The magnitude of this rotation increases progressively from the pelvis to the tibia. During normal walking over level ground the pelvis undergoes a maximum rotation in each gait cycle of about 6°, the hip rotation averages 8°,[19] while the tibia undergoes about 18° in the same period.[12]

12. What is the decelerating role of the short rotators in relation to medial pelvic and ipsilateral lower limb rotation beyond midstance phase of gait?

Gait is initiated by medial pelvic rotation, and may occur via concentric contraction of iliacus, and the short hip rotators of the swing leg. This medial pelvic rotation, which persists throughout early stance, is accomplished by concentric action of the short rotators and eccentric action of the internal rotators. During midstance phase of gait, the pelvis reverses direction and laterally rotates so as to allow for contralateral medial pelvic rotation so as to move forward with the opposite swing leg. This alternating sequence concentric contraction of lateral rotators and eccentric contraction of the medial rotators, and vice versa, is essentially a cocontraction of the rotators. The hip joint, characterized by three degrees of freedom, is thus modulated by a dynamic elimination of several degrees of freedom so as to prevent wobbling during ambulation. Cocontraction of the rotators acts to silence the expression of those degrees of freedom not essential an efficient gait.

This reversal from medial to lateral rotation of the lower stance limb is in keeping with the local kinesiology at the knee and foot. Once heel rise occurs, the femerotibial complex of the stance limb externally rotate in unison. The tibia externally rotates as a function of subtalar joint supination, which begins to manifest as pronation is progressively diminished at midstance. At the knee, extension is achieved during late stance at toe off in which the lower limb acts as a lever to forward-thrust the body and perpetuate a new cycle of locomotion. This cooperative lateral limb rotation is necessary for the synchronous action of the knee, hip, and pelvis.

Thus during late stance the contractile mode of the internal and external rotators of the hip joint alternate such that piriformis and the other short rotators eccentrically contract to decelerate the medial rotation of the femur on the pelvis,[25] whereas the anatomic internal rotators concentrically work to laterally rotate the stance-side pelvis.

13. How may a forefoot varus postural abnormality of the foot predispose for the development of piriformis syndrome?

The proximal biomechanical effects of forefoot varus (see p. 347) result from an internally generated rotary moment up along the tibial shaft commensurate with subtalar joint pronation. Pronation is occurring (beyond midstance) when the subtalar joint should ideally be supinating corresponding to lateral rotation of the upper and lower leg. This lateral limb rotation is necessary for the synchronous action of the knee, hip, and pelvis. If the lateral rotation component that accompanies subtalar joint supination is absent, the tibia will still laterally rotate, albeit not through its complete excursion, but only at foot flat as a function of the lateral terminal extension at the knee. However, synchronous function of the lower extremity complex is interrupted. The knee is faced with the biomechanical dilemma of negotiating the combined proximally derived lateral tibial rotation and distally derived medial tibial rotation. The knee cannot extend without lateral rotation, and does so as a result of permitting abnormal valgus opening at the knee. The price paid is in terms of compromising the various dynamic and static supporting structures at the knee. Thus damage may be incurred at the delicately balanced knee extensor mechanism.

The knee may, in part, avoid this dilemma by having the femur medially rotate along with the tibia thereby transferring the problem to a more proximal source. In the patient with a forefoot varus deformity, the femur will be subject to an internal rotary moment at the same time that the piriformis is working to externally rotate the femur. The net effect of these moments is to pull the bony attachments of the piriformis muscle in opposite directions[25] and distract the muscle along its origin and insertion simultaneously. Subsequently, the sciatic nerve, which courses through the piriformis, may compromise tension at the muscle insertion. Thus if the poorly timed rotation is transferred proximally, a piriformis muscle syndrome or sacroiliac joint dysfunction may occur.

14. What is the clinical presentation?

Palpation may show exquisite point tenderness in the midsubstance of the piriformis; alternately, patients may complain of a dull, aching pain in the buttock. Pain in the gluteal or sacral regions remains the most constant symptom.[16] Pain typically increases with sitting or walking and decreases when lying supine. The patient may present with a history of symptoms provoked following prolonged working at a computer or playing the piano for many hours. Resisted hip extension may be painful, as the piriformis is also a hip extensor. Pain may be increased during hip extension as the muscle bulk of the overlying gluteal mass balls up and impinges on the piriformis. Although resisted external hip rotation is painful, passive internal hip rotation and adduction superimposed on hip and knee flexion may also produce pain as it stretches the piriformis. Biasing the sciatic nerve for tension may be accomplished by superimposing ipsilateral hip adduction and medial rotation upon hip flexion during the straight leg raise test (Fig. 55-6).[4] As the piriformis lies behind the hip axis for flexion and extension, it functions as a hip extensor. Consequently, passive hip flexion will stretch the distal insertion of piriformis.

Pain and paresthesia may present along the entire sciatic nerve distribution. Paresthesia may include a burning sensation, hypesthesia, or anesthesia. Motor weakness and eventual atrophy may develop. Trophic skin changes may occur if the sympathetic branches accompanying the sciatic nerve are compressed.[16]

15. What is the differential diagnosis?

Because the piriformis is so close to the origin of the sciatic nerve origin at the nerve root levels, it is often difficult to differentiate a lumbosacral root lesion from a high proximal peripheral sciatic neuropathy.* Thus the recognition of piriformis syndrome remains one of uncertainty.[5] Diagnosis is based upon patient history and clinical examination and the elimination of other causes of sciatic nerve impingement or irritation.[16]

- *Radiculopathy.* It is often difficult to disentangle a diagnosis of peripheral sciatic neuropathy from sciatica secondary to a *lumbosacral root lesion*. This is especially so if there are concurrent symptoms or a history of back derangement. Although motor symptoms of sciatic radiculopathy may cause palpable gluteal muscle atrophy, sciatic neuropathy will spare these muscles. In addition, whereas a radicular source of sensory alteration is characterized along topographic dermatomes, peripheral nerve causes of altered sensation manifest along peripheral nerve sensory distributions. Radicular sensory alterations, unlike periph-

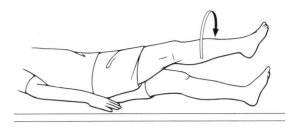

FIG. 55-6 Sciatic nerve compression from piriformis syndrome may be provoked by tensing the sciatic nerve. This is best accomplished by superimposing passive hip adduction and medial rotation upon hip flexion during the straight leg raise test.

eral neuropathy, often manifests as monoradicular symptoms in which the pain radiates as far distally to the lateral side of the foot and small toe (S1), the dorsum of the foot (L5), or to the medial part of the calf (L4). In addition, a root lesion due to a herniated disk often manifests as bilateral lower extremity symptoms in a positive contralateral crossed test. Moreover, pain of radicular origin is often accompanied by heightened thecal symptoms on coughing, laughing, sneezing, and during a bowel movement. Finally, patients with a herniated lumbosacral disk report pain relief in recumbency particularly with the knees and hips partially flexed.

- *Spinal stenosis.* Stenosis of the lumbar spine involves narrowing of the neural canal or foramen resulting in constriction of the dura and cauda equina in central stenosis and the nerve roots in lateral stenosis. Although central spine stenosis manifests as a diffuse dull lumbosacral ache, lateral spine stenosis may cause claudication-like pain to the calf muscles. Patients are typically beyond middle age and complain of pain on walking or standing that is relieved by forward flexing while erect as well as in the sitting and lying postures. A positive straight leg raise or bowstring test is uncommon. Dural signs such as pain on coughing, sneezing, and during a Valsalva maneuver do not exacerbate symptoms. Moreover, the radicular pain component associated with neurogenic claudication is that, unlike sciatic nerve entrapment, it does not delineate along a singe nerve root and does not dominate the historical presentation.

- *Diabetic neuropathy.* A diabetic neuropathy may result in sciatic pain. Symptoms are relatively acute in onset and develop over several days. Unlike patients with spinal disease these patients have no back pain.

---

*Before disk disease was proven to be a major cause of sciatica by Barr and Mixter in 1931, piriformis tenotomy was a popular operation.[3]

Some patients may demonstrate symptoms of other neuropathies and exhibit weakness or sensory loss in the femoral or saphenous nerve territories as well.

- *Peroneal nerve injury.* Peroneal nerve injury at the level of the knee may be confused with proximal common peroneal nerve compression at the piriformis muscle. However, because the peroneal component of the sciatic nerve innervates the short head of biceps femoris, positive electromyographic testing and a weakened grade during manual muscle testing of the biceps femoris imply a high lesion of the peroneal trunk and not an injury at the knee. Additionally, compression at the knee is often accompanied by a history of trauma.

- *Bursitis.* Bursitis overlying the posterior hip capsule is suspected in the absence of radicular pain, low back pain, or pain on active or resistive hip movements that imply a musculotendinous lesion. Suspicion of bursitis is strengthened by pain elicited by passive anterior hip extension. Management typically involves gluteal exercises, general lower extremity stretching program, nonsteroidal antiinflammatory medication, and an occasional injection of steroid or local anesthetic.[22]

- *Sacroiliac joint dysfunction.* The sacroiliac joint is a large joint of irregular contour that is not easily disturbed by mechanical derangement. Serious disruption of this joint may accompany pelvic fractures and separation of the pubic symphysis. The sacroiliac joint is often the first articulation of the axial skeleton to be affected by inflammatory disorders such as pelvic infection in women and prostatitis in men. The piriformis muscle has the distinction of being the only sacroiliac muscle as it is the only muscle to cross that joint. Like piriformis syndrome, pain resulting from sacroiliac (SI) dysfunction may follow trauma or may occur insidiously. However, SI dysfunction is often characterized by unilateral tenderness over the associated posterior superior iliac spine and along the sacral sulcus without motor, reflex, or sensory deficit. Furthermore, provocative tests for SI joint involvement are negative in piriformis dysfunction.

16. What therapeutic intervention is appropriate in management of piriformis syndrome?

- *Therapeutic exercise.* Malalignment of the lower extremity such as occurs with miserable malalignment syndrome must be addressed via *strengthening* of the hip internal rotators, *stretching* the external rotators (Fig. 55-7), and providing the appropriate *orthoses* to

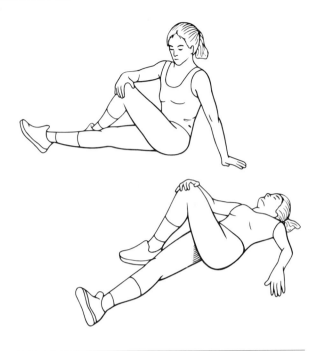

FIG. 55-7 Self-stretching of piriformis may be performed with the patient supine or long-sitting. With the patient in supine, raise the knee of the painful side up to waist level, cross it over the contralateral leg and anchor the foot against the knee. The knee is gently leaned toward the surface of the examination table.

address excessive pronation at the foot. This will also help to redress the *muscle imbalance* between the medial and lateral hamstrings by providing a stretch to the tightened semitendinosus and semimembranosus. It is important to provide simultaneous strengthening to the lateral hamstrings (biceps femoris).

- *Orthoses.* A forefoot varus deformity is orthotically addressed by fitting the patient with a medial forefoot post, and thereby minimize or eliminate the proximal effects of this foot deformity.

- *Postural training.* Postural imbalance due to hyperlordosis of the lumbar spine is addressed by strengthening of those muscles working antagonistic to the erector spinae and hip flexors. Strengthening must be directed at the hip extensor and abdominal muscle groups by way of selective strengthening and performing posterior pelvic tilting in the antigravity posture. Stretching of the overactive back and prefemoral muscles are an important adjunct to managing the postural basis for piriformis syndrome.

- *Modality usage.* The use of a heating modality such as *diathermy* or *ultrasound,* or *hydrotherapy* in a

Hubbard tank is appropriate at helping to relieve discomfort. The use of nonsteroidal antiinflammatory medications may be used, as well as judicious use of corticosteroid injection into the piriformis muscle. Reduction of muscle spasm is facilitated by *ice massage* in combination with ultrasound and electrical stimulation. The therapeutic effect may be enhanced by applying a low-load passive stretch to the piriformis (achieved by internal hip rotation). If the muscle is in spasm, it is important to *gently* stretch the muscle so as to avoid pain. The use of a *spray and stretch* technique using ethyl chloride spray over the involved buttock is appropriate following piriformis stretching. *Neuromuscular reeducation* may be an important adjunct of management; patients may be taught to relax pelvic floor musculature by way of biofeedback. Patients are instructed to avoid activities or postures that may aggravate or precipitate symptoms. The patient is advised not to wear their wallet in their back pocket. Prolonged sitting or excessive stair climbing activities are discouraged.

Patients who experience no significant relief of symptoms after several months of treatment may undergo surgery in which the entrapped nerve is freed by sectioning one of the heads of origin of the piriformis muscle.

RECOMMENDED READING

Pace JB, Nagle D: Piriformis syndrome, *West J Med* 124:435, 1976.

Pecina MM, Krmpotic-Nemanic J, Markiewitz AD: *Tunnel syndromes,* Boca Raton, Fla., 1991, CRC Press.

REFERENCES

1. Beaton LE, Anson BJ: *J Bone Joint Surg* 20, 686, 1938.
2. Berkol N, Mouchet A, Gogen H: *Annis Anat. Pathol* 12, 596, 1935.
3. Brody DM: Running injuries. In Nicholas JA, Hershman EB editors: *The lower extremity and spine,* ed 2, vol 2, St Louis, 1995, Mosby.
4. Butler DS: *Mobilisation of the nervous system,* Melbourne, 1991, Churchill Livingstone.
5. Dawson DM, Hallett M, Millender LH: *Entrapment neuropathies,* ed 2, Boston, 1990, Little, Brown and Company.
6. Hollinshead WH: *Anatomy for surgeons: back and limb,* ed 2, vol 3, New York, 1969, Harper & Row.
7. Ilic A, Mrvaljevic D, Blasotic M et al: *Acta Orthop (Yugosl)* 7, 163, 1976.
8. Inman VT, Ralston HJ, Todd F: *Human walking,* Baltimore, 1981, Williams & Wilkins.
9. Kopell HP, Thompson WAL: *Peripheral entrapment neuropathies,* New York, 1976, Robert E Krieger.
10. Lazorthes G: *Le systeme nerveux peripherique,* Paris, 1955, Masson.
11. Lillegard WA, Rucker KS: *Handbook of sports medicine: a symptom-oriented approach,* Boston, 1993, Andover Medical Publishers.
12. Manley MT: Biomechanics of the foot. In Helfet AJ, Gruembel Lee D editors: *Disorders of the foot,* Philadelphia, 1980, JB Lippincott.
13. Mouret J: *Montepell. Med* 2:230, 1893.
14. Odajima G, Kurihara T: *Excerpta Med* 17:9, 1963.
15. Pecina M: *Acta Anat.(Basel)* 105:181, 1979.
16. Pecina MM, Krmpotic-Nemanic J, Markiewitz AD: *Tunnel syndromes,* Boca Raton, Fla., 1991, CRC Press.
17. Pecina M: *Acta Orthop (Yugosl)* 6:196, 1975.
18. Pecina M: Ostecenja zivcanog stabla i ogranaka ishijadikusa uvjetovana posebnim topografskoanatomskim odnosima, disertacija, *Medicinski Fafultet, (Zagreb)* 1969.
19. Perry J: *Gait analysis: normal & pathological function,* Thorofare, NJ, 1992, Slack.
20. Pfeifer TH, Fitz WFK: The piriformis syndrome, *Z Orthop* 127:691, 1989.
21. Rodgers MM: *Dynamic biomechanics of the normal foot and ankle during walking and running,* Dayton, OH, Laboratory of Applied Physiology.
22. Sammarco GJ: Dance injuries. In Nicholas JA, Hershman EB editors: *The lower extremity and spine,* ed 2, vol 2, St Louis, 1995, Mosby.
23. Sim FH, Rock MG, Scott SG: Pelvis and hip injuries in athletes: anatomy and function. In Nicholas JA, Hershman EB editors: *The lower extremity and spine,* ed 2, vol 2, St Louis, 1995, Mosby.
24. Synek VM: The pyriformis syndrome: review and case presentation, *Clin Exp Neurol* 23:31, 1987.
25. Tiberio D: *Pathomechanics of structural foot deformities,* Conn., On-Site Biomechanical Education and Training.
26. Vallois HV: *CR Assoc Anat* 24:519, 1929.
27. Valmassy RL: *Clinical biomechanics of the lower extremities,* St Louis, 1996, Mosby.

56

Insidious Low Back Pain and Morning Stiffness of Greater than 3 Months Duration that Improves with Activity and Worsens with Rest in a Caucasian Man Below Age 40

A 28-year-old white, male, vicar complains of low back pain of insidious onset with a duration of more than 3 months. He complains of neck stiffness that makes driving an automobile difficult. He also reports morning stiffness that improves with activity and exercise. He also complains of a left swollen knee and right painful heel. Sitting through a long church sermon is uncomfortable. When asked, he admits that he often wakes up in the middle of the night to walk about or take a hot shower so as to relieve his pain. The patient presents you with a letter of referral from a rheumatologist that is accompanied by the results of several tests. Pulmonary function tests showed diminished vital capacity and total lung capacity, although residual and functional residual lung volumes were increased. Hematologic tests showed a mild normocytic anemia, and a normal peripheral white count. Erythrocyte sedimentation rate as well as alkaline and creatinine phosphatase were elevated. No rheumatoid factor was present.

OBSERVATION Posture shows flattening of the lumbar lordosis and a dorsal stoop with accentuation of thoracic kyphosis.

PALPATION Tenderness over the spinous processes of the lumbar and thoracic vertebrae. A bony spur is palpated at the right heel at the proximal insertion of the plantar fascia.

RANGE OF MOTION Severely diminished lateral flexion of the spine. Forward flexion and backward extension are decreased by one-half range. Both passive and active range of the left knee are diminished by 10°.

STRENGTH This is grossly normal throughout with exception to left knee flexion and extension, which are G−.

FLEXIBILITY Tightness noted in the left hamstring and triceps surae, as well as the right Achilles tendon.

SPECIAL TESTS There is a positive Gaenslen's test.

RADIOGRAPHS Calcific spurring present in the right heel.

CLUE Titer for HLA-B27 antigen was positive.

? **Q**uestions

1. What is most likely the cause of this patient's symptoms?
2. What are seronegative spondylarthropathies?
3. What is the pathogenic etiology of ankylosing spondylitis?
4. What is the prevalence of this disease?
5. How does ankylosing spondylitis differ from rheumatoid arthritis?
6. Which proximal and distal sites are typically affected with the spread of inflammation associated with AS?
7. What are the extraarticular manifestations of AS?
8. How does the radiographic appearance of AS change with the evolution of this disease?
9. What is spondylodiskitis?
10. What is the clinical presentation of these patients?
11. How is loss of spinal range of motion best assessed?
12. How is costovertebral involvement best assessed?
13. Which provocative clinical tests elicit sacroiliac tenderness due to sacroiliitis?
14. What are complications of AS?
15. What is the differential diagnosis of AS?
16. What physical therapy is appropriate in the management of this patient?
17. When is surgery appropriate in the management of AS?

1. What is most likely the cause of this patient's symptoms?

Ankylosing spondylitis (AS) is an inflammatory disorder of unknown etiology that primarily affects the spine, the axial skeleton, and the large proximal joints of the body including the sacroiliac joint, the symphysis pubis, and the hip, knee, and shoulder articulations leading to end-stage ankylosis (fusion) (Fig. 56-1). Asymmetric peripheral arthropathy occurs in one-fifth of all patients at presentation and one-third of patients at some later stage of the disease, and most often affects the lower limb.[18] The term "ankylosing spondylitis" etymologically derives from the Greek word *ankylos* (meaning bent or crooked), *spondylos* (vertebrae), and *itis,* meaning "inflammation of." This disease was considered to be a spinal form of rheumatoid arthritis and was alternately known as rheumatoid arthritis, Bechterew disease, and Marie Strumpel disease until the 1930s, after which it was recognized as a distinct pathologic and clinical entity. AS is characterized by a gradual, yet relentless, cephalad progression of fibrosis, secondary ossification, and ankylosis of the involved joints resulting in spinal immobility that may skip segments enroute to its upward migration to the occiput. Most patients, and women in particular, with symptomatic ankylosing spondylitis do not progress to solid fusion.[17] AS typically affects young men in their second through fourth decades, although young women may also, although less commonly, be affected.

The classic presentation of this disease occurs in a young male between 15 to 40 years of age complaining of insidious onset of intermittent or persistent low back pain and stiffness that is worse in the early morning hours or after prolonged rest. Pain is typically relieved by physical activity. Symptomatology of this disease may be mild and gradually progressive with minimal early morning stiffness, or may be severe and relentlessly progressive and crippling in the occasional patient (10%). In the latter patients death occurs from aortic insufficiency, uremia secondary to amyloidosis, or is due to atlantoaxial subluxation with cord compression. In some patients, skeletal involvement is limited to mild sacroiliitis and may not ever progress to severe spondylitis or ankylosis. Generally, the younger the patient the worse the prognosis.

2. What are seronegative spondylarthropathies?

AS is correctly categorized as a prototype of a spectrum of diseases sharing in common the presence of a specific histocompatability antigen, and lack of rheumatoid nodules, that are collectively known as *seronegative* (referring to the absence of serum Rh factor) *spondylarthropathies.* These include Reiter's syndrome, psoriatic arthritis,[24] rheumatoid arthritis, arthropathy result-

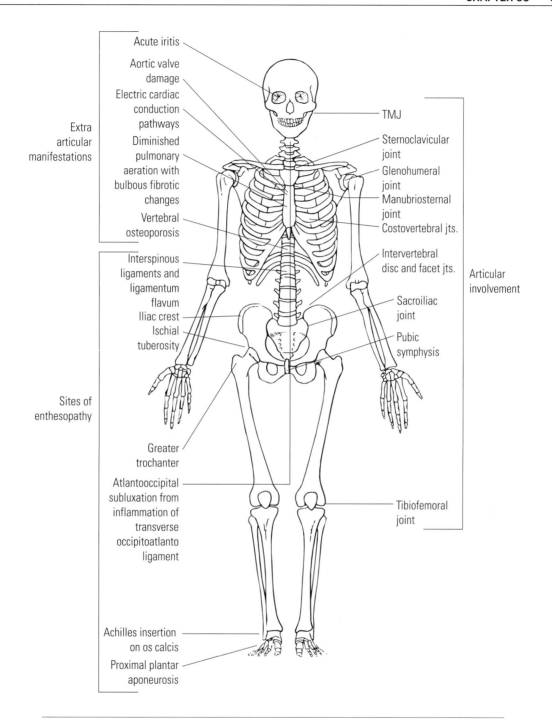

Extra articular manifestations

Acute iritis
Aortic valve damage
Electric cardiac conduction pathways
Diminished pulmonary aeration with bulbous fibrotic changes
Vertebral osteoporosis

Sites of enthesopathy

Interspinous ligaments and ligamentum flavum
Iliac crest
Ischial tuberosity

Greater trochanter

Atlantooccipital subluxation from inflammation of transverse occipitoatlanto ligament

Achilles insertion on os calcis
Proximal plantar aponeurosis

TMJ
Sternoclavicular joint
Glenohumeral joint
Manubriosternal joint
Costovertebral jts.
Intervertebral disc and facet jts.
Sacroiliac joint
Pubic symphysis

Tibiofemoral joint

Articular involvement

FIG. 56-1 Pathologic distribution of *ankylosing spondylitis*. Pathology includes articular involvement, enthesopathic sites, and extraarticular manifestations.

ing from ulcerative colitis and Crohn's disease, as well as those from systemic gastrointestinal bacterial infection such as *Yersinia, Shigella,* and *Salmonella,* which cause enteric arthritis.

3. What is the pathogenic etiology of ankylosing spondylitis?

In the 1970s a positive association between the HLA-B27 histocompatibility antigen and AS was discovered,[20] suggesting that the risk of disease is strongly, although not absolutely related to genetic risk. There is a 20 times greater incidence of AS among relatives with known AS, and these relatives have a much higher incidence of the B27 antigen than the normal population. Whether this antigen is the primary cause or whether it acts as a receptor for an infective and/or environmental agent that triggers the disease is unknown. However, because AS occurs in both white and black populations who are B27 negative, we may conclude that the antigen is not solely responsibly for the development of AS.

Although the etiology of AS is unknown, several theories exist that may account for the pathogenesis of this disease. An infectious etiology is postulated with *Klebsiella,* a ubiquitous organism, incriminated as a possible triggering infection before onset of the disease,[11] although definitive proof is lacking. In addition to the HLA-B27 link, raised level of complement inactive products, certain antiglobulins, and circulating immune complexes suggests an immunologic role in the pathogenesis of AS.[8] Conceivably, an infectious agent might interact with B27 positive cells to render them auto antigenic, leading to an autoimmune state.[1] The pathogenesis of AS may in fact be a complex interplay between genetic, autoimmune, antigenic, and infectious variables.

4. What is the prevalence of this disease?

The incidence of patients with clinical manifestation of AS is two to three per thousand[21] with an increased male to female ration of 2:1 to 10:1.[1] The sacroiliitis associated with AS is more prominent in males, and the disease is typically more progressive. Women tend to have more peripheral joint involvement and are sometimes misdiagnosed as having seronegative rheumatoid arthritis.[6] More often than not, men demonstrate a greater proportion of the spinal form of AS.[15] In American and African blacks[18] the overall prevalence of AS is approximately one-fourth that of Caucasians. Interestingly, although blacks do not have the B27 antigen,

they do have the related B7 antigen. Although the prevalence rate among native Japanese is less than that of Caucasian Americans, the prevalence in North American Indians (Pimas tribe) is very high, approaching 20% of their total male population.[1]

5. How does ankylosing spondylitis differ from rheumatoid arthritis?

The differences between these two seronegative spondylarthropathies may be traced to the predilection of inflammation in the type of connective tissue specific to each disease. All connective tissue derives from embryonic mesenchyme and is differentiated one type from the other by the triad of components comprising connective tissue. Those tissues affected by AS are primarily composed *of dense connective tissue,* whereas rheumatoid arthritis has a predilection for inflammation of *loose connective tissue.* Synovial tissue, being composed of mostly loose connective tissue, is thus the initial site of periarticular inflammation in rheumatoid arthritis. In contrast, fibrocartilage comprising the articular surfaces of the diarthrodial joint is the primary site of inflammation in AS. The synovitis of AS is secondary and spreads from adjacent inflammation of the cartilage, but resembles inflammation derived from rheumatoid arthritis, including pannus formation, although it is less necrotic.[1] Because periosteum and subchondral bone are composed of dense connective tissue, periostitis and osteitis, may occur in patients with AS. However, because muscles are composed of dense and loose connective tissue, muscle inflammation may occur in both AS and rheumatoid arthritis. Against this backdrop, these spondylarthropathies are considered diseases of connective tissue.

When comparing AS and rheumatoid arthritis we note more differences than similarities between both spondylarthropathies. AS is distinctly different from rheumatoid arthritis as a distinct clinical and pathologic entity in that it is predominant in young men, demonstrates absence of rheumatoid factor and nodules, and has a predilection for the axial skeleton (i.e., the spine and major, proximal joints.) Spinal involvement is total and ascending with AS, but only confined to the cervical spine in patients with rheumatoid arthritis. In AS, the distribution is racial, a positive family history is frequent, it is more frequently diagnosed in males, it involves the sacroiliac joint, aortic regurgitation may be present, and it has no nodules. In contrast, with rheumatoid arthritis distribution is worldwide, a family history is rare, it is more common in females, the sacroiliac joint is not involved, there is no aortic regurgitation, and nodules are typically present.[7] With AS, seldom is relief provided by salicylates, symptomatic relief is provided by phenylbutazone and indomethacin whereas these drugs are minimally effective in rheumatoid patients and no benefit is derived from gold therapy, aspirin, or administration of adrenocorticosteroids. In contrast, rheumatoid arthritis is more common in females and has a predilection to affect the joint of the appendicular skeleton. With AS, the main presenting clinical problems are gross fixed deformities, whereas in rheumatoid arthritis, the main problems are local joint destruction and instability.[21]

In addition, AS differs from rheumatoid arthritis as it is characterized by *enthesopathy,* extraarticular inflammation, and eventual ossification of the articular capsule, as well as ligament and tendon insertion into bone. AS and rheumatoid arthritis are not mutually exclusive in the sense that both conditions may manifest simultaneously in the same patient. Also, atlantoaxial subluxation and dislocation may occur in both diseases.

6. Which proximal and distal sites are typically affected with the spread of inflammation associated with AS?

Although, at first, the sites of inflammation associated with AS seem spread out over the musculoskeletal system they are in fact occurring as enthesopathy over a wide variety of sites. The most proximal site of involvement begins at the sacroiliac joint, specifically at the insertion of the sacrotuberous and sacrospinal ligaments, and eventually ossifying the sacroiliac ligaments.[13] Enthesopathy may then migrate throughout the pelvic basin to the iliac crest(s), the ischial tuberosity, and the pubic symphysis. Distal migration may occur at the greater trochanter, and has a predilection for the Achilles tendon insertion, and the proximal plantar aponeurosis from the calcaneus. Proximal migration of AS involves the annulus fibrosis, the anterior longitudinal ligament, and processes of each vertebrae. As AS migrates to the thoracic level, invariably enthesopathy spreads ventrally within the rib cage to involve the insertion of the costotransverse, manubriosternal, and sternoclavicular joints.

7. What are the extraarticular manifestations of AS?

Because fibrocartilage is comprised of dense connective tissue, it is the primary site of articular inflammation with AS. However, as fibrous tissue, composed of dense connective tissue is found throughout the body, AS is a systemic disease that has extraarticular manifestations, which develop as the duration of the disease increases.

- *Acute iritis.* Refers to inflammation of the iris of the eye, and is the commonest extraarticular manifestation of AS as it occurs in as much as 20% of spondylitic patients.[9] Iritis is a self-limiting condition that manifests as an irregular, patch-shaped pupil known as *synechiae.* This may result in impaired vision due to scarring or secondary granuloma with extensive ocular damage if not treated with topical corticosteroids. Iritis may affect one eye and then the other.
- *Aortic valve damage.* Damage occurs due to dilatation of the aortic ring. Present in as much as 5% of spondylitic patients and hemodynamically insignificant, it may progress to aortic insufficiency and valvular regurgitation that may culminate in severe aortic incompetence. Cardiovascular involvement may also result in cardiomegaly.[18]
- *Heart block.* Because fibrous tissues occasionally extend below the heart valves, inflammation of the aortic valve may migrate distally and invade tissue, including the electrical cardiac conduction pathways. Conduction defects occur in approximately 10% of patients and may lead to conduction abnormalities such as heart block, although pacemaker placement is rarely required.[1]
- *Pulmonary compromise.* This is caused by thoracic kyphosis and restriction of the thoracic cage during lung expansion at inspiration. Normal chest expansion (measured at the level of the fourth rib) is reduced from over 5 cm to 2 cm. Pulmonary function tests in these patients indicate diminished vital capacity and total lung capacity, although the residual and functional residual volumes are increased. This loss of chest mobility occurs early during the disease process owing to diffuse costovertebral involvement. Specifically, a progression of inflammation, fibrosis, and ossification occurs at the posterior costovertebral and costotransverse articulations, and the anterior costochondral junctions, manubriosternal junction, and the radiate ligament at the head of each rib. Thus any gain in respiratory capacity afforded by secondary respiratory muscles that increases the thoracic cage diameter in both the sagittal and frontal planes is lost. Fusion at these sites results in reduced lung volumes although gaseous exchange is not physiologically impaired as the diaphragm tolerates the increased work of breathing well. Nevertheless, those

apices of the lungs that are poorly aerated may account for the increased likelihood for development of chest infection in spondylitic patients.

- In addition, diminished apical aeration may also account for the development of bulbous fibrotic changes in the upper lobes that occur in approximately 1.5%[9] of all spondylitic patients. Known as apical lobe fibrobullous disease, these bullae are susceptible to the development of *aspergillomas* (i.e., colonized by the *Aspergillus* fungus) and appear as cavities and fibrosis on radiographs.[1] Here, parenchymal tissue becomes nodular (amyloid deposition), cavitated, and easily mistaken for tuberculosis on radiograph. This progression represents serious pulmonary pathology and, in contrast to the more benign pulmonary involvement mentioned above, does impair gas exchange. This, in turn, results in coughing, sputum production, and dyspnea.[12] Cavitation may lead to hemoptysis and death.

- *Osteoporosis.* Osteoporosis of the spine is an early, common finding that contributes to susceptibility of spinal fracture in the event of a fall or injury. Lack of trunk mobility makes the spondylitic patient prone to falls, and the rigid spine is vulnerable, with fracture often occurring through the bony bridges. Thus patients with ankylosed spines are more vulnerable to vertebral fractures and possible cord compression, particularly in the cervical spine following minimal or even trivial trauma.

8. How does the radiographic appearance of AS change with the evolution of this disease?

Any discussion of radiographic changes occurring during the evolution of AS must be prefaced by the concurrent pathologic changes occurring at the principal site of AS: synovial and fibrous joints. Pathologic changes at these articulations occur as chronic synovitis that is followed by a triad of fibrosis, calcification, and ossification. These changes occur as a triad of fibrosis, calcification, and ossification. The sacroiliac joints are always involved, whereas the intervertebral discs, symphysis pubis, and manubriosternal joints are frequently involved. Only in extremely rare cases, do spinal symptoms become radiologically discernible before pathologic sacroiliac signs.[10] In some patients, sacroiliitis may not radiologically manifest for 2 years after onset of AS, and radioscintigraphy with bone seeking isotopes is more helpful in cases of suspected diagnoses.[19]

The earliest radiographic changes occur at the sacroiliac joints in 99%[10] of all patients and are best de-

tected by an anteroposterior pelvic radiograph. Changes may occur throughout the sacroiliac joint but are initially seen in the lower two-thirds (synovial portion) of the joint. When present, changes are symmetrical, or minimally asymmetrical, although the patient may complain of symptoms on one side only. The presence of unilateral sacroiliac arthritis is incompatible with a diagnosis of AS. Radiographic changes include widening of the joint space known as pseudowidening, superficial bone erosions that have a "punched out" appearance, sclerosis of the adjacent bone, blurring of the joint space margins secondary to narrowing of the joint causing the bony borders of the sacroiliac joint to become indistinct, interosseous bridging of the joint, and eventual obliteration of the joint space as fusion occurs. These progressive changes are graded I to IV according to the degree of pathologic progression.[16]

Peripheral joint involvement involves inflammatory synovitis, especially at the ball-and-socket joints that is pathologically indistinguishable from other inflammatory arthropathies such as rheumatoid arthritis. On radiograph appearance, however, there is a greater tendency toward central articular erosion with AS. At the hip, AS is distinguished by concentric joint space narrowing and lateral femoral osteophytes.[1] Eventually, changes at the hip joint will result in protrusio acetabuli. At the glenohumeral joint, medial erosion of the humeral head is followed by bone deposition, narrowing of the glenohumeral joint space, upward migration of the humeral head, and impingement of the rotator cuff secondary to diminished subacromial space.

Extrapelvic periarticular spread occurs at the bone-ligament junction, known as the enthesis. *Enthesopathy* causes erosion of the bone and changes in the ligament. Inflammatory infiltration occurs in the vessels of the ligament followed by the body's reaction at attempted healing by way of bone deposition. This compensatory strategy of the musculoskeletal system is similar to callous formation of a broken bone in which the bloody hematoma surrounding the two ends of the fracture site is converted to bone as an attempt to stabilize the site of fracture. Similarly, healing in response to inflammatory infiltration occurs by bone deposition, which reduces inflammation at the expense of ligament destruction. This occurs at other tendon-bone or ligament-bone junctions as proliferative bony margins or whiskery spicules in the pelvis at the sacrotuberous and sacrospinal ligament insertions, the greater trochanter of the femur, fluffy erosions at the origins of the adductor muscles, and at either the distal Achilles tendon insertion or the proximal plantar fascia insertion. The manubriosternal joint may present as a biconcave appearance on radiograph.[14]

As inflammation spreads cephalad up the spine, a similar process occurs at the junction of the annulus fibrosus with the vertebral body. This results in vertebral chondritis and subchondral osteitis of the vertebral end plate that is followed by fibrosis and ossification similar to the sacroiliac joint. Erosive changes secondary to periostitis leads to early loss of the normal bony contour of the vertebra at the junction between the vertebra and the disc known as vertebral squaring. The *Romanus sign* is an erosion surrounded by sclerosis at the vertebral body margin. Although a lateral view of the normal lumbar spine shows vertebrae with a pronounced anterior concavity, periostitis from AS causes bone to fill in this concavity resulting in a square, sloped vertebra. This is known as *squaring of the vertebral body.*

Inflammation at the juncture between the annulus fibrosis and vertebral endplate occurs behind the leading edge of the upwardly migrating disease, leaving in its wake a reactionary bone formation radically different from the laterally projecting bone spurs of classic osteoarthritis. With AS, the spurs, known as bridging syndesmophytes are vertically oriented and typically occur at the L1 to L2 and T11 to T12 levels. A common site for the first syndesmophyte is at the thoracolumbar junction (L1 to L2).[9] These vertical spurs appear delicate at first and bridge together so as to give the characteristic "bamboo spine" appearance on radiograph. The spreading wave front of inflammation invariably affects the capsular facet joints and causes their ossification over time so that the spine is converted from a flexible structure into an immobile and rigidly fixed rod. Ossification then spreads to the interspinous ligaments and ligamenta flava, so that the end result is a conversion of the soft tissue of the spine into an ossified column of trabecular bone. With the exception of the neural elements and the nucleus pulposus, the metamorphosed soft tissue is much harder and stronger in caliber than the vertebral body. It is for this reason that fractures of the spine are more likely to occur through the vertebral body than through the adjacent, newly ossified bone.[21]

9. What is spondylodiskitis?

Just as early erosive sclerotic changes of the sacroiliac joints occur with AS, erosive sclerosis may involve the intervertebral disc endplate. *Spondylodiskitis* refers to vertebral endplate destruction due to this erosive sclerosis, and most commonly occurs in the lower thoracic spine with a 5% to 6% incidence.[21] Radiologically, this presents as considerable disc space narrowing and irregularity, with widening of the disc space and increased radiodensity of the surrounding bone. Spondylodiskitis is frequently asymptomatic but may become symptomatic as pain following minor injury or stress. This condition occurs when an isolated disc level remained unaffected by bony ankylosis. For some unknown reason, the cephalad migration of ossification skipped a spinal level, resulting in a consequent excess of movement at that point, and subsequent source of pain.[9]

10. What is the clinical presentation of these patients?

The sacroiliac joint is often the first joint of the axial skeleton to be affected by inflammatory disorders. Because AS is a disease of the spine and axial skeleton, and is characterized by a caudal-to-cephalad migration, it is not surprising that the sacroiliitis, often perceived as pain in the low back, is the very first manifestation of AS. Pain may center at the lumbosacral spine but may also occur in the buttocks and hips. Pain and stiffness are insidious in nature and may either be intermittent or persistent. These symptoms are often worse in the early morning hours or following prolonged rest, and typically relieved by physical activity. Complaints of difficulty sitting through a cinema showing or during church services are common. The patient may report rising from bed in the middle of the night and walking about so as to provide pain relief. A hot shower may provide relief.

Because the radiographic changes occurring with sacroiliitis secondary to AS may take years to become radiologically visible, clinical examination is the cornerstone of diagnosis. Thus when AS is clinically suspected, but not radiologically supported, the best choice is to consider the patient to have a presumed diagnosis of AS provided that other disease entities are ruled out. This, then, is followed by serial radiographs every few months in an attempt to confirm the diagnosis.

Sacroiliitis may present as an inflammatory type of back pain characterized by morning stiffness and pain recurring after periods of inactivity during the day. Pain around the chest wall may present early in the course of the disease and may be accompanied by a history of iritis. This nonspecific form of acute iritis may be recurrent and may cause scarring and even secondary glaucoma with each episode.

Early on in the disease, the patient may complain of chest wall discomfort when exertion necessitates deep breathing and encourages a progressive dorsal stoop that becomes ever more prominent. This is accompanied by secondary neck pain and stiffness that may make activities such as driving difficult. This is often what causes patients to seek medical help. The temporomandibular joints (TMJ) may be affected, leading to local pain and dental malocculsion.[1] Diffuse costovertebral fusion and secondary enthesitis (inflammation) of the muscular attachments to the ribs may present as anterior chest pain that may mimic angina pectoris. The patient may also complain of thoracic spine, shoulder, or neck pain and stiffness. In addition, enthesopathy, presenting as tenderness over bony prominences of the ischial tuberosity, greater trochanter, spinous processes, or at the os calcis as heel pain may be present. Peripheral joint involvement may occur, and when it does, typically presents with a swollen knee.[9] Asymmetric extraaxial joint involvement (hips, knees, and shoulders) tend to cause decreased passive and active range of motion, followed by early contractures. A heel spur may be palpable. Fever is seldom present, but may transiently occur during acute arthritic flares as may be accompanied by fatigue, weight loss, and anemia. The patient with severe AS assumes a characteristic posture (Fig. 56-2).

11. How is loss of spinal range of motion best assessed?

In many patients, loss of normal spinal curve as well as loss of spinal range of motion occurs before radiologic signs of the spinal manifestation of the disease are present. Typically, there is a loss of lumbar lordosis as the lumbosacral aspect of the spine assumes a flattened appearance, while the thoracic kyphosis is accentuated. All directions of lumbar spinal movement become restricted, although lateral flexion is reduced first. Thoracic spinal rotation may also be reduced and is visually assessed by having the patient seated on a surface to immobilize the pelvis while the shoulders are then rotated by the examiner.

- *Forward spinal flexion.* This may be assessed using the Schober method in which marks are made at two points along the spine. The first is made at the lumbosacral junction and the second at a point 10 cm above. The distance between the marks is measured when the patient maximally flexes forward. Distraction of less than 5 cm is considered abnormal.
- However, measurement of finger-to-floor distance in

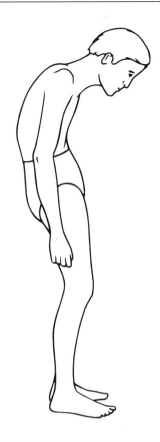

FIG. 56-2 Characteristic posture of patient with severe ankylosing spondylitis.

the assessment of forward flexion may yield a false negative response because a patient with a rigid or even fused spine may be able to touch their toes by using their hips. Measurement of forward flexion is usually assessed by using **Macrae's modification of Shober's method.** With the patient erect, the lumbosacral junction is identified between the dimples of Venus. A mark is made 10 cm above the lumbosacral junction and a second mark 5 cm below it. A tape measure is held along this 15-cm line. When the patient bends forward the distance between the marks increase. In this manner, diminishment of forward flexion range may be quantitated over time (Fig. 56-3).

- *Lateral spinal flexion.* This is measured with the patient standing. Two marks are made on the lateral trunk at the level of the xiphisternum and the iliac crest and distance between them is measured. The patient is asked to bend sideways away from the side with the marks, sliding their hand down the ipsilateral

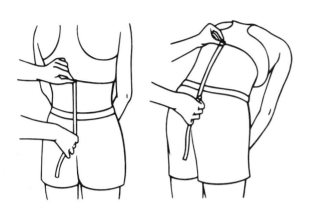

FIG. 56-3 Measurement of forward flexion.

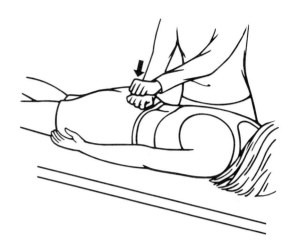

FIG. 56-4 Provocative testing of an inflamed sacroiliac joint may provoke pain by applying *direct pressure over the sacrum* with the patient lying prone.

thigh, and a new distance between the two marks is measured. A difference of less than 3 cm is considered abnormal and represents significant diminishment of lateral truncal flexion.

12. How is costovertebral involvement best assessed?

Each rib forms two synovial joints as it articulates with the vertebral column. A *costovertebral joint,* reinforced by a radiate ligament covering the anterior aspect of the joint, joins the head of the rib either with one vertebral body or with two vertebral bodies and an intervening intervertebral disc. A costotransverse joint joins the tubercle of the rib with the transverse process of the ipsisegmental vertebra, and is reinforced by the costotransverse and lateral costotransverse ligaments.

Costovertebral involvement with ossification of the radiate ligaments of the head of the ribs is reflected in decreased chest expansion. When assessing for diminished chest expansion the tape measure is at the fourth intercostal space in men (typically just above the nipple line) or under the breast in females. The normative value should consider the patient's age and gender and not simply consider an arbitrary 2.5 cm as the basis for comparison. Less than 5 cm of chest expansion during inspiration in the adult is considered a significant reduction.

13. Which provocative clinical tests elicit sacroiliac tenderness due to sacroiliitis?

Provocative testing of an inflamed sacroiliac joint may provoke pain by applying direct pressure over the sacrum with the patient lying prone (Fig. 56-4). Alter-

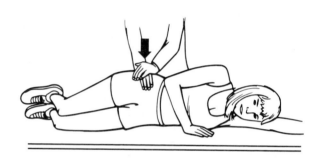

FIG. 56-5 The sacroiliac joint may be assessed by *lateral compression* of the pelvis.

nately, the pelvis may be compressed by the therapist's hands while the patient is side lying; this is known as *lateral side compression of the pelvis* (Fig. 56-5). *Pelvic springing* may be performed with the hands over the anterior superior iliac spine as the patient lies supine (Fig. 56-6). Alternately, with *Gaenslen's test* (Fig. 56-7), the patient lies supine over the edge of the examining table with the knees flexed and with one buttock over the edge. The patient then drops the unsupported leg off the table. This maneuver elicits pain in the contralateral sacroiliac joint by stretching it. In addition, an inflammatory lesion of the sacroiliac joint is painfully provoked by flexing the ipsilateral hip to 90° and then forcibly adducting the hip.[17]

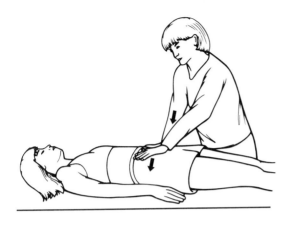

FIG. 56-6 *Pelvic springing* may be performed with the hands over the anterior superior iliac spine as the patient lies supine.

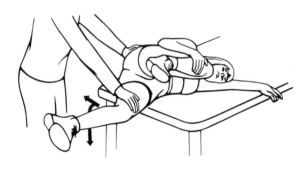

FIG. 56-7 *Gaenslen's test.* The patient lies supine over the edge of the examining table with the knees flexed and with one buttock over the edge. The patient then drops the unsupported leg off the table. This maneuver elicits pain in the contralateral sacroiliac joint by stretching it.

14. What are complications of AS?

Complications of AS include:

- *Atlantoaxial subluxation.* As AS progresses cephalad, increased stress at the craniocervical junction may occur due to the solid column of bone inferior to the atlantoaxial and atlantooccipital joints. Atlantoaxial instability is caused by inflammation of the transverse atlantooccipital-atlanto ligament.

  The first and second cervical vertebrae are respectively known as the *atlas* and *axis*. The atlas resembling no other vertebra, lacks a vertebral body and is a ring of bone that carries the skull while the axis forms a pivot around which the atlas and skull may rotate. Thus nodding occurs at the atlantooccipi-

tal joint whereas rotation occurs at the atlantoaxial joint.

The combination of this stress coupled with attritional effects of inflammation of the transverse ligaments and bony attachments associated with AS may cause severe pain, instability, anterior subluxation, and even dislocation in which the atlas may slide forward on the axis and impinge upon the spinal cord by the odontoid process. In some patients, progression may result in subluxation and then stabilize in the subluxated position without significant symptoms. In other patients, pain accompanied by rotatory and angular deformity may also accompany anterior subluxation. Conservative management is initially attempts to reduce pain, with caution administered not to injure the neck and head and avoidance of tumble-saw and similar activities. If this does not help, the deformity may be gradually reduced by a halo-dependent traction device. Routine flexion and extension lateral radiographs are thus essential to the patient with AS. Because of the danger of spinal cord compression from either dislocation or subaxial fracture,* surgical stabilization by occipital-cervical fusion may be required in some cases.

- *Cauda equina syndrome.* This results from encasement and stenosis of nerve roots in deformed vertebral bone causing bedwetting, impotence, diminished bladder and rectal sensation, buttock or lower extremity pain, or an absent ankle (S1) reflex.

- *Pathologic fracture.* As the pelvis, spine, and thorax become fixed into a single rigid bony union, the axial and proximal appendicular skeleton lose the energy dissipating capability afforded by the joints and soft tissue comprising the musculoskeletal system. In addition, the lessened activity accelerates the rate of osteoporosis in the skeletal system. The lack of trunk mobility increases the risk for falls and pathologic fracture.

15. What is the differential diagnosis of AS?

The differential diagnosis of AS represents a clinical challenge. Many patients with AS remain undiagnosed or are incorrectly diagnosed with neurosis, mechanical back pain, or seronegative rheumatoid arthritis, and inappropriately receive bed rest, improper exercises, or undergo a myelogram. The clinician must bear in mind

---

*Patients with ankylosed spines have increased susceptibility to vertebral compression fractures, particularly in the cervical regions, after falls or even minor trauma.

that lab tests are of limited diagnostic use. The B27 antigen is the single best laboratory clue as it is present in 95% of all white spondylitics. The erythrocyte sedimentation rate (ESR) is a measure of plasma viscosity and is often raised in spondylitic patients. There is moderately elevated serum alkaline and creatinine phosphatase,[5] and a negative rheumatoid factor. Diagnosis is suggested by patient history and examination, and corroborated by positive radiographs. If three or more of the following features are present,[18,22] a possibility of AS is strongly considered. However, a definite diagnosis of AS is pronounced if even one clinical criterion is accompanied by positive radiologic criterion.[22] This underscores the importance of radiographic confirmation in the diagnosis of AS:

- Age of onset is less than 40 years
- Insidious onset
- Duration of back pain and stiffness greater than 3 months that is unrelieved by rest
- Morning stiffness
- Improvement of stiffness with exercise
- Limitation of lumbar spinal motion in both sagittal and frontal planes
- Limitation of chest expansion

Conditions that must be distinguished from AS include:

- *Reiter's syndrome.* This is a relatively common cause of peripheral arthritis of greater than 1 month duration in young males that occurs in association with urethritis/cervicitis, conjunctivitis, and mucous membrane lesions. The latter refers to small, superficial, painless, grey-colored, oral ulcers seen on the tongue as well as painless, red ulcers on genital mucosa. Reiter's syndrome classically presents as a triad of arthritis, uveitis, and urethritis.[23] Patients may also develop hyperakeratotic skin lesions of the palms and sole around the nails, whereas hyperkeratosis may also occur. The latter refers to heaping of cornified material beneath the fingernail. In addition, the interphalangeal joints of the hands may be affected, most commonly in an asymmetric manner.

  The two recognized forms of Reiter's syndrome include the dysenteric form in which bowel inflammation is caused by different infectious agents, and the sexually transmitted form. The latter is thought to be associated and preceded by episodes of sexual intercourse with multiple partners. The full episodic attack of this disease may be accompanied by fever and anorexia. Arthritic onset is often abrupt and affects the weight bearing joint, especially the knees and ankles with muscle wasting around the joint(s), particularly the quadriceps. Back pain from sacroiliitis is not uncommon. Both forms of Reiter's syndrome may manifest in the spine as a particular type of syndesmophyte that is uniquely different from that of AS or the spurring associated with osteoarthritis of the spine. Here, bony outgrowth occurs from the lateral and anterior surfaces of the vertebral bodies; in contrast to AS in which osteophytes grow from the margins of the vertebral bodies. A positive association exists between Reiter's syndrome and AS because approximately 10% to 30% of patients with the former condition have associated AS.[17]

- *Septic sacroiliitis.* This is a form of infectious arthritis caused by a pathologic microbe infecting synovial tissue. The most commonly implicated pathogen is staphylococcus. Patient will complain of acute sacroiliac joint pain and stiffness, a warm and tender joint, and fever and chills that are often present. Because the sacroiliac joint may be rapidly destroyed if this condition is not promptly treated, acute bacterial arthritis is considered a medical emergency. Suspected septic sacroiliitis should undergo needle aspiration and culture.

- *Psoriatic arthritis.* Approximately 10% of patients affected with psoriasis of the skin or nails will also experience psoriatic arthritis, a skeletal manifestation of the disease. The classic skin lesions may either precede or follow articular involvement. Sacroiliitis develops in about one-third of patients with psoriatic arthritis.[2] Psoriatic arthritis differs from AS in that it is more common in females, whereas the syndesmophytes tend to be asymmetric. Moreover, the distal interphalangeal joints are especially affected as they undergo excessive destruction and become swollen and distorted in what is called *arthritis mutilans*. The toes may also exhibit a sausage-like swelling.

- *Osteoarthritis.* Osteoarthritis of the sacroiliac joint does occur although radiologic involvement is limited to the lower portion of the joints. This is not the case with AS in which radiologic involvement involves the entire joint.

- *Osteitis condensans ilii.* This is a sclerotic condition of one or both females of one or both iliac surfaces articulating with the sacrum. This condition, common to females, may be asymptomatic in multiparous women, or may present as back pain in both men and women runners secondary to leg length discrepancy[3] or running along a banked surface secondary to shearing action across the sacroiliac joint. This condition is radiographically characterized by sclerosis of the sacroiliac joint that differs from AS in that sclerosis is wedge-shaped and confined to the iliac side of the joint so that the joint margin is more clearly demarcated. This is not the case in with AS.

- *Lumbosacral disc disease.* This is easily differentiated from AS as the former is characterized by neurologic lumbar root compression signs such as sciatica that often extends distal to the knee, reflex diminishment, muscular weakness, and sensory changes. Moreover, lumbar disc disease is a mechanical rather than inflammatory condition whose clinical features include acute onset, local muscle spasm, neurodeficit, local tenderness, and asymmetrical loss of range of motion. In addition, lumbosacral nerve entrapment is worsened by exercise and made better by rest. These features are not present with AS, which is characterized by an opposite symptomatic pattern in which pain intensifies with rest and improves with exercise. Moreover, straight leg raising is normal, whereas onset is insidious. In addition, with AS lateral flexion is usually abnormally limited, and typically unaffected by lumbar disc disease. Finally, the tenderness in AS is diffuse, whereas diminished range of motion is symmetric.
- *Diffuse idiopathic skeletal hyperostosis (DISH).* DISH is synonymous with ankylosing hyperostosis and Forestier disease, and results from an abnormal tendency of the body to ossify excessively taut, fibrous connective tissue, typically occurring as ligaments, joint capsules, and tendons of the spine. This condition closely resembles and even clinically mimics AS, and differs only in that it occurs in elderly males greater than 50 years of age. Moreover, radiologically evident ligamentous calcification is limited to the cervical and lower thoracic spine but spares the sacroiliac and vertebral facet joints. With this condition, ossification of the anterior longitudinal ligament does occurs, whereas it does not occur in AS.[10] In addition, the ESR is normal and there is no link to the B27 antigen.
- *Oligoarticular arthritis.* Oligoarticular arthritis of the lower extremities, typically as heel pain, is often the early presentation of juvenile AS in older boys before evidence of radiographic sacroiliitis. Almost all children are B27 positive and this may mimic and often be confused with rheumatoid arthritis. However, with time the child develops the more typical features of the adult form of AS.
- *Acquired immune deficiency syndrome (AIDS).* There is a rapidly expanding list of rheumatic and musculo-skeletal problems associated with HIV infection. A reactive arthritis, as Reiter's syndrome and psoriatic arthritis are increasingly recognized as early manifestations of AIDS, particularly in patient who engage in unprotected sexual behavior and intravenous drug abuse.

16. What physical therapy is appropriate in the management of this patient?

Management of AS involves a race against time in which the therapist, in conjunction with the patient and family, attempts to institute an extension posture with regard to all of the activities of daily living for that patient. Eventually, the triad of fibrosis, calcification, and ossification will convert the entire axial skeleton into a rigid rod. Although therapy cannot alter the rate of this process, it can attempt to ensure that calcification occurs in as extended a spinal posture as possible so as to provide the patient with a normal life, which is possible once ossification is complete.

Essential to management of AS is early diagnosis so that intervention may be implemented before deformity and disability occur. All patient should be enrolled in a physical therapy program[1] as soon as possible so as to be able to maintain as normal a life as possible.[4] The therapist must inculcate in the patient a strict adherence to trunk and lower extremity extension so as to counter the kyphotic tendency. Good postural habits begin with a "think tall" attitude. Thus the patient is encouraged to maintain an erect posture in all activities including sitting, standing, walking, and lying down. Sleeping should occur with the patient in the prone or supine position on a firm mattress with a 1-inch thickness plywood board (cut to mattress size) placed between the mattress and boxspring for additional firmness. No pillow is recommended, or a flat, small one at most. When the patient must sit, he should place a lumbar support at the lumbar spine. Exercises may be preceded by a warm to hot shower or bath that may relieve symptoms. Antiinflammatory medications (such as indomethacin, naproxen, sulindac, or phenylbutazone) may be of help in managing the symptoms of AS. Salicylates, for unknown reasons do not provide relief to patients with AS.

Strengthening exercises of the extensor muscles of the back, hips, and shoulders may be performed by concentric and eccentric exercises; whole flexion exercises are avoided. The patient may lie prone, lift their head off the surface while squeezing their shoulder blades together and lifting the shoulders off the surface and count to five.

A walking exercise in a pool is helpful, although swimming should be performed with the backstroke. The patient should be taught to perform diaphragmatic breathing while supine with a 1- to 2-lb weight lying over the diaphragm (see Fig. 18-10). Forced deep breathing exercises will help maintain or improve chest extension. Manual mobilization may be helpful to maintain spinal and peripheral joint extension. It is important to teach body relaxation techniques and provide emotional support. Patient education includes avoidance of activities and occupations that cause kyphosis. As kyphosis progresses, the patient may require prismatic spectacles to see forward.

17. When is surgery appropriate in the management of AS?

In the relentlessly progressive form of the disease the deformity will cripple the patient so that the head becomes completely fixed chin-to-sternum, or the patient's head looks down and behind and may come to be postured between his legs so that the eyes may see backward. With the former deformity, as well as for the patient who has significant postural kyphosis, a vertebral wedge osteotomy may be performed at the C8-T1 juncture or at L3 so as to permit the patient to stand upright and see ahead. Surgical correction to improve function at other articulations includes joint arthroplasty for the hip, knee, and shoulder. Surgery may also be used for stabilization of atlantoaxial subluxation and condylar resections of ankylosed TMJ. The problem with surgery in the patient with AS is the tendency for ectopic bone formation and recurrence of bony ankylosis at the operative site.

RECOMMENDED READING

Beary JF III, Christian CL, Johanson NA editors: *Manual of rheumatology and outpatient orthopedic disorders: diagnosis and therapy,* ed 2, 1987, Boston, Little, Brown and Company.

Calin A: Ankylosing spondylitis, prognosis. In Fries JF, Ehrlich GE editors: *Prognosis: contemporary outcomes of disease,* Bowie, Md., 1981, Charles Press.

REFERENCES

1. Beary JF III, Christian CL, Johanson NA editors: *Manual of rheumatology and outpatient orthopedic disorders: diagnosis and therapy,* ed 2, 1987, Boston, Little, Brown and Company.
2. Benoist M: Inflammatory spondyloarthropathies. In Weinstein JN, Wiesel SW editors: *The lumbar spine,* Philadelphia, 1990, WB Saunders.
3. Brody DM: Running injuries, *Clin Symp* 39(3):1-36, 1987.
4. Calin A: Ankylosing spondylitis, prognosis. In Fries JF, Ehrlich GE editors: *Prognosis: contemporary outcomes of disease,* Bowie, Md., 1981, Charles Press.
5. Calin A: Creatine phosphkinase in ankylosing spondylitis, *Ann Rheum Dis* 34:244-248, 1975.
6. Calin A, Marks SH: The case against seronegative rheumatoid arthritis, *Am J Med* 70:992-994, 1981.
7. Calin A: Spondylarthritis, medicine, *Sci Am* 3:3, 1982.
8. Corrigal V, Panayi GS, Unger A et al: Detection of immune complexes in serum of patients with ankylosing spondylitis, *Ann Rheum Dis* 37:159-163, 1978.
9. Dieppe PA, Bacon PA: *Atlas of clinical rheumatology,* Philadelphia, 1986, Lea & Febiger.
10. Dihlmann W: *Radiologic atlas of rheumatic diseases,* Stuttgart, 1986, Georg Thieme Verlag.
11. Eastmond CJ, Calguneri M, Shinebaum R et al: A sequential study of the relationship between faecal Klebsiella aerogenes and the common clinical manifestation of ankylosing spondylitis, *Ann Rheum Dis* 41:15-20, 1982.
12. Editorial: The lungs in ankylosing spondylitis, *Br Med J* 3:492-493, 1971.
13. Keim HA, Kirkaldy-Willis WH: Low back pain, *Clin Symp* 39(6):37, 1987.
14. Macnab I: *Backache,* Baltimore, 1977, Williams & Wilkins.
15. Marks SH, Barnett M, Calin A: A case control study of juvenile- and adult-onset ankylosing spondylitis, *J Rheumatol* 9(5):739-747, 1982.
16. Moll JMH, Wright V: New York criteria for ankylosing spondylitis: a statistical evaluation, *Ann Rheum Dis* 32:354-358, 1973.
17. Porter RW: *Management of back pain,* ed 2, Edinburgh, 1993, Churchill Livingstone.
18. Rodnan GP (editor): *Primer of the rheumatic diseases,* ed 8, Atlanta, 1983, The Arthritis Foundation.
19. Rosenthall L, Libsona R: Role of radionuclide imaging in benign bone and joint disease of orthopaedic interest. In Freeman LM, Weissman HS editors: *Nuclear medicine annual,* New York, 1980, Raven Press.
20. Schlosstein L, Terasaki PI, Bluestone P et al: High association of anti HL-A antigen, W27, with ankylosing spondylitis, *N Engl J Med* 288:704, 1973.
21. Simmons EH: Arthritic spinal deformity-ankylosing spondylitis. In White AH, Schofferman JA (editors): *Spine care: operative treatment,* Vol 2, St Louis, Mosby.
22. Van der Linden S, Valkenburg HA, Cats A: Evaluation of diagnostic criteria for ankylosing spondylitis. A proposal for modification of the New York criteria, *Arth Rheum* 27:366, 1984.
23. Wilkens RF, Arnett FC, Bilter T et al: Reiter's syndrome. Evaluation of preliminary criteria for definite disease, *Arth Rheum* 24:844-849, 1981.
24. Wright V, Moll JMH: *Seronegative polyarthritis,* Amsterdam, 1976, North Holland Publishing.

57

Elderly Patient with Low Back Pain and Lower Limb (Neurogenic) Claudication Exacerbated by Lumbar Extension

CASE 1: A 63-year-old retired butcher complains of intermittent low back pain of several months' duration before his retirement 6 months ago. His work consisted of standing for many hours and preparing various portions and sizes of meat, which were later packaged, labeled, and priced. The patient describes his low back and buttock pain starting after standing for progressively shorter periods. Leaning forward over a chair for several minutes allowed the painful ache to subside, only to reappear some time later after resuming his work. When asked whether he exercises routinely, the patient replied that he was once an avid walker and enjoyed lengthy walks with his wife daily. However, approximately 10 months ago he began to experience the onset of buttock, and occasional calf pain during prolonged walking. Initially he is pain free, but after walking several blocks he feels pain in the low back which intensifies on continued walking and migrates into both buttocks, posterior thighs, and the lateral aspect of the right leg, but does not extend into the foot. Pain forces him to sit down at any available seat, and in the absence of a sitting surface, lifting his right leg up on a curb affords relief from the pain which abates after several minutes of rest; he then resumes walking another block until the cycle of pain repeats itself. As of late, he uses a walking cane as this seems to allow him to walk for longer periods before experiencing pain.

OBSERVATION Patient shows strong muscular features with a flattened lumbar back so that he is postured in −5° of hip extension.

PALPATION This yields no lower back or lower extremity tenderness, nor was there any palpable gap over his spinal process. His feet felt warm.

RANGE OF MOTION The patient was able to bend over with fingertips reaching to 20 cm from the floor without discomfort. Lateral flexion was 20° in either direction. Range of motion of the hip joint was full and painless. Maintaining lumbar hyperextension for greater than 25 seconds replicated painful symptoms.

STRENGTH Manual muscle testing showed normal strength grades relative to patient age and history of activity level.

FLEXIBILITY There is diminished hamstring extensibility bilaterally.

DEEP TENDON REFLEXES   There is diminished right patellar reflex. Brisk ankle jerks bilaterally.

SENSATION   This is intact to light touch, pinprick, pressure, temperature, and vibratory sense.

PULSES   This is intact in both feet.

SPECIAL TESTS   Negative straight leg raise and Lasègue's sign.

CLUE:

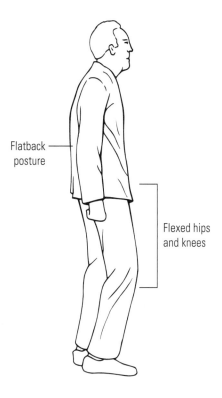

Flatback posture

Flexed hips and knees

The patient with neurogenic claudication secondary to spinal stenosis will eventually assume a characteristic simian standing posture of flexed hips and knees. The loss of lumbar lordosis results in flat or even convex back. Thus pressure on the cauda equina and resultant pain are relieved.

CASE 2: A 70-year-old retired female complains of lumbosacral pain with radiation down the posterior aspect of both thighs. The patient presents with a history of low back pain for the last 17 years but has persevered and continued with her regular activities despite steady deterioration. Over the past several weeks pain increased centrally and peripherally to radiate into the buttocks and posterior thighs as far as the knees. Transferring from a chair or bed is difficult, and walking has become increasingly difficult, with symptoms starting after a short distance. Pain is relieved by rest, after which she walks an even shorter distance before symptoms recur. Sitting and lying immobile afford relief. Turning over in bed aggravates pain, as does sneezing or coughing.

OBSERVATION   Normal.

PALPATION   A pronounced hollow is noted in the lumbar region and a "step" is readily palpable. There is no local tenderness.

RANGE OF MOTION   Forward flexion occurs until just below knee level with almost all of the movement at the hip joints. Both flexion and extension are uncomfortable, and extension following forward flexion is accompanied by a hitching movement.

STRENGTH   She stands on her heels and toes, walks on the borders of her feet, and squats without difficulty.

FLEXIBILITY   There is significant bilateral (60°) hamstring extensibility.

REFLEXES   Normal plantar responses.

SENSATION   Normal.

PULSES   The feet were warm with good pedal pulses.

SPECIAL TESTS   Prone press-ups have no effect on centralization or peripheralization of pain. Negative diurnal straight-leg raise, negative Gaenslen sign, and positive Thomas test bilaterally.

? Questions

1. What is the origin of these patients' symptoms?
2. What are central and lateral spinal stenoses?
3. What is the vertebral osteology of the lumbar spine?
4. What are the clinical implications of progressively increased pedicle thickening in the lumbar spine?
5. What is the local anatomy of the lumbar spinal cord?
6. How does the organization of the cell bodies of lower motor sensory and motor fibers emerging from the spinal cord differ?
7. What is the anatomic origin of the spinal nerve, and is its encroachment within the intervertebral foramen more likely to cause sensory deficit?
8. What is the structural and functional unit of the peripheral nervous system, and what are its cascading patterns of branching before becoming a specific peripheral nerve?
9. What are the membranous supportive tissues of the central nervous system?
10. What is the dura mater?
11. What is the nerve supply to the lumbar spine?
12. What are thecal signs?
13. What is the dural root sleeve?

14. At what site is the nerve root most vulnerable to traction injury?
15. What static and dynamic mechanisms and design strategy protect the emerging nerve roots from tensile traction?
16. What external dural connections stabilize neuromeningeal tissues?
17. What is the vasculature of the spinal cord and nerve roots?
18. What is the range of motion of the lumbar spine?
19. What length changes do the spinal and root canals undergo with normal movement?
20. What adaptive mechanisms exist in the neuraxis, nerve roots, and meninges that diminish tension derived from movement?
21. What variations in the spatial architecture of the vertebral canal predispose for central stenosis?
22. What factors influence the development of the vertebral canal?
23. Why do redundant nerve roots occur with normal aging and how do they diminish space within the spinal canal?
24. Why is the L5 nerve root more vulnerable to compression?

25. What is the structural degenerative cascade?
26. How may spondylitic facet arthrosis cause lateral canal stenosis?
27. What is degenerative disk disease and how may it result in central and lateral canal lumbar stenosis?
28. What is the role of soft-tissue encroachment upon the neural elements?
29. What is spondylolisthesis and how does it result in spinal stenosis?
30. What are the clinical and radiologic signs of degenerative spondylolisthesis?
31. What are the congenital and other acquired forms of lumbar spinal stenosis?
32. What is the pathophysiology of neurogenic claudication?
33. What is the clinical presentation of central and lateral stenosis?

34. How may the straight leg raise be interpreted to clinically differentiate between nerve root impingement deriving from spinal stenosis and disk pathology?
35. How may the diurnal straight-leg raising test be used to differentiate between nerve root irritability due to disk lesion versus spinal stenosis?
36. How are symptoms arising from spinal stenosis differentiated from acute disk pathology?
37. What imaging techniques are appropriate?
38. What is the differential diagnosis?
39. What rehabilitation strategy is most effective in the management of lumbar spinal stenosis?
40. What are the surgical indications for spinal stenosis?

---

1. What is the origin of these patients' symptoms?

Central spinal stenosis in Case 1 compressing the L5 and S1 nerve roots, and *lateral canal stenosis* due to subarticular entrapment in Case 2 compressing the L5 nerve root. The clue in Case 1 shows the eventual characteristic bent-over posture of the patient with central stenosis. The spine, hips, and knees are flexed, the back is flat, with an absence of normal lordotic curvature as this posture relieves pressure on the cauda equina. Bony or soft-tissue encroachment on the emerging root within the root canal may occur in any of the lumbar nerve roots, although the fifth lumbar root is most commonly involved. This is due to the frequency of degenerative change at the L5/S1 level and also because of the relatively long length of the root canal at L5 inferior to the broad pedicle. Thus the L5/S1 nerve root exposes relatively more of its length to the likelihood for encroachment.[69-73] Because the nerve root lies in the upper third of the intervertebral foramen,[18] osteophytic overgrowth from the superior facet compresses the emerging nerve root occurs beneath the facet joint as the root is tightly stretched against the pedicle in the lateral recess.[69-73] This is known as *subarticular entrapment* (Fig. 57-1).[69-73]

In Case 2, the "step" in the lumbar region on examination immediately suggests the presence of spondylolisthesis. Vascular claudication would be ruled out by good pedal pulses. The history of spinal claudication

during walking suggests that spinal stenosis may now be considered as a complicating feature of chronic low back pain secondary to degenerative spondylolisthesis and tertiary to degenerative disk disease and posterior facet arthrosis. Hyperlordosis, which often stems from tight hip flexor musculature and anterior pelvic tilt may result in central or spinal stenosis. Hyperlordosis narrows the intervertebral foramina, especially in the lateral recesses via impingement by the superior articular process of the inferior lumbar vertebrae. Hyperlordosis also narrows the central spinal canal via impingement by the inferior articular process of the superior lumbar vertebrae.[47] Thus either extreme of pelvic tilting may result in pathology, so that maintenance of a neutral pelvic posture and low back is essential and promoted by adequate soft-tissue extensibility of the pre- and postfemoral musculature.

Facet joint hypertrophy, deriving from degenerative spondylolisthesis, may result in both central and lateral canal stenoses causing neurogenic claudication or radicular encroachment, respectively. At some point in the forward migration, the disk collapses and the thickened ligamentum flavum becomes redundant, further contributing to both central and lateral stenosis. Radiographs demonstrate a grade II spondylolisthesis at L4/L5 with degeneration of the disk to the point of flattening. There was extensive lumbar spondylosis with osteophyte formation, marked narrowing of the L5/S1

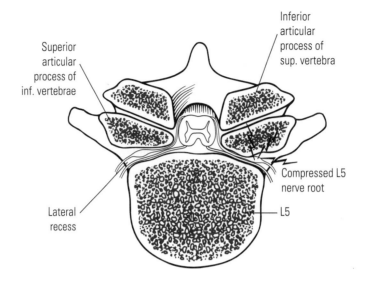

FIG. 57-1 *Lateral canal stenosis* deriving from subarticular entrapment of the L5 nerve root. Because the nerve root lies in the upper third of the intervertebral foramen,[18,43,61,69-73,76] osteophytic overgrowth from overhanging osteophytes from the superior facet of inferior vertebra compress the emerging nerve root beneath the facet joint as the root is tightly stretched against the pedicle in the lateral recess.

disk and a positive vacuum sign, and retrolisthesis with disk narrowing at the L2/L3 level. This patient has *degenerative spondylolisthesis* at L4/L5.

2. What are central and lateral spinal stenoses?

Lumbar *spinal stenosis* refers to narrowing of the vertebral canal, intervertebral foramen, or both.[51,*] When stenosis occurs centrally, the posteriorly located cauda equina may be compressed within the vertebral canal, so that a degenerative central disk protruding backward at L4-L5 is capable of compressing all the roots below L5. The most anterior roots, L5-S2, are most vulnerable, and the patient experiences neurogenic claudication of the cauda equina. Neurogenic claudication has its greatest prevalence in the sixth decade of life.[7]

Lateral canal stenosis constricts the laterally emerging nerve root causing singular claudication of a lumbar and/or nerve root secondary impingement in the intervertebral foramen.[3] In Case 2, the L5 nerve root is either compressed by a posterolateral L4 disk protrusion or from an inferior projecting osteophyte at the L5 facet joint margins or from a superior spur from the S1

facet joint. Alternately, osteophytic spurs from the vertebral body margins of the L5 or S1 vertebrae may compress on the L5 nerve root. Regardless of the cause of nerve root claudication, the patient experiences root symptoms when walking.

Stenosis is defined as a narrowing of either the anteroposterior or the transverse diameter of either the central or lateral canals. The source of compressive encroachment may be osseous or soft tissue in nature. Lumbar spinal stenosis is the most common preoperative diagnosis in persons over 65 years of age who undergo lumbar spinal surgery.[89] Approximately 1 in 1000 individuals over 65 years of age annually undergo spinal laminectomy in the United States for lumbar spinal stenosis with estimated costs of one billion dollars.[38]

3. What is the vertebral osteology of the lumbar spine?

Lumbar osteology is divided into a robust anterior vertebral body and a stout posterior vertebral arch (Fig. 57-2).† The vertebral body, wider transversely than

---

*The corollary is also true: degenerative spinal stenosis does not occur at a nonmobile level, so that despite the fact that the spinal canal is narrowest at T6, stenosis does not occur at that intervertebral level.

---

†The five lumbar vertebrae are distinguished by the absence of transverse foramina and costal facets.

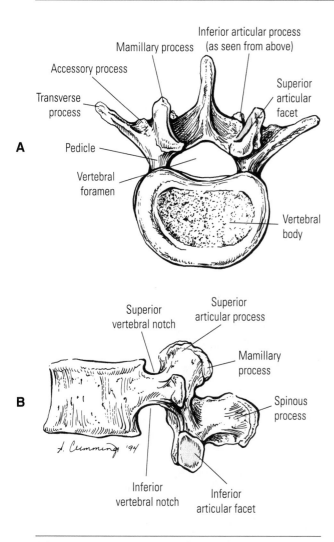

A

Inferior articular process
(as seen from above)

Mamillary process

Accessory process

Superior
articular
facet

Transverse
process

Pedicle

Vertebral
foramen

Vertebral
body

B

Superior
vertebral notch

Superior
articular process

Mamillary
process

Spinous
process

A. Cumming '94

Inferior
vertebral notch

Inferior
articular facet

FIG. 57-2 Typical lumbar vertebra. **A,** Superior view. **B,** Lateral view. (From Cramer GD, Darby SA: *Basic and clinical anatomy of the spine, spinal cord, and ANS,* St Louis, 1995, Mosby.)

from front to back, is designed to bear weight while the posterior elements comprising the vertebral arch form a triangular vertebral foramen that encases, and thereby protects the spinal cord like a ring of armor. The *vertebral foramen* forms an aperture, which when organized in series with the other vertebrae forms a *vertebral* (or *spinal,* or *central*) *canal* for the transmission of the neuraxis. The vertebral arch is a ring of bone formed by two pedicles, laminae, transverse processes, four articular processes that connect the vertebrae above and below, and one spinous process. The transverse processes emerge laterally, while the spinous process projects posteriorly from the center of the rings. The function of

both processes is to serve as attachment sites for ligaments and postural muscles, while acting as a series of levers for muscles.[96] The portion of the arch between the body and transverse processes is called the *pedicle* (Latin for little foot) and is short and thick in the lumbar spine.

The fifth lumbar vertebra is wedge shaped so that its anterior height exceeds its posterior height by 3 mm. The other lumbar vertebrae are each inclined backward with respect to the vertebrae below, endowing the lumbar spine with a lordotic shape. Lordosis is augmented by the wedge shape of the lumbosacral disk.

The portion of the arch between the transverse spinous process is the *laminae* (singular, lamina, and meaning flat plate). The junctional area between the pedicles and laminae has articular processes projecting vertically upward and downward on each side of the vertebrae. Thus the side of each vertebra has a superior and inferior articular process for a total of four articular processes. Although the superior facets embrace the inferior facets of the vertebra above, the inferior facets articulate with the superior facets of the vertebra below. The lumbar facets are oriented obliquely to the sagittal plane[79] and this limits motion in the low back to flexion and extension but little rotation (13°).[78]

A second major aperture of the spine is the *intervertebral foramen,* which is shaped like an inverted pear (Fig. 57-3). It is also known as the *nerve root canal,* and *lumbar radicular canal.* Because the pedicles are placed superior to the midpoint of the vertebral body and are smaller in size, a groove or *vertebral notch* is formed above and below (superior and inferior vertebral notches, respectively). The *superior vertebral notch* is shallower and smaller than the *inferior vertebral notch.* When two vertebrae articulate, the vertebral notches join together as two connecting half-rings that form an osseous tunnel. The resulting intervertebral foramen or lateral canal is primarily osseous, with exception to the facet joint capsule and ligamentum flavum posteriorly and the annulus fibrosus anteriorly.

The intervertebral foramen contains many structures including the spinal nerve, dorsal root ganglion,[79] dural root sleeve, the spinal branch of a segmental artery, intervertebral veins, lymphatic channels, adipose tissue, and two to five sinuvertebral nerves,[18] the latter of which occupy between a fourth and a third of available space in the upper half of the foramen.[39] The aperture of the intervertebral foramen is approximately 18 mm[68] although it enlarges with spinal flexion and diminishes with extension. The intervertebral foramen is

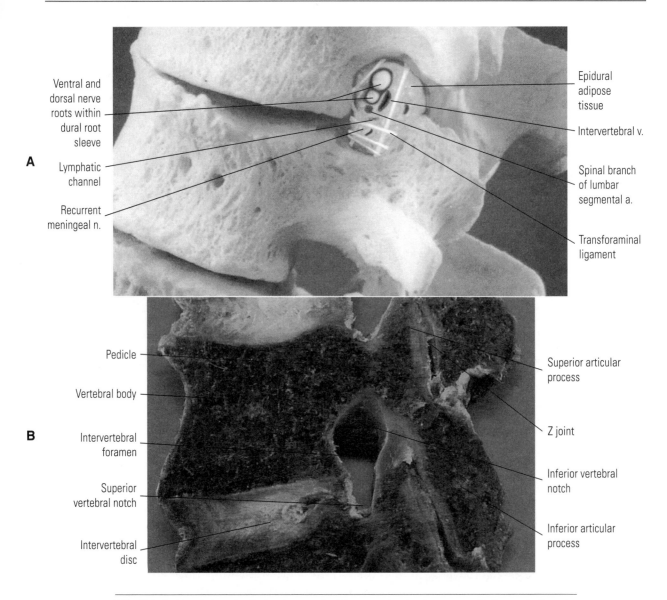

A,
Ventral and dorsal nerve roots within dural root sleeve

Lymphatic channel

Recurrent meningeal n.

Epidural adipose tissue

Intervertebral v.

Spinal branch of lumbar segmental a.

Transforaminal ligament

B,
Pedicle

Vertebral body

Intervertebral foramen

Superior vertebral notch

Intervertebral disc

Superior articular process

Z joint

Inferior vertebral notch

Inferior articular process

FIG. 57-3 A, Lateral view of a lumbar intervertebral foramen, showing its contents. **B,** Parasagittal section through the fourth lumbar intervertebral foramen. The foramen has the shape of an "inverted pear" when viewed from the side. (From Cramer GD, Darby SA: *Basic and clinical anatomy of the spine, spinal cord, and ANS,* St Louis, 1995, Mosby.)

unlike any other in the body in that the contents running through it pass through an aperture formed by two movable bones (vertebrae) and two articulations (anterior intervertebral and posterior facet joints).[2] It is clinically relevant that the posterior wall of the intervertebral foramen is comprised of the (anterior aspect of the) facet joints and part of the lamina whereas the (posterior aspect of the) intervertebral disk and the postero-inferior part of the vertebral body form the anterior wall, because degenerative changes of either may result in lateral stenosis. *The emerging nerve root is bounded above and below and laterally by pedicles.* The contents of this tunnel are confined within a fixed area so that encroachment on this space by a thickened ligamentum flavum, chronic disk bulges, acute disk herniations, osteophytes from arthritic facet joints, or combinations of these factors may crowd neural tissue and impede circulation of the neural elements.

4. What are the clinical implications of progressively increased pedicle thickening in the lumbar spine?

Increased broadening (thickening) of pedicle thickness is clinically relevant to the frequency of degenerative changes resulting in root canal encroachment. The pedicles become progressively broader caudally in response to its role in transmitting axial loading from the anterior to the posterior elements. As the pedicle forms the roof of the intervertebral foramen, a broader pedicle increases the length through which the emerging nerve root must travel before it exits freely as a peripheral nerve ramus. Subsequently, the L5 nerve root, which emerges below the L5 pedicle, is more likely to experience bony encroachment from hypertrophic bone spurs and posterolateral disk protrusions as it is held close to the compression zone for a longer length than the superiorly placed pedicles.[69-73]

5. What is the local anatomy of the lumbar spinal cord?

The *spinal cord* is comprised of 31 pairs of spinal nerves emerging from 31 spinal cord levels, which are numbered according to the number of the spinal nerve. A *spinal cord level* may be defined as the outwardly emerging paired dorsal and ventral rootlets from the cord, so that one pair of spinal nerves is associated with one cord segment. There are eight cervical, 12 thoracic, five lumbar, five sacral, and one coccygeal cord segments (Fig. 57-4). Roughly elliptical in cross section, the cord is wider from side to side than front to back. A furrow known as the dorsal median fissure runs down the back of the cord while a shallower depression, the ventral medial fissure (housing the anterior spinal artery) runs down the front. Together, both fissures, as in the brain, divide the cord into equal but opposite halves.

The spinal cord descends through the vertebrae approximately 45 cm (43 cm in females) and terminates at the first lumbar vertebra, specifically at the level of the L1 intervertebral disk, as the inferior tip of the cord known as the *conus medullaris*. The remainder of the lumbosacral spinal roots resembles a horse's tail and is therefore called the *cauda equina*. Those destined for more caudal locations lie medially and dorsally, while those about the leave the dural sac lie laterally and ventrally. The cauda equina is enclosed within a large sub-arachnoid space (when compared with that in the cervical and thoracic regions), which is a reservoir for cerebrospinal fluid.* Thus the cauda equina floats within a fluid medium within the subarachnoid space, which below the level of the L1 vertebra is called the *lumbar cistern.*

6. How does the organization of the cell bodies of lower motor sensory and motor fibers emerging from the spinal cord differ?

In contrast to the brain, which contains gray matter on the surface and white matter in the interior, the spinal cord is organized into an "H" or butterfly shaped central region of gray matter surrounded by myelinated ascending and descending axon tracts of *white matter.*† The central gray matter is composed of discrete collections of cell bodies of motor neurons located in the posterior (or dorsal) horns that are composed of central processes of sensory neurons. The cell bodies of sensory neurons are located outside the central nervous system in the dorsal roots of spinal nerves and hence termed *ganglions.*

7. What is the anatomic origin of the spinal nerve, and why is its encroachment within the intervertebral foramen more likely to cause sensory deficit?

Thirty-one pairs of spinal nerves emerge from the cord at regular segments between vertebra intervals, consistent with chordates. At each segment of the neuraxis, a pair of nerves emerges from the right and left of the vertical column. On the right side, for example, motor fibers emerge from the right ventral horn while sensory fibers emerge from the left dorsal horn. Before the joining of these fibers into a single mixed nerve, the sensory fibers merge into a bulbous ganglion within the intervertebral foramen. The dorsal root ganglion is situated in the upper third of the intervertebral foramen

---

*Although the *cerebrospinal fluid* has a primarily nutritive role, it also acts as a hydraulic cushion surrounding the cord and the proximal extensions of the laterally emergent nerve roots and offering protection during spinal motion, in much the same way amniotic fluid protects the growing neonate. Composed of high levels of sodium and magnesium and low levels of potassium, cerebrospinal fluid has an insulating effect on conduction of nerve impulses, as well as a role in removing metabolites. Cerebrospinal fluid also provides a relief mechanism for the increase in intracranial pressure that occurs with each arterial pulse of the blood to the brain.

†White matter appears white because of myelin sheathing.

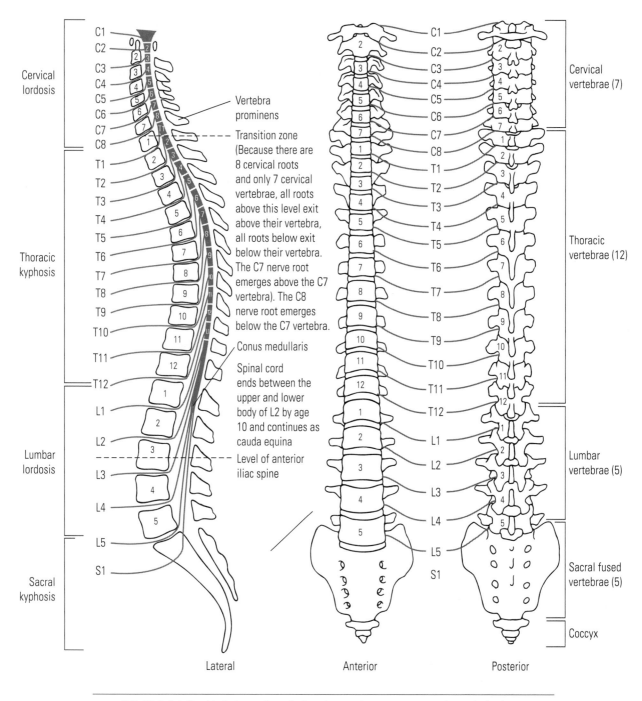

Cervical lordosis

Thoracic kyphosis

Lumbar lordosis

Sacral kyphosis

Vertebra prominens

Transition zone (Because there are 8 cervical roots and only 7 cervical vertebrae, all roots above this level exit above their vertebra, all roots below exit below their vertebra. The C7 nerve root emerges above the C7 vertebra). The C8 nerve root emerges below the C7 vertebra.

Conus medullaris

Spinal cord ends between the upper and lower body of L2 by age 10 and continues as cauda equina

Level of anterior iliac spine

Cervical vertebrae (7)

Thoracic vertebrae (12)

Lumbar vertebrae (5)

Sacral fused vertebrae (5)

Coccyx

Lateral   Anterior   Posterior

FIG. 57-4 Relationship between the spinal cord, emerging nerve roots, and vertebral column.

inferior to the pedicle, and because of its large size is more prone to compressive ischemia in degenerative spines.[74] Thus *because the preganglionic sensory fibers and ganglion take up more space within the interverte-bral foramen, encroachment of the foramen from osteo-phyte or disk protrusion is more likely to cause sensory than motor signs and symptoms.*[69-73] Thus the postgan-glionic sensory fibers and the motor fibers join a short distance from the cord to form a single fixed nerve root called the *intervertebral foramen.*

8. What is the structural and functional unit of the peripheral nervous system, and what are its cascading patterns of branching before becoming a specific peripheral nerve?

The peripheral nervous system consists of bundles of sensory (afferent) and motor (efferent) axons from the ventral (anterior) and dorsal (posterior) roots respectively, that merge into the *structural and functional unit of the peripheral nervous system:* the *spinal nerve.* These 31 pairs of nerves project laterally from the spinal cord in a segmental, bilateral manner and radiate to all parts of the body in a distribution pattern of rami, trunks, branches and terminal nerves. As each newly formed spinal nerve takes leave of the cord, it passes through the upper third of the intervertebral foramen to emerge beyond the foramen to divide into a posterior and anterior *ramus* corresponding to large first-order branchings of the peripheral nerve. The posterior ramus supplies the muscles and cutaneous distribution of the back. The posterior primary rami also supply the facet joints.

A more complex arrangement of nerves occurs at four plexi in the neck, upper and lower extremities, and pelvis as a strategy toward injury prevention, as these sites commonly undergo a variety of motion and thereby expose their peripheral nerves to greater injury. With the formation of each plexus, the anterior spinal roots graft onto each other in a tangle of complex interwoven axon networks called *plexi* (singular = plexus). With the brachial plexus, several anterior rami merge into *trunks,* which distally split into *divisions,* only to combine again to form *cords* before finally subdividing into individual motor and cutaneous *nerves.* The lumbosacral plexus has a slightly different configuration.

The advantage conferred by the interconnected design complex of the plexus and the fifth order branching (rami, trunks, divisions, cords, and nerve) is an architecture ideally suited to force distribution. Disruptive stretch to one branch is minimized by distribution throughout the entire plexus by means of tension transmission via elongation to all five-order branchings that enhances its ability to withstand (traction) injury.[14]

9. What are the membranous supportive tissues of the central nervous system?

The *meninges* (Greek for *membranes*) are the central nervous system equivalent of the epineurium, perineurium, and endoneurium, which cover the fascicles of the peripheral nerve. The purpose of the meningeal layers is to surround the spinal cord with a series of buffers and thus diminish the likelihood of neuraxis contact with the irregular bony surface of the internal spinal canal. The meninges include the thicker, outer *dura mater* covering the *leptomeninges,* comprised of the delicate *arachnoid* and *pia mater* (Fig. 57-5). A lattice arrangement of collagen fibers allows for stretch and compression without kinking, and thus offers protection to the neural elements while providing for movement.[12]

The *subarachnoid space* lying between the thin layer of arachnoid and innermost pia mater contains most of the vessels to the cord, and becomes the *dural sac* caudal to the termination of the spinal cord. Although the pia mater closely adheres to the spinal cord, it descends further caudally from the conus as the *filum terminale.* In contrast, the dura mater and arachnoid continue caudally to the second sacral vertebral level to form an enlarged subarachnoid space called the dural sac. The filum terminale, however, continues distally through the sac, picking up dural and arachnoid investment at this level and attaches to the first coccygeal level.

10. What is the dura mater?

The *spinal dura mater* (Latin for *hard mother*) is a protective sheath investing the central nervous system and is composed of both an outer and inner layer. The outer or periosteal layer of dura is closely adherent to the inner walls of the spinal canal, serving as its periosteum.[22] Continuous with the cranial dura mater, the inner *meningeal layer* of the dura mater forms a continuous closed tube within which the spinal cord and cauda equina are encased, running from the foramen magnum distally to its closed inferior end at the *filum terminale,* terminating at the level of the inferior border of the S2 vertebrae in adults.[56] The limited space between the inner and outer dural layers is called the epidural space and contains the internal vertebral venous plexus and adipose tissue. Also known as a *theca,*[25] the spinal dura mater is a tough, white, fibrous, and elastic membrane that is the toughest of all three meningeal layers.* The dura mater is an ideal

---

*The *Naffziger test* causing back or local pain from mechanical or inflammatory causes (such as meningitis) is based upon the close association of the meninges and the cerebrospinal fluid. The test is based upon the hypothesis that bilateral jugular compression increases cerebrospinal fluid pressure. The pressure increase in the subarachnoid space in the root canal may cause pain by irritating a local mechanical or inflammatory condition. This effect is heightened by asking the patient to cough, thereby increasing intrathecal pressure even more. (From White AA, Panjabi MM: *Clinical biomechanics of the spine,* Philadelphia, 1978, JB Lippincott.)

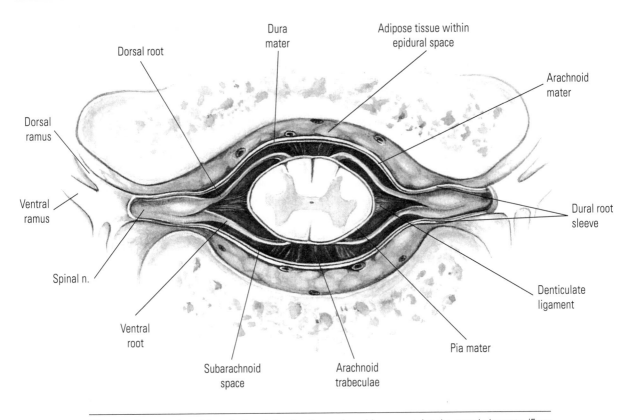

FIG. 57-5 Cross section of the spinal cord showing the meningeal layers covering the neural elements. (From Cramer GD, Darby SA: *Basic and clinical anatomy of the spine, spinal cord, and ANS*, St Louis, 1995, Mosby.)

protective tissue as it does not deteriorate with age and is so remarkably tough as to be suitable for heart valve replacement.[90]

11. What is the nerve supply to the lumbar spine?

The *recurrent meningeal nerve* or *sinuvertebral nerve of Von Luschka*[55] is found at each intervertebral foramen of the vertebral column (Fig. 57-6). These tiny nerves derive from the most proximal portion of the anterior primary ramus beyond the dorsal ganglion, immediately distal to the intervertebral foramen. After dividing from the anterior ramus they receive a sympathetic branch from the closest grey communicating ramus and turn back to reenter the anterior aspect of the intervertebral foramen close to the pedicle that forms the roof of this aperture. Several recurrent meningeal nerves may enter each intervertebral foramen and thereby contribute to crowding and may be a source of back pain (neuropathy) if compressed[27] by an arthritic facet or the ligamentum flavum. Upon entering the intervertebral foramen, the recurrent meningeal nerves give off ascending, descending, and transverse branches that anastomose with adjacent vertebral segments, including those on the opposite side of the spine.[40] In addition to supplying the dura, the sinuvertebral nerves innervate the posterior longitudinal ligament, the posterior portion of the annulus fibrosus,[92] periosteum of the posterior aspect of the vertebral bodies, the lamina, epidural venous plexus,[27] and the posterior longitudinal ligament. The posteromedial region of the spinal dura is not innervated and does not sense pain.[41] The aching pain accompanying spinal claudication from stenosis may derive from the sinuvertebral nerve secondary to venous congestion of the epidural venous plexus.

The facet joint capsules are supplied by branches from the medial division of each posterior primary ramus of the lumbar roots. The innervation pattern is organized so that the capsule is innervated by fibers arising from the nerve root at that level, and from the root from the level above. Thus a nerve from a given level supplies fibers to the inferior capsule of the posterior facet joint at that level, and the superior capsule of the joint at the next level.

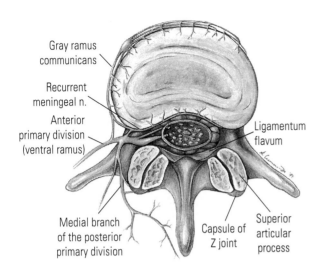

Gray ramus communicans

Recurrent meningeal n.

Anterior primary division (ventral ramus)

Ligamentum flavum

Medial branch of the posterior primary division

Capsule of Z joint

Superior articular process

FIG. 57-6 Superior view of lumbar vertebral and neural structures. The four primary sources of neural innervation to spinal structures include the anterior and posterior primary divisions, the recurrent meningeal nerve, and sensory fibers that course together with the sympathetic nervous system. Note that the recurrent meningeal nerve also innervates the posterior aspect of the intervertebral disc, the posterior longitudinal ligament, and the anterior aspect of the spinal dura mater. (From Cramer GD, Darby SA: *Basic and clinical anatomy of the spine, spinal cord, and ANS,* St Louis, 1995, Mosby.)

12. What are thecal signs?

Certain motions or space occupying lesions such as a posterolateral disk protrusion against the dural sleeve will cause dural sleeve-derived pain. Similarly osteophytes from degenerative joint disease of the facet joints may press against the dural sleeve with certain motions such as spinal extension. Moreover, coughing, sneezing, or straining during a bowel movement dilates the veins within the dura mater. Bending the head forward tenses the dura and pulls it closer to the dural sleeve. This same effect is distally achieved by a straight leg raise and Lasègue's test in which the ankle is sharply dorsiflexed.

13. What is the dural root sleeve?

As the nerve roots emerge laterally from the spinal cord they are invested by both dura and arachnoid membranes similar to a coat sleeve, as they emerge from the spinal canal to enter the intervertebral foramen. The motor and sensory fibers comprising the mixed nerve root unite within the funnel-shaped dural root sleeve.[26] The *dural root sleeve* is adherent to the periosteum lining the intervertebral foramen by internal restraints. Shortly beyond the intervertebral foramen the dura mater termi-

nates for a short length of span before coverage by epineurium* that protectively sheaths the newly formed spinal nerve beyond the foraminal aperture. Thus although the nerve root is allowed movement, excursion in the intervertebral foramen is limited by dural fixation.

14. At what site is the nerve root most vulnerable to traction injury?

Although the emergence of the spinal nerve roots from the cord represents the demarcation point between the central and peripheral nervous systems, nerve roots resemble the central nervous system in that they have a meningeal covering, lack of Schwann cells, and receive at least half of their nutrition from cerebrospinal fluid. Before becoming a peripheral nerve, the emerging *root-let* is unprotected for a short length as it is only covered by a delicate mesh of pia mater.[64] This *junctional area* between the termination of the meningeal sleeve and the supportive tissues enveloping the peripheral nerve is a relatively unprotected site. Nevertheless, nerve root avulsion from the spinal cord from excessive tension is uncommon.[36] Tension to the nerve roots from traction is diminished by denticulate ligaments,[82] which absorb force along their length, as well as being able to unfold their coiled structure and thereby relieve traction.[63,64] Nerve root injury more commonly occurs from neighboring structures such as osteophytic facet joints and protruding intervertebral disks.

15. What static and dynamic mechanisms and design strategy protect the emerging nerve roots from tensile traction?

The lumbar dura mater has internal attachments to adjacent vertebrae and ligaments at each segmental level that keep it tethered within the intervertebral foramen. Between the pia and dura mater are 21 pairs of *denticulate ligaments* that are classified as internal dural attachments (Fig. 57-7). These ligaments suspend the cord within the canal akin to the vertical support cables supporting the roadway of a suspension bridge.[22] The denticulate ligaments also separate the anterior and posterior nerve roots, and relieve traction on the nerve roots. Additionally, the denticulate ligaments prevent excessive cord elongation during trunk flexion.[30] The *lateral root ligament* is a band of connective tissue attaching the external dural root sleeve to the inferior pedicle of the intervertebral foramina and also offers resistance to traction force.[26] The dural root sleeve also

---

*The *epineurium* refers to the outermost supporting connective tissue of the peripheral nervous system.

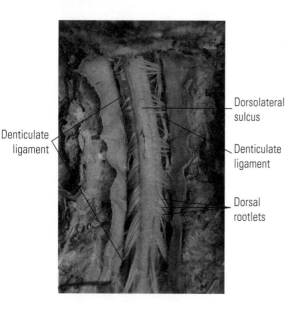

Denticulate ligament

Dorsolateral sulcus

Denticulate ligament

Dorsal rootlets

FIG. 57-7 Between the pia and dura mater are 21 pairs of *denticulate ligaments* that are classified as internal dural attachments. These ligaments suspend the cord within the canal akin to the vertical support cables supporting the roadway of a suspension bridge. The denticulate ligaments also separate the anterior and posterior nerve roots and tether the emergent nerve root within the intervertebral foramen and thereby relieve the disruptive pull of tensile traction upon the nerve roots. (From Cramer GD, Darby SA: *Basic and clinical anatomy of the spine, spinal cord, and ANS*, St Louis, 1995, Mosby.)

provides resistance to traction as it will first rupture before avulsion of the root occurs.

Dynamic protection of the emerging nerve roots from avulsion is offered by the psoas muscle. Although the anterior origin of psoas major attaches to the lumbar bodies and intervertebral disks, the posterior origin attaches anteriorly on the transverse processes. Thus the psoas major surrounds the lateral openings of the first four lumbar vertebrae so that the ventral rami from these levels merge to form the lumbosacral plexus within the substance of psoas major. In the event of hyperflexion or hyperextension of the hip, psoas may serve to absorb the traction forces before their causing injury proximal at the intervertebral foramen.[21]

16. What external dural connections stabilize neuromeningeal tissues?

The biomechanics of the neuromeningeal tissue are directly affected by the external connections of the dura in the body's attempt to protect the spinal cord. Proxi-

mally, there is a firm attachment at the foramen magnum, although the external filum terminale attaches the caudal end to the coccyx by a thin elastic tube that acts as a buffer to overstretching of the spinal cord.[84] In addition, a network of dural ligaments known as *Hoffman ligaments* (Fig. 57-8) tether the anterior dura to the posterior longitudinal ligament to the posterior vertebral periosteum, attaching the dura to the spinal canal. In the lumbar spine, these ligaments are well developed and tether the dura centrally. In contrast, corresponding attachments occur in the posterior aspect of the spinal canal between the flaval ligament and the posterior dura mater.[65] The significance of these ligaments lies in their providing the spinal cord and its protective coverings with a strong attachment to the spinal canal, and their role in force distribution.

17. What is the vasculature of the spinal cord and nerve roots?

Consisting of only 2% of body mass, the nervous system consumes 20% of available oxygen circulating in the blood stream.[24] Blood supplies the necessary energy for impulse conduction and for the intracellular movement of cytoplasmic and axoplasmic flow within the neuron. Neurons are particularly sensitive to alterations in blood flow, as an uninterrupted vascular supply is imperative to meet the metabolic demands of neural structures and normal axoplasmic transport. Toward this end, the vasculature pattern within the nervous system, termed the *vasa nervorum,* are designed with both intrinsic and extrinsic components that may operate independently. If a feeder vessel is compromised the internal system serves as a bypass that shunts enough blood for normal neural function.[14]

Three longitudinal vessels supply the spinal cord. The *anterior spinal artery,* arising as two vessels from the vertebral arteries in the foramen magnum descend within the *transverse foramen* of C1 to C6 vertebral transverse processes.* The anterior spinal artery is the longest identifiable artery in the body as it runs the length of the cord and supplies the anterior two-thirds of the neuraxis. The caliber of this artery is smallest in the midthoracic region of the cord resulting in an avascular water shed between the T4 to T9 vertebral levels.[24] The continuity of blood flow from the anterior spinal artery is reinforced by a series of six to eight

---

*The transverse foramen of the C7 vertebra only transmits the vertebral veins.

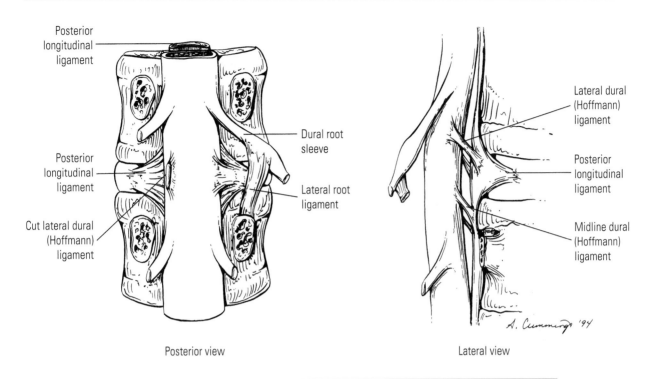

Posterior longitudinal ligament

Posterior longitudinal ligament

Cut lateral dural (Hoffmann) ligament

Dural root sleeve

Lateral root ligament

Lateral dural (Hoffmann) ligament

Posterior longitudinal ligament

Midline dural (Hoffmann) ligament

Posterior view

Lateral view

FIG. 57-8 *Hoffmann ligaments* are a network of dural ligaments that tether the anterior dura to the posterior longitudinal ligament and hence, to the posterior vertebral periosteum, thereby anchoring the dura, centrally, to the spinal canal. In the lumbar spine, these ligaments are well developed and tether the dura centrally. The significance of these ligaments lies in their providing the spinal cord and its protective coverings with a strong attachment to the spinal canal, and plays a role in force distribution. (From Cramer GD, Darby SA: *Basic and clinical anatomy of the spine, spinal cord, and ANS*, St Louis, 1995, Mosby. Adapted from Kirkaldy-Willis W: *Managing low back pain*, ed 2, New York, 1988, Churchill Livingstone.)

ventral, bilateral, *radicular* (*radix* meaning root) *arteries* arising from the intercostal, lumbar, and sacral arteries that replenish blood to ensure a constant supply. These segmental vessels originate outside the vertebral column and at the lumbar spine enter as branches of the aorta known as lumbar arteries. Each lumbar artery divides into three major branches: an anterior branch supplying the vertebral body, dura mater, and ligaments, an intermediate branch entering the spinal canal at the intervertebral foramen to divide into anterior* and posterior radicular arteries, and a posterior branch passing along the side of the pars articularis to supply the posterior elements (neural arch) of the spine.[50]

The anterior spinal artery gives off circumferential vessels, which lie on the surface of the cord, forming a surface plexus by anastomosing with branches of the posterior spinal arteries and supplying the periphery of the cord.[69-73] The paired *posterior spinal arteries* supply the posterior one-third of the spinal cord and form a plexus over the dorsal column, which they supply. At the level of the conus medullaris, a loop is formed as the anterior spinal artery anastomoses with the two posterior spinal arteries.[50]

The cauda equina receives its blood supply distally from the radicular arteries and also proximally from the cruciate anastomosis surrounding the conus medullaris. The proximal and distal vessels form an anastomosis at the junction of the proximal and middle thirds of the cauda equina roots. This watershed represents a critical zone of avascularity where the cauda equina is vulnerable to compression.[23]

The complicated valveless venous channels in the

*The larger of the two anterior radicular arteries supplying the lumbosacral enlargement of the cord typically arises on the left and is know as the *great radicular artery of Adamkiewicz*. This artery reinforces the anterior spinal artery, by providing the main blood supply to the inferior two thirds of the spinal cord.

extradural compartment of the vertebral canal is known as the *vertebral venous plexus,* or *Batson's plexus,*[10] and accompanies the emergent nerve roots through the intervertebral foramen. Because they are valveless, they are under little pressure, allowing flow reversibility, and an accommodating mechanism to sudden in-rushes of blood, as may occur from coughing, lifting, and straining.[67] Vasculature of the nerve roots is supplied by two afferent vessels, the proximal and distal radicular arteries.[63] Within the nerve root, the intraneural anastomosis allows for rapid shunting of blood despite the "piston-like" movement of nerve roots that occurs in the foramina during spinal movements.[83]

Nervous tissue is sensitive to a reduced oxygen intake. Compression of nerve roots blocks axoplasmic transport either mechanically, or via ischemia, as transport is an energy dependent process. As little as 5 to 10 mm Hg compression pressure may cause venous congestion of the intraneural microcirculation of nerve roots[59] and may cause radicular ischemia within the intervertebral foramen and consequent radicular signs.[33]

18. What is the range of motion of the lumbar spine?

Although each segment of the lumbar spine is capable of limited motion, the collective action of the lumbar spine allows for overall large movements. The lumbar spine is capable of flexion and extension, lateral bending, and axial rotation. Flexion and extension is greatest at the L4/L5 vertebral level with a mean value of 24°, whereas the L5/S1 and L3/L4 levels average 18°. Flexion for all the lumbar vertebrae is 53°, whereas total extension is 30°. Lateral bending is equal for either side and averages a total of 40° from one extreme to the other. Total rotation of the lumbar spine averages 16° with the L4/L5 and L5/S1 vertebral levels averaging 4° and capable of the greatest amount of rotation.[75] The range of lumbar spinal motion is reduced by approximately 30% between 20 and 70 years of age.[35]

19. What length changes do the spinal and root canals undergo with normal movement?

The spinal canal is spacious enough in all directions to allow for normal movement of the cord and meninges, as well as to accommodate for some normal spondylitic or disk changes without clinically detectable neurologic compromise. The spinal canal undergoes significant length changes during movement. From spinal extension to flexion, the spinal canal elongates as much as 5 to 9 cm with most of the elongation occurring in the cervical and lumbar regions.[54] During early spinal flexion, the cross-sectional area of the spinal canal increases due to an increase of its anteroposterior diameter, whereas the cross-section decreases with extension.[20] This explains why patients with central encroachment from a disk or osteophyte have exacerbation of symptoms while in extension. These patients seek relief by adopting a posture with several degrees of lumbar flexion. In contrast, extension of the lumbar region is accompanied by broadening of the cauda equina, slackening of the ligamentum flavum, and bulging of the intervertebral disks into the vertebral canal.[18] It is no wonder that spinal extension exacerbates central stenosis.

The walls of the vertebral canal do not move as one segment during movement. During spinal flexion, the posterior wall of the canal elongates more than the anterior wall, while the reverse occurs with spinal extension.[5] Similarly, lateral flexion elongates the convex side of the spinal canal while shortening the concave aspect.[12]

The effects of flexion and extension at the intervertebral foramen cause marked changes in the cross section of that aperture. Spinal flexion from neutral increases the cross-sectional area of the root canal by as much as 30%, while extension decreased the available space by 20%.[62] These changes are clinically significant in a canal that contains many neurovascular structures.[12] Thus in addition to exacerbating central stenosis, spinal extension will additionally exacerbate lateral stenosis.

20. What adaptive mechanisms exist in the neuraxis, nerve roots, and meninges that diminish tension derived from movement?

The spinal cord occupies roughly one-half of the space in the spinal canal in each direction.[45] This allows for room needed to maintain cord integrity in the event of sudden, extreme movement of the thorax. Nevertheless, the ascending tracts located in the periphery of the cord are more likely to suffer the possibility of mechanical injury from rubbing or impingement by the internal osseous cage comprising the spinal canal. Because the axis for flexion and extension is forward of the cord,[14] the posterior columns of the cord will undergo greater elongation during spinal flexion than the anterior side of the neuraxis as they move anteriorly within the spinal canal.[12] In extension, the anterior columns elongate as the neuraxis moves posteriorly. With lateral flexion movements, those ascending tracts on the convex side will stretch more than those on the concave side. Because axonal length is typically convoluted in folds and spirals, the axons comprising the ascending tracts on the convex side of the cord will protectively unfold as a strategy to reduce excessive tension. The posterior columns are more folded and twisted than the anterior columns because they are further away from the instantaneous axis of rotation and become taut during forward flexion.[95] Another neuroaxial adaptation to stretch is movement of the cord in relation to neighboring vertebral segments.[12]

21. What variations in the spatial architecture of the vertebral canal predispose for central stenosis?

Segmental variation in the shape of the spinal canal is appreciated from an axial view (from the head), which shows considerable variability in the aperture diameter of the canal (Fig. 57-9). The upper cervical canal is large and triangular in shape, whereas the thoracic spinal canal is smaller and more cylindrical. The lumbar vertebral canal is larger than the thoracic canal, dome-shaped, and lacks a lateral recess in the upper lumbar region, but becomes more triangular in shape caudally. The size of the lumbar vertebral canal ranges from 12 to 20 mm anteroposteriorly in the midsagittal plane and 18 to 27 mm in its transverse (interpedicular) diameter.[18]

In the lumbar spine, the dimensions of the vertebral canal become progressively less round and more triangular from the first to the fifth lumbar level.[72] Population differences in the size of the vertebral canal exist so that approximately 15%[71] of the population have a *trefoil shaped* lumbar vertebral foramen referring to a canal configuration in which the neural arch has a posterolateral indentation and two deep lateral recesses.[71] A *lateral recess* or *gutter* exists at each corner of the triangular base of the foramen and represents a site of potential constriction as a nerve root exits through each lateral recess to enter the intervertebral foramen. The trefoil shape is less common at L4, and rare at more proximal levels. A trefoil-shaped canal is at risk for central stenosis because its cross sectional area is less than that of nontrefoil canals,[72] whereas the L5 nerve roots are at greater risk for lateral stenosis from encroachment of posterolateral disk or osteophytes into the lateral recess.[29] Women have slightly wider canals than men,[29] which may account for why spinal stenosis more commonly affects males. Because the achondroplast* has short, thick pedicles, the anterior-posterior diameter of the canal is reduced.

Achondroplasia is a hereditary, congenital disturbance of epiphyseal growth resulting in a form of dwarfism.

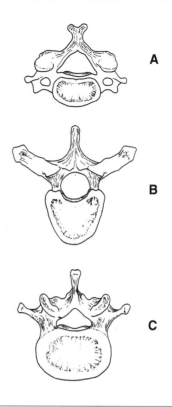

FIG. 57-9 Axial view of the typical cervical **(A)**, thoracic **(B)**, and **(C)** lumbar vertebrae. The cross-sectional area of the vertebral canal varies according to region. The upper cervical canal is large and triangular shaped, whereas the thoracic spinal canal is smaller and more cylindrical. The lumbar vertebral canal is larger than the thoracic canal, dome shaped, and lacking a lateral recess in the upper lumbar region but becoming more triangular in shape caudally. (From Watkins RG: *The spine in sports*, St Louis, 1995, Mosby.)

22. What factors influence the development of the vertebral canal?

Although changes in vertebral size may occur as a direct function of the normal aging process,[52] spinal stenosis appears to have strong links to prenatal and perinatal growth.[17] The vertebral canals of small children are remarkably large because canal growth is approximately 90% complete by late infancy. In utero, the neural arch may be epigenetically influenced by the growth of the spinal cord,[77] much as the brain determines the size of the skull in hydrocephalus and microcephalus.[53] Possible causes of neonatal malnutrition include smoking, alcohol, toxins, infections (both bacterial and viral), and placental insufficiency.[85] In the same way that maternal smoking has been shown to significantly reduce head circumference, the same phenomenon may occur with the vertebral canal.[17] It is postulated that an early adverse environment affects neuro-osseous development such that a small vertebral canal is matched to a small conus. Despite good nutrition that may follow, a critical period is passed and a normally sized cauda equina may become housed in a shallow vertebral canal left behind by an ascending cord. Thus the individual with this canal is predisposed to canal stenosis if the canal becomes pathologically compromised.[71] The growth curves of the thymus, the central nervous system,[42] cardiovascular system,[8] and liver[9] are similar to that of the neuro-osseous development, and are similarly affected by an early environment. The idea that a small canal is associated with poor health status due to immune deficiency is compatible with observations that adults with spinal stenosis more frequently visited their physicians with infections as children and adults than patients with wider canals.[69] There is also evidence that academic performance in children with wider vertebral canals at 16 years of age is better than their peers with smaller canals. Whether this is due to their socioeconomic status or their early neurological development is unknown.[71]

23. Why do redundant nerve roots occur with normal aging and how do they diminish space within the spinal canal?

Changes occurs in the size of the spinal[52] and lateral canals over time as part of the normal aging process. Beyond middle age, changes in the proteoglycan content of the nucleus pulposus of the intervertebral disk translate to a loss of water and hence disk height. Over the years the vertebrae shorten as much as 14 mm on average.[88] Reduction of superior-to-inferior length shortens the vertebral canal and causes redundancy of the nerve roots along the cauda equina. Redundancies are a common abnormality in degenerative spinal stenosis.[88] *Redundant nerve roots* refer to undulations within the longitudinal length of the nerve roots so that they may buckle or loop, causing them to fill the subarachnoid space more completely. Posterior osteophytes from the vertebral bodies or other constrictions within the vertebral canal are more likely to rub against the roots during movement resulting in friction neuritis, manifesting as either nerve root ischemia or central compression with intermittent claudication.

Moreover, as shrinkage occurs and the vertical dimension between the vertebrae is reduced, the spinal cord undergoes a slackening as the vertebrae approximate. This kinking of the cord occupies more space within the central canal, and is thus more likely to come

in contact with the inner osseous topography of the vertebral foramen, particularly if it is trefoil shaped. In addition, the dura becomes indented anteriorly at the disk level by a bulging annulus.[71] Because the posterolateral aspect of the annulus fibrosus represents the anterior wall of the intervertebral foramen, a decrease in disk height that accompanies increasing age will also result in a decrease of the vertical dimension of the intervertebral foramen and thereby decrease the available space for its contents.[19]

24. Why is the L5 nerve root more vulnerable to compression?

In the lumbar spine, the lumbosacral junction and L4-L5 level statistically account for some 95% of all cases of spinal injury. Of the three remaining lumbar joints, pathology at L3/L4 appears to be far more common than at the other two higher levels.[37] Exactly why this is so much relates to the anatomy of the L4-L5, and particularly the L5-S1 articulations. The lumbosacral articulation is composed of the L5 vertebrae superiorly and the sacrum inferiorly. The lateral recess at this level is narrower than the superior segments whereas the lateral root canal at this level is longer because it runs beneath a relatively wider (L5) pedicle. The L5 nerve root is the largest of the lumbar nerves, exiting the L5 intervertebral foramen, the smallest of the lumbar spine.[60] Another factor is the presence of the *corporotransverse ligament,* a tough, fibrous band that crosses the intervertebral foramen and is classified as a *transforaminal ligament.* This ligament runs between the vertebral body and the transverse process at the L5-S1 junction.[6] It is present in the lumbar foramen and may be a cause for root entrapment. The presence of this ligament occupies space within the foramen and may contribute to root entrapment.[16]

Because the orientation of the L5/S1 facet joints permits more axial rotation than the other lumbar levels, the L5/S1 articulation is the most movable of all lumbar joints possessing 5° of unilateral rotation, 3° of lateral bending, and 10° of flexion and extension. This greater movement increases the likelihood of injury to the annular fibers of the L5/S1 disk and subsequent prolapse. Thus the unique characteristics of the lumbosacral articulation make it extremely vulnerable to injury.

25. What is the structural degenerative cascade?

The *structural degenerative cascade* is a series of pathoanatomic changes that occur over time accounting for the majority of pain of spinal origin. This schema is based upon understanding the functional unit between the joints of the anterior and posterior elements of the spine. The intervertebral disk and the two facet joints between two adjacent vertebrae comprise a three-part complex, so that pathologic conditions or dysfunction in one component can adversely affect the others.[48] In this conception, the various conditions of the spine may be viewed as a spectrum of related pathologies along a continuum of degenerative structural changes.

Beginning most often with degenerative disk disease, the degenerative cascade begins with micro- or macro-trauma in the intervertebral disk or facet joints and results in structural alteration of the vertebral motion segment. One vertebral motion segment is defined as the intervertebral disk joint anteriorly and the two posteriorly located facet joints that define and limit the amount of movement at the disk joint. The degenerative cascade is similar to the degenerative process at other articular surfaces and occurs as a function of joint movement and the normal process of wear-and-tear of tissue. At some point in a patient's life, the amount of motion at the spinal motion segment causes more wear than can be tolerated leading to degenerative wear of soft and osseous tissues. As this process continues, structural degeneration may eventually manifest as disk degeneration or herniation, spinal instability, malalignment, facet arthrosis, lateral or central canal stenosis. However, because patients may or may not be symptomatic at any stage, and because of the many ways in which pathology may manifest, the degenerative cascade may lead to a variety of clinical presentations. Thus the degenerative cascade represents a spectrum of soft and osseous tissue degeneration of the spinal motion segment whose clinical presentation spans a host of pathological changes, each of which has its unique clinical presentation.[49]

26. How may spondylitic facet arthrosis cause lateral canal stenosis?

Lumbar spondylosis refers to degenerative joint disease of the articular facet joints causing osteophytic spurring from the margins of that joint that may constrict *both* the central and root canals.[71] Osteoarthritic changes due to spondylosis will primarily occur at those spinal levels that exhibit the greatest mobility.* Thus spondylosis

---

*The corollary is also true: degenerative spinal stenosis does not occur at a nonmobile level, so that despite the fact that the spinal canal is narrowest at T6, stenosis does not occur at that intervertebral level.

is most likely to occur at the L4/L5 interspace. Approximately 75% of lateral canal stenosis occurs at the L5/S1 level. *Central stenosis* may derive from impingement from osteophytic arthrosis from the *inferior articular process* comprising the lower hemi-facet joint. Because it faces anteriorly, marginal spurring will be directed toward the spinal cord. In contrast, the superior articular process faces backward and medially. Because the nerve root lies in the upper third of the intervertebral foramen,[18] osteophytic overgrowth from overhanging osteophytes encroach on the *superior articular process* comprising the superior facet, along the attachment of the ligamentum flavum[74] (which forms its joint capsule) is likely to cause *lateral canal stenosis.*[91] This is known as *subarticular entrapment* because encroachment of the emerging nerve root occurs beneath the facet joint as the root is tightly stretched against the pedicle in the lateral recess.[69-73] Bony spurring may also develop from the vertebral body along the attachment of the annulus fibrosus.

27. What is degenerative disk disease and how may it result in central and lateral canal lumbar stenosis?

Degenerative disk disease (see Chapter 58) refers to degeneration of the cartilaginous disks with secondary pathologic changes as a function of aging and loss of water content in the gelatinous central core making it hard and brittle. Bulging disks may compress the spinal nerves that exit behind them. Disk deterioration results in fissures of the annulus fibrosus through which the nucleus herniates. Disk fragments or the disk in its entirety may become displaced and press on the spinal nerve roots. Because the intervertebral disk forms the anterior border of the intervertebral foramen, a decrease in disk height affects the lateral canal by decreasing its vertical dimension.[19]

Root entrapment typically occurs from bony or soft-tissue encroachment in the root canal in the form of osteophytes from the margins of the apophyseal joints and occasionally in the central canal. In response to degeneration, the vertebral margins along the attachment of the annulus fibrosus grow bony spurs that protrude and occasionally form a bony bridge between the vertebrae in an attempt to stabilize that segment. When spurring occurs between the posterior margins of two vertebral bodies, the central and lateral canals may be compromised.[44] The dimensions of the central canal are also significantly reduced by hypertrophic bone formation of the inferior facet, especially if there is associated thickening and subsequent bulging of the ligamentum flavum.[79] Thus enlargement of the inferior facets is more likely to cause central canal stenosis, whereas enlargement of the superior facets often results in lateral canal stenosis. Bony or soft-tissue encroachment of the emerging root may occur in any of the lumbar nerve roots, although the fifth lumbar root is most commonly involved. This is due to the frequency of degenerative change at the L5/S1 level and also because of the relatively long length of the root canal at L5 inferior to the broad pedicle. Thus the L5/S1 nerve root exposes relatively more of its length to the likelihood for encroachment.[69-73]

28. What is the role of soft-tissue encroachment upon the neural elements?

Flecks of the annulus, following a disk protrusion, may become wedged in the lateral recess and result in further constriction of the nerve root. Extrusion or fibrosis of the sequestrated nucleus reduces the available space for the nerve root. The lumbar *ligamentum flavum* extends between the laminae of adjacent vertebrae throughout the lumbar region (Fig. 57-10) and acts to protect the spinal canal from encroachment by soft tis-

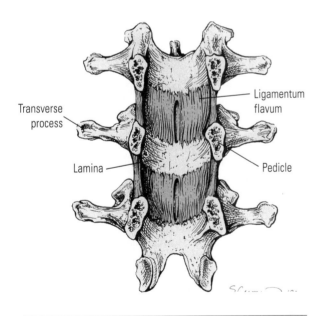

Transverse process

Lamina

Ligamentum flavum

Pedicle

FIG. 57-10 Anatomy of the ligamentum flavum. Pedicles have been sectioned in a coronal plane to show the ligamentum flavum passing between adjacent laminae. (From Cramer GD, Darby SA: *Basic and clinical anatomy of the spine, spinal cord, and ANS*, St Louis, 1995, Mosby.)

sue on flexion movements. Located posteriorly on the neural arch, the ligamentum flavum narrows the inferior aspect of the intervertebral foramen and helps form the posterior boundary of the intervertebral foramen.[56] The thickness of the ligamentum flavum ranges between 2 and 7 mm, and is thinnest when the spine is flexed, pulling the ligament taut. During spinal extension it is contracted and thick and occupies more space within the canal, in which case it will indent into the vertebral canal.[80] Because of disk space narrowing in degenerative disk disease, the vertebrae will approximate each other. This causes the ligamentum flavum to kink on itself, bulging further into the spinal canal and aggravating any tendency toward stenosis. In addition, this ligament may ossify,[86] particularly in vertebral hyperostosis and in Paget's disease.[94] Although the ligamentum flavum may infold, the posterior longitudinal ligament may thicken,[87] the apophyseal joint capsule may hypertrophy or bulge with synovial hyperplasia,[74] and the soft tissue of a lytic pars interarticularis may proliferate until space for the nerve root is minimal.[71]

The *corporotransverse ligament* is a tough, fibrous band that crosses the intervertebral foramen and is classified as a *transforaminal ligament*. This ligament runs between the vertebral body and the transverse process at the L5-S1 junction.[6] The presence of this ligament occupies space within the intervertebral foramen and may contribute to root entrapment.[16] Other factors that occupy space within the intervertebral foramen include venous engorgement with edema, epidural fibrosis following surgical trauma, infection, or hematoma.[69-73] Finally, the dorsal root ganglion is a bulbous enlargement that is a likely candidate for constriction within the intervertebral foramen.

29. What is spondylolisthesis and how does it result in spinal stenosis?

Spondylolisthesis occurs when a stress fracture of the lamina between the superior and inferior articular processes is accompanied by forward displacement of the superior on the vertebrae, causing central canal stenosis at the level of the pars interarticularis defect. If vertebral displacement occurs at L5, the L5 nerve root is impaired as it passes laterally and anterior to the pars interarticularis to exit the L5 intervertebral foramen. *Lateral canal stenosis* is caused by the portion of the pars located above the fracture site, entrapping the laterally emerging nerve root.

Degenerative spondylolisthesis is defined as forward slippage of one vertebra over the next as a result of degenerative change in the intervertebral disk and/or articular facet joint.* This occurs because erosion of the superior articular facet allows forward displacement of the upper vertebral body on the lower body, trapping the inferior nerve root that exists one level below between the inferior facet and the back of the vertebral body.[48] Commonly occurring at the fourth lumbar level, degenerative spondylolisthesis most likely occurs as a function of facet joint orientation and differs from the classic isthmic type of spondylolisthesis in that the former is characterized by an intact neural arch and lack of primary disk degeneration. It is alternately known as *pseudospondylolisthesis.* A fourfold increased incidence of sacralization is observed in these patients, which further increases the stress to this vulnerable L4/L5 disk level.[76] Degenerative spondylolisthesis predominantly occurs in females (3:2) greater than 50 years of age,[58] and causes the inferior articular processes of L4 to entrap the L5 and S1 nerve roots against the posterior aspect of the vertebral body of L5.[23,24] Compression of the cauda equina against the body of L5 may occur as the lamina and inferior articular process of L4 slide forward, and result in neurogenic claudication. Accordingly, degenerative spondylolisthesis may result in *central stenosis* with possible compromise of the cauda equina,[48,49] and compromise of the lateral nerve root causing *lateral stenosis.* Segmental spinal motion affects canal stenosis dynamically. Extension and rotation reduce the available space encroaching on the nerve root complex and radicular vessels.[71]

The pathologic process of degenerative spondylolisthesis begins with deterioration of the intervertebral disk[31] followed by malalignment of the facet joints as disk height is lost, and is accompanied by osteophyte formation and synovial hypertrophy of the synovial facet joints that become rounded and arthritic. This loss of vertical orientation of the facet joints undermines the stabilizing role provided by the posterior joints to the intervertebral disk joint, allowing for excessive forward displacement of the vertebra during flexion. Pain may arise at the degenerative disk and at the arthritic facet joints. Consequently, the superior vertebra (L4) begins

to migrate or "slip" and roll forward during lumbar flexion. Depending on the extent of slip, a "step" may be palpable. Unlike the spondylolytic variety, the step occurs between the spinous process of the affected vertebra and the one below. As the superior vertebral body shifts forward, the interposed disk undergoes shearing strain that further exacerbates and accelerates disk degeneration. The forward slippage of the fourth lumbar vertebra ceases when the intact lamina and inferior articular facets of L4 come to rest against the body of L5. Because of this, degenerative spondylolisthesis seldom exceeds a grade 1, or 25% slip.[57] As the slip progresses, the inferior facet of the cephalic vertebra erodes throughout the superior articular process of the caudal vertebra.

Facet joint hypertrophy results in both central and lateral canal stenosis. At some point in the forward migration, the disk collapses and the thickened ligamentum flavum becomes redundant, further contributing to both central and lateral stenosis. An *intrasynovial spinal cyst* may originate in the facet joint as a result of the degenerated facet joint changes in degenerative spondylolisthesis, and may act as a stenotic source.†

30. What are the clinical and radiologic signs of degenerative spondylolisthesis?

Signs and symptoms include a protracted history of low-grade back pain that is intermittently intense, but rarely causes severe disability. More commonly, the inferior articular process of L4 will entrap the L5 nerve root in the lateral recess and may result in sciatica.[32] Discomfort is related to disk degeneration and posterior facet arthrosis, or may be due to nerve root irritation or entrapment or symptoms of spinal stenosis. Hence, patients develop early morning aching and stiffness and often experience difficulty getting out of bed that improves following a hot shower. Once up and about the patient feels much better. Maintaining a flexed posture for long periods aggravates discomfort. Similarly, sitting in an upright hard chair is more comfortable than a soft, easy chair in which patients insist on sitting near the edge where they may sit upright. Although turning in bed can be annoying, walking is the least symptomatic of activities. The examination is mostly negative, and does not present with pinpoint tenderness as the lamina is not loose. Physical examination often shows a patient who is flexible and able to touch the floor on

---

*Alternately, the vertebra above displaces posteriorly on the one below. This is known as *retrolisthesis,* and invariably occurs secondary to degenerative disc disease and facet arthrosis. The pain pattern is opposite that of degenerative spondylolisthesis, and is aggravated by standing and any activity increasing lordosis, whereas mild flexion affords relief.

---

†Management of isolated intraspinal cysts includes aspiration, corticosteroid injection, or cyst rupture through injection.

forward flexion with their knees locked in extension, although maintaining this position cause marked discomfort. Discomfort is worse while extending the back into the erect position and is frequently associated with a "hitching" movement. Instead of a smooth resumption from flexion to extension the patient first extends the lumbar spine, fixing it in lordosis, and then extending at the hips until the erect position is regained; this is known as *hitching*. Patients may occasionally complain of pain both during flexion and extension. Degenerative spondylolisthesis rarely presents with acute symptoms; subacute or chronic discomfort is the typical presentation. Compression of the cauda equina against the body of L5 may occur as the lamina and inferior articular process of L4 slide forward, and results in neurogenic claudication.

Suspected degenerative spondylolisthesis is confirmed by anteroposterior, lateral, and oblique radiographs performed with the patient standing so as to axially load the spine and stress the slip.[28] This is then compared with supine radiographs, and a positive degenerative spondylolisthesis is identified for those patients exhibiting a proportionally greater slip on the standing radiograph. The severity of patient symptoms may not necessarily correlate with the amount of slip.[15] Associated, but nondiagnostic changes that may also be seen include hypertrophic changes of the facet joints, foraminal and disk-space narrowing, and impingement of the inferior articular process of L4 into the superior articular process of L5. Occasionally, a vacuum sign may be seen in the lumbar disk space on plain radiographs (and especially on computerized tomography) and is strongly suggestive of segmental instability.

Patients with minimal impairment and early stages of disk degeneration respond best to physical therapy, whereas the intermediate stages of degeneration respond to nonsteroidal antiinflammatory medications, facet injections of corticosteroids, or rarely, facet rhizotomy.[13] The advanced stages may respond to epidural or selective root injections. The major indication for surgery is incapacitating neurogenic claudication or persistent pain secondary to radiculopathy after a trial of conservative care.

31. What are the congenital and other acquired forms of lumbar spinal stenosis?

Congenital forms of spinal stenosis occur from forms of dwarfism such as achondroplasia, osteochondrodystrophy, and mucopolysaccharidosis, and other abnormalities such as osteogenesis imperfecta, acromegaly, and Down syndrome. Other acquired forms of lumbar spinal stenosis includes iatrogenic causes from surgery, hematoma, foreign body reaction, rough handling, or infection that may cause epidural fibrosis.[71] Other acquired forms of stenosis include:

- *Paget's disease.* Named after Sir James Paget, who first described osteitis deformans in 1876. This is a chronic disorder of the adult skeleton in which localized areas of hyperactive bone are replaced by softened and enlarged bone. Occurring in approximately 3% of patients over age 40, and having a 3:2 male to female predominance, this condition is most prevalent in England, the United States, Eastern and Western Europe, Australia, and New Zealand. Increasing in incidence to 10% by the ninth decade of life, the disease may affect any bone, and is usually asymmetric. Although the etiology is unknown, Paget's disease is thought to be caused by a virus. The bones most commonly affected include the pelvis, femur, skull, tibia, vertebra, clavicle, and humerus. The pathophysiology of this disease is primarily the osteoclastic resorption of bone, followed by osteoblastic repair that leads to structurally enlarged and weakened bone, despite the heavy calcification, and is prone to deformity and pathologic fracture. Macroscopic enlargement of the vertebrae results in impingements within the spinal canal and intervertebral foramen, and correspondingly causing spinal and lateral canal stenosis. Although there is no cure for Paget's disease, the hormone calcitonin directly blocks bone resorption by inhibiting osteoclastic activity. In some patients, spinal decompression may be necessary to decompress a stenosed spinal canal.[11]
- *Fluorosis.* This refers to excessive accumulation of fluorine that occurs in the skeletal system in populations ingesting excessive fluorine in their drinking water. Bony changes include osteosclerosis and exostosis of the spine and genu valgum, which may occur in adults following high fluorine intake.[11] Fluorosis may result in disk calcification.

32. What is the pathophysiology of neurogenic claudication?

The pathophysiology of neurogenic claudication relates to ischemia of the cauda equina due to mechanical encroachment that impairs venous drainage and leads to back pressure and *capillary stasis.* Posterior pressure against the cauda equina causes increased pressure over the venous system within the epidural space. The veins, unlike the arteries, have thin walls and therefore operate as a low-pressure system and tolerate compressive force poorly. This results in *blood flow back up* into the capillary system, which because of their smaller bore diameter causes increased resistance. This *venous congestion* will be maximal in the watershed areas of the central cord and at the *critical avascular zone of the cauda equina.* This pathophysiology is set in motion in the lordotic posture during walking as lordosis narrows the already tight spinal canal to the point of vascular embarrassment of the circulation of the cauda equina.

Walking leads to mechanical encroachment that compromises the cauda equina circulation. The resulting venous engorgement blocks the free-flow of cerebrospinal fluid around this bundle so that the nutritional needs of the nerve roots are unsatisfied resulting in ischemia. Moreover, noxious metabolic wastes build up in the constricted area. The subsequent ectopic nerve impulses produce numbness and painful cramping symptoms in one or both legs. On stooping and bending forward, sitting, or leaning against a support, the lumbar lordosis is decreased with consequent stretching and thinning of the ligamentum flavum and decreased pressure within the canal.

33. What is the clinical presentation of central and lateral stenosis?

The majority of patients with central stenosis are over the age of 50, and usually greater than 65 years of age. They often have a history of intermittent low back pain spanning several years. Patients seek medical advice because of a change in their symptoms, which presents as a dull ache across the lumbosacral region when standing for lengthy periods, and especially when walking. The classic description by the patient is to describe how symptoms are less aggravating in the supermarket as they are leaning forward while pushing a shopping cart. Pain in the form of a "heavy, dragging" feeling typically radiates from the lumbosacral region into both buttocks and proximal thighs, requiring them to stop and sit down, lean forward against a supporting structure, or bend forward slightly, resting their hands on their lower thighs. After a few minutes rest, they resume walking only to begin this cycle again after progressing a shorter distance. In the case of high lumbar involvement, symptoms will occur in the anterior thigh distribution. At night, patients frequently complain of nocturnal pain or cramping, especially when supine, due to increased lumbar lordosis. Symptoms are relieved by placing a large pillow under the knees to reduce the lordosis or by sleeping on either side in the fetal position. On examination, evidence of facet arthrosis, or spondylolisthesis may be present, or the examination may be completely normal. The knee-to-

chest position is usually comfortable, the straight leg raise often limited only by hamstring tightness, and the prone knee-bend test negative unless the L3 nerve root is involved. Walking uphill is easier than walking downhill. In the long-standing condition, the spine, hips, and knees are flexed, the back is flat, with an absence of normal lordotic curvature as this posture relieves pressure on the cauda equina. The history remains preeminent in making the diagnosis.

Bladder and bowel involvement is unusual in spinal stenosis because the conus medullaris is located at the lowest portion of the cord adjacent to the L1-L2 vertebrae where the cord ends. Hence stenosis of vertebral levels below this point "misses" the cord. This is not the case in the event of a cauda equinus lesion, which causes an ever enlarging lesion that occupies ever more space enlarging to the point where the nerve roots are compressed.

Lateral recess stenosis may result in jamming of the nerve root in the lateral recess by an impinging osteophyte that may be unremitting and virtually continuous at times, so that the patient may get up to walk about in an effort to relieve pain. This is because bony encroachment of the lateral recess is often unchanged by assuming a recumbent position. This is in direct contrast with radicular encroachment from a soft-tissue lesion such as a bulging disk in which the recumbent position often provides relief. The presence of motor, reflex, and sensation deficits depends on the degree of nerve root involvement.*

34. How may the straight leg raise be interpreted to clinically differentiate between nerve root impingement deriving from spinal stenosis and disk pathology?

Between 35° to 70° of straight leg raise (SLR) causes tensing of the lumbosacral nerve roots,[34] and the test may only be considered positive if symptoms are elicited within this range. When tension is applied to a nerve, the intraneural pressure increases as the cross-sectional area decreases. This increase in pressure results in both blood deprivation, which interferes with conduction, and effects on axonal transport within the sciatic tract.[14] Pain and limitation of SLR due to a claw osteophyte (spinal stenosis) will more likely reduce the available SLR minimally in comparison with a herni-

---

*Electromyographic testing of paraspinal musculature may detect multiple level radiculopathies not evident on extremity testing. This is of limited diagnostic use because these findings may also occur in metabolic disorders such as diabetes, and in subclinical neuropathies.

ated disk. This is because the traction spur represents a local tethering of the nerve root which limits the amount of sliding the nerve root may undergo. Nevertheless, the root may accommodate to impingement by undergoing elongation, in addition to some, albeit reduced, mobility. Thus lateral stenosis may be associated with a SLR greater than 50°.

In contrast, significant disk pathology in the form of a herniated disk may compress a relatively large portion of the nerve root and eliminate sliding of that portion of the sciatic tract emerging from that root. This may correspond to less available SLR. Thus a SLR between 25° and 50° is almost pathognomic for a disk lesion.[69-73]

35. How may the diurnal straight-leg raising test be used to differentiate between nerve root irritability due to disk lesion versus spinal stenosis?

The diurnal SLR may be used to differentiate between a limitation of SLR due to disk pathology or spinal stenosis. If the outer annular fibers are intact, the disk is considered competent as no nuclear material has extruded through the annulus. Because the disk is competent, its changing fluid content will affect root tension signs. Following as little as 2 hours of recumbency in bed or after a night sleep, the disk will reimbibe fluid. In the morning, the bulging disk will be tense, and clinically manifest as a diminished SLR angle as compared with the night before. After being up and around for 1 or 2 hours, the hydrostatic pressure induced by spinal compressive loading will cause fluid loss in the disk, and is demonstrated by an increased range in the degree of SLR. This phenomenon will not occur in the situation where the limitation of SLR derives from central or lateral canal stenosis.[73]

36. How are symptoms arising from spinal stenosis differentiated from acute disk pathology?

Radicular pain due to spinal stenosis is similar to that of disk pathology. Symptoms associated with central and lateral canal stenosis are unique in that pain is not symptomatic of just one level (as may occur with sciatica due to a herniated disk) but is reflective of pathology at multiple levels. Moreover, SLR is much less commonly positive, or only minimally positive as compared with disk. In addition, dural signs such as coughing, sneezing, or bearing down to move one's bowels do not usually cause exacerbated symptoms whereas they often do with disk pathology. In addition, the radicular component of symptoms accompanying spinal stenosis is often diffusely localized. If spinal stenotic pain uncommonly occurs along a single nerve root, unlike sciatica associated with disk pathology, it will not dominate the history. Finally, whereas root entrapment secondary to disk pathology is more common over 50 years of age, radicular symptoms are more common over age 50.

37. What imaging techniques are appropriate?

The diagnosis of central stenosis is made on the history and confirmed by imaging. Plain radiographs are unrevealing, although evidence of degenerative disk disease of mild spondylolisthesis can serve as a clue to possible stenosis. Myelography, which shows any abnormal protrusion of a herniated disk or other space occupying lesion into the spinal cord, nerve root, or cauda equina is helpful in diagnosing central stenosis. Multiplanar computerized tomography is also helpful in imaging central stenosis. Frequently, multiple levels are involved and usually span between L2 to L5. In contrast to acute disk rupture the L5/S1 level is rarely involved. Computerized tomography (CT) and magnetic resonance (MR) imaging is helpful in confirming a suspected diagnosis of lateral stenosis.[47] Some radiologists prefer CT myelography in which tomographic scanning is enhanced by intrathecal contrast, or nerve root injection that confirms the diagnosis if there are pain relief and prolonged steroid effect. If the lateral recess shows free space of 5 mm, stenosis may be ruled out at that level, although only 2 mm of height or an impinging osteophyte is evident pressing on the corresponding nerve root, and the diagnosis is more likely. Despite gross degenerative changes that are sometimes encountered in the lumbar spine, the nerve root tunnel may be reduced but never occluded. If computerized tomography should display a nonexistent canal, it is representing an underestimate of the aperture size due to an artifact of the mathematical display.[81] Spinal fluid protein levels are often elevated.

38. What is the differential diagnosis?

- *Peripheral atherosclerotic disease of the lower extremities.* This is an occlusive arterial disease due to atherosclerotic plaque. The initial symptom is intermittent arterial claudication—a deficient blood supply in exercising muscle, experienced as lower limb angina, typically as an ache in the calf, foot, thigh, hip, or buttocks in that order. Symptoms are quickly relieved after 1 to 5 minutes of rest, and sitting is not necessary to obtain relief.[11] The absence of pedal pulses does not prove that symptoms are due to arterial disease.[4] To complicate matters, neurogenic and intermittent claudication frequently coexist (see Table 57-1).[46]

- *Cauda equina syndrome.* This consists of damage to the cauda equina, which includes the terminal spinal cord and all the spinal roots from T12 to S5, within the spinal canal at any level below the T10 vertebra. The cause of cauda equina syndrome derives from a mass within the spinal canal that may occur from an extruded central disk, tumor of the filum terminale (ependymoma), lipoma (common with spina bifida or other dorsal defects), or neurofibroma. Symptoms may include low back, rectal, or genital pain, micturition disturbances, loss of bowel control, diminished perianal (S2-S5) sensation, atonic anus, perianal numbness, occasional pelvic and buttock pain,[93] and

TABLE 57-1

Pseudoclaudication due to spinal stenosis	Vascular intermittent claudication
Pain varies according to distance traveled	Pain brought on soon after walking
Distress worsened when walking downhill	Distress worsened by walking uphill
Dysesthesia present	No dysesthesia
Pain decreased with spinal flexion	Pain is not dependent upon spinal position
Relief time is slow	Pain abruptly stops after exercise
Standing and walking are painful	Walking is painful while standing is not
Pulses are normal	Pulses diminished or absent, while femoral bruits may be present
Good skin nutrition	Trophic skin changes
Pain is a heavy, aching, and dragging feeling that typically radiates distally	Pain is sharp and rarely radiates after onset
Incidence demonstrates a peak in the seventh decade	Affects age 40 and up

loss of potency. Diminished ankle reflexes and myotomal patterns of muscle weakness are often experienced. Perianal innervation is arranged in concentric rings, and may be assessed. The innermost ring is S5, surrounded by S4, then S3, and then S2 at the outer perimeter. The penis and scrotum receive sensory innervation from S2 and S3. Loss of perianal sensation may indicate an impending cauda equina syndrome. A high lesion may result in pyramidal signs below the lesion, manifesting as hyperreflexia, ankle clonus, and an extensor plantar (Babinski) response. Cauda equina syndrome is an indication for immediate surgery.

- *Leriche syndrome.* This refers to gradual occlusion of the terminal aortic bifurcation causing intermittent claudication in the buttocks, especially the gluteal muscles and the muscles of the thigh. The gluteus maximus muscles cramp and hurt, and the recovery is much longer than neurogenic claudication.[66] It may be accompanied by impotence in men. Treatment is by angioplasty or replacing occluded segments by vein grafts or prostheses.[11]

- *Abdominal aortic aneurysm.* The abdominal aorta bifurcates at the level of the L3 vertebra, and may undergo aneurysm predominantly in older persons over the age of 50. Abdominal aneurysm typically passes unnoticed until they become large enough to cause symptoms or be palpated as a pulsating mass. Rupture of an abdominal aneurysm is a surgical emergency that is the thirteenth most common cause of male death in the United States, especially over the age of 65. There are often no symptoms associated with an abdominal aneurysm, although patients may complain of a dull, nagging or severe low back pain due to erosion of the lumbar vertebrae by the aneurysm. Pressure from the pulsating vessel may cause excruciating pain in the abdomen or the back.

  Some patients typically have other associated diseases such as hypertension, high blood cholesterol, diabetes, and a history of smoking. Abdominal aneurysm may be caused by infection, syphilis, arteritis, Marfan's syndrome, and congenital abnormalities. Pain from abdominal aortic aneurysm may cause back pain that mimics a herniated lumbar disk. When suspected, it is essential to assess lower extremity pulses and skin temperature and palpate the abdomen for a pulsating mass, and auscultation for a bruit. When suspected, immediate referral to a vascular surgeon is mandatory.

- *Unstable isthmic spondylolisthesis.* This may cause back pain that is referred into the thighs when walking, mimicking neurogenic claudication. Radiographs will identify the unstable spine. Degenerative isthmic spondylolisthesis is more common in women.

39. What rehabilitation strategy is most effective in the management of lumbar spinal stenosis?

With developmental, spondylolisthesis, or congenital lumbar stenosis, symptoms may initially be handled conservatively. In some patients, the stenosis stabilizes and the patient may learn to adapt.[61] As hyperlordosis is associated with anterior pelvic tilt, patients may be able to learn to maintain their lumbar spine in flexion throughout the day by tipping the pelvis anteriorly. However, because anterior pelvic tilt may be limited by tight hip flexors, a flexibility program is an essential component of rehabilitation.

Hyperlordosis, which often stems from tightened hip flexor musculature and anterior pelvic tilt, may also cause central or spinal stenosis. Hyperlordosis narrows the intervertebral foramen, especially in the lateral recesses via impingement by the superior articular process of the inferior lumbar vertebrae. Hyperlordosis also narrows the central spinal canal via impingement by the inferior articular process of the superior lumbar vertebrae.[47] Thus either extreme of pelvic tilting may result in pathology, so that maintenance of a neutral posture of the pelvis and low back is essential and promoted by adequate soft-tissue extensibility of the pre- and postfemoral musculature.

Maintenance of the lumbar spine in anterior pelvic tilt may be helped by using a rigid lumbar orthosis. Abdominal strengthening exercises are also an essential part of the therapeutic regimen as they restore balance to the trunk musculature and help diminish lumbar lordosis. Excessive lordosis, which is associated with increased symptoms of spinal stenosis, may also be minimized by a weight reduction program. Aerobic conditioning is appropriate for the patient with spinal stenosis. Patient education includes instruction on correct postures for lifting and carrying.

Many patients with Paget's disease and spinal stenosis find a sudden and dramatic improvement in walking after taking calcitonin, and some patients may continue to improve after cessation of the drug.[70] Calcitonin is a peptide hormone produced by the thyroid gland that inhibits osteoclast resorption of bone and thereby prevents loss of calcium and phosphate to the blood. The mechanism of response to calcitonin is probably vascular in nature. Calcitonin reduces skeletal blood flow.[98] Venous blood drains from the vertebral bodies into Bat-

son's extradural plexus and presumably, if this is reduced, the neural elements will have more space.

40. What are the surgical indications for spinal stenosis?

Surgery is reserved for when symptoms are so severe as to interfere with normal leg movement despite physical therapy and calcitonin treatment. This may occur gradually or with sudden onset from an acute herniated nucleus pulposus so that what began as a mildly symptomatic condition causes significant disability characterized by back and leg pain and considerable reduction in SLR. The procedure involves a wide laminectomy to ensure a completely free dura,[97] typically over several levels, in which both laminae, ligamentum flava, the spinous process, and the nucleus pulposus are removed. If osteophytes are discovered pressing on a laterally emerging nerve root, they are also excised. Preservation of the facet joint on at least one side is essential to provide lumbar stability, although the medial third of the joint must often be removed and the facet undercut. Advanced age is no contraindication to decompression as it will often improve the quality of life for the elderly.[1] After surgery, many patients experience improved sensation in their legs and can soon walk long distances. However, many patients also relapse and walk progressively shorter distances as epidural scar tissue develops over the posterior dura. A potential complication following surgery is the formation of scar tissue forming around the nerve root and later impingement on neural structures. Extensive decompression may lead to segmental instability.

REFERENCES

1. Ami Hood S, Weigl K: Lumbar spinal stenosis: surgical intervention for the older person, *(Isr) J Med Sci* 19:169, 1983.
2. Amonoo-kuofi HS, el-Badawi MG, Fatani JA: Ligaments associated with lumbar intervertebral foramina. I. L1 to L4, *J Anat* 156:177-183, 1988.
3. Arnoldi CC, Brodsky AE, Cachoix J et al: Lumbar spinal stenosis and nerve root entrapment: syndromes, definition, and classification, *Clin Orthop* 115:4-5, 1976.
4. Aronheim JC: *Case studies in geriatrics for the house officer,* Baltimore, 1990, Williams & Wilkins.
5. Babin E, Capesium P: Etude radiologique des dimensions du canal rachidien cervical et de leurs variations au cours des epreuves fonctionelles, *Annas of Radiology* 19:457-462, 1976.
6. Bachop W, Janse J: The corporotransverse ligament at the L5 intervertebral foramen, *Anat Rec* 205, (Abstract) 1983.
7. Badley EM: Epidemiological aspects of the aging spine. In Hukins DWL, Nelson MA editors: *The aging spine,* Manchester, UK, 1987, Manchester University Press.

8. Barker DJP, Bull AR, Osmond C et al: Fetal and placental size and risk of hypertension in adult life, *Br Med J* 301:259-262, 1990.

9. Barker DJP, Meade TW, Fall CDH et al: Relation of fetal and infant growth to plasma fibrinogen and factor VII concentrations in adult life, *Br Med J* 304:148-152, 1992.

10. Batson OV: The function of the vertebral veins and their role in the spread of metastases, *Ann Surg* 112:138-149, 1940.

11. Berkow R: *The Merck manual of diagnosis and therapy,* ed 15, Rahway, N.J., 1987, Merck & Co.

12. Breig A: *Adverse mechanical tension in the central nervous system,* Stockholm, 1978, Almqvist & Wiksell.

13. Brown MD, Lockwood JM: *Degenerative spondylolisthesis, Intr Course Lect Am Acad Orthop Surg,* St Louis, 1983, Mosby.

14. Butler DS, Jones MA: *Mobilisation of the nervous system,* Melbourne, 1991, Churchill Livingstone.

15. Cauchoix J, Benoist M, Chassaing V: Degenerative spondylolisthesis, *Clin Orthop* 115:122, 1976.

16. Church CP, Buehler MT: Radiographic evaluation of the corportransverse ligament at the L5 intervertebral foramen: a cadaveric study, *J Manipulative Physiolog Therap* 14:240-248, 1991.

17. Clark GA, Panjabi MM, Wetzel FT et al: Can infant malnutrition cause adult vertebral stenosis? *Spine* 10:165-170, 1985.

18. Cramer GD, Darby SA: *Basic and clinical anatomy of the spine, spinal cord, and ANS,* St Louis, 1995, Mosby,

19. Crock HV: Normal and pathological anatomy of the lumbar spinal nerve root canals, *J Bone Joint Surg* 63, 1981.

20. Dai LY, Xu YK, Zhang WM et al: The effect of flexion-extension motion of the lumbar spine on the capacity of the spinal canal, *Spine* 1989, 14:523-525.

21. de Peretti F, Micalef JP, Bourgeon A et al: Biomechanics of the lumbar spinal nerve roots and the first sacral root within the intervertebral foramina, *Surg Radiol Anat* 11:221-225, 1989.

22. Diamond MC, Scheibel AB, Elson LM: *The human brain coloring book,* New York, 1985, Barnes & Noble Books.

23. Dommisse GF, Louw JA: Anatomy of the lumbar spine. In Floman Y editor: *Disorders of the lumbosacral spine,* Rockville, Md. and Tel Aviv, 1990, Aspen and Freund.

24. Dommisse GF: The blood supply of the spinal cord, *J Bone Joint Surg* 56B:225-235, 1974.

25. *Dorland's Illustrated Medical Dictionary,* ed 27, Philadelphia, 1988, WB Saunders.

26. Dupuis PR: The anatomy of the lumbosacral spine. In Kirkaldy-Willis W editor: *Managing low back pain,* ed 2, New York, 1988, Churchill Livingstone.

27. Edgar M, Ghadially J: Innervation of the lumbar spine, *Clin Orthop* 115, 1976.

28. Ehni G: Effects of certain degenerative disease of the spine, especially spondylosis and disk protrusion of the neural contents particular in the lumbar region: historical account, *Mayo Clin Proc* 50:327, 1976.

29. Eisenstein S: Morphometry and pathological anatomy of the lumbar spine in South African Negroes and Caucasoids with specific reference to spinal stenosis, *J Bone Joint Surg* 59B:173-180, 1977.

30. Epstein BS: An anatomical, myelographic and cinematographic study of the dentate ligaments, *Am J Roentgenography* 98:704-712, 1966.

31. Epstein JA, Epstein BS, Lavine L: Nerve root compression associated with narrowing of the lumbar spinal canal, *J Neurol Neurosurg Psychiat* 25:165, 1962.

32. Epstein NE, Epstein JA, Carras R et al: Degenerative spondylolisthesis with an intact neural arch: a review of 60 cases with an analysis of clinical findings and the development of surgical management, *Neurosurgery* 13:555, 1983.

33. Evans JG: Neurogenic intermittent claudication, *BMJ* 2:985, 1964.

34. Fahrni WG: Observations on straight leg-raising with special reference to nerve root adhesions, *Can J Surg* 9:44, 1966.

35. Fitzgerald GK, Wynveen KG, Rhealt W et al: Objective assessment with establishment of normal values for lumbar spinal range of motion, *Phys Ther* 63:1776, 1983.

36. Frykolm R: Lower cervical nerve roots and their investments, *Acta Chirugica Scandinavica* 101:457-471, 1951.

37. Gracovetsky S: Biomechanics of the spine. In White AH, Schofferman JA editors: *Spine care diagnosis and conservative treatment,* vol 1, St Louis, 1995, Mosby.

38. Graves EJ: Detailed diagnoses and procedures: National hospital discharge survey 1987: National Center of Health Statistics. *Vital Health Stat* 13 (100):151-194-195, 1989.

39. Grieve GP: *Common vertebral joint problems,* London, 1981, Churchill Livingstone.

40. Groen G, Baljet B, Drukker J: Nerves and nerve plexuses of the human vertebral column, *Am J Anat* 188:282-296, 1990.

41. Groen GJ, Baljet B, Drukker J: The innervation of the spinal dura mater: anatomy and clinical implications, *Acta Neurochir (Wien)* 92:39-46, 1988.

42. Hack M, Breslan N, Weissman B, et al: Effect of very low birth weight and subnormal head size on cognitive ability at school age, *New Engl J Med* 325:231-237, 1991.

43. Hanley EN: Decompression and distraction-derotation arthrodesis for degenerative spondylolisthesis, *Spine* 11:269, 1986.

44. Hasue M, Kikuchi S, Sakuyama Y et al: Anatomic study of the interrelation between lumbosacral nerve roots and their surrounding tissues, *Spine* 8(1):50-58, 1983.

45. Hollinshead WH, Jenkins DJ: *Functional anatomy of the limbs and back,* ed 5, Philadelphia, 1981, WB Saunders.

46. Johansson JE, Barrington TW, Ameli M: Combined vascular and neurogenic claudication. *Spine* 7(2):150-158, 1982.

47. Keim HA, Kirkaldy-Willis WH: *Clinical Symposia: Low Back Pain,* Bull 39, Number 6, Summit, N.J., 1987, CIBA-GEIGY.

48. Kirkaldy-Willis WH, Wedge JH, Yong-Hing K et al: Pathology and pathogenesis of lumbar spondylosis and stenosis, *Spine* 3(4):319-328, 1978.

49. Kirkaldy-Willis WH: *Managing low back pain,* ed 2, New York, 1988, Churchill Livingstone.

50. Lazorthes G, et al: Arterial vascularization of the spinal cord. *J Neurosurg* 35, 1971.

51. Lee CK, Rausschning W, Glenn W: Lateral lumbar spinal canal stenosis: classification, pathologic anatomy and surgical decompression, *Spine* 13:312-320, 1988.

52. Leiviska T, Videman T, Nurminen T et al: Radiographic versus direct measurements of the spinal canal at the lumbar vertebrae L3-L5 and their relations to age and body stature, *Acta Radiol Diagn* 26:403-411, 1985.

53. Lindborgh JV: The role of genetic and local environmental factors in the control of postnatal craniofacial morphogenesis. *Acta Morphol Neerlando-Scandinavia* 10:37-47.

54. Louis R: Vertebroradicular and vertebromedullar dynamics, *Anatomica Clinica* 3:1-11.

55. Luschka H von: *Die nerven des menschlichen eirbelkanales,* Tubingen, 1850, Laupp.

56. Moore KL: *Clinically oriented anatomy,* ed 2, Baltimore, 1985, Williams & Wilkins.

57. Newman PH, Stone KH: The etiology of spondylolisthesis with a special investigation, *J Bone Joint Surg* 45B:39, 1963.

58. Newman PH: Surgical treatment for spondylolisthesis in the adult, *Clin Orthop* 117:106, 1976.

59. Olmarker K, Rydevik B, Holm S et al: Effects of experimental, graded compression on blood flow in spinal nerve roots, *J Orthop Res* 7:817, 1989.

60. Olswski JM, Simmons EH, Kallen FC et al: Evidence from cadavers suggestive of entrapment of fifth lumbar spinal nerves by lumbosacral ligaments, *Spine* 16:336, 1991.

61. Onel D, Sari H, Donmex C: Lumbar spinal stenosis: clinical/radiologic therapeutic evaluation in 145 patients, *Spine* 18:291, 1993.

62. Panjabi MM, Takata K, Goel VK: Kinematics of lumbar intervertebral foramen, *Spine* 8:348-357, 1983.

63. Parke WW, Gammell K, Rothman RH: Arterial vascularization of the cauda equina, *J Bone Joint Surg* 63A:53-62, 1981.

64. Parke WW, Watanabe R: The intrinsic vasculature of the lumbosacral spinal nerve roots, *Spine* 10:508-515, 1985.

65. Parkin IG, Harrison GR: The topographical anatomy of the lumbar epidural space, *J Anat* 141:211-217, 1985.

66. Patten J: *Neurological differential diagnosis,* ed 2, Springer, 1996, London.

67. Penning L, Wilmink JT: Biomechanics of the lumbosacral dural sac: a study of flexion-extension myelography, *Spine* 6:398-408, 1981.

68. Pfaundler S: Pedicle origin and intervertebral compartment in the lumbar and upper sacral spine, *Acta Neurochir* 97:158-165, 1989.

69. Porter RW, Drinkall JN, Porter DE et al: The vertebral canal, part 2: health and academic status, *Spine* 12, 1987.

70. Porter RW, Hibbert C: Calcitonin treatment of neurogenic claudication, *Spine* 8:585, 1983.

71. Porter RW: *Management of back pain,* ed 2, Edinburgh, 1993, Churchill Livingstone.

72. Porter RW: Measurement of the lumbar spinal canal by diagnostic ultrasound, MD Thesis, 1980, University of Edinburgh.

73. Porter RW, Trailescu IF: Diurnal changes in straight leg raising, *Spine* 15:103, 1990.

74. Rauschning W: Normal and pathologic anatomy of the lumbar root canals, *Spine* 12:1008-1019, 1987.

75. Remer S, Neuwirth MG: Anatomy and biomechanics of the spine. In Nicholas JA, Hershman EB editors: *The lower extremity and spine in sports medicine,* ed 2, St Louis, 1995, Mosby.

76. Rosenberg NJ: Degenerative spondylolisthesis: predisposing factors, *J Bone Joint Surg* 57:467, 1975.

77. Rothman NR: The patho-physiology of disc degeneration, *Clin Neurosurg Proc Congress of Neurolog Surgeons,* 1972.

78. Rothman RH, Simeone FA: *Spine,* vol 1, Philadelphia, 1975, WB Saunders.

79. Selby DK: The lumbar spine. In White AH, Schofferman JA editors: *Spine care: diagnosis and conservative treatment,* vol 1, St Louis, 1995, Mosby.

80. Schonstrom NR, Hansson JH: Thickness of the human ligamentum flavum as a function of load: an in vitro experimental study, *Clin Biomechanics* 6.

81. Smith G, Aspden R, Porter RW: Measurement of vertebral foraminal dimensions using three-dimensional computerized tomography, *Spine,* 18:629, 1993.

82. Sunderland S: Meningeal-neural relations in the intervertebral foramen, *J Neurosurg* 40:756-763, 1974.

83. Sunderland S: *Nerves and nerve injuries,* ed 2, Edinburgh, 1978, Churchill Livingstone.

84. Tani S, Yamada S, Knighton RS: Extensibility of the lumbar and sacral cord: pathophysiology of the tethered spinal cord in cats, *J Neurosurg* 66:116-123, 1987.

85. Tanner JM: *Foetus into man,* ed 2, 1989, Castlemead Publications, Ware.

86. Tomita K, Kawahara N, Baba H et al: Circumspinal decompression for thoracic myelopathy due to combined ossification of the posterior longitudinal ligament and ligamentum flavum, *Spine* 15:1114-1120, 1990.

87. Towme EB, Reichert FL: Compression of the lumbosacral roots of the spinal cord by thickened ligamenta flava, *Ann Surg* 94, 1931.

88. Tsuji H, Tamaki T, Itoh T et al: Redundant nerve roots in patients with degenerative lumbar spinal stenosis, *Spine* 10:72-82, 1985.

89. Turner JA, Ersek M, Herron L et al: Surgery for lumbar spinal stenosis: an attempted meta-analysis of the literature, *Spine* 17:1-8, 1992.

90. Van Noort R, Black MM, Martin TRP et al: A study of the uniaxial mechanical properties of human dura mater preserved in glycerol, *Biomaterials* 2:41-45, 1981.

91. Vital JM, Lavignolle B, Grenier N et al: Anatomy of the lumbar radicular canal, *Anat Clin* 5:141-151, 1983.

92. Watkins RG: *The spine in sports,* St Louis, 1996, Mosby.

93. Weisberg LA, Garcia C, Strub R: *Essential of clinical neurology,* ed 3, St Louis, 1996, Mosby.

94. Weisz GM: Lumbar spinal canal stenosis in Paget's disease, *Spine* 8, 1983.

95. White AA, Panjabi MM: *Clinical biomechanics of the spine,* Philadelphia, 1978, JB Lippincott.

96. Williams PL, Gray H: *Gray's anatomy,* ed 37, Edinburgh, 1989, Churchill Livingstone.

97. Wiltse LL, Newman PH, Macnab I: Classification of spondylolysis and spondylolisthesis, *Clin Orthop Rel Res* 117:23 1976.

98. Wooton R, Tellez M, Green JR et al: Skeletal blood flow in Paget's disease of bone, *Metabolic Bone Disease and Related Research* 4 & 5:263, 1981.

RECOMMENDED READINGS

Arnoldi CC, Brodsky AE, Cachoix J et al: Lumbar spinal stenosis and nerve root entrapment: syndromes, definition, and classification, *Clin Orthop* 115:4-5, 1976.

Lee CK, Rausschning W, Glenn W: Lateral lumbar spinal canal stenosis: classification, pathologic anatomy and surgical decompression, *Spine* 13:312-320, 1988.

58

History of Fall on Buttocks During Childhood and Progressive Lumbosacral Ache, Pain, and Limitation of Flexion in Adulthood that is Aggravated by Jarring Motions and Relieved by a Hot Shower

CASE 1: A 49-year-old school gym teacher complains of lumbosacral ache for the past 16 years, which appears to steadily worsen over the past year. Lately, he finds the requirements of his job as sporting activities instructor cause jarring motions that aggravate pain. He recalls falling from a 12-foot-high brick wall and landing heavily on his buttocks when he was 15 years of age. At that time, he suffered severe low back pain, which required several days of bed rest before being allowed to return to school. When asked, he admits that symptoms following that incident subsided over the following several weeks, and he was able to resume full sport activities within 1 month. Up until his early thirties he did not experience any back discomfort, although once past age 35 he began to experience periodic mild discomfort that became chronic over time. He currently complains of pain every day, which begins as a stiff aching every morning as he attempts to get out of bed with extreme difficulty. Supine to short sitting transfer is accomplished by rolling onto his abdomen, and then standing erect slowly. After a hot shower and simple exercises, symptoms markedly improve within 30 minutes. Coughing is severely painful, as are any jarring movements. Walking is relatively pain-free, while sitting and recumbency are painless except when changing positions. Transferring in and out of the seated position, whether a car seat or couch, are uncomfortable. When performing work that requires forward bending he must support his body weight by resting his arms on the worktop. The day after strenuous work, or sporting activity, symptoms are considerably aggravated. Back pain has not radiated into the lower extremities, but is confined to the lumbosacral midline and the buttocks.

OBSERVATION The patient is muscular and healthy looking, and indicates the area of pain as being across the lumbosacral region.

PALPATION Tenderness present on firm pressure applied to the L5 spinous process.

RANGE OF MOTION The patient can almost touch his toes on forward flexion, although he bends at the hips and knees, thus avoiding movement at the waist. On resuming the upright posture, he first extends the lumbar spine, fixing it in lordosis, and then extends the hip joint until resuming the erect posture. Spinal extension and lateral bend are within normal limits to either side, and are performed without any discomfort whatsoever.

STRENGTH   Normal lower extremity muscle strength testing indicated by the ability to walk on heels, toes, and borders of both feet.

SENSORY   Normal cutaneous innervation.

DEEP TENDON REFLEXES   These are normal. Downward plantar responses.

PULSES   These are normal.

CIRCUMFERENTIAL MEASUREMENT   Normal girth for bilateral mid thigh and calf measurements.

SPECIAL TESTS   Positive stoop test, and strongly positive heel drop test. Straight leg raise is 75° bilaterally. Negative Lasègue, sacroiliac compression, Faber, and femoral nerve stretch tests.

CASE 2: A 40-year-old female accountant ran every day for the past 16 years and regularly participated in a local marathon. Nine years ago, after a particularly difficult labor, she developed sudden discomfort in the low back and right buttock region that slowly resolved by the time she completed her maternity leave from her employment. Soon after, she began to resume running, but would experience back spasms after running that increased in frequency. Lately, her running has become restricted by her symptoms that include sudden lumbosacral and buttock pain at 20-minute intervals although she continues to run through the pain. Several hours after the run, she experiences low back pain that makes it difficult to come to the standing position, and walks briskly for approximately 15 minutes before symptoms ease off. Taking a hot bath relieves symptoms after a run, and a hot shower after a night's sleep followed by 10 minutes of stretching eases stiffness. When brushing her teeth in the morning, she stoops over the wash basin and supports her torso by holding the sink counter with one hand. Walking long distances aggravates pain, as does standing for longer than 2 hours. Episodic spasmodic pain also occurs when she attempts to climb in and out of her car. Bending over her desk for several minutes or doing gardening activities causes marked discomfort. Symptoms are relieved by squatting and flexing forward, or by lying on her back with her hips and knees fully flexed. Sitting in a hard, straight-backed chair is tolerated although getting up from sitting is difficult after running. Recumbency relieves pain. There is no radiation of pain. Lately, she has been forced to diminish the length of her run by more than half, although wearing a lumbosacral corset helps relieve symptoms.

OBSERVATION   She stands erect with a slight convex lumbar curve. There is loss of normal lordosis and the low back appears flattened on side view.

PALPATION   Tenderness is present at the lumbosacral area. No palpable "step."

RANGE OF MOTION   During forward flexion, her fingers reach to just below knee level and she hitches her back as she assumes the upright posture. Spinal extension and lateral bend is greater than average and pain free.

STRENGTH   She can walk on her heels, toes, and lateral borders of her foot without difficulty.

FLEXIBILITY   Normal extensibility in bilateral hamstrings, quadriceps, and iliopsoas muscles. When asked, she claims that she could easily touch her toes in the past.

SENSATION   This is normal.

DEEP TENDON REFLEXES   This is normal.

PERIPHERAL CIRCULATION   This is intact.

PULSES   These are normal.

SPECIAL TESTS   Negative straight leg raise, Lasègue, femoral nerve stretch, squat, and sacroiliac compression tests. Positive heel drop test. Positive leg length discrepancy with the right lower extremity measuring 2 cm shorter than the contralateral leg.

CASE 3: A 67-year-old female complains of low back pain radiating to her buttocks and upper thighs, although the latter symptoms are less pronounced that back pain. Pain began gradually several years ago and has steadily increased with age. Symptoms of stiffness are present in the early morning but tend to ease after a hot shower and simple exercises. She can briefly bend to pick up objects, although maintaining a semiflexed position such as when washing dishes or pushing her shopping cart causes considerable discomfort, as does bending and resuming the upright posture. She can no longer bend down to pick up her infant grandchildren, and carrying groceries is extremely uncomfortable and difficult. Discomfort is less pronounced when sitting forward in a firm chair, walking on a level surface, and standing for short periods. Walking up inclines or up a staircase provokes symptoms, as does sitting in a soft, easy chair. Pain is relieved by recumbency, particularly when lying on a firm mattress in the supine position with a pillow under her knees. Coughing and sneezing aggravate her pain. She is aware of a crepitant sensation on movement.

OBSERVATION   There is mild thoracic kyphosis present.

PALPATION   There is localized tenderness on firm palpation to the lumbosacral region, and a "step" is palpable.

RANGE OF MOTION   The patient can touch her toes, although this is performed with discomfort and a hitching movement when straightening. Lateral bend with extension to either side is average and painless. Extension range is average, although painful at extremes.

STRENGTH   This is normal.

FLEXIBILITY   There are bilaterally tight hamstring muscles.

SENSATION   This is normal.

DEEP TENDON REFLEXES   This is normal.

PULSES   This is normal.

SPECIAL TESTS   Negative prone knee bend, negative straight leg raise, negative sacroiliac joint testing, and a negative squat test.

? Questions

1. What is most likely the cause of these patients' symptoms?
2. What is the structural degenerative cascade?
3. What is the spinal motion segment?
4. What are the functions of the anterior and posterior articulations comprising the trijoint spinal complex?
5. What is the anatomy of the facet joints?
6. What is the role of the facet joints in motion of the lumbar spine?
7. What are the biomechanical ramifications of incongruity of the facet joints?
8. What is the evolutionary sequence of the degenerative cascade?
9. What degenerative sequence occurs in the anterior elements of the spinal motion segment?
10. What is the relationship between hamstring tightness and disk degeneration?
11. How may hypertrophic bone formation of the anterior spinal joint result in nerve root compression?
12. What is a Schmorl node, how may it cause internal disk disruption, and how may this result in nerve root compression?
13. What is the evolutionary sequence of degeneration in the posterior elements of the spinal motion segment?
14. What is posterior facet arthrosis?
15. What is the sequential progression of degenerative tissue destruction during the evolution of the osteoarthritic facet joint?
16. Why is *degenerative spondylolisthesis* the end-stage pathology of the structural degenerative cascade?
17. What is the clinical and radiographic presentation of degenerative spondylolisthesis?
18. What is the clinical presentation of degenerative disk disease and posterior facet arthrosis?
19. Can posterior facet arthrosis occur without concurrent degenerative changes in the disk?
20. What are the two ways in which acute low back pain may occur in patients with degenerative changes in the posterior facet joints?
21. What is the *acute locked back?*
22. What are the radiographic signs of degenerative disk disease (DDD) and posterior facet arthrosis?
23. How is DDD differentiated from the clinical presentation of herniated disk?
24. What physical therapy is appropriate in the management of DDD and posterior facet arthrosis?

1. What is most likely the cause of these patients' symptoms?

The clinical and historical presentation of Case 1 is classic for chronic *degenerative disk disease* that was initially precipitated by the traumatic incident in his youth, which set the stage for disk degeneration that caused the progressive symptoms. The initial injury may have resulted in annular (annulus fibrosus) trauma that initiated the degenerative process of annular wear. The history is a most important feature in the diagnosis, and the clinician should not be misled by the excellent range of motion during the evaluation. The positive heel drop test substantiates the history as the jarring motion incurred by suddenly dropping on one's toes from the equinus position causes pain at that disk. Pa-

tients with osteoarthrosis of the facet joints or inflammation of the intervertebral disks resume the erect posture by "hitching" the spine. Normally, the return to flexion should be smooth and proceed cephalad to caudally. Hitching reflects a ratchety motion in which the pain first progresses to the lumbar spine, fixing it in lordosis, and then occurs at the hips until an erect posture is achieved. Following sporting activity or lifting furniture may provoke edema around and within the capsule and synovium of the arthritic facet joints that result in diminished movement such as difficulty getting out of bed, which may recur on standing should the patient sit or lie down for any lengthy period. Maintaining the stooped position for more than a few seconds is very uncomfortable as this increases tension of the degenerated annulus fibrosus that may either buckle, or cause nuclear material to migrate toward the periphery of the disk via radial and circumferential tears. Because the outer third of the annulus is innervated, this will provoke pain and ache. Radiographs further substantiate the suspected diagnosis, as they showed gross narrowing of the L4/L5 disk.

The history and clinical presentation of Case 2 without objective motor, sensory, or reflex deficit is classic for chronic degenerative *facet arthrosis.* Arthritic changes of the facet joints may certainly occur without the concurrent degenerative disk disease of the anteriorly located intervertebral disk joint, although they may often accompany it. The symptoms have been present for many years and are gradually worsening. The many forces acting on the lumbosacral junction during prolonged labor may have been an inciting factor in causing an acute flare-up following giving birth. The discomfort during running may result from the jarring effect on the facet joints, whereas the spasm may have occurred from a reactive splinting of the local paraspinal musculature in response to pain originating from a provoked osteoarthritic facet joint(s). The loss of lumbar lordosis on examination suggests concurrent narrowing (degenerative disk disease) at the lumbosacral junction, as this large disk is wedge shaped and significantly contributes to the normal lordotic contour of the low back. Spondylolysis or spondylolisthesis are ruled out because extension aggravates these two pathologies; moreover, patients with spondylolytic pathology prefer not to stand for even short periods. The sudden jarring motion caused by standing on tiptoe and then thudding heavily onto the heels transmits jarring to the spine, and will be painful for patients with facet arthrosis and inflammatory conditions. Pressure distribution among the facet joints is unequal secondary to pelvic obliquity or lumbar scoliosis in which the facet on the concavity of the curve bears the brunt of excessive load and hence develops radiographic evidence of degenerative change. Marked asymmetry between the left and right facet joints at a given segment may occur and provoke facet joint arthrosis secondary to incongruity between the facet joints. Symptomatic improvement following mobilization and a hot shower following a night's sleep suggests a low-grade inflammatory process such as chronic arthritis of the posterior facet joints. The radiographic findings corroborated the clinical impression as they showed significant right posterior facet arthrosis at L5/S1 and moderate left facet degeneration, and marked narrowing at the L5/S1 disk space whereas the adjacent disk spaces were well preserved. Traction osteophyte formation was evident on the inferior aspect of the body of L5 anteriorly.

The history and clinical presentation of Case 3 suggest a slowly progressive mechanical back problem. Symptoms relieved by ambulation exclude spinal stenosis, especially because the latter affords relief in the flexed position. Because there is no objective neurologic deficit, the possible etiology of this patient's symptoms could be either degenerative disk disease or spondylolisthesis. The presence of a step in the low back indicates the latter, and the pattern of specific aggravating and relieving factors favors a diagnosis of degenerative spondylolisthesis over spondylolytic spondylolisthesis. With isthmic spondylolisthesis, pinpoint tenderness would occur secondary to the loose lamina. Degenerative spondylolisthesis most commonly presents with subacute or chronic symptoms. Radiographs were indicated and showed gross narrowing of the L4/L5 disk with a grade I forward shift of L4 on L5 on a stress flexion view without a pars interarticularis defect, indicating *degenerative spondylolisthesis.* Degenerative spondylolisthesis is the endstage pathology of a degenerative cascade that begins anteriorly at the intervertebral disk and migrates posteriorly to encompass the posterior facet joints.

2. What is the structural degenerative cascade?

Painful degenerative disk disease may occur because of a single traumatic event that initiates the degenerative process, or may occur insidiously from a history of cumulative microtrauma known as the structural degenerative cascade. The *structural degenerative cascade*[28] is a series of structural changes that occur over time that accounts for the majority of pain of spinal origin. Beginning most often with degenerative disk disease at the anterior intervertebral joint, the degenerative cascade begins with micro or macro trauma in the intervertebral disk or facet joints and results in structural alteration of the vertebral motion segment. One *vertebral motion segment* is defined as the intervertebral disk joint anteriorly and to the two posteriorly located facet joints that define and limit the amount of movement at the disk joint. The degenerative cascade is similar to the degenerative process at other articular surfaces and occurs as a function of joint movement and the normal process of wear-and-tear of tissue. At some point in a patient's life, the amount of motion at the spinal motion segment causes more wear than can be tolerated leading to degenerative wear of the soft and osseous tissue comprising the spinal motion segment. As this process continues, structural degeneration may eventually manifest as disk degeneration or herniation, central and/or lateral canal stenosis, spinal instability, malalignment, and facet arthrosis as pathology migrates posteriorly across the posterior elements to affect the posterior facet joints. However, because patients may or may not be symptomatic at any stage, and because of the many ways in which pathology may manifest, the degenerative cascade may lead to a variety of clinical presentations. The degenerative cascade may be provoked or hastened by other factors including surgery or a previous history of disk pathology. Following diskectomy, the level at which the disk was removed often narrows, resulting in incongruity of the posterior facets with subsequent facet arthrosis. Alternately, degenerative disk disease may develop at the level of disk herniation following resolution of sciatica. This may occur because, as the disk narrowed anteriorly, the corresponding posterior facet joints do not fit perfectly together and facet arthrosis resulting in facet joint arthrosis. Heredity and obesity are also important factors in the degenerative etiology of the anterior and posterior joints of the spine. Thus the degenerative cascade represents a spectrum of soft and osseous tissue degeneration of the spinal motion segment whose clinical presentation spans a host of pathologic changes, each of which has its unique clinical presentation.

3. What is the spinal motion segment?

It is erroneous to conceptualize the spine and its pathology in terms of only the intervertebral disk, but rather understand each level of the spine in terms of trijoint unit. A *spinal motion segment* is a compound articulation comprised of a three-joint complex composed of an anterior symphysis and two posterior synovial facet joints. The intervertebral disk is located anteriorly between the endplates of two adjacent vertebral bodies and principally functions to bear axial load. The joints of the posterior spine are formed by the articular processes of the superior and inferior vertebrae and function to guide and limit the amount of motion at the anterior joint. As such, the motion segment is considered the basic kinematic unit of the spine and represents a partnership of articulations that protect the neural elements of the spine, while allowing for motion. A unique characteristic of a motion segment is that it exhibits *coupled motion* meaning that motion in one segment affects motion in the other segment.[37] This becomes significant when we consider normal motion and patho-

logic degradation of the spinal joints. Arthritic degradation of one component of the spinal trijoint complex leads to *segmental instability* of that spinal motion segment.

4. What are the functions of the anterior and posterior articulations comprising the trijoint spinal complex?

The upper and lower surfaces of the vertebral bodies are flat because they must function as weight-bearing pillars of the vertebrae in response to axial compression. The flat design presents a maximal surface area capable of withstanding longitudinal compressive forces. The flaw in this design strategy emerges when we consider that the spine must be capable of motion. During spinal movement, the flat inferior and superior surfaces of the vertebral bodies lack stabilizing features that would prevent their sliding over each other. This missing stability is provided by the posterior elements of the vertebrae, particularly the *zygapophyseal facet joints*. The inferior articular process (Fig. 58-1) of each vertebra constitutes "hooks" that engage the superior articular process of the next lower vertebra that resist forward sliding between vertebral bodies.

Thus the two posteriorly located facet joints represent the other portion of the trijoint complex comprising the motion segment and typically bear 16%[9] of weight-bearing capacity, when standing erect under in normal physiologic conditions. The primary function of the lumbar facet joint is to provide *torsional stability* of a motion segment.[15]

5. What is the anatomy of the facet joints?

The zygapophyseal facet joints are classified as true diarthrodial (synovial) as they have articular cartilage, synovial linings, and joint capsules. The facets correspond to the articular processes of each vertebra that are analogous to "hooks" in which the inferior articular processes of each vertebra engage the superior articular processes of the next lower vertebrae. The articular cartilage of a facet joint is relatively small and measures between 8 to 10 mm across,[19] whereas its cartilage thickness is 1 to 2 mm.[8] Facet joints are considered planar joints. Facets on the superior articular process are concave and have an anterior portion that faces backward and a posterior portion that faces medially. In contrast, the convex facets on the inferior articular process reciprocally face forward and laterally. The inferior facet of a superior vertebra and the superior facet of the vertebra below it form a facet joint. The shape of the

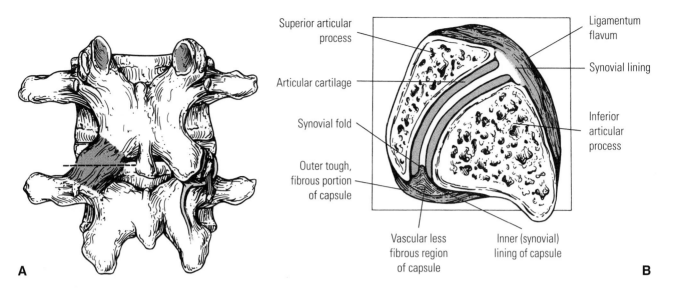

Superior articular process — **Articular cartilage** — **Synovial fold** — **Outer tough, fibrous portion of capsule** — **Ligamentum flavum** — **Synovial lining** — **Inferior articular process** — **Vascular less fibrous region of capsule** — **Inner (synovial) lining of capsule**

A   B

FIG. 58-1 The apophyseal facet joint indicated by *dotted line* in **A. B,** Note the ligamentum flavum anteriorly, and the facet joint capsule posteriorly. The lateral aspect of the capsule blends with the articular cartilage, whereas the medial aspect extends for a considerable distance along the posterior aspect of the inferior articular process. Notice the synovial fold extending into the joint space. (From Cramer GD, Darby SA: *Basic and clinical anatomy of the spine, spinal cord, and ANS,* St Louis, 1995, Mosby.)

superior facet conforms almost perfectly with the inferior articular facet of the vertebra above. The two orientations of each facet joint permit the facets to collectively resist forward displacement and axial rotation of the upper vertebral on the lower vertebra.

An *articular capsule* covers the posterior aspect of each facet joint, whereas the ligamentum flavum covers the anteromedial aspect of each joint. The articular capsule is tough, possesses a rich sensory innervation, and is well vascularized.[18] These capsules are so strong that during full flexion of the lumbar spine, capsules support approximately 40% of the body weight with a tensile strength of 319 N.[33] The *multifidus lumborum muscles* attach to the articular capsule, which lies just medial to the primary attachment of this muscle to the mamillary process and may acts in a *retractor capacity* to keep the capsule out of the joint space.[53] The anterior capsule of the facet joint is formed by the ligamentum flavum, which unlike other spinal ligaments is comprised of collagen and elastic fibers.

Intraarticular folds exist within the facet joint known as *meniscoid inclusions* comprised of fibroadipose tissue that is pain sensitive and may become trapped within the joint due to incongruity of the facets and result in a condition known as the *acute locked back*. Synovial lined extensions of the articular capsule projects into the joint space to provide adequate coverage for the hyaline cartilage of the facet joint. These too can become pinched with facet joint incongruity following decreased height of the intervertebral disk secondary to degenerative disk disease.[9]

Having a rich supply of sensory innervation, the facet joints are supplied by branches from the medial division of each posterior primary ramus of the lumbar roots. The innervation pattern is organized so that the facet joint capsule is innervated by fibers arising from the nerve root at that level, and from the root at the level above. Thus a nerve from a given level supplies fibers to the inferior capsule of the posterior facet joint at that level, and the superior capsule of the joint at the next level.[47] This multilevel innervation may account for why pain deriving from the facet joint frequently demonstrates a broad referral pattern.[25]

6. What is the role of the facet joints in motion of the lumbar spine?

Although motion between two adjacent vertebrae is minimal, the combined movement between many vertebral segments result in considerable motion including flexion, extension, side bending, and rotation. It is the orientation of the lumbar facet joints that determine the motion between adjacent vertebrae. Whereas the thoracic facet joints face anteriorly and are therefore prevented from moving one on the other, the facet joints between T12 and L1 and those facets inferior to that level face laterally so that the angle between the facet joints lie in the sagittal plane. Thus the lumbar facet joints permits considerably more flexion than the frontal alignment of the thoracic facet joints.[22] Having two principal movements, the facet joints either slide or gap. When they slide on both sides simultaneously, the result is forward bending, whereas when they slide on one side only, the result is side bending. Rotation may occur by distracting on the side of one facet, while the other facet serves as a fulcrum.[24]

The shape and size of the lumbar facet joints restrain forward lumbar flexion to approximately 60° before restraint of the lumbar facets.[53] In contrast, extension of the lumbar region is limited by the inferior articular process on each side of the lumbar vertebra contacting the pars interarticularis; the junction between the lamina and superior articular process.[8] Extension is also limited by the anterior longitudinal ligament and the facet joint capsular ligaments.[10]

Because the facets face in an almost lateromedial direction, they are therefore aligned in the sagittal plane,[45] which limits the total rotation in the lumbar spine. As a result of the superior and inferior orientation of the lumbar articular facets, lateral flexion of the lumbar spine is accompanied by axial rotation away from the side of lateral flexion. For example, left lateral flexion of the lumbar region is accompanied by right rotation of the vertebral bodies and left rotation of the spinous processes.[8] Degeneration is most likely to occur at the L4 and L5 levels because facet joints at these levels are obliquely aligned, making them susceptible to recurrent rotational strain. The wedge shape of the intervertebral disks here also increases the risk of degenerative change[26] as it accentuates the lumbar lordosis.

7. What are the biomechanical ramifications of incongruity of the facet joints?

The facet joints at any level are paired synovial joints that must fit congruously to maintain normal joint function. Should this normal anatomic congruity be lost, degenerative changes will occur. An analogy may be drawn to the knee joint, which is also a paired articulation consisting of the medial and lateral tibiofemoral joints. A bowlegged patient develops arthritic changes on the medial (loaded) aspect of the knee, whereas a

knock-knee deformity results in arthritic changes on the lateral side of the joint. Similarly, the facet joints are located to either side of midline and must undergo equal loading to function normally. Asymmetry of the facet joints may be congenital, result from trauma, or occur secondary to scoliotic deformity so that the facet on the concave (loaded) side of the curve develops arthritic changes. With degenerative disk disease, symmetric loading due to *narrowing* of the intervertebral disk causes an imperfect fit of the facet joints so that they begin to override each other. Over time, the joint space narrows, the capsule thickens, and osteophytes may develop anywhere around the periphery of the facet joints. Although large osteophytes may project posteriorly, others may grow on the anterior aspect of the joint and thereby encroach on the spinal canal and frequently narrow the existing foramen for the spinal nerves.[47]

8. What is the evolutionary sequence of the degenerative cascade?

The *degenerative cascade* of the spinal motion segment refers to a process that involves degradation and inflammation of the various segments of the motion segment, which in turn causes dysfunction in the adjacent segment. The beginning of the degenerative process usually affects the intervertebral disk, which shows signs of failure in the form of microtrauma derived from eccentric (off-center) and torsional loading that culminates in circumferential tears of the outer annular layers. This results in separation of the vertebral endplate which, in turn, interrupts the blood supply and leads to loss of nutritional supply to the intervertebral disk. This, in turn, begins a sequence of proteoglycan breakdown that lead to loss of water content within the disk. Progressive loss of mechanical competence translates in the loss of the ability of the trijoint complex to withstand the harmful effects of shear forces, which only hastens the degenerative process. Subsequently, progressive loss of disk height results in narrowing of the vertebral foramen in the cephalad-caudal direction. Because the intervertebral disk forms the anterior border of the intervertebral foramen, a decrease in disk height affects the lateral canal by decreasing its vertical dimension, and thereby results in lateral canal stenosis by compressing the laterally emerging nerve root (Fig. 58-2). Moreover, the presence of any extruded nuclear material in the epidural space may chemically irritate the nerve root, and contribute toward its ischemia by way of an inflammatory response.

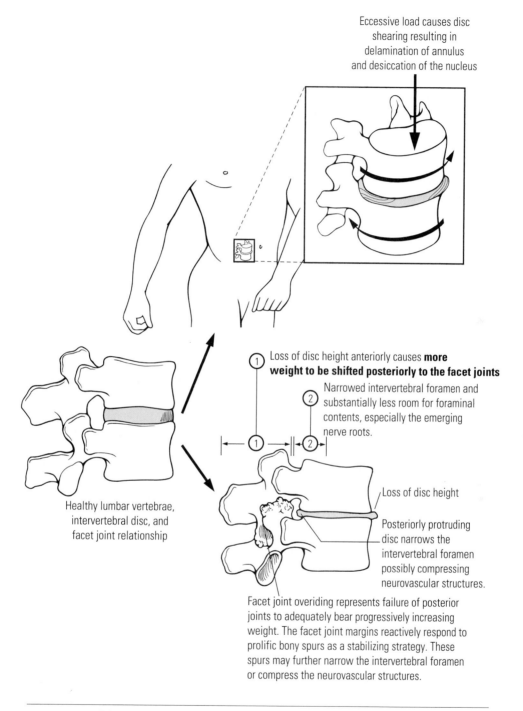

Eccessive load causes disc shearing resulting in delamination of annulus and desiccation of the nucleus

① Loss of disc height anteriorly causes **more weight to be shifted posteriorly to the facet joints**

② Narrowed intervertebral foramen and substantially less room for foraminal contents, especially the emerging nerve roots.

Healthy lumbar vertebrae, intervertebral disc, and facet joint relationship

Loss of disc height

Posteriorly protruding disc narrows the intervertebral foramen possibly compressing neurovascular structures.

Facet joint overriding represents failure of posterior joints to adequately bear progressively increasing weight. The facet joint margins reactively respond to prolific bony spurs as a stabilizing strategy. These spurs may further narrow the intervertebral foramen or compress the neurovascular structures.

FIG. 58-2 Sequential degenerative cascade of the spinal motion segment.

9. What degenerative sequence occurs in the anterior elements of the spinal motion segment?

With normal or accelerated aging, changes occur within the biochemical composition of the intervertebral disk so that it demonstrates a loss of hydrostatic properties. As a result, the disk becomes more susceptible to trauma by *delamination* of the laminae of the annulus fibrosis. Degeneration of the nucleus pulposis, which is accelerated by smoking and vibration,[2] may lead to a loss of disk height and altered load transmission, so that the instant center of rotation shifts posteriorly.[16] As a result, alteration of load transmission from disk degeneration transmits progressively more axial compression posteriorly across the vertebral arch to the posterior facet joints. Because the degenerated disk is less capable of absorbing superincumbent load, it is more likely to bulge[21] posteriorly because of the posterior shift in the center of rotation of the intervertebral disk. This bulging is prevented from occurring centrally by the rhomboidal shape[22] of the posterior longitudinal ligament, but follows the path of least resistance in the posterolateral direction. Once the bulge reaches a certain critical level it may exert direct pressure of the nerve root either in the lateral recess or the intervertebral foramen, causing radiculopathy.

10. What is the relationship between hamstring tightness and disk degeneration?

The large muscles which span significant lengths of the trunk or lower extremities affect the low back owing to their insertion on the pelvis. The hip flexors and extensors, in particular, should be stretched because tightness of these muscles will rotate the pelvis excessively,* and may negatively impact on both posture and the magnitude of lumbar lordosis. Hyperlordosis is associated with anterior pelvic tilt, which causes the pelvis to rotate forward due to tightened hip flexors. Tight hamstrings cause a pull on the pelvis to rotate it backwardly about the common hip axis as posterior pelvic tilt and therefore increase shear of L5 ("sliding down the hill") on S1. This increases the shear, which is already at a premium at the L4/L5 and L5/S1 segments because of the normal anatomy of this region, and pre-

---

*Pelvic rotation is known as *pelvic tilt,* which is defined in relation to the anterior superior iliac spine (ASIS). Anterior pelvic tilt, associated with tight iliopsoas and quadriceps muscles as well as hyperlordosis, involves the ASIS moving anteriorly and downward. In contrast, posterior pelvic tilt, associated with hypolordosis and tightened and tightened hamstring musculature, involves the ASIS moving posteriorly and upward.

disposes for accelerated disk and facet degeneration (Fig. 58-3).[47] Thus hamstring tightness is a predisposing factor in disk degeneration, and may reinforce progressive hypolordosis of the lumbosacral spine in conjunction with progressive posterior pelvic tilt. Subsequently, hamstring stretching is an integral part of management of degenerative disk disease and posterior facet arthrosis.

In contrast, hyperlordosis, which often stems from tight hip flexor musculature and anterior pelvic tilt may cause central or spinal stenosis. Hyperlordosis narrows the intervertebral foramina, especially in the lateral recesses via impingement by the superior articular process of the inferior lumbar vertebrae. Hyperlordosis also narrows the central spinal canal via impingement by the inferior articular process of the superior lumbar vertebrae (Fig. 58-4).[26] Thus either extreme of pelvic tilting may result in pathology, so that maintenance of a neural posture of the pelvis and low back is essential and promoted by adequate soft-tissue extensibility of the pre- and postfemoral musculature.

11. How may hypertrophic bone formation of the anterior spinal joint result in nerve root compression?

In response to degeneration, the vertebral margins along the attachment of the annulus fibrosus grow bony spurs in an attempt to stabilize the trijoint complex. This hypertrophic bone formation protrudes from the vertebral margin and occasionally form a bony bridge between the vertebra as an attempt to stabilize that segment. When spurring occurs between the posterior margins of two vertebral bodies, the central and lateral canals may be compromised.[20] The dimensions of the central canal are also significantly reduced by hypertrophic bone formation of the inferior facet, especially if there is associated thickening and subsequent bulging of the ligamentum flavum.[48]

As disk height is lost, mechanical competence of the disk is diminished, and the principal weight-bearing function of the anteriorly located disk is shifted posteriorly to the components of the neural arch. As transfer of axial loading to the posterior elements gradually occurs, the degenerative cascade spreads to the zygapophyseal facet joints. These diarthrodial articulations have articular and subchondral cartilage, a capsule and synovium lining the joint capsule, as well as a meniscus. Thus the facet joints are subject to the same degenerative and reparative changes characteristic of osteoarthritis that may occur at the hip or knee joints.[42]

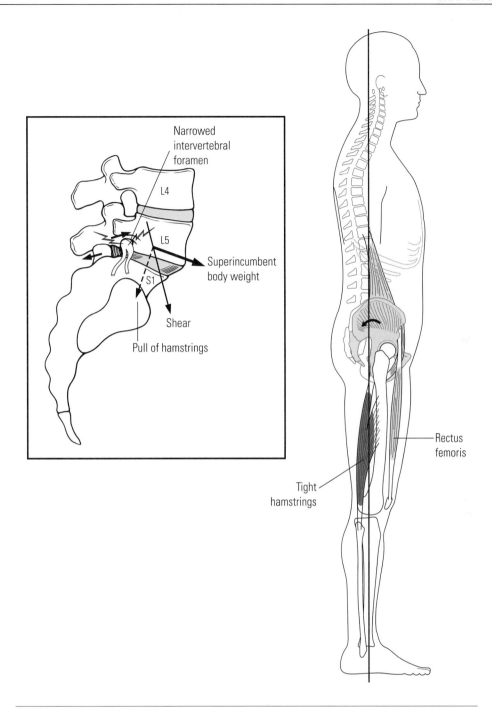

FIG. 58-3 Tight hamstrings cause a pull on the pelvis to rotate it backwardly about the common hip axis as posterior pelvic tilt and therefore increase shear of the L5 on S1 and predisposes for accelerated disk and facet degeneration.

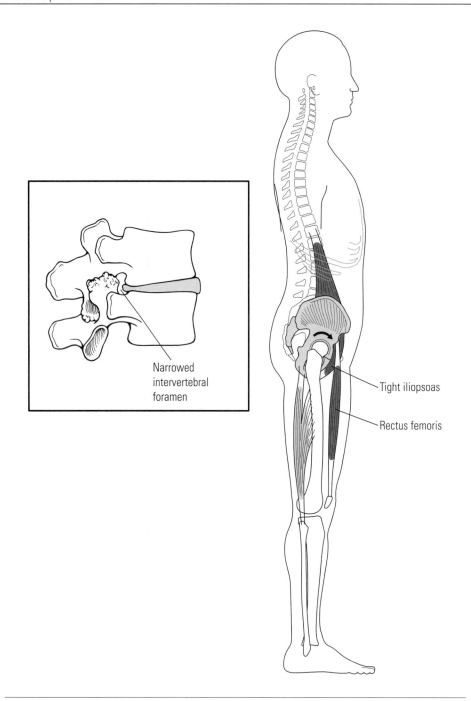

FIG. 58-4 The effect of tight hip flexor musculature on the low back. Anterior pelvic tilt caused by tight il-iopsoas and rectus femoris results in an extension posture of the lumbar vertebrae. This results in narrowing of the intervertebral foramen, making nerve root entrapment more likely.

12. What is a Schmorl node, how may it cause internal disk disruption, and how may this result in nerve root compression?

The *vertebral endplates* are comprised of two relatively flat and parallel surfaces that provide the source of nourishment to the avascular nucleus pulposus, and to the annulus via the vertebral sinusoids.* When the disk is loaded during axial compression, the vertebral end plate is the weakest structure among the three components of the intervertebral disk.[5] The healthy annulus can tolerate much greater compressive stress than the failure stress of the vertebral endplate. In youth, when the nucleus pulposus is well hydrated and relatively incompressible, the effects of longitudinal compressive force will result in failure of the bony endplate before failure of the disk. However, before endplate fracture, a protective mechanism occurs in which the nucleus loses 1 to 2 ml of fluid by way of exchange into the sinusoid as a way of reducing the impact of sudden, compressive force. If the compressive force is excessive, as may occur from a fall on the buttocks or when lifting heavy objects, the vertebral endplates will bulge initially before fracture. Thus axial compressive force will cause an endplate fracture before annular disruption, typically superiorly into the central substance of the adjacent vertebral body is what is termed a *Schmorl node*. These endplate herniations, occurring at the site of the central defect, are often located at the lower thoracic and upper lumbar levels,[3] in just over one-third of all spine, more typically in males, and occur at the thinnest aspect of the endplate. Occurring as frequently in adolescents as adults, Schmorl nodes are typically painless because of the relative lack of nociceptors at this site.† Thus the intervertebral disk can withstand compressive loads far beyond that which the vertebral body can withstand resulting in vertebral body fractures before disintegration of the disk itself.[43] The subsequent approximation of the upper and lower vertebral body alters the balance of forces between the posterior and anterior elements, which leads to more force to be borne by the anterior

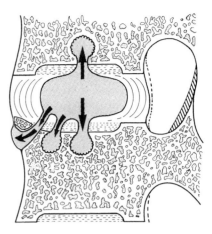

Schmorl's nodes

Limbus vertebra   Central anterior

FIG. 58-5 Schmorl's node. (From White AH, Schofferman JA, editors: *Spine care: diagnosis and conservative treatment,* St Louis, 1995, Mosby.)

intervertebral joints and posterior facet joints, and thereby hastening the degenerative process.[8]

Although an endplate fracture may heal without noticeable symptoms and pass unnoticed, it may set in motion a series of sequelae that may result in pain and degradation of the disk. The proteoglycans of the nucleus pulposis are biochemically similar to those of the vitreous humor, and in penetrating eye injuries, exposed lens protein may sensitize lymphocytes so that they exert a destructive inflammation if they reach the intact eye.‡ Similarly, the proteoglycans of the nucleus are foreign to the body and throughout its development, the nucleus is avascular and is never exposed to the body's circulation. Consequently, following a vertical endplate fracture, migration of nuclear material may expose the nuclear proteoglycans to the circulation, causing the immune system to mount an autoimmune response against the nuclear material. If the prolapsed nuclear material contacts the vertebral spongiosa following a traumatic Schmorl node (Fig 58-5),[30] it will come in contact with the body's blood supply and elicit an antigenic response.[17] This, in turn, triggers an inflammatory response that leads to progressive degradation of the nuclear matrix and alteration of its biophysical properties. The disk is less capable of binding water

---

*In comparison, this nourishment by diffusion has no analogue in the major synovial body joints as no fluid exchange occurs between the subchondral bony plate and the joint cavity. Instead, the source of nutrient diffusion is the synovial fluid.

†However, a secondary inflammatory cascade within the nucleus and subsequent nuclear degeneration and disruption may occur secondary to endplate herniation. This may be as an autoimmune response or because the endplate fracture activates endogenous proteolytic enzymes normally present in the disk and inhibited by proteinase inhibitors.

‡This condition is known as *sympathetic ophthalmia.*

in what is described as an *isolated disk resorption*[55] and gradually loses its ability to withstand axial compressive force. Subsequently, the role of weight bearing is borne by the annulus fibrosus, which may creep under compression, leading to buckling and bulging of the annulus and narrowing of the disk space, and result in *canal or foraminal stenosis*. Thus spinal stenosis represents the end stage of the sequence of internal disk disruption that follows an endplate herniation in which the nuclear material comes in contact with the systemic circulation.

13. What is the evolutionary sequence of degeneration in the posterior elements of the spinal motion segment?

The initial stage of facet degeneration occurs in response to increased loading, which may be accelerated if the applied load is asymmetrical and may derive from uneven loss of disk height anteriorly secondary to a disk protrusion that was not midline oriented. The first stage of degeneration of the facet joints begins as synovitis, which may result in nonspecific back pain that is made sensitive by extension motions of the spine. This is followed by progressive destruction of the cartilaginous articular surface, which, if unilateral, may cause incongruity of the posterior facet joints. This incongruity may lead to overriding of the facet joints and subluxation or dislocation on one side,[48] which results in an acute condition known as the *acute locked back*.[47]

Stretching and tearing of the facet joint capsule may accompany articular incongruity causing back pain due to the richly innervated capsule. Pain may also be generated from narrowing and motion in the lateral canal that may traumatize the nerve root and cause sciatica. The final step in the spectrum of the degenerative cascade, similar to marginal osteophytes of the anterior joint, manifests as bony overgrowth of the joints in an attempt to stabilize. Thus the facets increase in size as they progressively bear more weight in response to failure of the intervertebral joint. Progressive osteophytosis of the inferior articular facet will narrow the central canal, whereas enlargement of the superior articular facet will narrow the exit of one of the intervertebral foramina and cause lateral stenosis.[48]

14. What is posterior facet arthrosis?

Posterior facet joint arthrosis refers to degenerative joint disease of the articular facet joints causing osteophytic spurring from the margins of that joint that may

constrict *both* the central and root canals. The pathologic changes in the posterior elements of the trijoint complex usually begin with synovitis of the diarthrodial facet joints, followed by osteophytic overgrowth. *Central spinal stenosis* may derive from impingement from osteophytic arthrosis from the *inferior articular process* comprising the lower hemi-facet joint as it faces anterior and laterally. Because it faces anteriorly, marginal spurring will be directed toward the spinal cord. In contrast, the superior articular process faces backward and medially. Because the nerve root lies in the upper third of the intervertebral foramen,[8] osteophytic overgrowth from the *superior articular process* comprising the superior facet along the attachment of the ligamentum flavum[42] (which forms its joint capsule) is likely to cause *lateral canal stenosis.*[56] Thus although enlargement of the inferior facets is more likely to cause central canal stenosis, enlargement of the superior facets often results in lateral canal stenosis. Bony spurring may also form from the vertebral body along the attachment of the annulus fibrosus.

15. What is the sequential progression of degenerative tissue destruction during the evolution of the osteoarthritic facet joint?

The pathogenesis of degenerative arthrosis refers to the sequential degenerative changes of the posterior facet joints that may be provoked by any number of factors. Whether degenerative joint disease is primary or secondary, the pathologic sequence causing joint destruction is the same. Once the pore size of the surface layer of articular cartilage is altered through wear, proteoglycans leak out into the synovial fluid resulting in impaired chondrocyte nutrition. With loss of proteoglycan from the matrix, the collagen fibers become more susceptible to mechanical damage secondary to wear.[49] As a result, the elastic resilience of cartilage becomes impaired so that the articular surface becomes increasingly less able to withstand even minor stress. Moreover, the poorly nourished chondrocytes must bear the brunt of direct frictional stress. Protease, a lysosomal enzyme, is released due to chondrocyte damage. The chondrocytes, in turn, respond defensively by increasing the rate of proteoglycan synthesis in an effort to ward off the damage. However, the rate of mechanical wear outstrips any attempted repair in those sites subject to the greatest load bearing or shearing stress. Enzymatic degradation due to marked lysosomal activity[41] results in thwarting proteoglycan synthesis, and small fragments of abraded dead cartilage are released into the joint and swept about due to joint motion producing a reactionary synovitis.[7] What began as a purely degenerative process progresses to focal areas of secondary inflammatory synovitis. This results in villous hypertrophy and fibrosis of the synovium and subsequent moderate synovial effusion leading to greater viscosity. Changes in the synovial membrane are often accompanied by fraying and instability.[50] Moreover, as bone is lost the joint surfaces approximate and the ligaments become more lax. In addition, fibrosis and thickening spreads to the adjacent fibrous joint capsule, which further limits joint motion so that the endstage may be a fibrous ankylosis of the joint. The muscles adjacent to the affected joint demonstrate spasm in response to pain, and muscles, typically the hamstrings, undergo contracture and cause joint deformity and further restriction of motion. Thus osteoarthritis represents a failure in repair that occurs when chondrocyte proliferation and proteoglycan production cannot keep pace with the pace of destruction. This sets into motion a cascade of degeneration of the articular cartilage and surrounding soft tissue.

Once the tangential layer of the central, weight-bearing aspect of articular cartilage undergoes shredding, fraying and fibrillation of the weakened area, minor stress renders the cartilage matrix more susceptible to friction. *Fibrillation* refers to vertical splitting of the superficial portion of articular cartilage causing softening (malacia) as the surface becomes rough, resembling a shaggy carpet. The articular surface, which is normally a bluish-white, smooth and glistening, becomes yellow, granular, and dull with fibrillation. It is at this point that conservative intervention is most helpful in the form of nonsteroidal antiinflammatory medications, which inhibit prostaglandin synthesis by fibroblasts, as prostaglandin is an intermediary in releasing catabolic enzymes causing pain.[54]

If the degenerative process is not interrupted, fibrillation gives way to deep *fissures* or cracks representing partial-thickness defects within the articular surface. Clusters of chondrocytes proliferate clusters called *clones* around the fissures in an attempt to ward off impending disaster by metabolizing collagen and proteoglycan at a more rapid rate than usual. Despite these efforts, fissuring represents a point of no return in the degenerative process. Eventually, all four layers of articular cartilage are worn away and the joint is *denuded*. Once the fissures have grown deep enough to penetrate subcortical bone, an influx of marrow cells allows fibrocartilage to grow upward at an attempt at

repair. Healing of the surface defect at best occurs in the form of a scar comprised of fibrocartilage comprised of randomly oriented fibers unsuited for load bearing. In addition, because fibrocartilage is, unlike hyaline cartilage, a vascularized tissue, continued wearing of these defects causes bleeding into the joint, which further contributes to degradation of any remaining or adjacent articular cartilage. As weight bearing continues and fibrocartilage is progressively worn away, the subchondral bone serves at the joint surface causing raw bone to rub against raw bone. In response, the subchondral bone undergoes *eburnation* in which it becomes as smooth as polished ivory, and hypertrophies to the point of becoming *sclerotic* (having increased radiographic density) on radiograph. Sclerosis represents a healing process, similar to callus formation, of microfractures in subchondral bone.[40] In contrast, in the peripheral areas which are characterized by minimal stress, the subchondral bone atrophies and becomes radiographically *rarefied* (less dense). The trabeculae in these central areas of maximum stress and friction suffer fracture and heal with callus, which increases the rigidity of bone so that the bone becomes denser and less resilient. As the normal architecture of bone is lost, the trabeculae degenerate and are replaced by cystic areas of bone that are radiographically apparent just beneath the eburnated surface and may be filled with pockets of synovial fluid,[50] which leak in from the joint surface via defects in the subchondral bone. Eventually, continued wear through to these cysts appears as multiple pits on the eburnated surface.

Whereas the proportion of bone increases centrally, cartilage behaves differently in that it decreases centrally and increases peripherally. At the peripheral border of the joint, cartilage undergoes hypertrophy and hyperplasia to form a thickened rim of cartilage around the joint margin. This cartilaginous outgrowth is called a *chondrophyte* and ossifies to become a peripheral bony outgrowth known as a bone spur or *osteophyte* in an attempt to minimize joint motion and more broadly distribute loading forces. This change in the shape of bone at the joint margins involves stretching of the highly innervated periosteum that is painful. This new bone may even grow inwardly into the joint space. This loss of cartilage centrally and simultaneous growth peripherally represents a protective strategy to minimize joint motion. In the process, however, incongruity of the joint surfaces increases so that an alteration of the distribution and magnitude of the biomechanical stresses on the joint occurs. In this way, this form of remodeling may have the short-term benefit of minimizing pain by restricting motion, but does so at the expense of decreasing joint congruity which leads to progressive arthrosis of that joint. Thus the body's various attempts to ward off the effects of degeneration throughout the evolution of osteoarthrosis are met with increasing failure that only, in the long run, contributes to the ultimate demise of the joint, characteristic of a vicious cycle of degeneration.

16. Why is *degenerative spondylolisthesis* the endstage pathology of the structural degenerative cascade?

Progressive cartilaginous destruction and overriding of the facet joints represents a failure of the posterior elements to assume the weight for axial loading, a role which they were not designed for. This results in further narrowing of the disk space anteriorly and ligamentous laxity posteriorly with facet joint instability. If instability progresses, the spinal motion segment will undergo *segmental instability* and may culminate in *degenerative spondylolisthesis,* which corresponds to the endstage pathology of the structural cascade.

Degenerative spondylolisthesis is defined as forward slippage of one vertebra over the next as a result of degenerative change in the intervertebral disk and/or articular facet joint.* This occurs because erosion of the superior articular facet allows forward displacement of the upper vertebral body on the lower body, trapping the inferior nerve root that exists one level below and between the inferior facet and the back of the vertebral body.[27] Commonly occurring at the fourth lumbar level, degenerative spondylolisthesis most likely occurs as a function of facet joint orientation and differs from the classic isthmic type of spondylolisthesis in that the former is characterized by an intact neural arch and lack of primary disk degeneration; thus it is alternately known as *pseudospondylolisthesis.* A fourfold increased incidence of sacralization is observed in these patients, which further increases the stress to this vulnerable L4/L5 disk level. Degenerative spondylolisthesis predominantly occurs in females (3:2) greater than 50 years of age.[36]

The pathologic process begins with degeneration of the intervertebral disk[12] that is followed by malalignment of the facet joints as disk height is lost, and is accompanied by osteophyte formation and synovial hypertrophy of the facet joints that become rounded and arthritic. This loss of vertical orientation of the facet joints undermines the stabilizing role provided by the posterior joints to the intervertebral disk joint, allowing for excessive forward displacement of the vertebra during flexion. Pain may arise at the degenerative disk and at the arthritic facet joints. Consequently, the superior vertebra (L4) begins to migrate or "slip" forward on the L5 vertebra. This allows the upper vertebra to roll forward on the one below during lumbar flexion. Depending on the extent of slip, a "step" may be palpable. Unlike the spondylolytic variety, the step here occurs between the spinous process of the affected vertebra and the one below.[47] If a step is not distinctly palpable, spondylolisthesis may be suggested by a protruding lumbar spinous process, which may be tender upon percussion. As the superior vertebral body shifts forward, the interposed disk undergoes shearing strain that further exacerbates and accelerates disk degeneration. The forward slippage of the fourth lumbar vertebra ceases when the intact lamina and inferior articular facets of L4 come to rest against the body of L5. Because of this, degenerative spondylolisthesis seldom exceeds a grade 1, or 25% slip.[35] As the slip progresses, the inferior facet of the cephalic vertebra erodes through the superior articular process of the caudal vertebra.

Facet joint hypertrophy, deriving from degenerative spondylolisthesis, may result in both central and lateral canal stenoses causing neurogenic claudication or radicular encroachment, respectively. At some point in the forward migration, the disk collapses and the thickened ligamentum flavum becomes redundant, further contributing to both central and lateral stenosis. An *intrasynovial spinal cyst* may originate in the facet joint as a result of the degenerate facet joint changes in degenerative spondylolisthesis, and may act as a stenotic source.†

17. What is the clinical and radiographic presentation of degenerative spondylolisthesis?

Signs and symptoms include a protracted history of low-grade back pain that is intermittently intense, but rarely causes severe disability. More commonly, the in-

---

*Alternately, the vertebra above displaces posteriorly on the one below—this is known as *retrolisthesis,* and invariably occurs secondary to degenerative disc disease and facet arthrosis. The pain pattern is opposite that of degenerative spondylolisthesis, and is aggravated by standing and any activity increasing lordosis, whereas mild flexion affords relief.

---

†Management of isolated intraspinal cysts includes aspiration, corticosteroid injection, or cyst rupture through injection.

ferior articular process of L4 will entrap the L5 nerve root in the lateral recess and may result in sciatica.[13] Discomfort is related to disk degeneration and posterior facet arthrosis, or may be owing to nerve root irritation or entrapment or symptoms of spinal stenosis. Hence, patients develop early morning aching and stiffness and often experience difficulty getting out of bed that improves following a hot shower; alternately, once up and about they feel much better. Maintaining a flexed posture for long periods aggravates discomfort. Similarly, sitting in an upright hard chair is more comfortable than a soft, easy chair in which they insist on sitting near the edge where they may sit upright. Although turning in bed can be annoying, walking is the least symptomatic of activities. The examination is mostly negative, and does not present with pinpoint tenderness, as the lamina is not loose. Physical examination often shows a patient who is flexible and able to touch the floor on forward flexion with their knees locked in extension, although maintaining this position causes marked discomfort. Discomfort is worse on extending the back into the erect position and is frequently associated with a "hitching" movement. Instead of a smooth resumption from flexion to extension the patient first extends the lumbar spine, fixing it in lordosis, and then extending at the hips until the erect position is regained; this is known as *hitching*.[47] Patients may occasionally complain of pain both during flexion and extension.[47] Degenerative spondylolisthesis rarely presents with acute symptoms; subacute or chronic discomfort is the typical presentation.[47] Compression of the cauda equina against the body of L5 may occur as the lamina and inferior articular process of L4 slide forward, and result in neurogenic claudication.

Suspected degenerative spondylolisthesis is confirmed by anteroposterior, lateral, and oblique radiographs performed with the patient standing so as to axially load the spine and stress the slip.[11] This is then compared with supine radiographs, and a positive degenerative spondylolisthesis is identified for those patients exhibiting a proportionally greater slip on the standing radiograph. The severity of patient symptoms may not necessarily correlate the amount of slip.[6] Associated, but not diagnostic changes that may also be seen include hypertrophic changes of the facet joints, foramina and disk-space narrowing, and impingement of the inferior articular process of L4 into the superior articular process of L5. Occasionally, a vacuum sign may be seen in the lumbar disk space on plain radiographs (and especially on computerized

tomography) and is strongly suggestive of segmental instability.

Patients with minimal impairment and early stages of disk degeneration respond best to physical therapy, whereas the intermediate stages of degeneration respond to nonsteroidal antiinflammatory medications, facet injections of corticosteroids, or rarely, facet rhizotomy.[4] The advanced stages may respond to epidural or selective root injections. The major indication for surgery is incapacitating neurogenic claudication or persistent pain secondary to radiculopathy after a trial of conservative care.

18. What is the clinical presentation of degenerative disk disease and posterior facet arthrosis?

Degenerative disk disease may result from an inherent weakness of the annulus, injury, or simple wear and tear. The history and physical findings in osteoarthrosis of the posterior facet joints are virtually identical to those in degenerative disk disease.[47] Although some patients with degenerative disk disease and posterior facet arthrosis may have no history of previous injury, others may remember having acute low back pain at an early age due to a fall or some other trauma that served to initiate degenerative changes at a given segment. The L4/L5 disk is the most common symptomatic disk, followed by L5/S1. With either level, pain is localized to either side of midline of the lumbosacral region, and occasionally referred to the upper buttocks. Most patients walk into the office and sit down as though they have no back problem whatsoever. Moreover, examination may be entirely normal, with no tenderness, an intact neurologic examination, and excellent motion. Patients with degeneration localized to one level may have excellent range of motion because restriction at one level only will not noticeably affect the total range of motion. However, if these seemingly "normal" patients are asked to maintain a semistooped position for 1 to 2 minutes, most will complain of pain on holding this position as it considerably increases tension in the disks and also strains the capsular ligament of the facet joints. The fact that the patient has excellent range of spinal motion does not contradict a diagnosis of degenerative disk disease and facet arthrosis. Moreover, patients with osteoarthrosis of the facet joints or inflammation of the intervertebral disks resume the erect posture by "hitching" the spine. Normally, the return to flexion should be smooth and proceed cephalad to caudally. Hitching reflects a ratchety motion in which the pain first extends the lumbar spine, fixing it in lordosis,

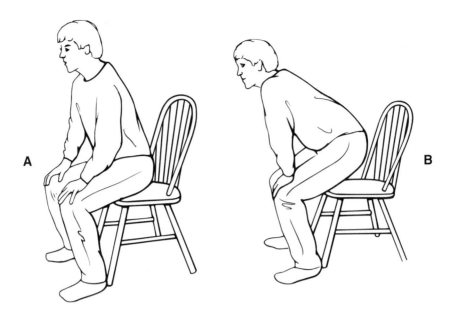

FIG. 58-6 A, When rising from a chair, a patient with degenerative disk or facet disease will flex the hips to move the center of gravity over the feet in an attempt to keep the spine straight. **B,** He will then use his hands for support when standing upright.

and then extends at the hips until the erect posture is achieved.* Alternately, patient will decrease their discomfort when straightening by "climbing up their leg" in a Gowers maneuver. This may also be noted when attempting to rise from a chair (Fig. 58-6).

The pattern of patient complaint is similar to that of osteoarthrosis of other synovial joints, varying from entirely asymptomatic to markedly symptomatic, and from marked motion to restriction to no loss of motion, with various gradations between these extremes. Patients will frequently complain of early morning stiffness and difficulty rising from bed. Because bending is difficult owing to stiffness and aching in the low back, patient usually leans on one arm to support their body weight when stooping over the wash basin. Discomfort eases with mobility and especially after a hot shower may disappear as the day goes on, despite vigorous activity such as work and sport, although symptoms may return after sitting for lengthy periods in soft easy chairs. Sitting in a firm chair is more comfortable. Stooping for any length of time is unbearable, but is relieved by placing one foot up on a step or box while standing. Standing for long periods is uncomfortable as

this increases the lumbar lordosis and further strains the osteoarthritic facet joints. Toward the end of the day, however, symptoms tend to return. Patients prefer a firm mattress to sleep on because a sagging mattress will cause excessive postures, each of which may aggravate the condition. Thus lying prone will increase lumbar lordosis, lying supine will increase lumbar kyphosis, while lying on the side will result in lateral lumbar curvature. Coughing, sneezing, and turning in bed may aggravate the pain when facet arthrosis is more advanced because of movement imposed on the facets. Patients with more advanced facet arthrosis and disk degeneration will often score positive for a *heel drop test* performed by asking the patient to stand on tiptoe in the erect position and thud heavily onto the heels. A positive test is indicated by pain from jarring of the spine.[47]

As the L4/L5 disk is the most commonly affected disk, the nerve root most often affected by degenerative disk disease is the L5 root in more complicated forms of this pathology. In this case of lateral stenosis, radiation of pain occurs across the buttock, down the posterolateral thigh, the lateral side of the leg and across the ankle joint, and along the dorsum and sole of the foot. Painful tingling down the lower extremity to the big toe typically occurs from an L5 root lesion.

---

*Hitching may also reflect unstable spondylolisthesis.

19. Can posterior facet arthrosis occur without concurrent degenerative changes in the disk?

Arthritic changes of the posterior facet joints may certainly occur without the concurrent degenerative disk disease of the anteriorly located intervertebral disk joint. Congenital anomalies, particularly at the L5/S1 level, may cause marked asymmetry between the left and right facet joints at a given segment and provoke facet joint arthrosis secondary to incongruity between the facet joints. Alternately, pressure distribution among the facet joints may be altered by the presence of pelvic obliquity or lumbar scoliosis in which the facet on the concavity of the curve bears the brunt of excessive load and hence develops radiographic evidence of degenerative change. Alternately, posttraumatic arthrosis of the facet joints may occur from compression of articular cartilage and joint surface disruption with or without loss of joint congruity. Idiopathic facet joint arthrosis may also occur. The history and physical finding of osteoarthrosis of the posterior facet joints are virtually identical to those with degenerative disk disease. Confirmation of suspected facet arthrosis at a particular segment might be confirmed with selective injection, preferably with guidance of computerized tomography, and relief of symptoms.[47]

20. What are the two ways in which acute low back pain may occur in patients with degenerative changes in posterior facet joints?

Although degenerative changes of the intervertebral and facet joints may occur gradually over the course of several years, and may or may not be precipitated by severe impact such as a fall onto the buttocks, acute low back pain may occur at the posterior facet joints in two different pathways. In the first, the patient may complain of acute discomfort following heavy physical activity such as shifting furniture. This may provoke edema around and within the capsule and synovium of the arthritic facet joint that results in diminished movement such as difficulty getting out of bed. After the patient mobilizes by way of light exercise and taking a hot shower, the aching and stiffness markedly diminish. Should the patient sit or lie down for any lengthy period, symptoms may recur on getting up again. Pain is experienced across the lumbosacral region and there may be mild tenderness to deep palpation over the facet joints. The heel drop test will be positive.[47] Symptoms usually resolve, with appropriate management, after several days. The other mode of acute onset of low back pain in patients with posterior facet arthrosis is the acute locked back.

21. What is the *acute locked back?*

In patients with posterior facet joint arthrosis, severe pain and discomfort may be provoked for something as trivial as bending over at the washbasin, or to one side to tie one's shoes, picking up a piece of paper, or from some unprotected movement in bed while sleeping, as this asymmetric motion shifts one of the facet joints at a specific segment out of its normally congruous relationship. Occurring during the bending-over motion, this movement represents a sudden unprotected motion that allows for nipping or "jamming" of the synovial meniscus, which is highly innervated. This triggers a reflex spasm of the overlying musculature, resulting in a "locking" of the back to minimize movements for fear of provoking intense discomfort and hence the term *acute locked back.* In one mode of onset the patient is seized with sudden agonizing pain in the low back that is so severe as to preclude standing erect. In another mode of onset, the patient is only aware of a mild discomfort that begins with a remembered triggering movement that intensifies to severity within a few hours. Pain is localized to the lumbosacral level slightly to one side of midline and may occasionally radiate to the upper ipsilateral thigh, but never as far as the knee. There may be a history of one or more similar episodes in the past and patients typically remain completely symptom free between incidents. The patient climbs onto the examination table with difficulty, for fear of inducing further severe pain. Although immobility relieves discomfort, change of position greatly aggravates it. Walking is moderately comfortable provided they take small steps and do not climb stairs. During coughing and sneezing, patients will attempt to firmly brace themselves so as to minimize the jarring impact. Although lateral flexion to one side is possible, it is virtually impossible to the contralateral side. Transferring from sit to stand is done gingerly, whereas a mild lateral scoliosis, without a rotational component, may be apparent in the upright position. This trunk list is an attempt to ease pain and stand in a manner that provides maximal relief. Tenderness at the source of pain, as pointed out by the patient, is absent or mild at best even on firm palpation because the facet joints and laminae are not readily palpable owing to the interposed muscles and fasciae.[14] The straight leg raise test will provoke acute discomfort in the region of the posterior superior iliac spine as it aggravates the subluxated facet and not because of neurologic reasons. The neurologic examination is entirely normal in these patients. Radiographs are not appropriate, as they will be misleading if the patient stands with a pronounced tilt. The diagnosis is primarily based on the patient history and presentation. Manipulation is an effective and immediate treatment in the management of the acute locked back.[47]

22. What are the radiographic signs of degenerative disk disease (DDD) and posterior facet arthrosis?

Regardless of the cause of the degenerative process, the disk will gradually begin to narrow and the edges of the vertebral bodies contiguous with the disk may become sclerotic, although radiologic evidence of degeneration may require several years to become evident and even longer for radiographic confirmation of facet arthrosis. At times, early narrowing of the most commonly affected disk (L4/L5), the widest disk of the entire spine, is missed because it still appears wide relative to the disk above and below. If L4/L5 is narrower than the L3/L4 disk, it is suggestive of early degeneration. A *vacuum phenomenon* is occasionally evident on radiographs and tomographic scans, and appears as a dark area within the disk reflecting marked degeneration. The "vacuum" refers to the space resulting from loss of disk substance. With DDD, a *limbus vertebra* may occasionally be seen and refers to where the disk has ruptured transosseously, separating off the anterosuperior corner of the vertebra, resulting in disk narrowing.[47]

Lumbar spondylosis refers to the radiologic presence of narrowed disks with osteophyte formation. Approximation of vertebral bodies may be accompanied by marginal osteophytes developing along the margins of bulging disks, which may project anteriorly, laterally, or posteriorly. In some patients, the minute anteroposterior shearing movements allowed from degeneration cause the bulging disk to overlap the edge of the vertebral body so that the osteophytes that form are horizontally oriented and not level with the disk surface of the vertebral body. Traction spurs develop a few millimeters from the upper and lower borders of the vertebral bodies and grow into the attachments of the anterior longitudinal ligament and annular fibers, and are associated with disk degeneration.[38] The presence of these *traction osteophytes* is suggestive of the to-and-fro movement occurring at that segment[47] and implies some degree of anteroposterior instability. Thus there is a spectrum of osteophytes, from claw to traction spurs. *Claw-type osteophytes* develop at the edge of the vertebral margin around the annulus and sometimes meet

and fuse adjacent vertebrae together, are commonly seen on the concave side of a scoliosis, and may or may not be associated with disk degeneration. Osteophyte formation may be small or extensive, and may occur at the margins of the apophyseal joints. Degenerative changes may be localized to one level or may diffusely extend over several adjacent segments. A caveat is offered to the clinician regarding the tenuous practice of diagnosing spinal pathology based upon radiographs. Often, patients with severe lumbar spondylosis may be completely asymptomatic, whereas others may be aware of mild discomfort at times or suffer from severe chronic pain and have radiographs that appear normal. Thus the severity of a patient's pain is not proportional to the extent of radiologic findings. The good clinician will rely on history and clinical acumen before routinely ordering and viewing spinal radiographs.

23. How is DDD differentiated from the clinical presentation of herniated disk?

Although many symptoms of DDD may be similar to disk herniation, they differ in several respects. Patients with disk pathology often complain that sitting in any type of chair, hard or soft, aggravates pain as this flexed posture increases intradiskal pressure, causing the extruded material to bulge even more so. This is further aggravated by distention of the posterior longitudinal ligament, which increases radicular pressure and pain. As a result, forward flexion motions will be restricted secondary to pain. In contrast, patients with degenerative disk disease seldom have restriction of forward spinal motion, and complain of aggravated symptoms only in the soft chair-variety, but have no difficulty in sitting in a chair with a hard back.[47]

24. What physical therapy is appropriate in the management of DDD and posterior facet arthrosis?

Treatment focuses upon functional restoration consisting of muscle strengthening, improved flexibility and patient education. Many patients with DDD have weak trunk extensor muscle and weak upper and lower abdominal muscles. Various exercises are available to help "off-load" the spine and transfer some of the burden to the musculature, and thereby improve symptoms. A rigid orthosis may also provide relief.

- *Bracing.* Bracing via spinal orthoses is for the purpose of supporting the lower back in neutral, improving posture, and minimizing movement to the lumbar vertebrae. In addition, an orthosis can decrease intradiskal pressure[34] and may provide relief by way of local warmth and stimulation of mechanoreceptors. If only the lumbosacral region (L4-S1) is to be immobilized, then a lumbosacral support is indicated, whereas if the lesion is in the mid or upper lumbar region, a longer appliance is necessary. Supports within the canvas corset in the form of metal stays placed in posterior pockets fasten in front and have side straps for adjusting tightness. These supported forms of spinal corsets provide better relief than the same canvas without support.[32] Custom made supports are molded to the shape of the torso and are most useful for patients whose body configuration is difficult to fit with conventional supports. Body casts, composed of plaster of Paris or fiberglass are used when patients required constant immobilization such as after some surgical procedures. Elasticized supports do not restrict spinal movement and mostly benefit patients with poor posture as they hold in the abdomen, reduce lumbar lordosis, and allow the patient to look and feel better. Bracing is appropriate for any low back condition in which movements that stress the joint increase the discomfort. This is particularly relevant in patients with posterior facet arthrosis, spondylolysis and either isthmic or degenerative spondylolisthesis, in which extremes of flexion or extension result in pain and discomfort. A lumbar support will restrict excessive movement and force the patient to compensate for flexion at the hips and knees. With spondylolisthesis, bracing reduces the to-and-fro movement associated with pathology and is accompanied by gratifying pain relief. Patients with acute disk pathology may benefit from a spinal orthosis if they must carry heavy weights, work in a semi-stooped posture, or be involved in sports that involve spinal flexion and extension. The use of surgical corsets is helpful in patients suffering from acute disk herniation as restriction of flexion minimizes intradiskal pressure, and may be worn for as long as 6 weeks following preliminary bed rest. Bracing is also indicated for patients with infections, and for elderly osteoporotic patients suffering from repeated compression fractures.[47]

- *Exercises.* These are particularly relevant for patients having poor posture, a protuberant abdomen, and who are overweight. Neither lumbar extension nor abdominal strengthening exercise is indicated for the patients with acute episodes of low back pain, regardless of etiology. Spondylolytic patients (i.e., with spondylolysis and spondylolisthesis) will also benefit from abdominal strengthening exercises and should avoid extension exercises as that will further stress the pars interarticularis. In contrast, patients with degenerative spondylolisthesis and chronic disk degeneration would benefit from spinal extension exercises. Graduated extension exercises are highly beneficial for patients with compression fractures, whereas flexion exercises are contraindicated.* Slow squatting exercises are excellent for strengthening leg and thigh musculature. The most important flexion exercise is contraction of the abdominal muscles against resistance and achieved by the patient performing sit-ups or lying supine and elevating the lower limbs a few inches for 4 to 5 seconds and repeating the exercise. Intradiskal pressure can be reduced if the patient performs the sit-up while keeping the hips and knees slightly flexed and then raising the torso until the outstretched hands reach the knees. Alternately, the patient lies supine and raises his/her head and shoulders several inches and holds that position for 3 to 5 seconds. To maintain the range of motion in the facet joints, the patient may flex the knees fully and bring their knees up to their chest. Toe-touching exercises are not advised.[47]

- *Dynamic lumbar stabilization.* These programs are based on the idea that patients with a painful back can be taught to function within a pain-free range of activity through muscular development and movement patterns that stabilize the spine.[46] This concept is centered on the premise than an injured lumbar motion segment creates a weak link that is predisposed to injury and reinjury, that by strengthening torso musculature, the patient can be taught to maintain cocontraction of abdominal and gluteal muscles to provide a corseting effect on the lumbar spine. The patient learns to maintain the lumbar lordosis while keeping spinal posture in a *neutral position,* defined as the midpoint of available range of motion between anterior and posterior pelvic tilt. This position is often the one of greatest comfort and represents the loose-packed position which decreases tension on ligaments and joints, and permits a more balanced segmental forced distribution between the anterior and posterior spinal joints. Optimal muscle strength can protect the spinal motion segment from chronic repetitive stress or acute overload. The muscular spinal stabilizers include the abdominal muscles (especially

---

*However, if any particular exercise aggravates a patient's symptoms, it should be omitted, regardless of all theories to the contrary.

the transversus abdominis and obliquus internus), latissimus dorsi, the spinal intersegmental muscles (i.e. the multifidi, rotators, and interspinalis), the iliopsoas, the erector spinae and the quadratus lumborum. Cocontraction is initially performed while standing and later advanced to sitting, jumping, supine lying, bridging, prone lying, and quadruped positions with and without alternating arm and leg raises. Thus once neutral spine stabilization is mastered, postion transition exercises while maintaining precise pelvic control (and avoidance of torsion and shear) are accomplished by the addition of extremity exercises. The use of a physioball may enhance these rehabilitation techniques. Stabilization is an eclectic management strategy in that it also incorporates all other aspects of conservative treatment including joint mobilization, patient education, work hardening, flexion and extension exercise regimens, and physioball activities.

- *Stretching.* Correction of soft-tissue inflexibility of trunk musculature and especially the lower extremity is imperative toward optimal maintenance of the low back. A key element in maintaining the lumbosacral spine at the midway neutral location between anterior and posterior pelvic tilt is adequate stretching of the hip flexor and extensor musculature. These large muscles which span across significant lengths of the trunk or lower extremities affect the low back due to their insertion on the pelvis. Posterior pelvic tilt often occurs because of tight hamstrings, acting to increase shear in the low back and predispose for facet and disk degeneration.[47] In contrast, excessive anterior pelvic tilt often occurs because shortening of the iliopsoas muscles may result in spinal and central stenosis by narrowing the intervertebral foramina and central spinal canal, respectively.[26] The hip flexors and extensors, in particular, should be stretched because tightness of these muscles will rotate the pelvis excessively,* and may negatively impact on both posture and the magnitude of lumbar lordosis. Hyperlordosis is associated with anterior pelvic tilt, which causes the pelvis to rotate forward due to tightened hip flexors. Tight hamstrings cause a pull on the pel-

---

*Pelvic rotation is known as *pelvic tilt* which is defined in relation to the anterior superior iliac spine (ASIS). Anterior pelvic tilt, associated with tight iliopsoas and quadriceps muscles as well as hyperlordosis, involves the ASIS moving anteriorly and downward. In contrast, posterior pelvic tilt is associated with hypolordosis and tightened and tightened hamstring musculature, and involves the ASIS moving posteriorly and upward.

vis to rotate it backwardly about the common hip axis as posterior pelvic tilt and therefore increase shear of L5 ("sliding down the hill") on S1.

- *Patient education.* This is a *central* concept in the management of low back pain and perhaps the most important component of any back care program including acute injury.[23] Patients need to be reassured that the majority of patient with low back pain recover following time and conservative treatment. Often, telling patients that they will be able to go back to work once they get better removes a great deal of anxiety.

Sitting—A firm straight-back chair is preferred by most patients as this supports the back and maintains a normal lumbar lordosis, whereas soft easy chairs and sofa induces flexion and may aggravate symptoms due to a reversal of the lordotic curve. The latter provide relief for patients with spinal stenosis because flexion relieves their discomfort. Chairs should preferable have armrests, and car seats should be slid as forward as possible so as to bring the legs closer to the foot pedals. In a seat situated far back, the spine must accentuate lordosis as the legs extend downward to reach the pedals, and this may induce low back pain. For patients with chronic back pain or osteoporosis with or without compression fracture, upright sitting must be avoided as it increases the tendency to compression collapse. The load on both the vertebrae, posterior and anterior elements are markedly reduced in the semi-reclining position when sitting on a recliner.

Standing—To avoid symptoms when standing for long periods, patients may find relief by raising one foot on a step or stool as this reduces lumbar lordosis. High heels are to be avoided in those patients in which increased lumbar lordosis worsens symptoms.

Walking more briskly is often more comfortable than walking slowly. Shoes may be fitted with Sorbothane inserts to reduce the concussive jarring effects of heel strike on the low back.

Bending—When flexing the spine from the upright position, the range of hip flexion indicates tightness (and hence flexibility) of the hamstrings, which is felt as a pulling sensation behind the knees. Because the hamstrings attach on the pelvis, hamstring strain may occur on further flexion. Also, excessive flexion considerably increases intradiskal pressure and may exacerbate an already painful condition. Patients with back pain can avoid this by bending at the hips and knees so as to maintain a normal lumbar curve.

Wearing a lumbosacral corset for several weeks assists the patient in habituating this type of bend.

Sleeping—The type of bed or recumbent posture used depends on the cause of back pathology. The objective of choosing a mattress is based upon one that maintains the spinal curves in as natural position as possible. Unnatural curves imposed upon the spine from a sagging mattress may cause patient to complain of aching, especially on getting up in the morning. A firm mattress with a nonsagging base is recommended. Patients with spondylolisthesis and many with degenerative facet arthrosis prefer not to sleep prone or lie on a soft and sagging mattress, as this increases the lumbar lordosis and aggravates their symptoms.

Carrying—Patient with low back pain should avoid carrying or lifting heavy weights whenever possible. If lifting is necessary, patient should never stretch forward to lift the weight as this excessively strains the lumbar spine by increasing the length of the lever arm from the fulcrum. Instead, patients should flex as the hip and knees and, with the back held straight, should keep the weight as close to the center of gravity located at the S2 level. Sudden loads should be avoided. Intradiskal pressure is less when objects are pushed, so that pushing is preferable to pulling.

- *Modalities.* The use of physical modalities may help relieve the pain associated with the acute phase. Cold therapy decreases spasm, inflammation, pain, and capillary blood flow, and is particularly helpful in cases of acute annular tear or ligament sprain. Although the skin cools quickly, the rate of muscle cooling is directly proportionate to the thickness of overlying fat and may range for 10 to 30 minutes.[29] The subacute or chronic states are preferably treated with thermotherapy such as deep heat (ultrasound, microwave, or short-wave) that minimizes spasm and pain. Electrostimulation in the form of transcutaneous electrical nerve stimulation (TENS) or high volt galvanic stimulation (HVGS) may reduce acute muscle spasm, decrease edema, and relieve pain.[44] The mechanism for pain relief from TENS involves raising the circulating levels of endogenous endorphins or by stimulating cutaneous afferents that block pain stimuli in the substantia gelatinosa.[31] Percutaneous dorsal column stimulators can also help patients with chronic back pain.[39]

- *Weight reduction.* Excessive weight may range from mild to morbid obesity and is often associated with poor posture. Because obesity aggravates symptom-atology of low back pain, regardless of the etiology, actual reduction in body mass is an essential component of conservative management.[47] Because of the protruding abdomen that often accompanies obesity, the lower back is postured in excessive lordosis, placing strain on the posteriorly located facet joints as they undergo excessive axial compression. Hyperlordosis of the lumbar spine in turn is accompanied by excessive anterior pelvic tilt, which causes foreshortening of the hip flexors, and serves to reinforce the lumbar lordosis. For many persons in industrialized countries who struggle with excessive weight, overeating, hormonal imbalances such as thyroid disease not withstanding, is often an issue of ennui and a sense of boredom. Being a universally difficult goal, patients requiring weight loss may well be referred to experts in that field.

- *Endurance training.* Cardiovascular and cardiopulmonary fitness are extremely important and may include brisk walking, jogging, swimming, tennis, and stationary bicycle activities. Many patients find that brisk walking eases their discomfort. Aerobic fitness activities should emphasize activities that avoid high-impact and ballistic-type spinal movements.

- *Pharmacology.* Pharmacologic treatments may be categorized into analgesics that relieve pain, antiinflammatory medications, and muscle relaxants. Antiinflammatory drugs have both an antiinflammatory and analgesic effect that promote healing by increasing circulation and bringing necessary nutrient into the inflamed area and eliminating toxic inflammatory substances, thereby allowing patients to more fully participate in physical therapy and activities of daily living. Antiinflammatory medications appear to be effective for relieving back pain if started within 2 days of onset of acute low back pain.[1] Muscle relaxants, whose site of action is either the muscle spindle or the central nervous system, operate from relieving skeletal muscle spasm in the back without interfering with muscular function. In this manner they promote greater mobility that is essential to the recuperative process. Opioid analgesics interact by binding to the body's opiate receptors for endorphins and enkephalins, and are appropriate for severely acute back pain. If used on a short-time contingency basis there is little chance for addiction.[52] Use of opioid analgesic for chronic back pain is discouraged because of the potential for addiction. Antidepressant drugs may elevate mood and increase pain tolerance in the emotionally depressed patient, reducing chronic low back pain.[58]

- *Selective injection.* Therapeutic short or long acting injection of steroids and anesthetics is often performed by an anesthesiologist into the epidural space, which surrounds the dural covering of the spinal cord, exiting spinal nerves, the nerve roots, facet joints, and trigger points.[59] Epidural steroid injections may be appropriate for disk related pathology such as annular tears, disk herniations, radiculopathy, and spinal stenosis.

Other forms of treatment include relaxation techniques,[51] therapeutic massage, myofascial release, as well as acupuncture, acupressure, and electroacupuncture along hypothetical body meridians.[57] For patients whose symptoms are recalcitrant to conservative management, the *pain clinic* may offer relief of pain.

RECOMMENDED READING

Seimon LP: *Low back pain: clinical diagnosis and management,* ed 2, New York, 1995, Demos Vermande.

White AH, Schofferman JA editors: *Spine care: diagnosis and conservative treatment,* St Louis, 1995, Mosby.

REFERENCES

1. Amlie E, Weber H, Holme I: Treatment of acute low back pain with Piroxicam: results of a double-blind placebo-controlled trial, *Spine* 12:473, 1987.
2. Boshinzen HC, Bongers PM, Hulshof CTJ: Self-reported back pain in fork-lift, container, tractor drivers exposed to whole body vibration, *Spine* 17:59 1992.
3. Boukris R, Becker KL: Schmorl's nodes and osteoporosis, *Clin Orthop* 104:275, 1974.
4. Brown MD, Lockwoood JM: *Degenerative spondylolisthesis, Intr Course Lect Am Acad Orthop Surg,* St Louis, 1983, Mosby.
5. Brown T, et al: Some mechanical tests on the lumbosacral spine with particular reference to the intervertebral disc, *J Bone Joint Surg* 39A;1135, 1937.
6. Cauchoix J, Benoist M, Chassaing V: Degenerative spondylolisthesis, *Clin Orthop* 115:122, 1976.
7. Chrisman OD: Biochemical aspect of degenerative joint disease, *Clin Orthop* 64:77, 1969.
8. Cramer GD, Darby SA: *Basic and clinical anatomy of the spine, spinal cord, and ANS,* St Louis, 1995, Mosby.
9. Dunlop RB, Adams MA, Hutton WC: Disc space narrowing and the lumbar facet joint, *J Bone Joint Surg* 66:706, 1984.
10. Dupuis PR, et al: Radiologic diagnosis of degenerative lumbar spinal instability, *Spine* 10:262, 1988.
11. Ehni G: Effects of certain degenerative disease of the spine, especially spondylolysis and disc protrusion of the neural contents particular in the lumbar region: historical account, *May Clin Proc* 50:327, 1976.
12. Epstein JA, Epstein BS, Lavine L: Nerve root compression associated with narrowing of the lumbar spinal canal, *J Neurol Neurosurg Psychiat* 25:165, 1962.
13. Epstein NE, Epstein JA, Carras R et al: Degenerative spondylolisthesis with an intact neural arch: a review of 60 cases with an analysis of clinical findings and the development of surgical management, *Neurosurgery* 13:555, 1983.
14. Fairband JC, Hall H: History taking and physical examination: Identification of syndromes of back pain. In Weinstein JN, Wiesel SW, editors: *The lumbar spine,* Philadelphia, 1990, WB Saunders.
15. Farfan HF, Cossette JW, Robertson GH et al: The effects of torsion of the lumbar intervertebral joints: the role of torsion in the production of disc degeneration, *J Bone Joint Surg* 52A:468, 1970.
16. Farfan HG: The pathological anatomy of degenerative spondylolisthesis: a cadaver study, *Spine* 5:412, 1980.
17. Gertzbein SD, Tile M, Gross A et al: Autoimmunity in degenerative disc disease of the lumbar spine, *Orthop Clin North Am* 6:67, 1975.
18. Giles LG, Taylor JR: Human zygapophyseal joint capsule and synovial fold innervation, *Br J Rheumatol* 26:93, 1987.
19. Giles LG: The pathophysiology of the zygapophyseal joints. In: Haldeman S editor: *Principles and practice of chiropractic,* ed 2, East Norwalk, Conn., 1992, Appleton & Lange.
20. Hasue M, Kikuchi S, Sakuyama Y et al: Anatomic study of the interrelation between lumbosacral nerve roots and their surrounding tissues, *Spine* 8:50-58 1983.
21. Hirsch C, Naehemson A: New observations on the mechanical behavior of lumbar discs, *Acta Orthop Scand* 23:254, 1954.
22. Hoppenfeld S: *Orthopaedic neurology: a diagnostic guide to neurologic levels,* Philadelphia, 1977, JB Lippincott.
23. Jackson CP: Historic perspectives on patient education and its place in acute spinal disorders. In Mayer TG, Mooney V, Gatchel RJ editors: *Contemporary conservative care for painful spinal disorders,* Philadelphia, 1991, Lea & Febiger.
24. Jackson DW, Lowery WD, Ciullo JV: Injuries of the spine. In Nicholas JA, Hershman EB editors: *The lower extremity and spine in sports medicine,* ed 2, St Louis, 1995, Mosby.
25. Jeffries B: Facet joint injections, *Spine: state of the art reviews* 2:409, 1988.
26. Keim HA, Kirkaldy-Willis WH: *Low back pain, clinical symposia,* vol 39, West Caldwell, NJ, 1987, CIBA-GEIGY.
27. Kirkaldy-Willis WH, Wedge JH, Yong-Hing K et al: Pathology and pathogenesis of lumbar spondylosis and stenosis, *Spine* 3:319, 1978.
28. Kirkaldy-Willis WH: *Managing low back pain,* ed 2, New York, 1988, Churchill Livingstone.
29. Lehman J: Therapeutic heat and cold, *Clin Orthop* 99:207, 1974.
30. McCall IW, Park WM, O'Brien JP et al: Acute traumatic intraosseous disc herniation, *Spine* 10:134, 1985.
31. Melzack R, Wall PD: Pain mechanisms: a new theory, *Science* 50:971, 1965.
32. Million R, Nilsen KH, Jayson MIV et al: Evaluation of low back pain and assessment of lumbar corsets without and without back supports, *Ann Rheum Dis* 40:449, 1981.
33. Myklebust JB, Pintar F, Yoganandan N et al: Tensile strength of spinal ligaments, *Spine* 13(5):526, 1988.
34. Nachemson A: Lumbar spine instability; a critical update and symposium summary, *Spine* 10:290, 1985.

35. Newman PH, Stone KH: The etiology of spondylolisthesis with a special investigation, *J Bone Joint Surg* 45B:39, 1963.

36. Newman PH: Surgical treatment for spondylolisthesis in the adult, *Clin Orthop* 117:106, 1976.

37. Pope MH, Wilder DG, Krag MH: Biomechanics of the lumbar spine. In Frymoyer JM editor: *The adult spine: principles and practice,* New York, 1991, Raven Press.

38. Quinnel RC, Stockdale HR: The significance of osteophytes on the lumbar vertebral bodies in relation to discographic findings, *Clin Radiol* 23:197, 1982.

39. Racz GB, McCarron RF, Talboys P: Percutaneous dorsal column stimulator for chronic pain control, *Spine* 14:1, 1989.

40. Radin EL, Rose RM: Role of subchondral bone in initiation and progress of cartilage damage, *Clin Orthop* 213:34, 1986.

41. Radin EL: The physiology and degeneration of joints, *Semin Arthritis Rheum* 2(3):245, 1972-1973.

42. Rauschning W: Normal and pathologic anatomy of the lumbar root canals, *Spine* 12, 1987.

43. Roaf R: A study of the mechanics of spinal injuries, *J Bone Joint Surg* 42B:810, 1960.

44. Roeser WM, Meeks LW, Venis R, et al: The use of transcutaneous nerve stimulation for pain control in athletic medicine: a preliminary report, *Am J Sports Med* 4:210-213, 1976.

45. Rothman RH, Simeone FA: *The spine,* vol 1, Philadelphia, 1975, WB Saunders.

46. Saal JA, Saal JS: Non operative treatment of herniated lumbar intervertebral disc with radiculopathy: an outcome study, *San Francisco Spine Institute,* August, 1988.

47. Seimon LP: *Low back pain—clinical diagnosis and management,* ed 2, New York, 1995, Demos Vermande.

48. Selby DK: The structural degenerative cascade. In White AH, Schofferman JA editors: *Spine care: diagnosis and treatment,* vol 1, St Louis, 1995, Mosby.

49. Sledge CB: Structure, development and function of joints, *Orthop Clin North Am* 6(3):619, 1975.

50. Sokoloff L: Pathology and pathogenesis of osteoarthritis. In McCarty DJ editor: *Arthritis and allied conditions,* Philadelphia, 1979, Lea & Febiger.

51. Sternbach RA: *Mastering pain,* New York, 1987, Putnam Books.

52. Stimmel B: Pain, analgesia, and addiction: an approach to the pharmacological management of pain, *Clin J Pain* 1:14, 1985.

53. Taylor JR, Twomey LT: Age changes in lumbar zygapophyseal joints: observations on structure and function, *Spine* 11:739, 1986.

54. Vane J: Inhibition of prostaglandin synthesis as a mechanism of action of aspirin-like drugs, *Nature New Biol* 231:232, 1971.

55. Venner RM, Crock HV: Clinical studies of isolated disc resorption in the lumbar spine, *J Bone Joint Surg* 63B:491, 1981.

56. Vital JM, Lavignolle B, Grenier N, et al: Anatomy of the lumbar radicular canal, *Anat Clin* 5:141-151, 1983.

57. Wallnofer H, von Rottauscher A: *Chinese folk medicine and acupuncture.* New York, 1965, Bell.

58. Ward NG: Tricyclic antidepressants for chronic low back pain: mechanisms of action and predictors of response, *Spine,* 11:661, 1986.

59. White AH, Derby R, Wynne G: Epidural injections for the diagnosis and treatment of low back pain, *Spine* 5:78, 1980.

59

Acute, Localized, Low Back Pain After Sudden Movement that Progressively Worsens and Accompanied by Palpable Tenderness Without Sensory, Motor, or Reflex Deficit

CASE 1: A 27-year-old triage nurse at a trauma hospital assisted emergency medical person-nel in lowering an injured patient from an ambulance onto the pavement outside the hospi-tal emergency room. Instead of facing the patient cot directly, she bent downward with a twist to one side and gave it a sudden tug to lift it, together with other personnel, off the floor. As it was unexpectedly heavy and caught her offguard, she felt something "snap" in her back and experienced severe mid-lumbar pain. For several minutes, she was "frozen" in the semi-flexed position, and gradually came upright. Pain remained intense for approxi-mately 5 minutes and then eased off only to increase again ½ hour later and became pro-gressively worse over the subsequent few hours. As any movement aggravates pain, bending in any direction is impossible. She reports marked relief when recumbent in the side-lying or supine position, although prone lying and turning over in bed aggravate symp-toms. Sitting relieves symptoms , although sit to stand transfer is performed gingerly, with the patient easing herself down very carefully taking the weight of her torso through her arms. This maneuver was repeated when she climbed onto the examination table. When asked to localize the maximal site of pain she points to the area of the L3 spinous process.

OBSERVATION   She is healthy looking with no obvious deformity.

PALPATION   Point tenderness at the L4/S5 region.

RANGE OF MOTION   Range of motion is untested secondary to back pain. Normal range of motion to bilateral lower extremities. Straight leg raising is 80° bilaterally.

STRENGTH   Patient stands on heels, toes, and borders of feet without difficulty.

DEEP TENDON REFLEXES   These are normal.

PERIPHERAL CIRCULATION   This is normal.

SPECIAL TESTS   Negative Lasègue, squat test, and sacroiliac compression/distraction tests.

RADIOGRAPHS   Oblique radiographs show intact pars interarticularis and no evidence of vertebral fracture.

CASE 2: A 50-year-old chief executive corporate officer set out on a Sunday afternoon, snow shovel in hand, to clear his driveway and sidewalk of the 4 inches of snow that fell earlier that day. This labor-intensive task took him approximately 1½ hours, after which he felt pleased with himself. On waking up the next morning he experienced severe pain in the low back and buttocks that caused him significant difficulty in rising from bed and going to the bathroom. He could not bend over to wash his face, nor could he bend over for the next 2 days. His chief complaint was an ache, which has not diminished in the 2 days since it began, although he feels mildly improved today. Sneezing and coughing provoke his aching. When asked whether he felt any pain or discomfort while shoveling he replied "no." He does not regularly exercise because of his many responsibilities at work which, he complains, leave no time for stretching or strengthening activities.

OBSERVATION   There is normal standing posture with no obvious deformity. The patient, slightly obese, walking into the examination area very carefully and with small steps. He diffusely indicates the thoracolumbar paravertebral region to indicate the area of maximal pain. Sit to stand transfer is performed gingerly, taking care to keep his back straight. He climbs onto the examination table with difficulty, appearing stiff. No swelling is observed.

PALPATION   Diffuse tenderness over the thoracolumbar paraspinal musculature.

RANGE OF MOTION   All lumbar movements are markedly decreased.

STRENGTH   This is normal to bilateral lower extremities.

FLEXIBILITY   There is moderate tightness noted in bilateral hamstrings, psoas, and hip adductors.

DEEP TENDON REFLEXES   There is no reflex deficit noted.

PULSES   These are normal.

SPECIAL TESTS   Negative straight leg raise, Lasègue's, hip scouring, pelvic spring, and squat tests.

CASE 3: A 44-year-old housewife presents with a chronic history of low back pain that has been present for at least 10 years duration. She has had 3 pregnancies in the last 4 years and is approximately 25 lbs overweight. She cannot trace onset of symptoms to a specific event, and whereas aching is usually mild, over the past 6 months it has increased in severity and has begun to interfere with her activities. Occasionally, she has severe episodes that last several days and later settle down. Symptoms are aggravated by activities that require her to bend over, such as washing the dishes, ironing clothes, or giving her infant a bath in the tub, as well as standing, sitting, and walking for greater than 1½ hours. She has never experienced pain in recumbency, or any peripheralization of pain. Discomfort is occasionally reported when she carries heavy packages. When asked, she says that coughing, sneezing, or other jarring movements do not aggravate symptoms. Prior to her marriage 6 years ago she regularly played tennis and swam, although she complains that she no longer has time to participate in these or any other sport-related activities.

OBSERVATION   She stands erect with no apparent deformity, except a mild increase in lumbar lordosis. Her abdomen is protruding and her buttocks are prominent.

PALPATION   There is mild midline tenderness over the lumbosacral region. No "step" or swelling noted.

RANGE OF MOTION   The patient can easily touch her toes. Her range of spinal motion is average.

STRENGTH   The patient can walk on her heels, toes, and bilateral borders of her feet.

FLEXIBILITY   There is moderate tightness noted in bilateral hip flexors.

SENSATION   Sensation is normal.

DEEP TENDON REFLEXES   These are normal.

PULSES   These are normal.

SPECIAL TESTS   Negative spring, scouring, Lasègue's, femoral nerve stretch tests. Positive Thomas test.

CLUE   Increased lumbosacral angle noted on radiographs.

? Questions

1. What is most likely the cause of these patients' symptoms?
2. What are the spine and vertebral column?
3. What are the components and function of the vertebral body?
4. What is the role of spinal torsion in human locomotion?
5. What advantage is conferred upon the spine by virtue of its sagittal curves?
6. What is the difference between ligamentous and muscle tissue with respect to injury and soft-tissue repair?
7. Which ligaments reinforce the anterior intervertebral joints and posterior facet joints at each segment?
8. What is the anatomy of the anterior longitudinal ligament?
9. What is the anatomy of the posterior longitudinal ligament?
10. How has the posterior longitudinal ligament become an anatomical risk factor for posterior disk pathology during the transition from the quadruped to the biped posture?
11. What is the anatomy and function of the ligamentum flavum?
12. What is the anatomy and function of the supraspinous and interspinous ligaments?
13. What is the anatomy of the thoracolumbar fascia?
14. What is the function of the thoracolumbar fascia?
15. What are shear and torsional forces, and what segment of the lumbar spine is most vulnerable to these forces?
16. Which osseous and soft-tissue structures are effective restrainers of shear forces in the low back?
17. What is the role of the musculoligamentous system in attenuating torsion forces in the low back?
18. What is the anatomy of the corporotransverse ligament and how may it contribute to pathologic root entrapment?
19. What is the organization and function of the muscles of the back?
20. What are the various layers of back musculature?
21. What are the "true" back muscles?
22. What are the anterolateral abdominal muscles and what is their role in stabilization of the spine?
23. What is the role of the psoas major and quadratus lumborum muscles in relation to the spine?
24. What other muscles of the lower extremity indirectly affect the spine by virtue of their effect on pelvic rotation?

25. How do the trunk and lower extremity muscles relate as biomechanical force couples?
26. What is the effect of pelvic tilt on lumbar lordosis and how is this mediated by the muscles of the trunk and lower extremity?
27. How do the muscles of the trunk act to eccentrically stabilize the spinal column?
28. What is correct posture, and how may faulty posture lead to musculoskeletal pathology?
29. What are common causes of excessive lordosis and kyphosis, and what are other common postural deformities of the spine?

30. What pathologic changes occur in the soft and articular tissues owing to faulty posture?
31. What are postural strain syndromes and what is their clinical and radiologic presentation?
32. What are the biomechanical and clinical definitions of *stress* and *strain?*
33. What is the clinical presentation of ligamentous sprain and muscular strain?
34. What is the differential diagnosis?
35. What physical therapy is appropriate in the management of these injuries?

1. What is most likely the cause of these patients' symptoms?

The history and clinical presentation of Case 1 of acute low back pain that was accompanied by a snapping sensation that increased in severity over the next few hours and then remained constant suggests either ligamentous sprain, annular tear, acute disk prolapse, or fracture of the pars interarticularis. Local tenderness could be accounted for by either local ligamentous injury or via referred movement to the fracture site on applying pressure to the spinous process. Nor is there any palpable "step" that so often accompanies spondylolisthesis. Radiographs showed an intact pars interarticularis. Vertebral compression fracture is ruled out by radiographs, and this patient is probably too young to have osteoporosis and has no history of bone disease. With an acute annulus tear, the annulus fibrosus is too deeply placed to cause provocation with pinpoint tenderness. The same may be said for acute disk prolapse. With the latter, there may be accompanying sciatica, and the patient with acute disk prolapse frequently cannot find a comfortable position, whereas the patient with ligamentous disruption, once having found a position of comfort, feels much better and loathes moving out of this position. Having ruled out several other possibilities, a presumed diagnosis of ligamentous sprain of the low back was concluded and confirmed by pain relief and improved range of motion for several hours following infiltration of 4 cc of local anesthetic. Any discussion of musculoligamentous pathology of the spine is predicated upon understanding the role of these soft tissues in maintaining spinal curvature, absorbing energy, maintaining posture, and facilitating as well as limiting spinal motion.

The history and clinical presentation of Case 2 suggests a muscular strain in which pain does not occur at the time of injury, but many hours later. When a patient is relatively deconditioned, their muscular circulation is incapable of coping with the sudden accumulation of noxious metabolic by-products (lactic acid) causing intramuscular irritation that is perceived as aching and stiffness. The patient in Case 2 is similar to the first time runner who, delighted to cover a mile of distance the first day, wakes up the next morning with legs so sore, stiff, and tender that he can barely walk to the bathroom. Muscular strain may also refer to tearing of muscle tissue. In contrast to ligamentous sprain, pain and tenderness derived from muscular strain generally extends over a very wide area.

The history and clinical presentation of Case 3 suggests *postural strain syndrome,* which is frequently encountered in patients who are chronically inactive, overweight, and who frequently maintain faulty posture or whose work environment involves maintenance of abnormal posture in the absence of objective motor, sensory, or reflex disturbance. The patient typically presents with chronic, mild low back pain, aggravated by prolonged sitting, walking, and especially standing, with relief in recumbency and when sitting for short periods. All spinal motions are typically within functional limits. Frequently, chores such as washing dishes, doing the laundry, and vacuuming aggravate discomfort. Although chronic degenerative disk disease with mild facet arthrosis may mimic this presentation, radiographs show no abnormalities with the exception of an increased lumbosacral angle. The patient often demonstrates a positive Thomas test. Symptoms in these patients generally result from chronically poor posture secondary to inadequate musculature.[78] The abdomen is prominent when standing and the lumbar lordosis is increased, which in turn strains the pain-sensitive soft tissues of the low back.

2. What are the spine and vertebral column?

The major portion of the axial skeleton located below the skull is the *spine*,[60] which may be defined as the vertebral column and its contents, and the adjacent soft tissue comprised of the muscles, ligaments, nerves, and blood vessels of the vertebral column. The osseous components of the spine comprise a series of articulated vertebrae that constitute the central, axial skeleton of the body. The phylum Chordata was an evolutionary success primarily because it offered an internal framework (endoskeleton) that was lighter, more flexible, and more versatile that the outer shells of other phyla, which were burdened by the sheer weight of a cumbersome exoskeleton.[3] As the subphylum Vertebrata in the animal kingdom compromises all animals that have a spinal column, the primary function of the *vertebral column* is to endow the body with longitudinal rigidity in a segmented manner. This relates to the protective role to the neurovascular components within the spine that is offered by the osseous components.

3. What are the components and function of the vertebral body?

The vertebral column is composed of segmental rings of bone known as *vertebrae* (see Fig. 57-2). The *vertebral body,* wider transversely than from front to back, is designed to bear weight while the posterior elements comprising the vertebral arch form a triangular vertebral foramen that encases, and thereby protects the spinal cord like a ring of armor. The vertebral or neural arch is a ring of bone formed by two pedicles, laminae, transverse processes, four articular processes that connect the vertebrae above and below, and one spinous process. The *neural arch* primarily serves to transmit the stabilizing forces from the articular and muscular processes posteriorly to the anterior intervertebral joint. Without the restraining action of the facet joints and soft tissues anteriorly, the interbody joint, which is essentially a ball bearing would become destabilized during bending movements. The transverse processes emerge laterally, while the spinous process projects posteriorly from the center of the rings. The function of both processes is to serve as attachment sites for ligaments and postural muscles, while acting as a series of levers so that muscles attaching to both sides perform active movement.[89]

In addition to constituting a firm base from which structures such as the ribs and abdominal muscles are suspended, the vertebrae function as a system of levers and articulate with each other via the posterior facet joints and anterior interbody disk joints that function as pivots. In this system of levers, the ligaments function as passive restraints, while the muscular attachments operate as activators.[88] Each segment, through the vertebral arches, forms a first class lever system where the articular processes serve as a fulcrum. Thus axial compressive loads are applied through the vertebral column with direct and passive absorption of load at the disk and indirect absorption by the muscles and ligaments.[40]

4. What is the role of spinal torsion in human locomotion?

The earliest vertebrates were the Pisces (Latin for *fishes*) and existed in a buoyant environment and had no requirement for their spine to assume a weight-bearing function. At most, the spine undulated to-and-fro as it does in fish and snakes, thus operating in a locomotive capacity to propel the organism through its environment. As the vertebral column was not initially designed for weight bearing, vertebrate design in humans has accommodated to the upright posture in a gravitational environment. Our vertebral column constitutes an arched, horizontal bridge between the four limbs that suspends the abdominal and thoracic cavities, while balancing a head atop the cervical spine that serves as a cantilever extension permitting the head to move about in space. The primary locomotive function of the spine in lower organisms has been preserved in humans as torsion of the axial skeleton during our uniquely alternating reciprocal bipedal gait.

Torsion confers a valuable advantage to bipedal gait. In early vertebrates, the spine was essential in locomotion. Indeed, that fishlike segmented amphioxus (i.e. lancelet), which so closely resembles the early human embryo, moved through its aquatic environment with fishlike undulations of its spine. Movement of the spine, preserved as torsion, may have been preserved through the evolutionary process if we conceive of a *spinal engine* that facilitates driving the pelvis forward in our reciprocal bipedal gait. Our spine may act to convert the primitive lateral bend of our fishlike ancestors into an axial torque.[51] Indeed, the reciprocal and opposite motions of the upper and lower extremities act as an energy storage and release mechanism. The locus of this mechanism is the spine, and is observed as reverse rotations between the shoulder and pelvic girdles during the gait cycle.[29]

5. What advantage is conferred upon the spine by virtue of its sagittal curves?

Although the normal spine appears rectilinear in the coronal plane, it has four curvatures in the sagittal plane (Fig. 59-1). The thoracic and sacral regions are kyphotic (concave forward), being present at birth and lie opposite the thoracic and pelvic visceral cavities. The two lordotic curves (convex forward) are located at the cervical and lumbar regions, arising during infancy as weight bearing occurs, and characterize the regions of the vertebral column with the greatest mobility. The 3 mobile curves, in and of themselves, convey an advantage to the erect spine to withstand compressive forces 10 times that of uniformly straight spine.[40] Axial compressive loading of the spine tends to accentuate

the spinal curvatures, and may be resisted, in part, by tension developed in the ligaments along the convex aspect of the curves. Thus although the curvatures endow the spine with a springlike capacity for absorbing energy and increasing flexibility, variations in compressive load may be statically attenuated by variations in ligamentous tension.

6. What is the difference between ligamentous and muscle tissue with respect to injury and soft-tissue repair?

Ligaments are noncontractile structures comprised of dense connective tissue, and are in the majority, inelastic, with a poor vascular supply. Although ligaments normally receive blood vessels from periarticular arterial plexuses that are easily damaged,[66] intraligamentous vessels are sparse, so that some degree of diffusion is necessary for midsubstance cellular nutrition. Consequently, ligaments heal poorly following injury. The biomechanical properties of ligaments are such that during a slow rate of loading, avulsion failure at the ligament insertion to bone is more likely, whereas during a rapid rate of loading, midsubstance ligament tears are common. In the spine, the numerous processes of the posterior elements serve to allow for both muscular and ligamentous attachment, whereas the longer (e.g., transverse) processes act as levers to enhance the actions of the attached muscles.

7. Which ligaments reinforce the anterior intervertebral joints and posterior facet joints at each segment?

The anteriorly located intervertebral joints are reinforced by the anterior and posterior longitudinal ligaments spanning their ventral and dorsal aspects. The anterior and posterior longitudinal ligaments are also known as the *intercentral ligaments* because they connect the anterior and posterior surfaces of adjacent vertebral bodies (centra).[30] These ligaments also serve to attach the vertebral bodies to the intervertebral disks. Although the longitudinal ligaments reinforce the anterior interbody joint at each segment, the *posterior ligaments of the vertebral arches* support the posterior zygapophyseal facet joints and include the ligamentum flavum, the interspinous ligament, and the supraspinous ligament. A second classification of spinal ligaments organizes them as either continuous or interrupted. The continuous ligaments include the anterior and posterior longitudinal ligaments, and the supraspinous ligament. The interrupted ligaments include

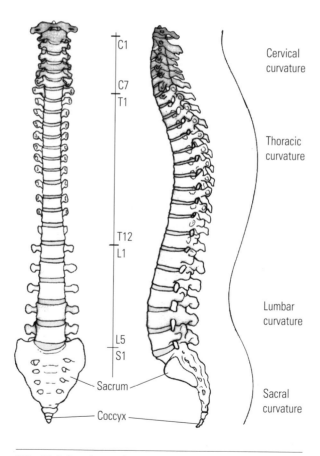

FIG. 59-1 Complete spine. Anterior and lateral views. (From Mathers LH et al: *Clinical anatomy principles*, St Louis, 1996, Mosby.)

the ligamentum flavum and the interspinous ligament (Fig. 59-2).

8. What is the anatomy of the anterior longitudinal ligament?

The *anterior longitudinal ligament,* providing anterior stability to the spine, extends the full length of the spine from the occiput to the sacrum. Beginning at the anterior tubercle at the atlas, and rather narrow at the level of C2, the anterior longitudinal ligament broadens as it descends and firmly adheres to the anterior margins of the vertebral bodies and disks. This ligament consists of a superficial layer consisting of long fibers that span as many as 5 vertebrae, and a deep layer that is intimately blended with the anterior vertebral periosteum and outer-anterior fibers of the annulus fibrosus. The anterior longitudinal ligament has a tensile strength of 676 N[61] or nearly 3000[22] psi functions to resist vertical separation of the anterior margins of the bodies, limits flexion and prevents hyperflexion, acts to support by

reinforcement of the anterior disks during the lifting of heavy loads,[27] and may be torn during extension injuries of the spine. The anterior longitudinal ligament receives sensory (nociceptive and proprioceptive) innervation from branches of the gray communicating rami of the lumbar sympathetic trunk, so that damage to this ligament during extension injuries may be a direct source of pain.

9. What is the anatomy of the posterior longitudinal ligament?

The *posterior longitudinal ligament,* providing posterior stability to the spine, is considerably less sturdy than its anterior counterpart and extends from the axis to the sacrum. Proximally, its upper end is continuous with the tectorial membrane in the high cervical region serving to separate the basivertebral plexus from the dural sac of the spinal cord. Broader above than below, the posterior longitudinal ligament descends as a narrow band along the posterior surface of the vertebrae and interbody joints. Although the posterior longitudinal ligament adheres to the intervertebral disks at each level, it is not attached to the dorsal surface of the vertebral bodies due to the interposition of the basivertebral veins that join the anterior internal vertebral venous plexus. Although having relatively thick attachments centrally, they are serrated in appearance as they extend laterally. Possessing a denticulated appearance, the posterior longitudinal ligament flares laterally at each intervertebral disk where it attaches to the posterior aspect of the annulus fibrosus. The ligament is essentially bowstrung across the posterior aspect of the vertebral column, resulting in a small, thin attachment laterally within a rhomboidal area posterolaterally. The serrated outline of the ligament renders it unlikely to have any substantial mechanical role, and it is indeed, identified as an anatomic risk factor for posterolateral disk protrusion and herniation. Of the 2 layers comprising the posterior longitudinal ligament, the deeper layer spans only 2 articulations, whereas the fibers of the more superficial layer span as many as five vertebras. The posterior longitudinal ligament, running inside and posterior to the vertebral canal, prevents hyperextension and allows for flexion of the spine. Substance P, a sensory neurotransmitter associated with pain sensation and enkephalins,[46] a neuromodulator, has been found in the lumbar posterior longitudinal ligament, which suggests that this area is extremely sensitive to pain. Mechanical irritation of this ligament, as may occur with a midline herniation, causes pain to

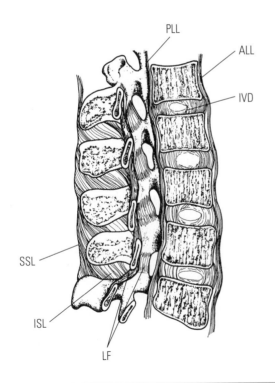

FIG. 59-2 Lateral view of the principal ligaments of the spine. *SSL,* Supraspinous ligament; *ISL,* interspinous ligament; *LF,* ligamentum flavum; *PLL,* posterior longitudinal ligament; *IVD,* intervertebral disc; *ALL,* anterior longitudinal ligament. (From Watkins RG: *The spine in sports,* St Louis, 1995, Mosby.)

be felt in the midline and radiate into the low back and superior aspect of the buttock.[17]

10. How has the posterior longitudinal ligament become an anatomical risk factor for posterior disk pathology during the transition from the quadruped to the biped posture?

In the quadruped position, there is little opportunity for posterior disk herniation as the forces responsible for such pathology occur secondary to axial compression in the upright biped posture. Indeed, the anterior longitudinal ligament is vastly more capable in resisting anterior disk protrusion that may come from the sagging spine of a mature quadruped. Deficient posterolaterally, the posterior longitudinal ligament is ill suited to erect posture and may be said to be at risk for the development of posterior disk pathology. Indeed, the fibers of the posterior longitudinal ligament seem to do little more than resist separation of the posterior ends of the vertebral bodies and thereby limit flexion.

11. What is the anatomy and function of the ligamentum flavum?

The lumbar *ligamentum flavum* is a paired structure at each level, joining the laminae of adjacent vertebrae between the C2/C3 to L5/S1 levels, and acts to protect the spinal canal from encroachment by soft tissue on flexion movements. As its name implies, this elastic containing yellow ligament is unique, as up to 80% of its fibers have elastic properties. Correspondingly, it has a tensile strength of only 113 N.[61] Although offering some resistance to separation of the laminae in flexion of the vertebral column, the ligament is too distensible secondary to its elastic nature to limit this motion. Located posteriorly, the ligamentum flavum narrows the inferior aspect of the intervertebral foramen and helps form the posterior boundary of the intervertebral foramen.[60] In the lumbar spine, this ligament forms the more anterior portion of the facet joint within the intervertebral foramen, and comes in direct contact with the exiting dorsal and ventral nerve roots.[32] The primary function of the ligamentum flavum is to provide a smooth posterior wall to the vertebral canal that accommodates large changes in interlaminar distance during flexion and extension of the vertebral column without buckling.[83] The ligaments increase in thickness from the cervical to the lumbar region, and extend laterally to the facet joints at each segment throughout the spine. The thickness of the ligamentum flavum ranges between 2 mm and 7 mm; the ligament is thinnest when the spine is flexed, as this posture pulls the ligament taut. During spinal extension it is contracted and thick and occupies more space within the canal,[78] in which case it will indent into the vertebral canal.[76] Because of disk space narrowing in degenerative disk disease, the vertebrae will approximate each other. This causes the ligamentum flavum to infold or kink on itself, bulging further into the spinal canal and aggravating any tendency to stenosis,[78] and thereby serve as a secondary source of low back pain. In addition, this ligament can ossify,[82] particularly in vertebral hyperostosis and in Paget's disease.[87]

12. What is the anatomy and function of the supraspinous and interspinous ligaments?

The *supraspinal ligament* is a loose extension of the nuchal ligament of the cervical spine that lies in the midline and interconnects the tips of the spinous process from C7 to the sacrum. Becoming broader as it descends, the supraspinal ligament is the most superficial of all spinal ligaments and therefore farthest from the axis of flexion. Because of this, as well as having low stiffness and failing at very low loads,[70] the supraspinal ligament has greater potential for sprain.[39] Being a distinctly fatty structure with no single, continuous longitudinal structure, it may provide a protective cushion over the spinous processes.[34] This ligament is assisted in its ability to restrain excessive spinal flexion passively by the interspinous ligament and dynamically by the spinalis portion of the erector spinae muscle. The *interspinal ligaments* are obliquely running fibers composed of ventral, middle, and dorsal fibers that also connect adjacent spinous processes, filling the gap along the length of these processes. Only the anterior two thirds of each ligament is truly ligamentous, and passes around the supraspinous ligament to merge with the thoracolumbar fascia and thereby help anchor the latter to the spine.[81] The posterior third represents terminal tendons of the erector spinae muscle finding attachment to a spinous process.[6-9] The supraspinous ligament and interspinous ligaments together statically limit the end range of lumbar flexion and are the first to undergo sprain during hyperflexion of the lumbar region.[35] Interspinous ligament failure may act as the precursor of eventual disk injury by permitting an unacceptable degree of segmental flexion, subsequently overloading the disk.[1] Disruption of the interspinous and supraspinous ligament may also precede degenerative spondylolisthesis.[34] Hence, soft tissue injury may serve as a precursor to segmental instability.

13. What is the anatomy of the thoracolumbar fascia?

The *thoracolumbar fascia* is a thick, strong, and transparent structure that envelops the paravertebral musculature, quadratus lumborum, and psoas major, spanning an area between the iliac crest and sacrum up to the thoracic cage. The thoracolumbar fascia forms a thin covering over the erector spinae in the thoracic region, whereas in the lumbar region it is thick and trilaminar,[6] and acts in the capacity of a dynamic ligament that can generate nearly 2000 psi[21-24] in maintaining stability in the spine.[53] Attached securely to bone at its upper and lower ends, its three layers, comprised of vertical, oblique, and horizontal fibers wrap around the trunk, corsetlike, by forming lateral attachments to the three layers of the abdominal musculature and the latissimus dorsi and glutei. Thus the tension in this fascial sheet is affected both by the angle of flexion of the spine, and muscle contraction. Its vertical fibers, located anteriorly and separating the anterior and middle groups of back muscles, are derived from the fascia of the quadratus lumborum and attach medially to the anterior surface of the lumbar transverse processes. The vertical fibers are tensed by gluteus maximus during lifting activities. The horizontal fibers are tensed through forces applied by the transversus abdominis and internal obliques, which exert an extension force on the spinous process.[28,80] The oblique fibers derive from the aponeurosis of the latissimus dorsi muscle and comprise the posterior layer of the thoracolumbar fascia, and allow translation of forces coming into the back by lifting an object with the upper extremities.

14. What is the function of the thoracolumbar fascia?

The thoracolumbar fascia is believed to play an important role in minimizing the effects of shear forces to the low back generated during the lifting of heavy loads. Because of its wrap-around distribution, the cocontraction of the abdominal and trunk musculature that accompanied lifting generates tension in the thoracolumbar fascia that resists flexion and thereby reduces shear at the lumbar spine. Flexion will instead occur at the hips. Dampening shear is accomplished by amplifying the dampening of shear forces attempted by the trunk musculature. As a person bends forward, the increasing moment of body weight is supported by muscle, until the ligament stretch is sufficient for the moment. Beyond this point, the ligaments support the moment while the muscles relax. On full flexion, as the paraver-

tebral muscles becomes mechanically disadvantaged and electrically silent, the thoracolumbar fascia becomes the major resisting factor against further flexion.[52] Moving from the full-flexed position to the upright posture, the pelvis is first rotated backward, raising the spine and stretching the ligaments to the tension required to support the moment. Once the paravertebral muscles are restored to their mechanically advantageous length, they can assume support of the moment so that the back is straightened and lumbar lordosis is restored. Picking up a heavy object will necessitate rotating the pelvis back even further to the angle at which the muscles can assume the increased moment. On extension from a full flexed position, the gluteus maximus and hamstring muscles act in concert in a closed kinetic chain to generate passive tension in the thoracolumbar fascia of up to 15,000 pounds per square inch. This initiates the extension movement by posturing the pelvis in posterior tilt and thereby minimizing exposure of the lumbosacral spine to shear forces, particularly when lifting a heavy object.

15. What are shear and torsional forces, and what segment of the lumbar spine is most vulnerable to these forces?

Inadequately restrained shear forces in the low back represents a major cause of back pain. *Shear* refers to two uniplanar forces working in opposite directions with some distance between them and causing oblique distortion of the interposed tissue, namely the intervertebral disk. Alternately, the lumbosacral spine may be exposed to torsion in an unguarded moment. *Torsion* may be defined as multiplanar forces working in opposite directions that impart a rotatory force to the disk, and may occur from excessive axial rotation of the spine. The motions of the lumbar spine are defined by the coronal orientation of the facet joints, which allow for anterior and posterior flexion and extension, lateral deviation, and right and left rotation. However, the facet orientation in the lumbar spine allows for only minimal rotation and is compensated for by shearing force.[55] The facet joints of the lumbar spine have three degrees of motion.

In the upright posture the L3/L4 disk space is horizontal.[24] In contrast, the L4/L5 and L5/S1 intervertebral segments and disk are progressively inclined and therefore particularly subject to sagittal shearing forces. Shear is generated through the disk when the direction of thrust is not perpendicular to the vertebral.[56] Excessive shear is determined by factors such as the degree of lordosis due to pelvic tilt, which is itself determined by trunk and lower extremity muscular extensibility, and the presence of transitional vertebrae.[21] The primary resistance to shear in the low back is the facet joints which, by virtue of their orientation, act to restrain shear. In the event of overload, the disk annulus is stretched and torn off its attachment to the vertebral end plate. Annular injury is often the precursor of many degenerative and mechanical causes of low back pain. Moreover, while one facet joint is compressed and suffers damage to its articular surface on one side, the ligaments of the other facet joint are subjected to traction injury.[23] A single episode of overwhelming force may cause this injury, but more frequently it results from several minor episodes.[24]

16. Which osseous and soft-tissue structures are effective restrainers of shear forces in the low back?

Annular injury is often the precursor of many degenerative and mechanical causes of low back pain. The role of preventing annular injury falls upon those structures responsible for restraining shear, namely, the apophyseal joints, the musculoligamentous structures, the thoracolumbar fascia, intraabdominal pressure and the intervertebral disk itself. The latter is resistant to shear and torsion by virtue of the oblique cross-fibers of the annulus. The restraints to shear are normally adequate to prevent segmental displacement. In the appendicular skeleton, ligamentous injury will result in an unstable joint, whereas weakened muscle makes the adjacent joint more likely to suffer ligamentous injury. Similarly, spinal ligamentous injury may cause segmental instability in the axial skeleton.

The inclination of the upper lumbar levels prevents rotation better than the lower lumbar levels because the apophyseal joints are oriented toward the sagittal plane, which permits flexion and extension but restrains rotation. In contrast, the facet joints of the lower lumbar spine are oriented in the coronal plane so that shear is restrained at the expense of torsion.[37] At L5, torque is buttressed by the broad pedicles of L5. The 90° orientation of the lumbar facet joints allows only 2° to 3° of pure rotation, thereby protecting the annulus from excessive torsion by maintaining the amount of exposure within a "safe range." However, because of the unique facet orientation at the lumbosacral junction, a rotation at the L5-S1 level greater than 3° may result in frank sprain of the annulus, facet fracture, injury to the pars interarticularis such as a pars stress reaction or fracture

(spondylosis),[62,77] sprain of the facet capsule, interposition of the meniscoid, or subluxation of a unilateral facet (acute locked back).

17. What is the role of the musculoligamentous system in attenuating torsion forces in the low back?

When the lumbar spine is extended, the facet joints are in the close-packed position with the male and female surfaces of the joints fitting point-for-point. In contrast, during lumbar flexion, the joints are in the loose-packed position with incongruity of the two surfaces. This incongruity occurs because the convex surface has a smaller curvature than the concave surface so that both surfaces articulate at one point. The annulus is vulnerable to excessive rotational strain but is protected by the configuration of the facet joints. The flexed spine disengages the apophyseal joints, and exposes the unprotected annulus to sprain from concurrent rotation. *In the loose-packed flexion position, the principal protection preventing excessive rotation is the musculoligamentous system that splits the trunk to avoid rotation by way of the spinal ligaments and lumbar fascia, the intraabdominal pressure via the diaphragm, and by the dynamic action of the trunk and abdominal musculature.*[4] Once flexion is added to axial lumbar rotation, the collagen fibers of the annulus undergo torsion and may be stretched beyond their limits resulting in microtearing of the lamellae comprising the annulus. This is most likely to occur in an unguarded moment such as a stumble, fall, misstep, or violent sneeze that combines flexion and rotation during attempted recovery and injury prevention.[72]

18. What is the anatomy of the corporotransverse ligament and how may it contribute to pathologic root entrapment?

The *corporotransverse ligament* is a tough, fibrous band that crosses the intervertebral foramen and is classified as a *transforaminal ligament.* This ligament runs from the vertebral body and intervertebral disk of L5 to the transverse process of L5.[13] Running directly over the anterior primary division of L5,[67] the corporotransverse ligament creates an osteoligamentous tunnel through which the L5 nerve runs and is therefore more likely to be come entrapped within.[11] Traditional imaging is negative and requires far lateral parasagittal magnetic resonance imaging scans that are farther lateral than standard magnetic resonance protocols to show the relationship between the L5 nerve and the cor-

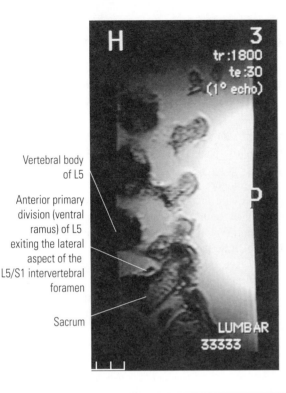

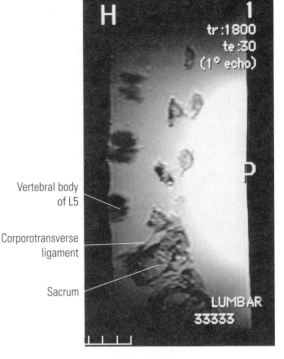

A

Vertebral body of L5

Anterior primary division (ventral ramus) of L5 exiting the lateral aspect of the L5/S1 intervertebral foramen

Sacrum

B

Vertebral body of L5

Corporotransverse ligament

Sacrum

FIG. 59-3 Parasagittal MRI scans showing **A,** The anterior primary division (ventral ramus), and **B,** The corporotransverse ligament. (From Cramer GD, Darby SA: *Basic and clinical anatomy of the spine, spinal cord, and ANS,* St Louis, 1995, Mosby.)

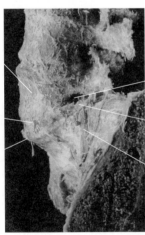

Vertebral body of L5

L5/S1 intervertebral disc

Sacral promontory

L5/S1 intervertebral foramen

Corporotransverse ligament

Anterior primary division (ventral ramus) of L5

FIG. 59-4 Lateral view of a cadaveric lumbar spine. The two pin heads are inserted beneath the corporotransverse ligament that spans the left L5/S1 intervertebral foramen. The anterior primary division (ventral ramus) passes beneath this ligament and between the two pin heads. (From Cramer GD, Darby SA: *Basic and clinical anatomy of the spine, spinal cord, and ANS,* St Louis, 1995, Mosby.)

porotransverse ligament (Fig. 59-3).[86] This may be a cause for root entrapment, particularly with L5 isthmic spondylolisthesis in which the corporotransverse ligament has a guillotine-like effect as it descends on the anterior primary division of L5, trapping it between the transverse process of L5 and the sacral ala (Fig. 59-4). The presence of this ligament occupies space within the interforamen and may contribute to root entrapment.[27]

19. What is the organization and function of the muscles of the back?

The entire vertebral column is surrounded by muscle posteriorly, but only the cervical and lumbar regions are covered by muscles both anteriorly and laterally, whereas the thoracic region lacks any lateral or prevertebral musculature. The contractile tissues of the spine consist of muscle, the musculotendinous junction, the tendon (when present), and the insertion of tendon into bone through the periosteum via Sharpey's fibers.[13] In addition to moving the spine, the back and trunk muscles function as shock absorbers, acting to disperse and thereby attenuate applied loads to the spine. The

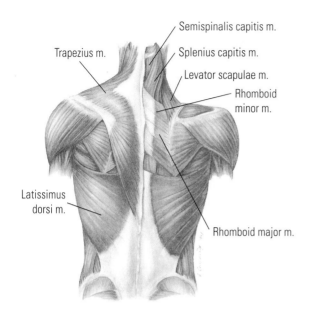

FIG. 59-5 Anatomy of the first and second layer muscles of the back. (From Cramer GD, Darby SA: *Basic and clinical anatomy of the spine, spinal cord, and ANS*, St Louis, 1995, Mosby.)

posterior back muscles are the "true" back muscles, collectively known as the paraspinals. These deeply located muscles are bilaterally symmetric to the left or right sides of the medial axis of the vertebral column. In addition, they lie behind the plane of the transverse process, are segmentally supplied by the posterior primary rami, and may be subdivided into deep, middle, and superficial groupings. In addition to topographic location, the muscles of the vertebral column may be classified according to size. Small, unisegmental muscles connecting consecutive vertebrae are covered by muscles of various lengths lying posterior, anterior, and lateral to different regions of the spine.

20. What are the various layers of back musculature?

Several superficial layers of back muscles exist, the most superficial of which are associated with the shoulder and upper limb. Thus the most superficial layers consist of the trapezius and latissimus dorsi muscles, which, when combined span the entire spine from the occiput to the sacrum (Fig. 59-5). Although primarily acting on the shoulder joints, they also function to distribute the upper extremity load across the entire span of the back rather than concentrating force in the upper thoracic area.[54] The second, deeper layers in-

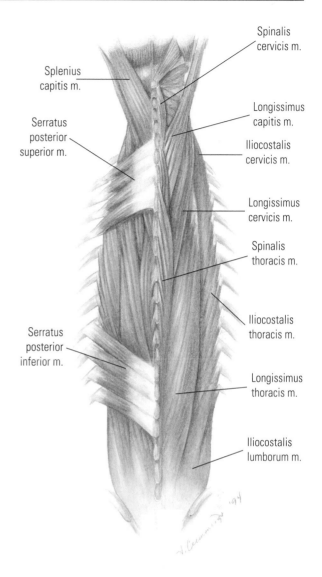

FIG. 59-6 Third, fourth, and fifth layers of back muscles. (From Cramer GD, Darby SA: *Basic and clinical anatomy of the spine, spinal cord, and ANS*, St Louis, 1995, Mosby.)

clude the rhomboid major, rhomboid minor, and levator scapulae muscles. The third layer consists of two thin, almost quadrangular muscles, namely the serratus posterior, superior, and inferior. Moving more deeply one encounters the splenius capitis and cervicis muscles. The fifth layer of muscles is the largest group and is composed of the erector spinae group (Fig. 59-6). The sixth layer of back muscles (Fig. 59-7) is called the transversospinalis group because they originate from the transverse processes and insert onto spinous pro-

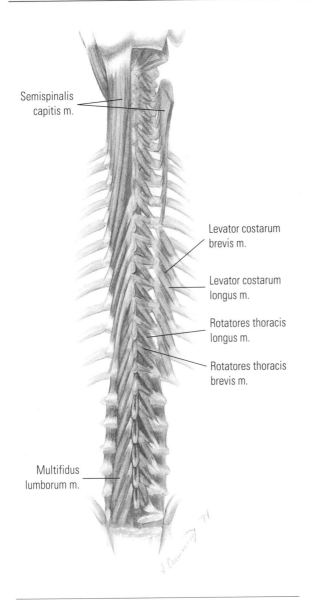

Semispinalis capitis m.

Levator costarum brevis m.

Levator costarum longus m.

Rotatores thoracis longus m.

Rotatores thoracis brevis m.

Multifidus lumborum m.

FIG. 59-7 Sixth, and deepest, layer of back muscles. (From Cramer GD, Darby SA: *Basic and clinical anatomy of the spine, spinal cord, and ANS,* St Louis, 1995, Mosby.)

cesses. The transverso spinalis muscles include the rotatores, multifidus, and semispinalis and are so arranged that from superficial to deep, the length of the muscles becomes progressively shorter. In contrast to the erector spinae, which, because of their relative distance to the axis of motion are considered primary movers of the spine, the muscles of the transversospinalis group, located close to the axis of rotation for the spine are thought to function as spinal stabilizers, adjusting and

fine-tuning the motion between individual vertebrae during spinal motion. The most deeply placed short muscles function primarily in a posture role as stabilizers, rather than as prime movers of the spine.[8]

21. What are the "true" back muscles?

The "true" back muscles is the appellation given by standard anatomy texts to the muscles known as the posterior group and include in superficial to deep order:

- *Sacrospinalis.* These are long, polysegmental muscles that are also known as the *erector spinae,* and have a vertical orientation allowing them to run parallel with the spine. Located within the vertebrocostal groove of the back and lying under the posterior layer of the thoracolumbar fascia, these massive extensor muscles, whose fiber orientation of span is medial to lateral as they move upward, are organized into three groups that are aligned with the coronal plane. These groups include the lateral *iliocostalis,* the middle *longissimus,* and the medial *spinalis.* Collectively, the erector spinae hold the spine erect and thereby stabilize the body when contracting bilaterally. When contracting unilaterally, these muscles act to laterally flex the spine. Also, because iliocostalis is laterally placed, its distance from the axis for lateral flexion is further from the medially placed spinalis and therefore has greater mechanical advantage to perform side bending.

- *Iliocostalis.* This is the most lateral portion of the sacrospinalis muscles and is well developed in the thoracic region. Iliocostalis lumborum is composed of a thoracic and lumbar component.[13] Beginning at the crest of the ilium and inserting on the angle of the lower sixth or seventh rib, the iliocostalis lumborum muscle spans the lumbar spine without gaining attachment to it and acts to increase lumbar lordosis during bilateral contraction and axial rotation of the lumbar spine.

- *Longissimus.* The name of this muscle derives from its considerable length. The largest division of longissimus is the longissimus thoracis, located medial to the iliocostalis group, and has many fibers originating from the transverse and accessory processes of the lumbar vertebrae. These fibers converge to a common tendon that inserts into the medial aspect of the posterior superior iliac spine.[9] When acting unilaterally, it laterally flexes the spine. When acting bilaterally, this muscle holds the spine erect.

- *Spinalis.* This muscle connects the spinous processes and is divided into three parts, namely, the spinalis capitis, the spinalis cervicis, and the spinalis thoracis. The spinalis is the most medial division of the erector spinae and is the thinnest and most poorly defined portion.

- *Transversospinales.* The name of this muscle group implies its proximal and distal insertions and is composed of the posterior *rotatores,* middle *multifidus,* and anterior *semispinalis,* all of which obliquely run lateromedial as they ascend the spine.

- *Multifidi.* These are a series of multipennate muscles extending over the entire length of the vertebral column between the sacrum and axis, lying beneath the semispinalis muscles, where they fill the groove between the transverse and spinous processes of the vertebrae. These muscles cover the laminae of the vertebral column, each originating on the transverse or mamillary process[43] and travel lateromedially before inserting on the spinous process one to four segments above that level. The multifidi insert onto all the vertebrae except the atlas. Thickest in the lumbar region, this muscle primarily extends the vertebral column when acting bilaterally. When acting unilaterally, the fibers of multifidi pull down on the spinous process from which they arise, laterally flex the spine and also execute posterior sagittal rotation of their vertebra of origin. Rotation in the lumbar spine, however, is minimal as significant rotation is precluded by the orientation of the facet joints. When the oblique abdominal muscles contract to produce trunk rotation, some trunk flexion also occurs. The multifidi oppose this flexion component and maintain pure axial rotation, and thereby act as stabilizers during trunk rotation.

- *Semispinalis.* This muscle is not present in the lumbar spine, but is confined to the cervical and thoracic regions and overlies the multifidus. The semispinalis consists of three parts including the semispinalis capitis,[42] cervicis, and thoracis, all of which act to extend the spine.

- *Rotatores.* These are the shortest representatives of the transversospinal group and, located deep to the multifidus group, constitute the deepest muscle fasciculi located in the groove between the spinous and transverse processes. The rotatores longus and brevis help extend the spine when acting bilaterally. When acting unilaterally, contraction yields spinal rotation such that the vertebral bodies move away from the side contracted.[27] Like the unisegmental muscles, the rotatores act to stabilize the vertebral column.

- *Unisegmental muscles.* These muscles are the intertransversarii and the interspinales. The *intertrans-*

verse muscles are short pairs of muscles connecting adjacent transverse processes of the cervical and lumbar vertebrae and function to laterally flex the spine by approximating adjacent transverse processes. Similarly, the *interspinalis* are small muscles connecting the adjacent spinous process. Because their orientation of span is short and lie close to the axes of motion for lateral flexion and rotation of the spine, they are at considerable mechanical disadvantage with regard to being primary movers of the spine. Of all the muscles of the body, third only to those of the eye and hand, the unisegmental muscles of the vertebral column carry the highest density of muscles spindles, and six times more muscle spindles than other deep back muscles.[31] Thus these muscles may serve in a sensory capacity as proprioceptive transducers, providing afferent information for spinal and supraspinal circuits, thereby facilitating erect posture and smooth movements of the spine.

22. What are the anterolateral abdominal muscles and what is their role in stabilization of the spine?

Forming the anterior and lateral walls of the abdominal cavity, the *abdominal muscles,* in addition to functioning as supporters of the abdominal viscera, work together with the muscles of the back via the thoracolumbar fascia to create a semirigid column. Although antagonistically placed in relation to the paraspinal musculature, the abdominal muscles work in synergy with the erector spinae and other muscles of the back to envelop the viscera anteriorly and the spine posteriorly. Together, they provide a corset that permits motion within safe limits and without compromise to the neural elements of the spine. Thus the four muscles comprising the anterolateral abdominal wall do not have direct attachments to the spine; they nevertheless contribute to motions of the trunk including flexion, side bending, and rotation.

The abdominal muscles consist of large muscle sheaths in several layers whose fibers are strengthened by virtue of their running in different directions. These muscles include the external abdominal oblique, internal abdominal oblique, rectus abdominis, and transversus abdominis muscle; they contribute to flexion and rotation of the torso, and are active in sit-up exercises. These muscles are considered postural muscles, and during straining and heavy lifting, act to increase intraabdominal pressure and thereby increase external support.[43] This is important for parturition, expiration, emptying the bowel and bladder, and vomiting.

- *Rectus abdominis.* This is a superficial, long, straplike muscle with longitudinally oriented fibers extending the entire length of the anterior abdominal wall, consisting of two portions, one on either side of the linea alba (Fig. 59-8). Forming the medial border of rectus abdominis, the *linea alba* is a fibrous band (raphe) running in the midline of the abdominal region, ex-

tending from the xiphoid process above to the symphysis pubis and uniting the aponeuroses of the muscles on the right and left sides. Rectus abdominis spans between the xiphoid process and fifth through the seventh costal cartilage to the pubic crest. During flexion of the trunk, rectus abdominis is active and may be viewed anteriorly, on either side of midline, when isometrically contracted as protruding "hills" in a well-muscled individual. Bilateral contraction of

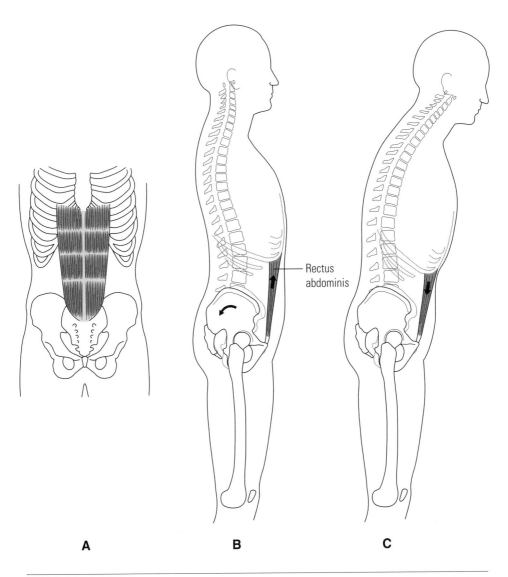

Rectus
abdominis

A   **B**   **C**

FIG. 59-8 *Rectus abdominis,* spanning between the xiphoid process and fifth through the seventh costal cartilages to the pubic crest, is a superficial, long, straplike muscle with longitudinally oriented fibers extending the entire length of the anterior abdominal wall, consisting of two portions, one on either side of the linea alba. **A,** Frontal view. **B,** Lateral view. Bilateral contraction of the recti flexes the lumbar spine when the pelvis is fixed; while **C,** posteriorly tilting the pelvis if the thorax is fixed.

the recti flexes the lumbar spine, whereas unilateral contraction results in lateral flexion to that side. If the thorax is fixed, bilateral contraction of rectus abdominis posteriorly tilts the pelvis.

- *External abdominal oblique.* This is located lateral to the rectus abdominis and covers the anterior and lateral abdominal regions, it constitutes the largest and most superficial layer of the abdominal wall (Fig. 59-9). The external abdominal oblique is actually composed of anterior and lateral fibers. Bilateral action helps to produce forward trunk flexion. Because of their orientation of span, like the sterno-cleidomastoid in the neck, unilateral contraction of the external abdominal oblique rotates the trunk to the opposite side when the pelvis is fixed. To activate the muscle on the right side, the trunk is actively rotated to the left; the muscle on the left side contract in trunk rotation to the right. Bilateral acts of the lateral fibers tilts the pelvis posteriorly as a function of its attachment on the inguinal ligament into the anterior superior spine and pubic tubercle.[27]

- *Internal abdominal oblique.* These are composed of the upper and lower anterior fibers, and lateral fibers. They are located (Fig. 59-10) immediately deep to the

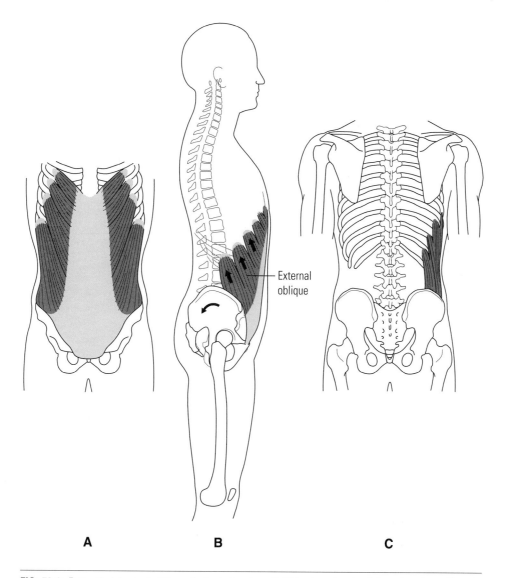

External oblique

A   **B**   **C**

FIG. 59-9 *External abdominal oblique.* **A,** Posterior view. **B,** Side view showing bilateral action pulling the pelvis into posterior tilt and accompanying hypolordosis of the lumbosacral spine. **C,** Anterior view.

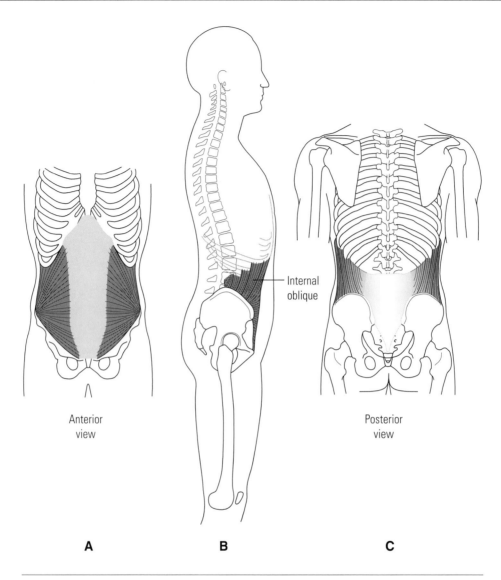

Anterior
view

Internal
oblique

Posterior
view

A   **B**   **C**

FIG. 59-10 Anatomy of the internal abdominal oblique muscles. **A,** Anterior view. **B,** Lateral view. **C,** Posterior view.

external oblique and run in the opposite oblique direction of the externus abdominis, so that if the trunk is actively rotated to the left, the left internal abdominal oblique is active, along with the right external oblique muscle to produce rotation. Both oblique muscles are oriented 90° to each other and correspond to the internal and external intercostal muscles.[7] Thus as both muscles are apparent anatomic antagonists, they act in synergy from a kinesiologic standpoint to rotate the trunk in either direction. The internus fibers attach to the thoracolumbar fascia and are believed to actively bring about spinal extension via tension on that fascia.[25]

• *Transversus abdominis.* These compose the innermost layer of the abdominal wall and hug the abdominal cavity like a corset (Fig. 59-11). Its transverse fibers form an important tie between the muscle-fascia column formed posteriorly by the sacrospinalis muscle and thoracolumbar fascia. Transverse force applied the transversus abdominis is thought to extend the spine through tension on the thoracolumbar fascia.[27] The fibers of transversus abdominis act like a girdle that flatten the abdominal wall and compress the abdominal viscera. Muscle weakness invariably follows obesity, which stretches the muscle to the point of diminishing its physiologic

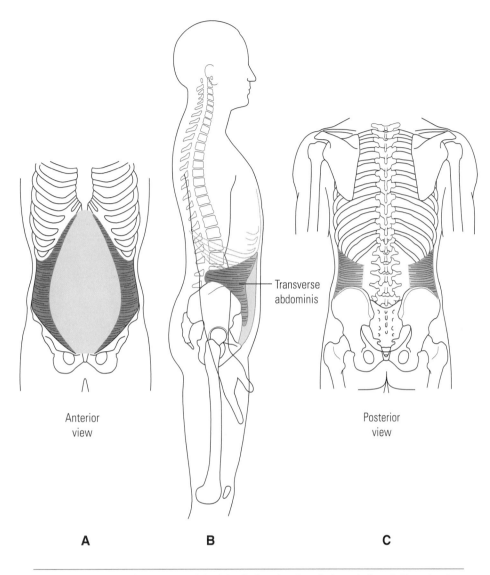

FIG. 59-11 Anatomy of transversus abdominis. **A,** Anterior view. **B,** Lateral view. **C,** Posterior view.

advantage and indirectly tends to effect an increase in lordosis.[89]

23. What is the role of the psoas major and quadratus lumborum muscles in relation to the spine?

Although both the psoas major and quadratus lumborum affect the lumbar spine either through direct attachment or indirectly via attachment on the pelvis, the former is considered a middle group muscle whereas the latter is an anterior group muscle. The anterior group muscles, such as the psoas major and minor, include those muscles that lie anterior to the plane of the transverse process and are supplied segmentally by

both anterior primary rami. In contrast the middle group musculature, such as the quadratus lumborum, is attached in the plane of the transverse processes. Although psoas provides anterior-posterior support to the lumbar spine, quadratus lumborum provides medial-lateral support. Thus both muscles, by virtue of their proximal insertions, work together during co-contraction to stabilize the lumbar spine[15] in the sagittal and frontal planes and dynamically attenuate the effects of shear and torsion.

• *Psoas.* The psoas (Greek for loins—*psoa*) major, a fusiform muscle, arises from the transverse processes, the intervertebral disks, and vertebral bodies of the lumbar spine and forms a common tendon that

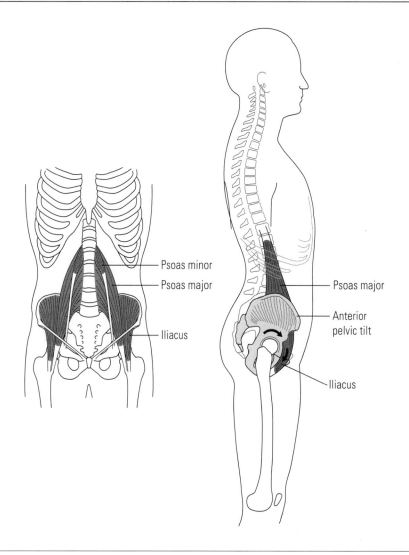

FIG. 59-12 Iliopsoas contraction acts to initially anteriorly tilt the pelvis and accentuate lumbar lordosis, as well as flex the trunk forward.

inserts onto the lesser trochanter of the femur (Fig. 59-12). As psoas merges with the unipennate iliacus muscle to form the iliopsoas muscle, both muscles have differing origins and share a common distal attachment. The prime function of this muscle is to flex the hip in the open kinetic chain. Because its insertion onto the greater trochanter is on the posterior medial side of the femur, psoas also acts as an external rotator. Although its fascicles lie too close to the axis of rotation of the lumbar vertebrae to exert a moment comparable to their effect on the hip joint,[36] bilateral psoas contraction with the lower limb stabilized in the closed kinetic chain exerts a substantial compres-

sive force that accentuates lordosis by anteriorly tilting the pelvis and flexing the trunk. Thus when the lower limbs are fixed psoas acts as a primary flexor of the lumbar spine.[8] When unilaterally contracting, psoas may result in a scoliosis.[27] The psoas minor muscle is absent in approximately 40% of the population.[89] It arises from the T12-L1 disk and blends with the psoas fascia distally.

The psoas major muscle offers a dynamic role in protection of the emerging nerve roots from nerve root avulsion. Although the anterior origin of psoas major attaches to the lumbar bodies and intervertebral disks, the posterior origin attaches anterior to the transverse process. Thus the psoas major surrounds the lateral openings of the first four lumbar vertebrae so that the ventral rami from these levels merge into divisions to form the lumbosacral plexus within the substance of psoas major. In the event of hyperflexion or hyperextension of the hip, psoas may serve to absorb the traction forces before causing injury proximally at the intervertebral foramen.[43]

- *Quadratus lumborum.* This is a flat, quadrangular-shaped muscle forming part of the posterior abdominal wall and spanning the iliac crest to the last rib (Fig. 59-13). It is difficult to palpate this muscle, as it lies deep to the erector spinae. As a respiratory muscle, quadratus lumborum functions to stabilize the twelfth rib during inspiration so that the diaphragm may function optimally. During open kinetic chain motion of the lower extremity, quadratus lumborum acts as a hip hiker during swing phase as it actively holds the pelvis in a neutral position.[13] When the pelvis is fixed as in the closed kinetic chain, quadratus lumborum, by virtue of its attachment to the transverse processes of the lumbar vertebra, provides mediolateral support, and acts as a lateral flexor of the spine when contracting unilaterally,[49] extends the spine when contracting bilaterally, and provides resistance to shear forces acting at the lumbosacral junction.[38,73] When the pelvis is stabilized, quadratus lumborum acts to posteriorly tilt the pelvis on the femur.

24. What other muscles of the lower extremity indirectly affect the spine by virtue of their effect on pelvic rotation?

HAMSTRING MUSCLES

These define the posterior group of thigh muscles and are comprised of three muscles, in order from medial to lateral, the semimembranosus, semitendinosus, and biceps femoris muscle. The latter has two heads of origin known as the long (medial) and short (lateral) heads. The hamstrings, with the exception of the short head of biceps femoris, have their proximal attachments on the ischial tuberosity and collectively insert on the tibia and fibula. In the lower extremity, these muscles extend the hip and flex the knee joints. There is also minimal rotary action on the tibia. The "semi" muscles rotate the flexed leg medially whereas the biceps femoris muscle rotates it laterally. When the thigh is fixed or flexed, the hamstring muscles posteriorly tilt the pelvis backward on the femur (Fig. 59-14).

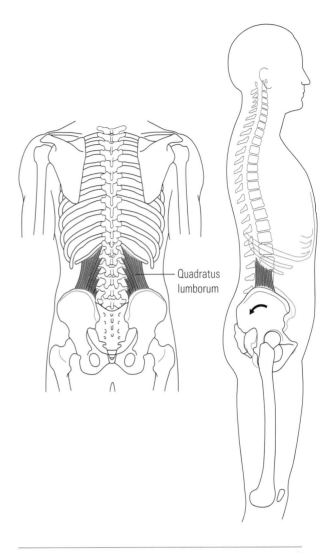

Quadratus lumborum

FIG. 59-13 *Quadratus lumborum* is a flat, quadrangular-shaped muscle forming the posterior abdominal wall and spanning the iliac crest to the last rib. Among its other functions, this muscle acts to posteriorly tilt the pelvis on the femur.

GLUTEUS MAXIMUS

This is the largest muscle in the body and is the most superficial of the muscles in the gluteal (Greek, *gloutos,* buttock) region (Fig. 59-15). Often an inch or more thick, the large size of this muscle is a uniquely human characteristic of gluteal musculature and is attributed to mankind's role in attaining an upright posture.[43] Its fibers run inferolaterally from the ilium, coccyx, and aponeurosis of the erector spinae and distally attach to the iliotibial tract of the fascia lata and the gluteal tuberosity of the femur. Like the quadriceps muscles, it

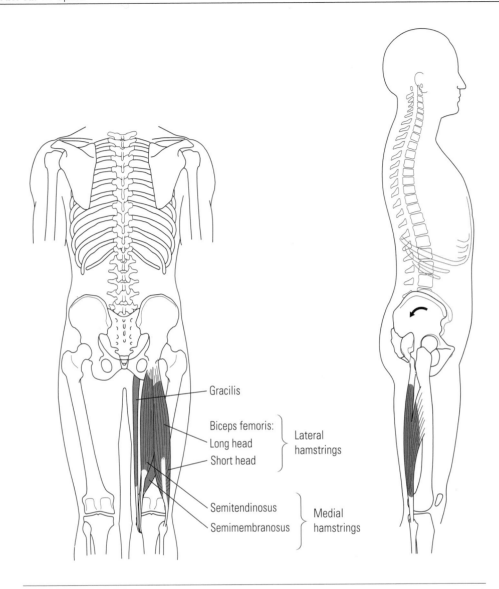

FIG. 59-14 The *hamstring muscles* are comprised of three muscles, namely in order from medial to lateral, the *semimembranosus, semitendinosus,* and *biceps femoris* muscle. The latter has two heads of origin known as the long (medial) and short (lateral) heads. Because of it relation to the pelvic axis of rotation, the hamstring muscles posteriorly tilt the pelvis backward on the femur.

may be contracted by "setting" it without any joint motion being carried out. Its orientation of span and relation to the hip joint axis endow it with the ability to extend and externally rotate the hip. Functionally, it primarily contracts during stair climbing, running, and jumping. Through its insertion into the iliotibial tract, it helps stabilize the femur on the tibia by maintaining the knee joint in extension. If the thigh is stabilized, as it is

in the closed kinetic chain, contraction of gluteus maximus rotates the pelvis posteriorly on the femoral head.

LATISSIMUS DORSI

This is a thin, broad, superficial muscle covering the lower quarter of the back. Having an extensive origin that includes the spinous processes from T11 to L5, the

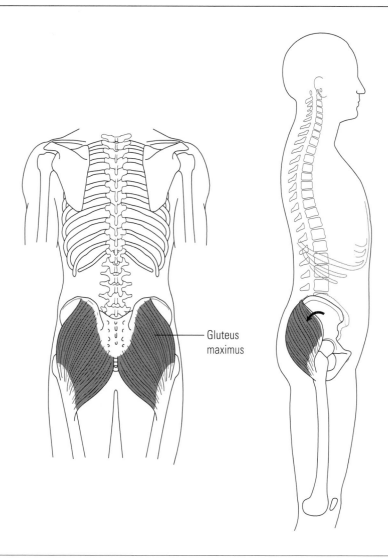

FIG. 59-15 *Gluteus maximus* fibers run inferolaterally from the ilium, coccyx, and aponeurosis of the erector spinae and distally attach to the iliotibial tract of the fascia lata and the gluteal tuberosity of the femur. If the thigh is stabilized, as it is in the closed kinetic chain, contraction of gluteus maximus rotates the pelvis posteriorly on the femoral head.

posterior third of the iliac crest, the inferior angle of the scapula (in approximately one half of the population), and the thoracolumbar fascia. Its fibers pass anteriorly, superiorly, and laterally to insert on the crest of the lesser humeral tubercle. With its origin fixed, the function of latissimus dorsi is defined in reference to shoulder movement, as it is a strong shoulder girdle depressor, hyperextensor, internal rotator, horizontal abductor, and vertical adductor. With its insertion fixed, it tilts the pelvis anteriorly when acting bilaterally (Fig. 59-16). When contracting unilaterally, it tilts the pelvis later-

ally. The latissimus dorsi is innervated by the thoracodorsal nerve which is a branch of the posterior cord of the brachial plexus.

25. How do the trunk and lower extremity muscles relate as biomechanical force couples?

A *force couple* is defined as two forces working in opposite directions, but acting on a single object and physically separated so as to cause a rotational movement of that object. Despite the anatomic antagonism between the abdominals, erector spinae, and lower ex-

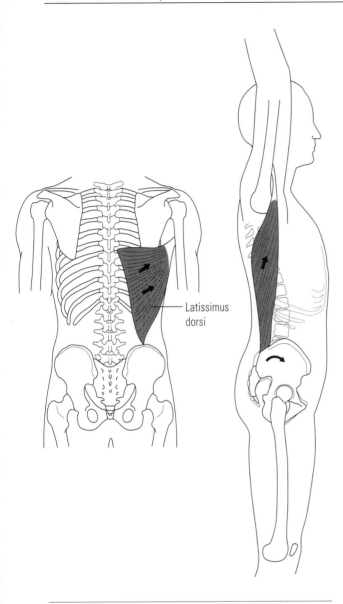

Latissimus
dorsi

tremity muscles, cocontraction manifests as a kinesiologic synergy among these muscle groups. For example, during flexion of the lumbar spine from the supine posture, as in the performance of a sit-up, the psoas major and rectus abdominis muscles concentrically act as prime movers, while the erector spinae simultaneously undergoes an eccentric contraction toward the end of the sit-up. The muscles all work in synergy, and the erector spinae works in a secondary,

albeit necessary, capacity to allow for a graceful and safe performance of this movement.

26. What is the effect of pelvic tilt on lumbar lordosis and how is this mediated by the muscles of the trunk and lower extremity?

Pelvic rotation in the sagittal plane is known as *pelvic tilt,* which is defined in relation to the anterior superior iliac spine (ASIS). *Anterior pelvic tilt,* associated with tight iliopsoas and quadriceps muscles and hyperlordosis, involves the ASIS moving anteriorly and downward. Hyperlordosis is associated with anterior pelvic tilt, which causes the pelvis to rotate forward because of tightened hip flexors. Hyperlordosis is an essentially extended position of the lumbar facet joints and causes marked narrowing of the spinal canal and intervertebral foramen. In contrast, *posterior pelvic tilt,* which is associated with hypolordosis (flat back) and tightened hamstring musculature, involves the ASIS moving posteriorly and upward. Tight hamstrings cause a pull on the pelvis to rotate it backwardly about the common hip axis as posterior pelvic tilt and therefore increase shear of L5 ("sliding down the hill") on S1.

Various muscles of the trunk and lower extremity affect the degree of lumbar lordosis by virtue of their insertion on the pelvis. Contraction of these muscles will alternately either rotate the pelvis anteriorly or posteriorly, depending on the site of insertion. The iliopsoas muscles located ventrally but below the pelvis and the erector spinae muscles located dorsally and above the pelvis work in synergy as a force couple to tilt the pelvis anteriorly and increase lordosis of the lumbar spine. In contrast, the gluteus maximus and hamstring muscles are located dorsally and below the pelvis couple with the rectus abdominis, oblique externus[59] located ventrally and above the pelvis to tilt the pelvis posteriorly and thereby flatten the lumbar lordosis.[8,47] Quadratus lumborum also tilts the pelvis posteriorly. Imbalance of the muscles responsible for pelvic tilt is implicated in many persons with low back pain. These individuals may have various combinations of shortening and lengthening that either increases shear at the lumbosacral spine or diminishes space of the exiting nerve roots out of the intervertebral foramen.

27. How do the muscles of the trunk act to eccentrically stabilize the spinal column?

The muscles of the trunk, including the abdominals, erector spinae, psoas, quadratus, as well as the muscles of the neck all serve as stabilizing guy wires. Together they provide dynamic control against the force of gravity as the weight of various segments shifts away from the base of support. As the trunk shifts or sways in one direction, contralateral muscles contract and function as guy wires to restrain excessive drift. Extreme or sustained deviations are supported by inert (ligamentous) structures. When the line of gravity shifts forward, the extensor muscles such as the erector spinae, and posterior cervical muscles such as the upper trapezius provide eccentric control. When the line of gravity shifts backward, stabilization is eccentrically provided by the flexor muscles including the abdominals and intercostal muscles, as well as psoas major, anterior scalenes, the capitis musculature, and sternocleidomastoid. When the line of gravity shifts laterally, the contralateral musculature provides stabilization and includes psoas, quadratus lumborum, erector spinae, the internal and external obliques, the sternomastoid, scalenes, and intercostal muscles (Sprangford E, 1982, personal communication).[14,84]

28. What is correct posture, and how may faulty posture lead to musculoskeletal pathology?

Correct posture may be simply defined as the position in which minimum stress is applied to each joint. In contrast, any posture that increases stress to a given articulation may be considered faulty. The appropriate postural alignment is significantly dependent upon the soft tissue spanning each joint. With regard to contractile tissue adjacent to each articulation, either excessive shortening or diminished extensibility may be culpable in abnormal posture of that joint and may result in some form of pathology. The abnormal stress to that joint, if repeated over a period of time, may result in articular wearing of joint surfaces and reactionary osteophytic traction spurs that attempt to minimize postural malalignment. When occurring in the spine, traction spurs may encroach upon nerve roots or the supporting ligamentous structures,[43] causing pain and dysfunction. Moreover, the soft tissue surrounding the joint, including muscles and ligaments, may become weakened, stretched, or traumatized by increased stress.

29. What are common causes of excessive lordosis and kyphosis, and what are other common postural deformities of the spine?

Prior to discussing faulty posture it is essential to define ideal postural alignment (Fig. 59-17), which may be defined by holding a plumb line laterally so that it bisects the following surface landmarks in the ideal posture:

the lobe of the ear, through the shoulder joint, through the bodies of the vertebral bodies, through the greater femoral trochanter, slightly anterior to the knee joint, and slightly anterior to the lateral malleolus. In this postural alignment, the pelvis is balanced anteriorly and posteriorly. Anteriorly, the abdominal muscles exert an upward pull that is balanced by the downward pull of the hip flexors. Posteriorly, the back muscles exert an upward pull that is counterbalanced by the downward pull of the hip extensors.[45]

Causes of increased *hyperlordosis,* defined as excessive anterior curvature of the spine, include postural deformity, lax abdominal musculature, a heavy abdomen due to pregnancy or obesity, hip flexion contracture, wearing high heeled shoes, spondylolisthesis, congenital hip dysplasia, failure of segmentation of the neural arch of a facet joint segment, or as a compensatory mechanism secondary to another deformity such as kyphosis. In contrast, *kyphosis* (meaning *humpback* in Greek), defined as excessive posterior spinal curvature, may derive from pathology such as vertebral compression fractures, Scheuermann's disease, ankylosing spondylitis, senile osteoporosis, tumors, tuberculosis, congenital anomalies, or as a compensatory mechanism secondary to excessive lordosis.[43]

There are various patterns of faulty posture of the spine, which, if not addressed may result in postural strain syndrome, chronic degenerative changes, or sudden, acute injury to the low back in the form of annular rupture and disk pathology. The origin of postural pain syndrome stems from the muscles not used to provide support, so that the axial skeleton yields to the effects of gravity. Because of this, the passive structures (such as ligaments and joint capsules) stretched to the limit at the end of each joint range, and bony approximation, provide stability. Muscles and ligaments maintained under prolonged tension will adaptively lengthen while those maintained under prolonged relaxation will adaptively contract. When this occurs in contractile tissue, the ability of muscles to contract becomes physiologically advantaged, resulting in a loss of protective muscular contribution to staving off soft-tissue injury. The cumulative effects of these soft-tissue changes result in overstretching of certain soft tissues and contracture of others, which, together with excessive articular pressure of the spinal joints at their end range, stresses the soft and osseous tissues of the axial skeleton. The musculoligamentous supporting structures of the lumbar spine are innervated by the lateral, intermediate, and medial branches of the primary dorsal rami. The pain-

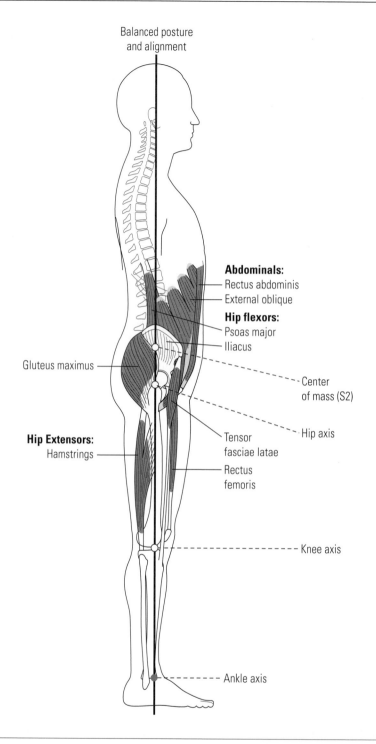

FIG. 59-17 *Ideal posture* referenced to a plumb line alignment on side view that corresponds to the gravitational force line. In this postural alignment, the pelvis is balanced anteriorly and posteriorly because of a muscular balance among the various muscles affecting the pelvis. Anteriorly, the abdominal muscles exert an upward pull that is balanced by the downward pull of the hip flexors. Posteriorly, the back muscles exert an upward pull that is counterbalanced by the downward pull of the hip extensors.

producing areas of these tissues may primarily be located at the muscle-tendon and ligament-bone junctions as well as the neurovascular bundle sites.[41] Although patients with postural pain are often pain free after a good night's rest, maintaining faulty posture throughout the day may lead to backache. Alterations in the sagittal plane curvatures of the spine distally is often proximally expressed as a cervical postural alteration known as a *forward head posture* and accompanies many of the following postures[43]:

- *Hyperlordotic posture.* Also known as the *kypholordotic posture,*[45] is characterized by an increase in lumbar lordosis that is accompanied by anterior pelvic tilt, and hip flexor tightness (Fig. 59-18). This posture, typical in the last trimester of pregnancy, may also occur in obese persons, or those having weak abdominal muscles. Radiographically, the patient will demonstrate an increase in the *lumbosacral angle.*[43] This posture stresses the anterior longitudinal ligament, approximates the articular facets, and narrows the posterior disk space and intervertebral foramina.[26] Muscle imbalances observed include tight hip flexors and erector spinae, as well as stretched abdominal muscles and hamstrings, the latter noted by a good angle during straight leg raising. Clinically, the patient demonstrates a positive *Thomas test.*

- *Swayback posture.* This is often mistaken for the hyperlordotic posture, but is uniquely characterized by posterior pelvic rotation, forward hip displacement, a flattened lower lumbar spine, a slight lordosis of the upper lumbar spine, increased thoracic kyphosis,[33] and is often accompanied by a forward head (Fig. 59-19). This posture is a relaxed one and causes stress to the iliofemoral ligaments, the anterior and posterior longitudinal ligaments of the upper lumbar and thoracic spine, narrowing of the intervertebral foramina and facet approximation in the lower lumbar spine. The strong *iliofemoral ligament,* also known as the "Y" ligament of Bigelow because it resembles an inverted Y at its stem, courses from the lower aspect of the anterior inferior iliac spine with divergent bands attaching along the length of the intertrochanteric line of the femur. Because it lies on the anterior side of the hip joint, it passively limits hyperextension of the hip joint[43] and one may literally stand in such a posture so as to balance themselves by passive stretch of these ligaments.[78] In this position, the body's weight tends to roll the pelvis backward on the femoral heads. The posterior pelvic tilt accompanying the

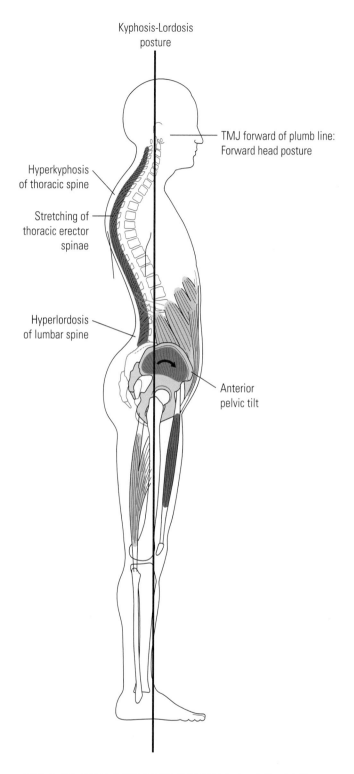

Kyphosis-Lordosis posture

TMJ forward of plumb line: Forward head posture

Hyperkyphosis of thoracic spine

Stretching of thoracic erector spinae

Hyperlordosis of lumbar spine

Anterior pelvic tilt

FIG. 59-18 The *kypholordotic posture* is characterized by an increase in lumbar lordosis that is accompanied by anterior pelvic tilt, and hip flexor tightness, stretching of the abdominal and hamstring muscles, and forward head posture.

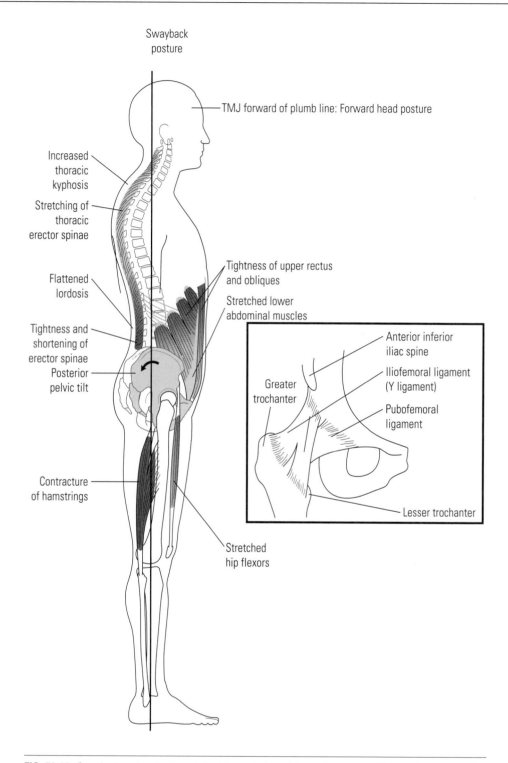

Swayback
posture

TMJ forward of plumb line: Forward head posture

Increased
thoracic
kyphosis

Stretching of
thoracic
erector spinae

Flattened
lordosis

Tightness and
shortening of
erector spinae

Posterior
pelvic tilt

Contracture
of hamstrings

Tightness of upper rectus
and obliques

Stretched lower
abdominal muscles

Anterior inferior
iliac spine

Iliofemoral ligament
(Y ligament)

Pubofemoral
ligament

Greater
trochanter

Lesser trochanter

Stretched
hip flexors

FIG. 59-19 *Swayback posture* is characterized by posterior pelvic rotation, forward hip displacement, a flattened lower lumbar spine, a slight lordosis of the upper lumbar spine, increased thoracic kyphosis, hamstring, erector spinae and upper abdominal tightness, stretching of the lower abdominal and hip flexors, and forward head posture.

swayback posture places this ligament on stretch. Muscle imbalances accompanying the swayback posture include tightness of the upper abdominal muscles and upper segments of the rectus abdominis and obliques, internal intercostal, hip extensors, lower lumbar extensor musculature, and the hamstrings; as well as stretched lower abdominal muscles, extensor muscles of the lower thoracic region, and the hip flexor muscles. The cause of this posture may derive from muscle weakness and may also relate to emotional affect,[5] reflecting a defeated attitude.

- *Flat back posture.* This is characterized by decreased lumbosacral angle and consequently lumbar lordosis (hypolordosis) and posterior pelvic tilt (Fig. 59-20). The lack of the normal physiologic shock-absorbing lordosis predisposes the low back to injury, while stressing the posterior longitudinal ligament. Muscle imbalances observed include tightness of the trunk flexors, namely the rectus abdominis and intercostals and hip extensor muscles, as well as stretched and weakened lumbar extensor and hip flexor musculature,[78] although tight hamstrings and weak hip flexors are the most consistent findings. Slight knee flexion may also occur because of excessive hamstring tightness.[20]

30. What pathologic changes occur in the soft and articular tissues because of faulty posture?

The muscles and ligaments surrounding a joint optimally function in a state of normal posture of that joint. Postural malalignment results in stretching of soft tissue on one side of the joint with concomitant shortening of soft tissue on the other side of the joint. For example, with hyperlordosis of the lumbar spine, the erector spinae shorten and the pelvis assumes an anterior posture due to tightness or contracture of the hip flexion musculature. Correspondingly, the abdominal musculature is over stretched, especially if the individual is obese, while the hamstring musculature is slackened. Muscles that are habitually kept in a shortened position tend to lose their elasticity and test strongly in the shortened position and become weak as they are lengthened[78] in what is known as *tight weakness.*[44] In contrast, *stretch weakness* refers to muscles that weaken because they are habitually kept in a stretched position beyond the physiologic resting postion.[65,75]

For muscles to contract optimally, they must remain within narrow physiologic parameters to generate an adequate contraction. If either excessively shortened

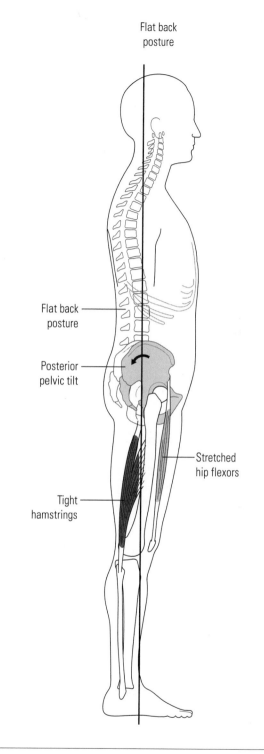

FIG. 59-20 *Flat back posture* is characterized by hamstring tightness that pull the pelvis into posterior tilt and accompanying flat lumbar back, as well as weakness of the hip flexors.

or extensible, muscles become mechanically disadvantaged and rapidly lose their ability to generate force. Thus the individual with faulty posture loses the beneficial protection to the spine afforded by the musculoligamentous system and is at increased risk for acute injury such as acute annular tear. Pathology may also occur gradually in the form of degenerative disk disease or posterior facet arthrosis due to the chronic effects of faulty posture. Alternately, if mechanical stress exceeds the supporting capabilities of the periarticular tissues, breakdown may occur. If this continues without adequate healing, over use syndromes with inflammation and pain may occur as postural pain syndrome, which affects function without apparent injury.

31. What are postural strain syndromes and what is their clinical and radiologic presentation?

Postural strain syndromes are frequently encountered and represent patients who are chronically inactive, overweight, and who frequently maintain faulty posture or whose work environment involves maintenance of abnormal posture in the absence of radicular symptoms. The faulty spinal postures that may lead to postural strain include hyperlordosis, kypholordosis or the flat back posture.

With hyperlordosis or kypholordosis, all movements are within functional limits, and the patient demonstrates no objective motor, sensory, or reflex disturbance. The patient typically presents with chronic, mild low back pain, aggravated by prolonged sitting, walking, and especially standing, with relief in recumbency and when sitting for short periods. Frequently, chores such as washing dishes, doing the laundry, and vacuuming aggravate discomfort. Although chronic degenerative disk disease with mild facet arthrosis may mimic this presentation, radiographs show no abnormalities with the exception of an increased lumbosacral angle. The patient often demonstrates a positive Thomas test. Symptoms in these patients generally result from chronically poor posture secondary to *inadequate musculature*.[78] The abdomen is prominent when standing and the lumbar lordosis is increased, which in turn strains the pain-sensitive soft tissues of the low back.

32. What are the biomechanical and clinical definitions of *stress* and *strain*?

Stress and *strain* both have a biomechanical and clinical definition. From an engineering standpoint, *stress* refers to an internal force generated in a material in response to an external load whereas *strain* refers to the

changes or deformation of a material or structure as a result of that strength, and is referred to as the stress/strain characteristics of the material. If the strain is within the elastic limit, then the deformed material will return to its preformed state. However, if the strain exceeds the elastic limit of the material, then permanent or plastic deformity occurs, so that the material eventually fails with further stress (Fig. 59-21). This applies to all soft tissues including the annulus, ligament, muscle, fascia, tendon nerves, skin, fat, and vessels. With soft tissue, the elastic limit varies with the speed of applied stress, the duration of the load, and the frequency of load. If the force is applied rapidly and/or repetitively, then the tissue is fatigued by repetitive loading. Once the elastic limit of soft tissue is exceeded, it is only a matter of time before the tissues fail by disruption with continuous strain. In contrast, the clinical term *strain* refers to the excessive deformation of the muscle-tendon unit or fascia beyond their elastic limit,[78] whereas *sprain* refers to excessive deformation of the ligamentous unit surrounding a joint. Both clinical forms of disruption result in partial or complete disruption of tissues. Whereas disruption of muscle carries a good prognosis, the fibrous repair following ligamentous sprain carries a poor prognosis as the meager vascular supply of ligament results in scar tissue formation that is a poor substitute for restraint.

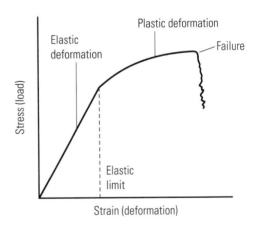

FIG. 59-21 A *stress/strain graph* showing how a material is deformed with increasing stress. Initially, the deformed material returns to its preformed state. However, when the elastic limit is reached plastic deformation will occur, so that the material becomes permanently deformed even when the stress is reduced or eliminated. The material eventually fails with further stress.

33. What is the clinical presentation of ligamentous sprain and muscular strain?

During the acute phase, all soft tissue injuries present a similar clinical picture of pain, localized swelling, and tenderness on palpation. Differentiating between a muscle versus ligament injury is primarily based upon patient history. There may be protective muscle guarding regardless of whether the injured tissue is inert or contractile.

The distinguishing clinical features of acute ligamentous sprain include a history in which injury is almost always overt, and may be accompanied by a 'snapping' sound, and acute localized tenderness that is readily accessible to the probing finger. In addition, pain begins immediately at the time of injury and gradually worsens. Finally, localized swelling may not always be observed because if the injured ligament were deeply located, edema would not be readily apparent. The predisposing movement causing ligamentous sprain is not restricted to extension, but may also occur when bending over in flexion and twisting to one side, as may occur from lifting an object that was heavier than anticipated.

With muscular strain, pain does not occur at the time of injury, but many hours later. When the patient is relatively deconditioned, their muscular circulation is incapable of coping with the sudden accumulation of noxious metabolic by-products (lactic acid) causing intramuscular irritation that is perceived as ache and stiffness. The patient in Case 2 is similar to the first time runner who, delighted to cover a mile of distance the first day, wakes up the next morning with legs so sore, stiff, and tender that he can barely walk to the bathroom. In contrast to ligamentous sprain, pain and tenderness derived from muscular strain generally extends over a very wide area.

34. What is the differential diagnosis?

- *Spinal stenosis.* Spinal stenosis derives from osseous compression of the cauda equina or nerve roots(s) because of a narrow spinal canal in the former and osteophytic compression in the latter. Central compression of the cauda equina often produces neurogenic claudication of the thighs or calves that, unlike like nerve root pathology from disk disease, is often relieved by the stooped posture. Differentiation of osteophytic nerve root entrapment from nerve root compression derived from disk pathology is based upon interpretation of the straight leg raise (see previous section).

- *Degenerative disk disease.* This disease differs from disk herniations in several respects. Whereas with disk herniation, the patient frequently complains that pain is aggravated when sitting in any type of chair, whether soft or hard, with degenerative disk disease (DDD) the patient avoids the soft chair but often feels comfortable in the hard chair. With DDD, flexion is not usually restricted, and symptoms gradually diminish with activity. In contrast, patients with disk pathology have marked restriction of lumbar flexion, and experience increasing discomfort as the day wears on.

- *Acute annular tear.* This must be differentiated from a spinal ligamentous sprain. Although an acute annular tear is deeply located and not provoked by pinpoint tenderness, localization is often possible on palpation with a ligamentous tear. With a ligamentous sprain, pain is constant from the outset, particularly during spinal movement, and usually eases off for a short while only to recur and persist without remission unless the patient is recumbent. In contrast, the patient with acute disk prolapse cannot entirely alleviate pain in recumbency, particularly if disk material compresses on the posterior longitudinal ligament, in which case pain will be unremitting even while lying down.[19]

- *Acute locked back syndrome.* In patients with posterior facet joint arthrosis, severe pain and discomfort may be provoked by bending over as at the washbasin, or to one side to tie one's shoes, picking up a piece of paper, or from some unprotected movement in bed while sleeping. This asymmetric motion shifts one of the facet joints at a specific segment out of its normally congruous relationship. Occurring during the bending-over motion, this movement represents a sudden unprotected motion that allows for nipping or "jamming" of the synovial meniscus, which is highly innervated. This triggers a reflex spasm of the overlying musculature, resulting in a "locking" of the back to minimize movement for fear of provoking intense discomfort and hence the term *acute locked back*. In one mode of onset the patient is seized with sudden agonizing pain in the low back that is so severe as to preclude standing erect. In another mode of onset, the patient is only aware of a mild discomfort that begins with a remembered triggering movement that intensifies in severity within a few hours. Pain is localized to the lumbosacral level slightly to one side of midline and may occasionally radiate to upper ipsilateral thigh, but never as far as the knee. There may be a history of one or more similar episodes in the past and patients typically remain completely symptom free between incidents. The patient climbs onto the examination table with difficulty, for fear of inducing further severe pain. Although immobility relieves discomfort, change of position greatly aggravates it. Walking is moderately comfortable provided they take small steps and do not climb stairs. During coughing and sneezing, patients will attempt to firmly brace themselves so as to minimize the jarring impact. Although lateral flexion to one side is possible, it is virtually impossible to the contralateral side. Transferring from sitting to standing is done gingerly, whereas a mild lateral scoliosis, without a rotational component, may be apparent in the upright position. This trunk list is an attempt to ease pain and stand in a manner that provides maximal relief. Tenderness at the source of pain, as pointed out by the patient, is absent or mild at best even on firm palpation because the facet joints and laminae are not readily palpable owing to the interposed muscles and fasciae.[78] The straight leg raise test will provoke acute discomfort in the region of the posterior superior iliac spine as it aggravates the subluxated facet and not because of neurologic reasons. The neurologic examination is entirely normal in these patients. Radiographs are not appropriate, as they will be misleading if the patient stands with a pronounced tilt. The diagnosis is primarily based on the patient history and presentation. Manipulation is an effective and immediate treatment in the management of the acute locked back.[78]

- *Degenerative spondylolisthesis.* This is defined as forward slippage of one vertebra over the next as a result of degenerative change in the intervertebral disk and/or articular facet joint.[78] This occurs because erosion of the superior articular facet allows forward displacement of the upper vertebral body on the lower body, trapping the inferior nerve root that exists one level below between the inferior facet and the back of the vertebral body.[12] Degenerative spondylolisthesis predominantly occurs in females (3:2) greater than 50 years of age.[70] Commonly occurring at the fourth lumbar level, degenerative spondylolisthesis most likely occurs as a function of facet joint orientation and differs from the classic isthmic type of spondylolisthesis in that the former is characterized by an intact neural arch and lack of primary disk degeneration; thus it is alternately known as *pseudospondylolisthesis.* With degenerative spondylolisthesis, the superior vertebra (L4) begins to mi-

grate or "slip" forward on the L5 vertebra. This allows the upper vertebra to roll forward on the one below during lumbar flexion. Depending on the extent of slip, a "step" may be palpable. Unlike the spondylitic variety, the step here occurs between the spinous process of the affected vertebra and the one below.[78] If a step is not distinctly palpable, spondylolisthesis may be suggested by a protruding lumbar spinous process, which may be tender upon percussion. As the superior vertebral body shifts forward, the interposed disk undergoes shearing strain that further exacerbates and accelerates disk degeneration.

Degenerative spondylolisthesis rarely presents with acute symptoms; subacute or chronic discomfort are the typical presentation.[78] Signs and symptoms include a protracted history of low-grade back pain that is intermittently intense, but rarely causes severe disability. More commonly, the inferior articular process of L4 will commonly entrap the L5 nerve root in the lateral recess and may result in sciatica.[37] Discomfort is related to disk degeneration and posterior facet arthrosis, or to nerve root irritation or entrapment with symptoms similar to spinal stenosis. Hence, patients develop early morning ache and stiffness and often experience difficulty getting out of bed, which improves following a hot shower, but once up and about they feel much better. Maintaining a flexed posture for long periods aggravates discomfort. Similarly, sitting in an upright hard chair is more comfortable than a soft, easy chair in which they insist on sitting near the edge where they may sit upright. Although turning in bed can be annoying, walking is the least symptomatic of activities. The examination is mostly negative, and does not present with pinpoint tenderness as the lamina is not loose. Physical examination often shows a patient who is flexible and able to touch the floor on forward flexion with their knees locked in extension, although maintaining this position causes marked discomfort. Discomfort is worse on extending the back into the erect position and is frequently associated with a "hitching" movement. Instead of a smooth resumption from flexion to extension the patient first extends the lumbar spine, fixing it in lordosis, and then extending at the hips until the erect position is regained; this is known as *hitching.*[70] Patients may occasionally complain of pain during both flexion and extension.[78]

- *Pars interarticularis fracture.* This is also known as *spondylolysis* and refers to a stress fracture to the pars interarticularis without shift of the vertebral body that may be detected on an oblique radiographic view. Hamstring tightness is often associated with spondylolysis of a painful nature and may be an etiologic factor by increasing tension to the low back during flexion.[78] The *one-legged hyperextension test* provokes pain at the site of the fractured pars and is performed by asking the patient to stand on one leg and arch the back backward. In a positive test, the patient localizes the site of the lesion by pointing to it. Local tenderness occurs from movement of the probing finger transmitted through the spinous processes of the affected segment to the fracture site. Because the L5 nerve root runs directly anterior to the site of the defect, the hyperextended position may elicit sciatica, a symptom absent with an isolated ligament injury. These patients dislike standing and lying prone, both of which increase the lumbar lordosis. This is because the lordotic position angulates the loose lamina even more at the defect side, and thereby increases pressure of the nerve root.

- *Isthmic spondylolisthesis.* This is the classic pars interarticularis fracture due to a nonunited stress fracture and demonstrates a male to female ratio of involvement of 2:1. In those patients with bilateral pars interarticularis defects, the integrity of posterior elements becomes destabilized as the defect grows causing the superior vertebral body and transverse process to shift forward on the vertebral body below, while the spinous process and lamina remain behind in their normal position. Isthmic spondylolisthesis affects approximately 6% of the general population. The L5 vertebra normally is rectangular with a trefoil canal shape. Those persons with a trapezoidal shape and having a dome shaped canal are associated with a higher incidence of lysis[70] and vertebral shift.[10] Although the incidence of pars defects is higher in boys, the incidence of progressive vertebral slippage is four times[69] higher in girls,[16] and often progresses between the ages of 9 and 13. In contrast to degenerative spondylolisthesis (see p. 926), isthmic spondylolisthesis most commonly occurs at the L5/S1 levels and is only occasionally seen at the L4/L5 level. It rarely occurs above that level. The L5 vertebra normally is rectangular with a trefoil canal shape. Those persons with a trapezoidal shape and a dome shaped canal are associated with a higher incidence of lysis[48] and vertebral shift.[74] The history and findings in patients with spondylolisthesis are similar to spondylolysis, and when mild, present a clinical picture that is almost identical to disk degeneration,[57] although spondylolisthesis may be asymptomatic.[71] High-grade slips, as in a palpable step-off when palpating the tips of the spinous processes may also be visible. The greater the degree of slippage, the more prominent the "hollow" palpated between the spinous process of the affected vertebra and the one above. However, the step may not be readily palpable in obese persons. Pressure over the spinous process of the loose lamina will elicit pain. Pain is often aggravated by lying in the prone position. Serious disruption of the interspinous ligament may result in a palpable gap between adjacent spinous processes,[64] and may be differentiated from isthmic spondylolisthesis by an oblique radiograph.

- *Spinal muscle compartment syndrome.*[58] This is extremely uncommon, but may present as a cause of low back pain. The origin of this pathology derives from exercise induced low back pain that causes flattening of the lumbar lordosis,[63] is relieved by rest, and has no lower limb neurologic deficit. More common in athletes, this condition occurs because of raised intramuscular pressure which does not normalize after 20 minutes of rest. Compartment syndrome due to edema within the erector spinae muscles occurs as the posterior and middle layers of the thoracolumbar fascia envelop the erector spinae muscle and represent a closed compartment. Magnetic resonance imaging supports the diagnosis.[18] Fasciotomy may be indicated to normalize pressure.

35. What physical therapy is appropriate in the management of these injuries?

- *Modalities.* The use of physical modalities may help relieve the pain associated with the acute phase. Cold therapy in the form of an ice compress or ice massage, decreases spasm, inflammation, pain, and capillary blood flow, and is particularly helpful in cases of acute annular tear or ligament sprain. Although the skin cools quickly, the rate of muscle cooling is directly proportionate to the thickness of overlying fat and may range for 10 to 30 minutes.[68] The subacute or chronic states are preferably treated with thermotherapy such as deep heat (ultrasound, microwave, or shortwave) and, like heat, also minimize spasm and pain. Electrostimulation in the form of transcutaneous electrical nerve stimulation (TENS) or high volt galvanic stimulation (HVGS) may reduce acute muscle spasm, decrease edema, and relieve pain.[50] The

mechanism for pain relief from TENS involves raising the circulating levels of endogenous endorphins
or stimulating cutaneous afferents that block pain
stimuli in the substantia gelatinosa.[2] Percutaneous
dorsal column stimulators can also help patients with
chronic back pain. Phonophoresis or iontophoresis
with hydrocortisone, lidocaine, or salicylate may help
validate a suspected superficial ligamentous injury,
while providing immediate, albeit temporary, relief.
Gentle intermittent traction for ligament sprain, with
forces less than that required to separate the individual lumbar vertebrae (less than half of body
weight) may help the inhibition of transmission of
pain stimuli. Traction is not indicated for patients
with muscular strain.

- *Bracing.* Bracing via spinal orthoses is for the purpose of supporting the lower back in neutral, improving posture, and minimizing movement to the lumbar
vertebrae. The purpose of a lumbosacral corset or
lumbar support is to help prevent postural changes as
the ligament attempts to undergo repair. The corset
also helps to minimize hypermobility to that segment
so that scar tissue growing in between the two ends of
the frayed ligament does so with the ligament in a
shortened position.

    A lumbosacral orthosis may decrease intradiskal
pressure[79] and may also provide relief by way of local warmth and stimulation of mechanoreceptors.
Bracing is appropriate for any low back condition in
which movements that stress the joint increase the
discomfort. If only the lumbosacral region (L4-S1) is
to be immobilized, then a lumbosacral support is indicated, whereas if the lesion is in the mid or upper
lumbar region, a longer appliance is necessary. Supports within the canvas corset in the form of metal
stays placed in posterior pockets fasten in front and
have side straps for adjusting tightness. These supported forms of spinal corsets provide better relief
than the same canvas without support.[85] Elasticized
supports do not restrict spinal movement and mostly
benefit the patient with poor posture as they hold in
the abdomen and reduce lumbar lordosis allowing the
patient to look and feel better.

- *Strengthening.* Patients with postural strain syndrome
should exercise those weakened muscles that demonstrate excessive extensibility. Thus the patient with
excessive hyperlordosis, in addition to stretching the
tight psoas and paraspinal musculature, should
strengthen the abdominal and hamstrings muscles.
Performing sit-up exercises with the hips and knees

flexed activates the abdominal muscles, but should
not be performed through a large range as this will
increase pressure on the lumbar disk. These *trunk
curls* are best performed in a limited range of motion
so that the scapular just clears the floor, and thereby
minimize strain to the lumbar spine while effectively
recruiting abdominal musculature. A *reverse trunk-
curl* is performed with the hips and knees flexed so
that the knees are brought to the chest. This also
strengthens the abdominal muscles while limiting
stress to the lumbar spine. In contrast to sit-ups, leg
lifts may place increasing strain on the psoas muscle
which, when strongly contracted, pulls the pelvis into
anterior pelvic tilt and thereby increases the load to
the low back via hyperlordosis. With ligament sprain,
spinal flexion exercise is contraindicated, as they will
stress the injured ligaments. Strengthening of the
erector spinae may be performed in the prone position as extension exercises. To minimize increased
pressure placed on the lumbar disks with hyperextension, a pillow may be placed under the abdomen as a
support and contraction of the paraspinal musculature
may be done isometrically. With muscular strain, spinal extension exercises are contraindicated, as they
will stress the injured muscle(s).

- *Stretching.* Correction of soft tissue inflexibility of
trunk musculature and especially the lower extremity
is imperative toward optimal maintenance of the low
back. These large muscles which span across significant lengths of the trunk or lower extremity affects
the low back due to their insertion on the pelvis. The
hip flexors and extensors, in particular, should be
stretched because tightness of these muscles will rotate the pelvis excessively, and may negatively impact on both posture and the magnitude of lumbar
lordosis. Hyperlordosis is associated with anterior
pelvic tilt, which causes the pelvis to rotate forward
due to tightened hip flexors. Tight hamstrings cause a
pull on the pelvis to rotate it backwardly about the
common hip axis as posterior pelvic tilt and therefore
increase shear of L5 ("sliding down the hill") on S1.

- *Endurance training.* Cardiovascular and cardiopulmonary fitness are extremely important and may include brisk walking, jogging, swimming, tennis, and
stationary bicycle activities. Many patients find that
brisk walking eases their discomfort. Aerobic fitness
activities should emphasize activities that avoid high-
impact and ballistic-type spinal movements.

- *Pharmacology.* Pharmacologic treatments may be
categorized into analgesics that relieve pain, antiin-

flammatory medications, and muscle relaxants. Anti-inflammatory drugs have both an antiinflammatory and analgesic effect that promote healing by increasing circulation and bringing necessary nutrients into the inflamed area and eliminating toxic inflammatory substances, thereby allowing patients to more fully participate in physical therapy and activities of daily living. Antiinflammatory medications appear to be effective for relieving back pain if started within two days of onset of acute low back pain. Muscle relaxants, whose site of action is either the muscle spindle or the central nervous system, operate by relieving skeletal muscle spasm in the back without interfering with muscular function. In this manner they promote greater mobility that is essential to the recuperative process. Opioid analgesics interact by binding to the body's opiate receptors for endorphins and enkephalins, and are appropriate for severely acute back pain. If used on a short-term contingency basis there is little chance for addiction. Use of opioid analgesic for chronic back pain is discouraged because of the potential for addiction. Antidepressant drugs may elevate mood and increase pain tolerance in the emotionally depressed patient, reducing chronic low back pain.

* *Selective injection.* Therapeutic short- or long-acting injection of steroids and anesthetics into the area in which ligament disruption occurred may provide relief.

RECOMMENDED READING

Seimon LP: *Low back pain: clinical diagnosis and management,* ed 2, New York, 1995, Demos Vermande.

White AA, Panjabi MM editors: *Clinical biomechanics of the spine,* ed 2, Philadelphia, 1990, JB Lippincott.

REFERENCES

1. Adams MA, Hutton WC: Prolapsed intervertebral disk—a hyperflexion injury, *Spine* 7:184, 1982.
2. Amlie E, Weber H, Holme I: Treatment of acute low back pain with Piroxicam: results of a double-blind placebo-controlled trial, *Spine* 12:473, 1987.
3. Asimov I: *The wellsprings of life,* New York, 1960, New American Library.
4. Bachop W, Janse J: The corporotransverse ligament at the L5 intervertebral foramen, *Anat Rec* 205, (Abstract) 1983.
5. Baker BE: Current concept in the diagnosis and treatment of musculo-tendinous injuries, *Med Sci Sports Exercise* 16:323, 1984.
6. Bogduk N, Macintosh JE: The applied anatomy of the thoracolumbar fascia, *Spine* 9:164, 1984.
7. Bogduk N, Pearch MM, Hadfield G: The anatomy and biomechanics of psoas major, *Clin Biomechanics* 7:109, 1992.
8. Bogduk N, Twomey LT: *Clinical anatomy of the lumbar spine,* ed 2, Melbourne, 1991, Churchill Livingstone.
9. Bogduk N, Tynan W, Wilson AS: The nerve supply to the human lumbar intervertebral discs, *J Anatomy* 132:39, 1981.
10. Carr D, Frymoyer JW, Krag MH et al: The lumbo-dorsal fascial compartment, *Transamerican Orthop Res Soc* 9:252, 1984.
11. Church CP, Buehler MT: Radiographic evaluation of the corportransverse ligament at the L5 intervertebral foramen: a cadaveric study, *J Manipulative Physiol Therap* 14:240-248, 1991.
12. Ciullo JV, Jackson DW: Pars interarticularis stress reaction, spondylolysis, and spondylolisthesis in gymnasts, *Clin Sports Med* 4:95, 1985.
13. Cramer GD, Darby SA: *Basic and clinical anatomy of the spine, spinal cord, and ANS,* St Louis, 1995, Mosby.
14. Cyrix J: *Textbook of orthopaedic medicine: diagnosis of soft tissue lesions,* vol 1, ed 8, London, 1982, Bailliere-Tindall.
15. de Peretti F, Micalef JP, Bourgeon A et al: Biomechanics of the lumbar spinal nerve roots and the first sacral root within the intervertebral foramina, *Surg Radiol Anat* 11:221-225, 1989.
16. Difazio FA, Barth RA, Frymoyer JW: Acute lumbar paraspinal compartment syndrome, *J Bone Joint Surg* 73-A:1101, 1991.
17. Edgar M, Ghadially J: Innervation of the lumbar spine, *Clin Orthop* 115:35, 1976.
18. Ekholm J, Arborelius U, Fahlcrantz A et al: Activation of abdominal muscles during some physiotherapeutic exercise, *Scan J Rehabil Med* 11:75, 1979.
19. Epstein NE, Epstein JA, Carras R et al: Degenerative spondylolisthesis with an intact neural arch: a review of 60 cases with an analysis of clinical findings and the development of surgical management, *Neurosurgery* 13:555, 1983.
20. Fairband JC, Hall H: History taking and physical examination: identification of syndromes of back pain. In Weinstein JN, Wiesel SW, editors: *The lumbar spine,* Philadelphia, 1990, WB Saunders.
21. Farfan HF: Biomechanics of the spine in sports. In Watkins RG editor: *The spine in sports,* St Louis, 1996, Mosby,
22. Farfan HG: *Mechanical disorders of the low back,* Philadelphia, 1973, Lea & Febiger.
23. Farfan HF: Reorientation in the surgical approach to degenerative lumbar intervertebral joint disease, *Orthop Clin North Am* 8:9, 1977.
24. Farfan HF: The biomechanical advantage of lordosis and hip extension for upright man as compared with other anthropoids, *Spine* 3:336, 1978.
25. Gargan MF, Fairband JCT: Anatomy of the spine. In Watkins RG editor: *The spine in sports,* St Louis, 1996, Mosby.
26. Gossman M, Sahrmann S, Rose S: Review of length-associated changes in muscle, *Phys Ther* 62:1977, 1982.
27. Gould JA III: *Orthopaedic and sports physical therapy,* ed 2, St Louis, 1990, Mosby.
28. Gracovetsky S, Farfan HF, Helleur C: The abdominal mechanism, *Spine* 10:317, 1985.
29. Gracovetsky S: *The spinal engine,* Vienna, 1988, Springer-Verlag.
30. Grenier N, Greselle JF, Vital JM et al: Normal and disrupted lumbar longitudinal ligaments. Correlative MR and anatomic study, *Radiology* 171:197, 1989.

31. Hamilton WJ, editor: *Textbook of human anatomy,* ed 2, St Louis, 1976, Mosby.

32. Hasue M, Kikuchi S, Sakuyama Y et al: Anatomic study of the interrelation between lumbosacral nerve roots and their surrounding tissues, *Spine* 8:50, 1983.

33. Huges P: *Advanced upper extremity course. Workshop notes,* St Louis, 1979, Mosby.

34. Hukins DWL, Kirby MC, Sikoryn TA, et al: Comparison of structure, mechanical properties and functions of lumbar spinal ligaments, *Spine* 15:787, 1990.

35. Hutton WC: The forces acting on a lumbar intervertebral joint, *J Manual Med* 5:66, 1990.

36. Inman VT, Ralston HJ, Todd F et al: *Human walking,* Baltimore, 1981, Williams & Wilkins.

37. Jackson DW, Wiltse LL, Cirincione RJ: Spondylolysis in the female gymnast, *Clin Orthop* 117:68, 1976.

38. Jackson R: *The cervical syndrome,* Springfield, 1977, Charles C Thomas.

39. Kapandji IA: *The physiology of the joints,* vol 3, ed 2, London, 1974, Churchill Livingstone.

40. Kapandji I: *The physiology of the joints: the trunk and vertebral column,* vol 2, ed 2, New York, 1974, Churchill-Livingstone.

41. Kapandji IA: The physiology of joints: lower limb, vol 2, ed 2, London, 1970, ES Livingstone.

42. Kapit W, Elson LM: *The anatomy coloring book,* New York, 1977, Harper & Row.

43. Kendall FP, McCreary EK: *Muscles: testing and function,* ed 3, Baltimore, 1983, Williams & Wilkins.

44. Kirkaldy-Willis WH, Wedge JH, Yong-Hing K et al: Pathology and pathogenesis of lumbar spondylosis and stenosis, *Spine* 3:319, 1978.

45. Kisner C, Colby LA: *Therapeutic exercise: foundations and techniques,* ed 2, Philadelphia, 1990, FA Davis.

46. Korkala O, Gronblad M, Liesi P et al: Immunohistochemical demonstration of nociceptors in the ligament structures of the lumbar spine, *Spine* 10:156, 1985.

47. Kuslich SD, Ulstrom CL, Michael CJ: The tissue origin of low back pain and sciatica: a report of pain response to tissue stimulation during operations on the lumbar spine using local anesthesia, *Orthop Clin North Am* 22:181, 1991.

48. Lehman J: Therapeutic heat and cold, *Clin Orthop* 99:207, 1974.

49. Lehmkuhl LD, Smith LK: *Brunnstrom's clinical kinesiology,* ed 4, Philadelphia, 1983, FA Davis.

50. Lindh M: Biomechanics of the lumbar spine. In Nordin M, Frankel VH editors: *Basic biomechanics of the musculoskeletal system,* ed 2, Philadelphia, 1989, Lea & Febiger.

51. Lovett AW: A contribution to the study of the mechanics of the spine, *Am J Anat* 2:457, 1903.

52. MacConaill MA, Basmajian JV: *Muscles and movement,* Baltimore, 1969, Williams & Wilkins.

53. Macintosh JE, Bogduk N, Graccovetsky S: The biomechanics of the thoracolumbar fascia, *Clin Biomechanics* 2:78, 1987.

54. Macintosh JE, Bogduk N: The morphology of the lumbar erector spinae, *Spine* 12:658, 1987.

55. Magee DJ: *Orthopedic physical assessment,* Philadelphia, 1987, WB Saunders.

56. McGill SM, Normal RW: Effects of anatomically detailed erector spinae model of L4/L5 disc compression and shear, *J Biomechanics* 20:591, 1987.

57. Melzack R, Wall PD: Pain mechanisms: a new theory, *Science* 50:971, 1965.

58. Million R, Nilsen KH, Jayson MIV et al: Evaluation of low back pain and assessment of lumbar corsets without and without back supports, *Ann Rheum Dis* 40:449, 1981.

59. Moe JH, Bradford DS, Winter RB et al: *Scoliosis and other spinal deformities,* Philadelphia, 1978, WB Saunders.

60. Moore RL: *Clinically oriented anatomy,* Baltimore, 1980, Williams & Wilkins.

61. Myklebust JB, Pintar F, Yoganandan N et al: Tensile strength of spinal ligaments, *Spine* 13(5):526, 1988.

62. Nachemson A: Electromyographic studies on the vertebral of the psoas muscle, *Acta Orthop Scand* 37:177, 1966.

63. Nachemson A, Elfstrom G: *Intravital dynamic pressure measurements in lumbar discs: a study of common movements, maneuvers, and exercises,* Stockholm, 1970, Almqvist & Wiksell.

64. Nachemson A: Lumbar spine instability; a critical update and symposium summary, *Spine* 10:290, 1985.

65. Newman PH: Surgical treatment for spondylolisthesis in the adult, *Clin Orthop* 117:106, 1976.

66. Nimini ME: Collagen: structure, function and metabolism in normal and fibrotic tissues, *Semin Arthritis Rheum* 13:1, 1983.

67. Norwicki BH, Haughton VM: Ligaments of the lumbar neural foramina: a sectional anatomic study, *Clin Anat* 5:126, 1992.

68. Partridge MJ, Walters CE: Participation of the abdominal muscles in various movements of the trunk in man: an electromyographic study, *Phys Ther* 39:791, 1959.

69. Peck D, Nicholls PJ, Beard C et al: Are there compartment syndromes in some patient with idiopathic back pain? *Spine* 11:468, 1986.

70. Porter RW: *Management of back pain,* ed 2, Melbourne, 1993, Churchill Livingstone.

71. Racz GB, McCarron RF, Talboys P: Percutaneous dorsal column stimulator for chronic pain control, *Spine* 14:1, 1989.

72. Rauschning W: Normal and pathologic anatomy of the lumbar root canals, *Spine* 12:1008, 1987.

73. Rocabado M: *Physical therapy and dentistry I and II.* Course notes. 1979 and 1981.

74. Roeser WM, Meeks LW, Venis R et al: The use of transcutaneous nerve stimulation for pain control in athletic medicine: a preliminary report, *Am J Sports Med* 4:210, 1976.

75. Rosenberg NJ: Degenerative spondylolisthesis: predisposing factors, *J Bone Joint Surg* 57:467, 1975.

76. Schonstrom NR, Hansson TH: Thickness of the human ligamentum flavum as a function of load: an in vitro experimental study, *Clin Biomechanics,* 6.

77. Schultz AB, Andersson GBJ, Haderspeck K et al: Analysis and measurement of lumbar trunk loads in tasks involving bends and twists, *J Biomechanics* 15:669, 1982.

78. Seimon LP: *Low back pain: clinical diagnosis and management,* ed 2, New York, 1995, Demos Vermande.

79. Stimmel B: Pain, analgesia, and addiction: an approach to the pharmacological management of pain, *Clin J Pain* 1:14, 1985.

80. Tesh D, Dunn L, Evans J: The abdominal muscles and vertebral stability, *Spine* 12:501, 1987.

81. Tesh KM, Shaw-Dunn J, Evans JH: The abdominal muscles and vertebral stability, *Spine* 12:501, 1987.

82. Tomita K, Kawahara N, Baba H et al: Circumspinal decompression for thoracic myelopathy due to combined ossification of the posterior longitudinal ligament and ligamentum flavum, *Spine* 15.1990.

83. Twomey LT: *Clinical anatomy of the lumbar spine,* ed 2, Melbourne, 1981, Churchill Livingstone.

84. Waitz E: The lateral bending sign, *Spine* 6:388, 1981.

85. Ward NG: Tricyclic antidepressants for chronic low back pain: mechanisms of action and predictors of response, *Spine,* 11:661, 1986.

86. Warwick R, Williams P: *Gray's anatomy,* ed 35, (Br), Philadelphia, 1973, WB Saunders.

87. Weisz GM: Lumbar spinal canal stenosis in Paget's disease, *Spine* 8, 1983.

88. White AA, Panjabi MM editors: *Clinical biomechanics of the spine,* ed 2, Philadelphia, 1990, JB Lippincott.

89. Williams PL, Gray H: *Gray's anatomy,* ed 37, 1989, Edinburgh, Churchill Livingstone.

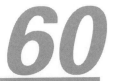

60

Spontaneous Low Back Pain Aggravated by Flexion and Straining, Relieved by Recumbency, that Decreases with Concurrent Peripheralization of Pain

CASE 1: A 51-year-old male construction worker with no previous history of back pain experienced sudden stabbing pain emanating from the low back several weeks ago after lifting a heavy hose. He dropped the hose and could not immediately straighten due to severe pain. After 10 minutes, pain had subsided somewhat and he continued working, using a 45-lb jackhammer in a flexed posture. After ½ hour operating the jackhammer his back pain recurred and became increasingly severe over the next several hours to the point where he could not bend or straighten. A coworker drove him home and he went to bed as lying down, while still painful, felt more comfortable than standing or sitting. After several days in bed, he was able to get up for trips to the toilet and meals, although sitting in either a hard or soft chair aggravated pain. Ten days after the onset of symptoms he was walking up a hill and experienced sudden severe pain in the middle of the right buttock with radiation down the posterolateral aspect of the thigh and lateral aspect of the leg and ankle as corresponding to diminishment of back pain. Once leg symptoms became dominant, pain was aggravated by sitting and changing position and relieved when standing and walking. Coughing, sneezing, laughing, and straining during bowel movements aggravated buttock pain.

OBSERVATION   The patient is strong and muscular and normally stands erect without deformity. No muscle wasting observed. A loss of lumbar lordosis is noted.

PALPATION   A mild tenderness is present on firm palpation in the lumbosacral region. There is no palpable step at the lumbosacral junction.

RANGE OF MOTION   Spinal flexion is markedly restricted and causes radiating pain to the right buttock. Extension is negative, as is bilateral lateral bend, although pain occurs in the right buttock when bending to that side.

STRENGTH   Patient walks on heels, toes, and the lateral and medial borders of his feet without difficulty. The right extensor hallucis longus (EHL) is slightly weaker than the left. The right gluteus medius muscle is graded Good minus.

FLEXIBILITY   There is normal soft tissue extensibility in the lower extremity musculature.

CIRCUMFERENTIAL MEASUREMENTS   There is no muscle wasting evident at the mid thigh or mid calf level.

SENSATION   There is normal sensation in both lower limbs except for a small area over the dorsomedial aspect of the right forefoot, where there is diminution to pinprick.

DEEP TENDON REFLEXES   Knee and ankle reflexes are brisk and equal, whereas plantar response is downward. Mild diminution of the right tibialis posterior reflex.

SACROILIAC AND HIP JOINTS   Negative Gaenslen test and Faber maneuver.

PERIPHERAL CIRCULATION   The lower extremity pulses are intact.

SPECIAL TESTS   The right straight leg raise (SLR) is limited to 30°and there is a positive Lasègue sign with pain radiating down the posterior aspect of the thigh. Left SLR is 75° and a negative Lasègue. With the patient in a sitting position, the right leg was passively extended slowly; the patient leaned backward to a position equivalent to a 30° SLR. Femoral stretch test is bilaterally negative. A prone press up somewhat relieves and centralizes pain.

CLUE   Electromyographic testing yielded fibrillation potentials and positive sharp waves in the right gluteus medius and toe extensors, particularly extensor hallucis longus.

CASE 2:   A 40-year-old female physician presents with low back pain, right sciatica, and the following history. During the last 3 of her 4 pregnancies she experienced left sciatica that resolved with subsequent low back pain and subsequent mild and occasional low back discomfort. The latter did not restrict her activities until approximately 8 months ago when she experienced greater pain than usual, which required 9 days of bed rest until symptoms decreased. Several weeks ago she experienced a second bout of spontaneous back pain but, as she could not take off work, remained at her job. Pain was aggravated by bending, sitting in a soft chair, or while straining, and was relieved by recumbency, sitting in a firm, upright chair, and when walking. After several days the pain eased off although she suddenly developed severe pain radiating down from her low back to her left buttock, ischial tuberosity, and down the posterior aspect of her left thigh and leg as well as lateral aspect of her foot. She believes this started when she bent down to pick up a heavy object. When asked, she admits that the latter area feels numb and tingles at times. Now, sitting in any type of chair aggravates pain, as does sneezing or coughing, and walking, in addition to bending and lifting objects. Back symptoms are relieved considerably by recumbency in the supine posture with her left knee bent and supported by a pillow, although leg symptoms persisted.

OBSERVATION   A left trunk list is observed in the direction of the sciatica that is abolished when the patient lies down. There is significant flattening of the lumbar spine. No swelling noted.

PALPATION   There is mild lumbosacral tenderness; no "step" is palpable. The paraspinal muscles feel "tight" and in spasm.

RANGE OF MOTION   Although lateral bending and extension are unremarkable, forward spinal flexion is markedly restricted and aggravates pain. The patient claims that before the recent symptoms she was able to touch her toes with ease.

STRENGTH   She walks on tiptoe but is unable to maintain the equinus posture on the left due to weakness of gastrocnemius. She can walk on her heels and on the lateral but not medial borders of left foot. Mild weakness in the left gluteus maximus and hamstring musculature compared with the right. The left extensor hallucis is normal. There is a suggestion of mild resisted knee flexion on the left.

FLEXIBILITY   The prone bend test for psoas muscle extensibility shows diminished flexibility on the left side, indicated by a higher, more protruding left buttock. Positive Thomas test bilaterally.

SENSATION   There is blunting to pinprick over the left heel and lateral border of the foot including the lateral two toes.

DEEP TENDON REFLEXES   Although both knee jerks are brisk and equal, both ankle jerks are present, although the left is diminished. Additionally, the distal medial and lateral hamstring reflexes are diminished on the left. Unsustained clonus of the left ankle noted. Plantar responses are downward.

PULSES   These are intact.

CIRCUMFERENTIAL MEASUREMENTS   The left thigh and calf demonstrate a difference in girth of 1 and 1.5 cm, respectively, as compared with the right lower extremity.

SPECIAL TESTS   Although the right SLR is 70°, the left is 45°. When seen a few days later, her left SLR had improved to 65°. Positive Lasègue on the left but not right. Positive bowstring sign and Brudzinski test on left. Left heel drop test is weakly positive. Squatting is normal. Positive diurnal SLR and crossed-leg sign.

CASE 3:   A 17-year-old male reports that 9 months ago he was deep sea fishing with his father when his boat was caught in the wake of another vessel while approaching port. He was flung into the air and came down landing heavily on his back. He screamed and lay motionless. His father immediately brought him to the nearest hospital where he was cleared for any fracture and allowed to go home as within several hours he was much better and has continued to make good progress. Since that time he continues to experience pain in the low back, specifically in the lumbosacral region, that is brought on by bending and especially when coming upright after working in a flexed position for some time or lifting objects in a flexed position. Pain does not radiate to the buttocks or lower limbs. Apart from this, his back does not bother him. He can run, jump, and sit for as long as he likes without any discomfort in recumbency.

OBSERVATION   He is a healthy looking young man with excellent posture. He stands erect, with the pelvis and shoulders level. He climbs onto the examining plinth with ease.

PALPATION   Tenderness is present in the midline of the midlumbar level. There is no "step" or any evidence of a palpable mass.

RANGE OF MOTION   Lumbar flexion is performed easily with fingertips reaching to 10 cm from the floor. Lateral bend to either side is normal, as is spinal extension. Lateral bend to the right in combination with flexion provokes slight discomfort.

STRENGTH   He can walk on his heels and toes, and either border of his feet without hindrance.

FLEXIBILITY   There are tight hamstrings suggested by bilateral limitation of straight leg raising to 40° with pain proximal to the popliteal space. No tightness noted in the quadriceps and iliopsoas musculature.

DEEP TENDON REFLEXES   These are normal.

PULSES   These are normal.

SACROILIAC AND HIP JOINTS   Negative sacroiliac compression and Patrick test.

SPECIAL TESTS   Negative straight leg raising bilaterally, and negative Lasègue's tests.

RADIOGRAPHS   These are normal.

CLUE   Computerized tomography was positive for internal disk disruption.

CASE 4: A 32-year-old powerfully built underwater welder was taking down heavy pipes from a shelf at full arms' stretch and twisted toward one side as he lowered them down. He felt something "give" in his low back, which felt like a twinge of pain. He ignored this until the following day when he lifted a scuba tank and again felt a twinge of pain in the lumbosacral area, which this time radiated toward his buttocks. The next day, while sitting, he developed increasing pain radiating to the posterior aspect of his upper thighs that made walking very difficult. Symptoms were aggravated by sneezing, coughing, and turning over in bed. Pain was most severe when sitting in any kind of chair or when standing in a slightly stooped position. Flexing his neck would only worsen symptoms. The most comfortable position was lying supine with both hips and knees flexed over a large bolster, although this did not entirely alleviate the dull, aching pain. When asked, the patient does not report any acute urine retention.

OBSERVATION   The patient is muscular and stands erect without evidence of spinal deformity.

PALPATION   There is mild tenderness in the lumbosacral region. No "step" palpable. Paraspinal musculature is tight and in spasm.

RANGE OF MOTION   Forward flexion is markedly limited with fingers barely reaching knee level. Extension and lateral flexion are average and pain free.

STRENGTH   He is capable of walking on tiptoe, heels, and the borders of his feet without difficulty.

FLEXIBILITY   Negative Thomas test and prone knee bend. Hamstring flexibility untested secondary to pain, although the patient reports being able to touch his toes with ease before symptoms.

SENSATION   This is normal.

DEEP TENDON REFLEXES   These are normal.

PULSES   These are normal.

SPECIAL TESTS   Positive bilateral SLR of 30° with marked discomfort in the low back, but no referred pain down the lower extremities. Negative Lasègue test, bilaterally. Splaying and compression of the sacroiliac joints prove negative.

CASE 5: A 31-year-old tall and muscular auto mechanic complains of low back pain since the age of 16 and is aware of aching when waking up on most mornings. Several times per year, particularly after strenuous activity, symptoms are more pronounced while range-of-motion is markedly restricted, although they usually settle down after a few days rest. He regularly plays basketball, cricket, and splits firewood. Six weeks ago he awoke one morning and could hardly transfer out of bed secondary to severe low back pain that was aggravated by any change of position such as sitting, getting in and out of a car, and while turning around while sitting. He is relatively comfortable when walking slowly, and experiences complete abatement of pain when completely immobile. When asked, the patient localizes the area of maximum discomfort to the right lumbosacral region.

OBSERVATION   The patient stands upright and no visible "step" is apparent. He has no difficulty climbing onto the examination table.

PALPATION   The L5 spinous process is palpably prominent. No localized tenderness with exception to mild tenderness with pinpoint pressure over the L5 spinous process.

RANGE OF MOTION   Flexion is restricted to one half of full range with pain at the right posterior iliac superior spine. Before this incident, the patient claims he could almost touch his toes. Although extension and left lateral bend are negative, right lateral bend is painful, especially when simultaneously extending.

STRENGTH   The patient walks on his heels, toes, and borders of his feet without difficulty.

FLEXIBILITY   Bilaterally tight hamstrings.

DEEP TENDON REFLEXES   This is normal.

PULSES   These are normal.

SPECIAL TESTS   Negative SLR, Lasègue, femoral stretch and heel drop tests.

? Questions

1. What is most likely the cause of these patients' symptoms?
2. What is the spectrum of mechanical causes of low back pain?
3. What is lumbar disk disease?
4. What are the clinical implications of a growth differential between the spinal cord and vertebral elements?
5. What are the implications of the differential growth of the spinal cord and vertebrae to the orientation of nerve roots below the cervical spine?
6. What are the intercentral ligaments of the spine?
7. What are the components of the intervertebral disk?
8. What are the structural components of the intervertebral disk?
9. What is the innervation of the intervertebral disk?
10. What are vertebral endplates and what is their role in fluid inflow and outflow?
11. What is the annulus fibrosus?
12. What structural properties are endowed to the annulus by the oblique organization of its concentric lamellae?

13. Which portion of the annulus is weakest and what is the clinical significance?

14. What is the nucleus pulposus and how do its constituent properties change with age?

15. How do the proteoglycan molecules within the disk matrix contribute to regulation of the flow of water within the matrix of the intervertebral disk?

16. How does disk hydration vary with the erect posture and diurnal changes?

17. Why does the amount of water within the vertebral disk vary with age?

18. What are endplate herniations and why are they more common in the younger population?

19. How may progressive deterioration of the nuclear matrix known as *internal disk disruption* result from an endplate herniation?

20. How does internal disk disruption serve as a primary source of low back pain?

21. What two endstage pathologies may result secondary to internal disk disruption?

22. Why does disk degeneration that accompanies aging result in horizontal as opposed to vertical endplate herniations?

23. What is the relationship between degenerative disk disease and disk prolapse?

24. What is the protective role of the facet joints and musculoligamentous system in relation to the intervertebral disk?

25. How may a circumferential tear of the annulus fibrosus in the absence of nuclear migration serve as a primary source of back pain?

26. What is the difference between circumferential and radial tears of the annulus fibrosus?

27. How is the location of the instantaneous center of the intervertebral disk related to disk pathology?

28. Why do disks herniate posterolaterally?

29. What is a far lateral disk herniation?

30. What is the progressive sequence of disk prolapse?

31. What is the pathogenesis of radicular pain following disk prolapse?

32. Why is the L5 nerve root more vulnerable to compression?

33. What is the relationship between the spinal nerves and the intervertebral disks in the lumbar spine?

34. What are the various patterns of nerve root compression at any given lumbar level?

35. What are the relevant nerve root innervations to the dermatomes and myotomes of the lower extremities?

36. What are the reflexes of the lower extremity and what is their diagnostic value?

37. What are deep tendon reflexes of the lower extremity and how are they elicited?

38. What is the clinical presentation of disk pathology?

39. What is a trunk list?

40. What is the *straight leg raise* (SLR) and what does a positive test signify?

41. How may the SLR be interpreted so as to clinically differentiate between nerve root impingement deriving from spinal stenosis and disk pathology?

42. What is the diurnal SLR test and what is its clinical significance?

43. What is the crossover sign and what does it signify?

44. In addition to the motor, sensory, and reflex assessment, what are other essential components of the examination?

45. What factor does vertebral canal size play in symptomatology following a disk lesion?

46. What are nonorganic forms of back pain?

47. What is the differential diagnosis of low back pain?

48. What are pars interarticularis lesions?

49. What is the most common form of spondylolisthesis?

50. How is spondylolysis differentiated from disk pathology?

51. What is the relationship between isthmic spondylolisthesis and acute locked back?

52. What therapeutic intervention is most appropriate in the conservative rehabilitation of patients with disk pathology?

53. What are the indications for surgery?

1. What is most likely the cause of these patients' symptoms?

L5 nerve root compression in Case 1, S1 nerve root compression in Case 2, acute annular tear in Case 3, midline herniation in Case 4, and spondylitic pathology in Case 5. Because of the anatomy of the lumbar nerve roots in relation to the lumbar vertebrae, L4/L5 disk herniations most commonly affect the L5 nerve root, whereas L5/S1 protrusions affect the S1 nerve root.

The historical and clinical presentation of Case 1 is classic for a *lumbar disk herniation*. The initial sudden sharp pain corresponds to annular cracking that progresses to extrusion through the annular crack by increased intradiskal pressure from the flexed lumbar posture that facilitates posterior migration of the nuclear material out of the annulus. The recurring and increasingly severe back pain that subsequently occurred stemmed from pressure of the extruded material on the innervated posterior longitudinal ligament, causing protective muscle spasm that markedly restricts range of motion, particularly flexion. Recumbency somewhat relieves symptoms as it diminishes the axial compression of the disk and temporarily arrests the posterior nuclear migration. Symptoms were somewhat relieved as the sensory receptors acclimate to the volley of afferent pain impulses. Ten days later, the sustained activity of walking up an incline corresponds to sustained lumbar flexion and increased intradiskal pressure causing lateralization of symptoms. The sudden alleviation of back pain and increased leg pain corresponds to the extruded material migrating posterolaterally along the path of least resistance beyond the rhomboidal shaped posterior longitudinal ligament to chemically irritate or mechanically compress the right L5 spinal nerve root. Alternately, the protrusion may burst through the posterior longitudinal ligament, relieving tension on that ligament with subsequent diminishment of back pain, with the extruded material now pressing on the L5 nerve root. L5 radiculopathy was suggested by the subsequent clinical findings such as marked limitation in lumbar flexion, positive right straight leg raise (SLR) and Lasègue, positive thecal signs, weakness of the right extensor hallucis longus (EHL), a diminished tibialis posterior reflex, and mild diminution of pinprick in the region of the right big toe medially. Loss of lumbar lordosis occurs secondary to local muscle spasm because lordosis causes narrowing of both the spinal canal and intervertebral foramen, whereas flattening

provides more space to the neural elements and relieves pain. Radiographs show mild narrowing of the L4/L5 disk space and gross narrowing of the L5/S1 disk space with osteophyte formation. The increased narrowing of the disk below was worse due to years accumulation of disk and facet joint degeneration secondary to shear across the lumbosacral junction from heavy manual labor. This altered the local biomechanics of the spinal motion segment above the lumbosacral junction and predisposed disk pathology (annular weakening) of the L4/L5 level. Compressive forces on the L5 nerve root from an L4/L5 disk herniation increase with flexion of the L4/L5 motion segment resulting in increased tension on the nerve root, whereas extension decreases the compressive force. Thus *centralization of symptoms* during press-ups correlates with a good prognostic outcome and suggests that rehabilitation should bias extension over flexion as a primary thrust of physical therapy.

The historical presentation in Case 2 of low back pain, subsequently easing with concomitant development of left sciatica accompanied by signs and symptoms of an S1 radiculopathy suggests a clinical diagnosis of an *L5/S1 disk herniation* involving the *left S1 nerve root*. In this classic history of a disk herniation at the L5/S1 disk interspace, the initial back pain was attributed to stretching of the posterior longitudinal ligament by the herniated material. The sudden radiation of pain peripherally, which coincided with diminished low back pain, probably resulted from the disk rupturing through the posterior longitudinal ligament, relieving the tension, but now pressing on the S1 nerve root. When looking for evidence of an S1 root lesion, *eversion* of the foot is the best choice for motor assessment. The S1 motor contribution to other muscles includes the gluteus maximi, the hamstrings, and the gastrocnemius-soleus muscles. However, as the former two are large and powerful muscles with multiple root supply, weakness and wasting may be difficult to detect in the presence of a single root lesion. Clinical muscle testing of gastroc-soleus may be performed by having the patient walk on their toes, and weakness of the left was suggested by a positive heel drop test. Hypoesthesia in the S1 cutaneous distribution is consistent with S1 radiculopathy. The presence of unsustained *clonus* may be a normal variant and may occur from anxiety, medication, or drug withdrawal. Sciatic pain secondary to disk pathology typically results in positive *thecal signs* in which coughing, sneezing, laughing, or straining aggravates the nerve root within the dural sleeve enveloping the root.

The presence of a negative femoral stretch test and positive prone knee bend is not contradictory. Although the former tests for nerve root compression of L3 by stretching the femoral nerve, the latter, performed identically, tests for extensibility of psoas tightness. Nerve root compression would manifest as increased back and/ or anterior thigh pain, whereas tightness of the hip flexors is a distinctly different "pulling" sensation along the hip flexors. A *list* occurs as a protective response that reflexively postures the back in a position that eases the root away from the prolapsed disk and thereby eases root irritation. The muscles responsible for generating the list include the psoas major and spinal muscles. When the herniation is medial to the nerve root, the list is toward the side of the sciatica because tilting away would irritate the root and provoke pain. Abolition of the list may be accomplished by lying down or hanging from a bar. The lumbar area will become flattened owing to *loss of normal lumbar lordosis.* This is due to associated muscle spasm, which may range from moderate to severe, and acts to diminish extension of the spine because hyperlordosis causes narrowing of both the spinal canal and intervertebral foramen. With regard to the *positive diurnal SLR,* following as little as 2 hours of lying in bed or after a night's sleep, the disk will reimbibe fluid. In the morning, the bulging disk will be tense and clinically manifest as diminished straight leg raising as compared with the night before. After being up and around for 1 or 2 hours, the hydrostatic pressure of axial spinal compressive load will cause fluid loss from within the disk and is demonstrated by an increased range in the degree of straight leg raising. The *Thomas test,* indicating a fixed *hip flexion contracture,* refers to the inability to fully extend the leg without arching the thoracolumbar spine. The shortness of these anterior muscles on the pelvis causes an anterior pelvic tilt that accentuates the lumbar lordosis and results in greater strain to the motion segment. A positive *crossover sign* refers to pain that is symptomatically worsened by raising the contralateral lower extremity and suggests a situation where the disk material lies medial to the nerve root. Thus contralateral leg raising has the effect of depressing the affected nerve root and moving it toward midline, which increases root tension and provokes pain. This test may cause pain on both sides as it may stretch both the ipsilateral and contralateral nerve roots.

The historical and clinical presentation of Case 3 of sudden acute back pain in a young person with no previous history and no accompanying neurological signs suggests either an *acute annular* or ligament *tear.* However, the mechanism of injury suggests a cleavage through the annulus, which occurs from excessive axial compressive force or the combination motions of flexion and torsion. This was later confirmed by computerized tomography (CT) diskography. The initial pain was purely diskal in origin and corresponded to the combination of sudden annular and circumferential tears of the central lamellae that extended peripherally into the outer third of the annulus and stimulated nociceptors there. Classified under *internal disk disruption,* the pain associated with annular sprain is intensified by any factor that increases disk compression and increases disk stress; hence, flexion would be painful. Two endstage pathologies may evolve in years to come following internal disk disruption. Damage having occurred to the disk, gradual deterioration sets in as the disk is less capable of binding water and loses its cohesive properties and can poorly withstand compressive force. Disk resorption after injury causes the weight at that motion segment to be borne by the annulus, which eventually buckles under compression and manifests on radiographs years later as a narrowing of the disk space. This shifts the weight-bearing role at that segment posterior to the facet joints, which respond by osteoarthritic hypertrophy. Alternately, following the initial annular tear, the circumferential tears of adjacent lamella may connect via radial tears so that a channel is created from the deep, central aspect of the disk to its periphery through successive layers of the annulus. This channel serves as a potential path for expression of the nucleus pulposus and the evolution of disk pathology that, with gradual nuclear deterioration over time, may cause radiculitis during an unguarded movement involving torsion or flexion. This young man's tight hamstrings will posteriorly tilt his pelvis and result in a decreased lordotic curve. This relative flexion may aggravate pressures of the lower lumbar disks. As such, in addition to education concerning proper bending and lifting, an essential part of rehabilitative management would be hamstring stretching.

The history and presentation of Case 4 suggests a patient with a large *midline disk herniation* without evidence of radiculopathy. The initial and secondary twinge may have corresponded to annular tearing and enlargement of the initial tear, which is so vulnerable to torsion derived from the combined motions of flexion and rotation. The positive thecal signs of pain exacerbated by sneezing and coughing suggest herniation of a disk with tense pressure against the posterior longitudinal ligament causing unremitting pain, that is reduced by the supine lying posture with the flexed hips and knees. A ligamentous injury should not cause constant pain with bed rest, but would cause restriction of all motions but would not demonstrate a positive SLR. Because the large herniation is confined by the posterior longitudinal ligament, no radicular compression has occurred and consequently, the Lasègue sign, which tenses the sciatic nerve tract, would be negative as no neural elements are compromised. A bilateral positive SLR is highly suggestive of an acute midline disk herniation.

The historical and clinical presentation of Case 5 with no antecedent history of trauma, spontaneous low back pain since the age of 16 and periodic exacerbations, combined with no objective motor, sensory, or reflex deficit, is highly suggestive of *spondylitic pathology*. The recent episode of pain after waking up from a night's sleep presented as an acute locked back due to an unguarded movement that caused a perturbation of the right pars interarticularis or right facet joint. The palpable prominence of the L5 spinous process substantiates the diagnosis of spondylolisthesis as this sign is almost pathognomic for forward slippage of L4 (which is less prominent) on L5 (which is relatively prominent in relation to L4). Radiographs confirmed the suspected diagnosis by showing a *grade 1 isthmic spondylolisthesis of L4 on L5* with bilateral defects of the pars interarticularis.

2. What is the spectrum of mechanical causes of low back pain?

Low back pain includes the variety of mechanical disease entities and spans the pathologic spectrum from degenerative disk disease to disk pathology, acute locked back, spondylitic pathology, and spinal stenosis. In the United States during the decade from 1971 to 1981, the number of individuals suffering by low back pain grew at a rate 14 times that of the population growth.[100] Low back pain causes innumerable loss of time from work and is so common as to almost be considered a variation of normal.[198] Back pain is estimated to occur in 80% of adults at some point in their lives and is possibly the most common complaint related to industrial injury and compensation claims. It is estimated to constitute the majority of patients seen for evaluation and treatment in orthopaedic physical therapy clinics,[45] and accounts for annual hospital costs estimated at one billion dollars per year.[49] The magnitude of the overall economic burden has been estimated at 40 to 50 billion dollars annually, which includes medical, compensation, legal, vocational retraining, and lost productivity costs.[100] Patients with symptomatic lower lumbar disk lesions suffer peak prevalence in the fourth decade, instability in the fifth decade, neurogenic claudication with or without root entrapment in the sixth decade, and a steady decline in presentation of these pathologies thereafter.[151]

3. What is lumbar disk disease?

Acute lumbar disk herniation goes by a variety of synonyms such as disk prolapse, disk rupture, acute sciatica, and slipped disk. In 1934, Mixter and Barr[136] introduced the concept of neurologic compression of the nerve roots due to a mechanical cause such as a herniated disk. Indeed, they made sense of the clinical affliction known for centuries and referred to by Shakespeare's Timon of Athens as "Thou cold sciatica cripple our senators."[34] The colloquial term "slipped disk" is inaccurate in that this name implies the intervertebral disk in its entirety slips like a coin from a slot. Disk lesions may either be hard or soft, although both may cause nerve root compression. The hard type refers to a loose, cartilaginous fragment of annulus that bulges outward near a neural structure, or actually breaks free and compresses a neural structure. The soft disk pathology refers to the inner nucleus pulposus extruding through the outer annulus fibrosus and compressing a neural structure. Moreover, a disk herniation may result in a previously healthy disk following a particularly severe strain such as when lifting a heavy weight. Alternately, herniation may occur from relatively lesser strains in previously damaged or degenerative disks.[174]

The frequency of lumbar disk disease at various levels varies considerably. Lesions affecting the L5 and S1 nerve roots account for 85% of disk pathology, whereas lesions affecting L2, L3, and L4 account for the remainder, most of these occurring at the L4 level. It follows that root lesions of the L2 and L3 nerve roots, as well as the S2, S3, S4, and S5 roots are more likely to result from other pathologies and mandate urgent investigation. Epidemiologically, symptomatic disk lesions more commonly occur in the male during the fourth decade of life.[178] Thus disk disease occurs in middle age, whereas the outcrops of bone that progressively cup the spine with increasing age offer the benefit of increased stability to the anterior and posterior joints of the spine and correspondingly protect against excessive spinal motion that would injure the annulus and provoke nuclear prolapse. Hence, the frequency of disk-related backache is greatest between the ages of 40 and 50, diminishes between 50 and 60, and reduces by two thirds between 60 and 70 years of age.[42] There is a positive familial relationship in patients with disk protrusions. More than twice as many have first degree relatives with back pain than might otherwise be expected,[153] and identical symptoms in teenage twins also suggest a familial factor.[70]

4. What are the clinical implications of a growth differential between the spinal cord and vertebral elements?

If the spinal cord and column were of the same length, then we could expect the cord segments at each level (represented by the emergent nerve roots for that level) to be adjacent to the vertebrae and each successive nerve would emerge straight out, horizontally. However, because of a growth differential in the neonate between the rate of osseous and neural tissue, this corresponding relationship is lost below the cervical spine. The vertebral column and dura mater lengthen more rapidly than does the neural tube, so that the terminal end of the spinal cord gradually assumes a relatively higher level than the termination of the osseous spine.* The effect of this growth differential impacts on the orientation of span of the emerging nerve roots such that the cord segments are not located at the same level as their corresponding vertebrae. The cervical nerve roots are minimally affected and have a slight downward angulation along their exit span. At birth, the caudal tip of the spinal cord (conus medularis) lies at the level of the L3 vertebral body and continues to move upward as the child grows into an adult so that the conus is usually located anywhere between the T12 and L2 disk.[56] The L1 through the coccygeal cord segments (and emergent nerve root) are housed by vertebrae T9 through L1. The clinical implications of this anatomic difference between the cervical and lumbar spine is that because the spinal cord ends opposite the L1 vertebra, lumbar disk lesions can **only** cause root syndromes and cannot compress the cord and cause spastic paraparesis.

5. What are the implications of the differential growth of the spinal cord and vertebrae to the orientation of nerve roots below the cervical spine?

As a result of this unequal growth between the spinal cord and its osseous cover, the portion of the cord giving rise to emergent root pairs at each level is higher than the corresponding intervertebral foramen through which the corresponding nerve exits. This obliquity varies throughout the length of the vertebral column and becomes progressively oblique toward its inferior end. The *spinal cord level* refers to that level of the cord from which the nerve roots emerge. The spinal cord levels and vertebral levels do not coincide below the cervical cord.†

The lumbar, sacral, and coccygeal spinal cord levels (corresponding to 10 pairs of spinal nerve roots) emerge between the spinous processes of T10 and L1, where the spinal cord ends as the conus medullaris, and descend within the subarachnoid space (lumbar cistern) of the lumbar canal. The caudal course of this vertical mass of parallel nerve roots is the *cauda equina.* Each nerve root pair emerges at their respective vertebral levels.

6. What are the intercentral ligaments of the spine?

The *anterior* and *posterior longitudinal ligaments* are collectively known as the *intercentral ligaments* because they connect the anterior and posterior surfaces of adjacent vertebral bodies (centra) (see Fig. 59-2).[68] These ligaments also serve to attach the vertebral bodies to the intervertebral disks. During flexion the posterior longitudinal ligament limits flexion, while the anterior longitudinal ligament limits spinal extension. The posterior longitudinal ligament is clinically significant to disk pathology as a function of its rhomboidal shape. Possessing a denticulated appearance, the posterior longitudinal ligament flares laterally at each intervertebral disk where it attaches to the posterior aspect of the annulus fibrosus. Receiving innervation from the sinuvertebral nerve, the posterior longitudinal ligament is sensitive to pain, so that a midline herniated disk results in midline pain that radiates into the superior aspect of the buttock.[50]

---

*A normal growth differential appears to be dependent upon adequate neonatal and postnatal nutrition.

†The cervical spinal cord levels lie at intervals between the foramen magnum and the spinous process of C6. The upper six thoracic spinal cord levels are located between the spinous processes of C6 and T4, whereas the lower six thoracic spinal cord levels correspond to the spinous processes of T4 and T9.

7. What are the components of the intervertebral disk?

Between the bodies of each two spinal vertebrae lies an *intervertebral disk,* except at the uppermost two cervical joints (Fig. 60-1). First described by the great Belgian anatomist Andreas Vesalius in 1555, there are 23 vertebrae and 23 intervertebral disks spanning from C2 to the space between L5 and the first sacral segment. No disk is present between the occiput and the atlas or the atlas and the axis, although a small disk does exist between the sacrum and the coccyx. The 24 disks include 6 cervical, 12 thoracic, 5 lumbar, and 1 sacrococcygeal disk. Classified as a symphysis[207] and considered the largest avascular structure in the body, the intervertebral disk is a nonsynovial structure that obtains nutrition through diffusion and fluid flow.[24] Similar in function to the symphysis pubis or the menisci at the knee, the intervertebral disks comprise approximately one-fourth of the height of the vertebral column (about 6 inches).[37] In addition to facilitating spinal movement, the intervertebral disk serves as a major absorber of compressive force.

The intervertebral disk is usually named with reference to the two vertebrae that surround it. Alternately, a disk may also be referred to with respect to the vertebra directly above the disk and may be easily remembered by imagining a vertebral body "sitting" on its respective disk. Composed of 3 component structures, the disk has an inner nucleus pulposus surrounded by an annulus fibrosus which, in turn, are covered above and below by cartilaginous vertebral endplates. The lumbar intervertebral disks are the thickest in the spine and are thicker anteriorly than posteriorly. Approximately one-third the height of the lumbar vertebral bodies, their wedge shape contributes to the formation of the lumbar lordosis. The anterior and posterior aspects of the intervertebral disks are supported by the anterior and posterior longitudinal ligaments, respectively. During flexion the anterior aspects of the disks are compressed, while during lateral flexion the sides of the ipsilated intervertebral disks are compressed.

8. What are the structural components of the intervertebral disk?

The major structural components comprising the intervertebral disk are proteoglycan, collagen, and water and compose up to 95% of the volume of a normal disk. The disk also contains stratified cells and noncollagenous proteins. Cells within the annulus are cigar-shaped while those within the nucleus pulposus are round.[7] The cells form proteoglycans, primarily by way of glycolysis, although the oxidative pathway for aerobic respiration occurs as well. Typically lactic acid by-products build up within the disk from the anaerobic pathway and lower the pH in the central portion.[147] Normally, an enzymatic homeostasis exists within a lumbar disk, which prevents the unintended degradation of the outer annular fibers by collagenase and elastase.[141] Water, most of which is extracellular, is the main constituent of the disk occupying the majority of the tissue volume.[158]

9. What is the innervation of the intervertebral disk?

The outer third of the annulus, particularly the posterior border and less so the lateral and anterior borders, have sensory nerve endings in the form of encapsulated and free nerve endings, implying both proprioceptive and nociceptive functions.[116] Although the posterior aspect of each disk receives innervation from the sinuvertebral (recurrent meningeal) nerve, the lateral border and small portion of the anterior aspect of the disk are supplied by the branches of the gray communicating rami of the lumbar sympathetic trunk.[50] The clinical significance of this innervation is that disk disturbance may represent a primary source of lower back pain. The remainder of the annulus and the nucleus have no innervation.[36] The intervertebral disks are dynamic structures that are capable of self-repair and considerable self-regeneration.[143]

10. What are vertebral endplates and what is their role in fluid inflow and outflow?

Although some consider the *vertebral endplate* as the superior and inferior portions of the vertebral body, most authorities[17] consider the endplate as an integral portion of the intervertebral disk.[37] Approximately 1 mm thick peripherally and 3 mm thick centrally, the endplates demonstrate a funnel-shaped defect centrally where the longitudinal notochord track formerly penetrated the developing disk, but disappeared with maturation. This clinically significant channel represents a potentially weak area.

Composed of hyaline cartilage along the vertebral body, the side of the endplate resting along the disk is composed of fibrocartilage. Providing a comparable function to subchondral bone in a synovial joint, the vertebral endplates serve to disperse the load absorbed by the disk it houses. However, unlike subchondral bone, the vertebral endplate is very porous and does

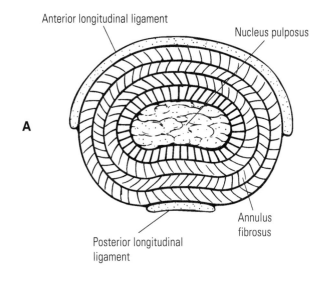

A

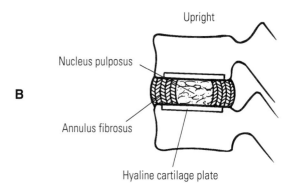

B

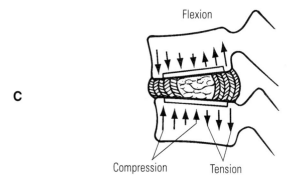

C

FIG. 60-1 Intervertebral disk. **A,** Transverse section of intervertebral disk and its reinforcing ligaments. **B,** and **C,** Sagittal sections of intervertebral disk in upright and flexed positions, respectively. (From White AH, Schofferman JA, editors: *Spine care: diagnosis and conservative treatment*, St Louis, 1995, Mosby.)

permit fluid exchange and hence diffusion of nutrients to the nucleus pulposus and annulus fibrosus by way of blood vessels within the vertebral bodies known as *vertebral sinusoids*.* Thus the disk obtains nutrition through diffusion and fluid flow[23-25] through the osmotic disk-bone interface[96] as well as through the annulus, which is vascularized and permeable along its periphery.[81] The direction of fluid flow from the disk to the sinusoids within the endplates occurs in a similar fashion to articular cartilage of weight-bearing joints. The direction of fluid flow occurs in response to compressive loads.[118] When the load on the disk increases, there is fluid outflow and the disk deforms. Upon removal of load, the fluid that was squeezed out returns carrying solute particles. Correspondingly, with influx of fluid, the turgor—defined as stiffness of the disk—will proportionally increase.

11. What is the annulus fibrosus?

The *annulus fibrosus* surrounds the nucleus pulposus, bears approximately one-fourth of axial compressive load, and is composed of two distinct layers. The outer annulus is comprised of type I collagen (also found in tendon) and inserts into the vertebral body via Sharpey fibers and offers the disk resistance to bending. The inner annulus encapsulates the nucleus pulposus and is comprised of type II collagen (also found in hyaline cartilage) and is thus considered an extension of the vertebral endplate. The architectural organization of the fibrocartilage comprising the annulus is ringlike lamellae, comprised of closely packed collagen fibrils, which are convex externally. In addition to collagen fibers, the annulus is also composed of a small percentage (10%) of elastic fibers.[16,17]

The mechanical properties of the annulus that resist compression derive from collagen fibers and proteoglycan. The intralamellar spaces within the annulus are filled with abundant proteoglycans that bind with collagen fibers and water. The annulus is the most important disk structure in transmission of vertical weight-bearing forces,[101] provides maximal stability

---

*Vibration, so common in occupations such as drivers of trucks, tractors, and trains, are at relatively greater risk of back pain (Weinstein J, Pope M, Schmidt R et al: Neuropharmacologic effects of vibration on the dorsal root ganglion, *Spine* 13:521, 1988.) because disk exposure to vibrations at 5 hz for 25 minutes results in significant disk dehydration owing to spasm in the vessels of the vertebral endplate. (Pope MH, Jayson MIV, Blau AD et al: The effect of vibration on serum levels of von Willebrand's factors. Presented to the International Society for the Study of the Lumbar Spine, Heidelberg, May 1991.)

against horizontal displacement,[62] and provides a significant amount of torsional stability.[55] With aging and degenerative changes of proteoglycans the disk becomes more susceptible to trauma by delamination of the annulus fibrosus.

12. What structural properties are endowed to the annulus by the oblique organization of its concentric lamellae?

Both the inner and outer annulus have their collagen organized into 15 to 25[188] concentric *lamellae,* arranged much like the layers of an onion[42] and aligned at acute angles with alternate layers of fibers running in opposite directions.[73] This alternating layered structure is so arranged that each adjacent layer is oriented in an opposite direction and endows the annulus with a *radial ply effect* that withstands considerable axial compressive force. The lamellae expand obliquely across the disk space between the vertebral end plates and afford the intervertebral disk ability similar to the menisci in the knee that is well suited to resist compressive force. The orientation of the lamellae is organized so that two adjoining layers course in opposite direction causing their fibers to cross each other at 120°. The significance of the alternating organization of lamellae is similar to metal hoops around a wooden barrel that resist elongation and thereby resist barrel expansion. The oblique orientation of one set of fibers running tangentially to the others serve as "ties" that provide structural rigidity preventing longitudinal splitting resulting from excessive compression. Thus the vertical compressive load of superincumbent body weight is applied to the disk whose fiber orientation absorbs centripetal load by translation of force into tensile or circumferential stresses. In this fashion, *hoop tension* generated within the annulus as a function of annular collagen fiber orientation serves as a constraint, like hoops on a barrel, preventing peripheral annular displacement. These "hoop" forces are then transmitted to the vertebral endplates above and below and absorbed along their relatively flat surfaces. This organization endows the annulus with stiffness,[60] low deformation, and maximal energy dissipation.[62]

13. Which portion of the annulus is weakest and what is the clinical significance?

The anterior and lateral portions of the annulus are composed of more than 20 moderately thick lamellae. The outer lamellae are attached to the stronger anterior longitudinal ligament. In contrast, the posterior and posterolateral portions of the annulus are considerably thinner as they are composed of only 12 to 15, more closely arranged, thinner lamellae that fuse with the posterior longitudinal ligament.[65] Thus the lamellar reinforcement of the anterior aspect of the disk is strongest, whereas the posterolateral region is most poorly reinforced. Subsequently, the posterolateral aspect of the intervertebral disk is susceptible to disk pathology.[38]

14. What is the nucleus pulposus and how do its constituent properties change with age?

The *nucleus pulposus* is a remnant of the embryologic notochord, and by virtue of its incompressible viscous substance, bears ¾ of the compressive load to the spine. Normally, the nucleus pulposus is located near, although slightly posterior to the geometric center of the disk owing to the lumbar lordosis. Composing ⅔ of the surface area of the disk, the nucleus is composed of 90% water from youth into the third decade of life. Having no cells, the matrix of the nucleus pulposus consists of a three-dimensional network of collagen fibers (mainly type II in a healthy nucleus) embedded within a mucoprotein gel.[80] The fluid characteristics of the nucleus are likened to an incompressible "marble" that acts as a ball bearing between vertebrae with spinal motion. The intranuclear water content gradually diminishes to approximately 60% over the subsequent 4 decades, and the subsequent loss of hydrostatic properties renders the nucleus less homogenous with age. The reduction of hydration occurs in proportion to the amount and type of proteoglycan content within the disk.

15. How do the proteoglycan molecules within the disk matrix contribute to regulation of the flow of water within the matrix of the intervertebral disk?

The matrix of the intervertebral disk is principally comprised of collagen fibers in a proteoglycan-water gel. This matrix may be described as being *hyperhydrated;* as a result of proteoglycan aggregates imbibing water in the matrix. Synthesized by chondrocytes within the nucleus, proteoglycans are the largest macromolecules in the body and have a remarkable capacity to imbibe water so that their weight may increase by approximately 250%.[172] The proteoglycan aggregates of the intervertebral disk are of a smaller size and somewhat different composition (with regard to their sulfated chains) than those found in articular cartilage.[26] These megamolecules have chemical and electrical properties that endow them with the ability to sequester water.

The side chains of the proteoglycan aggregate, comprised of proteoglycan monomers contain many electronegative surface charges (on the sulfated sugars and carboxyl groups) that repel each other, causing the molecules to attempt to unwind and enlarge within the cartilaginous extracellular matrix. The water molecules in the extracellular fluid act as dipoles: the positively charged hydrogen atoms are attracted to the negatively charged sulfated groups, whereas the negatively charged oxygen atoms comprising the water molecules repel one another. The net effect of these reactions is the attraction of water molecules in-between the monomers, which serve as a molecular sponge. Moreover, because the proteoglycan aggregates within the extracellular matrix are larger than the hyaluronidase molecules within synovial fluid, a *concentration gradient* is created in the direction of the extracellular matrix so that water tends to flow from the vascular supply within the vertebral endplates into the disk as a function of *simple passive diffusion*. Thus both the size and the electrochemical properties of the proteoglycan molecule aggregates act like a hydrophilic "pump." This tendency to *imbibe water* creates a swelling pressure within the disk, which acts as an enormous hydration sphere surrounding the proteoglycan aggregates within the extracellular matrix. The intervertebral disk is thus pressurized by water and uses its incompressibility to protect against the deleterious effects of axial loading of the spine.

16. How does disk hydration vary with erect posture and diurnal changes?

The dynamics of fluid flow in and out of the intervertebral disk occur in response to application and removal of compressive load.[118] Optimal health of the disk is maintained by movement and erect posture, which insures proper hydration, whereas disk degeneration strongly correlates with decreased axial loading and diminished movement.[189] Fluid flow into the disk provides nutrition and internal resistive force to axial compression. During weight bearing, the external pressures secondary to superincumbent body weight and ground reaction force collide at the articulating surfaces of the intervertebral joint. This is known as *axial compression* and is transmitted to the intervertebral disk by the car-

tilaginous plates above and below the disk. The effect of this vertical-weight bearing force deforms the disk and causes fluid to flow outward so that the disk become shorter during the day while carrying the load of the torso. When joint compression occurs during weight bearing, water is forced out of the extracellular matrix against the concentration gradient, across the vertebral endplate and into vertebral blood vessels synovial fluid. Although the disk loses water with axial loading, it retains sodium and potassium ions. This increase in electrolyte concentration creates an osmotic gradient that results in rapid rehydration when the disk is unloaded.[108]

After removal of the load, the fluid that was squeezed out returns carrying solute particles. This endows the disk with an internal resistive force in the form of *osmotic pressure* that withstands the vertical compressive forces of the upright spine. With the collective loss of fluid from all 23 disks incurred from weight bearing while in the erect posture by day, and with advancing age, there is progressive loss of height. Water is reimbibed by the disk while in the recumbent position and occurs every night during sleep. Thus diurnal changes are accompanied by changes in disk hydration in which the disks swell with water they have lost during waking hours.* Disks rehydrate to gain their optimal turgor after approximately 5 hours of sleep.[189]

Neither excessive compression nor rest is beneficial for the optimal health of the intervertebral disk. In the absence of erect posture and weight bearing with normal muscular activity, the disks do not develop their normal thickness; the vertebral endplates do not change from their infantile convexity to a flat or concave shape. In contrast, a decrease in disk hydration may occur in as little as 5 weeks of bed rest.[109]

17. Why does the amount of water within the vertebral disk vary with age?

The changes in structure and composition that are common to all forms of cartilage with aging occur earlier and to a greater extent with the intervertebral disk.[10] The core protein of the proteoglycan monomer is divided into sulfated groups including chondroiton-2 and keretan-4 sulfate bound to a backbone of hyaluronic

---

*Astronauts who returned to Earth after approximately 80 days or more in space were found to be a full 1½ to 2 inches taller than at liftoff.

acid core protein in varying proportions consistent with the age of the individual. Peak disk hydration occurs at approximately age 30, whereas the progress of degeneration begins shortly thereafter.[37] With increasing age and degeneration, the proportion of chondroitin sulfate falls and that of keratosulfate rises,[3] corresponding to the diminution of metabolic activity of chondrocytes. Keratosulfate, because of its decreased molecular weight and fewer side chains, has a diminished ability to sequester water and, correspondingly, the water content and hence the turgor of the disk decreases with age. Whereas the amount of water within the disk is approximately 85% in preadolescent age, it diminishes to approximately 70% in middle age adults.[158]

As age and degeneration progress the total proteoglycan content decreases, the fixed charge density is reduced,[193] the total proteoglycan content decreases, and the keratin–sulfate:chondroitin–sulfate ratio increases. A dehydrated disk has densely packed proteoglycan with a small pore size between the molecules that reduces fluid diffusion. The net sum of these changes translates into a reduction of the water-imbibing ability of the intervertebral disk, particularly within the nucleus pulposus.[113] Subsequently, the disk undergoes the most marked age-related changes in both composition and structure of all connective tissue.

At least 7[52] of the 12 different types of collagen[124] are found in the intervertebral disk, although mainly types I and II are present. Connective tissue changes include an alteration of subtypes so that type II collagen is replaced by type I and type II,[76] and is accompanied by irreducible collagen cross linking.[97] This results in a decreased ability of the disk to absorb fluid and leads to a decreased ability of the disk to withstand compressive loads. The sum of these changes makes the disk more vulnerable to prolapse in middle life. Moreover, in response to compressive load, the disk degenerates and narrows in its superior-to-inferior dimension and adjacent vertebral bodies that may become thickened and opaque on x-ray (sclerotic.) Because the intervertebral disk forms the anterior border of the intervertebral foramen, a decrease in disk height results in a decrease of the vertical dimension of the foramen,[40] and tends to compress the emergent nerve root.

18. What are endplate herniations and why are they more common in the younger population?

The vertebral endplates are comprised of two relatively flat and parallel surfaces that provide the source of nourishment for the avascular nucleus pulposus, and to the annulus via the vertebral sinusoids.* When the disk is loaded during axial compression, the vertebral endplate is the weakest structure of the three components of the intervertebral disk.[25] The healthy annulus can tolerate much greater compressive load than the vertebral endplate. In youth, when the nucleus pulposus is maximally hydrated and relatively incompressible, the effects of longitudinal compressive force will result in failure of the bony endplate before failure of the disk. However, before endplate fracture, a protective mechanism occurs in which the nucleus loses 1 to 2 ml of fluid into the sinusoid as a way of reducing the impact of sudden, compressive force. If the compressive force is excessive, as may occur from a fall on the buttocks or when lifting heavy objects, the vertebral endplates will bulge and fracture before annular failure typically superiorly into the central area of the adjacent vertebral body in what is termed a *Schmorl's node*. These endplate herniations, occurring at the site of the central defect are often located at the lower thoracic and upper lumbar levels,[20] in just over ⅓ of all spines, more typically in males, and occur at the thinnest part of the endplate. Over time, ingrowth of vascular granulation tissue through the fracture into the disk nucleus erodes the disk from inside out so that progressive loss of disk height eventually culminates in subluxation of the posterior facet joints.[61]

Occurring as frequently in adolescents as adults, *Schmorl's nodes* are typically painless because of the relative lack of nociceptors at this site.† Thus the intervertebral disk can withstand compressive loads far greater than the vertebral body resulting in vertebral bodies fractures before disintegration of the disk itself.[160] The subsequent approximation of the upper and lower vertebral body alters the balance of forces between the posterior and anterior elements and leads to more force to be borne by the anterior intervertebral joints and posterior facet joints, thereby hastening the degenerative process.[38]

---

*In comparison, this nourishment by diffusion has no analogue in the major synovial body joints as no fluid exchange occurs between the subchondral bony plate and the joint cavity. Instead, the source of nutrient diffusion is the synovial fluid.

†However, a secondary inflammatory cascade within the nucleus and subsequent nuclear degeneration and disruption may occur secondary to endplate herniation. This may manifest as an autoimmune response because the endplate fracture activates endogenous proteolytic enzymes normal present in the disk and inhibited by proteinase inhibitors.

19. How may progressive deterioration of the nuclear matrix known as *internal disk disruption* result from an endplate herniation?

Although an endplate fracture may heal without symptoms and pass unnoticed, it may set in motion a series of events that result in pain and degradation of the disk. The proteoglycans of the nucleus pulposus are biochemically similar to those of the vitreous humor in the eye, and in penetrating eye injuries, exposed lens protein may sensitize lymphocytes so that they exert a destructive inflammation if they reach the intact eye.* Similarly, the proteoglycans of the nucleus are foreign to the body and throughout its development, the nucleus is avascular and is never exposed to the body's circulation. Consequently, following a vertical endplate fracture, migration of nuclear material may expose the nuclear proteoglycans to the vertebral body circulation, triggering a repair response. The unfamiliar nuclear proteoglycans are treated as if they are a foreign body and cause the immune system to mount an autoimmune response against the nuclear material.[16]

Thus if the prolapsed nuclear material contacts the vertebral spongiosa following trauma to a Schmorl's node,[125] it will come in contact with the body's blood supply and elicit an antigenic response.[64] Contact triggers an inflammatory response that leads to progressive degradation of the nuclear matrix and alteration of its biophysical properties.

Destruction of the proteoglycan aggregates and monomers composing the disk occurs and is termed *internal disk disruption*.[102] This nomenclature implies an abnormal state of the disk in which the nucleus and inner annulus are disrupted, the outer perimeter of the disk remains intact and normal in contour. There is no element of disk bulge or herniation at this stage, and initially, the disk has no means of being symptomatic. This is because nerve endings are absent from these inner portions of the disk, whereas the chemical degradation of the nuclear material are undetected by the nervous system.

20. How does internal disk disruption serve as a primary source of low back pain?

Pain that is of purely diskal origin may clinically manifest as low back pain and may result from progression of the internally disrupted disk. Pain may be chemically induced and derive from spreading of the inflamed nucleus outwardly, so that it eventually spreads to the outer third of the annulus and directly stimulates the nociceptors there. Alternately, as the inner lamellae of the annulus break down, the tears spread peripherally and eventually reach the nociceptors in the outer third where they cause mechanically derived pain. Both mechanisms of pain production may occur simultaneously.[16]

Normally, an enzymatic homeostasis exists within the lumbar disk which prevents the unintended breakdown of the outer annular fibers by collagenase and elastase.[141] However, the acidic environment accompanying disk injury may alter the expression of these enzymes and thereby expose the annulus to degradation. The clinical features of internal disk disruption include constant and deep aching low back pain that may be aggravated by any movement that mechanically stresses the affected disk. Pain may intensify with any increase in disk compression. Muscle guarding may be present and neurologic signs would be conspicuously normal because the lesion does not involve nerve root irritation or compression. The standard radiographic examination, myelography, and CT are often all normal. The suspected internally disrupted disk is confirmed by CT diskography.[39]

21. What two endstage pathologies may result secondary to internal disk disruption?

The internally disrupted disk is less capable of binding water in what is described as an *isolated disk resorption*.[196] Additionally, it loses its cohesiveness and gradually its ability to withstand axial compressive force. Subsequently, weight is borne by the annulus fibrosus, which may creep under compression, leading to buckling and bulging of the annulus and narrowing of the disk space, resulting in *canal or foraminal stenosis*.

Alternately, as the annulus undergoes progressive axial loading without the benefit of a healthy, hydrated disk, it may undergo circumferential and radial tearing of its lamellae. The radial fissure provides a channel through the annulus, whereas degradation of the nuclear matrix destroys its intrinsic cohesiveness and renders the nucleus expressible. A disk bulge may occur at this time. Thus the stage is set for disk prolapse which may occur from an excessively strong compressive load or combination of movements such as flexion and rotation. This would propel the nuclear material out of the annulus and into the spinal canal or intervertebral foramen where it may irritate or compress nerve roots.

---

*This condition is known as *sympathetic ophthalmia*.

22. Why does disk degeneration that accompanies aging result in horizontal as opposed to vertical endplate herniations?

With aging, or accelerated degeneration due to chronic manual labor during early adulthood, the changes in proteoglycan content result in low osmotic pressure within the nucleus causing loss of turgor and disk height.[154] Loss of height, in turn, causes a physical deformation of the outer layer of the annulus, which compromises its physiologic strength. Stress on the collagen fibers composing the annulus is termed *delamination*. Disk degeneration often begins in males during the second decade of life and a decade later in females. By age 50, virtually all lumbar disks degenerate.[132] Thus as humans age, the disk degenerates, losing water content from the nucleus pulposus and elastic resilience from the annular fibers.[23] Eventually, the annulus becomes progressively weaker while the endplate is hardened by skeletal maturity.

The effects of increased axial compressive load on the strained annulus causes its outer layer to bulge out in what is described as a *buckling phenomenon*. This may cause pain by stimulation of the nociceptive endings contained within the outer layers and may result in direct pressure on the nerve root, resulting in radiculopathy. Because disk changes occur as a function of structural degeneration that most commonly accompanies aging, intervertebral disk injuries primarily occur in the fourth decade of life and are uncommon in adolescents.[143] The nerve roots comprising the cauda equina housed within the lumbar vertebral canal are more frequently affected by disk protrusions than in the cervical and thoracic regions.[33]

23. What is the relationship between degenerative disk disease and disk prolapse?

Disk herniation typically results from the chronic wear and tear characteristic of degenerative disk disease, provoked by a sudden aggravating factor such as lifting an excessively heavy weight. This is most commonly seen in patients spanning the 35 to 50 year old range, before the development of osteophytes that stabilize the spine beyond middle age. Alternately the patient underwent a sudden violent impact that caused a cleavage or crack of the annulus many years previously and now experiences a disk herniation due to lifting an excessively heavy load. These patients are typically in there early or mid twenties and have radiologic evidence of localized degenerative disk disease.[171]

Degenerative disk disease typically begins at the most mobile levels of the lumbar spine (L4/L5 and L5/S1) and is referred to as *segmental instability*. Motion at these lower two segments in flexion and extension is approximately 20° and is defined by an *instantaneous axis of rotation* that, similar to the glenohumeral joint, must be maintained to ensure proper joint function and stability. The multiple axes of rotation of a joint follow a line in three dimensions, defined by the points of the instantaneous axes of rotation, known as a *centrode*.[65] As vertebrae move from extension to flexion, motion is mathematically reduced to small sequential increments corresponding to an instantaneous axis of rotation. These axes describe a circular path of a small diameter corresponding to the centrode. In the healthy, the centrode of a spinal motion segment is small and uniform. With early disk degeneration, the centrode becomes long and irregular, as the vertebral segment moves in an excessive and erratic manner predisposing toward disk pathology and injury.[17] The spine, in turn, protectively responds by developing traction osteophytes that act to counter segmental instability by directly limiting the motion between adjacent vertebrae. With increasing age, the centrode reduces in length and once again becomes small and regular accounting for why disk pathology most often occurs during middle age and not beyond this time.

24. What is the protective role of the facet joints and musculoligamentous system in relation to the intervertebral disk?

When the lumbar spine is extended, the facet joints are in a close-packed position with the male and female surfaces of the joints fitting point-for-point. In contrast, during lumbar flexion, the joints are in the loose-packed position with incongruity of the two joint surfaces. This incongruity occurs because the convex surface has a smaller curvature than the concave surface so that both surfaces articulate at one point. The annulus is vulnerable to excessive rotational strain but is protected by the configuration of the facet joints. The flexed spine disengages the apophyseal joints and exposes the unprotected annulus to sprain from simultaneous rotation. In flexion, the principal protection against restraining excessive shear and preventing excessive rotation is the musculoligamentous system (spinal ligaments and lumbar fascia) that splints the trunk to avoid rotation. In addition, other muscles provide a dampening effect on spinal motion in three axes of rotation including the intraabdominal pressure via the diaphragm, and the dynamic action of the trunk and abdominal musculature.

Inadequate muscular dampening may result in an over-swing, or dangerous combined movements such as flexion and rotation. Once flexion occurs with lumbar rotation, the collagen fibers of the annulus undergo torsion and may be stretched beyond their limits resulting in microtearing of the lamellae comprising the annulus. This is most likely to occur from an erratic movement or during an unguarded motion such as a stumble or fall that combines flexion and rotation during attempted recovery and injury prevention.*

25. How may a circumferential tear of the annulus fibrosus in the absence of nuclear migration serve as a primary source of back pain?

Annular fissures occur when physical deformation (strain) occurs beyond its physiologic limit,† and may occur gradually from the inner to the outer layers, or all at once in the event of an acute, severe disk injury. Normally, annular tearing does not occur because the collagen fibers of the lumbar disk are capable of withstanding more than three degrees of axial rotation without undergoing stretch beyond their capacity. Combined movements of the lumbar spine carry the highest injury potential, so that the spine that is forward flexed and rotated is at the greatest risk for disk injury.[127]

When the lumbar spine is extended, the facet joints are in the close-packed position with the male and female surfaces of the joints fitting point-for-point. In contrast, during lumbar flexion, the joints are in the loose-packed position with incongruity of the two surfaces. This incongruity occurs because the convex surface has a smaller curvature than the concave surface so that both surfaces articulate at one point. The annulus is vulnerable to excessive rotational strain but is protected by the configuration of the facet joints. The flexed spine disengages the apophyseal joints and exposes the unprotected annulus to sprain from concomitant rotation. In the loose-packed flexion position, the principal protection preventing excessive rotation is the musculoligamentous system that splits the trunk to avoid rotation by way of the spinal ligaments and lumbar fascia,

the intraabdominal pressure via the diaphragm, and by the dynamic action of the trunk and abdominal musculature. Once flexion is added to axial lumbar rotation, the collagen fibers of the annulus undergo torsion and may be stretched beyond their limits resulting in microtearing of the lamellae comprising the annulus. This is most likely to occur in an unguarded moment such as a stumble or fall that combines flexion and rotation during attempted recovery and injury prevention.

Torsion injury is defined as excessive axial rotation of the spine.‡ With as little as 3° of rotation, the annulus undergoes microtearing that increases up to 12°, beyond which the annulus undergoes frank failure[78] and is avulsed from the endplate and its laminae separate and tear. The same mechanism of injury causing an *acute annular tear* may also injure the capsular ligaments of the facet joints.

The 90° orientation of the lumbar facet joints allows only 2° to 3° of pure rotation, thereby protecting the annulus from excessive torsion within a "safe range." However, because of the unique facet orientation at the lumbosacral junction, failure of the annulus, facet fracture, or injury to the pars interarticularis such as a pars stress reaction or fracture (spondylosis) may occur.[89] The safe range of movement may be exceeded more easily without the benefit of normal muscular splinting that may occur during positioning while under general anesthesia.

26. What is the difference between circumferential and radial tears of the annulus fibrosus?

Sprain of the annulus occurs sequentially with circumferential tears preceding radial tears.[87] Both tears represent forms of internal disk disruption. A *circumferential*

---

*It is for this reason that lifting should be performed with a lordotic spine flat or in extension.

†*Strain* has both a biomechanical and clinical definition. Biomechanically, *strain* refers to the deformation of structures caused by forces applied upon them, resulting in *stress*. This refers to the stress/strain characteristics of the material comprising the annulus. In contrast, the clinical term *strain* refers to the excessive deformation of the muscle-tendon unit, whereas *sprain* refers to excessive deformation of the ligamentous unit.

---

‡It is postulated that the reason the body did not evolve a mechanism that would protect against the damaging effects of torsion is because of the advantage conferred by such motion to bipedal gait. In early vertebrates, the spine was essential in locomotion. Indeed, that fishlike amphioxus (i.e., lancelet), which so closely resembles the early human embryo, moved through its aquatic environment with fishlike undulations of its spine. Movement of the spine, preserved as torsion, may have been preserved through evolution if we conceive of a spinal engine that facilitates driving the pelvis forward in our reciprocal bipedal gait. Our spine may act to convert the primitive lateral bend of our fishlike ancestors into an axial torque. (Lovett AW: A contribution to the study of the mechanics of the spine, *Am J Anat* 2:457, 1903.) Indeed, the reciprocal and opposite motions of the upper and lower extremities act as an energy storage and release mechanism. The locus of this mechanism is the spine, and is observed as reverse rotations between the shoulder and pelvic girdles. (Gracovetsky S: *The spinal engine,* Vienna, 1988, Springer-Verlag.)

tear represents a separation of adjacent lamellae that is circular or circumferential and may cause the lamellae involved to tear away from their vertebral attachments. These tears may occur following torsion or the combined motions of lumbar flexion and rotation. Because of the nociceptive innervation of the outer third of the disk, these tears may result in a primary source of pain.

With repeated episodes of trunk flexion and rotation, other circumferential tears of several adjacent lamellae of the annulus fibrosus are likely to occur. The overall effect of adjacent lamellar tearing is that a path, known as a *radial tear,* is created within the annulus from its deep, central aspect to its periphery through successive layers of annulus. A radial tear represents the connecting path between various circumferential tears, providing a channel through which the gelatinous nucleus may migrate from the geometric center of the disk to the periphery. In the degenerated disk, the instant center of rotation shifts posteriorly,[54] and so the nuclear material will typically aggregate along the posterior border of the disk. Continued spinal motion will cause the disk to bulge. Once this has occurred, continued torsion, or perhaps mere flexion alone may cause tearing of the outer annulus. Annular tears occur posteriorly, just lateral to the posterior longitudinal ligament where the elliptical disk geometry concentrates stress at the site of maximum convexity.[79] Annular fragments or nuclear material herniate laterally or posterolaterally into the vertebral canal or intervertebral foramen causing entrapment or stretching of the nerve roots.

27. How is the location of the instantaneous center of the intervertebral disk related to disk pathology?

The gelatinous nucleus pulposus is located near, but slightly posterior to the geometric center of the intervertebral disk. Acting like a ball bearing, when the vertebral bodies roll over the disk during flexion and extension, the center of rotation changes instantaneously, depending on the position of the spine.[162] Because spinal flexion occurs more commonly during the activities of daily living, the instant center of rotation tends to be situated posterior to the geometric center of the disk and degenerative changes within the disk also result in posterior migration. Thus flexion results in preferential loading of the disk anteriorly, resulting in posterior displacement of nuclear material.[108a]

28. Why do disks herniate posterolaterally?

Bulging or herniation of the lumbar intervertebral disk more likely results in a posterolateral protrusion. The annulus fibrosus is intact and strong anteriorly whereas it is relatively weak posteriorly. This is because the annulus, being narrower posteriorly and broader anteriorly, is inherently weaker in the lumbar spine.[171] Increased tensile force within the posterior annular collagen fibers are poorly tolerated, and with forward bending and rotation the posterolateral margin of the annulus is at risk for failure. Furthermore, the anterior longitudinal ligament is anatomically broader and stronger than the narrower posterior ligament. Because a disk usually herniates under pressure, it will break through the annulus in the direction of least resistance—posteriorly. However, midline herniations are less common because the posterior longitudinal ligament is strongest posteriorly. Because of the rhomboidal shape of the posterior longitudinal ligament, the weakest portion of the ligament is posterolaterally where it is thinnest, so that the bulge or herniation will most likely occur to either side of midline at the posterolateral margin.[83]

29. What is a far lateral disk herniation?

Another type of disk injury includes the far (out) lateral disk herniation in which the location of the nerve root impingement is at the foraminal exit zone or extraforaminally.[90] Thus an ensuing radiculopathy involves the nerve root from the level above. For example, a far lateral herniation at L5/S1 affects the L5 nerve root. This form of herniation does not usually result in lower back pain.[171] Instead, this problem clinically manifests as lower extremity pain, sensory disturbance and/or weakness in the L3, L4, or L5 myotomes. Symptoms are often worse with standing or walking, and are occasionally reduced with sitting. Thecal signs are absent because a far lateral disk affects the nerve beyond the dural sleeve.[151] Straight leg raises or reverse SLR is either negative or minimally positive despite severity of symptoms. Radiculopathy of the S1 nerve root cannot occur from a true far lateral disk herniation unless an S1-S2 disk is present congenitally or there is an extra (L6) lumbar vertebra.[106] Far lateral protrusions are not visualized by myelography.[171]

30. What is the progressive sequence of disk prolapse?

Once the structural integrity of the nucleus pulposus and annulus fibrosus are compromised, disk pathology may progress from a simple bulge to complete *extrusion* of nuclear material outside the annulus. Thus the nucleus pulposus may cause bulging of the outer annular fibers or may herniate through the annulus.[136] An analogy may be drawn to an automobile tire and inner tube in which the former, being thick and strong, represents the annulus, and the soft and compressible inner tube may represent the inner nucleus. A defect in the tough, outer rubber tire may derive from a variety of causes including a factory defect, gradual wear and tear, or injury from a hard object in which the sudden violent impact caused a cleavage within the outer tire. Regardless of the cause of the defective area, the pressure within the tube will push against this site, so that over time, the tire will begin to bulge and ultimately burst.[171] A similar process may occur in the intervertebral disk.

Migration of disk material toward the spinal canal and intervertebral foramen may occur as a smooth uniform *disk bulge* without focal protrusion. Bulging is usually associated with heavy lifting or trauma.[119] A state of *disk protrusion* refers to a focal prolapse when either the outer fibers of the annulus are intact, or compromised. If the lamellae compromising the outer annular fibers are torn or separated, a protrusion will increase in size and nuclear material will rupture through the outer fibers as a *nuclear hernia*. If the herniation has herniated through the outer annulus, but not through the posterior longitudinal ligament, it is considered an *extruded disk*. Moreover, with an extruded disk, the nuclear material within the vertebral canal is still connected to material within the disk. When extruded disk material breaks free as one or more fragments it is considered *sequestrated*.[151-153] The sequestrated fragment, lying between the vertebra and the posterior longitudinal ligament, is often prevented from migrating freely into the canal by the posterior longitudinal ligament. Central disk herniation may result in back pain without radiating signs or symptoms.[78] However, the fragment may break through the posterior longitudinal ligament and lie posterior to it.[171] Alternately, because of the effective barrier to midline herniations offered by the posterior longitudinal ligament, the herniated material may follow the path of least resistance and migrate laterally or posterolaterally toward the lateral recess or intervertebral foramen (Fig. 60-2).

31. What is the pathogenesis of radicular pain following disk prolapse?

There is no likely single cause of pain following disk herniation, but rather mechanical, vascular, biochemical, and neurochemical factors all contribute to the clinical syndromes of low back pain and radiculopathy. The pain that results radiates in a dermatomal pattern regardless of whether it derives from mechanical pressure or chemical irritation on the emerging nerve root. This pain is termed radicular pain because of its origin from the dorsal root (radix) or dorsal root ganglion.* The discovery that pain is referred segmentally along specific dermatomes was made by Sir Thomas Lewis in 1936. Thus a *dermatome* refers to an area of skin and subcutaneous tissue innervated by a spinal nerve.†

Of all the peripheral nerves, the nerve root is the least tolerant to compressive force, most likely because of the relative lack of epineurial tissue.[185] Mechanical compression of the nerve root may lead to focal demyelination and edema with impairment of axoplasmic transport, whereas compression of epidural, radicular veins results in dilation of noncompressed veins, venous hypertension with obstruction to normal capillary flow, and perineurial fibrosis and atrophy.[94] The vascular role in the pathogenesis of nerve root damage may be of particular significance because epidural veins have been shown to have a lower compressive threshold than other neurovascular structures, so that compression may result in a vascular induced hypoxic injury.[145] Moreover, the lumbar nerve root is more susceptible to rapid compression, whereas the sensory nerve root appears to be more rapidly affected than the motor nerve root. In contrast, sensory nerve roots recover more rapidly than their motor counterparts.[144] Finally, a chemical radiculitis may occur in the presence of nonmechanical radicular pain in which proteoglycans leaking out of an annular tear may cause pain by creating a chemical irritation of the exiting nerve roots.

The inflammatory response to injury, including sensitization of the sensory nerve fibers to painful stimuli, is ultimately a protective mechanism.[78] Thus radicular pain may occur from mechanical impingement of disk material directly upon neurovascular structures before, or within the confines of the intervertebral foramen.‡ Alternately, radicular pain may result from released neuropeptides from within the disk that sensitize the sensory nerve fibers to painful stimuli.

---

*During fetal development, those nerves innervating various organ and body systems emerge from the spinal cord adjacent to where those systems developed in the small fetal body. During subsequent fetal growth and elongation, organ and body systems migrate and "take" their nerves with them, although they still emerge from the spinal cord at the original level.

†Dermatomes overlap and their borders are not distinct. Additionally, injury to a nociceptor may sensitize adjacent nociceptor and produce hyperalgesia or hyperesthesia in adjacent receptor fields. (From Fields H: *Pain,* New York, 1987, McGraw-Hill.)

‡Radicular pain may also result from direct compression due to narrowing of the lateral recess of osteophytic impingement characteristic of lateral canal stenosis.

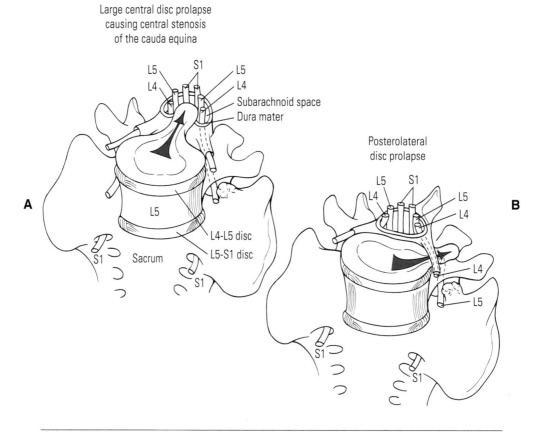

Large central disc prolapse
causing central stenosis
of the cauda equina

Posterolateral
disc prolapse

FIG. 60-2 Central and posterolateral disk prolapse. **A,** Large central disk prolapse of the L4-L5 disk is capable of damaging L5 and all roots below it. The L4 nerve root will most likely escape compression by virtue of its being situated within the lateral recess at this level. L5 may also be compressed by lumbosacral facet joint osteophytes. **B,** Posterolateral disk prolapse of the L4-L5 disk predominantly compresses the L5 nerve root.

These chemical pain mediators include phospholipase A2,[164] prostagladins, serotonin, histamine, and bradykinin. They act to sensitize nociceptive receptors directly; alter nerve transmission; sensitize neurons to mechanical stimulation; cause vascular congestion and neural ischemia; possibly stimulate histamine release from mast cells; and attract polymorphonuclear cells and monocytes.[78]

32. Why is the L5 nerve root more vulnerable to compression?

In the lumbar spine, the lumbosacral junction and L4-L5 level statistically accounts for some 95% of all cases of spinal injury. Of the three remaining lumbar joints, pathology at L3/L4 appears to be far more common than at the other two higher levels.[61]

The lumbosacral junction is comprised of the L5 vertebrae superiorly and the sacrum inferiorly. The lateral recess at this level is narrower than the superior segments whereas the lateral canal at this level is longer. The L5 nerve root is the largest of the lumbar nerves and exits the L5 intervertebral foramina, which is the smallest intervertebral foramen of the lumbar spine.[146]

The *corporotransverse ligament* is a tough, fibrous band that crosses the intervertebral foramen and is classified as a *transforaminal ligament*. This ligament runs between the vertebral body and the transverse process at the L5-S1 junction,[9] is present in the lumbar foramen, and may be a cause of root entrapment.[31]

Because the orientation of the L5/S1 facet joints permit more axial rotation than the other lumbar levels, the L5/S1 articulation is the most movable of all lumbar joints permitting unilateral rotation, lateral bending,

TABLE 60-1

Nerve Root	Disk	Muscles	Sensation	Reflex
L2	L1-L2	Psoas major	Mid anterior thigh	Cremasteric
L3	L2-L3	Quadriceps	Distal anterior thigh	Adductor jerk
L4	L3-L4	Adductor magnus	Medial leg	Knee jerk
L5	L4-L5	Extensor hallucis longus	Lateral leg and dorsum of foot	Tibialis posterior reflex
S1	L5-S1	Peronei	Lateral foot	Hamstrings and Achilles tendon

and flexion and extension. Greater potential motion increases the likelihood of injury to the annular fibers of the L5/S1 intervertebral disk with subsequent disk prolapse likely.

33. What is the relationship between the spinal nerves and the intervertebral disks in the lumbar spine?

The lumbosacral spinal nerve roots angle more obliquely as they approach the terminal cord and descend vertically as the cauda equina to emerge at their corresponding exit points. After reaching their respective intervertebral foramina, the emergent nerve roots turn 45° around the inferior aspect of the pedicle to exit very high in the intervertebral foramen. Because the pedicle is situated near the upper third of the vertebral body, the nerve root, tethered to that pedicle, never crosses the disk space below and does not lie in the path of a herniating disk. However, a nerve root may suffer compression from a disk located above its exit point because the nerve root descends posteriorly behind several intervertebral disks as part of the cauda equina. For example, the L5 nerve root crosses the disk space between the L4 and L5 vertebrae, and then winds around the L5 pedicle and exits the spinal canal via the neural foramen above the margin of the L5-S1 disk space. However, the L5 nerve root might also be compressed by an L3-L4 disk herniation as the L5 nerve root crosses behind the L3-L4 disk as part of the vertical nerves descending with the cauda equina. Herniations closer to the midline at the L4/L5 disk might affect both the L5 and S1 nerve roots. Similarly, if the disk protrudes in the midline at L5/S1 it may compress the S1 (and possibly S2) nerve root supply to both lower extremities. More commonly, nuclear extrusion presents on one side of the midline.[171] A lumbar disk

usually damages the root this is passing to the interspace below, so that a disk lesion at L4/5 will usually damage the L5 root and a disk at L5/S1 will damage the S1 root. However, if the disk protrusion is very large, or if the bulge is more laterally situated, it may also compress the L5 nerve root as well.[171]

34. What are the various patterns of nerve root compression at any given lumbar level?

A disk lesion may damage a nerve root *anywhere* between its origin from the spinal cord and its exit through the intervertebral foramen. Disk lesions, more commonly compress the adjacent root just below that level. However, there are numerous patterns of nerve root compression based on the level of compression, direction of disk bulge, and origin of osteophytic growth. Alternately, if herniation is midline, a single disk may involve two nerve roots.[83]

Clinical determination of the exact level and cause of a lesion may then be confirmed by electromyography and appropriate imaging, including magnetic resonance imaging, computerized tomography, or myelogram. Straight radiographs appear normal in most patients with acute disk herniation, as disk narrowing is not a feature of acute herniation. Disk narrowing will only present in the event of massive herniation or when the herniation as a result of a previous long standing degenerated disk.

35. What are the relevant nerve root innervations to the dermatomes and myotomes of the lower extremities?

The student must commit to memory the nerve root innervation for muscles (myotomes), cutaneous (dermatome) distributions, and deep tendon reflexes of the lower extremity. This is summarized in Table 60-1. Al-

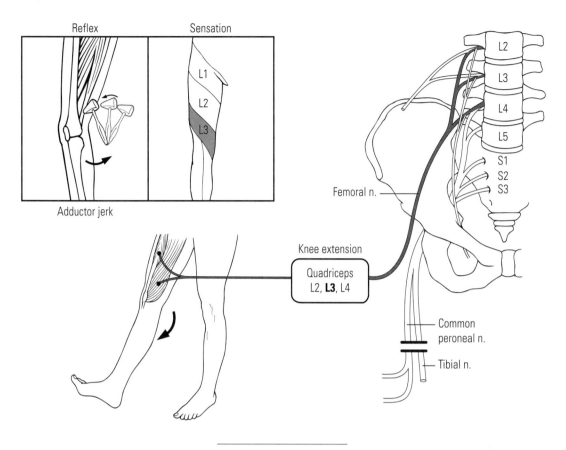

FIG. 60-3 L3 neurologic level.

though it is important to learn the many root contributions to each lower extremity muscle, it is most simple to assess for smaller muscles that are almost exclusively innervated by a single nerve root. Weakness or atrophy of these muscles suggests a specific nerve root lesion. Clinical confirmation may be facilitated by electromyographic data and a myelogram or other imaging. Neurophysiologic testing such as *electromyography* (EMG) accurately measures motor potentials. Approximately 2 weeks after nerve injury or nerve root lesion, abnormal spontaneous electrical discharges known as *fibrillation potentials* and *positive sharp waves* appear in the resting muscle (such as the anterior spinal muscles or muscles of the lower extremity) and represent evidence of muscle denervation supplied by that root. Nerve conduction studies may show delayed or absent late waves (H or F waves) consistent with interruption of the sensory arc. These abnormal findings are evidence of muscle denervation that can result from herniated disks, nerve root avulsions, plexus or cord lesions, and peripheral nerve lesions. A myelogram will demonstrate a bulge in the spinal cord adjacent to that disk space.

The L2 root is predominantly responsible for hip flexion and makes a major contribution to thigh adduction, whereas the L3 root makes a major contribution to both knee extension (i.e., the quadriceps muscles) and thigh adduction (Fig. 60-3). Interestingly, although the knee jerk is conveyed through the L4 nerve root, it contributes minimally to the quadriceps. Instead, the motor contribution of the L4 root is primarily below the knee and almost exclusively supplies the invertors of the foot, namely tibialis anterior and posterior via the peroneal and tibial nerves respectively. Thus the patient with an L4 nerve root lesion will demonstrate marked weakness of inversion of the foot and be incapable of walking on the lateral border of the affected foot (Fig. 60-4). The L4 root is the highest root commonly affected by disk disease, although compared with the L5 and S1 roots, it is relatively unusual. With L5 nerve root lesions, it is detectable in gluteus medius at the hip, the toe extensors, and extensor hallucis longus (Fig. 60-5). The latter two are functionally tested by asking the patient to walk on the heels with their ankles in neutral. When looking for evidence of an S1 root lesion, ever-

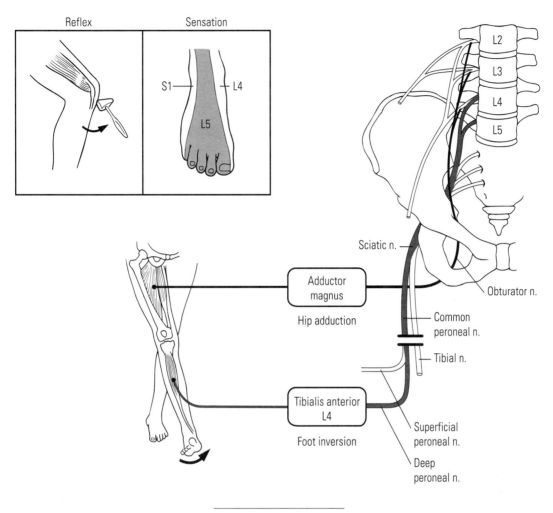

FIG. 60-4 L4 neurologic level.

sion of the foot is the best choice for motor assessment. The S1 motor contribution to other muscles includes the gluteus maximus, the hamstrings, and the gastrocnemius-soleus muscles (Fig. 60-6). However, as the former two are large and powerful muscles with multiple root supply, weakness and wasting may be difficult to detect in the presence of a single root lesion. Clinical muscle testing of gastrocnemius-soleus may be performed by having the patient walk on their toes.[82]

36. What are the reflexes of the lower extremity and what is their diagnostic value?

The term *reflex* means "bending back" in Latin because it refers to a sensory impulse that travels to the central nervous system only to "bend back" away from the central nervous system along a motor nerve to bring about a response. The specific nerve cell connections along

which the nerve impulse travels from the initial sensation to the final response is the reflex arc. Most reflex arcs involve a three-neuron complex, in which a receptor neuron is connected to an effector neuron by means of an intermediate neuron called the connector neuron, which lies wholly within the central nervous system. Thus most spinal reflexes are *polysynaptic* in nature.

The *reflex arc* is automatic and involuntary and because of its simplicity, operates with no added input from higher cortical levels.* The *patellar reflex* is unusual in its simplicity as it only consists of two neurons, the sensory and the motor, without the benefit of the connector neuron. As such, the two-neuron reflex arc is primarily contained within the peripheral nervous

---

*The independence of spinal reflexes from the brain is demonstrated by abnormal reflex preservation in quadriplegics.

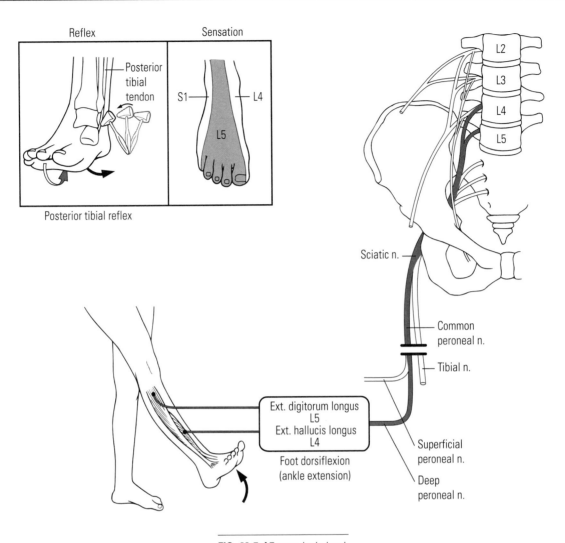

FIG. 60-5 L5 neurologic level.

system and may be said to be monosynaptic. The patellar reflex, otherwise known as the knee jerk, is tested by having the patient cross one leg over the other, thereby allowing the tested leg to hang limply. This has the effect of placing the tendon on slight stretch. By tapping the tendon with a reflex hammer, the tendon stretches acutely to the point that the proprioceptive muscle spindles within the tendon fire and cause initiation of the reflex arc. The dendrites of the sensory nerve carry the impulse to the sensory cell body within the dorsal root ganglion, whereas the axons of that same nerve cell enter the anterior horn of the spinal cord where they synapse with dendrites of a motor cell whose body lies within the cord. The impulse is then carried across the motor axon of this same neuron through the emerging

L4 nerve root and is conveyed through the femoral nerve which causes the quadriceps to contract and the foot to fly upward.

Nonappearance of the patellar reflex implies a disorder involving the portion of the nervous system through which the reflex arc travels. The disorders may be due to a disturbance in the muscle spindle, the muscle fibers, the peripheral nerve, or the spinal cord synapse. If compression of the nerve root occurs from a disk herniation or from osteophytic compression it may cause *hyporeflexia* which is defined as a diminishment of the reflex intensity. Bilateral comparison is essential because the degree of reflex activity varies from person to person. Reflexes may be documented as normal, increased, or decreased.

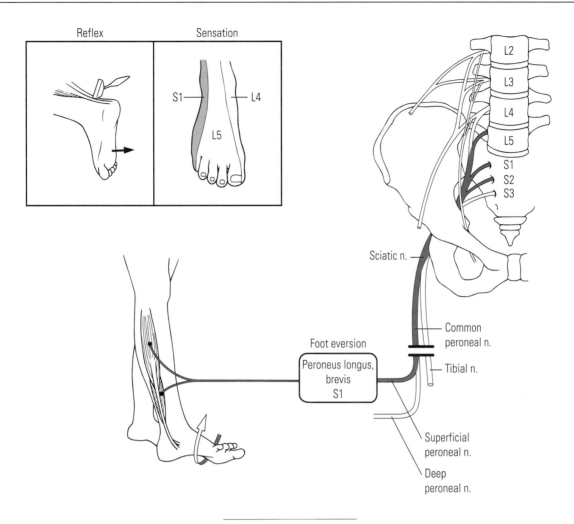

FIG. 60-6 S1 neurologic level.

37. What are deep tendon reflexes of the lower extremity and how are they elicited?

Including the knee jerk, there are a total of four reflexes* of diagnostic significance that may be elicited in the lower extremity.

---

*Although high lumbar disk lesions are extremely unlikely, if not rare, the cremasteric reflex is mediated through the L2 root. In addition to supplying the cutaneous supply over the femoral triangle via the genitofemoral nerve, the L1/L2 nerves provides motor innervation to the cremaster muscle in the spermatic cord. Present only in males and classified as a superficial reflex, the *cremasteric reflex* is provoked by lightly stroking the skin along the inner proximal thigh causes retraction of the testicle on that side. The *anal wink* is mediated through the S2-S3-S4 roots, whereas the *bulbocavernous reflex* is mediated through the S3-S4 nerve roots. Here, the patient will complain of pins and needles at the lower sacrum and perineal numbness. There is a negative straight leg raise here because the fourth sacral root does not run down the leg.

ADDUCTOR JERK

This is an L3 reflex conveyed through the obturator nerve and is the highest reflex that may be elicited in the lower extremity. The obturator nerve supplies the obturator externus (a lateral thigh rotator) and all the hip adductor musculature. Before emerging through the obturator foramen in the medial compartment of the thigh the obturator nerve runs adjacent to the uterus in the pelvis, and is thus vulnerable to peripheral nerve lesions during obstetric and gynecological procedures. Either a peripheral nerve lesion or damage to the L2, but mostly L3 nerve root may result in abolition of this reflex. With the patient's thigh in slight external rotation and the knees slightly flexed, the fingers are placed over the adductor tendon in the distal medial thigh. The reflex hammer then taps the tendon and the muscle will be felt to contract as the thigh adducts.

TIBIALIS POSTERIOR REFLEX

This is ascertained by holding the forefoot in several degrees of eversion and dorsiflexion and tapping the tendon of the tibialis posterior on the medial aspect of the foot just before it inserts into the navicular tuberosity. Although difficult to elicit routinely, a positive response results in a slight plantar inversion motion.[83]

ANKLE JERK

This is conveyed in the tibial nerve through the S1 nerve root. It is necessary to place the Achilles tendon on slight stretch by slightly dorsiflexing the ankle. The tendon is then struck with a reflex hammer and the calf muscle contracts as the ankle plantarflexes.

HAMSTRING REFLEX

This may be elicited at the distal, medial, and lateral hamstring tendons before their insertion. Both reflexes are conveyed through the S1 nerve root, although it is of clinical significance that the medial reflex, like the ankle reflex, is carried in the tibial division of the sciatic nerve whereas the lateral hamstring reflex is in the peroneal division. In other words, the tibial nerve supplies the long head of biceps femoris, whereas the peroneal nerve innervates the short head. The latter may be of value in establishing the level of a peroneal nerve lesion and will be preserved if the lesion is at or below the knee, which is usually the case. The hamstring reflexes are assessed with the patient in the same posture as used to elicit the knee jerk. With the fingers placed on the medial and lateral hamstring tendons, respectively, a sharp tap of the reflex hammer should readily elicit both reflexes.

38. What is the clinical presentation of disk pathology?

The patient may report a tearing sensation or the feeling of "something give" corresponding to annular disruption that precedes egress of the nucleus pulposus. The extruded material initially presses upon the posterior longitudinal ligament and this stretching provokes considerable centralized lower back pain. With *midline herniations,* the pain will be more severe than posterolateral herniations. Midline disk lesions may irritate roots to both limbs and should be suspected in the case where the pain is felt initially in one buttock and subsequently shifts to the opposite side, or when a positive bilateral straight leg raising is present.

With *posterolateral protrusions* and *herniations,* as the stretch becomes chronic over time, the sensory receptors become gradually acclimated to the continuous volley of painful signals and low back pain slowly diminishes. However, as the disk protrusion increases in size it begins to mechanically compress or chemically irritate a nerve root so that the patient begins to complain of limb pain. Although lower back pain is often the first symptom, it is the monoradicular pain that suggests disk pathology. With disk lesions, the radicular limb pain is often more prominent than the low back pain.[171] At times, polyradicular pain may occur from a large disk lesion, which compresses more than one nerve root.

The term *sciatica* refers to pain at the sciatic distribution, which may take one of several forms, depending on the nerve root compressed by the intervertebral disk. The pattern of radicular pain differs for the L5 and S1 nerve roots. L5 nerve root lesions present with pain and/or paresthesia radiating down the posterolateral aspect of the thigh, continuing down the lateral aspect of the leg, and then over the anterolateral aspect of the distal third, and continuing over the dorsum of the foot to the first and second toes. Symptoms are most prominent over the distal half of the leg anterolaterally and the patient may rub the area while presenting the history. With an L5 root lesion, the tibialis posterior reflex will be diminished. In contrast, an S1 nerve root lesion manifests as pain radiating from the buttock to the ischial tuberosity, down the posterior aspect of the thigh and leg to the heel and outer border of the foot. Here, symptoms are most prominent over the posterior thigh and calf, although patients frequently complain of numbness in the lateral three toes. With an S1 nerve root lesion, the hamstring and Achilles reflexes will be diminished. Dermatomal sensory loss may be assessed* with fingertips or wisps of cotton.† Range of motion of the lumbar spine will possibly be limited. Flexion will be most restricted because pressure increases greatly within the intervertebral disk during this movement. Following limited forward flexion from, say brushing

---

*A pinwheel should not be used unless it is sterilized between patients, because of the potential risk of transmission of hepatitis of HIV viruses.

†Perianal innervation is arranged in concentric rings, and may be assessed. The innermost ring is S5, surrounded by S4, then S3, and then S2 at the outer perimeter. The penis and scrotum receive sensory innervation from S2 and S3. Loss of perianal sensation may indicate an impending *cauda equina syndrome.*

one's teeth or washing one's face, the patient may become locked in the stooped position that takes time and gentle help to come to extension.[151] It is important to scan for evidence of muscle wasting. Circumferential measurements of both calves and thighs are appropriate. For the thigh, measurements should be taken 20 and 12 cm proximal to the medial joint line, and on the calf, 12 cm to the distal joint line.

The lumbar area will become flattened owing to loss of normal lumbar lordosis.[85] This is because the associated muscle spasm, which may range from moderate to severe, acts to diminish extension of the spine because hyperlordosis causes narrowing of both the spinal canal and intervertebral foramen.

Sciatic pain secondary to disk pathology typically results in positive *thecal signs* in which coughing, sneezing, laughing, or straining aggravates the nerve root within the dural sleeve enveloping the root. This occurs because these activities dilate the veins on the inner aspect of the dural tube and causes a momentary rise in the cerebrospinal fluid pressure.[41,42] Tests that are similar to the SLR in their ability to provoke dural irritation and thereby indicate nerve root involvement are Brudzinski's and Kernig's signs. *Brudzinski's sign* involves passive flexion of the patient's head causing flexion of the thighs and legs. Here, cephalic dural tension provokes compensation at the caudal end to ease tension and hence pain on the dural tract. *Kernig's sign* involves flexing the hips and knees, and having the patient slowly attempt to extend their knee; a positive sign is indicated by an inability to straighten the knees without accompanying hamstring spasm and pain. Here, the source of caudal tension to the theca is prevented by protective hamstring spasm.[21]

Sciatic pain is accentuated by forward bending and is associated with moderate-to-severe muscle spasm. Leg pain is more severe in the upright posture because the tension of a protrusion is greater in a loaded disk. Sitting in a soft or hard chair will aggravate pain because back flexion will cause considerably more pressure on the disk and encourage increased nerve root compression. When rising from a chair, the patient may flex the hips to move the center of gravity over his feet, and then use his hands for support when standing upright. When recumbent, most patients will prefer to lie with their hips and knees flexed. The pain from a herniated disk is often relieved by lying down because this relieves the axial compression on the disk, and hence the nerve root compressed by the disk.[85] This is so despite the fact that after several hours of recumbency the disk becomes more swollen owing to reimbibing fluid. Many patients experience difficulty in donning their shoes and socks and find it easier to lie in bed and flex their hips to their chest, one leg at a time, to reach their toes rather than simulate a SLR by bending over while sitting in a chair. Similarly, patients prefer short sitting to the long-sitting posture for the same reason.

The presence of *clonus* may be assessed by holding the knee flexed to approximately 30° and applying a sharp dorsiflexion moment to the ankle joint. Hyperreflexia and clonus may be a normal variant and may occur from anxiety, medication, or drug withdrawal. Clonus is more readily detected in the child than the adult with lumbar spinal pathology. This is to be differentiated from the sustained clonus and hyperreflexia associated with disease of the central nervous system.[169]

39. What is a trunk list?

Approximately one third of all patients with disk protrusion demonstrate a gravity-induced *trunk list* or *tilt,* alternately known as *sciatic scoliosis,* in which the pelvis remains horizontal with the floor while the lumbar spine deviates to one side with a "wind-swept" appearance. A list may be defined as lumbar curvature present in the standing position that is gone when the patient is recumbent.[102] A list shifts the center of gravity away from the central plane, thereby altering the distribution of weight while standing. Occurring as a function of reflex muscle spasm, a list develops in response to an acute onset low back pain secondary to disk protrusion,[170] herniation, or torn annulus.[169] A list occurs as a protective response that reflexively postures the spine so as to ease the root away from the prolapsed disk[148] and thereby ease root irritation. The muscles responsible for generating the list include the psoas[69] and spinal muscles. In some cases, the list is on the same side as the sciatica, whereas at other times it is toward the opposite side. When the herniated disk is lateral to the nerve root, a list to that same side would provoke pain, whereas a list to the opposite side would ease tension off the nerve root. In contrast, when the herniation is medial to the nerve root, the list is toward the side of the sciatica because tilting away would irritate the root and provoke pain.[204] Abolition of the list may be accomplished by lying down or hanging from a bar.[151] In contrast, idiopathic scoliosis is more visible with the patient standing or bending forward and does not abate when the patient is prone.

40. What is the *straight leg raise* (SLR) and what does a positive test signify?

The *SLR* as a clinical provocative test for the presence of sciatica was first described by a pupil (i.e., Forst) of the Paris neurologist Ernest Charles Lasègue (1816-1883) who ascribed it to his teacher.[178] The SLR may be considered the most important clinical sign for the diagnosis of disk herniation as its limitation is a sign of root tension and is rarely encountered in any other pathology.[151-153] The mechanical basis of the SLR is movement of the low lumbar and high sacral nerve roots and particularly the pain-sensitive dura mater investing the roots. Thus the SLR is a clinical measure for neural irritability. The SLR may also be used as a clinical yardstick in measuring improvement following the acute state in which the ipsilateral leg rises higher as the condition improves.[171]

During a unilateral SLR, the lumbosacral nerve roots move caudal in relation to their respective intervertebral foramen and in a caudal direction within the pelvis.[67] Although pain provoked before 20° is often considered nonphysiologic, pain experienced beyond 60° is considered nonspecific.[169] During the first 35° of elevation there is rarely pain as slack is taken up within the sciatic arborization. Tension is applied to the sciatic nerve roots at 35° and above. The L5 and S1 nerve roots undergo an excursion of between 2 and 6 mm, so that full stretch of these roots occurs at 70°.[167] When performing a unilateral SLR, 80° to 90° of hip flexion is considered normal, although beyond 70° pain may result from passive stretch of the musculoligamentous structures whereas neural tension is not increased.[78] Thus although complete elongation of the sciatic tract occurs at 70° of hip flexion, the additional 10° to 20° characterizing the normal range of hip flexion is accomplished by a sliding movement of the sciatic tract in relation to its surrounding soft and osseous tissue.[27]

The SLR is a passive test performed with the patient relaxed in the sitting or supine position with the hip medially rotated and the knee extended as the hip is flexed. It is important that the patient be completely relaxed[115] before beginning the test because resistance in the form of limitation may occur as a reflex to prevent root tension.[86] Care must be taken to prevent posterior pelvic rotation in the seated position, which may result in false-positive findings. At this point, the examiner slowly drops the limb down to just short of the tolerance point. The patient's ankle is then passively dorsiflexed, or the patient is asked to forward-flex his neck so as to touch his chin to his chest. This superimposition of neck motion component is known as *Brudzinski's* (or *Hyndman's*) *sign.* Alternately, the latter two may be performed simultaneously.

The SLR sign is considered positive if it produces sciatic pain radiating below the knee in conjunction with a diminished leg-raise angle. Pain proximal to the popliteal space is more likely indicative of hamstring tightness. It is essential to differentiate true sciatica from mere hamstring tightness. Typically, a positive SLR results in approximately 45° lower limb elevation on the involved side while the other side exhibits full range of motion. However, persons with tight hamstrings may not even reach 45° of elevation, so that if a patient cannot elevate to 45°, it does not necessarily indicate a positive SLR. With hamstring tightness, leg pain occurs at about the same angle for both legs, and pain is confined to the posterior thigh and does not extend distal to the knee. In patient with tight hamstrings and suspected disk pathology, back pain that is produced before reaching the point of hamstring tightness is suggestive of a disk herniation (Fig. 60-7).[171] A patient may experience a *painful arc* during the SLR that often coincides with a painful arc during forward spinal flexion. A painful arc corresponds to a maximal point of discomfort as the nerve root catches or rubs across the cause of impingement, be it a bulging or sequestrated disk, or osteophytes. A painful arc may occur in the midrange in either elevation or depression of the leg, or the patient may suddenly deviate laterally during forward spinal flexion and return to a symmetrical posture as soon as this painful juncture is passed.[41]

A positive SLR neither predicts the size nor the location (e.g., lateral recess, central) of a disk herniation.[190] The SLR may also be used as a guide to prognosis because the first sign of a receding disk displacement* is the increased range of straight-leg raising.[42] Although a negative SLR does not rule out the presence of disk pathology, a positive response in conjunction with a positive history and supplementary signs, allows for a presumptive diagnosis of a lumbar intervertebral disk lesion.[151-153] A bilat-

---

*A bulging disk may back up into the disk space whereas extruded disk material may simply become resorbed over time. Other signs of improvement that accompany resorption or recession include abatement of visible spinal deformity, trunk list, improved lumbar spine motion, centralization of sciatica, and return of normal motor and neurologic signs.

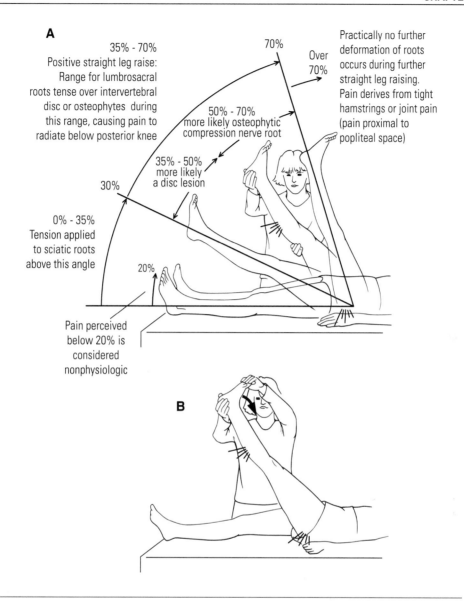

A,

35% - 70%
Positive straight leg raise:
Range for lumbrosacral
roots tense over intervertebral
disc or osteophytes during
this range, causing pain to
radiate below posterior knee

70%

Over
70%

Practically no further
deformation of roots
occurs during further
straight leg raising.
Pain derives from tight
hamstrings or joint pain
(pain proximal to
popliteal space)

50% - 70%
more likely osteophytic
compression nerve root

35% - 50%
more likely
a disc lesion

30%

0% - 35%
Tension applied
to sciatic roots
above this angle

20%

Pain perceived
below 20% is
considered
nonphysiologic

B

FIG. 60-7 A, The *straight leg raising test.* **B,** *Lasègue test.* Positive tests implicate the L5 and/or S1 nerve roots.

eral positive SLR may occur with central (midline) herniations.

In addition to nerve roots moving distally during a SLR, they also translate laterally. Their lateral translation will cause them to collide with a posterolateral protrusion and thereby strain the root(s). Subsequently, the lateral translation moves the roots away from a central disk lesion, so that a patient with midline disk pathology may not experience sciatica during straight leg raising.[175]

Modifications of this neural tension test may be reproduced by the *Lasègue test** in which the hip is flexed to 90°, and the knee is slowly extended to the point of limitation or sciatic pain. This test is less valuable than the classic SLR.[169] The *bowstring sign* is produced by applying digital pressure to the sciatic tract at

---

*The *Lasègue test* is alternately known to some clinicians as sharply dorsiflexing the ipsilateral ankle joint just below the point of maximal elevation of the involved leg.

the midline of the popliteal space while it is maximally elongated.[114] The clinician's pressure upon the already maximally stretched sciatic tract represents an artificially superimposed double crush and is positive in the presence of pain.

The SLR does not identify tension on any nerve root rostral to L5. These proximal nerve roots (particularly, the L3 root) are tension-tested by a reverse-straight leg raise known as the *femoral stretch test* or *prone knee bend* (Fig. 60-8). Symmetrical limitation of bilateral lower extremities indicates quadriceps tightness. A patient who complains of low back pain radiating down the anterior aspect of the thigh and who has difficulty squatting may have a mid-lumbar disk herniation, as the ability to squat normally reflects on the power of the quadriceps and gluteal muscles. A mid-lumbar nerve root lesion may be considered once spinal stenosis and hip joint pathology are ruled out. Sciatic pain during the prone knee bend is thought to be diagnostic of an L4/L5 herniated nucleus pulposus.[30]

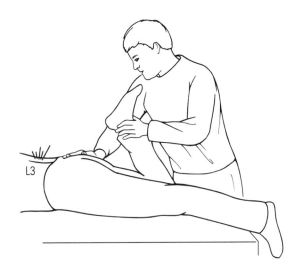

FIG. 60-8 *Prone knee bend test.* Although pain of the ipsilateral anterior thigh indicates tightness of the iliopsoas, pain in the lumbar area is positive for lumbar nerve root pathology rostral to L5.

41. How may the SLR be interpreted so as to clinically differentiate between nerve root impingement deriving from spinal stenosis and disk pathology?

Between 35° and 70° of SLR represents tensing of the lumbosacral nerve roots,[53] and the test may only be considered positive if symptoms are elicited within this range.[78] When tension is applied to a nerve, the intraneural pressure increases as the cross-sectional area decreases. This increase in pressure results in both blood deprivation, which interferes with nerve conduction, and also effects axonal transport within the sciatic tract.[27] Pain and limitation of SLR due to a claw osteophyte (spinal stenosis) will more likely reduce the available straight leg raising minimally in comparison with a herniated disk. This is because the traction spur represents a local tethering of the nerve root, which limits the amount of sliding the nerve root may undergo. Nevertheless, the root may accommodate to impingement by undergoing elongation, in addition to some, albeit, reduced mobility. Thus lateral stenosis may be associated with an SLR greater than 50°.

In contrast, significant disk pathology in the form of a herniated disk may compress a relatively large portion of the nerve root and effectively eliminate sliding of that portion of the sciatic tract emerging from that root. This may correspond to less available straight leg raising. Thus an SLR between 25° and 50° is almost pathognomic of a disk lesion.[151]

42. What is the diurnal SLR test and what is its clinical significance?

If the outer annular fibers are intact, the disk is considered competent as no nuclear material has been expressed through the annulus. Because the disk is competent, its changing fluid content will affect root tension signs. Following as little as 2 hours of recumbency in bed or after a night's sleep, the disk will reimbibe fluid. In the morning, the bulging disk will be tense and clinically manifest as a diminished angle of straight leg raising as compared with the night before. After being up and around for 1 or 2 hours, the hydrostatic pressure of axial spinal compressive load will cause fluid loss from within the disk and is demonstrated by an increased range in the degree of straight leg raising. This phenomenon will not occur in the situation where the limitation of SLR derives from central or lateral canal stenosis.[152]

Thus the diurnal SLR may be used to differentiate between a limitation of SLR due to disk pathology and spinal stenosis; to test the competence of the disk; and to distinguish whether there is a tense protrusion or a complete rupture of the annulus. A complete and thorough annular tear causing nerve root compression either due to impingement from an annular fragment or sequestered nuclear material will result in no change in the SLR regardless of the time of day testing occurred.

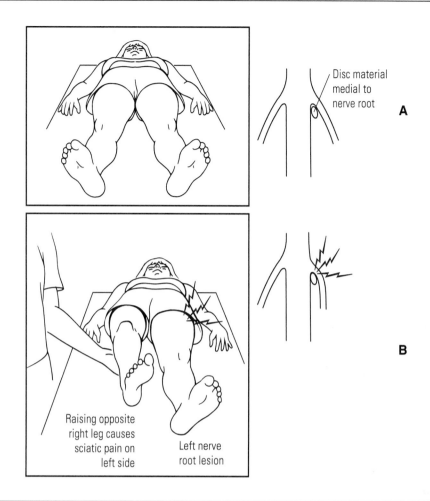

Disc material
medial to
nerve root

A

Raising opposite
right leg causes
sciatic pain on
left side

Left nerve
root lesion

B

FIG. 60-9 *Crossed straight leg raise test*—if the patient complains of thigh or calf pain on the opposite side, it is indicative of a high degree of nerve root irritation secondary to a large lateral intervertebral disk protrusion or herniation medial to the nerve at the L4-L5 level. If the fragmented annulus or extruded nucleus lay lateral to a given nerve root, a contralateral SLR would not have any effect on the disk lesion. However, because the disk material lies medial to the nerve root, contralateral leg raising has the effect of depressing the affected nerve root and moving it toward midline, which has the overall effect of increasing root tension and provoking pain. **A,** When the leg is raised on the unaffected side, the roots on the opposite side slide downward and toward midline. **B,** In the presence of a disk lesion medial to the contralateral nerve root, this movement increases root tension and pain by compressing the nerve root against the disk material.

43. What is the crossover sign and what does it signify?

If one lower limb undergoes a SLR and the patient complains of thigh or calf pain on the opposite side, it is indicative severe nerve root irritation secondary to a large lateral intervertebral disk protrusion or herniation medial to the nerve root[167] at the L4/L5 level.[30] If the fragmented annulus or extruded nucleus lay lateral to a given nerve root, a contralateral SLR would not have any effect on the disk lesion. However, because the disk material lies medial to the nerve root, contralateral leg raising has the effect of depressing the affected root and moving it toward midline, which has the overall effect of increasing root tension and provoking pain (Fig. 60-9).[44] Tension to the entire sciatic tract, accompanied by pain, my be accomplished by superimposing passive hip adduction and medial rotation upon hip flexion during the SLR test.

Pain in the symptomatic leg worsened by raising the contralateral lower extremity* goes by a variety of names known as the *crossed SLR*, the *well leg raise test of Fajersztajn*,[209] as well as the prostrate leg raise test, the sciatic phenomenon, and the cross over sign.[84] This test may cause pain on both sides as it may stretch both the ipsilateral and contralateral nerve roots.[115] The presence of this sign may indicate disk pathology too severe to respond to conservative management.[51]

44. In addition to the motor, sensory, and reflex assessment, what are other essential components of the examination?

Pain is characteristically centered in the lumbar area, but may also radiate over the buttocks, thigh, calf, leg, and foot. Evidence of nerve root impingement by disk material is obviated by weakness, numbness, pain, paresthesia, reflex changes, and positive provocative signs. Other components of a comprehensive evaluation include:

• *Ruling out hip pathology.* Because gluteal pain is the classic pattern of referred pain from the lower back, patients who complain of "hip pain" should have their lower extremities evaluated. Range of motion of the hip should be assessed with the patient supine as the Faber maneuver is applied to the joint. This consists of 90° flexion, abduction, and external rotation of the involved leg so that it lies in a "frog-legged" posture. This maneuver should be painless and unrestricted in the patient with sciatic radiculopathy because flexion of the lower limb places the lumbosacral nerve roots on slack and relieves the painful stretch of the involved nerve root.[202] Therefore if inguinal pain is provoked during this maneuver, hip pathology should be considered. Negative results are indicated by the leg falling in parallel with the opposite leg, whereas a positive test is indicated when the leg remains above the opposite leg. Although the role of sacroiliac joint in the production of lumbar pain is controversial, the Maitland[126] and Gaenslen tests (see Fig. 56-7) assess for sacroiliac joint dysfunction. The Faber test may also be used to stress and thereby assess the sacroiliac joint. This is accomplished by simultaneously pressing down on the ipsilateral knee and contralateral anterior superior iliac spine. Complaints of increasing pain suggest pathology of the sacroiliac joint (Fig. 60-10).[83] Thus pain in the front

is associated with hip pathology, whereas pain in the back is associated with pathology originating at the sacroiliac joint. Hip arthritis may also be ruled out by the scouring test in which the femur is forcibly pushed into the acetabulum as the flexed hip and knee are circumducted through the hip range of motion. This test "scours" throughout the range for arthritis by assessing the inner joint surface.

• *Press ups.* Compressive forces on the L5 nerve root from an L4/L5 disk herniation increase with flexion of the L4/L5 motion segment resulting in increased tension on the nerve root, whereas extension decreases the compressive force.[168] Press-ups, part of the diagnostic and therapeutic regime of McKenzie, may improve pain in the event of an annular tear, bulge, or small herniated nucleus pulposus. In patients with herniated nucleus pulposus with distal referral, pain that recedes from its peripheral location to become centralized closer to the low back during press-ups strongly correlates with successful conservative care, whereas failure of pain to centralize may correlate with poor prognostic outcome.[35] Moreover, *centralization of symptoms* during press-ups suggests that rehabilitation should bias extension over flexion as a primary thrust of physical therapy.

• *Flexibility.* Flexibility of the lower extremity muscle groups, particularly the hip flexors. Passive assessment for tightness of the iliopsoas and quadriceps muscles is accomplished with the Thomas test in which the inability to fully extend the leg without arching the thoracolumbar spine indicates a fixed hip flexion contracture. The shortness of these anterior muscles on the pelvis causes an anterior pelvic tilt that accentuates the lumbar lordosis and results in greater strain to the motion segment.

45. What factor does vertebral canal size play in symptomatology following a disk lesion?

Magnetic resonance imaging studies have shown that approximately 20% of the population have space occupying disk protrusions by age 60, although most of these are symptomless.[15] This may be directly related to the size of the vertebral canal, so that a disk prolapse into a restricted space is more likely to produce troublesome symptoms than protrusion into a wider canal.[107] These patients may be as likely to develop disk pathology at various sites as do persons with small canals, but may not experience root symptoms because of sufficient space within the canal for the roots to avoid compression.[149] This is supported by data indicating that

---

*Curiously, cross-leg femoral stretch of the upper lumbar nerve roots has yet to be described or investigated.

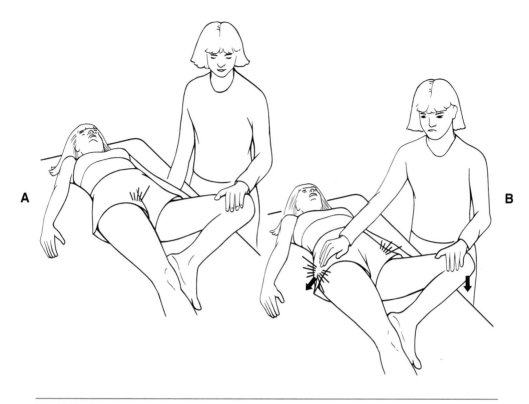

FIG. 60-10 *Faber test* to detect pathology of the hip and sacroiliac joint. **A,** With the patient supine, the foot of the involved side is placed on the opposite knee, causing the hip joint to be flexed, abducted, and externally rotated. Inguinal pain in this position is a positive sign. **B,** The sacroiliac joint is assessed by simultaneously pressing down on the contralateral pelvis and ipsilateral knee. Pathology of the sacroiliac joint is suggested by increasing pain.

nearly one half of patients with root symptoms and signs of acute disk protrusion demonstrate canal diameter measurements in the bottom 10% of the population.[131] Thus the degree of disability caused by a herniated disk depends on several factors including how much disk material has entered the spinal canal, how many nerve roots have been affected, and the space within the spinal canal. Although patients with very narrow canals may have severe symptoms with even a small disk lesion, those with wider canals may experience fewer or in some cases, no symptoms whatsoever from the same size herniation.[99]

Because of the variability of vertebral canal size in the general population, some patients will not demonstrate root-related symptoms associated with disk disruption, although a more generalized back pain, muscle spasm, and diminished range of motion may occur if the protrusion stretches the posterior longitudinal ligament or causes dural irritation. Thus although a small dome shaped canal may be troublesome, a small trefoil shaped canal may be very problematic. A large canal with a trefoil shape may not be a problem unless the disk extends out laterally and compresses the nerve root in the lateral recess.[151-153]

46. What are nonorganic forms of back pain?

Malingering is defined as a conscious and deliberate attempted to deceive, which is motivated by a secondary gain, based upon an ulterior motive such as financial gain, evading criminal prosecution, or avoiding military duties. Tangible secondary gain refers to monetary compensation relating to a work-related injury (workman's compensation or disability insurance) or civil litigation from an automobile accident, fall, or assault, in which the possibility of a large financial settlement plus the bonus of avoiding unpleasant work is tempting enough to motivate some persons to claim fictitious and extensive disabilities. The patient may also be seeking other forms of reinforcement from family, co-workers, and employers. The malingerer attempts to create the impression that symptoms are persistent and incapacitating.

The hallmark of malingering is the production of grossly exaggerated physical symptoms. Upon walking into the office, malingering patients may ambulate with a bizarre gait that is inconsistent with physical findings, often without a smile, but with a blank and despondent expression. Some grunt and groan as they sit down or climb aboard the examination table. Patients provide a vague history and may try to confuse the examiner by avoiding specific details of their symptoms and being intentionally vague in their answers with the exception that the source of pain is always identified as happening immediately after the accident. Everything they do hurts including sitting, standing, walking, lying, or bending. After bending forward, they may return to the erect posture groaning and complaining of increased pain in a cogwheel fashion. Symptoms have begun on the date of the injury and remain constant indefinitely. This is in direct contrast to patients with genuine mechanical low back problems such as disk pathology or other pathology who normally have fluctuations in the level of their discomfort, whereas those with true organic pathology have steadily increasing symptoms.

During gentle palpation of the low back, an exaggerated acute response will be evoked in which the malingerer will pull away from the examiner with an exclamation of "oohs and ahhs." In contrast, although the genuine patient may claim that palpation elicits tenderness or even hurts, they do not pull away. When attempting to assess spinal motions, all movement will be restricted although the patient exhibits no difficulty donning or doffing their shoes, or climbing onto the examination table. Manual muscle testing shows weakness, although asking the patient to sustain body weight while on tiptoe, on their heels, or the borders of their feet is easily managed. Muscle strength may present as a jerklike motion (cogwheel) or sudden release and inconsistencies will arise between different muscles with the same innervation. Inconsistencies may also occur when testing the same muscle isometrically and isotonically. A dynamometer may provide objective evidence of poor cooperation and overreaction of symptoms evidenced by trials of the same test.[177] Muscle atrophy may be absent and the patient may be well built and muscular. Sensory loss, if present, may not correspond to a dermatomal distribution and may occur in a glove-and-stocking distribution. Reflexes remain normal as they are not under conscious control. Although a patient with legitimate low back pain does not resist straight leg raising until the point at which the pain is induced, the malingerer actively resists elevation from the outset, or at best, no more than 25° to 30° and often winces with pain while pushing downward against the examiner's effort to prevent the limb from being further elevated. Long sitting (i.e., full knee extension while the patient sits upright) is equivalent to a 90° SLR, and would never occur in genuine sciatica with positive straight leg raising; instead, malingerers will lean the torso backward so as to restrict the degree of straight leg raising. However, the malingerer tolerates straight leg raising while seated, but not in the recumbent position.

The *Hoover test* is applicable for the patient who claims that he/she cannot raise their leg at all and is based on the normal SLR in which the contralateral leg presses downward on the examination surface in an attempt to stabilize and gain leverage in lifting the weaker leg. The examiner cups one hand under the contralateral heel. An absence of downward pressure under the contralateral calcaneus suggests that the patient is feigning symptoms and attempting to manipulate the examination.[8]

Malingering probably occurs much more frequently than it is diagnosed.[58] Inconsistencies may also be discovered when comparing the findings of physical examination of various health care providers who evaluated the same malingerer. A good way of confirming suspected malingering is the employment of investigators by legal counsel who, using video cameras and other vehicles, document over a period of time clear evidence of major discrepancies in claimed functional impairment.[49] It is not advisable to inform the patient of a malingering diagnosis as it can lead to legal action against the clinician for character defamation. The best course is to state that "no organic basis can be found for the patient's symptoms[99] and that there is nothing further you have to offer." Ordering unnecessary investigations or treatment only strengthens the patient's case, as it could be argued that results of these tests or therapies would not be sought unless real pathology was suspected.[171]

Several psychological conditions masquerade as low back pain including conversion disorders, depression, hypochondriasis, somatization and somatoform pain disorders, and Munchausen syndrome, to name just a few. This group does not experience fictitious back pain, does not intentionally produce symptoms, and does not represent malingering.

47. What is the differential diagnosis of low back pain?

Although disk pathology secondary to mechanical causes or chemical irritation may often be diagnosed on the basis of history and examination alone,[99] the clinician must be aware of the many possible sources of low back pain to know when to refer the patient to the primary physician for further studies. Except for compression fractures from osteopenia or cancer, medical causes of low back pain do not usually have a traumatic onset. Medical causes of low back pain most often occur in the elderly, who typically complain of progressively worsening pain that is not relieved by sleep, recumbency, or change in position. A history of infection elsewhere in the body (particularly the urinary tract), alcoholism, intravenous drug use, or recent invasive or surgical procedures may be related to infection of the vertebrae or disk space. Malignancy is the most feared cause of spinal pain, and metastatic disease to the spine must be suspected in any patient with even a remote history of malignancy.[169] The first symptoms of retroperitoneal mass or colon or prostate carcinoma may be low back pain.[75] However, with metastatic lesions, decrease of low back pain with onset of radicular symptoms is uncommon. The most common malignant lesions in the pediatric spine include leukemia, osteosarcoma, Ewing's sarcoma, and non-Hodgkin's lymphoma and often present with pain, neurologic deficit, and pathologic fracture. The symptoms associated with tumor include well-localized pain that frequently worsens at night, and is neither associated with activity nor relieved by rest. Diseases of the viscera may cause radicular pain, whereas those which may produce back pain include posterior wall cardiac ischemia or infarction, ulceration of the stomach wall causing pain in the right posterior chest wall, gallbladder, biliary tree, and pancreatic disease, pelvic disease in the form of tumor, mass, or inflammation, and retroperitoneal mass or hemorrhage in which nerve root symptoms are often present at the lesion level.[202] The differential diagnosis of low back pain includes several categories, including degenerative disorders, infection, circulatory disorders, cancer, inflammatory causes, and metabolic disorders:

DEGENERATIVE DISORDERS

- *Spinal stenosis.* This derives from osseous compression of the cauda equina or nerve root(s) due to a narrow spinal canal in the former and osteophytic compression in the latter. Central compression of the cauda equina often produces neurogenic claudication of the thighs or calves that, unlike nerve root pathology from disk disease, is often relieved by a stooped posture. Differentiation of osteophytic nerve root entrapment from nerve root compression derived from disk pathology is based upon interpretation of the SLR (see previous section).

- *Degenerative disk disease.* This differs from disk herniation in several respects. Whereas with disk herniation, patients frequently complain that pain is aggravated when sitting in any type of chair, with degenerative disk disease (DDD) patients avoid the soft chair but often feel comfortable in a hard one. With DDD, flexion is not usually restricted and symptoms gradually diminish with activity. In contrast, patients with disk pathology have marked restriction of lumbar flexion and experience increasing discomfort as the day wears on.

- *Ligament sprain.* This must be differentiated from an acute annular tear. Although an acute annular tear is deeply located and not provoked by pinpoint tenderness, localization is often possible on palpation with a ligamentous tear. With a sprain, pain would have been constant from the outset, particularly during spinal movement and usually eases off for a short while only to recur and persist without remission unless the patient is recumbent. In contrast, patients with acute disk prolapse cannot entirely alleviate pain while recumbent, particularly if disk material compresses the posterior longitudinal ligament, in which case pain will be unremitting even while lying down.[171]

INFECTION

- *Diskitis.* This refers to a low grade bacterial infection (most commonly *Staphylococcus aureus*) of the pediatric intervertebral disk space between the adjacent endplates often involving the lower thoracic or upper lumbar levels (most commonly L4/L5) in infants and children. Average age of incidence is between 2 and 7 years, although the peak age of onset is 6 years. The lumbar spine is typically affected.[151-153] Occasionally, more than one level is involved. Clinical findings are age-related and include low grade fever, limpness, irritability, stiff back, unwillingness to stand or ambulate, abdominal, gluteal, or hip pain, and vomiting in the infant. The adolescent may complain of vague and poorly localized back pain that is accompanied by a stiff back and elevated erythrocyte sedimentation rate.[203] Signs include a diminished range of straight leg raising, a decrease or increase in lumbar lordosis, while examination in the prone position with the knees flexed 90° may elicit pain and spasm with alternating hyperextension of the hips. No neurologic deficit is evident. Early on, a bone scan may show increased uptake over multiple vertebral levels, whereas disk space narrowing[151-153] and mild irregularity and sclerosis of the vertebral endplates[122] are seen on a lateral radiographic view after 3 weeks. Diskitis is accompanied by an elevated erythrocyte sedimentation rate (ESR) and may be differentiated from vertebral osteomyelitis using magnetic resonance imaging. Diskitis usually spontaneously resolves with 6 to 12 weeks of rest, although oral antibiotics are appropriate if the child is systemically ill[132] or if the child is not relieved by rest. Immobilization in a "panty spica" or brace for 4 to 6 weeks may significantly reduce the child's discomfort. Although residual narrowing and occasional fusion of the disk space may follow, late disability is rare.

- *Vertebral osteomyelitis.* This is more commonly seen in the elderly, immunosuppressed, or diabetic population, and is rare in children under 9 years of age.[5] Most commonly caused by hematogenous spread of *S. aureus* and a wide range of other bacteria, fungi, or anaerobes,[173] infection may also be introduced during spinal surgery, epidural injections, myelography, or from adjacent infectious lesions. Whereas the responsible pathogen is usually staphylococci in the younger population, it is the gram negative organisms that affect the elderly spine where most are commonly derived from the urinary tract.[173] The highest incidence of vertebral osteomyelitis occurs in the third decade, which may relate to the fact that the lumbar intraosseous arteries are end arteries (supplying a segment of bone) in adults and adolescents.[157] Following endplate destruction, the disk is rapidly destroyed by proteolytic enzymes of the pyogenic organism and may spread to adjacent vertebrae. The major symptom is gradual onset of localized low back pain that is progressively unremitting and worse at night.[202] Other symptoms include fever, malaise, vague abdominal complaints, paravertebral muscle spasm, spinal rigidity, and frequently more muscle spasm than is usually encountered with a disk lesion.[156] Although loss of appetite and weight may accompany spinal infection, pathology is often not suspected until a late stage.[57] Pain is not alleviated by bed rest or antiinflammatory medication, is continu-

ous, and is accentuated by movement. Point tenderness occurs at the level of the infected vertebra and is made worse with percussion. The frequently accompanying scoliosis of vertebral osteomyelitis is fixed, whereas the sciatic scoliosis deriving from a disk protrusion is induced by gravity and abolished by lying down. There may be an increase in white blood cell count and ESR, whereas blood culture is positive in the acute phase and often negative when back pain becomes subacute or chronic. A vertebral biopsy is often performed when blood cultures prove negative and determines the form of antibiotic therapy. During the first 3 weeks of the disease progressive collapse of the vertebral body occurs that is only radiographically obvious after 3 weeks when it is accompanied by endplate destruction and possibly kyphosis. Radioisotope scanning and magnetic resonance imaging may be helpful in identifying this pathology in the early stages. The prognosis for recovery is good provided appropriate management occurs consisting of antibiotic therapy, rest, and immobilization. The disease process is followed by intense bony regeneration in the form of bone bridging in 80% of cases. Some patients are identified in retrospect as they recover without treatment.[181]

- *Acute pyogenic infection.* Pyogenic means "pus forming." These infections are usually blood borne from a primary source elsewhere in the body, either the respiratory tract (in younger persons), the urinary tract (in older persons), or from postoperative wound infections in all ages. Spinal tuberculosis is still a cause of back pain in underdeveloped countries.

- *Epidural abscess.* This is rarely encountered, but may occur in a patient with underlying infection that may be remote (dental abscess) or adjacent (vertebral osteomyelitis, sacral decubitus ulcer, pelvic inflammatory disease, or retroperitoneal abscess), or may arise spontaneously. The most common causative organisms include *S. aureus, Escherichia coli,* and various anaerobes. The patient complains of severe and localized thoracic or lumbar back pain, which may radiate. In the event of cord compression, paraparesis or paraplegia may progress over the course of hours to days in the event of abscesses, or within minutes to several hours with *spinal epidural hematoma.* Patients with abscess are usually feverish. Diagnosis is via myelography and antibiotic therapy should be started following blood cultures, and preferably before surgery. Surgical decompression and abscess removal must be immediately performed.[11]

- *Sacroiliac joint infection.* Pyogenic (pus forming) arthritis of the sacroiliac joint is uncommon but may cause localized pain in the lumbar, gluteal, or adductor areas that is relieved with exercise and worsened with rest. A definitive clinical sign involves reproducing pain by raising the ipsilateral leg and flexing the hip with adduction across the opposite leg. Alternately, pathology is suggested by forced bilateral hip abduction. Treatment is by aspiration and drainage of the abscess followed by recumbency and immobilization.

CIRCULATORY DISORDERS

- *Abdominal aortic aneurysm.* The abdominal aorta begins to bifurcate at the level of the L3 vertebra where it may undergo aneurysm predominantly in persons over the age of 50. Rupture of an abdominal aneurysm is a surgical emergency that is the thirteenth most common cause of male death in the United States, especially over the age of 65. There are often no symptoms associated with an abdominal aneurysm, although patients may complain of a dull, nagging or severe low back pain due to erosion of the lumbar vertebrae by the expanding vessel. Some patients typically have other associated diseases such as hypertension, high blood cholesterol, diabetes, and a history of smoking. Abdominal aneurysm may be caused by infection, syphilis, arteritis, Marfan's syndrome, and congenital abnormality. Pain from abdominal aortic aneurysm may cause back pain that mimics a herniated lumbar disk. When suspected, it is essential to assess lower extremity pulses and skin temperature and inspect and palpate the abdomen for a pulsating mass, and auscultating for a bruit. When suspected, immediate referral to a vascular surgeon is required.
- *Leriche syndrome.* This involves *thrombotic occlusion of the terminal aorta* and may simulate a herniated disk. Pain in the back, buttocks, thighs, and legs typically accompanies exercise. Fatigue, weakness, and muscle atrophy occur, as well as impotence in males. Arterial pulses below the aortic bifurcation may be palpated as a result of the segmental arteriosclerotic occlusion.[99]

CANCER

- *Benign tumors.* Tumors of the spinal canal are usually benign and are classified as *intradural* or *extradural*.

The former may be *intramedullary* (involving the spinal cord) or *extramedullary* (inside the dura but not involving the cord.) Intradural extramedullary tumors include meningioma, neurofibroma, and schwannoma. Although benign, these tumors may destroy the spinal cord by expansion and pressure. Vertebral hemangioma may occur in the vertebral body and causes trabeculae to appear longitudinal on radiographs.

- *Osteoid osteoma.* This is a benign tumor that typically involves long bone, but may involve the vertebrae and cause back pain and a fixed scoliosis. This form of tumor, like osteoblastoma, characteristically occurs in the second and third decades of life and produces night pain that is dramatically relieved by aspirin. It is best visualized on bone scans, but may be radiographically imaged as a small radiolucent zone surrounded by a large sclerotic zone. Treatment is surgical removal. In contrast to osteoid osteoma, spinal cord tumor is rare in children.[180] In adults, malignancy or infection is classically chronic, steadily progressive, and painfully unremitting.
- *Malignant tumors.* These tumors may be classified as *primary* or *metastatic.* Metastatic tumors spread from other adjacent or distant portions of the body that have a primary tumor. The spine is the most common site for skeletal metastatic tumors because of the rich venous supply to the vertebral bodies—especially from the vertebral venous plexus. As much as 30% of the vertebral mass may be destroyed before detection with plain radiographs. The common primary sites of malignant migration include the lung, breast, prostate, kidney, and thyroid. Metastatic disease is classified as osteolytic (hypernephroma, breast, thyroid, and large bowel) or osteoblastic (lung, breast, prostate). Metastatic tumors include adenocarcinoma of the pancreas, and rectal carcinoma. Primary tumors arise locally in a specific bone or neural structure and include:
- *Multiple myeloma.* This is also known as *plasmacytoma* and is a common spine tumor, usually seen in males over age 50. This form of neoplastic disease is characterized by marrow plasma cell tumors that most frequently involve the spine, pelvis, ribs, or skull. This malignant primary bone neoplasm invades and replaces trabecular bone. Signs and symptoms include persistent back pain, malaise, fatigue, weight loss, and anemia, recurrent bacterial infections and renal failure. Lab results and radiographic findings corroborate suspicions.

INFLAMMATORY CAUSES

- *Ankylosing spondylitis.* This (see Chapter 56) is a seronegative arthropathy that usually presents between a range of 15 and 40 years of age as an insidious onset of low back or gluteal pain in most patients. Pain and stiffness are most pronounced in the morning hours or after periods of inactivity, and improves with activity. The patient typically undergoes progressive loss of spinal extension as the spine becomes calcified from the caudal end proximally. Provocative sacroiliac joint testing is often positive. Laboratory findings typically include an elevated sedimentation rate, and the majority of patients score positively for the presence of the HLA-B27 antigen.

METABOLIC CAUSES

Diabetic amyotrophy. Also known as *neuralgic amyotrophy,* this is a frequently misdiagnosed complication of diabetes that affects either the L2, L3, and L4 nerve roots, or the femoral nerve which derives from these roots. Typically affecting males with noninsulin dependent diabetes mellitus, this condition is characterized by onset of excruciating pain down the front of the thigh, which often radiates down the medial border of the leg to the medial malleolus. A prodrome of general ill health and history of rapid weight loss often occur before onset. Within several days of onset, pain abates and the patient suddenly develops rapid weakness and wasting of the quadriceps muscles, so that walking becomes impossible. Six months may elapse before recovery, and full recovery may require 18 to 24 months.

48. What are pars interarticularis lesions?

The *pars interarticularis,* otherwise known as the *isthmus,* refers to that part of the neural arch in the region of the lumbar lamina located between the superior and inferior articular processes, or more precisely, the point at which the inferior articulating process approaches the pedicle.[83] Lesions of the pars include *spondylolysis* and *spondylolisthesis* and are frequent causes of teenage backache, particularly following sport-related activities.[83]

Why posterior element defects occur at or adjacent to the lumbosacral junction relates to the facet orientation and the magnitude of *shear forces* at that level. At the lumbosacral (L5/S1) junction the facet joints abruptly change their orientation from the sagittal plane somewhat obliquely into the frontal plane. This endows the lumbosacral articulation with the ability to be the most movable of all lumbar joints[28] and capable of 10° of extension, 12° of flexion, 5° of unilateral rotation, and 3° of bending. The L4/L5 junction is also quite mobile. Despite the amount of motion occurring at L5/S1, the tight apposition of facet surfaces provides the principal counterbalance to the enormous shear forces present at the lumbosacral junction.[95]

The term *spondylolysis* refers to a unilateral* or bilateral defect in the form of a crack across the pars interarticularis, but without shift of the vertebral body. Although rare before ages 5 or 6, spondylolysis often occurs in young athletes involved in gymnastics, board diving, weight training, serving in tennis, blocking and hitting in American football linemen, ice hockey, baseball pitching, wrestling, pole vaulting,[91] or partnering during ballet, in which a male dancer lifts his female partner at arm's length.[29] The common denominator in these activities is repetitive postural stress, in which jarring forces combined with hyperextension and rotation cause the inferior facet proximally and the superior facet of the vertebra distally to the affected vertebral to produce a pistoning shearlike effect on the pars interarticularis culminating in a stress fracture. The incidence of spondylolysis is approximately 4.4% in children and 6.0% in adults.[59] Although neural arch defects most commonly occur between the ages of 5 and 7, forward vertebral slippage most frequently occurs between the ages of 10 and 15, but rarely increases after age 20.[114]

Spondylolysis may be symptomatic or asymptomatic[171] and may manifest as one of two modes of clinical presentations. The patient may or may not remember an episode of acute discomfort when the defect occurred characterized by sudden and spontaneous episodic pain. In contrast, a fatigue fracture of the pars may result in persistent, unexplained lumbar pain in the young athlete that is typically unilateral and aggravated by twisting and hyperextension motion. Alternately, the patient may experience intermittent discomfort and pain that often develops insidiously during adolescence or the late teens. Patients may have remission of symptoms lasting from weeks to many years in which they can participate in all normal activities. Hamstring tightness is often associated with spondylolysis of a painful nature and may be an etiologic factor by increasing tension to the low back during flexion.[171] The *one-legged hyperextension test* provokes pain at the site of the frac-

---

Unilateral spondylolysis occurs in less than 1% of the population and is more common on the right side. (Willis T: The separate neural arch, *J Bone Joint Surg* 13:709, 1931.)

tured pars and is performed by asking the patient to stand on one leg and arch the back backward. In a positive test, the patient localizes the site of the lesion by pointing to it.[32]

Fatigue fractures of the pars result in lysis of the isthmus and is therefore called spondylo*lysis,* and may occur gradually or suddenly. When occurring gradually, patients usually complain of intermittent or chronic symptoms and may remember a fall downstairs, or from a wall or tree some years ago. When occurring acutely, the patient may describe a feeling or may even hear a "crack" or snapping sound following an acute strain such as flexing forward and lifting a heavy weight. Similar to all acute fractures, all movements will aggravate discomfort and immobility relieves pain. Based on history, an acute pars defect is clinically differentiated from an acute annular tear or ligament sprain in that pain is usually intensified by hyperextension with the former and flexion with the latter. Lying prone increases discomfort as it postures the low back in relative extension. Findings are usually confined to the low back with no evidence of neurologic deficit. However, because the L5 nerve root runs directly anterior to the site of an L5 pars defect, the hyperextended posture may cause nerve root impingement due to the loose lamina irritating the underlying nerve root at the site of defect, and is relieved by coming out of the extended position. In contrast, nerve impingement due to a torn annulus and nuclear protrusion is worsened by flexion.

With stress fractures of the pars, point tenderness over the spinous process of the affected lamina may occur as pressure from the examiner's hand moves the fracture site. Acute discomfort often subsides after a few days. When the pars defect is well established for many months or even years, acute discomfort may be induced by acute strains imposed on this region.

Unlike stress fractures in other parts of the body, spondylolysis does not exhibit new periosteal bone formation and subsequent fibrous union because the factors that produced it in the first place are still present and thereby preclude union. Instead, the body attempts to repair the defect by fibrocartilaginous tissue filling the space and often proliferating beyond the site of the lesion. Subsequently, fibrocartilaginous proliferation may impinge on the nerve root that lies deep to the site of the pars interarticularis defect.[171] The site of nonunion becomes an established pseudarthrosis and contributes to symptoms, especially on the morning following intense activity such as digging or lifting

weights. As with pseudarthroses in other parts of the body, symptoms may be aggravated by sudden acute or chronic strains. An acute strain may occur while the patient engages in vigorous activity and experiences no pain until a sudden twisting motion strains the area and causes discomfort. These patients dislike standing and lying prone, both of which increase the lumbar lordosis. This is because the lordotic position angulates the loose lamina even more at the defect side, and thereby increases pressure on the nerve root. Relief is gained during slight lumbar flexion, which reduces the lordosis. Radiography of the lumbar spine on straight lateral and different degrees of obliquity often shows the lesion, although tomographic studies and bone scanning often identify the lesion. Whereas pars defects do not preclude patient participation in sports, flexibility, back, and abdominal strengthening exercises should be encouraged. The average time for return to pain-free competition following an acute pars interarticularis stress fracture is approximately 7 months.[92]

In some patients with bilateral pars interarticularis defects, the integrity of posterior elements becomes destabilized as the defect grows causing the superior vertebral body and transverse process to shift forward on the vertebral body below, while the spinous process and lamina remain behind in their normal position. This is known as *spondylolisthesis* and affects approximately 6% of the general population.[171] The extent of forward slippage is classified by grades and degree of slippage and is measured clinically by the relationship of the superior vertebra to the inferior vertebra. If the anteroposterior diameter of the lower vertebral body is divided into quarters, a grade I slip reflects up to a quarter forward shift; a grade II a half a slip; a grade III three quarters; and a grade IV a total displacement, which may be associated with spinal stenosis. The latter may be referred to as a *spondylolisthesis crisis.* The degree of pain does not necessarily correlate with the degree of slippage, so that a patient with a slip of up to 25% may feel greater pain than the patient with greater than 75% slippage, who may, in fact, feel no pain.[83] The L4 and L5 vertebrae are most often affected. The L5 vertebra normally is somewhat rectangular with a trefoil canal shape. Those persons with a trapezoidal shape and having a dome shaped canal are associated with a higher incidence of lysis[151-153] and vertebral shift.[171] Although the incidence of pars defects is higher in boys, the incidence of progressive vertebral slippage is four times[171] higher in girls,[91] and often progresses between the ages of 9 and 13.

49. What is the most common form of spondylolisthesis?

Spondylolisthesis was first recognized by obstetricians in the eighteenth[77] and nineteenth centuries who erroneously ascribed the condition to females only following obstruction of the birth canal during labor secondary to spondylolisthesis.[77,103] This is the classic pars interarticularis fracture due to a nonunited stress fracture and demonstrates a male to female ratio of involvement of 2:1. Inherent weakness of the pars occurs more commonly in certain population groups, such as the Eskimo,[180] Australian aborigines, and South African bushmen. Although the incidence of isthmic spondylolisthesis is as high as 6% in North American males of European descent, oriental females have the lowest incidence of all ethnic groups. Nevertheless, it appears that adolescent females have a strong disposition toward developing high-grade slips.[159] Isthmic spondylolisthesis is linked to both genetic[187] and developmental causes.* The pars defect typically occurs at age 6, whereas the forward slip commences during the adolescent growth spurt, which is earlier for girls (11 to 13 years) than boys (13 to 15 years.) Displacement may progress up to skeletal maturity and rarely beyond age 20. In contrast to degenerative spondylolisthesis (see p. 926), isthmic spondylolisthesis most commonly occurs at the L5/S1 levels and is only occasionally seen at the L4/L5 level. It rarely occurs above that level.

The history and findings in patients with spondylolisthesis are similar to spondylolysis, and when mild, present a clinical picture that is almost identical to disk degeneration,[171] although spondylolisthesis may be asymptomatic.[114] The physical findings and typical deformity of patients with high slippage include the classic spondylolisthesis build of a shortened torso, heart-shaped buttocks, and a rib cage that appears low, along with high iliac crests, an abdominal crease, and a vertical sacrum. The latter does not permit the hips to fully extend, whereas stance is altered by tight hamstrings. Hamstring spasm may result in associated *short-strided gait.*[202] The iliac crest appears abnormally high and imparts a short-waisted appearance secondary to decreased vertical height of the lumbar spine due to displacement. This form of marked deformity at the lumbosacral junction is associated with high-grade slips, as is a palpable step-off when palpating the tips of the spinous processes, which may also be visible. The greater the degree of slippage, the more prominent the

"hollow" palpated between the spinous process of the affected vertebra and the one above. However, the step may not be readily palpable in obese persons. Pressure over the spinous process of the loose lamina will elicit pain. Pain is aggravated by lying in the prone position. The intervertebral foramen may be markedly reduced in size, and the nerve root coursing around the inferior edge of the pedicle is pulled taut as the vertebral body slips forward causing the patient to complain of unremitting sciatica and finding it difficult to locate a position of comfort.[171] A frequent finding in patients with spondylolisthesis with involvement of the L5/S1 nerve roots is hamstring spasm as a direct function of the medial and lateral hamstrings supplied by the L5 and S1 nerve roots, respectively.[83]

Disk pathology and spondylolisthesis may coexist, especially because a shearing strain on the disk occurs as the vertebral body shifts forward.[171] Although the intact disk is itself a restraint against shear, it eventually succumbs to pathologic change. Because of this, the incidence of herniated disk is greater in patients with spondylolisthesis than in the general population. The disk herniation usually occurs one level above the bony pathology.[83] Thus radicular symptoms may occur directly from spondylolisthesis or from an adjacent pathologic disk. Far out stenosis often occurs in patients with grade II or greater spondylolisthesis of the L5/S1 level that traps the L5 nerve root between the transverse process and the sacral ala.[208]

Posterolateral (oblique) views of the lumbar spine give a radiographic outline of a "Scottie dog" comprising the posterior elements. The dog appears to be wearing a collar in spondylolysis without spondylolisthesis. With dysplastic spondylolisthesis the pars becomes attenuated as if it was pulled taffy and the posterior elements take on the appearance of a greyhound characterized by the pars appearing like an elongated neck. With isthmic spondylolisthesis, the anterior luxation of L5 on the sacrum due to fracture of the isthmus appears as a wide gap at the neck causing the "Scottie dog" to appear decapitated (Fig. 60-11). Patients with symptoms of nerve root compression should be considered for magnetic resonance imaging. A displaced vertebra may be easily recognized by ultrasound examination.[151-153]

Isthmic spondylolisthesis is successfully managed in most patients by conservative measures. The goal of treatment is to prevent childhood slips from progressing beyond grade II,[74] as well as symptoms resolution. When a pars injury is due to significant injury that occurred within the past months, it is appropriate to immobilize the patient in a body jacket or the Boston

---

*Patients who have never walked, as well as newborns, have a zero incidence of isthmic spondylolisthesis.

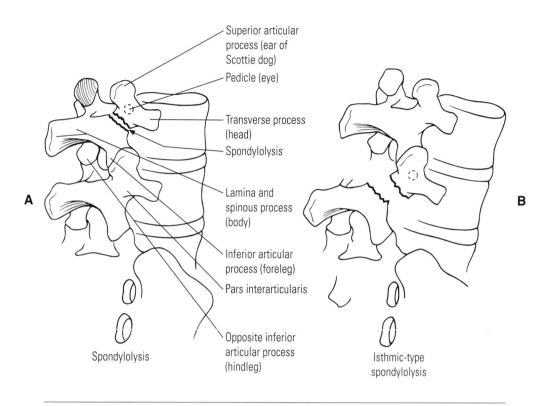

Superior articular
process (ear of
Scottie dog)

Pedicle (eye)

Transverse process
(head)

Spondylolysis

Lamina and
spinous process
(body)

Inferior articular
process (foreleg)

Pars interarticularis

Opposite inferior
articular process
(hindleg)

A

B

Spondylolysis

Isthmic-type
spondylolysis

FIG. 60-11 Schematic drawing of an oblique radiograph of the lumbar spine showing the formation of the characteristic "scottie dog" appearance of the posterior elements. **A,** With spondylolysis, the dog appears to be wearing a collar. **B,** With isthmic-type spondylolisthesis, anterior luxation of L5 on the sacrum occurs because of fractures of the pars. Note that the gap between the head and body of the dog is wider and the dog appears decapitated.

brace to promote union of the fracture, although only a small percentage of patients undergo spontaneous union of their pars fracture.[182] Adults may find symptomatic relief from a lumbosacral corset. Exercises may stabilize or improve a patient's symptoms, although stabilization exercises with a flexion bias have been shown to achieve better results in patients with spondylolisthesis.[174] Adults who experience leg pain may receive selective root injections for pain relief. Women of childbearing age with a known lysis of the pars should receive precautionary advice during pregnancy as they are at risk of developing instability particularly if overweight. Patients should rest frequently, particularly in the third trimester, and should avoid unnecessary lifting and carrying.[117]

The skeletally immature athlete with an established grade I or II lesion is permitted to be active as long as they remain asymptomatic. Although the likelihood of further slippage is low, the patient should be monitored with serial radiographs for progression. Patients with

grade III slips are at higher risk for further activities and should avoid activities that place the spine at further risk. Grade IV slips preclude the participation in athletic activity. The latter two gradations are candidates for operative stabilization. Additionally, patients with cauda equinus compression, nerve root compression or persistent pain despite adequate rest and conservative measures should be managed with fusion and attempted reduction of the high-grade slip. Operative stabilization with elimination of pain is very successful[180] although pseudoarthrosis of that segmental level may later set in and present as similar to degenerative disk disease and facet arthrosis.

50. How is spondylolysis differentiated from disk pathology?

The question arises as to how nerve root impingement is differentiated from spondylitic pathology versus a disk lesion. This becomes particularly relevant in the case in which the history and findings are typical of disk herniation but radiographs show a classic spondylolysis or even spondylolisthesis. Whereas patients having back and radicular pain from herniated disks experience worsening symptoms on walking and standing, symptoms secondary to spondylolysis are worse on standing but are frequently relieved by walking. Although sitting aggravates the herniated disk, it relieves spondylitic discomfort. Spondylitic patients, in contrast to patients with disk herniation, generally have a good range of flexion, although holding the flexed posture for more than several seconds induces pain. The SLR is usually negative and may only be limited secondary to tight hamstrings, a common finding in spondylitic patients. Thus nerve root compression from a spondylitic source, unlike that of a herniated disk, does not elicit a positive SLR because the irritation of the nerve root is from behind and not in front, as with a disk herniation.[171] Also, with spondylitic pathology, a trunk list, typically as a result of disk prolapse, is rarely seen.[151-153]

51. What is the relationship between isthmic spondylolisthesis and acute locked back?

It is conjectured that patients with isthmic spondylolisthesis may be prone to episodes of the acute locked back because the lamina of the affected vertebra is loose. An acute locked back condition may either occur from minor unilateral displacement at the site of the defect or from unilateral subluxation of a facet joint at the level of the pars defect. Severe pain and discomfort may be provoked by something as trivial as bending over at the washbasin, or to one side to tie one's shoes, picking up a piece of paper or tennis ball, or from some unprotected movement in bed while sleeping. Asymmetric motion shifts one of the facet joints at a specific segment out of its normally congruous relationship. Occurring during the bending-over motion, this movement represents a sudden unprotected motion that allows for nipping or "jamming" of the synovial meniscus, which is highly innervated. This triggers a reflex spasm of the overlying musculature, resulting in a "locking" of the back to minimize movements for fear of provoking intense discomfort and hence the term *acute locked back.* In one mode of onset the patient is seized with sudden, agonizing pain in the low back that is so severe as to prevent standing erect. In another mode of onset, the patient is only aware of a mild discomfort that begins with a triggering movement that intensifies in severity within a few hours. Pain is localized to the lumbosacral level slightly to one side of midline and may occasionally radiate to the upper ipsilateral thigh, but never as far as the knee. There may be a history of one or more similar episodes in the past and patients typically remain completely symptom-free between incidents. The patient climbs onto the examination table with difficulty, for fear of inducing further severe pain. While immobility relieves discomfort, change of position greatly aggravates it. Walking is moderately comfortable provided they take small steps and do not climb stairs. During coughing and sneezing, patients will attempt to firmly brace themselves to minimize the jarring impact. Although lateral flexion to one side is possible, it is virtually impossible to the contralateral side. Transferring from sit to stand is done gingerly, whereas a mild lateral scoliosis, without a rotational component, may be apparent in the upright position. This trunk list is an attempt to ease pain and stand in a manner that provides maximal relief. Tenderness at the source of pain is absent or mild at best even on firm palpation because the facet joints and laminae are not readily palpable owing to the interposed muscles and fasciae.[54] The SLR test will provoke acute discomfort in the region of the posterior superior iliac spine as it aggravates the subluxed facet and not because of neurologic reasons. The neurologic examination is entirely normal in these patients. Radiographs are not appropriate, as they will be misleading if the patient stands with a pronounced tilt. The diagnosis is primarily based on the patient history and presentation. Manipulation is an effective and immediate treatment in the management of the acute locked back.[171]

52. What therapeutic intervention is most appropriate in the conservative rehabilitation of patients with disk pathology?

Conservative management is effective is at least 90%[99] of patient with low back pain and should always be attempted before considering surgery. Improvement occurs within 6 to 12 weeks in 85% to 90% of low back injured patients.[1,175,194] Physical therapy is often helpful in relieving symptoms with disk herniations, including large extruded fragments. Because of this, reassurance that low back pain is most often benign and a self-limited condition will have a calming and fear-reducing effect on patients. This is essential as patients may see their current condition as a crippling one that will not progress beyond the point of their current pain and incapacity. Failure to receive an adequate and early explanation of the back pain problem is a major source of patient dissatisfaction.[46] The personal attention and interest of a physical therapist may play a significant role in hastening recovery.[93] If physical therapy becomes prolonged or assumes an indefinite course, it may have the effect of reinforcing dependence and lack of ownership and control over their condition.

- *Bed rest.* Many patients with low back pain benefit from short-term bed rest. The objective of rest is to allow edema around the area of injury to subside and for the extruded material to gradually shrink, thereby relieving pressure of the posterior longitudinal ligament and nerve root(s).[171] Shrinkage and resorption of extruded disk material may take as long as a year in some cases,[42] although pain may diminish within relatively short period after the acute state from acclimation to the volley of pain impulse. In the latter, there may be increased mechanoreceptor input activating the pain gate mechanism.[131] Acute low back pain is markedly reduced in the supine position with the hips and knees flexed over a large pillow or bolster, while sitting upright in bed is contraindicated because this increases intradiskal pressure and may exacerbate symptoms. The patient may lie on their side if they prefer.[151] Bed rest for acute low back pain with or without sciatica should not continue longer that 7 to 10 days because too much rest is counterproductive and reinforces a sense of illness. Moreover, excessive recumbency weakens the musculoskeletal system[195] as well as causing debilitating effects on strength, flexibility, bone density, cardiovascular fitness,[19] disk nutrition, and increases segmental spinal stiffness.[193]

- *Bracing.* Spinal orthosis supports the lower back in neutral, improves posture, and minimizes movement of the lumbar vertebrae. Additionally, an orthosis may decrease intradiskal pressure[139] and provide relief by way of local warmth and stimulation of mechanoreceptors. If only the lumbosacral region (L4-S1) is to be immobilized, then a lumbosacral support is indicated, whereas if the lesion is in the mid or upper lumbar region, a longer appliance is necessary. Supports within a canvas corset in the form of metal stays placed in posterior pockets fasten in front and have side straps for adjusting tightness. These reinforced types of spinal corsets provide better relief than those without support.[135] Custom-made supports are molded to the shape of the torso and most useful for patients whose body configuration is difficult to fit with conventional supports. Body casts, comprised of plaster of Paris or fiberglass are used when patients require constant immobilization such as after some

surgical procedures. Elasticized supports do not restrict spinal movement and benefit patients with poor posture as they hold in the abdomen and reduce lumbar lordosis, allowing the patient to look and feel better.

Bracing is appropriate for any low back condition in which movements that stress the joint increase the discomfort. This is particularly relevant in patients with posterior facet arthrosis, spondylolysis, and either isthmic or degenerative spondylolisthesis, in which extremes of flexion or extension result in pain and discomfort. A lumbar support will restrict excessive movement and force the patient to compensate for flexion at the hips and knees. With spondylolisthesis, bracing reduces the to-and-fro movement associated with pathology and is accompanied by gratifying pain relief. Patients with acute disk pathology may benefit from a spinal orthosis if they must carry heavy weights, work in a semi-stooped posture, or be involved in sports that involve spinal flexion and extension. Surgical corsets are very helpful in patients suffering from acute disk herniation, as restriction of flexion minimizes intradiskal pressure, and may be worn for as long as 6 weeks following preliminary bed rest. Bracing is also indicated for patients with infections, and for elderly osteoporotic patients suffering from repeated compression fractures.[171]

- *McKenzie method.* This is a conservative care program of diagnosis and treatment based upon a principle of *centralization*[130] in which patients are evaluated to determine which spinal motion causes pain to shift from a peripheral location such as the leg towards the midline of the back. The effect of lumbar extension may reduce edema and anterior nuclear migration through an annular tear, reduce intradiskal pressure,[138] decrease tension on the nerve root,[168] or may realign incongruous facets. Lumbar flexion exercises may be added later when the patient has full spinal range of motion. Because this method works best for acute back pain that responds to lumbar extension, the McKenzie technique has been erroneously labeled an extension exercise program. In fact, McKenzie advocates positions (i.e., modified resting positions for lying, sitting, and standing) and movement patterns that best relieve the patient's symptoms including flexion or lateral bending. The patient may progress as tolerated to prone-lying without support, prone-lying with support under the chest, prone-on-elbows, and press-ups.[128] Once those movements (usually extension and lateral bending) that decrease peripheral symptoms are discovered, the patient is taught to perform an individualized exercise program in the direction of the least painful movement. Given the permutations of movement combinations that may potentially centralize symptoms, McKenzie defined more than 40 different exercise regimens that may be customized to the needs of the patient. In contrast, maneuvers that peripheralize or exacerbate symptoms are discontinued. Through trial and error, those positions and movement patterns are discovered which, if repeated, presumably correct the underlying disk pathology. For a movement to eventually centralize pain, it must be performed repetitively. Treatment consists of cyclic application of these postures and movement patterns that alter the perceived location of pain from referred to centralized so that, gradually, function may be restored. Centralization occurs most rapidly if the initial movements are performed passively to the passive end range, provided that distal pain continues to diminish.[22]

- *Williams flexion exercises.* This is a flexion regimen of six exercises developed by Paul Williams in the 1930s that widen the intervertebral foramen and thereby minimize nerve root compression; decrease compressive load on the posterior margin of the disk; stretch hip flexors and back extensors; and strengthen abdominal and gluteal musculature. The problem with this management approach is that three of the six exercises increase intradiskal pressure to approximately 210%[137] over standing posture. Consequently, because these latter exercises may exacerbate symptoms in patient with disk protrusion, they are contraindicated for patients with an acutely herniated disk.

- *Exercises.* These are indicated for patients having poor posture, a protuberant abdomen, and who are overweight. Neither lumbar extension nor abdominal strengthening exercises are indicated for the patient with acute episodes of low back pain, regardless of etiology. Spondylolytic patients (i.e., with spondylolysis and spondylolisthesis) will also benefit from abdominal strengthening and should avoid extension exercises that stress the pars interarticularis. In contrast, patients with degenerative spondylolisthesis and chronic disk degeneration may benefit from spinal extension exercises. Graduated extension exercises are beneficial for patients with compression fractures, whereas flexion exercises are contraindi-

cated.* Slow squatting exercises are excellent for strengthening leg and thigh musculature. The most important flexion exercise is contraction of the abdominal muscles against resistance and is achieved by the patient performing sit-ups or lying supine and elevating the lower limbs a few inches for 4 to 5 seconds and repeating the exercise. Intradiskal pressure may be reduced if the patient performs the sit-up while keeping the hips and knees slightly flexed and then raising the torso until the outstretched hands reach the knees. Alternately, the patient lies supine and raises his or her head and shoulders several inches and holds that position for 3 to 5 seconds. To maintain the range of motion in the facet joints, the patient may flex the knees fully and bring their knees up to their chest. Toe touching exercises are not advised.[171]

- *Dynamic lumbar stabilization.* These programs are based on the idea that patients with a painful back can be taught to function within a pain-free range of activity through muscular development and movement patterns that stabilize the spine.[163] This concept is centered on the premise than an injured lumbar motion segment creates a weak link that is predisposed to injury and re-injury, and that by strengthening torso musculature, the patient may be taught to maintain cocontraction of abdominal and gluteal muscles providing a corseting effect on the lumbar spine. The patient learns to maintain the lumbar lordosis while keeping spinal posture in a *neutral position,* defined as the midpoint of available range of motion between an anterior and posterior pelvic tilt. This position is often the one of greatest comfort and represents the loose-packed position, which decreases tension on ligaments and joints, and permits a more balanced segmental forced distribution between the anterior and posterior spinal joints. Optimal muscle strength will protect the spinal motion segment from chronic repetitive stress or acute overload. The muscular spinal stabilizers include the abdominal muscles (especially the tranversus abdominis and internal obliques), latissimus dorsi, the spinal intersegmental muscles (i.e., the multifidi, rotators, and interspinalis), the iliopsoas, the erector spinae and the quadratus lumborum. Cocontraction is initially performed while standing and later advanced to sitting, jumping, supine lying, bridging, prone-lying, and quadruped positions with and without alternating arm and leg

---

*However, if any particular exercise aggravates a patient's symptoms, it should be omitted, regardless of all theories to the contrary.

raises. The use of a physio-ball may enhance these rehabilitation techniques. Stabilization is an eclectic management strategy in that it also incorporates all other aspects of conservative treatment including joint mobilization, patient education, work hardening, flexion and extension exercise regimens, and physio-ball activities.

- *Stretching.* Correction of soft tissue inflexibility of trunk musculature and especially the lower extremities is important to maintain the low back. A key element is to maintain the lumbosacral spine in a neutral position between an anterior and posterior pelvic tilt to adequately stretch the hip flexor and extensor musculature. These large muscles, which span significant areas of the trunk or lower extremities, affect the low back owing to their insertion on the pelvis. Posterior pelvic tilting often occurs because of tight hamstrings acting to increase shear in the low back and predispose facet and disk degeneration.[171] In contrast, excessive anterior pelvic tilting often occurs because of shortening of the iliopsoas and may result in spinal and central stenosis by narrowing the intervertebral foramina and central spinal canal, respectively.[99] The hip flexors and extensors, in particular, should be stretched because tightness of these muscles will rotate the pelvis excessively,* and may negatively impact on both posture and the magnitude of lumbar lordosis. Hyperlordosis is associated with anterior pelvic tilt due to contractured hip flexors. Tight hamstrings rotate the pelvis backward about the common hip and increase shear of L5 ("sliding down the hill") on S1.

- *Joint mobilization.* This involves graded manual force applied to joints in an oscillatory manner with or without joint distraction stretching the capsule surrounding that articulation. With regard to the spine, oscillatory movements are applied to the spinous processes at the affected level, rotating away from the side pain.

- *Manipulative therapy.* This is used by osteopaths, the occasional orthopedist,[171] physical therapists, and chiropractors and attempts to realign a subluxated facet joint or reduce a hard annular fragment away from the nerve root in much the same way a fragment of meniscus is relocated in the knee. Occasionally, manual traction is applied to the lumbar joints.[42] The contraindications to spinal manipulation include situations where the limb symptoms predominate over the back symptoms; if pain radiates below the knee[171]; or if the protrusion is excessively large, awkwardly placed, or too long standing.[41,42] The use of manipulative treatment in the presence of acute radiculopathy is controversial and has been associated with complications.[18]

- *Spinal traction.* This may be intermittent or continuous, and applied manually, or automatically preset. Indications for spinal traction include spinal nerve root impingement secondary to a herniated nucleus pulposus, or encroachment secondary to foraminal stenosis.[165] To achieve distraction of the vertebral bodies with the body in the horizontal position, a traction force of at least 25% of body weight must be exerted.[18] The purpose of traction is to produce a negative pressure within the intervertebral joint to reduce extruded material back into the disk through the annular defect. Additionally, the effects of traction include increasing the size of the intervertebral foramina; decreasing intradiskal pressure; and tensing both the posterior longitudinal ligament and annular fibers; alternately, by reducing intradiskal pressure, the pressure on the nerve root is diminished.[121] Although the effect of vertebral gapping is temporary (approximately 20 minutes), the accompanying relief may be sufficient to interrupt the reflex pain cycle.[105] Negative pressure is realized with painless traction that stretches the back musculature. In this way, fatigue and relaxation occur after approximately 2 minutes and the vertebral distraction commences.[41,42]

If symptoms are predominantly diskogenic in nature, traction may be applied in a prone-lying position, which helps maintain neutral or extended lumbar postures. However, if symptoms appear to be related to the posterior facet joints, traction may be applied in flexion.[78] When vertebral distraction is released following traction, a reverse and adverse phenomenon may occur in which intradiskal pressure is increased if sustained traction is maintained greater than 10 minutes.[105] Contraindications to traction include acute ligament sprains, muscular strains, or inflammation due to a disease process such as rheumatoid arthritis or infection.[165] Inversion gravity traction may also promote distraction of the vertebral bodies by 0.3 to 4.0 mm, although potential side ef-

---

*Pelvic rotation is known as *pelvic tilt,* which is defined in relation to the anterior superior iliac spine (ASIS). Anterior pelvic tilt, associated with tight iliopsoas and quadriceps muscles as well as hyperlordosis, involves the ASIS moving anteriorly and downward. In contrast, posterior pelvic tilt is associated with hypolordosis and tightened hamstring musculature and involves the ASIS moving posteriorly and upward.

fects include hypertension, tachycardia, gastrointestinal reflux, and berry aneurysm rupture.[66]

- *Patient education.* This is a *central* element in the management of low back pain and perhaps the most important component of any back care program including acute injury.[88] Patients need to be reassured that the majority of those with low back pain recover following time and conservative treatment. Often, telling patients that they will be able to go back to work once they get better removes a great deal of anxiety.

Sitting—A firm straightback chair is preferred by most patients as this supports the back and maintains a normal lumbar lordosis, whereas soft easy chairs or sofas induce flexion and may aggravate symptoms due to a reversal of the lordotic curve. The latter provide relief for patients with spinal stenosis because flexion relieves their discomfort. Chairs should preferably have armrests, and car seats should be slid as far forward as possible to bring the legs closer to the foot pedals. In a far-back seat, the spine must accentuate lordosis as the legs extend downward to reach the pedals, inducing back pain. For patients with chronic back pain or osteoporosis, with or without compression fracture, upright sitting must be avoided as this increases the potential for compression collapse. The load on both the vertebrae, posterior and anterior elements is markedly reduced in the semi-reclining position when sitting on a recliner.

Standing—To avoid symptoms when standing for long periods, patients may find relief by raising one foot on a step or stool to reduce lumbar lordosis. High heels should be avoided. *Walking* more briskly is often more comfortable that walking slowly. Shoes may be fitted with energy-absorbing inserts to reduce the concussive jarring effects of heel strike on the low back.

Bending—Because the hamstrings attach on the pelvis, hamstring strain may occur with excessive flexion. Also, excessive flexion considerably increases intradiskal pressure and may exacerbate an already painful condition. Patients with back pain can avoid this by bending at the hips and knees so as to maintain a normal lumbar curve. Wearing a lumbosacral corset for several weeks assists the patient in habituating this type of bend.

Sleeping—The type of bed or recumbent posture used depends on the cause of back pathology. Choosing the correct mattress helps maintain the spinal curves in as natural position as possible. Unnatural curves imposed upon the spine from a sagging mattress may cause patients to complain of aching back pain, especially on getting up in the morning. A firm mattress with a non-sagging base is recommended. Patients with spondylolisthesis, and many with degenerative facet arthrosis, prefer not to sleep prone or lie on a soft and sagging mattress, as this increases the lumbar lordosis and aggravates their symptoms.

Carrying—Patient with low back pain should avoid carrying or lifting heavy weights whenever possible. If lifting is necessary, patients should never lean forward to lift the weight as this excessively strains the lumbar spine. Instead, patients should flex at the hip and knees, with the back held slightly arched and the weight kept as close to the center of gravity as possible. Sudden loading should be avoided. Intradiskal pressure is less when objects are pushed versus pulled.

- *Modalities.* The utilization of physical modalities may help relieve the pain associated with the acute phase of back pain. Cold therapy decreases spasm, inflammation, pain, and capillary blood flow, and is particularly helpful in cases of acute annular tear or ligament sprain. Although the skin cools quickly, the rate of muscle cooling is directly proportional to the thickness of overlying fat and may range for 10 to 30 minutes.[110] The subacute or chronic states are preferably treated with thermotherapy such as deep heat (ultrasound, or short-wave) that, like heat, also minimizes spasm and pain. Electrostimulation in the form of transcutaneous electrical nerve stimulation (TENS) or high volt galvanic stimulation (HVGS) may reduce acute muscle spasm, decrease edema, and relieve pain.[161] The mechanism for pain relief from TENS involves raising the circulating levels of endogenous endorphins or stimulating cutaneous afferents that block pain stimuli in the substantia gelatinosa.[131] Percutaneous dorsal column stimulators can also help patients with chronic back pain.[155]

- *Weight reduction.* Excessive weight may range from mild to morbid obesity and is often associated with poor posture. Because obesity aggravates the symptomology of low back pain, regardless of the etiology, reduction in body mass is an important component of conservative management.[171] Because of a protruding abdomen that often accompanies obesity, the lower back is postured in excessive lordosis, placing strain on the posteriorly located facet joints as they undergo excessive axial compression. Hyperlordosis of the lumbar spine in turn is accompanied by excessive anterior pelvic tilt, which causes foreshortening of the hip flexors, and serves to reinforce the lumbar lordosis.

- *Endurance training.* Cardiovascular and cardiopulmonary fitness is important and may include brisk walking, jogging, swimming, tennis, and stationary bicycle activities. Many patients find that brisk walking eases their discomfort. Aerobic fitness activities should avoid high-impact and ballistic-type spinal movements.
- *Biofeedback.* This may be auditory or visual in which the magnitude of muscular contraction is conveyed to the patient through a speaker as high pitched sounds, or graphically displayed. With this feedback, the patient learns how to decrease or increase muscular tension, and develop heightened awareness at a threshold that might not otherwise be possible. Electromyographic (EMG) biofeedback is helpful in teaching patients to inhibit excessive or unbalanced muscle activity by lowering muscular tension and thereby reducing pain intensity.[98] The benefits of EMG biofeedback for patients with low back pain include increased mobility, greater tolerance for exercise, and preservation of gain even at an 18-month follow up.[140]
- *Imaging.* Utilizing imagery[201] as a strategy for pain management is based on the premise that mental presentations exert a profound influence on physical processes, emotions, and behavior.[2] Because pain increases muscular tension, visualizing relaxing muscles may be helpful in relieving pain. Imaging may also be distracting as one visualizes a pleasant experience. Patient can be taught that "seeing pain go away" may help make it less prominent in their lives.[49] Success with imagery is thought to positively affect disease processes through a psychoimmunologic mechanism.[4]
- *Back school.* This refers to a structured intervention program for a group of individuals that began in Scandinavia and has spread across the industrialized world.[210] Some back schools incorporate exercises into their program,[205] and a tailor-made program can reduce absenteeism by at least 5 days per year per employee and is therefore considered a cost-effective program to industry.[197] The goals of back school include teaching to prevent low back injury, and instructing the injured individual on how to speed their recovery and prevent relapse. Patient education regarding anatomy and biomechanics of the spine, is a critical component of this treatment regimen.

- *Functional rehabilitation.* This is based on the idea that many patients operate under the misconception that they must avoid all activities that may provoke anticipated pain rather than an actual experience of pain.[111] Passive avoidance prevents patients from full recovery from an acute episode of back pain because it promotes deconditioning and psychologically reinforces an invalid status. Functional rehabilitation attempts to reverse this situation by improving physical fitness and disk nutrition, assisting in healing of connective tissues, and increasing endorphins.[43] Indeed, functional rehabilitation is also helpful for patients with chronic back pain who have found little relief from conventional therapies and who are not surgical candidates as it helps them return to work.[123]
- *Work hardening.* This refers to a program that introduces progressive work-related activities performed under the guidance of a therapist so that proper posture and body mechanics are maintained.[13,120] Before beginning work hardening, patients may undergo a functional capacity assessment to determine physical and functional abilities. Physical therapy in work hardening addresses physical deconditioning (i.e., strength and endurance parameters) through a structured program of progressive resistive exercises that is tailored to the patient's work task.
- *Psychological counseling.* This is often appropriate in patients with chronic low back pain as some of their pain may represent a psychological overlay of personal problems and attitudes toward adversity that magnify symptoms out of proportion. Chronic back pain does not occur in a vacuum and each person's reaction to pain may be influenced by his or her environment or genetic makeup. A relatively high proportion of patients with chronic low back pain have psychologic or psychiatric disturbance.[112] Psychosocial variables for low back pain and musculoskeletal aches and pain include preexisting personality factors[63] where back pain becomes an expression of old unresolved and unrecognized dependency needs.[14] Indeed, many patients who report chronic unresolved pain have an early dysfunctional family history, parental divorce, alcoholism, and emotional impoverishment.[72,130,133,150,166,186] Psychological factors are known to have a great influence on the patient's perception of low back pain, and a patient's psyche has an important effect on the outcome of physical treatment.[12]

A cognitive behavioral approach to low back pain involving behavior modification in which "abnormal" behavior is actively discouraged whereas acceptable behavior is reinforced. *Cognitive therapy* teaches patients to recognize the effects of negative thinking by understanding the type of thinking errors (known as cognitive distortions) and ineffective coping strategies that accompany chronic pain, while emphasizing positive thinking and self-affirmation. Cognitive therapy is helpful in the treatment of mood disorders, and by extension, chronic pain conditions.[191]

- *Pharmacology.* Pharmacologic treatments may be categorized into analgesics that relieve pain, antiinflammatory medications, and muscle relaxants. Antiinflammatory drugs have both an antiinflammatory and analgesic effect that promote healing by increasing circulation and bringing necessary nutrient into the inflamed area and eliminating toxic inflammatory substances, thereby allowing patients to more fully participate in physical therapy and activities of daily living. Antiinflammatory medications appear to be effective if started within 2 days of onset of acute low back pain.[6] Muscle relaxants, whose site of action is either the muscle spindle or the central nervous system,[18] operate by relieving skeletal muscle spasm without interfering with muscular function. In this manner they promote greater mobility that is essential to the recuperative process. Opioid analgesics interact by binding to the body's opiate receptors for endorphins and enkephalins, and are indicated for severely acute back pain. If used on a short-term basis there is little chance for addiction.[184] Use of opioid analgesic for chronic back pain is discouraged because of the potential for addiction. Antidepressant drugs may elevate mood and increase pain tolerance in the emotionally depressed patient, reducing chronic low back pain.[200]

- *Selective injection.* Therapeutic short- or long-acting injection of steroids and anesthetics is performed by an anesthesiologist into the epidural space that surrounds the dural covering of the spinal cord, exiting spinal nerves, the nerve roots, facet joints, and trigger points.[206] Epidural steroid injections may be appropriate for disk related pathology such as annular tears, disk herniations, radiculopathy, and spinal stenosis.[78]

Other forms of treatment include relaxation techniques,[183] therapeutic massage, myofascial release, as well as acupuncture, acupressure, and electroacupuncture along hypothetical body meridians.[199] For patients whose symptoms are recalcitrant to conservative management, the *pain clinic* may offer relief of pain.

53. What are the indications for surgery?

The clearest indication for immediate surgery is when bladder or bowel dysfunction follows a massive disk prolapse of almost the entire nucleus pulposus, because failure to operate right away will result in a neurogenic bladder.* In addition to acute urine retention, flaccid paralysis of the lower extremity following sudden onset of severe low back pain secondary to *cauda equina syndrome* represents a true surgical emergency. Certain physical signs may assist in the prognostication of the outcome of disk herniation, and permit early recognition of herniation that may be refractory to nonsurgical management. In addition to failed conservative therapy, other factors that suggest surgery include the patient with a trunk list, as its presence increases the chances of a patient with disk symptoms that require surgery.[102] Persistent peripheralization of pain and an absence of centralization and distal-to-proximal return migration from the distal extremity to the lower back may indicate a poor prognosis.[47] Similarly, a positive cross-leg pain may be a predictor for possible surgery.[51] A competent disk is characterized by intact peripheral annular fibers that may show diurnal changes in straight leg raising by as much as 30°. However, diurnal changes, as evidenced by straight leg raising is suggested in the event that a free fragment has extruded or sequestered through an annular tear and suggests a poor outcome from conservative management.[152] However, the degree of limitation of straight leg raising, nor positive neurologic signs such as areflexia, motor weakness, wasting or sensory loss, are not a reason to operate as the patient may still recover. Similarly, merely identifying a disk lesion by imaging is no reason to operate as many patients have obvious disk lesions on imaging with no symptoms whatsoever.

Only a small percentage of patients suffering from mechanical forms of low back pain require surgical treatment. For most patients, symptoms abate with conservative management. Surgical procedures include diskectomy, microsurgical diskectomy, percutaneous diskectomy, spinal fusion, decompression, and combined procedures. The iliac crest is a excellent choice for a bone graft donor site. *Arachnoiditis* is a complicating sequel that refers to an inflammatory reaction of the arachnoid and subsequent adhesions among the

---

*Cauda equina syndrome may also result in bowel dysfunction.

arachnoid, the nerve roots, and the dura. This results in chronic scarring and constriction of the dura and tethering of nerve roots. Patients often complain of chronic low back pain radiating to the buttocks and occasionally down one or both legs. Pain may be burning or dull and aching, may present as cramping in the calves, and is present during activity and at rest (bed.) Management is surgical and involves microdissection of all intradural adhesions and grafting of the dura with a plastic replacement tissue.[171] A long-term sequel to disk excision is the inevitable and gradual disk narrowing of the excised disk space, which, in turn leads to overriding of the facet joints with the development of osteoarthritis.[171]

RECOMMENDED READING

Cramer GD, Darby SA: *Basic and clinical anatomy of the spine, spinal cord, and ANS,* St Louis, 1995, Mosby.

Porter RW: *Management of back pain,* ed 2, Edinburgh, 1993, Churchill Livingstone.

Seimon LP: *Low back pain: clinical diagnosis and management,* ed 2, New York, 1995, Demos Vermande.

REFERENCES

1. Abenhaim L, Suissa S: Importance and economic burden of occupational back pain: a study of 2500 cases representative of Quebec, *J Occupational Medicine* 29:670, 1987.
2. Achterberg J: *Imagery in healing,* Boston, 1985, New Science Library.
3. Adams P, Muir H: Qualitative changes with age of proteoglycans of human lumbar disks, *Ann Rheum Dis* 35:289, 1976.
4. Adler R editor: *Psychoneuroimmunology,* New York, 1981, Academic Press.
5. Allen EH, Cosgrave D, Mullard FJC: The radiological changes in infections of the spinal and their diagnostic value, *Clin Radiol* 29:31, 1978.
6. Amlie E, Weber H, Holme I: Treatment of acute low back pain with Piroxicam: results of a double-blind placebo-controlled trial, *Spine* 12:473, 1987.
7. Anddersson GBJ, Ortengren R, Nachemson A: Quantitative studies of back loads in lifting, *Spine* 1:178, 1976.
8. Archibald KC, Wiechec F: A reappraisal of Hoover's test, *Arch Phys Med Rehab* 51:234, 1970.
9. Bachop W, Janse J: The corporotransverse ligament at the L5 intervertebral foramen, *Anat Rec* 205, (Abstract) 1983.
10. Bayliss M, et al: Proteoglycan synthesis in the human intervertebral disc: variation with age, region, and pathology, *Spine* 13:972, 1988.
11. Berkow, R, Fletcher AJ editors: *The Merck manual of diagnosis and therapy,* ed 15, Rahway, N.J., 1987, Merck & Co.
12. Bigos SJ, Battie MC, Fisher LD et al. The prospective study of risk factors for the report of industrial back problems: a univariate analysis. Presented at the ISSLS meeting; April 13-17, 1988, Miami, FL.
13. Blakenship KL: *Work capacity and industrial consultation. Course manual,* Macon, Ga., 1984, American Therapeutics.
14. Blumer D, Heilbronn M: Chronic pain as a variant of depressive disease, *J Nervous Mental Dis* 170:381, 1982.
15. Boden SD, Davis DO, Dina TS et al: Abnormal magnetic-resonance imaging scans of the lumbar spine in asymptomatic subjects, *J Bone Joint Surg* 72A:403, 1990.
16. Boduk N: Pathology of lumbar disc pain, *Manual Med* 5:72, 1990.
17. Boduk N, Twomey LT: *Clinical anatomy of the lumbar spine,* London, 1991, Churchill Livingstone.
18. Borenstein D, Wiesel S: *Low back pain: medical diagnosis and comprehensive management,* Philadelphia, 1989, WB Saunders.
19. Bortz W: The disuse syndrome, *West J Med* 141:169, 1984.
20. Boukris R, Becker KL: Schmorl's nodes and osteoporosis, *Clin Orthop* 104:275, 1974.
21. Brody IA, Williams RH: The signs of Kernig and Brudzinski, *Arch Neurol* 21:215, 1969.
22. Brontzman SB: *Clinical orthopaedic rehabilitation,* St Louis, 1996, Mosby.
23. Brown AD, Tsaltis T: Studies on the permeability of intervertebral disc during skeletal maturation, *Spine* 1:240, 1982.
24. Brown MD, Tsaltos TT: Studies in permeability of the intervertebral disc during skeletal maturation, *Spine* 1:240, 1976.
25. Brown T, et al: Some mechanical tests on the lumbosacral spine with particular reference to the intervertebral disc, *J Bone Joint Surg* 39A:1135, 1937.
26. Buckwalter J, Smith KC, Kazarien LE et al: Articular cartilage and intervertebral disc proteoglycans differ in structure: an electron microscopic study, *J Orthop Res* 7:146, 1989.
27. Butler DS: *Mobilisation of the nervous system,* Edinburgh, 1991, Churchill Livingstone.
28. Cailliet R: *Low back pain syndrome,* ed 2, Philadelphia, 1982, FA Davis.
29. Callander J: The dancer's spine. Paper presented at the fourth annual Dance Medicine Seminar, Cincinnati, 1982.
30. Christodoulides AN: Ipsilateral sciatica on femoral nerve stretch test is pathognomic of an L4:L5 disc protrusion, *J Bone Joint Surg* 71B:88, 1989.
31. Church CP, Buehler MT: Radiographic evaluation of the corportransverse ligament at the L5 intervertebral foramen: a cadaveric study, *J Manipulative Physiol Therap* 14, 1991.
32. Ciullo JV, Jackson DW: Pars interarticularis stress reaction, spondylolysis, and spondylolisthesis in gymnasts, *Clin Sports Med* 4:95, 1985.
33. Clark GA, Panjabi MM, Wetzel FT: Can infant malnutrition cause adult vertebral stenosis? *Spine* 10:165.
34. Clarke WG, Wright WA editors: The plays and sonnets of William Shakespeare, vol 2, Chicago, 1952, William Benton, *Encyclopaedia Britannica.*
35. Conelson R, Silva G, Murphy K: Centralization phenomenon: its usefulness in evaluating and treating referred pain, *Spine* 15:211, 1990.
36. Coppes MH, Marani E, Thomeer RT et al: Innervation of annulus fibrosis in low back pain, *Lancet* 336:189, 1990.

37. Coventry MB: Anatomy of the intervertebral disc, *Clin Orthop* 67:9, 1969.
38. Cramer GD, Darby SA: *Basic and clinical anatomy of the spine, spinal cord, and ANS,* St Louis, 1995, Mosby.
39. Crock HV: Internal disc disruption: a challenge to disc prolapse fifty years on, *Spine* 11:650, 1986.
40. Crock HV: Normal and pathological anatomy of the lumbar spinal nerve root canals, *J Bone Joint Surg* 63:487, 1981.
41. Cyriax J: *Textbook of orthopaedic medicine,* vol 1, *Diagnosis of soft tissue lesions,* ed 8, London, 1982, Bailliere Tindall.
42. Cyriax J: *The slipped disc,* ed 3, New York, 1980, Charles Scribner.
43. Dale D, Fleetwood JA, Weddell A et al: Endorphine: a factor in 'fun run' collapse? *Br Med J* 294:1004, 1987.
44. De Palma AF, Rothman RH: *The intervertebral disc,* Philadelphia, 1970, WB Saunders.
45. De Rosa CP, Porterfield JA: A physical therapy model for the treatment of low back pain, *Phys Ther* 72(4):261-272, 1992.
46. Deyo RA, Diehl AK: Patient satisfaction with medical care for low back pain, *Spine* 11:28. 1986.
47. Donelson R, Silva G, Murphy K: The centralization phenomenon: its usefulness in evaluating and treating referred pain, *Spine* 15:21, 1990.
48. Reference moved to 108a.
49. Drukteinis AM: *The psychology of back pain: a clinical and legal handbook,* Springfield, Ill., 1996, Charles C Thomas.
50. Edgar M, Ghadially J: Innervation of the lumbar spine, *Clin Orthop* 115:35, 1976.
51. Eismant FJ, Currier B: Current concepts review. Surgical management of lumbar intervertebral disc disease, *J Bone Joint Surg* 71A:1266, 1989.
52. Eyre DR: The intervertebral disc. In *New perspective on low-back pain,* 1989, American Academy of Orthopedic Surgery.
53. Fahrni WH: Observations on straight leg-raising with special reference to nerve root adhesions, *Can J Surg* 9:44-48, 1966.
54. Fairband JC, Hall H: History taking and physical examination: identification of syndromes of back pain. In Weinstein JN, Wiesel SW, editors: *The lumbar spine,* Philadelphia, 1990, WB Saunders.
55. Farfan HF, Cossette JW, Robertson GH et al: The effects of torsion on the lumbar intervertebral joints: the role of torsion in the production of disc degeneration, *J Bone Joint Surg* 52A:468, 1970.
56. Fitzgerald MJT: *Neuroanatomy: basic and applied,* London, 1985, Bailliere Tindall.
57. Flood BM, Deacon P, Dickson RA: Spinal disease presenting as acute abdominal pain, *Br Med J* 287:16, 1983.
58. Ford CV: The somatizing disorders, *Psychosomatics* 27:327, 1986.
59. Frederickson BC, et al: The natural history of spondylolysis and spondylolisthesis, *J Bone Joint Surg* 66A(5):699, 1984.
60. Fung YB: Biomechanics: its scope, history, and some problems of centenuum mechanics in physiology, *Appl Mech Rev* 21:1, 1968.
61. Gacovetsky S: Biomechanics of the spine. In White AH, Schofferman JA, editors: *Spine care,* vol 1, *Diagnosis and conservative treatment,* St Louis, 1995, Mosby.
62. Galante JL: Tensile properties of the human lumbar annulus fibrosus, *Acta Orthop Scand* (suppl) 100, 1967.
63. Gamsa A: The role of psychological factors in chronic pain II. A critical appraisal, *Pain* 57:17, 1994.
64. Gertzbein SD, Seligman JV, Holtby R et al: Centrode patterns and segmental instability in degenerate disc disease, *Spine* 10:256, 1985.
65. Ghosh PK: Basic biochemistry of the intervertebral disc and its variation with aging and degeneration, *J Manual Medicine* 5:48, 1990.
66. Gianakopoulos G, Waylonis GW, Grant PA et al: Inversion devices: their role in producing lumbar distraction, *Arch Phy Med Rehab* 66:100, 1985.
67. Goddard MD, Reid JD: Movements induced by straight leg raising in the lumbosacral roots, nerves and plexuses and in the intra-pelvic section of the sciatic nerve, *J Neurol Neurosurg Psychiatry* 28:12, 1965.
68. Grenier N, Greselle JF, Vital JM et al: Normal and disrupted lumbar longitudinal ligaments. Correlative MR and anatomic study, *Radiology* 171:197, 1989.
69. Grieve GP: Treating backache—a topical comment, *Physiotherapy* 69:316, 1983.
70. Gunzburg R, Fraser RD, Fraser GA: Lumbar intervertebral disc prolapse in teenage twins, *J Bone Joint Surg* 72(5):914, 1990.
71. Reference deleted.
72. Han JS, Terenius L: Neurochemical basis of acupuncture analgesia, *Ann Rev Pharmacol Toxicol* 22:193, 1982.
73. Happy F: A biophysical study of the human intervertebral disc. In Jayson M, editor: *The lumbar spine and back pain,* New York, 1976, Grune & Stratton.
74. Harris IE, Weinstein SL: Long term follow up of patients with grade II and IV spondylolisthesis treatment with and without posterior fusion, *J Bone Joint Surg* 69A:960, 1987.
75. Hauser SL, Levitt LP, Weiner HL: *Case studies in neurology for the house officer,* Baltimore, 1986, Williams & Wilkins.
76. Hebert CM, Lindberg KA, Jayson MIV et al: Changes in the collagen of human intervertebral discs during aging and degenerative disc disease, *J Molec Med* 1:79, 1975.
77. Herbineaux G: *Traite sur divers accouchments laborieux, et sur les polypes de la matrice,* Brussels, 1782, JL DeBoubers.
78. Herring SA, Weinstein SM: Assessment and nonsurgical management of athletic low back. In Nicholas JA, Hershman EB, editors: *The lower extremity and spine in sports medicine,* ed 2, St Louis, 1995, Mosby.
79. Hickey DS, Hukins DWL: Relation between the structure of the annulus fibrosus and the function and failure of the intervertebral disc, *Spine* 5:106, 1980.
80. Hirsch C, et al: Biophysical and physiological investigation on cartilage and other mesenchymal tissues. VI. Characteristics of human nuclei pulposi during aging, *Acta Orthop Scand* 22:179, 1952.
81. Holm S, Nachemson A: Cellularity of the lumbar intervertebral disc and its relevance to nutrition, *Orthop Trans* 7:457, 1983.

82. Hoppenfeld S: *Orthopaedic neurology: a diagnostic guide to neurologic levels,* Philadelphia, 1977, JB Lippincott.

83. Hoppenfeld S: *Physical examination of the spine and extremities,* Norwalk, Conn, 1976, Appleton-Century Crofts.

84. Hudgins WR: The crossed-straight-leg-raising test, *N Engl J Med* 297:1127, 1977.

85. Hugo AK, Kirkaldy-Willis WH: *Low back pain: clinical symposia,* West Caldwell, N.J., 1987, CIBA-GEIGY.

86. Ismaiel AHMA, Porter RW: Effect of straight leg raising on blood pressure, *Spine* 17:1117, 1992.

87. Ito S, Yamada Y, Tsuboi S et al: An observation of ruptured annulus fibrosus in lumbar discs, *J Spin Discord* 4:462, 1991.

88. Jackson CP: Historic perspectives on patient education and its place in acute spinal disorders. In Mayer TG, Mooney V, Gatchel RJ, editors: *Contemporary conservative care for painful spinal disorders,* Philadelphia, 1991, Lea & Febiger.

89. Jackson DW, Lowery WD, Ciullo JV: Injuries of the spine. In Nicholas JA, Hershman EB, editors: *The lower extremity and spine in sports medicine,* St Louis, 1995, Mosby.

90. Jackson RP, Glah JJ: Foraminal and extraforaminal lumbar disc herniation: diagnosis and treatment, *Spine* 12:577, 1987.

91. Jackson DW, Wiltse LL, Cirincione RJ: Spondylolysis in the female gymnast, *Clin Orthop* 117:68, 1976.

92. Jackson DW, Wiltse L: Treatment of spondylolisthesis and spondylolysis in children, *Clin Orthop* 117:92, 1976.

93. Jayson MIV: A limited role for manipulation, *Br Med J* 293:1454, 1986.

94. Jayson MIV: The role of vascular damage and fibrosis in the pathogenesis of nerve root damage, *Clin Orthop* 279:40, 1992.

95. Kapjandji I: *The physiology of the joints. the trunk and the vertebral column,* vol 3, ed 2, New York, 1974, Churchill-Livingstone.

96. Katz MM, Hargens AR, Garfin SR: Intervertebral disc nutrition: diffusion versus convection, *Clin Orthop* 210:243, 1986.

97. Kawakami M, Chatani K, Weinstein JN: Anatomy, biochemistry, and physiology of low-back pain. In White AH, Schofferman JA: *Spine care: diagnosis and conservative treatment,* vol 1, St Louis, 1995, Mosby.

98. Keefe FJ, Black AR, William RB Jr et al: Behavioral treatment of chronic low back pain: clinical outcome and individual differences in pain relief, *Pain* 11:221, 1981.

99. Keim HA, Kirkaldy-Willis WH: *Low back pain—clinical symposia,* 1987, CIBA-GEIGY.

100. Kelsey JL: *Epidemiology of musculoskeletal disorders,* New York, 1982, Oxford University Press.

101. Keogh B, Ebbs S: *Normal surface anatomy,* London, 1984, William Heinemann Medical Books.

102. Khuffash B, Porter RW: Cross leg pain and trunk list, *Spine* 14:1602, 1989.

103. Kilian JF: Schilderungen neuer Backenformen und Ihrer Verhalten im Leben, *Isthmic spondylolisthesis,* Mannheim, 1854, Basserman und Mathy.

104. Kirkaldy-Willis WH, Wedge JH, Yong-Hing K, et al: Pathology and pathogenesis of lumbar spondylosis and stenosis, *Spine* 3:319, 1978.

105. Kisner C, Colby LA: *Therapeutic exercise: foundations and techniques,* ed 2, Philadelphia, 1990, FA Davis.

106. Kornberg M: Extreme lateral lumbar disc herniation: clinical syndrome and computed tomography recognition, *Spine* 12:586, 1987.

107. Kornverg M, Rechtine GR: Quantitative assessment of the fifth lumbar spinal canal by computed tomography in symptomatic L4/L5 disc disease, *Spine* 10:328, 1985.

108. Kraemer J, Kolditz D, Gowin R et al.: Water and electrolyte content of human intervertebral discs under variable load, *Spine* 10, 69-71, 1985.

108a. Krag MH, Seroussi RE, Wilder DG, et al : Internal displacement distribution from in vitro loading of human thoracic and lumbar spinal motion segments: experimental results and theoretical predictions, *Spine* 12:1001, 1987.

109. LeBlanc AD, Schonfeld E, Schneider VS et al: The spine: changes in T2 relaxation times from disuse, *Radiology* 169:105, 1988.

110. Lehman J: Therapeutic heat and cold, *Clin Orthop* 99:207, 1974.

111. Linton SJ: The relationship between activity and chronic back pain, *Pain* 21:289, 1985.

112. Lloyd GG, Wolkin SN, Greenwood R: A psychiatric study of patients with persistent low back pain, *Rheumatol Rehab* 18:30, 1979.

113. Lyons G, Eistenstein SM, Sweet MBE: Biochemical changes in intervertebral disc degeneration, *Biochem Biophy Acta* 673:443, 1981.

114. MacNab I: *Backache,* Baltimore, 1977, Williams & Wilkins.

115. Magee DJ: *Orthopedic physical assessment,* Philadelphia, 1987, WB Saunders.

116. Malinsky J: The ontogenetic development of nerve terminations in the intervertebral discs of man, *Acta Anat (Basel)* 38:96, 1959.

117. Maring-Klug R: Reducing low back pain during pregnancy, *Nurse Practitioner* 7:18, 1982.

118. Markolf KL, Morris JM: The structural components of the intervertebral disc, *J Bone Joint Surg* 56A:675, 1974.

119. Martin G: The role of trauma in disc protrusion, *N Z Med Journal,* March:208, 1978.

120. Matheson LN, Ogden LD, Biolette K et al: Work hardening: occupational therapy in industrial rehabilitation, *Am J Occupational Ther* 39:314, 1985.

121. Matthews J: The effects of spinal traction, *Physiotherapy* 58:64, 1972.

122. Matthews S, Wiltse L, Karbelnig M: A destructive lesion involving the intervertebral disc in children, *Clin Orthop* 9:162, 1957.

123. Mayer TG, Gatchel RJ, Mayer H et al: A prospective two year study of functional restoration in industrial low back injury, *JAMA* 258:1763, 1987.

124. Mayne R, Burgeon R: *Structure and function of collagen types,* New York, 1987, Academic Press.

125. McCall IW, Park WM, O'Brien JP et al: Acute traumatic intraosseous disc herniation, *Spine* 10:134, 1985.

126. McCombe PF, Fairbank JC, Cockersole BC, et al: 1989 Volvo Award in clinical sciences. Reproducibility of physical signs in low-back pain, *Spine* 14:908, 1989.

127. McGill SM: The influence of lordosis on axial trunk torque and trunk muscle myoelectric activity, *Spine* 17:1187, 1992.

128. McKenzie RA: Prophylaxis in recurrent low back pain, *N Z Med J* 89:22, 1979.

129. McKenzie RA: *The lumbar spine: mechanical diagnosis and therapy,* Waikanae, N.Z., 1981, Spinal Publication.

130. McWilliams JR, McWilliams P: *You can't afford the luxury of a negative thought,* Los Angeles, 1988, Prelude Press.

131. Melzack R, Wall PD: Pain mechanisms: a new theory, *Science* 150:971, 1965.

132. Menelaus MB: Diskitis: an inflammation affecting the intervertebral disks in children, *J Bone Joint Surg* 46B:16, 1964.

133. Merskey H, Boyd D: Emotional adjustment and chronic pain, *Pain* 5:73, 1978.

134. Miller JAA, Schmatz C, Schultz AB: Lumbar disc degeneration: correlation with age, sex, and spine level in 600 autopsy specimens, *Spine* 13(2):173, 1988.

135. Million R, Nilsen KH, Jayson MIV et al: Evaluation of low back pain and assessment of lumbar corsets without and without back supports, *Ann Rheum Dis* 40:449, 1981.

136. Mixter WJ, Barr JS: Rupture of the intervertebral disc with involvement of the spinal canal, *New Engl J Med* 211:210, 1934.

137. Nachemson A: Disc pressure measurements, *Spine* 6:93, 1981.

138. Nachemson A, Elfstrom G: Intravital dynamic pressure measurements in lumbar discs: a study of common movements, maneuvers, and exercises, *Scand J Rehabil Med* (suppl) 1:1, 1970.

139. Nachemson A: Lumbar spine instability; a critical update and symposium summary, *Spine* 10:290, 1985.

140. Newman RI, Seres JL, Yospe LP et al: Multidisciplinary treatment of chronic pain: long term follow-up of low back pain patients, *Pain* 4:283, 1978.

141. Ng SC, Weiss JB, Quennel R et al: Abnormal connective tissue degrading enzyme patterns in prolapsed intervertebral discs, *Spine* 11:695, 1986.

142. Nitobe T, Harata S, Okamoto T et al: Degradation and biosynthesis of proteoglycans in the nucleus pulposus of canine intervertebral disc after chymopapain treatment, *Spine* 11:1332, 1988.

143. Nuber GW, Bowen MK, Schafer MF: Diagnosis and treatment of lumbar and thoracic spine injuries. In Nicholas JA, Hershman EB, editors: *The lower extremity and spine in sports medicine,* ed 2, vol 2, St Louis, 1995, Mosby.

144. Olmarker K, Rydevik B, Holm S: Edema formation in spinal nerve roots induced by experimental, graded compression: an experimental study of pic cauda equina with special reference to differences in effects between rapid and slow onset of compression, *Spine* 14:569, 1989.

145. Olmarker K, Rydevik B: Pathophysiology of sciatica, *Orthop Clin North Am* 22:223, 1991.

146. Olsewski JM, Simmons EH, Kallen FC et al: Evidence from cadavers suggestive of entrapment of fifth lumbar spinal nerves by lumbosacral ligaments, *Spine* 16:336, 1991.

147. Parke WW: Development of the spine. In Rothman RH, Simeone FA, editors: *The spine,* ed 3, Philadelphia, 1992, WB Saunders.

148. Patzold U, Haller P, Engelhardt P et al: Zur fehlahltung der Lenden Wirbelsanle beim lumbalen. Baldscheiben voofall, *Zeitschrift fur Orthopadie* 113:909, 1975.

149. Penning L: Functional pathology of lumbar spinal stenosis, *Clin Biomechanics* 7:3, 1992.

150. Ponte JT, Jensen GJ, Kent VE: A preliminary report on the use of the McKenzie protocol versus William's protocol in the treatment of low back pain, *J Orthop Sports Phys Therapy* 6130, 1984.

151. Porter RW: *Management of back pain,* ed 2, Edinburgh, 1993, Churchill Livingstone.

152. Porter RW, Trailescu IF: Diurnal changes in straight leg raising, *Spine* 15:103, 1990.

153. Porter RWW, Oakshott GHL: Familiar aspects of disc protrusion, *J Orthop Rheum* 1:173 1988.

154. Puschel J: Derwssergehald normalerr and degenerieter zweischenwirbel scheiben, *Bietr Path Anat* 84:123, 1930.

155. Racz GB, McCarron RF, Talboys P: Percutaneous dorsal column stimulator for chronic pain control, *Spine* 14:1, 1989.

156. Rae PS, Waddell C, Benner RW: A simple technique for measuring lumbar spinal flexion, *J Royal Coll Surg Edinburgh* 29:281, 1984.

157. Ratcliffe JF: An evaluation of the intra-osseous arterial anastomoses in the human vertebral body at different ages. A microarteriographic study, *J Anat* 134:373, 1982.

158. Remer S, Neuwirth MG: Anatomy and biomechanics of the spine. In Nicholas JA, Hershman EB, editors: *The lower extremity and spine in sports medicine,* ed 2, St Louis, 1995, Mosby.

159. Reynolds JB, Banta C, Wiltse LL: High grade spondylolisthesis in the young: a long term follow up of in situ fusion. Presented at the 59th annual meeting of the American Association of Orthopedic Surgeons, Washington, DC, Feb. 20-25, 1992.

160. Roaf R: A study of the mechanics of spinal injuries, *J Bone Joint Surg* 42B:810, 1960.

161. Roeser W, Meeks LW, Venis R et al: The use of transcutaneous nerve stimulation for pain control in athletic medicine: a preliminary report, *Am J Sports Med* 4:210, 1976.

162. Rolander SD: Motion of the spine with special reference to stabilizing effect of posterior fusion, *Acta Orthop Scand* 90(suppl):1-144, 1966.

163. Saal JA, Saal JS: Non operative treatment of herniated lumbar intervertebral disc with radiculopathy: an outcome study, *Spine* 14:431, 1989.

164. Saal JS, Franson RC, Dobrow R et al: High levels of inflammatory phospholipase A2 activity in lumbar spine disc herniation, *Spine* 15:674, 1990.

165. Saunders H: Lumbar traction, *J Sports Phys Ther* 1:36, 1979.

166. Schachter CL, Stalker CA, Teram E: Toward sensitive practice: issues for physical therapist working with survivors of childhood sexual abuse. *Phys Ther* 79(3), 1999.

167. Schaum SM, Taylor TKF: Tension signs in lumbar disc prolapse, *Clin Orthop Relat Res* 75:195, 1971.

168. Schnebel BE, Watkins RG, Dillin W: The role of spinal flexion and extension in changing nerve root compression in disc herniations, *Spine* 14:835, 1989.

169. Schofferman JA: Physical examination. In White AH, Schofferman JA, editors: *Spine care,* vol 1, *Diagnosis and conservative treatment,* St Louis, 1995, Mosby.

170. Scott JHS: The spine. In Macleod J, editor: *Clinical examination,* ed 6, Edinburgh, 1983, Churchill Livingstone.

171. Seimon RL, Sprengler D: Significance of lumbar spondylolysis in college football players, *Spine* 6:72, 1981.

172. Selby D: The structural degenerative cascade. In White AH, Schofferman JA, editors: *Spine care: diagnosis and conservative treatment,* vol 1, St Louis, 1995, Mosby.

173. Silverhorn KG, Gillespie WJ: Pyogenic osteomyelitis: a review of 61 cases, *NZ Med J* 99:62, 1986.

174. Sinaki M, Luttness MP, Ilstrup DM et al: Lumbar spondylolisthesis: retrospective comparison and three-year follow up of two conservative treatment programs, *Arch Phys Med Rehab* 70:594, 1989.

175. Smith SA, Massie JB, Chesnut R et al: Straight leg raising: anatomical effects on the spinal nerve root with and without fusion, *Spine* 18:992, 1993.

176. Spedler D, Bigos S, Martin N et al: Back injuries in industry: a retrospective study, *Spine* 11:241, 1986.

177. Spengler DM: Newer assessment approaches for the patient with low back pain. In Rothman RH, Simeone FA, editors: *The spine,* Philadelphia, WB Saunders, 1999.

178. Spillane JD, Spillane JA: *An atlas of clinical neurology,* ed 3, 1982, Oxford University Press.

179. Sprankfort EV: The lumbar disc herniation: a computer aided analysis of 2,504 operations, *Acta Orthop Scand* (Suppl 142):1, 1972.

180. Staheli LT: *Fundamental of pediatric orthopedics,* New York, 1992, Raven Press.

181. Stauffer R: Pyogenic vertebral osteomyelitis, *Orthop Clin North Am* 6:1015, 1975.

182. Steiner ME, Micheli LJ: Treatment of symptomatic spondylolysis and spondylolisthesis with the modified Boston brace, *Spine* 10:937, 1985.

183. Sternbach RA: *Mastering pain,* New York, 1987, Putnam Books.

184. Stimmel B: Pain, analgesia, and addiction: an approach to the pharmacological management of pain, *Clin J Pain* 1:14, 1985.

185. Sunderland S: *Nerves and nerve injuries,* ed 2, New York, 1978, Churchill Livingstone.

186. Swanson DW, Swenson WM, Maruba T: The dissatisfied patient with chronic pain, *Pain* 4:367, 1978.

187. Synne-Davies R, Scott JHS: Inheritance and spondylolisthesis: a radiographic family survey, *J Bone Joint Surg* 61B:301, 1979.

188. Taylor JR: The development and adult structure of lumbar intervertebral discs, *J Manual Med* 5:43, 1990.

189. Taylor JR, Twomey LT: Age changes in lumbar zygapophyseal joints: Observations on structure and function, *Spine* 11:739, 1986.

190. Thelander U, Fagerlund M, Friberg S, et al: Straight leg raising test versus radiologic size, shape, and position of lumbar disc hernias, *Spine* 17:395, 1992.

191. Turner JA, Romano JM: Cognitive-behavioral therapy. In Bonica JJJ: *The management of pain,* ed 2, Philadelphia, 1990, Lea & Febiger.

192. Urban J, McMullin J: Swelling pressure of lumbar intervertebral discs: influence of age, spinal level, composition, and degeneration, *Spine* 13:179, 1988.

193. Urban JPG, Holm S, Marouidas A: Diffusion of small solutes into the intervertebral disc: an in vivo study, *Biorheology* 16:447, 1978.

194. Vallfors B: Acute, subacute and chronic low back pain: clinical symptoms, absenteeism and working environment, *Scand J Rehab Med* II (suppl):I, 1985.

195. Van der Wiel HE, Lips P, Nauta J et al: Biochemical parameters of bone turnover during ten days of bed rest and subsequent mobilization, *Bone Mineralization* 13:123, 1991.

196. Venner RM, Crock HV: Clinical studies of isolated disc resorption in the lumbar spine, *J Bone Joint Surg* 63B:491, 1981.

197. Versloot JM, Rozeman A, van Son AM et al: The cost-effectiveness of a back school program in industry, *Spine* 17:22, 1992.

198. Waddell G: A new clinical model for the treatment of low-back pain, *Spine* 12:632, 1987.

199. Wallnofer H, vonRottauscher A: *Chinese folk medicine and acupuncture,* New York, 1965, Bell.

200. Ward NG: Tricyclic antidepressants for chronic low back pain: mechanisms of action and predictors of response, *Spine* 11:661, 1986.

201. Warner L, McNeill ME: Mental imagery and its potential for physical therapy, *Phys Ther* 68(4), 1988.

202. Weisberg LA, Garcia C, Strub R: *Essentials of clinical neurology,* ed 3, St Louis, 1996, Mosby.

203. Wenger DR, Bobechko WP, Gilday DL: The spectrum of intervertebral disk-space infection in children, *J Bone Joint Surg* 1978; 60A:100.

204. White AA, Panjabi MM: *Clinical biomechanics of the spine,* Philadelphia, 1978, JB Lippincott.

205. White AH: *Back school and other conservative approaches to low back pain,* St Louis, 1983, Mosby.

206. White AH, Derby R, Wynne G: Epidural injections for the diagnosis and treatment of low back pain, *Spine* 5:78, 1980.

207. Williams PL, Gray H et al: *Gray's anatomy,* ed 37, Edinburgh, 1989, Churchill Livingstone.

208. Wiltse LL, Guyer RD, Spencer CW et al: Alar transverse process impingement of the L5 spinal nerve: the far-out syndrome, *Spine* 9:31, 1984.

209. Woodhall R, Hayes GJ: The well-leg-raising test of Fajersztjan in the diagnosis of ruptured lumbar intervertebral disc, *J Bone Joint Surg* 32A:786, 1950.

210. Zachrisson-Forsell M: *Low back pain school,* Sweden, 1972, Danderyds Hospital.

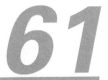

61

Lateral Spinal Curvature in a Senescent Woman with Low Back and Leg Pain During Standing and Walking that is Relieved by Recumbency

An 87-year-old female of average height complains of a history of scoliotic back pain over the last 10 years. She offers that her condition began in childhood, but was unattended until she became multiparous at an early age. Pregnancy was very difficult for her owing to serious back pain, which was only relieved by daily massage to her low back. For the last 47 years she avoided symptoms by going swimming for at least an hour 3 to 4 times a week. Over the last decade she has not gone swimming as she is unable to go to the pool because her loss of balance requires her to ambulate with a rolling walker or shopping cart at all times. While walking in the street, she uses her shopping cart to bend over slightly and thus avoid leg pain that might otherwise occur. Despite this, she complains of persistent left buttock and leg pain when standing or walking for long periods. Pain radiates to the lateral aspect of the left thigh and the anterior aspect of the left leg. The pain is not intense, and is not aggravated by bending, coughing, or sneezing. Relief is found by lying in bed once she has found a comfortable position.

OBSERVATION   A right primary thoracolumbar curve is seen when viewing the patient from behind and a large and prominent razorback rib hump deformity is noted. A compensatory curve is present above the major curve in the cervical spine and causes distortion of the neck-shoulder angle. The right shoulder and scapula appear more prominent. The patient presents with an uneven waistline due to an apparent difference in iliac crest height. The thoracic cage appears distorted and ovoid owing to the ribs on the left protruding anteriorly and recessed posteriorly. The thoracic spine appears excessively kyphotic while the lumbar spine appears hyperlordotic. There is no evidence of cafe-au-lait spots or hair over the midline of the middle or lower back.

TRUNK ALIGNMENT   Using a plumb line from the occiput to the gluteal cleft shows significant displacement to the right.

PALPATION   The site of the primary curve demonstrates rotation of the spinous processes toward the left. The ribs on the convex side are widely separated, whereas those on the concave side are in contact with each other.

RANGE OF MOTION   During forward spinal flexion, the patient's fingertips reach to knee level. All other spinal movements were less than average.

STRENGTH   The patient can walk on her toes and heels without difficulty.

FLEXIBILITY   The patient can perform 75° range of straight leg raising.

REFLEXES   There is brisk right knee jerk while the left is mildly diminished. Both ankle jerks are moderately diminished, while plantar responses are normal.

SPECIAL TESTS   An apparent leg length discrepancy is present although true limb length measurement is normal. The forward bending test does not eliminate the rib hump. Assessment for spinal curve flexibility by having the patient laterally bend into the convexity of the curve does not diminish the magnitude of the curve. Negative heel drop and Laségue tests. The femoral stretch test is weakly positive on the left.

PULSES   The feet are cool, but the pulses are readily palpable.

RADIOGRAPHS   A single anteroposterior radiograph shows a 58° right thoracolumbar curve. Significant narrowing of the left lower thoracic and upper lumbar intervertebral spaces is evident. In addition, advanced degenerative disk and facet disease was apparent at all levels and included marginal sclerosis, facet and vertebral body osteophytes, and vacuum phenomena. There was no evidence of any destructive lesion.

CLUE:

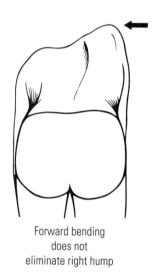

Forward bending
does not
eliminate right hump

? Questions

1. What is the cause of this patient's spinal deformity?
2. What terminology is essential to defining the various types of scoliotic curvature?
3. What is the etiology of idiopathic scoliosis?
4. What is the difference between structural and functional scoliotic curves?
5. How is scoliosis classified according to peak periods of onset?
6. What are the four distinct idiopathic curve patterns of adolescent idiopathic scoliosis?
7. What pathologic structural changes typically occur in idiopathic scoliosis?

8. **What is the clinical presentation of idiopathic scoliosis?**

9. **Which signs should alert the clinician to the presence of underlying disease?**

10. **What degree of spinal curvature is associated with compromised cardiopulmonary function?**

11. **What radiographs are appropriate in the scoliotic patient?**

12. **What is the prognosis for adolescent idiopathic scoliosis?**

13. **What is the differential diagnosis?**

14. **What are other forms of scoliosis?**

15. **What management strategy is most effective in treatment of scoliosis?**

16. **What is the role of exercises in the treatment of idiopathic scoliosis?**

17. **What is the role of electrical stimulation in the management of idiopathic adolescent scoliosis?**

18. **What is the treatment for scoliosis in adults?**

19. **When is surgery an appropriate treatment option for scoliotic patients?**

---

1. What is the cause of this patient's spinal deformity?

The patient has chronic thoracolumbar *adult scoliosis* with a recent onset of lumbar ache and radiculitis affecting the L3 or L4 nerve root on the left. Typically, in elderly persons with longstanding scoliosis, the radicular symptoms almost invariably present on the concavity side of the curve.[50] The symptoms and findings during the examination are consistent with mechanically induced pain. The patient had scoliosis for as long as she can remember, and unfortunately, it remained untreated and progressed beyond skeletal maturity.

Idiopathic scoliosis of the structural type comprises 85% of all types of scoliosis that occurs in approximately 0.5% of the population.[47] *Idiopathic adolescent scoliosis* is a spinal deformity that begins slowly, insidiously, and painlessly, and if untreated may progress to *adult scoliosis* causing significant pain and deformity. Minor scoliosis may be considered a variation of normal and, to some degree, is a function of handedness, so that a right-handed person will show a slight right convex curve. This occurs because the repetitive preference of the dominant upper extremity causes asymmetric contraction and peak muscular forces on the nondominant side.[57] In contrast, *pathologic scoliosis* is the most common back deformity and is characterized by a lateral curvature of the spine in the frontal plane that is accompanied by concurrent vertebral rotation due to sagittal and transverse plane malalignment. Scoliosis describes a state of deformity of the spine rather than a specific disease state or spinal disorder. As a deformity, the pattern of curvature and rotation takes a variety of forms depending upon its etiology as well as the age of onset. Scoliosis most often affects the thoracic spine, although deformities of the more flexible portions of the spine such as the lumbar, thoracolumbar, and cervical curves may also occur.

The spinal columns of patients with idiopathic scoliosis are usually normal at birth. Because idiopathic scoliosis begins slowly, insidiously, and painlessly, most patients are not aware of the curvature in the early stages of development, especially as clothing conceals the deformity. Indeed, many curves begin just before puberty, at age 10 or 11, and are very small and not easily detected. Often, by the time the curvature has sufficiently progressed to elicit clinical detection, it has already reached 30°.

2. What terminology is essential to defining the various types of scoliotic curvature?

Evaluation and management of scoliosis is predicated upon the understanding of terminology relating to this deformity. The terms *major curve* and *primary curve* are synonymous and refer to the most significant abnormal lateral curvature. This typically occurs in the thoracic spine, and may be accompanied by *compensating secondary curves* that develop in the opposite direction above the primary site in the cervical spine, as well as below in the lumbar spine. Compensating curves may be structural or functional in nature. The development of secondary curves allows for scoliosis to be *compensated* and refers to the fact that the shoulders are level and positioned directly above the pelvis. Scoliosis is said to be *decompensated* when the sum of the compensatory curves is less than the degree of deformity of the major curve, resulting in shoulders that are not level and accompanied by a lateral shift or "list" of the trunk to one side. The designations of right and left scoliosis refer to the convex side of the major curve.[47]

Normal sagittal plane alignment is determined by hanging a plumb line from the tip of the odontoid to the S1 vertebral body in a skeletal model. In the normal population the plumb line usually drops 1 cm anterior to the S1 vertebral body indicating a balanced spine in the sagittal plane. Lateral curvature due to scoliosis will alter this balance. When performing this procedure on the patient, the plumb line normally falls between the buttocks and bisects the S1 spinous process. The presence of a lateral curvature will shift the plumb line either to the left or right. A right thoracolumbar curve shifts the plumb line to the right of the vertical buttock dimple (Fig. 61-1). *Spinal decompensation* refers to the state in which the severity of primary lateral curvature causes a loss of balance of the torso in relation to the head and is radiographically quantified by measuring the horizontal distance between the plumb line and a line descending from the sacrum. Spinal compensation is likely accompanied by *secondary minor curves* operating as a *compensatory mechanism* to help keep the head aligned over the pelvis. When the head is not adequately aligned over the pelvis, the scoliosis is termed *decompensated*. Spinal curvature flexibility refers to the ability of a spinal curvature to be straightened. This cannot occur with a primary structural curve, but may occur with secondary compensatory curves. Straightening may also occur in a primary functional curve deriving from pelvic obliquity due to leg length discrepancy or muscle spasm. *Spinal curvature flexibility* is assessed either by traction, lateral side bending into the convexity, or radiographs. In addition to curve severity, curve flexibility is an important determinant of curve prognosis and response to treatment.

3. What is the etiology of idiopathic scoliosis?

Scoliosis appears to be familial and hence is believed to be a genetically linked deformity.[51] The mode of inheritance is not certain, but spinal curvature is thought to be a sex-linked trait that may be transmitted by a mother to either a son or daughter, but may only be transmitted from a carrier father to his daughter. The scoliotic trait may demonstrate incomplete penetrance meaning that it may skip generations, as well as have variable expression, meaning that it may cause a severe curve in a parent and only mild curves in a child. If a person with idiopathic scoliosis has offspring, approximately one third of their children will have scoliosis. If both parents carry scoliotic genes, the likelihood of their children to develop scoliosis is even greater, even if one of the parents does not exhibit the disease.

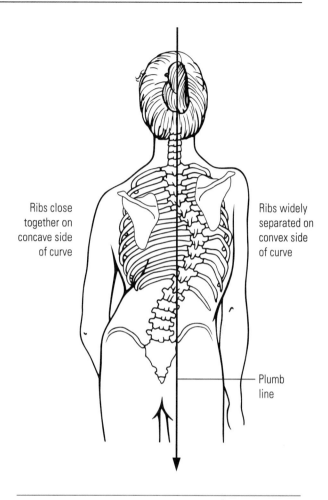

Ribs close together on concave side of curve

Ribs widely separated on convex side of curve

Plumb line

FIG. 61-1 Normal sagittal plane alignment is determined by hanging a plumb line from the tip of the odontoid to the S1 vertebral body in a skeletal model. Normally the plumb line falls between the buttocks and bisects the S1 spinous process. The presence of a lateral curvature will shift the plumb line either to the left or right. A right thoracolumbar curve shifts the plumb line to the right of the vertical buttock dimple.

Alternately, scoliosis may represent a dysfunction of the vestibular balancing system or a brainstem lesion of the posterior columns because minor abnormalities in vestibular function and vibratory sensitivity are commonly associated with idiopathic scoliosis. This suggests a reduction of the brain's ability to decode sensory clues, so that a deficiency of interpretation of how the body rights itself occurs. In response, the spine assumes an S or C shape. Thus scoliosis is a deformity that is not primarily a musculoskeletal problem, but rather a disruption in neuromuscular balance that may be accompanied by decreased vibratory sensation in the limbs.[24]

Proprioceptive dysfunction due to abnormal distribution of muscle spindles in paraspinal musculature[20] has been identified in patients with adolescent idiopathic scoliosis.[19] In addition, asymmetric muscle weakness[45] has also been found in these patients. It is unknown whether the anomalies described above are the cause or the result of idiopathic scoliosis. Thus the specific cause of idiopathic scoliosis remains unknown.[13]

4. What is the difference between structural and functional scoliotic curves?

Scoliosis may be broadly classified according to whether the spinal curves are structural or functional. *Structural scoliosis* refers to an irreversible lateral curvature of the spine due to bony changes. As a result, rotation of the vertebral bodies occurs in the area of the primary curve so that the lateral spinal curve fails to correct with side bending. Thus early loss of spinal flexibility is the first sign of structural scoliosis. In contrast, a functional curve is nonstructural and no bony changes are present. Consequently, rotation may be absent or minimal and the dynamic curve may be eliminated by correcting the underlying cause or by asking the patient to bend sideways and thereby distract the curve into a straightened posture. The common causes of *functional scoliosis,* also known as *postural scoliosis,*[25] are leg length inequality or muscle spasm,[10] which often cause positional changes and alignment of the pelvis or spine.

5. How is scoliosis classified according to peak periods of onset?

The classification of idiopathic scoliosis is based upon the peak age of onset. The actual distinctions between these classifications are blurry as the age difference may only relate to when the curvature was first noticed.

INFANTILE IDIOPATHIC SCOLIOSIS

This occurs between birth and 3 years of age, is predominant in boys, manifests as a left thoracic curve, and resolves spontaneously in nearly 90% of all patients by age 1 to 2 years of age.[51] Existing mostly in England or in those of British descent, the etiology of these curves in unknown although it is postulated that they derive from uterine molding. In addition to the *self resolving-type curve,* a second curve may occur in 10%

to 15% of the population that is *rapidly progressive* and leads to an extremely severe curvature despite treatment. Generally, the patient with the benign form of infantile idiopathic scoliosis does not have a curve greater than 35° and no intervention is needed due to spontaneous regression of the curve. In contrast, the treatment of choice for the rapidly progressive curve is early and aggressive intervention that involves serial casting followed by a Milwaukee brace to prevent the development of severely rigid structural curves later on.

JUVENILE IDIOPATHIC SCOLIOSIS

This occurs after age 3, and spans childhood up until the age of puberty, which typically begins at age 10. Unless early standing and side bending radiographs are available, it is practically impossible to distinguish cases of late infantile onset from early juvenile onset scoliosis. Similarly, the age difference between late onset of juvenile idiopathic scoliosis and early onset adolescent idiopathic scoliosis is not sharply demarcated. The difference between infantile and juvenile idiopathic scoliosis is that the curvature in the latter does not spontaneously resolve. Juvenile idiopathic scoliosis is more common in girls, is likely to be a right thoracic curve, and is typically progressive and therefore requires treatment. Any patient with a curve of 20° or more should be treated with a Milwaukee brace.[18]

ADOLESCENT IDIOPATHIC SCOLIOSIS

This is the classic form of scoliosis and diagnosed when the curve is noticed between the ages of 10 years and skeletal maturity. In fact, many of the adolescent curves first noticed after age 10 stem from undetected juvenile curves that were not recognized until the adolescent growth spurt. Although this form of scoliosis occurs in equal numbers in both boys and girls, progressive curves that are severe enough to warrant treatment occur about eight times more frequently in girls. The right thoracic curve is the most common pattern of spinal curvature.

6. What are the four distinct idiopathic curve patterns of adolescent idiopathic scoliosis?

Idiopathic scoliosis is characterized by four distinct patterns of curvature (Fig. 61-2):
• *Right thoracic curve.* This refers to containment of curvature entirely within the thoracic spine, usually

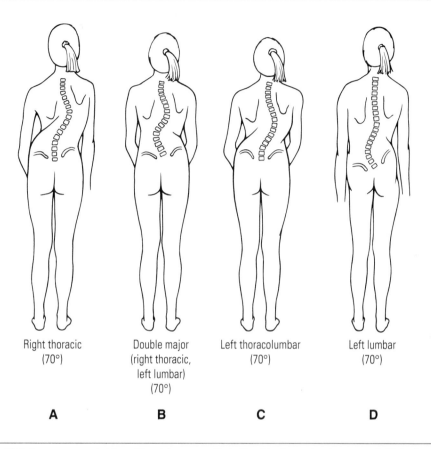

Right thoracic (70°)	Double major (right thoracic, left lumbar) (70°)	Left thoracolumbar (70°)	Left lumbar (70°)
A	**B**	**C**	**D**

FIG. 61-2 Curve patterns in idiopathic adolescent scoliosis listed in decreasing frequency. **A,** Right thoracic curve. **B,** Double major curve. **C,** Thoracolumbar curve. **D,** Lumbar major curve.

between T4 and T12, and the convexity on the right.* The right thoracic curve pattern is the most commonly encountered scoliotic curvature in adolescent girls, and is always the major curve that may or may not be accompanied by secondary minor curves above or below the major curves as a compensatory strategy to keep the head aligned over the pelvis. Approximately 80% of thoracic curves are to the right, and typically do not correct with side bending. Because of the significant concurrent vertebral rotation, the right ribs on the convex side are prominent posteriorly and recessed anteriorly whereas the left ribs decline dorsally and are prominent ventrally. Moreover, the rotated vertebrae demonstrate spinous processes and pedicles toward the left concavity. In addition, the ribs are widely separated on the right convex side and close together, if not touching, on the left

concave side. Because of this, the costal angles change so that the prominent posterior right ribs manifest as a rib hump when the patient forward-flexes the spine. During standing, the right scapula is more prominent, the right shoulder higher, and the left hip protrudes more than the right. Moreover, the right upper extremity is adducted, whereas the left upper extremity hangs in abduction further away from the torso. Thus a right thoracic curve yields a serious cosmetic defect as well as significant impairment of cardiopulmonary function. Because right thoracic curves can rapidly develop and progress, intervention must be initiated early. Beware of a left thoracic curve as it necessitates additional studies to rule out a lesion of the spinal cord.[51]

• *Thoracolumbar curve.* This refers to a curvature pattern in which the primary curve occurs across the thoracolumbar junction. This relatively common curvature pattern may be either to the right or left and is considerably longer in length than the more common

---

*This may be simulated in the person with a normal spine by lateral bending to one's left.

right thoracic curve. Extending between T4 and L4, the thoracolumbar curve is typically less cosmetically deforming than the thoracic curve, although it may cause severe rib and flank distortion due to vertebral rotation. Uneven waistline and apparent difference in iliac crest height are the most prominent findings.

- *Lumbar curve.* Here the curvature is mostly confined to the lumbar spine between T12 to L5. These curves are quite common and occur with a convexity to the left. Characteristic features include waistline asymmetry, apparent leg length discrepancy, and spinal decompensation (the majority of which are to the left). Often associated with pelvic obliquity, the patient with lumbar scoliosis attempts to align the pelvis during gait to compensate for obliquity by circumducting during swing phase or vaulting during stance phase of gait.[51] This strategy, while enabling the patient to ambulate, causes the spine to be thrown out of balance with each gait cycle, which has the cumulative long-term effect of marked degenerative spinal changes in later life.[26] While not initially very deforming, lumbar curves may become quite rigid, leading to severe pain during pregnancy and arthritic pain later in life. Over time, gradual deterioration of the disks and facets above and below the level of the scoliosis, especially in the concavity of the curve, results in arthritis that may trap emerging nerve roots and result in radicular pain.[50] Moreover, recent data indicate that these curves may progress 1° to 2° with each advancing adult year, so that a patient with a 30° curvature at age 21 may have a 50° or 60° curve at age 40.
- *Double primary curve.* This refers to two structural curves of almost equal prominence that occur as a number of thoracolumbar combinations. The most common presentation is a convex thoracic curve and convex lumbar curve. The double major curves balance each other so that the shoulders are level over the pelvis while the rib and lumbar prominences are not too severe. The major deformity here is trunk shortening.

7. What pathologic structural changes typically occur in idiopathic scoliosis?

The fundamental aspect of the pathogenesis of scoliotic deformity is its progression with skeletal growth, so that as lateral curvature and vertebral rotation occur secondary changes develop in the vertebrae and ribs. Progression of lateral curvature causes rotation of the vertebrae, pedicles, and spinous processes in the area of the major curve toward the concavity of the curve. The

rotating vertebrae impinge upon the ribs on the concave side, causing them to crowd together while those on the convex side are widely separated. As the deformity progresses, the entire thoracic cage becomes ovoid, causing the ribs on the concave side to protrude anteriorly and become recessed posteriorly (Fig. 61-3). Kyphosis and lordosis may often accompany the scoliotic deformity.[39]

In addition to lateral and rotational deformities, scoliosis causes pathologic changes in the intervertebral and facet joints at the site of structural change. The disk spaces on the concave side of the curve become narrower, the pedicles and laminae are shorter and thinner, while the vertebral canal is narrower. A lateral displacement of the nucleus pulposus may occur on the concave side.[16] Moreover, *claw type osteophytes,* in distinction from traction spurs associated with disk degeneration,[42] develop on the concave side of the scoliotic curve at the edge of the vertebral body margin around the annulus and may sometimes meet and fuse the two vertebrae together (Fig. 61-4).[32] On the convex side of the curve the disk spaces become wider as well as wedged (thicker).

The synovial posterior facet joints are paired, one on either side of the midline for each spinal segment, and must be symmetrically aligned to maintain congruity. Symmetrical congruity of the facet joints is dependent upon the intervertebral disk joint. If the intervertebral disk, located anterior to the facet joints, maintains adequate height between the vertebral bodies then both facets are equally loaded. However, as the disk space becomes narrowed on the concave (loaded) side of the curve, the superior and inferior articular surfaces of the facet joints on that side undergo osteoarthritic changes as they become overloaded and override each other. This facet incongruity causes capsular thickening and osteophytic growth posteriorly as well as anteriorly along the facet joint margins. Anteriorly projecting osteophytes may encroach on the spinal canal and narrow the exit for the spinal nerves in the intervertebral foramen, and thereby cause both forms of spinal stenosis.[50]

Many elderly patients frequently present in the fifth or sixth decade with complaints of back pain and radicular symptoms. The majority of these patients have left lumbar curves (i.e., convexity toward the left). The facets on the concave (right) side bear the brunt of load and develop arthrosis with radicular symptoms on the concave side of the curve. Radicular involvement most commonly involves the L2 or L3 nerve root, with pain felt over the iliac crest and anterolateral aspects of

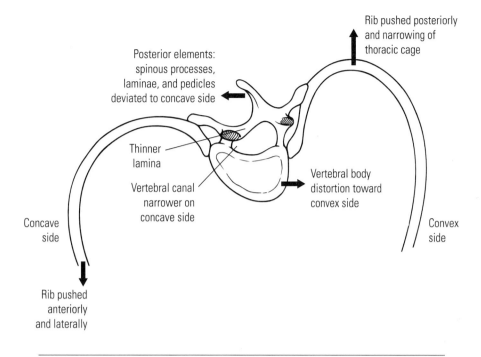

Posterior elements:
spinous processes,
laminae, and pedicles
deviated to concave side

Rib pushed posteriorly
and narrowing of
thoracic cage

Thinner
lamina

Vertebral canal
narrower on
concave side

Vertebral body
distortion toward
convex side

Concave
side

Convex
side

Rib pushed
anteriorly
and laterally

FIG. 61-3 Inferior view of pathologic distortion of the vertebrae and ribs in thoracic scoliosis.

the thigh. Symptoms are most commonly pronounced while sitting, although relief is obtained during recumbency.[50]

8. What is the clinical presentation of idiopathic scoliosis?

Examination of the scoliotic patient begins with a visual inspection from behind for back and trunk symmetry, differences in shoulder height, scapular prominence, flank crease, pelvic asymmetry, and discrepancy of the arms or legs. Scapular prominence occurs on the side of the convexity. The neck-shoulder angle may be distorted by asymmetry of the trapezius muscle secondary to high thoracic or cervical curves.[39] Uneven flanks are known as *lumbar humps.* It is important to notice whether the development of secondary sexual characteristics has begun, and whether anterior rib or breast asymmetry is present.[39] Any major and compensatory curves, as well as vertebral rotation in the area of the primary curve, should be noted. The loss of thoracic kyphosis manifesting as a flattening precedes or accompanies the development of the lateral curve. The earliest manifestation of developing structural scoliosis is often a *rotational prominence* that causes unevenness in the paravertebral area known as a *rib hump,* with or with-

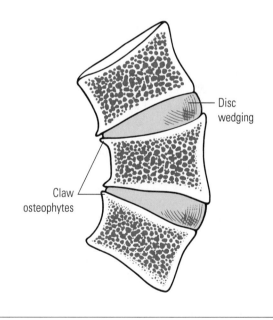

Disc
wedging

Claw
osteophytes

FIG. 61-4 Section through scoliotic vertebrae showing pathologic changes accompanying lateral curvature.

out an accompanying loss of thoracic kyphosis. A particularly large and angular rib hump causes deformity of the thoracic cage and is called a *razorback*.

Spinal rotation is most noticeable when the patient is asked to bend forward. The *forward bending test* is important for detecting truncal and spinal asymmetry. The patient is asked to slowly bend forward while keeping both palms together and outstretched as well as hanging freely. This eliminates the chance of error in determining if a rib hump is derived from a true structural scoliosis or simply from active rotation of the spine.[49] The clinician then visually scans each level of the spine to assess for symmetry. The forward bending test is performed to determine whether the curve straightens out as the child bends forward to determine if a visible, rotational rib cage deformity exists. If a rib hump is present, the resultant angular tilt of the trunk is measured with a *scoliometer.*

Spinal curve flexibility may be assessed by having the patient side bending into the convexity of the curve. By asking the patient to turn their trunk from side to side while in the forward flexed posture (Fig. 61-5), the flexible curve will unwind whereas the structural curve will not. The *lateral bending test*[17] is performed to determine whether the curve corrects or reverses as the child laterally flexes the trunk toward the convex side of the curve. Asymmetric side bending is an early sign that structural spinal changes may have already begun to develop.[10] Alternately, curvature flexibility may be assessed by traction in which the clinician gently lifts the patient by the head so as to distract the curve and thereby assess the degree of curvature flexibility or rigidity. Curve flexibility is an important determinant of curve prognosis and response to treatment.

Trunk alignment is assessed by using a tape measure as a plumb line held from the occiput. Displacement of the lower portion of the tape from the gluteal cleft (i.e., buttock crease) is recorded and indicates that the head and trunk are not aligned.

9. Which signs should alert the clinician to the presence of underlying disease?

If the patient is very tall, *Marfan's syndrome* should be ruled out. It is important to note the presence of *café-au-lait* spots of *neurofibromatosis* or the presence of hairy patches that accompany *spina bifida.*[14] The lumbar spine should be examined for pigmented areas or patches of hair indicating an underlying congenital condition, such as spina bifida or diastematomyelia.[48] The latter is a spinal condition that is accompanied by sen-

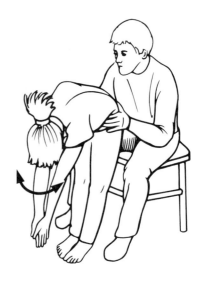

FIG. 61-5 *Forward* and *lateral bending tests* are performed by having the patient bend forward at the hips while holding their palms together, and then evaluating if the curve resolves or unwinds as the child turns the trunk from side to side. These tests assess spinal flexibility by determining whether the curvature is structural or functional.

sory or motor loss. It is of particular importance to detect the presence of these signs during the examination, which, if present, suggest an underlying disease and warrant additional studies. A left thoracic curve is quite unusual and suggests a spinal cord lesion. Excessive pain or stiffness suggests tumor or inflammation, while a midline skin lesion suggests spinal dysraphism.[51] Painful scoliosis suggests the possibility of osteoid osteoma, spinal cord tumors, spondylolysis, spondylolisthesis, or infection.[39]

10. What degree of spinal curvature is associated with compromised cardiopulmonary function?

The majority of patients with idiopathic scoliotic curves under 40° have normal cardiopulmonary function. Pulmonary function tests, electrocardiogram, and measurement of arterial blood gas levels should be taken to establish a baseline in patients with curvatures greater than 45°. A decrease in vital capacity and total lung capacity often occurs in patients with moderate and severe curves.[29] Curve progression between 90° and 100° causes pulmonary and spinal column dysfunction that is accompanied by a significant humpback disfigurement.

11. What radiographs are appropriate in the scoliotic patient?

Radiographs are indicated if the scoliometer reading is greater than 5° or if progression is likely given the presence of other factors such as family history, significant curves in other family members, and patient age. Radiographic screening involves a single anteroposterior (AP) radiograph from the occiput to the iliac crest taken standing on a 36-inch film.[51] Shielding of the thyroid, breasts, and gonads is mandatory. Radiographic examination reveals a lateral curve that is always more acute than would be expected from the external physical appearance of the patient.[47] Radiographs are also important to rule out congenital anomalies such as malformed vertebrae, absent disks, or fused or absent ribs.[34]

Side-bending radiographs are taken to distinguish structural from functional curves. Right side-bending allows a right thoracic curve to uncoil, so that a radiograph taken in this posture provides evidence of the suppleness of the ligaments and other soft-tissue structures. Similarly, left side bending uncoils a left lumbar curve and provides evidence of a nonstructural scoliosis.

The internationally accepted approach[31] of measuring the initial AP radiographs is the *Cobb method** which assesses the coronal plane magnitude of spinal curvature by relying upon the determination of the upper and lower end-vertebrae of the curve. The accuracy of the Cobb method depends on choosing the superior and inferior levels with the greatest tilt. These levels are respectively known as the superior and inferior *apical vertebra†* and represent the upper and lower limits of the end-vertebrae that tilt most acutely *toward* the concavity of the curve. A single line is drawn perpendicular to the upper margin of the vertebra that inclines most toward the curve, and a second straight line on the inferior border of the lower vertebra with the greatest angulation toward the curve. Once the straight lines have been drawn, perpendicular lines are then drawn from each of the horizontal lines so that a right angle is drawn superiorly and inferiorly. The angle created by the intersecting lines indicates the Cobb degree of curvature. A radiographic curvature of less than 10° is considered to be within normal[47] whereas curves greater than 15° are clinically significant.

In addition, vertebral rotation is most accurately assessed by estimating the amount of pedicle rotation on an AP radiograph. Skeletal maturation‡ may also be determined radiographically by pelvic radiographs that determine the degree of iliac crest excursion. Maturation is considered nearly complete when the iliac crest meets the sacroiliac joint and firmly seals to the ilium.

An alternative to radiographic exposure to the young adult involves Moire fringe topography,[46] a form of photography that may be used to document curve severity by detecting asymmetry on opaque surfaces. This technique involves using ordinary point light as projected through special grids to produce a pattern of shadows on the patient's back showing changes in symmetry. This detection technique is more sensitive than the forward bending test.[1]

12. What is the prognosis for adolescent idiopathic scoliosis?

Any discussion of prognosis for idiopathic scoliosis must be prefaced with a grading of curvature severity. Mild scoliosis is generally defined as having a curvature less than 20° to 25°, whereas moderate scoliosis is between 40° and 45°. Severe scoliosis is characterized by a curvature greater than 45°.

Early detection is extremely important in the prognosis of idiopathic scoliosis and has been spurred by standard scoliosis screening in the United States and sponsored by the National Scoliosis Foundation. School screening begins in fifth grade for both boys and girls who should be examined every 6 to 9 months.[3] If a lateral curvature is discovered, the child should be referred to an orthopedist.

The prognosis for adolescent idiopathic scoliosis relates to those risk factors that directly relate to the rate of curvature progression. In some patients the curve remains constant, whereas it may worsen or regress in others. There is no method for accurately predicting in a 10-year-old whether or not a given curve will progress, resolve, or remain static other than considering the presence of risk factors. Risk factors for progression include skeletal age at onset, gender, curve location, magnitude of curvature, a girl's age at menarche, and curve flexibility. Age at onset is particularly

---

*A second method of angle determination is known as the *Risser-Ferguson method,* although it is less commonly employed.

†*Transitional vertebra* refers to the neutral vertebra at each end of the curve that makes the transition from one curve to another, whereas the *apex* of the scoliotic curve is identified by the vertebra that is the greatest distance from the midline of the spine. It is referred to as the *apical vertebra.*

‡Maturation in girls generally occurs at about 16½ years of age, while it occurs approximately 15 to 18 months later in boys.

important in determining prognosis as it assesses the amount of growth that remains and hence the likelihood for increasing deformity.[54] Generally, structural curves have a strong tendency to rapidly progress during the adolescent growth spurt, whereas small, functional curves may remain flexible for long periods of time.[9] While adolescent curves may progress at a rate as high as 10° annually, typical structural curves in adults progress at a rate of 1° to 2° per year if the curve is greater than 60° at skeletal maturity. Moreover, the younger the child is when the structural curve develops, the less favorable the prognosis and the more likely it will increase.[2] Factors such as family history, compensation, and quantity of lordosis or kyphosis do not correlate with likelihood for curve progression.[30] A radiographic index for determining the likelihood for progression is the *Risser sign* that assesses maturation level by the extent of ossification of the iliac apophysis.[30] Generally, a curve that is less that 30° at age 25 is unlikely to progress.[39] In many adults, scoliosis progresses to pain and disability. Curves greater than 80° are at risk for cor pulmonale.*

13. What is the differential diagnosis?

The differential diagnosis includes:

- *Syringomyelia.* This refers to a fluid filled cavity (syrinx) within the substance of the spinal cord that expands during the teens or young adult years and interrupts pain and temperature fibers crossing from one side of the spinal cord to the other side. The patient typically experiences a painless burn or cut. A capelike sensory defect over the shoulders and back is common.[6] Syringomyelia often produces a curve that mimics idiopathic scoliosis, and is differentiated from the latter by magnetic resonance imaging or a myelogram.
- *Marfan's syndrome.* This is an inheritable disorder of connective tissue that is transmitted as an autosomal dominant trait that involves three major organ systems: vision, cardiovascular and musculoskeletal. The latter involvement presents as a tall and thin body habitus with skeletal disproportion. Scoliotic deformity is present in these patients who, because of their tall height, present with curves that may become severe.[41]
- *Osteogenesis imperfecta.* This refers to abnormal, congenital fragility of bones that results in a history

of multiple fractures throughout childhood secondary to trivial-to-minimal trauma. The most common pattern is familial. In the spine, the extreme brittleness of bones causes an accumulation of hundreds of spinal microfractures that eventually result in a mild scoliotic deformity secondary to wedging of the vertebral bodies. These children have blue sclera in the eyes, and often demonstrate tibial bowing, a barrel or pigeon chest, opalescent teeth, less than normal height, and deafness in adulthood.[56]

- *Neurofibromatosis.* This was first fully described by von Recklinghausen as an autosomal dominant disturbance of the supportive tissue of the nervous system that produces skin and nerve tumors as well as subcutaneous and bony deformities. Although roughly one third of patients are asymptomatic, approximately 30% initially complain of cosmetic problems. The characteristic skin lesions include the presence of six or greater café-au-lait (medium brown) patches over the trunk, pelvis, and flexor creases of the elbows and knees, which are present is over 90% of all patients. A few to several thousand flesh-colored lesions of the skin that manifest as hanging, velvety soft skin may appear in late childhood. Neurofibromas refer to tumors of Schwann cells and nerve fibroblasts that may develop along the course of subcutaneous peripheral nerves following puberty and may require excision. Intraspinal neurofibromas may cause spinal cord compression. Scoliosis is the most common bone lesion in neurofibromatosis and occurs in approximately 60% of all patients.[11] Changes in pulmonary and cardiac efficiency may also occur especially in the later stages of the disease.
- *Diskitis.* This refers to a low-grade bacterial infection (most commonly *Staphylococcus aureus*) of the pediatric intervertebral disk space between the adjacent endplates often involving the lower thoracic or upper lumbar levels in infants and children. The peak age of onset is 6 years and the lumbar spine is typically affected. Clinical features include low-grade fever, limpness, irritability, unwillingness to stand or ambulate, abdominal or hip pain, and vomiting in the infant. The adolescent may complain of vague and poorly localized back pain that is accompanied by a stiff back and an elevated erythrocyte sedimentation rate.[55] Early on, a bone scan may show increased uptake over multiple vertebral levels, whereas disk space narrowing is seen on a lateral radiographic view after 2 to 3 weeks. Diskitis usually spontaneously resolves with rest from circulating antibodies,

---

Cor pulmonale refers to a form of heart disease due to pulmonary hypertension secondary to disease of the lung or the vessels supplying the lung, that results in hypertrophy of the right ventricle.

although oral antibiotics are appropriate if the child is systemically ill.[35]

- *Osteoid osteoma.* This is a benign tumor that typically involves long bone, but may involve the vertebrae and cause back pain and a fixed scoliosis. This form of tumor characteristically produces night pain that is relieved by aspirin. It is best demonstrated on bone scans, but may be radiographically imaged as a small radiolucent zone surrounded by a large sclerotic zone. The treatment is surgical removal. In contrast to osteoid osteoma, spinal cord tumor is rare in children.[51] In adults, malignancy or infection is classically chronic, steadily progressive, and painfully unremitting.

14. What are other forms of scoliosis?

SCIATIC SCOLIOSIS

This refers to the protective posture assumed by the muscles of the back and trunk that causes the patient to stand with a tilted posture to alleviate pain. This lateral pelvic shift is known as a deviation and is often due to a posterolateral disk protrusion that occurs away from the painful side. If sciatic pain is aggravated by bending to one side, the patient will reflexively stand laterally flexed in the other direction.[50] Thus the spine curves to reduce pressure on a nerve root from a herniated disk or narrowed intervertebral foramen. Scoliosis will abate once the underlying disorder is corrected.

POSTURAL SCOLIOSIS

This derives from habitual poor posture or may compensate for a short leg and is simple to correct with a heel lift. This form of scoliosis is nonstructural in nature, and may also derive from unilateral muscle spasm to reduce pressure on a nerve root from a herniated disk (see previous section). The spasm and resultant curvature occur reflexively to reduce pressure on a nerve root from an impinging intervertebral disk or bony encroachment. When the cause of functional scoliosis is leg length discrepancy, the scoliosis is only present when the patient stands on both feet, but disappears during lying, sitting, and walking.

OSTEOPATHIC SCOLIOSIS

This refers to lateral curvature that may be congenital (see previous section) or may be acquired in nature. *Acquired scoliosis* includes curves stemming from traumatic and pathological fractures, as well as dislocations of the spine. Alternately, scoliosis may be acquired in the patient with rickets, osteomalacia, emphysema, or patient with unilateral chest operations.

CONGENITAL SCOLIOSIS

This refers to structural spinal curves derived from congenital vertebral defects secondary to an abnormality of the zygote or embryo. Because many organ systems develop simultaneously, children with congenital scoliosis of the thoracolumbar region often have urinary tract anomalies and should undergo an ultrasound evaluation of the urinary system.[51] Curve progression depends upon the type of bony defect, which may present as a *wedge vertebra, hemivertebra,*[33] *congenital bar, block vertebra,* or bizarre congenital combinations. The structural curves deriving from these morphological vertebral changes are not corrected by lying down. With hemivertebrae, the anomalous vertebrae grow and cause the spine to lengthen on the concave side. Similarly, unilateral bars may also result in spinal curvature. When congenital scoliosis is progressive, spinal fusion is best performed as soon as the curve progression is noted.[44]

NEUROMUSCULAR SCOLIOSIS

This is caused by a variety of disorders including upper motor neuron disorders such as cerebral palsy, syringomyelia, and Friedreich ataxia, as well as lower motor neuron* disorders such as poliomyelitis, spinal bifida, and spinal muscular atrophy. These conditions all result in severe, long C-shaped curves that may extend from the sacrum to the lower cervical regions. Myopathic forms of neuromuscular scoliosis include muscular dystrophy.

15. What management strategy is most effective in treatment of scoliosis?

The most important factor in effective management remains an accurate early detection.[51] The goal of treatment in adolescent scoliosis is to prevent progression of

---

*Upper motor neuron refers to neurons in the cerebral cortex that conducts impulses from the motor cortex to motor nuclei of cerebral nerves or the ventral gray columns of the spinal cord. An upper motor neuron lesion may result in hypotonia (flaccidity) due to loss of excitation to descending motor (alpha and gamma) neurons. *Lower motor neuron* refers to peripheral neurons whose cell bodies lie in the ventral gray columns of the spinal cord and whose terminations occur in skeletal muscles. A lower motor neuron lesion can produce symptoms of muscle paresis, paralysis, hypotonia, and hyporeflexia (from an interrupted reflex arc, muscle atrophy, and fasciculation).

a mild scoliosis and correct and stabilize a more severe deformity. The treatment of adolescent idiopathic scoliosis is by observation, bracing, or surgery. Exercise alone, without the benefit of bracing has shown to be ineffective in stopping curve progression,[52] although when used in conjunction with bracing it has been shown to be beneficial.[7] Surface electrical stimulation has similarly been shown to be an ineffective management strategy for moderate to severe scoliosis.[40] For patients with mild scoliosis, the only intervention is re-monitoring of the curve progression every 6 months. Effective bracing has limited application and is appropriate for children with curves of 20° to 40° (mild to moderate curves) with 2 or more years of anticipated growth (so that the curve is small and flexible), and is worn from the age the curve is identified until the end of skeletal growth. If the curve is below 20°, a brace may be unnecessary, as many of these curves are nonprogressive and often spontaneously resolve. In contrast, curves greater than 45° tend to respond poorly to an orthosis, especially if the child has reached the later stages of puberty, but may be braced early on. In these patients, bracing may be attempted on a trial basis so that if at least 30% improvement is not obtained during the first 6 months, surgery should be considered without excessive delay. Curves between 20° and 29° are usually not braced until progression has been documented,[37] whereas curves between 30° and 40° are usually braced immediately.

Bracing serves to stabilize a curve and may prevent worsening of the curve that normally occurs with the adolescent growth spurt. During the juvenile years, the spine is more flexible and hence correctable than later on, although there is no way of predicting if a curve will successfully respond to bracing. While some adolescents may gain permanent spinal straightening from bracing, many children have stiff curves that do not correct despite orthotic intervention. A few children have curves that progress despite bracing. In some cases, curves that have been corrected by bracing may regress to a prebracing level of curvature or even slightly worse.

Developed in 1945, the *Milwaukee brace* is the standard orthosis for the treatment of adolescent upper thoracic idiopathic scoliosis. Various holding pads may be attached so as to treat a variety of curve patterns. Based upon the "three-point principle of fixation," the most critical part of the brace is a well formed pelvic girdle that is deeply indented above the iliac crests so as to maintain a solid foundation. The brace has two pos-

terior uprights and a single anterior upright as well as a neck ring with a throat mold at the upper end. Pads are placed on the convex aspect of the curve. Bracing is often difficult for the adolescent girl owing to the cosmetic stigma associated with wearing the orthosis and may adversely affect self-image during these formative years. It is important to consider the coping ability of the adolescent because exceeding the tolerance limit will result in noncompliance. For patients with scoliosis at lower levels, a thoracolumbar sacral orthosis (TLSO) is more appropriate. The *Boston brace,* effective for thoracolumbar and lumbar curves, is a considerable cosmetic improvement over the Milwaukee brace as it eliminates the metal superstructure and is consequently hidden by ordinary clothes.[47] The low profile Boston brace is a molded plastic jacket extending from both axillae to the pelvis and is not recommended for curves with apices above T8.[53] The patient should be started on a full-time basis for several years and not be weaned off the brace as the latter only prolongs the adjustment period.[22] The brace should be worn both day and night and may be taken off for an hour each to perform exercises to maintain strength[21] and flexibility of the spinal muscles.[12] Neither the Milwaukee nor the Boston brace, both of which apply a laterally directed force, are effective for curves above T6.

16. What is the role of exercise in the treatment of idiopathic scoliosis?

While exercises may not inherently affect the progression of the curve, they may enhance a sense of well being and may require the intervention of physical therapy. Exercises should be performed both in and out of the brace. The role of therapy in treatment may make the difference between a compliant adolescent and an adolescent who quickly reaches their tolerance limit. In addition to maintaining trunk and hip strength and flexibility, as well as monitoring the patient's progress, the therapist also provides emotional support during a rather difficult period of adolescence.[51]

Appropriate exercises include chest retraction, asymmetrical exercises, push-ups, knee bends, deep breathing, and encouragement to participate in noncontact athletic activities.[38] Scapular retraction and protraction exercises are important in maintaining the scapula as a floating origin for the optimal mechanical efficiency of the muscles that control the glenohumeral joint. Deep breathing exercises should emphasize diaphragmatic breathing during abdominal strengthening exercises and during bilateral stretch of the pectoralis muscles. Also, segmental breathing to expand the lungs on the concave side of the curve during unilateral trunk stretching is helpful.[27] Several muscle groups become tight in scoliotic patients and include the sternocleidomastoids, scalenes, pectorals, erector spinae, as well as the hip flexors and hamstrings muscles.[27] With a left scoliotic curve, faulty alignment will occur among the muscles of the trunk and lower extremities (Fig. 61-6).

Thus stretching and strengthening activities are essential to an eclectic treatment program.

Other exercises performed out of the brace include: posterior pelvic tilt in supine with the hips and knees flexed as well as extended; posterior pelvic tilting while standing; trunk extension while prone; and partial sit ups with the knees flexed. Exercises performed while wearing the brace include those same exercises performed out of the brace, as well as active distraction

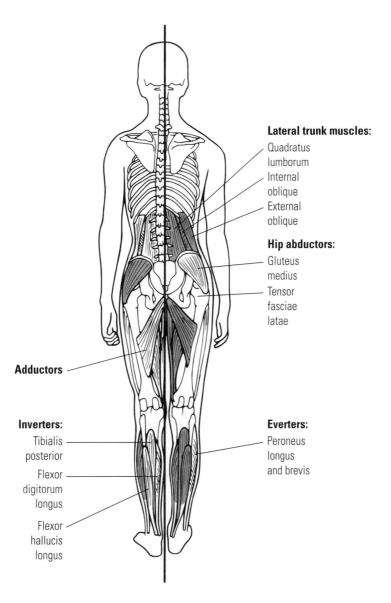

Lateral trunk muscles:
Quadratus lumborum
Internal oblique
External oblique

Hip abductors:
Gluteus medius
Tensor fasciae latae

Adductors

Inverters:
Tibialis posterior
Flexor digitorum longus
Flexor hallucis longus

Everters:
Peroneus longus and brevis

FIG. 61-6 Muscle imbalance of the trunk, pelvic, and lower extremity musculature deriving from a left scoliotic curve. The lighter shader corresponds to stretched muscles, while the darker color corresponds to shortened muscles.

from the thoracic pad at the posterior rib hump, and lateral trunk shift away from the thoracic pad to correct the major thoracic curve. If a lumbar pad is present, the patient may shift away from it. Also, the patient actively distracts away from the throat mold and attempts to 'become taller' (axial extension) in the brace by elongating their spine.[7]

17. What is the role of electrical stimulation in the management of idiopathic adolescent scoliosis?

For patients with mild to moderate curves (20° to 40°) and 2 years or more of growth remaining, implantation of electrospinal intramuscular electrodes[23] within the spinal muscles on the convex side of the curve have been shown successful in halting the progression of major curves in more than 80% of the mild and moderate curves.[8] This approach has fallen into disfavor because of its invasive surgical nature.

An alternative to surgical implantation is the use of surface electrospinal stimulation on the lateral convex aspect of the curve over the mid-axillary line causing the lateral trunk muscles to contract and cause the adjacent ribs to approximate.[15] Because the ribs articulate with the vertebrae, the corrective force is transferred to the spine, which causes straightening of the curvature. This approach may be used at night while the patient sleeps.[5] On the first day, the patient receives one half-hour stimulation 3 times. For the first half-hour, the device may be set at 30 to 40 mA, and increased to between 50 and 70 mA. On the second day, the patient may have two ½ hour sessions, and incrementally increase by 1 hour each subsequent day until 8 hours are tolerated, after which the patient is ready to be stimulated during sleep.[38] While this approach has been justifiably criticized because it tends to stimulate the more superficial muscles, it has been successful in halting the progression of mild to moderate curves.[4]

18. What is the treatment for scoliosis in the adult?

Treatment for adults with scoliosis should involve a strengthening and stretching program, as well as a daily walking or stationary bicycle program to maintain cardiopulmonary endurance while providing exercise to the extremities. Appropriate exercises include chest retraction, asymmetrical exercises, push ups, knee bends, and deep breathing. Breathing exercises should emphasize diaphragmatic breathing during abdominal strengthening exercises and with bilateral stretch to the pectoral muscles. Segmental breathing to expand the lungs on the concave side of the curve during unilateral trunk stretching may also be helpful. During pregnancy, lumbar curves may provoke particularly disturbing pain that may be relieved with soft-tissue massage. For the older adult, walking or swimming across a pool several times a week is an excellent means of maintaining strength and flexibility and may considerably help diminish many of the painful symptoms associated with adult scoliosis. If successful, exercise is a proactive experience that allows the patient to address their scoliosis and return to their home with less pain and the satisfaction of having empowerment over their scoliosis. Adults (but not senescent) with extreme curves may require surgical intervention if they interfere with cardiopulmonary function or are expected to do so in the future.

19. When is surgery an appropriate treatment option for scoliotic patients?

Operative management should not be considered as the last treatment alternative because surgery is a safe and reliable solution to many patients with scoliosis. Generally, when curves are greater than 50°, regardless of the curve pattern present, surgical stabilization is recommended. Patients with significant curves at the end of growth will often develop curves of up to 70° to 100° in as few as 20 to 30 years later and result in serious decline in pulmonary function secondary to respiratory insufficiency. Correction of the curvatures in the adult seldom yields significant improvement of respiratory function. Thus operative management in patients with curves greater than 50° is a prophylactic strategy.[36]

Other surgical criteria include: relentless curve progression; significant thoracic and lumbar pain; progressive thoracic lordosis; progressive loss of pulmonary function; significant cosmetic asymmetry in the shoulders and trunk; and significant curve progression despite bracing. The goal of surgery is to produce an arthrodesis of a balanced spine in the frontal and sagittal planes over a level pelvis.[28] Spinal fusion surgery involves inserting a rod along the spine to straighten it followed by bone grafts. The most common technique involves Harrington rod insertion named after Dr. Paul Harrington who developed this segmental fixation in 1962.[43] The spinal bone is decorticated so that the body reacts as if the bones were broken and attempts to heal them in conjunction with pelvic autografts added. The inserted steel rod is permanent and placed across the concavity of the primary curve so as to "jack" the spine as straight as possible. With the Luque technique, the spine is straightened with two rods attached with wires. The Cotrel-Dubousset technique employs two rods coupled together with transverse traction rods and hooks that offer the additional advantage of derotating the spine and correcting the rib hump. The major intraoperative risks for complication are very low and include wound infection; instrumentation failure; paralysis; pseudoarthrosis; and anesthetic complication.[51] Intraoperative monitoring of sensory-evoked potentials from the feet to the cerebral cortex has reduced the risk of irreversible spinal cord injury.[34]

RECOMMENDED READING

Rogala EJ, Drummond DS, Gurr J: Scoliosis: Incidence and natural history: a prospective epidemiological study, *J Bone Joint Surg* 71A:173-176, 1989.

Tachdijian MO: *Pediatric orthopedics,* ed 2, Philadelphia, 1990, WB Saunders.

REFERENCES

1. Adair IV, VanWijk MC, Armstrong GWD: Moire topography in scoliosis screening, *Clin Orthop* 129:1665, 1977.
2. Ascani E, Barolozzi P, Logroscino CA et al : Natural history of untreated idiopathic scoliosis after skeletal maturity, *Spine* 11:784-789, 1986.
3. Ashworth MA editor: Symposium on school screening for scoliosis: Scoliosis Research Society and British Scoliosis Society, *Spine* 13:1177-1200, 1988.
4. Axelgaard J, Brown JC: Lateral electrical surface stimulation for the treatment of progressive idiopathic scoliosis, *Spine* 8:242, 1983.
5. Axelgaard J, Brown JC, Nordwall A et al: Correction of spinal curvature by transcutaneous electrical muscle stimulation, *Spine* 8:463, 1983.
6. Berkow R: *The Merck manual of diagnosis and therapy,* Rahway, N.J., 1987, Merck & Co.
7. Blount WP, Bolinske J: Physical therapy in the nonoperative treatment of scoliosis, *Phys Ther* 47:919, 1967.
8. Bobechko WP, Herbert MA, Friedman HG: Electrospinal instrumentation for scoliosis: current status, *Orthop Clin North Am* 10:927, 1979.
9. Bunnell WP: The natural history of idiopathic scoliosis before skeletal maturity, *Spine* 11:773-776, 1986.
10. Calliet R: *Scoliosis,* Philadelphia, 1975, FA Davis.
11. Calvert PT, Edgar MA, Webb PJ: Scoliosis in neurofibromatosis: the natural history with and without operation, *J Bone Joint Surg* 71B:246-251, 1989.
12. Carr WA, Moe JH, Winter RB et al: Treatment of idiopathic scoliosis in the Milwaukee brace, *J Bone Joint Surg* 62A:599-612, 1980.
13. Cook SD, Harding AF, Burke SW et al: Upper extremity proprioception in idiopathic scoliosis, *Clin Orthop* 213:118, 1986.
14. Dandy DJ: *Essential orthopaedics and trauma,* Edinburgh, 1989, Churchill Livingstone.
15. Eckerson L, Axelgaard J: Lateral electrical surface stimulation as an alternative to bracing in the treatment of idiopathic scoliosis: treatment, protocol and patient acceptance, *Phys Ther* 64:483, 1984.
16. Engler GL: Scoliosis. In Nickel VL editor: *Orthopedic rehabilitation,* New York, 1982, Churchill Livingstone.
17. Farady JA: Current principles in the nonoperative management of structural adolescent idiopathic scoliosis, *Phys Ther* 63:512, 1983.
18. Figueiredo UM, James JI: Juvenile idiopathic scoliosis, *J Bone Joint Surg* 63B:61-66, 1981.
19. Ford DM, Bagnall KM, Clements CA et al: Muscle spindles in the paraspinal musculature of patients with adolescent idiopathic scoliosis, *Spine* 13:461, 1988.
20. Ford DM, Bagnall KM, McFadden KD et al: Paraspinal muscle imbalance in adolescent idiopathic scoliosis, *Spine* 9(4):373, 1984.
21. Granata C, Merlini L, Magni E et al: Spinal muscular atrophy: natural history and orthopaedic treatment of scoliosis, *Spine* 14:760-770, 1989.
22. Green NE: Part-time bracing of adolescent idiopathic scoliosis, *J Bone Joint Surg* 6A:738-742, 1986.
23. Herbert MA, Bobechko WP: Paraspinal muscle stimulation for the treatment of idiopathic scoliosis in children, *Orthopedics* 10(8), 1987.
24. Herman R, Mixon J, Fisher A et al: Idiopathic scoliosis and the central nervous system: a motor control problem. The Harrington lecture, 1983. Scoliosis Research Society, *Spine* 10:1-14, 1985.
25. Jensen GM, Wilson KB: Horizontal postrotatory nystagmus response in female subjects with adolescent idiopathic scoliosis, *Phys Ther* 59:1226, 1979.
26. Keim HA, Kirkaldy-Willis WH: Low back pain. *Clinical Symposia,* Summit, N.J., 1987, CIBA-GEIGY.
27. Kisner C, Colby LA: *Therapeutic exercise—foundations and techniques,* ed 2, Philadelphia, 1990, FA Davis.
28. Kostuik JP: Current concept review. Operative treatment of idiopathic scoliosis, *J Bone Joint Surg* 72A:1108-1113, 1990.
29. Levine DB: Influence of spinal deformities on chest function, *Phys Ther* 48:968, 1968.
30. Lonstein JE, Carlson JM: The prediction of curve progression in untreated idiopathic scoliosis during growth, *J Bone Joint Surg* 66A:1061-1071, 1984.
31. Lovell WW, Winter RB, editors: *Pediatric orthopedics,* ed 2, Philadelphia, 1986, JB Lippincott.
32. Macnab I: The traction spur, *J Bone Joint Surg* 53A:663-670, 1971.
33. McMaster MJ, David CV: Hemivertebra as a cause of scoliosis: a study of 104 patients, *J Bone Joint Surg* 68B:588-595, 1986.
34. Meals RA: *One hundred orthopaedic conditions every doctor should understand,* St Louis, 1992, Quality Medical Publishing.
35. Menelaus MB: Diskitis: an inflammation affecting the intervertebral disks in children, *J Bone Joint Surg* 46B:16, 1964.
36. Mielke CH, Lonstein JE, Denis F et al: Surgical treatment of adolescent idiopathic scoliosis: a comparative analysis, *J Bone Joint Surg* 71A:1117-1177, 1989.
37. Miller JA, Nachemson AL, Schultz AF: Effectiveness of braces in mild idiopathic scoliosis, *Spine* 9:632-635, 1984.

38. Moffat M: Lecture series outline from therapeutic exercise course materials. October, 1990. New York University Medical bookstore.

39. Netter FH: *The Ciba collection of medical illustrations,* vol 8, Musculoskeletal System, Part II: *Developmental disorders, tumors, rheumatic diseases, and joint replacement,* Summit, N.J., 1990, CIBA-GEIGY.

40. O'Donnell CS, Bunnell WP, Betz RR et al: Electrical stimulation in the treatment of idiopathic scoliosis, *Clin Orthop* 229:107-113, 1988.

41. Pyeritz RE, McKusick VA: The Marfan syndrome: diagnosis and management, *N Engl J Med* 300(14):772-777, 1979.

42. Quinnell RC, Stockdale HR: The significance of osteophytes on the lumbar vertebral bodies in relation to discographic findings, *Clin Radiology* 23:197-203, 1982.

43. Reichley ML: Clinicians take straightforward approach in treating people with scoliosis, *Adv Phys Ther* July 5, 1993.

44. Renshaw TS: *Congenital spinal deformity.* In: White AH, Schofferman JA, editors: *Spinal care,* Part VII, St Louis, 1995, Mosby.

45. Riddle H, Roaf R: Muscle imbalance in the causation of scoliosis, *Lancet* 1:1245, 1955.

46. Ruggerone M, Austin JHM: Moire topography in scoliosis: correlations with vertebral lateral curvature as determined by radiography, *Phys Ther* 66:1072, 1986.

47. Salter RB: *Textbook of disorders and injuries of the musculoskeletal system,* ed 2, Baltimore, 1983, Williams & Wilkins.

48. Samuelsson L, Eklof O: Scoliosis in myelomeningocele, *Acta Orthop Scand* 59:122-127, 1988.

49. Saunders HD: *Evaluation, treatment and prevention of musculoskeletal disorders,* Bloomington, Minn., 1985, Education Opportunities.

50. Seimon LP: *Low back pain—clinical diagnosis and management,* ed 2, New York, 1995, Demos Vermande.

51. Staheli LT: *Fundamentals of pediatric orthopedics,* New York, 1992, Raven Press.

52. Stone B, Beekman C, Hall V et al: The effect of an exercise program on change in curve in adolescents with minimal idiopathic scoliosis: a preliminary study, *Phys Ther* 59:759-763, 1979.

53. Uden A, Wilner S, Pettersson H: Initial correction with the Boston thoracic brace, *Acta Orthop Scand* 53:907, 1982.

54. Weinstein SL, Ponseti IV: Curve progression in idiopathic scoliosis, *J Bone Joint Surg* 65A:455-477, 1983.

55. Wenger DR, Bobechko WP, Gilday DL: The spectrum of intervertebral disk-space infection in children, *J Bone Joint Surg* 60A:100, 1978.

56. Wynne-Davies R, Gormley J: Clinical and genetic patterns in osteogenesis imperfecta, *Clin Orthop* 159:26-35, 1981.

57. Yeater R, Martin RB, White MK et al: Tethered swimming forces in the crawl, breast, and back strokes and their relationship to competitive performance, *J Biomech* 14:527, 1981.

62

Sudden, Intense, Mid-Level Back Pain in a Middle-Aged Female while Lifting a Heavy Object

CASE 1: A 52-year-old white female of slight build complains of back pain that began 4 days ago. While busy with her spring-cleaning she lifted a dinette table with both hands with the help of her daughter, and felt an acute pain in the middle of her back. The pain did not radiate and was aggravated whenever she lifted a half-gallon milk container to pour into her coffee. There was no report of night pain and the patient admits to sleeping well. She also reports good health since she kicked a smoking habit last year. She has a history of seizures, but no family history of arthritis. When asked, she admits to having had a problem with alcohol abuse, which is now under control. She freely offers that she became menopausal last year. In addition, she does not regularly exercise, and reports a childhood allergy to dairy products. Her only medication was long-term use of phenobarbital.

OBSERVATION   A lateral view of the torso suggests hyperlordosis of the cervical and lumbar spine.

PALPATION   There is point tenderness of the T9 vertebra. The paraspinal musculature offers a hard, taut feeling to the touch in the vicinity of T9.

RANGE OF MOTION   Both passive and active back range of movement is painful beyond midrange of motion.

STRENGTH   Strength of the trunk musculature was untested secondary to pain.

FLEXIBILITY   Mild tightness of bilateral hamstrings and pectoralis muscle groups noted.

RADIOGRAPHS   Lateral views of the thoracic and lumbar spine indicate anterior thoracic (T9) wedging and ballooning of the lumbar vertebral interspaces.

CLUE   A gibbus-type deformity is viewed and palpated at the ninth thoracic vertebra.

CASE 2: A 64-year-old retired male with a history of asthma for the past 15 years complains of acute low back pain that began 6 days ago when bending forward over a table. The patient complained of hearing a cracking noise followed by agonizing pain, causing him to grip the table for support until he called for help. When lying down pain eased off considerably, although it was still present. For several days the patient remained in bed and got up only to go to the bathroom, which was also painful. Over the last 2 days, pain has gradually eased. When asked, the patient admits to having similar prior episodes as well as long term prednisone therapy. Wearing his old spinal brace from the last episode provided significant relief.

OBSERVATION   This was normal.

PALPATION   Pinpoint pain at the L1 lumbar vertebra. The paraspinal musculature offers a hard, taut feeling to the touch in the vicinity of T1.

RANGE OF MOTION   Both passive and active low back range of movement is painful greater than the entire one-half range of available motion.

STRENGTH   Trunk musculature strength was untested secondary to pain. Normal lower extremity muscle strength.

FLEXIBILITY   Mild tightness of bilateral hamstrings.

RADIOGRAPHS   These reveal generalized osteoporosis in the low thoracic and high lumbar spine, and compression fracture at L1.

? Questions

1. What is the most likely cause of these patients' symptoms?
2. What are osteoporosis and osteopenia?
3. How does bone develop and what are the functions of osseous tissue?
4. What is the composition of osseous tissue?
5. What are the cellular elements of bone?
6. What is the structure of bone?
7. What is the significance of hormonal regulation of bone resorption and deposition?
8. Which two antagonistic hormones are responsible for maintenance of calcium homeostasis?
9. What is the homeostatic mechanism for regulating calcium?
10. What indirect role do systemic hormones have with respect to bone metabolism?
11. What hydraulic role do muscles offer in preventing bone fracture?
12. What is the mechanism by which mechanical deformation is transduced into electric potential that directs new bone deposition?
13. What is the relationship between applied load and bone morphology?
14. What mechanisms are required for maintenance of normal bone-mineral content?
15. How does bone remodeling vary with age?
16. What is the classification of osteoporosis?
17. What are the associated risk factors for osteoporosis?
18. Where do fractures most commonly occur in the appendicular and axial skeleton?
19. What is the clinical presentation?
20. What does radiographic imaging of osteoporosis delineate?
21. What two fracture patterns of the vertebrae may occur from osteoporosis?
22. What rehabilitative management is appropriate to patients with osteoporosis?
23. What is the role of good nutrition and supplementation therapies on bone integrity?

1. What is the most likely cause of these patients' symptoms?

A T9 vertebral compression fracture secondary to involutional osteoporosis in Case 1. In Case 2, the patient suffered a vertebral compression fracture at L1 secondary to long-term steroid therapy that induced osteoporosis. The history, combined with severe and sudden onset of pain, aggravated by movement and considerable relief while recumbent, suggests the diagnosis.

2. What are osteoporosis and osteopenia?

Osteoporosis is an age-related bone disorder characterized by loss of bone density due to a predominance of bone resorption (versus deposition), and subsequent structural weakness deriving from an enlarged medullary (marrow) and osteonal space and reduced cortical thickness. Osteoporosis is the most common skeletal disorder and is second only to arthritis as a leading cause of musculoskeletal morbidity in the elderly population. Characterized by loss of bone mass, or *osteopenia,* this disorder primarily affects the aged, particularly women over age 50, with a consequent tendency to sustain fractures from minor stress. Bone fracture is the primary complication of this disease with a predilection for *vertebral crush fractures* of the weight-bearing vertebrae (T8 and below) consisting primarily of trabecular bone, and fractures of the femoral neck and distal radius (consisting of both cortical and trabecular bone). Osteoporosis involves a greater proportional loss of trabecular than compact bone, especially horizontal trabeculae in postmenopausal women showing a considerable reduction in both thickness and number of trabecular cross-bridges.

The statistics regarding osteoporosis are staggering. Approximately 20 million Americans suffer from this silent disease, and greater than 1.2 million fractures[31] occur annually in the United States,[36] which costs nearly $14 billion per year.[52] At present, some 40 million American women are expected to reach menopause during the upcoming decade and have a life expectancy of 30 years following menopause.[56] Epidemiologic studies suggest that 1 of every 3 women over the age of 65 may be expected to have a vertebral fracture.[54] Given the expected epidemic proportions in the rise of this disease, osteoporosis is expected to be a significant cause of morbidity and mortality in the elderly.

Normally, resorption of both the organic and inorganic components of bone occurs as a function of re-

modeling of the skeletal system and because of the body's need to draw upon the calcium stores in bone for maintenance of vital body functions. The process of continuous bone remodeling results in the loss of several hundred milligrams of calcium each day through excretion. After age 25, the adult skeleton will typically undergo complete replacement every 7 years. We normally replenish calcium through appropriate dietary intake. If, however, the body has insufficient supplies of calcium due to factors such as inefficient absorption by the gut, which accompanies aging, dietary deficiency of calcium, or because of hormonal imbalance, the body will draw upon calcium reserves in bone despite the consequences of bone loss. Osteoporosis is an imbalance of calcium homeostasis due to accelerated bone loss despite the fact that the rate of bone formation is normal. Because bone resorption occurs much more quickly than formation, this individual will suffer a net loss of bone mass that leaves bones porous and full of resorption cavities due to osteoclastic activity; hence, the term osteo *(bone)* -porosis *(porous,* or full of holes.) The resulting weaker skeleton becomes biomechanically incompetent[18] and may respond to accumulated micro-stress with defective remodeling due to a shortage of calcium. The remodeling units within bone are thus incapable of keeping pace with propagation of micro-damage that occurs every day, and a critical point is reached in which bone fails under trivial loading.[17] Before discussing osteoporosis of the vertebrae and resulting compression fracture, it is appropriate to preface this process with a general discussion of structure, composition, function, and physiology of osseous tissue.

3. How does bone develop and what are the functions of osseous tissue?

Before discussing the structure of osseous tissue it is important to note that there are two types of bone tissue. Flat bones, such as the skull and scapula are very dense and thin and develop via *membranous ossification.* The other bones comprising the skeletal system are long, short, and irregular bones such as vertebrae and mature into bone from a cartilaginous state in a process known as *endochondral ossification.*

Bone provides for *mechanical support, regulation of mineral homeostasis,* as well as *hematopoiesis.* The latter role occurs in bone marrow in which red blood cells, platelets, and white blood cells are produced. In its role as an *endoskeleton,* the bones of the body serve as a structural frame that provides support, and in conjunction with skeletal muscles, as a *musculoskeletal system* of levers that allows for movement in a gravity dependent environment. Despite its deceptively inanimate appearance, bone is metabolically active in its role of regulating mineral homeostasis. Bone matrix serves as a reservoir of essential inorganic ions such as calcium, phosphate, magnesium, carbonate and sodium for use within osseous tissue as well as maintaining specific ionic concentrations in cells and blood throughout the body. The regulation of these ionic balances is mostly dependent upon hormones and mechanical stress.

4. What is the composition of osseous tissue?

Dense (cortical) bone excludes blood and fat within the bone marrow and is composed of 30% organic material and 70% inorganic minerals in adults. The organic component of bone matrix (osteoid) is composed of primarily type I collagen fiber (a fibrous protein arranged in long bundles, which is deposited along lines of mechanical stress in accordance with Wolff's law). The collagen fibrils possess high elasticity, tolerate compressive force poorly, endow bone with an ability to withstand tensile forces and serve as a template for bone crystal nucleation. Inorganic salts comprise the majority of the dry weight of bone and are flat crystal needlelike complexes of calcium carbonate and phosphate known as *hydroxyapatite* or bone apatite, account for bone's hardness and rigidity, and endow bone with the ability to withstand compressive force of up to 20,000 to 30,000 pounds per square inch.[13] Hydroxyapatite is arranged in alternating, yet asymmetric rows within a matrix bed of protein filaments similar to the composition of a clamshell. Clinically significant, the structure of these *large tricalcium phosphate crystals* is imperfect, and possesses the ability to incorporate magnesium, sodium, chloride, fluoride, and other bone-seeking radioactive elements. The advantage offered by this irregular organization is that it acts to ward off the deepening extension of stress-derived cracking so common to symmetrical constructions. The combined tensile and compressive strength offered by both the organic and inorganic components confers on bone many of the general properties exhibited by *two phase materials* such as fiberglass and bamboo, and endows osseous tissue with strength analogous to steel-reinforced concrete.

5. What are the cellular elements of bone?

Three types of cells are present in bony tissue. *Osteoblasts,* essential to formation and deposition of bone, synthesize the organic matrix, both collagen and ground substance and facilitate formation of a template upon which crystalline (inorganic) nucleation may then occur. Thus osteoblasts have the responsibility of biosynthesis and maturation of collagen into a longitudinal array of fibers, directing precipitation of crystal nuclei, and binding of the calcium to collagen that is parallel with the long axes of the collagen bundles. Bone formation, or ossification begins when osteoblasts secrete a matrix substance called *osteoid,* a gelatinous substance comprised of collagen (from the Greek word *kolla* meaning "glue" and *gen* meaning "forming") and mucopolysaccharide, organic glue. Osteoblasts are cuboidal shaped cells[16] located on the external and internal surfaces of bone that relay information via numerous filamentous channels known as *canaliculi* that transport oxygen, nutrients, and ions. In contrast, *osteocytes* are former osteoblasts that become embedded in newly formed bone matrix. These oval shaped cells reside within slitlike openings known as *lacunae* and are thought to be responsible for regulation of mineral homeostasis. Similar to their previous osteoblastic role, osteocytes maintain communication by an elaborate system of interconnecting canaliculi. Calcification results from a complex interplay between osteoblasts and osteocytes in which the latter are instrumental in seeding crystalline salts and facilitating their impregnation (deposition) within the ground substance secreted by the osteoblasts.

The mechanism by which bone cells transform mechanical or bioelectric signals into the unique configuration of bone consistent with applied stress is thought to be governed by *nucleation.* Following the principles of physical chemistry, when the concentration of solute in solution reaches a critical mass, the dynamic equilibrium between solute and solvent is upset and a nucleus of solid crystal calcium phosphate precipitates out of solution. In the body, precipitation of crystal in the blood stream is undesirable and prevented by a low pH and carbon dioxide levels.[62] In bone, the same principle applies with the osteoblasts regulating nucleation by releasing an enzyme (phosphatase) that promotes calcium phosphate nucleation, despite adverse levels of pH and carbon dioxide. This nuclear seeding serves as a core for further, rapid salt precipitation and is similar to the formation of a pearl within an oyster.

In contrast, *osteoclasts* are large, multinucleated phagocytotic-type cells that are highly mobile and are responsible for bone resorption and hence, regulate plasma-calcium concentrations. Containing proteolytic lysosomal enzymes, osteoclasts, which reside in shallow depression in trabecular bone known as *Howship's lacunae,* resorb bone by digesting the organic matrix causing dissolution of bone crystals. Resorption is a much more rapid process than bone formation, and occurs when clusters of cells erode free bone surfaces or form cutting cones that tunnel through compact bone and leave cylindrical cavities in their wake. Osteoblasts live for a few days to several weeks at most. All types of bone cells arise from undifferentiated osteogenic cells known as *mesenchymal cells* that give rise, under appropriate stimuli to either osteoblasts or osteoclasts in accordance with the needs of bone.

6. What is the structure of bone?

The adult skeleton contains two histologically different types of bone identified by their relative density. These two categories of bone are represented in a typical long bone such as the femur, tibia, or humerus, which contain *cancellous* or *trabecular* or *spongy bone* concentrated at each end, and *compact bone* forming the longitudinal walls of the shaft. Although trabecular bone is composed of an irregular network of mineralized bars of bony tissue, compact bone is composed of tubular units called *osteons.* The femoral shaft, for example, is a thick hollow tube of compact bone surrounding the longitudinal marrow cavity. The proximal and distal ends are primarily trabecular bone covered by a thin shell of compact bone.

The functional and structural unit of *cortical (compact) bone* is the microscopic *osteon,* or *Haversian system* that is oriented along the long axis of bone and named after the English anatomist Clopton Havers (1691). Similar to the rings in a tree trunk, the Haversian system consists of concentric layers of bony layers or *lamellae* that surround an innermost cylindrical *Haversian canal* containing the blood and nerves supplying that bone. The lamellae, in turn, are comprised of longitudinally oriented collagen fibrils impregnated with mineral crystals. Buried deep within small caverns called *lacunae* are live osteocytes that communicate with each other by minute channels, or *canaliculi,* which serve as vehicles of transport for oxygen, nutrients, and for communication.

In mature bone, extensive remodeling continuously occurs causing destruction and formation of many generations of osteons. Similar to the rings of a tree trunk, the newest osteons may be identified by their peripheral location on the outermost circumference of bone. Run-

ning perpendicular to the Haversian canals are bony channels known as *Volkmann's canals*[35] containing blood vessels and nerves that communicate with the periosteum and endosteum.

Periosteum is a fibrous vascular layer of tissue that covers bone except at its articular ends. The inner lining of periosteum (an osteogenic layer) is lined with osteoblasts that deposit new bone. The *endosteum* is a thin layer of connective tissue lining the walls of bone cavities in both cancellous and compact bone. The ends of long bones, and the spinal vertebrae are primarily composed of *cancellous (spongy)* or *trabecular bone* whose structure is comprised of an interlacing sponge-like network of *trabeculae,* which enclose cavities containing either red or yellow marrow. Red marrow is typically found in the embryonic state and in the newborn, but converts to yellow marrow in the adult. In the adult, red marrow is only found in the cavities of flat bones such as the ribs, sternum, and skull, and in the epiphyses of two long bones, the femur and humerus.

Cancellous bone lacks osteons and is comprised of an interlacing network of intersecting plates and spicules that form threadlike bars of bone known as *trabeculae,* which enclose space filled with blood vessels and marrow. These honeycomb-like cavities are less dense than compact bone, and are organized parallel with the direction and magnitude of major mechanical stresses. For example, in the proximal femur, three different forces account for a trabecular pattern. The strong *arcuate system,* resisting tensile forces, runs along the thick lateral cortex and arches up to the inferior border of the head and neck of the femur. The relatively straight, strong *medial system* runs along the medial cortex of the femoral neck to the superior surface of the head, and negotiates compressive forces. A weaker *lateral system* extends from the area of the lesser trochanter to the greater trochanter, and resists weaker forces of tension and compression.[51]

The external surfaces of vertebral bodies are formed by compact, cortical bone. The load bearing function of the vertebrae is derived from their external and internal structure, and may be understood by analogy to foam filling, which is used in the construction industry. This is analogous to a paper card holding up a weight. The card, corresponding to the superior vertebral endplate represents cortical bone that would readily deform from the brunt of weight. Similarly, if the weight were to bear down on a thick piece of sponge, corresponding to the cancellous bone within the vertebra, it will also deform under load. However, when the same load is applied to a composite sandwich of the materials—a sponge between two sheets of cards, there is minimal deformation despite the load. Thus it is both the external cortical as well as internal trabecular coupling of bone that endows vertebrae with light weight and strength.[50]

From an engineering perspective, trabeculae within vertebral bodies are analogous to a complex series of cross-braced struts that are organized to endow bone with maximal strength with minimal material. Despite its apparent porosity and relatively small volume, trabecular bone is remarkably well suited to resists compressive force, a major function of the vertebral body.

When bone is stressed by either tensile or compressive forces, the concave side of the bone (subjected to compression) becomes negatively charged, while the convex side of bone (subjected to compression) becomes electropositive. Thus stress-generated potentials are instrumental in bone formation at the electropositive convex aspect and bone resorption at the electronegative concave side. With regard to the vertebral body, formation and resorption is dependent upon the anatomy of the vertebra as well as postural considerations so that deposition of new bone by osteoblasts is counterbalanced by removal of bone by osteoclasts from the opposite trabecular surface. Thus the position of trabeculae within bone can shift as a function of coordinated resorption and deposition. The mechanism by which bone cells transform mechanical or bioelectric signals into the unique configuration of bone consistent with applied stress is not fully understood.

7. What is the significance of hormonal regulation of bone resorption and deposition?

The skeleton acts as a *dynamic mineral reserve* regulating the concentration of ionized calcium and phosphorus in the bloodstream. Living bone is never metabolically at rest as it constantly remodels and appropriates its mineral stores dictated by areas of stress within bone as well as the need for ionic concentrations in the blood and cells throughout the body. The extracellular needs for ions are critically important for numerous life-sustaining processes that include enzymatic reactions, mitochondrial function, cell membrane maintenance, muscle contraction, blood clotting, cell motility, neuromuscular transmission, and intercellular and interneuronal transmission and communication. A chemical equilibrium* between free ions in solution and ionic deposition within body, known as *skeletal metabolism,* is regulated by three groups of hormones: (1) hormones that regulate calcium include parathyroid hormone, vitamin D, and calcitonin; (2) systemic hormones such as growth hormone, insulin, thyroxin, estrogen, testosterone, and glucocorticoids; and (3) hormone-like factors and local factors such as somatomedins, prostaglandins, and bone growth factor. Although some of these hormones mediate osteoblasts, others mediate osteoclastic activity.

8. Which two antagonistic hormones are responsible for maintenance of calcium homeostasis?

Approximately 99% of total body calcium and 85% of total body phosphorus reside as mineral deposits within bone.[45] Bone is uniquely situated to mediate adjustment in concentration of calcium (a positive anion) and phosphate (negative cation) circulating in body fluids. Regularly fine-tuning of levels of these ionic salts is humerally controlled by two hormonal control loops (control systems with feedback): *parathyroid hormone* (PTH) and *calcitonin* (CT), both of which are concerned with regulation of calcium ion concentration. Calcium homeostasis is, therefore, a continuum of interactions among stored calcium precipitate, plasma calcium, and intracellular calcium.

9. What is the homeostatic mechanism for regulating calcium?

The basis for maintaining calcium homeostasis between soluble and precipitous calcium is governed by a feedback process. Thus bone is broken down and built up by interplay of two negative feedback systems regulating levels of blood calcium that operate antagonistically as two competing processes. Bone deposition leads to a build-up of calcium stores in the bone matrix. When serum calcium levels are low, bone is broken down by a

---

Calcium equilibrium refers to maintenance of a balance between calcium precipitate in bones and blood-plasma calcium within the confines of a narrow range. Excessive plasma calcium (caused by a tumor of the parathyroids) depresses the central nervous system, causes muscular weakness, and may cause cardiac arrest in systole. Calcium equilibrium represents a homeostatic strategy to protect against the dangers of hypocalcemia or hypercalcemia in a body that is extremely sensitive to even minor deviation of ionic calcium concentration. Thus need to regulate the level of calcium within narrow parameters is imperative to life.

process called osteogenic osteolysis in which thyrocalcitonin activates osteoclasts. In their activated state, osteoclasts break down bone matrix via enzymatic processes and liberate calcium (bone resorption), which is taken up by the blood thereby raising serum calcium levels. When calcium levels are high enough to sustain calcium-driven metabolic functions parathyroid hormone damps down and deactivates osteoclastic osteogenesis, resulting in bone deposition and calcium to be bound up (stored) in bone matrix.

Stated simply, thyroid *calcitonin* activates osteoclasts causing a release of calcium into the blood stream via osteolysis, whereas *parathyroid hormone* deactivates osteoclasts and thus terminates osteolysis. Parathyroid hormone, having a long-term effect, is to the calcium level in blood as glucagon is to the glucose level. Being very sensitive to the amount of plasma calcium, parathyroid hormone will be released and act to raise blood calcium by stimulating osteoclastic bone resorption. Low levels of plasma calcium may be caused by inadequate dietary intake of calcium, pregnancy, poor intestinal calcium absorption because of an excessive amount of other competing minerals, or from inadequate amounts of vitamin D.* Although calcitonin section is directly related to calcium ion concentration, parathyroid hormone is inversely related to calcium ion concentration. Calcitonin, being fast-acting and of short duration, acts in opposition to parathyroid hormone, as insulin acts in opposition to glucagon.[62]

10. What indirect role do systemic hormones have with respect to bone metabolism?

In addition to parathyroid hormone and thyrocalcitonin directly regulating bone formation and resorption, other endocrine hormones indirectly modify this process. *Growth hormone* regulates the deposition of collagen and chondroitin sulfate, as well as accelerating division of osteoblasts, thereby lengthening and widening bone before epiphyseal closure. Once the epiphyses have closed, growth hormone acts to increase bone girth (thickness).† *Insulin,* an anabolic hormone, acts in synergy with growth hormone to stimulate bone and carti-

lage directly and indirectly by way of *somatomedins* (pituitary-dependent growth factors). Thus children with juvenile-onset diabetes will frequently present with diminished bone mass. *Thyroxine* is a thyroid hormone essential for normal bone development. Whereas hyperthyroidism increases osteoclastic resorption, hypothyroidism will result in impaired bone growth and maturation. Prostaglandins are potent hormone-like molecules that play a number of systemic and local roles. *Prostaglandins* are powerful stimulators of bone resorption and are released as part of the pain cycle associated with degenerative joint disease.

The *sex hormones* include estrogen and testosterone, which promote longitudinal growth of bones as well as epiphyseal closure. Because levels of these hormones are elevated at puberty, growth of long bones terminates several years following puberty. Because estrogen is more effective than testosterone in closing the epiphyses, females usually stop growing in height before males. In contrast, testosterone promotes bone growth and continued calcium deposition so that male bones are relatively thicker and stronger.

With regard to osteoporosis, estrogen has a significant role in protecting both the axial and appendicular skeleton from osteopenia. Following menopause, estrogen deficiency leads to an increase in the rate of bone turnover, with resorption dominating formation such that each cycle of normal bone remodeling following menopause puts back less bone than it takes out, resulting in diminished bone mass. Estrogen is postulated to play an important role in prevention of calcium loss by exerting a tonic inhibitory effect on the skeletal action of parathormone[3] as well as a role of preventing loss of vitamin D at the kidney tubule.[62] Administration of estrogen to postmenopausal women may improve their proclivity to poor calcium absorption, and may increase bone sensitivity to parathyroid hormone and thus improve calcium deposition.[28]

11. What hydraulic role do muscles offer in preventing bone fracture?

Muscles play an indispensable role in prevention of fracture to adjacent bone by way of offering impedance of fluid outflow in cancellous bone. Because blood is a liquid, it is subject to the laws of hydraulics. In contrast to the gaseous state, liquids such as blood are categorized as inelastic fluids, which may be subjected to significant stress and experience negligible volume changes so as to be virtually incompressible. This has physiologic implications regarding the role intramedul-

---

*Provitamin D is either ingested or synthesized from cholesterol in the liver and stored in the skin. Sunlight in the ultraviolet frequency range activates provitamin D into vitamin D (cholecalciferol), a steroid, which is then stored in the liver until needed. Vitamin D enhances active transport of calcium through the intestinal cells.

†Excessive secretion of growth hormone before epiphyseal ossification causes *gigantism,* whereas some types of *dwarfism* are associated with an abnormally low level of growth hormone secretion.

lary blood has upon bone during osseous compression. Because one of the primary roles of bone marrow is the formation of blood cells, blood is normally present within cancellous endosteal bone. Normally, when bones undergo compression, blood contained within the cancellous bone as well as other fluids from the marrow cavity are forced out of bone through small foramina in the bone surface. However, the state of contraction of the surrounding musculature causes impedance of fluid outflow from the marrow cavity. In this normal state, the presence of contained fluid at increased pressure represents a hydraulic mechanism to attenuate compressive forces that may otherwise be potentially destructive to bone. This system works to dissipate the considerable magnitude of forces on bone that might result in fracture. In contrast, if the surrounding musculature is relaxed or paralyzed at the time of contraction, there is little or no impedance of intramedullary fluid outflow, bone marrow pressure remains depressed, and excessive force may be transmitted to the bone. Thus the ability of the surrounding muscles to develop an effective degree of hydraulic support is dependent on strong and timely contraction of the surrounding muscles. Older persons have a diminished capacity to activate this hydraulic bone sparing strategy because of the progressive loss in muscle strength with age. By the seventh decade of life, the average maximum voluntary contraction is at least 20% lower than in young adults. As a result, older persons are more susceptible to bone failure secondary to diminished impedance of intramedullary fluid outflow.

12. What is the mechanism by which mechanical deformation is transduced into electric potential that directs new bone deposition?

Bone is remarkably active despite its apparent inanimate nature. In the adult, for example, 3% to 5% of the total skeleton is being actively remodeled to adjust to the changing environmental and physiological demands at any one time. How is it that mechanical stress is interpreted by osseous tissue as a stimulus for bone formation and resorption? The mechanism by which bone formation and resorption are postulated to occur is a direct function of induced local electric fields that generate *bioelectric potentials* across osseous tissue. It is believed that these local electrical fields mediate the information exchange regarding lines of stress that regulate bone cells. Microelectric potentials are generated in the connective tissue within bone by both a *piezoelec-*

tric effect and *flow potentials.* The latter refers to generation of micropotentials (flow potentials) created within bone as the result of an increased rate of blood flow through vessels in bone, caused by intermittent contraction of overlying muscles. Although the net micropotentials deriving from either source are inadequate in producing a significant effect upon bone when considered separately, the cumulative effects of micropotentials from both sources generate enough potential to stimulate both secretion of procollagen by osteoblasts as well as deposition of bone crystals and calcium salts within bone matrix.[29]

Many nonconducting crystals or semicrystalline materials are comprised of both positively and negatively charged particles in equal distribution. Certain crystals, such as Feldspar quartz, tourmaline, Rochelle salt, and ceramic materials have an intrinsic separation of positive and negative charges giving rise to potential differences across the crystal. If mechanical energy in the form of pressure is applied to such crystals, the potential energy inherent in the crystal is expressed as an electromotive force, or voltage is induced.* Mechanical pressure polarizes the crystal by separating the center of positive charge from the negative charge so that equal and unlike charges build up on the opposite faces of the crystal. This effect was first discovered by the brothers Pierre and Jacques Curie in 1880[2] who named this phenomenon *piezoelectricity* (meaning electricity through pressure.) The potential difference (voltage) between the opposite crystal faces causes induction of an electric field. Bone is similarly comprised of (inorganic) hydroxyapatite crystals as well as (organic) collagen, which together endow osseous tissue with a piezoelectric ability. Deformation of bone by mechanical force induces a millivolt charge proportional to the applied force.

Bone modeling, growth and resorption, occurs as a direct function of the forces transmitted to bone. These forces generate small micropotentials in the connective tissue throughout bone. The piezoelectric phenomenon within living bone directs both osteoblastic and osteo-

---

*The reverse is true as well. When placing a piezoelectric crystal within an electric field, the crystal alters its shape. If the potential difference is applied and terminated repeatedly, the crystal is induced to vibrate and produce sound waves. This interconversion between electrical and acoustic energy may be amplified as they are in record players, microphones, submarine sonar, wave filters in telephone communication systems, or for emission of ultrasonic frequencies within the transducer heads of diagnostic or therapeutic ultrasound.

clastic activity. Regions under tension serve as *anode* whereas compressed regions represent a *cathode.* Bone accumulates about the cathode as the microcurrent aligns collagen fibrils and organic salts as they aggregate out of solution. When bone undergoes deformational stress the mechanical energy is transducted into a microvoltage that stimulates osteoblast activity at the negative end[62] and osteoclastic activity at the positive end of current flow.[45]

13. What is the relationship between applied load and bone morphology?

Galileo, in 1683, was the first individual credited for recognizing a relationship between body weight and bone. Although subsequent investigators noted that bone undergoes remodeling, the *direct relationship between bone morphology and applied load* was mathematically described by the German anatomist Julius Wolff. In his Law of Bone Transformation in 1892 he noted that changes in bone mass accompanied changes in load through a process of skeletal remodeling. In other words, *form follows function.* Bone formation will occur in areas where bone undergoes the greatest stress, whereas a bone that is underutilized, such as an immobilized leg, will undergo resorption.

The most remarkable example of *Wolff's law* clarifies the relationship between form and function when we consider the role of gravity upon the musculoskeletal system. During the early American Gemini and Apollo space flights as well as the 84-day Skylab mission, studies of the calcareous tissue of astronauts indicated a rapid and extensive cortical and trabecular bone loss akin to osteoporosis, as well as a decrease in muscle mass incurred during even brief periods of weightlessness. With prolonged weightlessness, however, full recovery of bone is less likely because of irreversible loss of trabecular scaffolding necessary for bone strength. The intersecting network of trabeculae is a biomechanical response to the sum of compressive and tensile forces derived from internally generated muscular contraction, and external forces such as superincumbent body weight and ground reaction forces. Thus both the inorganic as well as organic components of bone are deposited along lines of mechanical stress in accordance with Wolff's law. In contrast, physical activity may increase both bone volume and density as in the case of cavalrymen, who have been known to develop new bone in the thighs and buttocks (ischium) as a result of excessive horse riding.[62]

14. What mechanisms are required for maintenance of normal bone-mineral content?

Weight bearing alone, however, is an inadequate stimulus for maintenance of bone-mineral content. For astronauts as well as individuals confined to bed, rapid decalcification will occur despite performance of rigorous exercises. This is borne out by individuals with poliomyelitis of the calf musculature who, during the course of their day, stand for many hours but fail to demonstrate any increase in bone and muscle density in the affected leg. Thus both compression of bone and simultaneous activity of overlying muscles are needed to prevent loss of bone and facilitate stimulation of new bone growth.

15. How does bone remodeling vary with age?

Bone remodeling is most active during those childhood years of active growth, when skeletal growth results in bone deposition that outpaces the rate of resorption. Once skeletal maturity is reached during adolescence deposition and resorption remain in balance until approximately age 35. With aging, the balance between the rate of bone formation and resorption changes, leading to a net decrease in bone mass that differs in males and females. As a general rule, normal aging in males manifests as a decrease in formation of bone, whereas women are subject to increased bone resorption.[38] From the fourth decade the resorption rate exceeds the formation rate resulting in a loss of bone mass of five to ten percent per decade[49] regardless of gender. A decrease in bone mass may be noted in normal human females by their mid-forties,[49] and in the mid-fifties in males. As bone mass diminishes, the bone is remodeled to distribute its mass as far as possible from the central axis of the bone. This has the effect of increasing the load to failure, especially when bone is loaded in torsion. Cortical thickness also decreases linearly with age.[2] Blacks have a larger bone mass at maturity than whites.[62] In males of all ages, and in females over the age of 65, reduction of bone density occurs in both cortical and trabecular bone.[45]

16. What is the classification of osteoporosis?

The most common type of osteoporosis is known as primary, *evolutional,* or the *involutional* forms of the disease that may, in turn, be subdivided into two types. Type I is *postmenopausal osteoporosis* and occurs in females aged 51 to 75 years. Estrogen deficiency is implicated as a primary causative factor. This form of osteoporosis affects trabecular bone primarily in the appendicular skeleton, and manifests as vertebral and Colles fractures. The type II form of the disease, known as *senile osteoporosis* occurs as a direct function of the aging process and presents in males and females over 70 years old, manifesting as fractures of the hip, pelvis, and proximal humerus and tibia. The two forms of the disease differ in that osteopenia associated with type I form of the disease is disproportionate to, and more extensive than the osteopenia associated with type II osteoporosis.[4]

17. What are the associated risk factors for osteoporosis?

Those factors that predispose some individuals to osteoporosis may be considered *risk factors*. The most significant factor in the development of osteoporosis in postmenopausal females is *estrogen deficiency. Age* is also considered a significant risk factor as the imbalance between the rate of bone formation and the rate of resorption leads to a net loss of bone. *Endocrine abnormalities* secondary to hypogonadism, ovariectomy, hyperthyroidism, hyperparathyroidism, or hyperadrenalism (Cushing's syndrome) may lead to a profound loss of bone mass. *Drug-induced* bone loss such as long term use of the anticoagulant agent heparin or steroids such as prednisone may cause significant osteopenia. *Disuse osteoporosis* may result from either focal or generalized *immobilization*. Focal disuse osteoporosis involves a single bone or limb, which is affected by arthritis or bone fracture. With generalized immobilization, profound bone loss in the appendicular skeleton may result from prolonged bed rest or paralysis. *Nutritional deficiency* also plays an important role in the development of osteoporosis. *Alcoholism,* and associated poor diet, are the most common causes of bone loss in young adolescent men, as it directly depresses osteoblastic activity.[10] With advancing age, calcium and vitamin D absorption from the upper gastrointestinal tract becomes less efficient, necessitating more dietary calcium in older persons to maintain an adequate calcium balance. Moreover, elderly persons typically have meager exposure to sunlight and decreased intake of milk and other dairy products causing mild *vitamin D and calcium deficiency,* respectively. Patients who have undergone gastrectomy may demonstrate diminished calcium absorption. Increased protein intake accelerates calcium excretion by the kidney, which may account for the prevalence of osteoporosis in western industrialized countries where *a high-protein diet* is common.

Lack of sufficient *vitamin C intake* (an essential cofactor in collagen metabolism) may also result in decreased bone mass. *Anorexia nervosa* is an important cause of osteopenia in young women.[12] There is a higher incidence of osteoporotic hip and spinal fractures among smokers, as *smoking* may indirectly increase bone loss by enhancing the degradation of estrogen.[10] *Caffeine* has also been shown to increase the risk of osteoporotic fractures in middle-aged women.[63] Other risk factors include the Caucasian or Asian races, early menopause (as from premature ovarian failure), being underweight, living a sedentary lifestyle, lactose intolerance, family history of osteoporosis, a history of gastric or small bowel resection, long-term anticonvulsant therapy, and having freckles, blond or red hair,[49] multiparity, and breast feeding.[26]

18. Where do fractures most commonly occur in the appendicular and axial skeleton?

Osteoporotic compression fractures occur when the cumulative effects of osteopenia are sufficiently advanced that the structural integrity of trabecular bone can no longer tolerate simple mechanical stress. Reduction of bone mineral density by one-third reduces compressive strength of the vertebral body to one-ninth of normal, whereas reduction by one-half reduces compressive strength to one-quarter of normal.[6] Fracture may occur throughout the axial and appendicular skeleton, particularly at sites of trabecular bone remodeling such as the femoral neck, the proximal humerus, the distal radius and ulna, and especially, the thoracic and lumbar vertebrae. In fact, women who suffer a Colles fracture during middle age have a significantly higher risk of femoral neck fracture later in life.[20]

19. What is the clinical presentation?

The clinically silent form of osteoporotic vertebrae refers to patients whose vertebrae undergo a gradual series of micro-fractures over a protracted time period who are asymptomatic or at most complain of chronic back pain.[45] Radiographs of osteoporotic vertebrae reveal a definite pattern of bone atrophy characterized by a striking deficiency of horizontal trabeculae and preservation of vertically oriented trabeculae. As the horizontal trabeculae provide cross-bracing support that resists compressive loading, considerable loss of bone strength will occur.

More commonly, the earliest manifestation of osteoporosis is acute regional back pain secondary to a low thoracic or high lumbar vertebral compression fracture precipitated by routine activities such as standing-up, bending, or lifting. Pain may last from several days up to three to four weeks,[66] and may be referred to the low lumbar and lumbosacral region. Although vertebral compression fractures are usually stable injuries, associated structural changes may disturb the facet joints and alter the size of the intervertebral foramina leading to radiculopathy, although radicular pain to the lower extremities is rare. More likely, thoracic or high lumbar compression fractures will cause either unilateral or bilateral pain radiating anteriorly along the costal margins of the affective nerve root.[30] In the event of a coexistent spinal stenosis, neurogenic claudication may worsen owing to diminished space within the neural canal.[54]

Other associated symptoms include radiation of pain anteriorly or into the flank, nausea, abdominal pain, chest pain, strain-exacerbated pain such as coughing, sneezing and straining to move the bowels,[34] loss of appetite, abdominal distention, and ileus secondary to retroperitoneal hemorrhage. The resulting thoracic kyphosis displaces the body's center of gravity forward, and results in compensatory hyperlordosis of the cervical and lumbar curves. These compensatory changes in the curve of the spine, both above as well as below the level of the fracture site, result in a cascade of symptoms. This period of accommodation lasts about 9 months after which the patient becomes asymptomatic. However, some patients have persistent back pain for as long as 6 months after the fracture.[25]

Fracture may occur following a trivial movement such as turning over in bed, lifting a weight, coughing, sneezing, bending forward to pick an object off the floor or tie one's shoe, rising from a chair, a minor slip or twist, or as a result of a fall. Generally, the more cephalad vertebrae (thoracic) are endowed with less bone mineral content, and are thus predisposed to the greater likelihood of fracture than the lower (lumbar) vertebrae.[49] There is generally localized tenderness to pressure over the spinous process as well as associated muscle spasm. Spinal movements are severely restricted. Although pain intensifies from weight bearing, that is, from the sitting or standing posture, considerable relief is afforded by bed rest in the fully recumbent position.

A vertebral crush fracture results in both loss of height and forward tilt causing a *dowager's hump* and having the characteristic radiographic appearance of anterior thoracic wedging and ballooning of the lumbar vertebral interspaces.[50] Multiple compression fractures may lead to a posture of progressive *dorsal kyphosis,*

and secondary cervical and lumbar hyperlordosis. The patient's height may decrease between 2 and 4 cm with each episode of segmental vertebral collapse. Once vertebral collapse has progressed to the lower segments, the ribs rest on the iliac crest and further loss is unlikely. Impingement of the twelfth rib on the iliac crest may be a source of cosmetic embarrassment as well as back and girdle pain to some patients. Here, palpation between the rib and pelvis is difficult in the seated patient. The offending rib is tender and excision may yield welcome relief.[19] In this late stage of the disease, the side effects of kyphosis and diminished height are decreased size of the thoracic and abdominal cavities, which cause early satiety and restrictive hypoventilation. Circumferential abdominal skin folds develop at the costal and pelvic margins as the disease progresses.[45] The associated lumbar hyperlordosis is accompanied by abdominal protrusion and manifests as a chronic dull, aching pain due to stress placed upon the lumbar spinal muscles and ligaments.[50] Sequential vertebral fracture may culminate in structural changes so severe as to be almost indistinguishable from idiopathic scoliosis.[47] In very severe cases of osteopenia, a fracture may recur in a previously compressed and healed vertebral body.

20. What does radiographic imaging of osteoporosis delineate?

Often, an unsuspected reduction in bone density, signifying loss of mineral content, may be revealed during routine radiographic screening, although apparent density may be influenced by a number of technical factors. In some cases, radiographs may not show loss of bone mass until the disease process is advanced. This is because the radiological signs of demineralization are not readily apparent because up to one-third of skeletal mass is typically lost before evidence of bone rarefaction on plain radiographs.[55] Radiographs are valuable when they detect structural changes of the spine caused by osteopenia secondary to disuse osteoporosis that include: biconcavity and wedging of the vertebrae on lateral films of the thoracic and lumbar spine; prominence of the vertebral endplates; osteophytic absence; and vertical striations secondary to loss of horizontal trabeculae and preservation of horizontal trabeculae that may in some instances become thicker than normal.[49] In contrast to a benign concave deformity indicating osteopenia, an angular deformity is more likely to denote an underlying malignancy.[5] A thick dense band of increased horizontal density or pseudocallus adjacent to the fractured end plates caused by persistence of calcified cartilage suggests Cushing's syndrome.[49] The latter disease is characterized by an abnormally high secretion of corticosteroids, resulting in bone loss and subsequent fracture. Bone scanning is useful in documenting new compression fracture in persons with preexisting vertebral collapse. In uncomplicated postmenopausal osteoporosis, results of routine laboratory tests are normal.

21. What two fracture patterns of the vertebrae may occur from osteoporosis?

Vertebral compression fractures may be radiographically subdivided into those that manifest as wedging of the vertebral body and those that do not. Vertebrae with relatively high bone mineral content are more prone to central compression fractures, whereas wedge fractures are more likely to occur in vertebrae with low mineral content.[45]

ANTERIOR WEDGE COMPRESSION FRACTURES

When vertebrae experience vertical compressive force, trabecular damage to the horizontal trabeculae occurs in a sequential manner, followed by the oblique and vertical trabeculae, and finally succumbing to fracture of the bone cortex. The latter usually occurs at the anterior or anterolateral aspect of the vertebral body, resulting in anterior or anterolateral *wedging* of the bone, producing the characteristic kyphus. This type of fracture pattern, most commonly in the lower thoracic or upper lumbar spine, results in a sudden, severe episode of incapacitating back pain. This fracture pattern may also occur from forced spinal flexion from a blow across the shoulders that imparts a vertical compressive forces distally along the vertebrae.[5] Wedge fractures, most common in postmenopausal osteoporosis, cause increased mechanical strain upon spinal segments above and below the fracture site, with stretching of the ligaments of the apophyseal joints, the ligamenta flavum, the supraspinous ligament, and paravertebral muscles. Consequently, an alteration in the diameter of the intervertebral foramen at or adjacent to that spinal level may result in compression or stretching of one or more nerve roots.

BICONCAVE CENTRAL END PLATE COMPRESSION FRACTURE

This is demonstrated evidence of microfracture on radiographic review despite the fact that the vertebral bone cortex remains intact and no displacement occurs.

Microfractures are observed as small, local condensations of the trabecular network, most often as short, horizontal, pencil-thin marks that interrupt the regular honeycomb pattern typical of normal cancellous bone. The intervertebral disk develops a biconcave appearance as subcortical microfractures cause the disk to encroach into the adjacent vertebrae and is described as a "cod fish vertebra."[27] This fracture pattern most commonly occurs in the lumbar spine.

SYMMETRIC TRANSVERSE COMPRESSION FRACTURE

Collapse of the vertebral body causes it to assume a waferlike appearance that is so compressed as to be thinner than the intervertebral disk. When occurring at a single vertebral segment exclusively, this fracture pattern suggests a condition other than osteoporosis, such as metastatic disease, hemangioma or eosinophilic granuloma. Collapse may occur suddenly and spontaneously and is associated with sudden and severe pain.[61]

22. What rehabilitative management is appropriate to patients with osteoporosis?

The role of prevention of the osteoporotic disease process is paramount. Although cortical bone retains its capacity to repair or replace bone throughout life, trabecular bone does not. Loss of cancellous bone involves both a reduction in the thickness of trabeculae and an irrevocable loss of horizontal trabeculae, so that repair is limited to merely buttressing those trabecular bridges that remain intact. Thus even if normal bone density is once again achieved via exercise, hormonal therapy, and diet, trabecular loss remains permanent and represents significant loss of mechanical strength of bone. Several therapeutic regimens have been shown to reduce demineralization, and some may even increase total body calcium, including hormone replacement therapy, calcium, vitamin D, anabolic steroids, fluoride, calcitonin, and bisphosphonates. Nevertheless, it has yet to be proven that supplemental therapy can reduce the incidence of subsequent fractures. Because of this, early detection as well as early halting of the progression of osteoporosis is important and the role of physical therapy in the management of osteoporosis is both preventative as well as therapeutic.

Although osteoporotic compression fracture may cause significant short-term morbidity, healing occurs quickly, even in significantly osteopenic bone. The goals of therapy include pain relief, provision of an orthosis to improve spinal support, improvement of daily living activities, prevention of musculoskeletal and cardiopulmonary decompensation from excessive bed rest, and providing reassurance and encouragement to the patient. Management following compression fracture may be subdivided into preambulatory and postambulatory periods.

PREAMBULATORY PERIOD

This usually takes up to a 2-week period of bed rest for severe pain to subside as healing of damaged tissue commences. Many patients require short term analgesics or narcotic medication, particularly when muscle spasm is prominent, but side-effects may include respiratory depression, urinary retention, and constipation. These problems as well as disuse muscle and bone atrophy[60] from bed rest are countered by antigravity active limb and breathing exercises. The patient should preferably lie in the supine position with a pillow beneath bent knees to relieve lower back strain as well as a single pillow under the head, unless a cardiopulmonary condition is present. A firm mattress will prevent spinal flexion, which may aggravate a traumatic kyphosis. Use of a sheepskin mattress cover will reduce the risk of pressure sores over bony (spinous) processes. Transcutaneous electrical stimulation (TENS) applications may help alleviate pain, but should be set at a low frequency so as to avoid strong paravertebral muscle contractions. Gentle massage and moist heat may also provide pain relief. Once the acute pain begins to subside, the patient may initiate bed mobility exercises as well as short sitting for 10 to 15 minutes several times per day whereas continuing intermittent bed rest. During this period of recumbence the patient should perform deep breathing pursed-lip exercises so as to keep the lungs ventilated properly. Breathing exercises to strengthen the diaphragm may help counter respiratory problems that may occur from diminished thoracic expansion in the individual with multiple vertebral compression fracture.

If fracture of L1 or L2 has occurred, the celiac sympathetic ganglion may be affected and cause upset to the sympathetic nervous system that may manifest as paralytic ileus and orthostatic hypertension. Although the former often resolves after several days without treatment or by simply drinking large quantities of fluid, the latter may be more persistent and present as more of an obstacle in returning the patient to her premorbid functional level. Orthostatic hypertension may also occur from inactivity and being confined to bed and partly due to digestive difficulties. Thus before allowing the patient to stand, a tilt table is used that gradually (i.e., in increments of 10°) places the patient in an increasingly vertically position. The patient should be able to tolerate the erect posture for at least 5 minutes, without accompanying nausea or syncope, before attempting weight bearing.[57] Once this is accomplished, the patient may sit in a chair close to the bed for longer intervals until the patient is capable of spending most of the day sitting.

Bracing is necessary as it helps control pain by immobilizing the thorax and relieving the stress of aching spinal muscles and ligaments adjacent to the fracture site while enabling healing to progress. Bracing should be worn on attempted weight bearing, until the fracture is healed. A rigid thoracolumbar hyperextension orthosis provides external support and alleviates flexion forces on the affected vertebral segments. Because many patients find this type of brace cumbersome and restrictive, a more comfortable three-point semirigid thoracolumbar extension orthosis with porous cloth and Velcro fastenings discourages kyphosis and may be substituted. Alternately, a brace with a shoulder harness is readily washable, and may be worn under patient clothing.

AMBULATORY PERIOD

This may commence once the patient can get out of bed. Assisted standing and ambulation should begin using a walker, which, if too short, may place unnecessary strain on the fractured vertebral segment. Low-heeled and soft-soled shoes with foam inserts act to cushion the concussive forces transmitted to the spine during ambulation. The patient should progress to a less dependent assistive device proportionate with her pain, endurance, and confidence level. A daily program of active spinal extension exercises rehabilitates the paravertebral musculature and serves to decrease deforming flexion forces on the spine. Flexion exercises of the trunk are contraindicated as they may risk re-fracture of the already damaged vertebra or cause new fractures. A cardiopulmonary endurance program to increase stamina is appropriate at this time and swimming using the backstroke is an excellent rehabilitative exercise. After 6 to 8 weeks, many patients are relatively pain free and may resume normal activity.

PATIENT EDUCATION

Patient education is an essential part of therapy in the management of osteoporosis. The patient must be counseled regarding the importance of activity with regard to the musculoskeletal and cardiopulmonary systems, as well as strategies to reduce the progressive loss of bone. Patients must be instructed how to avoid unnecessary spinal compressive forces during lifting and bending. Instead of carrying heavy groceries, recommend that they use a shopping wagon or go with a friend who can help carry packages. It is important to assess the patient's home environment for the presence of throw rugs, which should be eliminated, whereas night lights, handrails, and shower mats should be recommended. Patients should have their eyesight checked and be advised to reduce or eliminate alcohol consumption, carbonated drinks, and smoking.

As older persons cannot tolerate cold as well as younger people can, prolonged exposure to cold may cause body temperatures to drop, leading to dizziness and falling. Because of this it is important to ensure that the thermostat at home is set no lower than 65° at night. Vision and hearing tests should be tested regularly. The use of an assistive device in patients who complain of feeling unsteady is wise, particularly at night when they wake up. It is important to inspect the patient's home for clutter or barriers that may cause the patient to fall. Lines and extension cords must be hidden away from walkways where they can cause someone to trip and fall. In the kitchen, items used every day should be placed within easy reach so as to avoid unnecessary bending or stooping. If a second floor is present, sturdy handrails should be installed on both sides of the stairwell to help break a fall. The first and last step should be marked with bright tape and light switches should be installed at the top and bottom of stairways. Nightlights should be present in hallways, bedrooms, and bathrooms. A nonskid rubber underliner should be placed under all area rugs, whereas linoleum floors should have a regular application of nonskid floor wax. Grab bars should be installed on the walls of the tub and shower, and beside the toilet. Nonskid mats are recommended on all standing surfaces that may become wet. It is essential to wear a nonskid (rubber) sole and low-heeled shoes. Wearing only socks or smooth-soled shoes or slippers, especially on waxed floors makes it very easy to slip and fall. Special caution should be taken in walking outdoors on wet and icy pavement. The patient with hypotension should take care to rise up out of the sitting position slowly to avoid dizziness with sudden change of posture.[43]

EXERCISE

As exercise is vital for normal bone, a daily program of walking, bicycling, rowing, or swimming is recommended, whereas activities that twist the back such as bowling and tennis are discouraged. Exercises should be enjoyable and should aim to maintain good posture, cardiorespiratory fitness, and should include low-impact aerobics, walking, stationary bicycle activities, and extension exercises. The intensity of exercise, the frequency of attendance, and the duration of the program all appear to be strongly and positively correlated with beneficial changes to bone density.[25] A 30-minute exercise consisting of walking, jogging, or dancing, or an exercise strengthening program of 10 to 15 minutes of isometric or isotonic muscle contraction of the extremities, or trunk muscle with weights attached to the ankles and wrists can improve bone density.[49] As little as 1 hour of aerobic exercises per day, 2[53] or 3[45] times a week, can prevent bone loss. Stretching exercises for all the major muscle groups, especially the pectoral musculature, before strength training is very important to maintain proper flexibility. Prophylactic exercise should not be considered as a substitute for drug treatment, but rather an adjunct to an eclectic management strategy of osteoporosis. When osteoporosis is severe or extensive, care should be taken to select an exercise program in which the mechanical forces transmitted through the weight-bearing bones do not cause pathological fracture.

An activity program may well result in changes in bone density. In most persons, an *exercise program* may slow the rate of reduction due to bone loss, whereas in some cases, bone loss may be completely halted or even increased.[39] Whereas normal bone, governed by Wolff's law increases density and cortical thickness is always associated with an increase in bone strength, this does not occur in the same manner in osteoporotic bone. In the latter, increased bone deposition is confined to the endosteal surface and in building up those remaining trabecular bridges. Thus restoration of bone density, whether in astronauts who have returned to Earth after a prolonged space flight or in osteoporotic persons who have taken an aggressive approach to combat their disease, at best regains near normal bone density while lacking the original mechanical strength of bone due to irrevocably lost trabecular bridging.

23. What is the role of good nutrition and supplementation therapies on bone integrity?

High oral *calcium supplementation,*[49] especially in the early postmenopausal years acts to primarily buttress cortical bone[44] and has no effect on trabecular bone loss.[49] Because a calcium intake of up to 1500 mg per day, the equivalent of six glasses of milk, may significantly reduce bone loss if combined with a low estrogen dose (of 0.3 mg per day) calcium intake is highly recommended.[8] The recommended dietary calcium dose is 1000 mg per day for patients on estrogen therapy, 1200-1500 mg per day for post-menopausal women who do not take supplemental estrogen, and 1000 mg per day for men.[37] There is greater bioavailability of calcium from calcium citrate or gluconate than from calcium carbonate.[1] Moreover, the latter may cause bloating and constipation. One glass of milk contains approximately 300 mg of elemental calcium.[49] Low fat (2%) milk is preferable as it will additionally help reduce cholesterol intake in atherosclerosis minded patients. Calcium-rich foods include milk products and fish such as oysters, sardines, salmon, and shrimp. Vegetables high in calcium include broccoli, soybeans, turnip greens, kidney beans, collards, and Chinese cabbage (bok choy.) Other sources of high-calcium foods include tofu, orange juice, dried figs, and sesame and sunflower seeds.[11] Too much calcium in the diet may result in the development of kidney stones. Care should be exercised by patients with a personal or family history of kidney stones to prevent excessive daily ingestion of calcium.[32]

During pregnancy and lactation, the demands for calcium sharply rise. If not enough dietary calcium is available for the skeletal system of the growing fetus, calcium will be supplied in sufficient amounts through the placenta against a concentration gradient so that the fetus is provided its needed share at the expense of the stored calcium from the maternal skeletal system. The severity of this depletion intensifies during lactation when 330 to 400 mg of calcium is lost daily via breast milk. Unless this amount is replaced, the maternal skeleton will suffer damage.[21] Thus supplemental calcium intake is recommended at 2000 mg per day for lactating women.[41]

Vitamin D supplementation therapy is indicated when there is calcium malabsorption or coexisting vitamin D deficiency. Vitamin D, considered a steroid hormone in its mode of action, facilitates increased intestinal calcium absorption in the elderly. Supplemental intake should be at least 400 IUD per day. In addition,

patients should seek increased body surface exposure to sunlight. Few food sources are good sources of vitamin D. Only cod liver oil and some fatty fish, such as salmon and mackerel are good sources. Fluoride treatment for osteoporosis is widely used in Europe, and femoral neck fractures are less common in populations drinking fluoridated water than in people consuming nonfluoridated drinking water.[10] Fluoride stimulates osteoblastic formation of new bone matrix and increased bone formation[46] in cancellous (but not cortical) bone resulting in newly generated trabecular crossbridging, and hence an increased strength of trabecular bone.[58] The recommended dose in 0.5 to 1.0 mg per kilogram of body weight (30 to 80 mg per day.) However, fluoride therapy without concomitant intake of calcium and vitamin D may lead to severe osteomalacia of bone.[48]

Exogenous *estrogen replacement therapy* may be administered transdermally or orally and confers an almost 50% reduction in the incidence of fractures,[58] as well as relieving menopausal symptoms. Estrogen acts to restore bone mass to its premenopausal level, and when combined with progesterone serves to facilitate substantial gain of bone mass in both the appendicular and axial skeleton.[62] Estrogen replacement therapy should preferably be administered close to menopause to obtain the maximal beneficial effect and should be continued for 10 to 15 years.* However, because estrogen administration is associated with an increased risk of endometrial carcinoma[10] in women with intact uteri, simultaneous ingestion of progesterone should also be taken. The latter reduces the possibility of cancer by inducing endometrial sloughing. Estrogen may be helpful in protecting against the likelihood of coronary heart disease, as it improves serum atherosclerotic risk factors. Total cholesterol and low-density lipoproteins are reduced, whereas high-density lipoprotein cholesterol is increased.[59] In contrast, estrogen replacement therapy may be related with a higher incidence of gallstones, hypertension, pulmonary embolism, and venous thrombosis as it exposes the liver to higher estrogen concentrations in the portal vein. The risk of breast cancer resulting from estrogen administration for osteoporosis is controversial. Estrogen replacement therapy is contraindicated in the presence of breast or endometrial cancer, as well as osteosclerosis. Relative contraindica-

---

*Exogenous estrogen is often prescribed in the form of birth control pills for amenorrheic athletes. This is problematic as the level of estrogen in birth control pills is below that produced during the normal menstrual cycle.

tions include a history of jaundice or liver disease, diabetes mellitus, hypertension, history of phlebothrombosis, endometriosis, uterine fibrosis, obesity, tobacco use, or a family history of breast cancer.[15]

Calcitonin has a direct action on bone consisting of inhibiting osteoclastic resorption and in this manner prevents loss of calcium and phosphate to the blood. Its indirect action occurs by decreasing resorption of calcium, phosphate, sodium, and water at the kidney tubule.[64] Long term supplemental calcitonin therapy in postmenopausal osteoporosis promotes a net gain of bone mineral in the axial skeleton, a slowing of bone loss in the appendicular skeleton,[45] and an increase in total body calcium and trabecular bone mass.[14] The recommended dose is 50 to 100 MRC units every other day delivered by self-injection, or nasal spray calcitonin. Because of antibody formation to salmon calcitonin, which limits the period of efficacy to several months, synthetic human calcitonin is preferable.[42] The use of parathyroid hormone is under investigation for its potential ability to increase bone mass.[40]

Chemically related to natural androgens, *anabolic steroids* exert a powerful protein anabolic effect and may promote bone formation by stimulating collagen synthesis in osteoporosis. Typically nandrolone decanoate is recommended at 50 mg IM every 3 to 4 weeks. This low dose should minimize the effect of liver dysfunction, hoarseness, male-pattern baldness, muscularization, and hirsutism. Usage is contraindicated in patient with cardiorenal failure or liver disease with impaired bilirubin excretion.

There are currently five medications approved by the U.S. Food and Drug Administration (FDA) to prevent or treat osteoporosis: calcitonin, estrogen, alendronate sodium (Fosamax), risedronate sodium (Actonel), and raloxifene (Evista).

SUGGESTED READING

Krolner B, Toft B, Pors Nielsen Set al: Physical exercise as a prophylactic against involutional bone loss—a controlled trial, *Clin Sci* 64:541-546,1983.

Sinaki M: Postmenopausal spinal osteoporosis—physical therapy and rehabilitation principles, *Mayo Clin Proc* 57:699-703, 1982.

Smith EL: Exercise for prevention of osteoporosis—a review, *Physician Sports Med* 10:72-83, 1982.

REFERENCES

1. Aloia J, Cohn S, Babu T: Skeletal man and body competition in marathon runners, *Metabolism* 27:1793, 1978.
2. Asimov I: *The history of physics,* New York, 1966, Walker and Company.
3. Asimov I: *The human brain: its capacities and functions,* New York, 1965, New American Library.
4. Barnard C editor: *The body machine: your health in perspective,* New York, 1981, Crown Publishers.
5. Berkow R editor: *The Merck manual,* ed 15, Rahway, NJ, 1987, Merck & Co.
6. Bikle DD, Genant HK, Cann C et al: Bone disease in alcohol abuse, *Ann Inter Med* 103:42, 1985.
7. Bush TL, Miller VT: Effects of pharmacologic agents used during menopause: impact on lipids and lipoproteins. In Mishell DR Jr editor: *Menopause: physiology and pharmacology,* Chicago, 1987, Year Book Medical Publishers.
8. Chow R, Harrison J, Notairins C: Effect of two randomized exercise programs on bone man of healthy postmenopausal women, *BMJ* 295:1441, 1987.
9. Civitelli R, Gonnelli S, Zacchei F et al: Bone turnover in post-menopausal osteoporosis: effect of calcitonin treatment, *J Clin Invest* 82(4):1268, 1988.
10. Connell MD, Jokl P: The aging athlete. In Nicholas JA, Hershman EB editors, *The lower extremity and spine in sports medicine,* St Louis, 1995, Mosby.
11. Cumming RG: Calcium intake and bone mass: a quantitative review of the evidence, *Calcif Tissue Int* 47(4):194, 1990.
12. Duncan H, Parfitt AM: The biology of aging bone. In Nelson CL, Dwyer AP: *The aging musculoskeletal system,* Lexington, Mass., 1984, The Collamore Press.
13. *Encyclopaedia Britannica* CD 1999, Chicago, 1999, Encyclopaedia Britannica, Inc.
14. Ettinger B, Genant HI, Cann CE: Long-term estrogen replacement therapy prevents bone loss and fractures, *Ann Intern Med* 102:319, 1985.
15. Farley JR, Mergedal JE, Baylink DJ: Fluoride directly stimulates proliferation and alkaline phosphatase activity of bone-forming cells, *Science* 222:330, 1983.
16. Fawcett DW: *A textbook of histology,* ed 7, Philadelphia, 1986, WB Saunders.
17. Frost HM: *Bone remodeling dynamics,* Springfield, IL, 1963, Charles C Thomas.
18. Frost HM: Coherence treatment of osteoporosis, *Orthp Clin North Am* 12:649, 1981.
19. Frost HM: The spinal osteoporosis: mechanism of pathogenesis and pathophysiology, *J Clin Endocrinol Metab* 2:257, 1973.
20. Fujita T, Handa N et al: Age-dependent bone loss after gastrectomy, *J Am Geriatr Soc* 19:840, 1971.
21. Gennari C et al: Comparative effects on bone mineral content of calcium and calcium plus salmon calcitonin given in two different regimens in post-menopausal osteoporosis, *Curr Ther Res Clin Exp* 38:455, 1985.
22. Gruber HE, Ivey JL, Baylink DJ et al: Long-term calcitonin therapy in postmenopausal osteoporosis, *Metabolism* 33:295, 1984.
23. Hadjipavlon A, Brooks EC: Etude de Paction de la calcitonin sur le rein, *L'Union Med Canada* 105:915, 1976.
24. Hadjipavlou AG, Lander PH: Osteoporosis of the spine and its management. In White AH editor: *Spine care: diagnosis and conservative treatment,* St Louis, 1995, Mosby.
25. Hanson T, Roos B: The relation between bone mineral content, experimental compression fractures, and disc degeneration in lumbar vertebrae, *Spine* 6:147, 1981.

26. Harma M, Parviainen M, Koskinen T et al: Bone density, histomorphometry and biochemistry in patient with fractures of hip or spine, *Ann Clin Res* 19(6):378, 1987.

27. Healy JH, Lane JM: Structural scoliosis in osteoporotic women, *Clin Orthop* 195:216, 1985.

28. Heaney RP: Unified concept of the pathogenesis of osteoporosis. In DeLuca HF editor: *Osteoporosis: recent advances in pathogenesis and treatment,* Baltimore, 1981, University Park Press.

29. Heidrich FE, Stergachin A, Gross KM: Diuretic drug use and the risk for hip fracture, *Ann Intern Med* 15:1, 1991.

30. Hernandez-Avila M , Colditz GA, Stampfer MJ et al: Caffeine, moderate alcohol intake, and risk of fractures of the hip and forearm in middle-aged women, *Am J Clin Nutr* 54(1):157, 1991.

31. Holbrook TL et al: The frequency of occurrence, impact, and cost of musculoskeletal conditions in the United States, *Am Acad Orthop Surg* Chicago, 1984.

32. Horsman A, Gallagher JC, Simpson M et al: Prospective trial of oestrogen and calcium in postmenopausal women, *BMJ* 2:289, 1977.

33. Jick SS, Walker AM, Jick H et al: Replacement estrogens and endometrial cancer, *N Engl J Med* 300:218, 1979.

34. Jowsey J: *Osteoporosis in the aging musculoskeletal system,* Lexington, Mass., 1984, The Collamore Press.

35. Kelly DE, Wood RL, Enders AC: *Bailey's textbook of microscopic anatomy,* ed 8, Baltimore, 1984, Williams & Wilkins.

36. Kelsey JF: Osteoporosis: prevalence and incidence. In *Proceedings of the NIH Consensus Development Conference,* April 2-4, 1984.

37. Krolner B, Toft B, Pors Nielsen S et al: Physical exercise as prophylaxis against involutional vertebral bone loss: a controlled trial, *Clin Sci* 64:541, 1983.

38. Kumar S, David PR, Pickles B: Bone marrow pressure and bone strength, *Acta Orthop Scand* 50:507-512, 1979.

39. Lane NE, Sanchez S, Modin GW et al: Parathyroid hormone can reverse steroid-induced osteoporosis, *J Med Investigations* 102(8):1627-1633, 1998.

40. Leblanc AD, Schneider VS, Evans HJ et al: Bone mineral loss and recovery after 17 weeks of bed rest, *J Bone Mineral Res* 5:843-850, 1990.

41. Lindsay R, Hart DM, Clark DM: The minimum effective dose of estrogen for prevention of post-menopausal bone loss, *Obstet Gynecol* 63:759, 1984.

42. Munk-Jensen N, Pors Nielsen S, Obel EB et al: Reversal of post-menopausal vertebral bone loss by estrogen and progestogen: a double-blind placebo controlled study, *BMJ* 296(6630):1150, 1988.

43. Murray RO: Radiological bone changes in Cushing's syndrome and steroid therapy, *Br J Radiol* 33:1, 1960.

44. National Osteoporosis Foundation guide and facts, Washington DC, 1995.

45. Netter FH: The Ciba collection of medical illustrations, vol 8, Musculoskeletal system, Part I, *Anatomy, physiology, and metabolic disorders,* Summit, NJ, 1987, CIBA-GEIGY.

46. Nicar MJ, Pak CYC: Calcium bioavailability from calcium carbonate and calcium citrate, *J Clin Endocrinol Metab* 61:391, 1985.

47. Patel U, Skingle S, Campbell GA et al: Clinical profile of acute vertebral compression fractures in osteoporosis, *Br J Rheumatol* 30(6):418, 1991.

48. Pennington JAT: *Valued of portions commonly used food,* ed 15, New York, 1989, Harper Collins.

49. Pickles B: Osteoporosis and exercise. In Peat M, editor: *Current physical therapy,* Toronto, 1988, BC Decker.

50. Porter RW: *Management of back pain,* ed 2, Edinburgh, 1993, Churchill Livingstone.

51. Ramamurti C. In Tinker R editor: *Orthopaedics in primary care,* Baltimore, 1979, Williams & Wilkins.

52. Ray NF, Chan JK, Thamer M et al: Medical expenditures for the treatment of osteoporotic fractures in the United States in 1995: report from the National Osteoporosis Foundation, *J Bone Miner Res* 12(1):24-35, 1997.

53. Resnick DL: Fish vertebrae, *Arthritis Rheum,* 1982. 25:322-325.

54. Riggs BL, Melton LJ III: Involutional osteoporosis, *N Engl J Med,* 314:1676, 1986.

55. Ringe JD: Clinical evaluation of salmon calcitonin in bone pain. In Christiansen C, editor: *Osteoporosis,* 1987, Proceedings of the International Symposium of Osteoporosis, vol 2, 662-666.

56. Sarrel PM: Estrogen replacement therapy, *Obstet Gynecol* 72(suppl):25, 1988.

57. Sartoris DJ, Clopton P, Nemcek A et al: Vertebral body collapse in focal and diffuse disease: patterns of pathological processes, *Radiology* 160:479, 1986.

58. Schumacher HR, Bomalaski JS: *Case studies in rheumatology for the house officer,* Baltimore, 1990, Williams & Wilkins.

59. Simonen O, Laitinen O: Does fluoridation of drinking water prevent bone fragility and osteoporosis? *Lancet* 2:432, 1985.

60. Steinbach HL: The roentgen appearance of osteoporosis, *Radiol Clin North Am* 2:191, 1964.

61. Stevenson JL, Whitehead MI: Calcitonin section and postmenopausal osteoporosis (letter), *Lancet* 1(8275):804, 1982.

62. Strand FL: *Physiology: a regulatory systems approach,* ed 2, New York, 1983, Macmillian.

63. Trotter M, Broman GE, Peterson RR: Densities of bone of white and negro skeleton, *J Bone Joint Surg* 42A:50, 1960.

64. Vesterby A, Gundersen HJ, Melsen F et al: Marrow space star volume in the iliac crest decreases in osteoporotic patients after continuous treatment with fluoride, calcium, and vitamin D for five years, *Bone* 12(2):99, 1991.

65. Wasnich RD, Benfante RJ, Yano K et al: Thiazide effect on the mineral content of bone, *N Engl J Med* 309:344, 1983.

66. Wilson DWF, Garisson RJ, Castell WP: Post menopausal estrogen use, cigarette smoking, and cardiovascular morbidity in women over 50: the Framingham study, *N Engl J Med* 313:1038, 1985.

63

Sudden Cervical Hyperextension Followed by Progressively Stiff and Painful Neck, Loss of Cervical Lordosis, Headache, and Tingling Sensation of the Upper Extremities

CASE 1: A 55-year-old male was driving home more carefully than usual on returning from a defensive driving course and came to a full stop at a red light before making a right turn. His vehicle was struck from behind by a car traveling, as was later determined by the insurance company, at 25 miles per hour. The patient did not hit his head nor did he complain of any immediate symptoms, but agreed to be taken by paramedics to a local hospital where, following unremarkable radiographs, he was released. He returned home and took a long nap and woke up with severe pain and stiff shoulders. He complains of a headache and is able to move his neck slightly with considerable pain and difficulty. When asked, he denies difficulty swallowing, eating, or speaking and feeling nauseous. He reports a history of bilateral carpal tunnel syndrome that resolved with surgery several years ago, and notes a tingling sensation in both arms when elevating his shoulders. There are no complaints of vertigo, blurring, dizziness, tinnitus, swallowing difficulties, or unsteadiness of gait although sleep is disturbed and the patient complains of a lack of ability to concentrate.

OBSERVATION   The neck musculature, particularly the scalenes and sternomastoid are prominent. The cervical lordotic curve appears straightened. There is no bruising evident.

PALPATION   Bilateral sternomastoid muscle spasm as well as "tight" upper trapezius muscles. Point tenderness in the mid sternomastoid as well as the upper and lower trapezius muscles.

RANGE OF MOTION   Active and passive range is limited in all directions with pain at the end of the range.

STRENGTH   Neck untested secondary to pain. Normal muscle strength in upper extremities bilaterally.

FLEXIBILITY   Tight pectoralis and latissimus dorsi musculature.

DEEP TENDON REFLEXES   These are normal.

SPECIAL TESTS   Negative tests for shoulder pathology. Cervical distraction increases the headache, while compression neither increases nor decreases patient pain. Positive shoulder depression test.

RADIOGRAPHS   Soft tissues are within normal limits, and the retrotracheal and retropharyngeal spaces are within normal limits.

CLUE:

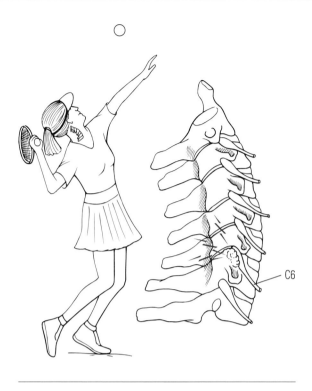

C6

CASE 2: A 45-year-old female presented with complaints of neck ache, and right arm pain that began 2 years ago when she suffered a whiplash injury while involved in a motor vehicle accident. Her symptoms abated approximately 1 year ago, and when asked to localize where the pain used to reside, she indicated an area corresponding to the superior medial angle and medial border of the scapula. Last week while playing tennis with her husband she felt acute right arm pain beginning after forcefully serving the ball that gradually worsened over the next hour. On subsequent days symptoms were generally worse when waking up in the morning and gradually eased after a hot shower and some mobility exercises. The pain pattern involved diminishment of centralized pain with progressive peripheralization to the distal extremity as well as medial scapular pain and headache. Neck extension and lateral flexion, and especially rotation to the right were extremely difficult as they exacerbated pain.

OBSERVATION   The right scalene and sternomastoid appear more prominent on the right. A forward head posture is apparent on side view and no muscle wasting is apparent in the scapular or shoulder regions.

PALPATION   The right scalenes, sternomastoid, and upper trapezius muscles appear to be in spasm. The right inferior aspect of the neck is tender.

RANGE OF MOTION   This is limited by one-half range in extension and right lateral bending, both of which provoked symptoms. The neck was otherwise stiff.

STRENGTH   G— muscle strength noted in the right biceps, brachialis, and brachioradialis muscles.

DEEP TENDON REFLEXES   There is diminished right supinator jerk.

PULSES   These are normal.

SPECIAL TESTS   Positive compression/distraction, shoulder depression test, and Spurling maneuver, causing peripheralization of pain.

RADIOGRAPHS   Oblique radiographs showed a narrowed, figure-of-eight appearance to the intervertebral foramen, bilaterally, with marginal osteophytes of the uncinate processes and articular facet joints.

CLUE   Normal nerve conduction velocity testing of C6 myotomes.

? Questions

1. What is most likely the cause of the patient's symptoms in Case 1?
2. What is a whiplash injury?
3. What is the mechanism for injury in whiplash related cervical injury?
4. What is the role of cervical muscles on the type of injury outcome following whiplash?
5. What is most likely the source of the patient's pain in Case 2?
6. What is the osteology of the lower cervical spine?
7. What type of articulation is formed by the uncinate processes of the cervical spine?
8. How do the cervical pedicles differ from the thoracolumbar pedicles?
9. What is the anatomy of the transverse processes of the cervical spine?
10. What are three weight-bearing pillars of the cervical spine?
11. What is the orientation of the facet joints of the cervical spine?
12. What are the intraarticular inclusions of the facet joints?
13. What is the anatomy of the cervical spinous processes?
14. What is the structure of the cervical intervertebral disk and what are the functions of their vertical and horizontal lamellae?
15. What hydraulic mechanism is offered by the intervertebral disk?
16. How do the intervertebral disks of the cervical region differ from the lumbar region?
17. What is the range of motion in the cervical spine?
18. What are the static stabilizers of the cervical spine?
19. What is the musculature of the cervical spine?
20. What is the role of the uncinate process in axial rotation of the cervical spine?
21. What are the uncovertebral joints and how does their development result in degenerative changes in the cervical spine?
22. Why does degeneration of the cervical disk often begin laterally, just medial to the uncinate process?
23. Why is intervertebral disk herniation less common in the cervical spine than the lumbar spine?
24. What is the structural degenerative cascade?
25. What is the pathophysiology of cervical spine disease?
26. How does the pathophysiology of cervical spine disease result in mechanical disturbance of the cervical motion segment?
27. What reactive stabilization strategy occurs in the cervical spine during cervical disk disease?
28. How may cervical spondylosis evolve into cervical spinal stenosis?
29. What length changes do the spinal and root canals undergo with normal movement?
30. What is a possible endstage pathology of cervical spondylosis?

31. Why are there more cervical nerve roots than cervical vertebrae?

32. What is the orientation between the upper and lower emerging cervical spinal nerves and their corresponding vertebrae?

33. What is the anatomical origin of the spinal nerve, and why is encroachment within the intervertebral foramen more likely to cause sensory deficit?

34. What are the relevant nerve root innervations to the dermatomes and myotomes of the upper extremities?

35. What are the reflexes of the upper extremity and what is their diagnostic value?

36. What are the deep tendon reflexes of the upper extremity and how are they elicited?

37. What is the differential diagnosis of cervical disk disease?

38. What is spinal cord neurapraxia?

39. What is nerve-root neurapraxia?

40. What is the clinical presentation of cervical spine disease and cervical sprain/strain?

41. What is the prognosis for cervical spine disease and cervical sprain/strain?

42. What imaging is indicated for patients with cervical spine disease?

43. What physical therapy is indicated in the management of these patients?

1. What is most likely the cause of the patient's symptoms in Case 1?

The history and clinical presentation of Case 1 suggest a classic whiplash injury due to cervical muscle and ligament sprain. The history and clinical presentation of Case 2 suggest cervical spondylosis confirmed by radiographic evidence of bilateral foraminal stenosis. The latter represents a classic case of upper extremity radiculitis secondary to cervical spondylosis that may have begun years ago with cervical disk disease that worsened with the previous whiplash, which, although stabilized, did so at the expense of osteophytic overgrowth at the bony margins of the exiting nerve roots. The sudden hyperextension during the tennis serve was the final insult to the C6 nerve root that emerged through an intervertebral foramen that was considerably reduced in diameter. This, in turn, resulted in encroachment and subsequent swelling of the nerve, which caused further ischemia of the nerve in the osseous canal of the foramen. Thus neck extension, lateral bending, or rotation worsens symptoms as these motions further narrow the aperture of the intervertebral foramen. Symptoms that improve following a hot morning shower and mobility are suggestive of a degenerative inflammatory process, consistent with cervical disk degeneration and reactive ossification. With radiculitis of the C6 nerve root, elbow flexion in both the supinated (achieved by biceps and brachialis via the musculocutaneous nerve) and the half-pronated position of the forearm (accomplished by brachioradialis via the radial nerve) will be weakened, whereas a peripheral nerve lesion of either the musculocutaneous or radial nerve will cause a more limited pattern of muscle weakness. Here, the pattern of muscle weakness was consistent with the C6 myotome, as well as diminishment of cutaneous sensation in the C6 dermatome as well as a diminished supinator jerk (C6). Nerve conduction tests are almost always normal in cases of uncomplicated radiculopathy, while electromyographic (EMG) tests show a myotomal pattern of involvement as well as denervation of the paraspinous musculature.

2. What is a whiplash injury?

Whiplash injury represents a rapid linear displacement of the head relative to the upper torso, typically in the sagittal plane that represents an injury classified as cervical muscle and/or ligament sprain.[65] Injury statistics in the United States indicate that almost every fourth injury to automobile occupants is related to rear-end crashes, and that three quarters of these injuries involve the neck.[23] The term whiplash was first coined by Crowe in 1928[24] and refers to an acceleration-deceleration mechanism[18] from diving accidents, or shaken-baby syndrome, but most often occurs as a result of motor vehicular trauma.[52] It may result from rear-end, front-end, or side-impact motor vehicle collisions or from collisions while in a go-cart or bumper car, and cause bony and/or soft-tissue injury. The mass and speed of the vehicle determine momentum and are essential factors in determining the magnitude of injury, as does whether the patient was using an adequately adjusted headrest. Headrest supports must come up at least to the occiput to prevent a severe hyperextension injury.[32] Elderly persons are especially vulnerable to hyperextension injuries because chronic disk degeneration and osteophytic overgrowth of the facets and uncinate processes may substantially reduce the diameter of the spinal and intervertebral canals, leaving both the cord and emerging nerve roots very little room for displacement during neck movement or for posttraumatic swelling of the cord or nerve roots.[77]

3. What is the mechanism for injury in whiplash related cervical injury?

Rear end collisions typically occur in dense traffic conditions. During the collision, the struck vehicle undergoes a forceful forward acceleration so that the car occupants are suddenly pushed forward by the seat backs. In the absence of a head restraint, the head will lag behind the body and undergo a swift rearward bending of the neck that continues until it reaches its end range of motion with violent overpressure beyond the end range. Thereafter, the head rebounds in the other direction, which is limited by the chin striking the chest (Fig. 63-1). Rotation may also have occurred. While hyperflexion may result in profound midline disk herniation and muscular strain of the posterior muscles, hyperextension may strain the anterior musculature and sprain the spinal ligaments.[122] The acute, rapid stretching of neck musculature causes a strong stretch reflex manifesting as sustained muscular contraction in the form of spasm, which may flatten the normal cervical lordosis. Tearing of ligaments, particularly the anterior longitudinal ligament will result in bleeding between the ligament and vertebrae, and may cause enough retropharyngeal swelling to provoke dysphagia several hours after the accident.[86] Moreover, facets may fracture and cause vertebral body dislocation and hemorrhage under the anterior or posterior longitudinal ligament, while muscles may be torn or stretched.[22] Additionally, the temporomandibular joints may suffer trauma. More than 80% of this type of accident results in severe soft-tissue injuries without involvement of osseous structures; otherwise, injury may lead to fracture with or without neurological deficit.[122] Tearing of the cervical sympathetic trunk and ganglia may occur during the extension phase of whiplash as these structures lie forward of the axis of flexion and extension.[31,33] Injury to the sympathetic trunk will produce ipsilateral Horner's syndrome. With severe hyperextension of the cervical spine, central cord syndrome may occur.[72] Spinal cord injuries may occur from whiplash injury, and the brain may be injured,[100] presumably by a coup-contra-coup type mechanism, resulting in concussion or worse. In very violent cervical trauma, death may occur from evulsion[85] of the medullopontine junction.[122] Soft and osseous tissue injury may also occur from whiplash following a head-on collision.

4. What is the role of cervical muscles on the type of injury outcome following whiplash?

The most common mechanism of whiplash injury involves an unaware victim in a stationary vehicle being struck from behind, causing forced hyperextension and forced hyperflexion in quick succession. These two phases may occur in opposite order in the

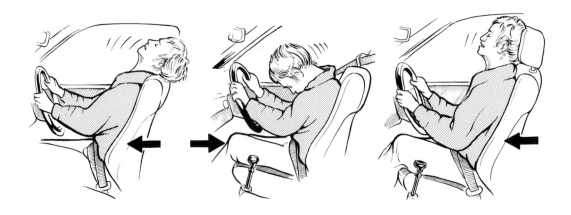

FIG. 63-1 Mechanism of whiplash injury to the cervical spine. Head movement is limited by a head restraint. (From Dandy DJ: *Essential orthopaedics and trauma*, ed 2, Edinburgh, 1993, Churchill Livingstone.)

event of a head-on collision. Various types of soft and osseous tissue injury may occur, depending on the amount of anticipation of the person with the injured neck. Generally, high bending moments to the neck will be accompanied by reflexive compressive forces arising from the neck musculature as they contract in an attempt to dampen the magnitude and speed of bending.

If the collision is unexpected, the neck and shoulder muscles will not have ample time to protectively contract and brace against the subsequent violent neck movement. Here, a bending moment dominates any compressive force. In this case, the muscles and ligaments are more likely to sustain injury, with the anterior structures being at risk during the hyperextension phase and the posterior structures during the hyperflexion phase. If the collision was partially anticipated, then the impact, resulting in both high compressive and bending stresses to the neck, may cause posterior disk prolapse during the hyperflexion phase. If the driver is alerted to the impending collisions, perhaps by the squeal of braking or the brake lights of the car in front, then the neck muscles may have time to adequately contract vigorously enough so that the ratio of compression to bending will be high, and result in damage to the vertebral endplate and body.[2]

5. What is most likely the source of the patient's pain in Case 2?

The history and clinical presentation of Case 2 suggests acute cervical spondylosis. The C6 nerve root may have been acutely compromised 2 years ago following the whiplash injury and subsequently stabilized with osteophytic proliferation of both the uncinate processes and facet joints. Thus the aperture of the intervertebral foramen at that level was significantly reduced by reactive bone formation following the initial injury that stabilized, although it remained predisposed toward compression. Here the preexisting spondylotic changes, which have developed because of the whiplash injury, are of critical significance in the pathogenesis of cervical spondylosis. Severe hyperextension of the neck during the tennis serve resulted in acute encroachment of the nerve root. Symptoms worsened with time as reactive edema of the traumatized nerve root and resulted in the classic presentation of C6 radiculopathy, namely decreased sensation to the lateral forearm, muscle weakness of the wrist extensor, and an absent brachioradialis reflex.

6. What is the osteology of the lower cervical spine?

The *lower cervical spine* includes the lower five cervical vertebrae, which share many common features. C1 and C2 are considered atypical vertebrae, while C7 is unique, so that the intermediate four vertebrae are considered *typical cervical vertebrae* (Fig. 63-2) having in common many features including a vertebral body, two laminae, two pedicles, a spinous process, two transverse processes, transverse foramina, and superior and inferior articular facets. The vertebral bodies of the cervical spine, oval or reniform[11] in shape when viewed from above, are smaller than the triangular spinal canal, and are also relatively small compared with the thoracic and lumbar vertebrae because they bear relatively less superincumbent body weight. The body generally increases in size from C3 to C7 to accommodate the increasing superincumbent load. Their mediolateral dimensions are greater than their anteroposterior dimensions. Because their anterior and posterior surfaces are of equal superior-inferior dimension, the normal cervical lordosis is produced by wedge-shaped intervertebral disks rather than by wedge-shaped vertebral bodies. The vertebral foramina have a rounded triangular shape, which is relatively narrower in the lower cervical spine than the upper cervical spine. The C2 through C7 cervical vertebrae are endowed with two synovial joints posteriorly and the intervertebral disk joint anteriorly.

7. What type of articulation is formed by the uncinate processes of the cervical spine?

The superior surface of the vertebral body is concave owing to two cranially projecting flanges, known as the *uncinate processes,* projecting upward from their lateral and posterolateral edges. The mediolateral concavity is most marked along the medial border of the uncinate process. The superior surface is also convex from the back because of the beveling (slanting) of the anterior surface. In contrast, there is a reciprocal mediolateral convexity on the lateral margin of the inferior surface of the next higher vertebral body. Because the anterior lip of the inferior surface of the vertebral body projects inferiorly, the lower surface is described as having a slight concavity in the sagittal plane, that is, from anterior to posterior. The interbody joint between typical cervical vertebrae therefore accommodates two orthogonally shaped concave surfaces, which qualifies it as a typical *saddle joint.* The advantage conferred on the

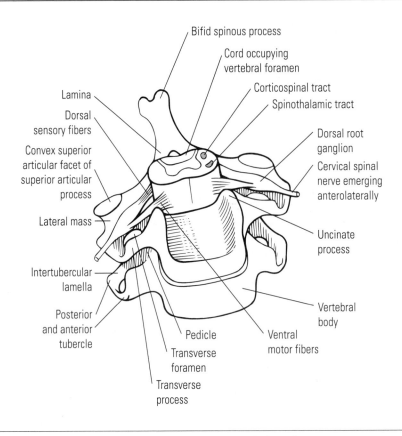

FIG. 63-2 Anatomy of a typical cervical vertebra.

cervical spine by the uncinate processes is that flexion and extension are unhindered while stability is maximized. Thus the inferior surface of one vertebral body fits onto the superior surface of the next vertebral body in an interlocking fashion that tends to resist translation movements in any direction.

8. How do the cervical pedicles differ from the thoracolumbar pedicles?

The relatively small pedicles of the typical cervical vertebrae differ from those of the thoracic and lumbar vertebrae in several respects. Because they arise midway between the inferior and superior surfaces of the vertebral body, they are equally grooved on their superior and inferior surfaces and correspondingly form superior and inferior vertebral notches of approximately equal size endowing the intervertebral foramina with substantial symmetry. The cervical intervertebral foramina are part of the anterolateral wall of the spinal canal, so that the emerging nerve roots course anterolaterally as they exit their dural sac to become nerve roots. The pedicles thus form the intervertebral foramina by connecting the superior and inferior notches along adjacent vertebrae. Unlike the thoracolumbar pedicles, which originate from the posterior aspect of the vertebral body, the cervical pedicles originate from the posterolateral aspect of the body. The cervical pedicles are directed posterolaterally causing the intervertebral foramina to face obliquely anterolaterally. Thus both the posterolateral origin and inclination of the pedicles tends to increase the mediolateral dimensions of the cervical spinal canal to permit better accommodation of the elliptical cervical spinal cord, which has its major dimension mediolaterally.

9. What is the anatomy of the transverse processes of the cervical spine?

The cervical transverse process is comprised of two distinct processes separated by a *transverse foramen*, both directed anterolaterally and inferiorly. The floor of the transverse processes from levels C1 to C6 exhibits a large transverse foramen that transmits the vertebral artery. The *anterior spinal artery* arises as two vessels from the vertebral arteries in the foramen magnum that descend within the *transverse foramen* of C1-C6 vertebral transverse process.[87] The uncovertebral joints offer the benefit of limiting excessive lateral bending of the cervical spine, which helps prevent kinking of the vertebral artery as it traverses through the transverse foramen.[68]

It is the presence of the transverse foramen that subdivides the transverse process into its three parts: a ventral bar in front of the foramen terminating as an anterior tubercle, a dorsal bar behind the foramen ending as a posterior tubercle, and an intertubercular lamella, lying lateral to the foramen and connecting the two tubercles. Thus the transverse process is composed of two separate portions known as anterior and posterior tubercles and connected by a bar known as the *costotransverse bar.* The *anterior tubercle* serves as the attachment site for the longus and anterior scalene muscles, while the *posterior tubercle* serves as the attachment site for the splenius cervicis, iliocostalis, cervicis, and the longissimus cervicis muscles. In a superior view, the transverse processes exhibit a U shape in cross section and form a gutter for the transmission of the primary ventral rami of the spinal nerves that emerge above the vertebrae. The anterior tubercles of C6 are large and termed the carotid tubercles because the common carotid arteries lie just anteriorly and may be compressed against them. The sympathetic trunk runs longitudinally along the anterior aspect of the anterior tubercles where it is vulnerable to trauma from a whiplash type injury.

10. What are three weight-bearing pillars of the cervical spine?

The junction of the pedicles and laminae are lateral, oval, projections comprising the articular facet joints. While the superior facets face up and backward, the inferior facets face down and forward. The superior surface is convex, while the inferior surface is concave. Stacked atop each other, the series of cervical articular facet joints have the appearance of one long, stout, pillar along each side of the cervical spine. The relative horizontal position and thickness of the articular pillars of the facet joint imply a greater role in weight bearing than facets in other regions of the spine, and act to support the weight of the head and neck.[90] Thus weight bearing in the cervical region is carried out by three longitudinal columns: the anterior column running through the vertebral bodies and disks, and the right and left articular pillars.[83]

11. What is the orientation of the facet joints of the cervical spine?

Whereas the facet joints of the upper cervical spine lie at an approximate 35° angle to the horizontal plane, those of the middle cervical spine lie at a 45° angle,[33] while those of the inferior cervical spine form a 65° angle with the horizontal plane.[8] Thus the oblique orientation of the facet joints increases at descending levels of the cervical spine, and approaches near vertical at C7. The angulation of the facet joints allows for movement in flexion, extension, lateral flexion, and axial rotation of the intervertebral joint. In addition to defining the amount and type of motion in the cervical region, the oblique plane allows the facet joints to participate in weight bearing, in addition to restricting anterior translation of the upper vertebral in any pair. Endowed with the most horizontal orientation of any of the spinal facet joints, these cervical facets may more easily become unilaterally or bilaterally dislocated without fracture. The synovial facet joints are located between the vertebral arches and are supported by their articular capsule and a number of extrinsic ligaments, including the ligamenta flavum, interspinal, supraspinal, nuchal, and intertransverse ligaments. Pain arising from injuries to the cervical facet joint may refer symptoms distal to the affected articulation.[126] The two most common patterns of pain referral are neck and head pain arising from the C2-C3 facet joints, as well as neck and shoulder pain deriving from the C5-C6 facet joints.[88]

12. What are the intraarticular inclusions of the facet joints?

Each articular facet is lined by hyaline cartilage and enclosed by a highly innervated fibrous capsule. *Intraarticular inclusions* within the facets include fat pads, fibroadipose menisci, and capsular rims. Various types of meniscosynovial folds, according to the age and degeneration at that segmental level, project into the facet joints at all levels.[125] Fibroadipose menisci and intra articular fat pads occur at the poles of the articulation where the capsule is relatively loose and help accommodate the normal joint luxation that accompanies movement. While the fat pads fill as joint fillers, the fibroadipose menisci intervene between the joint surfaces. Both act to spread a film of synovial fluid throughout the recesses of the joint during movement. Capsular rims are simply adventitious thickening of the articular capsule that fill the recesses between the curved edges of articular cartilage.

13. What is the anatomy of the cervical spinous processes?

The medially directed laminae are thin and relatively long and fuse posterior to form the *spinous processes.* The lower cervical spinous processes are short, although wide and bifid. *Bifid* means separated by a cleft into two equal parts, and refers to the spinous process developing from two separate secondary centers of ossification. The length of the spinous processes decreases from C2 to C4 and then increases from C4 to C7.[15] Their thickness and bifid nature provides a large surface area for the attachment of the ligamentum nuchae and many muscles that attach to them, including the rotatores, semispinalis cervicis, multifidi cervicis, and interspinal cervicis muscles. The advantage conferred by their shortness is that they are not likely to interfere with extension. The spinous process of the C7 is not bifid and being larger and more prominent than other cervical vertebrae is palpable and visible at the back of the neck. It is known as the *vertebra prominens.*

14. What is the structure of the cervical intervertebral disk and what are the functions of their vertical and horizontal lamellae?

Between the bodies of each two spinal vertebrae lies an *intervertebral disk,* except at the uppermost two cervical joints. In the young healthy spine, the intervertebral disks contribute about 22% of the length of the cervical spine. Classified as a symphysis[124] type joint and considered the largest avascular structure in the body, the intervertebral disk is a nonsynovial joint that obtains nutrition through diffusion and fluid flow.[10] The disk is usually named with reference to the two vertebrae that surround it. Alternately, a disk may also be referred to with reference to the vertebra directly above the disk, and may be easily remembered by imagining a vertebral body "sitting" on its respective disk. Comprised of three component structures, the disk is composed of an inner nucleus pulposus surrounded by an annulus fibrosus, which, in turn, are covered above and below by cartilaginous vertebral endplates.

The annulus fibrosus consists of many concentric lamellae of collagen fibers running obliquely in opposite directions. The fibers of each layer form a horizontal angle of 120° with a vertical angle of 60° with the fibers in the next layer.[105] The vertical component of fibers endows the annulus with the ability to counter tension during flexion-extension and lateral bending motions, while the horizontal component resists the tensile stress of rotatory motions of the spine. Two distinct portions are identified within the annulus. The outermost lamellae attach to the ring apophysis of the two vertebrae and constitute the ligamentous part of the annulus,[82] whereas the inner lamellae, rather than attaching to the vertebral endplates, insert into the vertebral endplates above and below the nucleus and form a spherical envelope around the nucleus (see Fig. 60-1).

15. What hydraulic mechanism is offered by the intervertebral disk?

The nucleus pulposus within the annulus fibrosus acts as a mass of incompressible fluid, which by way of analogy is like a balloon filled with water. As such, it will obey *Pascal's law,* which states that given a fluid inside a completely closed container, if pressure is increased on one site along the wall of the container (e.g., pressing the balloon with a finger) then that local pressure increase will transmit undiminished over the entire wall of the container. In the cervical spine, bending over in any direction increases compressive load to the concave side of the annulus and nucleus causing it to bulge outward (see Fig. 60-1*C*). This generates corresponding tensile force on the opposite convex side of the curve. Thus the young cervical intervertebral disk serves in the capacity of a self-contained fluid-elastic system that by way of a hydraulic mechanism deriving from its unique structure, permits motion, absorbs shock, and reduces pressure by distributing loads over a large surface area.

16. How do the intervertebral disks of the cervical region differ from the lumbar region?

The nucleus pulposus of the cervical disk represents a much smaller component of the disk than in the lumbar region. The nucleus pulposus of the lumbar disk constitutes about 50% of its cross-sectional areas and volume, whereas, in a typical cervical disk it is approximately 25%.[106] In infants, children, and adolescents, the nucleus pulposus of a cervical spine is like that of the lumbar disks. Once past age 20, the adult nucleus pulposus becomes quite fibrous and more like an interosseous ligament than the hydrodynamic structure of the adult lumbar disk.[5] Finally, transverse fissures across the posterior half of the cervical disks occur as a normal variant of increasing age.[69]

17. What is the range of motion in the cervical spine?

The cervical spine has the greatest range of motion of the total spine.[27] The range of motion below C2 includes flexion, extension, lateral flexion, and axial rotation between vertebrae.[73] Flexion and extension are greatest at the C5/C6 and C6/C7 interspaces, and total 17° and 16°, respectively. There is almost as much movement at C4/C5. Greater motion causes a greater potential for wear and tear. Thus the large amount of flexion-extension at the C5-C6 interval is potential cause for the high incidence of degenerative changes occurring at this segment.[90] Between C3 and C7, 40° of flexion and 24° of extension is possible. Lateral bending and rotation are maximal at the C3/C4 and C4/C5 levels where they total 11° to 12° of lateral bending.

Approximately 90° of axial rotation occurs between C3 and C7 with 45° to each side of neutral. If unilateral rotation reaches or exceeds 45°,[79] kinking of the ipsilateral vertebral or carotid artery may result in syncope or other symptoms in what is described as *subclavian steal syndrome.*[37] Because of the obliquity of the facet joints, lateral bending and rotation tend to be coupled. During lateral bending to the right, the superior facet slides downward and backward and the left superior facet slides upward and forward, causing the face to rotate toward the right. In the cervical spine, in direct contrast to the lumbar spine, lateral flexion and rotation occur in the same directions (Fig. 63-3).

18. What are the static stabilizers of the cervical spine?

ANTERIOR LONGITUDINAL LIGAMENT

This provides anterior stability to the spine, and extends the full length of the spine from the occiput to the sacrum. Beginning at the anterior tubercle at the atlas, and rather narrow at level of C2, the *anterior longitudinal ligament* broadens as it descends and firmly adheres to the anterior margins of the vertebral bodies and disks. Approximately 3.8 cm wide in the upper cervical spine, the anterior longitudinal ligament increases in width to 7.5 cm in the lower cervical spine.[45] This ligament consists of a superficial layer of long fibers that span as many as five vertebrae, and a deep layer that blends with the anterior vertebral periosteum and outer-anterior fibers of the annulus fibrosus. The anterior longitudinal ligament has a tensile strength of 676 N[9] or nearly 3000[7] psi, functions to resist vertical separation of the anterior margins of the bodies, limits flexion and prevents hyperflexion, acts to support by reinforcement of the anterior disks during the lifting of heavy loads,[63] and may be torn during extension injuries of the spine. The anterior longitudinal ligament receives sensory (nociceptive and proprioceptive) innervation from

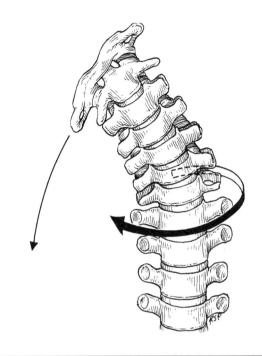

FIG. 63-3 Coupled motions of the cervical spine. Lateral flexion is coupled to rotation in the same direction. (From Malone TR, McPoil T, Nitz AJ: *Orthopedic and sports physical therapy,* ed 3, St Louis, 1997, Mosby.)

branches of the gray communicating rami of the lumbar sympathetic trunk, so that damage to this ligament during extension injuries may be a direct source of pain.

POSTERIOR LONGITUDINAL LIGAMENT

This is the inferior continuation of the tectorial ligament and provides posterior stability to the spine. The *posterior longitudinal ligament* extends from the axis to the sacrum and is considerably less sturdy than its anterior counterpart. Proximally, its upper end is continuous with the tectorial membrane in the high cervical region separating the basivertebral plexus from the dural sac of the spinal cord. Broader above than below, the posterior longitudinal ligament descends as a narrow band along the posterior surface of the vertebrae and interbody joints. The posterior longitudinal ligament is substantially thicker in the cervical region, and is approximately 3 to 4 times thicker in the cervical region than in the thoracic or lumbar regions.[79] While the posterior longitudinal ligament adheres to the intervertebral disks at each level, it is not attached to the dorsal surface of the vertebral bodies owing to the interposition of the basivertebral veins that join the anterior internal verte- bral venous plexus. While having relatively thick at- tachments centrally, it appears serrated in appearance laterally. The posterior longitudinal ligament flares lat- erally at each intervertebral disk where it attaches to the posterior aspect of the annulus fibrosus. The ligament is essentially bowstrung across the posterior aspect of the vertebral column, resulting in a small, thin attachment laterally within a rhomboidal-shaped area posterolater- ally. The serrated outline of the ligament renders it un- likely to have any substantial mechanical role, and it is indeed, identified as an anatomic risk factor for pos- terolateral disk protrusion and herniation. Of the two layers comprising the posterior longitudinal ligament, the deeper layer spans only two articulations, while the fibers of the more superficial layer span as many as five vertebrae. The posterior longitudinal ligament, running inside and anterior to the vertebral canal, prevents hy- perextension and allows for flexion of the spine. Sub- stance P, a sensory neurotransmitter associated with pain sensation, and enkephalins, a neuromodulator of pain, have been found in the lumbar posterior longitu- dinal ligament and suggest that it is extremely sensitive to pain. The posterior longitudinal is more likely to os- sify in the cervical spine than any other region, and may thus serve as source of spinal cord compression.[49]

LIGAMENTUM FLAVUM

This is a paired structure at each level, joining the lami- nae of adjacent vertebrae between the C2/C3 and L5/S1 levels, and acts to protect the spinal canal from encroachment by soft tissue on flexion movements. As its name implies, this elastic containing yellow liga- ment is unique, as up to 80% of its fibers have elastic properties. Correspondingly, it has a tensile strength of only 113 N.[115] While offering some resistance to sepa- ration of the laminae in flexion of the vertebral column, the ligament is too distensible secondary to its elastic nature to limit this motion. Located posteriorly, the *ligamentum flavum* narrows the inferior aspect of the intervertebral foramen and helps form the posterior boundary of the intervertebral foramen.[90] In the lumbar spine, this ligament forms the more anterior portion of the facet joint within the intervertebral foramen, and comes in direct contact with the exiting dorsal and ven- tral nerve roots. The primary function of the ligamentum flavum is to provide a smooth posterior wall to the verte- bral canal that accommodates large changes in inter- laminar distance during flexion and extension of the ver- tebral column without buckling[99] into the spinal canal.

The ligaments increase in thickness from the cervical to the lumbar region, and extend laterally to the facet joints at each segment throughout the spine. The thickness of the ligamentum flavum varies between 5 mm from an- terior to posterior. The ligament is thinnest when the spine is flexed, as this posture pulls the ligament taut. During spinal extension the ligamentum flavum is con- tracted and thick and occupies more space within the canal,[54] in which case it will indent into the vertebral canal.[108] Because of disk space narrowing in degenera- tive disk disease, the vertebrae will approximate each other. This causes the ligamentum flavum to infold or kink on itself, bulging further into the spinal canal and aggravating any tendency to stenosis.[123] The ligamen- tum flavum may undergo degeneration after trauma or with increasing age in which it increases its thickness and may either calcify* or become infiltrated with fat.[93] Additionally, this ligament can ossify,[57] particularly in vertebral hyperostosis and in Paget's disease.[55]

LIGAMENTUM NUCHAE

Instead of a definitive interspinous ligament, which is lacking in the cervical spine, the cervical interspinous space is occupied by the *ligamentum nuchae*. This fas- cial membrane is a thin, flat, structure consisting of midline raphe† formed by the interlacing tendinous fi- bers of the trapezius, splenius, and rhomboid minor, ex- tending from the external occipital protuberance to the tip of the C7 spinous process. Thus the ligamentum nu- chae may be described as the homologue of the inter- spinous ligaments of the thoracolumbar regions of the spine.

SUPRASPINOUS LIGAMENT

This is a loose extension of the nuchal ligament of the cervical spine that lies in the midline and interconnects the tips of the spinous process from C7 to the sacrum. Becoming broader as it descends, the supraspinal liga- ment is the most superficial of all spinal ligaments and therefore farthest from the axis of flexion. Because of this, as well as having low stiffness and failing at very low loads,[107] the *supraspinal ligament* has greater po- tential for sprain.[89] Being a distinctly fatty structure with no single, continuous longitudinal structure, it

---

*Calcification of the ligamentum flavum most commonly occurs in the thoracic spine.
†*Raphe* means "seam" and refers to the midline formed by the union of halves of various symmetrical structures.

may provide a protective cushion over the spinous processes.[47] This ligament is assisted in its ability to passively restrain excessive spinal flexion by the interspinous ligament and dynamically, by the spinalis portion of the erector spinae muscle. The *interspinal ligaments* are obliquely running fibers composed of ventral, middle, and dorsal fibers that also connect adjacent spinous processes, filling the gap along their length. Only the anterior two thirds of each ligament is truly ligamentous, and passes around the supraspinous ligament to merge with the thoracolumbar fascia and thereby help anchor the latter to the spine. The interspinous ligaments are poorly developed in the cervical region, consisting of a thin, membranous translucent septum deriving from the ligamentum nuchae.

19. What is the musculature of the cervical spine?

Two groups of muscles move and stabilize the spine. The larger muscles produce spinal motion because they are farther from the axis of rotation, have longer moment arms, and hence produce more force, whereas the smaller muscles have a short moment arm and serve to stabilize the adjacent spinal segments during gross motion. The muscles responsible for stabilizing and moving the cervical spine may be conceptualized as lying on either side of the midsagittal plane and hence divided into anterior and posterior groups. Because all muscles are situated on one aspect of the midsagittal plane they will laterally bend the spine to the ipsilateral side during concentric contraction, while the contralateral muscles protectively dampen this motion by eccentrically contracting. Hence, the anterior musculature will flex the spine concentrically whereas the posterior musculature flexes the spine eccentrically. Moreover, because almost all of the cervical spine musculature has a somewhat oblique orientation of span, they will rotate the spine and turn the face to either the ipsilateral or contralateral side. All these muscles may be injured by cervical spine trauma.

ANTERIOR MUSCULATURE (Fig. 63-4)

- *Longus colli.* This is also known as the longus cervicis. It is located along the anterior aspect of the cervical vertebrae, and is a three-part triangular muscle arising from the bodies of the transverse processes of the lower cervical vertebrae and inserting into the transverse processes of the higher cervical vertebrae. The superior portion passes between the middle and cervical transverse processes and the upper cervical vertebral bodies. The inferior portion passes between

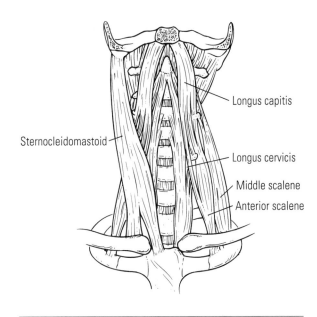

FIG. 63-4 Anterior musculature of the cervical spine. (From White AH, Schofferman JA, editors: *Spine care: diagnosis and conservative treatment*, St Louis, 1995, Mosby.)

the middle cervical transverse processes and the lower cervical and upper thoracic vertebral bodies. The middle, vertical portion connects the upper and lower cervical vertebral bodies. The vertical and two oblique components of the muscle flex the neck. The inferior and superior oblique help to laterally flex the neck, and the inferior oblique acts to rotate the neck to the opposite side. This muscle is innervated by branches of the anterior primary rami of C2 to C6.

- *Longus capitis.* This is located anterior and slightly lateral to the longus colli that originates as a series of thin tendons of the transverse process of C3 to C6 that unite and insert onto the basilar portion of the occipital bone. Longus capitis flexes the neck and is also innervated by the branches from the C1 to C6 anterior rami. Both longus muscles are not strong neck flexors because their lines of action lie close to the axes of sagittal rotation of the cervical vertebrae. They may function to control small amplitude movements of the head and neck in the sagittal plane.

- *Rectus capitis anterior.* This is a short, small muscle located deep to the inserting fibers of the longus capitis muscle and attaches to the lateral mass and transverse process of the atlas and inserts onto the occiput. It stabilizes and flexes the head at the atlanto-occipital joints and is innervated by the anterior primary rami of the first and second cervical nerves.

- *Rectus capitis lateralis.* This is also a short, small muscle originating from the transverse process of the atlas and inserts onto the jugular process of the occipital bone. It functions to stabilize the head and laterally flexes the occiput on the atlas, and is innervated by the C1 and C2 anterior rami.
- *Scalene muscles* (meaning "uneven" in Greek—*skalenos,* and referring to a triangle with uneven sides). These triangular shaped muscles comprise the lateral cervical muscles and are composed of anterior, middle, and posterior portions all of which arise from the transverse processes of the cervical vertebrae and insert on the first and second ribs. Scalenus anterior extends from the first rib to the anterior tubercles of the transverse processes of C3 to C6. The middle scalene courses from the first rib to the posterior tubercles of the C2 through C7 transverse processes, while scalenus posterior extends from the second rib to the posterior tubercles of the transverse processes of C4 through C6. Acting from above, the scalenes collectively function as secondary respiratory muscles by raising the first two ribs. Acting from below, the scalenes laterally flex the cervical spine. Additionally, the anterior scalene flexes, and rotates the face contralaterally, while posterior scalene may extend and rotate the face to the same side. These muscles are innervated by branches from the C3 to C8 anterior rami.
- *Sternomastoid.* This is a prominent and important muscle of the cervical region that is composed of two major divisions known as the sternal and clavicular heads, each of which has its own subdivisions (see Fig. 22-1). While each division possesses a separate head of origin distally, all subdivisions merge to insert proximally as a composite head. The proper (e.g., full) name of this interesting muscle, *sternocleidomastoid,* bespeaks the two distal origins of that muscle, namely, the manubrium of the sternum and medial clavicle, and proximally inserts on the tip of the mastoid process. The primary function of sternomastoid is to rotate the face to the opposite side. Contraction of one side turns the face to the opposite side. Simultaneous contraction of both muscles extends the neck. In both instances, this superficial muscle boldly stands out, clearly defining the neck's contour. Unilateral sternomastoid contraction is opposed by contralateral trapezius activity, so that right turning is opposed by left trapezius. If both muscles contract ipsilaterally, the face and head will then rotate. Sternomastoid also laterally bends the neck to the same side, flexes the cervical spine, and aids respiration by el-

evating the thoracic cage. The main motor supply for sternomastoid is from the spinal accessory nerve, with segmental input from the C2-C3 spinal cord level.

POSTERIOR MUSCULATURE (Fig. 63-5)

- *Trapezius.* The upper trapezius extends from the clavicle and acromion upward and medially to the C7 spinous process and ligamentum nuchae. The action of trapezius differs depending on whether the head/neck or scapula are stabilized. While the primary function of upper trapezius is shoulder elevation by way of its distal clavicular attachment, unilateral contraction with the scapula stabilized rotates the face to the opposite direction, while bilateral contraction extends the head and neck.[40] Trapezius is innervated by the spinal portion of the accessory nerve, with segmental proprioceptive input from the third and fourth cervical anterior rami.
- *Rhomboids.* These consist of rhomboideus major and minor, which are separated by a small fascial cleft, that course from the lower medial scapular border to the upper thoracic and lower cervical spinous processes. They retract the scapula or rotate the cervical spine to the same side. Both trapezius and the rhomboids rotate the face to the opposite direction because they attach to the skull or spinous processes. The

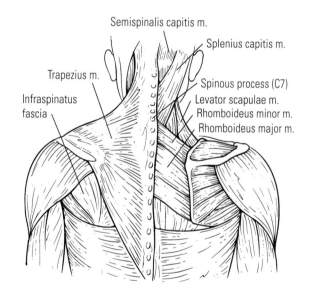

FIG. 63-5 Posterior musculature of the cervical spine. The most superficial muscles include trapezius, levator scapulae, and rhomboids. (From White AH, Schofferman JA, editors: *Spine care: diagnosis and conservative treatment,* St Louis, 1995, Mosby.)

rhomboids are innervated by the dorsal scapular nerve via the C5 nerve root.

- *Levator scapulae.* This muscle originates on the transverse processes of the first four cervical vertebrae and inserts medially on the superior scapular angle. Its primary function is implied in its name—it elevates the scapula with its origin fixed. When its insertion is fixed, it unilaterally flexes the cervical vertebrae and rotates their spines, and hence the face, toward the same side. Rotation, in contradistinction to that produced by trapezius and the rhomboids, is to the same side because the levator scapulae attaches to the transverse processes and not the spinous processes. Acting bilaterally, levator scapulae helps extend the spine. It is innervated by the dorsal scapular nerve.[48]

- *Levator costarum.* These arise from the tips of the transverse processes of C7 to T11 and run inferolaterally to attach on the ribs beneath their origin. These muscles, innervated by the posterior primary divisions of the spinal nerves, elevate the ribs and may laterally flex and rotate the trunk to the same side.

- *Splenius.* The splenius cervicis and the splenius capitis arise from the cervical and upper thoracic spinous processes. *Splenius cervicis* inserts into the cervical transverse processes, and *splenius capitis* inserts into the superior nuchal line and mastoid process of the skull. Wrapping around the posterior and lateral aspects of the neck, this muscle covers the other posterior neck muscles with the exception of upper trapezius and acts an extensor, lateral flexor of the neck, and rotates the face to the same side when acting bilaterally. Unilaterally, the splenius acts in synergy with the opposite sternomastoid muscles to rotate the head and neck. The splenii are innervated by the lateral branches of middle and lower cervical posterior rami.

- *Iliocostalis cervicis.* This is a small muscle that arises from the angles of the upper ribs to the posterior tubercles of the transverse processes of C4-C6. This muscle laterally flexes and extends the lower cervical region and is innervated by the posterior rami of the upper thoracic and lower cervical spinal nerves.

- *Longissimus.* Consists of two portions, namely, longissimus capitis and cervicis, which are part of the erector spinae. *Longissimus cervicis* spans between the upper thoracic transverse processes and the posterior tubercles of the transverse processes of C2 to C6. *Longissimus capitis* spans between the upper thoracic transverse processes and articular processes of C4 through C7 and inserts onto the mastoid process of the temporal bone. Both muscles extend, laterally bend, and rotate the face to the same side. Longissimus is innervated by the lateral branches of the cervical and upper thoracic posterior rami.

- *Semispinalis.* Consists of three parts including the semispinalis capitis, cervicis, and thoracis, all of which act to extend the spine. The *semispinalis capitis* is the largest muscle mass in the back of the neck and lies beneath the upper fibers of the trapezius muscle. This powerful muscles arise from upper transverse processes and run vertically upward to insert onto the occipital bone between its superior and inferior nuchal lines. It is innervated by the posterior rami of the first through sixth cervical spinal nerves. The *semispinalis cervicis* is the largest neck muscle and arises from the upper thoracic spinous processes to run upward and medially, inserting on the C2-C5 spinous processes. Running almost vertically between its two attachments, it is innervated by the posterior primary rami of the C6 to C8 spinal nerves. The semispinalis muscles, like multifidus, and the rotatory muscles are bilateral extensors, unilateral benders and rotate the face to the opposite side.

- *Multifidus cervicis.* This is a series of multipennate muscles extending over the entire length of the vertebral column between the sacrum and axis, lying beneath the semispinalis muscles, where they fill the groove between the transverse and spinous processes of the vertebrae. This muscle covers the laminae of the vertebral column, each originating on the articular processes of the lower four cervical vertebrae and transverse processes and traveling lateromedial before inserting on the spinous process one to four segments above that level. Multifidi insert onto all the vertebrae except the atlas. Thickest in the lumbar region, this muscle primarily extends the vertebral column when acting bilaterally. When acting unilaterally, the fibers of multifidus pull down on the spinous process from which they arise, laterally flex the spine and also execute posterior sagittal rotation of their vertebra of origin.

- *Rotatori.* These are the shortest representatives of the transversospinal group and, located deep to the multifidus group, constitute the deepest muscle fasciculi located in the groove between the spinous and transverse processes. These muscles are best represented in the thoracic region and poorly developed in the cervical and lumbar regions. The rotatores longus and brevis help extend the spine when acting bilaterally. When acting unilaterally, contraction yields spinal rotation such that the vertebral bodies move away from the side contracted.[91] Like the unisegmental muscles, the rotatores act to stabilize the vertebral column.

- *Suboccipital muscles.* Four deep suboccipital muscles interconnect the posterior aspect of the axis, atlas, and occipital bone. Innervated by the C1 dorsal ramus (suboccipital nerve), the rectus capitis posterior major and minor extends and rotates the face to the same side. The obliquus capitis inferior also rotates the atlas to turn the face to the same side, while the obliquus capitis superior extends and laterally bends the head.

20. What is the role of the uncinate process in axial rotation of the cervical spine?

The *uncinate process* acts, among its several functions, to limit lateral translation. Uncinate processes are unnecessary at the thoracic and lumbar levels, where lateral translation is limited, respectively, by the rib cage and the sagittal orientation of the lumbar facet joints. The uncinate processes also serve as a guiding mechanism for flexion and extension and for anteroposterior translation. A primary function of the uncinate process is to control rotation of the cervical spine. Consider the typical lumbar disk in which the axis of rotation lies within the midsubstance of the intervertebral disk. If this persisted in the cervical spine, then the uncinate processes would act as obstructions to motion. Because of this, the axis of rotation lies above the disk[47] so that uncinate motion occurs unobstructed. Control of axial interbody rotation in the cervical spine is shared by both the facet joint and the uncinate processes. Of the two, facet rotation plays a lesser role in controlling rotation. Facet rotation involves forward flexion of the contralateral facet over the inferior facet below with retraction of the ipsilateral side. However, these facets appear to be in lateral flexion in the frontal view. Lateral flexion of the facet joints results in rotation not because of facet orientation, but because of the position of the uncus that is controlling rotation. Thus rotational movements occur as a function of the intervertebral disk joint, uncus, and facet joints.[57,118]

21. What are the uncovertebral joints and how does their development result in degenerative changes in the cervical spine?

Because of the primary role the uncinate processes play in rotation of the cervical spine, over time degenerative changes occur in the posterolateral aspect of the annulus fibrosus just medial to the uncinate processes, sec-

ondary to accumulated friction. Adventitious uncovertebral clefts develop between the uncinate process and the annulus fibrosus representing reflected layers of split collagen fibers of the annulus that have undergone cartilaginous metaplasia. Two clefts occur in each intervertebral disk between the uncinate processes of the vertebrae above and below that disk that forms a joint between each uncinate process and the inferior lateral surface of the vertebral body. The convexity of the uncinate process above that disk forms a convex cleft with the disk called the *anvil* or *enchancrure* (notch), while the same disk forms a concave cleft called an *uncus* with the uncinate process below. There is no evidence of these clefts at birth, or in infants or children. By adolescence bilateral degenerative clefts have developed in the posterolateral portion of the annulus medial to the uncinate process, between C3 and T1, and may develop into synovial joints known as *neurocentral* or the *uncovertebral joint of Luschka* (Fig. 63-6).[94] The exact site of these joints is between the uncinate process of the inferior vertebral body (superolateral plateau) and the

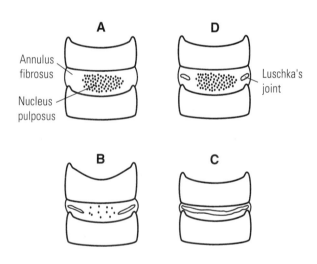

FIG. 63-6 Development of the *uncovertebral joints of Luschka* occurs as a function of aging of the intervertebral disk and ordinary motion at the cervical spine. **A,** In the newborn there is no evidence of degenerative clefts. **B,** By adolescence, degenerative clefts corresponding to the future site of Luschka joints have developed in the posterolateral annulus just medial to the uncinate processes. **C,** By 20 to 35 years of age, these degenerative clefts have enlarged and spread medially toward dehydrating the nucleus pulposus. **D,** Between the ages of 40 and 60, the clefts have met in midline and the intervertebral disk is severely desiccated, degraded, and has lost significant height. (From White AH, Schofferman JA, editors: *Spine care: diagnosis and conservative treatment*, St Louis, 1995, Mosby.)

semilunar facets of the vertebral body above[47] (infero-lateral plateau).[105] It is the development and maturation of these joints, typically occurring after age 30,[7] which causes erosion of the intervertebral disk that results in insidious dehydration of the intervertebral disk and provokes the degenerative cascade that pathologically alters the normal biomechanics of that spinal segment. Thus what began as metaplastic clefts during rotational motion eventually matures and desiccates the disk so that by middle age, these clefts extend through the disk midline. The disk suffers significant volume loss as its center has been largely replaced by ligamentous and fibrocartilage-like tissue. This leads to osteophytic proliferation of both the uncinate processes and the facet joints leading to a spectrum of pathology involving osseous encroachment on the neural elements of the spine.

22. Why does degeneration of the cervical disk often begin laterally, just medial to the uncinate process?

Degenerative disk disease initiates the degenerative cascade in the anterior interbody joint of the cervical spine and spreads posteriorly to involve the uncinate processes and the posterior facet joints. Degeneration of the cervical disk begins at the posterolateral aspect of the annulus fibrosus just medial to the uncinate processes, secondary to accumulated friction from the uncovertebral junction. This site of union between the uncinate process and the anterior inferior lip of the vertebral body above[59] happens to coincide with that portion of the annulus that is thinnest and therefore subject to the greatest strain. The biomechanical definition of strain is the change of length of an objection (deformation) under load divided by the original length. Hence, for the same displacement of the cervical spine in various directions, the portion of annulus that is thinnest is most likely to sustain the greatest percentage change in length. As a result, it will be subject to the greatest strain and more likely to fail. It is for this reason that transverse fissures across the posterior half of the cervical disk occur by age 30, with such regularity that they constitute a normal feature of cervical anatomy.[104]

23. Why is intervertebral disk herniation less common in the cervical spine than the lumbar spine?

Intervertebral disk herniation is less common at cervical levels than lumbar levels for a number of reasons. First, superincumbent loads are substantially less at the cervical levels. Second, the posterior longitudinal liga-ment is substantially thicker in the cervical region, and is approximately three to four times thicker in the cervical region than in the thoracic or lumbar regions.[51] Subsequently, the posterior longitudinal ligament serves as a barrier that is better suited to withstand pressure from a bulging disk. Additionally, the uncinate processes, by virtue of their interposed placement between the nerve roots and disks, act as a natural barrier to protect against lateral and posterolateral herniations. Moreover, the cervical posterior longitudinal ligament offers considerably more posterior reinforcement because of its substantially greater width and thickness, as compared with the lumbar spine. Finally, because degenerative changes appear earlier in the cervical intervertebral disks, the accompanying nuclear desiccation reduces the probability of nuclear herniation. Symptomatic cervical disk herniations are most common in the fourth decade of life and occur in a male/female ratio of 1.4 : 1. Risk factors include frequent lifting, cigarette smoking, and diving from a board.[53] Nuclear prolapse may occur intraforaminally, ventrolaterally, or in the midline,[60] although the former is the most common.[61] Asymptomatic disk bulges with subligamentous herniation are common in older patients, particularly at the C6-C7 disk.[36] Disk herniation may also occur in the younger person from a whiplash related injury or in conjunction with spinal cord neurapraxia.

24. What is the structural degenerative cascade?

The *structural degenerative cascade* is a series of pathoanatomic changes that occur over time that accounts for the majority of pain of spinal origin. This schema is based upon understanding the functional unit of the spine as a unit of function between the joints of the anterior and posterior elements of the spine. A *spinal motion segment* is a compound articulation comprised of a three-joint complex composed of an anterior symphysis and two posterior synovial facet joints, so that pathologic conditions or dysfunction in one component can adversely affect the others.[116] Various conditions of the spine may be viewed as a spectrum of related pathologies along a continuum of degenerative structural changes.

Beginning most often with degenerative disk disease, the degenerative cascade begins with micro or macro trauma in the intervertebral disk anteriorly migrating posteriorly across the uncinate process and vertebral arch to alter facet joint alignment. This results in structural alteration of the vertebral motion segment that, in turn, provokes marginal osteophytes. One *verte-

bral motion segment is defined as the intervertebral disk joint anteriorly and the two posteriorly located facet joints that define and limit the amount of movement at the disk joint. The degenerative cascade is similar to the degenerative process in other articular surfaces and occurs as a function of joint movement and the normal process of wear-and-tear of tissue. At some point in a patient's life, the amount of motion at the spinal motion segment causes more wear than can be tolerated leading to degenerative wear of the soft and osseous tissue comprising the spinal motion segment. In the case of the cervical spine, this process is hastened by the uncovertebral joint of Luschka, which, being ubiquitous to the normal cervical spine, ushers in this degenerative process early on. Over time, structural degeneration may eventually manifest as disk degeneration or herniation, spinal instability, malalignment, facet arthrosis, lateral canal stenosis, or central canal stenosis with or without myeloma. However, because patients may or may not be symptomatic at any stage, and because of the many ways in which pathology may manifest, the degenerative cascade may lead to a variety of clinical presentations. Thus the degenerative cascade represents a spectrum of soft and osseous tissue degeneration of the spinal motion segment that represents a range of pathological changes, each of which has its unique clinical presentation.[82]

25. What is the pathophysiology of cervical spine disease?

Degenerative disk disease of the cervical spine is termed *cervical disk disease* and occurs secondary to wear at the thinnest, posterolateral aspect of the annulus fibrosus just medial to the uncinate processes, secondary to several factors including accumulated friction from the uncovertebral junction. Torsion forces imposed on normal movement of a lower cervical motion segment cause lamellar unraveling of the annulus.[53] Annular delamination also occurs from repetitive loading in flexion and extension.[26] Coupled with degenerative changes at the uncovertebral joint, this process begins during early adult life as a normal variant of cervical disk anatomy and leads to early desiccation of the inner nucleus due to the development of transverse fissures across the posterior half of the cervical disk. Simultaneously, the disk undergoes proteoglycan changes involving the ratio of keratin to chondroitin sulfate, and diminishing its ability to imbibe fluid. At the same time, a lack of nutrition with calcification of the vertebral endplate occurs, so that osmosis of nutri-

ents from the vessels within the endplate to the avascular cervical disk is minimized by age twenty. By age forty, 70% of the endplate undergoes calcification and even ossification, whereas at age 70, endplate degeneration is almost complete.[70]

26. How does the pathophysiology of cervical spine disease result in mechanical disturbance of the cervical motion segment?

Fissuring heralds fibrillation of the cartilaginous lamellae comprising the annulus, as well as loss of disk height due to accelerated loss of water content. Loss of disk height initiates a disturbance between the weight-bearing functions of the anterior and posterior columns of the spine at that motion segment, and initiates a series of changes in the components comprising that segment. The accumulated microtrauma of these *minor annular tears* to the intervertebral disk anteriorly, represents a failure in the weight-bearing function of the anterior interbody joint, so that the responsibility for weight-bearing shifts posteriorly to the uncinate processes and facet joints. Moreover, the accompanying loss of height stemming from disk desiccation causes asymmetrical facet loading, causing incongruity in the fit of the facet joints. Unequal loading results in early degenerative changes such as *facet synovitis* on the more heavily loaded side, provoking a reactive *muscular response* in the form of increased tone or spasm as a protective attempt to dynamically stabilize the region and prevent future excessive motion. This degenerative process may be hastened by excessive motion and forces applied to the cervical spine, especially rotational strain.

27. What reactive stabilization strategy occurs in the cervical spine during cervical disk disease?

The cumulative pathophysiologic pathways leading to cervical spondylosis affects the spinal motion segment resulting in loss of motion segment height, loss of cervical lordosis and hypertrophy of the spinal elements. Chondro-ossification of the osseous elements of the cervical spinal segment is the body's attempt toward stabilization of the motion segment. Thus the vertebral endplates, as well as the uncovertebral and zygapophyseal joints respond to altered biomechanical segment motion by proliferating osteophytic bone spurs. Uncinate process enlargement secondary to osteoarthritis is most often found at the C5 and C6 vertebrae.[21]

Osteophytosis often begins with hypertrophy of the anterior and posterior surfaces of the vertebral endplate and the uncinate processes. Anterior vertebral osteophytes may cause dysphagia. Lateral osteophytes from the uncovertebral joints may cause vertebral artery compression, resulting in dizziness, intermittent visual changes, and retroocular pain. More commonly, degenerative osteophytes in the form of "ridges" from the uncovertebral joints extend posteriorly.

Reactive hyperostosis may progress to the point where the osteophytic lip of the posterior endplate and the uncinate spur coalesce in a "spondylitis bar." As segmental instability migrates posteriorly, the facet joints undergo cartilage destruction, failure of the joint capsule, end-plate hypertrophy, and facet arthrosis with osteophytes projecting into the lateral recess of the spinal canal and intervertebral foramen. Once osteophytic overgrowth has involved the facet joints, the intervertebral foramen is at risk for cervical spondylosis because encroachment on the nerve root may occur anteriorly from the uncinate processes and posteriorly from the apophyseal facet joints. If this occurs, the patient will experience stenotic radiculopathy.

28. How may cervical spondylosis evolve into cervical spinal stenosis?

In addition to the hypertrophic bone formation associated with cervical spondylosis, other changes occur that may directly compress the spinal cord. Primarily, osteophytic bone spurs from the posterior margin of the disk cause diminished space in the spinal canal. The loss of motion segment height and lordosis further decrease the space available for the cord and exiting nerve roots. With progressive loss of height, the posterior longitudinal ligament is stretched thin along its length. A reactive spondylolytic bar forms underneath the bucked longitudinal ligament and permanently tents the cord anteriorly and flattens it. With loss of height, the ligamentum flavum thickens. Moreover, lamina hypertrophy occurs. With forward flexion the anteroposterior diameter of the cord is decreased as the cord is stretched across the anterior elements. The cumulative effect of these changes on the central spinal canal has a pincer effect on the cervical cord, resulting in spinal stenosis and cervical myelopathy.

29. What length changes do the spinal and root canals undergo with normal movement?

The mobility of the neck makes significant demands on the cervical cord. The spinal canal undergoes significant length changes during movement and the spinal cord and adjacent soft tissue must accommodate these changes or else suffer encroachment, particularly during extension and lateral bending. The length of the cervical spinal canal increases with flexion and decreases with extension. The spinal cord and nerve roots are stretched and lengthened during cervical flexion and relaxed and pleated during extension.[13] From spinal extension to flexion, the spinal canal elongates by as much as 5 to 9 cm with most of the elongation occurring in the cervical and lumbar regions. During forward flexion, the length of the spinal canal is increased by approximately 2 cm and the cervical cord must stretch* by elongation. During early spinal flexion, the cross-sectional area of the spinal canal increases due to an increase of the anteroposterior diameter. During hyperextension of the neck the central canal shortens while its cross-section decreases with extension.[4] During hyperextension the cord slackens and undergoes shortening, while the ligamentum flavum buckles, protruding into the canal and decreasing the cross-sectional area within the cervical canal.[13] Because of disk space narrowing accompanying cervical disk disease, the vertebrae will approximate each other. This causes the ligamentum flavum to infold or kink on itself, bulging further into the spinal canal and aggravating any tendency toward stenosis.[92] This explains why patients with central encroachment from a disk or osteophyte have exacerbation of symptoms while in extension and hyperextension, as this posture crowds the spinal canal and narrows the intervertebral foramen. If a spondylotic bar is present anteriorly, hyperextension of the neck may compress the cervical cord anteriorly, especially as the buckled ligamentum flavum will occupy any remaining room within the canal, posteriorly. These patients seek relief by adopting a posture with several degrees of cervical flexion, which promotes forward-head posture.

The walls of the vertebral canal do not move as one segment during movement. During flexion motion of the spine, the posterior wall of the canal elongates more than the anterior wall, while the reverse occurs with spinal extension.[14,29] Similarly, lateral flexion movements elongate the convex side of the spinal canal while shortening the concave aspect.[92] Because of this, lateral bending may provoke pain by encroaching upon an emerging nerve root, which in the neutral-head position is pain free. With a thickened ligamentum flavum, lateral flexion may cause encroachment as the ligament buckles and occupies the medial aspect of the intervertebral foramen.

---

*This most likely accounts for the transient cord symptoms known as *Lhermitte's sign.*

30. What is a possible endstage pathology of cervical spondylosis?

Cervical myelopathy, more prevalent in the older population, may derive from disk herniation, ossification of the posterior longitudinal ligament, a congenitally narrow cervical spinal canal, and most commonly cervical spondylosis due to spur formation of the uncovertebral and zygapophyseal joints. The usual sagittal diameter of the trefoil-shaped cervical canal ranges from 15 to 20 mm, and patients with a diameter of 13 mm or less are at risk for developing cord compression with mild degrees of degenerative spondylosis.[122] Spinal cord impingement initially results in compromise of the blood supply (radicular arteries) as well as axoplasmic flow of neural tissue. Vascular compromise is believed to most readily occur in the small intramedullary arterioles of grey matter.[92] Continued compression leads to demyelination of the white matter, which is probably still a recoverable lesion, whereas subsequent changes of grey matter leading to infarction and gliosis* may become irreversible. Spondylotic myelopathy can only occur in the cervical and thoracic levels; the equivalent of myelopathy in the lumbar spine is compression of the cauda equina.†

Compressive *cervical myelopathy* occurs less frequently than cervical spondylosis, although when it occurs, it often coexists with cervical spondylosis. In patients with slow chronic compression from cervical spondylosis, the spinal cord may undergo considerable compression and still function normally. Patients with a congenitally narrow canal may be predisposed to central canal compression that manifests as a slowly progressive spastic paraparesis. The acute onset may precipitate following a fall onto the back of the head producing a sharp hyperflexion of the neck.[50] This may also occur following a severe whiplash injury, chiropractice manipulation, or from sitting with the neck hyperextended in a barber's chair. The most common levels of the cord affected are C5/C6 and C6/C7.[50]

The clinical presentation of cervical myelopathy includes many of the signs and symptoms of cervical spondylosis in addition to gait or balance complaints, hyperreflexia with long tract signs, weakness, spasticity, sensory loss, and complaints of arm and neck pain, and leg weakness. Lower extremity spasticity is more evident than weakness in patients with cervical spondylosis. Neck motion, particularly extension provokes pain, so that patients may present with a positive Lhermitte's sign.‡ The presence of an *inverted radial reflex* is almost pathognomic for cervical spondylosis with myelopathy and presents as diminished or absent C5 (biceps) and C6 (supinator) deep tendon reflexes, while the C7 (triceps) reflex is brisk. This indicates that the roots and cord are compressed at the C5/C6 interspace.[64] Focal hyporeflexia of a nerve root may be present if radicular compression coexists, or if there is anterior horn cell loss from severe spinal cord compression. Deep tendon reflexes are usually absent in acute cord compression (spinal shock), although the corresponding sensory level is often present.[92] Muscle atrophy and sphincter loss is a late sign,§ the latter indicating severe myelopathy. Diagnostic imaging appropriate for confirmation of suspected cervical myelopathy includes plain films with flexion and extension views, cervical myelograthy, CT myelography, or magnetic resonance imaging. Acute cord compression represents a surgical emergency, as the prognosis depends upon how long after significant encroachment posterior compression occurred. If imaging proves negative in the chronic presentation, different diagnostic entities such as spinal cord tumor, dural hematoma, epidural abscess, chronic progressive multiple sclerosis, syringomyelia, or vitamin B_{12} deficiency should be considered.[25]

Gliosis refers to a proliferation of astroglia in damaged areas of the central nervous system.

†The spinal cord is roughly elliptical in cross section, being wider from right to left than from front to back. A furrow known as the dorsal median fissure runs down the back of the cord while a shallower depression, the ventral medial fissure (housing the anterior spinal artery) runs down the front. Together, both fissures, as in the brain, divide the cord into equal but opposite halves. The cervical spinal cord levels lie at intervals between the foramen magnum and the spinous process of C6. The upper six spinal cord levels and thoracic spinal cord levels are located between the spinous processes of C6 and T4. At birth, the caudal tip of the spinal cord (conus medullaris) lies at the level of the L3 vertebral body and continues to move upward as a child grows into an adult so that the conus is usually located anywhere between the L2 and T12 disk. The L1 through the coccygeal cord segments (and emergent nerve root) are housed by vertebrae T9 through L1. The clinical implications of this anatomical difference between the cervical and lumbar spine is that because the spinal cord ends opposite the L1 vertebra, lumbar disk lesions can *only* cause root syndromes, and cannot compress the cord and cause spastic paraparesis. In contrast, central canal compression at the level of the cervical spine causes direct compression of the spinal cord and may result in myelopathy.

---

‡*Lhermitte's sign* consists of tingling in all four limbs or down the back on flexing the neck in patients with cervical spondylitic myelopathy, or any other condition that distorts or inflames the cervical spinal cord.

§Bladder and bowel abnormalities occur late with cervical spondylitic myelopathy and early with spinal cord neoplasms or demyelinating disease.

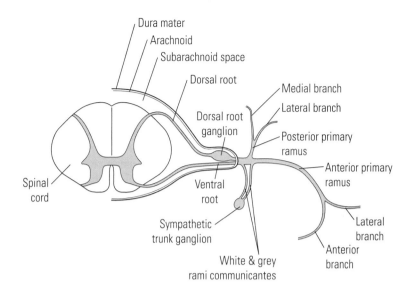

FIG. 63-7 Diagram of typical *spinal nerve root.*

31. Why are there more cervical nerve roots than cervical vertebrae?

The *cervical spinal cord* consists of eight cervical segments and each segment gives rise to a pair of posterior and anterior nerve roots, which converge and leave the dural sac as a spinal nerve (Fig. 63-7). Each pair of spinal nerve roots exits away from the spinal cord from in between adjacent vertebrae. The C1 spinal nerve rests on the posterior arch of the atlas, while the C2 spinal nerve lies behind or slightly below the lateral atlanto-axial joint. The first pair exits between the skull and first vertebrae, the second pair between the first and second vertebrae, the third pair between the second and third vertebrae, and so on. This organization is complete by the third fetal month in which the spinal cord extends the entire length of the embryo and respective spinal nerves exit their corresponding intervertebral foramina at their level or origin.[53]

The first eight pairs of *cervical spinal nerves,* the first of which passes *above* the first vertebra, to the eighth spinal nerve, which passes below the seventh vertebra, maintain their relationship to the vertebral bodies beyond neonatal life and into adulthood. Thus the cervical spinal nerves occupy and exit the intervertebral foramina lying above their ipsisegmental vertebrae, on top of the ipsisegmental pedicle, except for the C8 spinal nerve. Nerve roots inferior to C8, which also lie below their ipsisegmental vertebrae, exit below their respective ipsisegmental vertebrae. In this location, nerve roots C1 through C7 lie below the level of the intervertebral disk. This arrangement allows for one more cervical spinal nerve than cervical vertebrae, and also alters the relationships of the root to the vertebral interspace below the level of T1 (Fig. 63-8).* The clinical implication of this is that a lesion of the C5/C6 disk produces a C6 radiculopathy.

32. What is the orientation between the upper and lower emerging cervical spinal nerves and their corresponding vertebrae?

If the spinal cord and column were same length, then we could expect the cord segments at each level (represented by the emergent nerve roots for that level) to run level with the vertebrae, and each successive nerve would emerge straight out, horizontally. However, because of a growth differential within the neonate between the rate of osseous and neural tissue development, this corresponding relationship is lost below the cervical spine. The vertebral column and dura mater lengthen more rapidly than does the neural tube, so that the terminal end of the spinal cord gradually assumes a relatively higher level than the termination of the osseous spine.† The effect of this growth differential impacts on the orientation of span of the emerging thoracolumbar

---

*As a result, for example, the lumbar roots emerge *below* their respective vertebrae, so that the L4 nerve root emerges at the L4/5 interspace.

†A normal growth differential appears to be dependent upon adequate neonatal and postnatal nutrition.

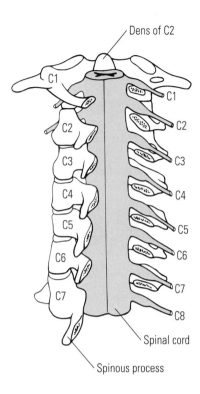

Dens of C2

C1
C2
C3
C4
C5
C6
C7

C1
C2
C3
C4
C5
C6
C7
C8

Spinal cord

Spinous process

FIG. 63-8 The relationship of the emerging nerve roots to the ipsisegmental vertebrae between C1 and C7 differs from the C8, and thoracolumbar levels. The first eight pairs of *cervical spinal nerves,* the first of which passes *above* the first vertebra, to the eighth spinal nerve, which passes below the seventh vertebra, maintain their relationship to the vertebral bodies beyond neonatal life and into adulthood. Thus the cervical spinal nerves occupy and exit the intervertebral foramen lying above their ipsisegmental vertebrae, on top of the ipsisegmental pedicle, except for the C8 spinal nerve and nerve roots inferior to C8, which also lie below their ipsisegmental vertebrae, and egress below their respective ipsisegmental vertebrae. In this location, nerve roots C1 through C7 lie below the level of the intervertebral disk.

nerve roots such that the cord segments are not located at the same level as their corresponding vertebrae. The cervical nerve roots are minimally affected and have a slight downward angulation that progresses more so at the lower end of the cervical spine. Thus within the dural sac the upper cervical nerve roots tend to pass upward to converge into their spinal nerve, the middle cervical spine roots pass transversely, while the lower roots pass slightly downward.

The orientation of the cervical spinal nerve roots is nearly horizontal as they exit the cord and intervertebral foramina, especially in the upper cervical spine. It is

this horizontal orientation of span of the cervical roots that accounts for the relatively horizontal course of the upper, middle, and lower trunks of the brachial plexus. Thus the relationship between the cord, emergent nerve roots, and corresponding vertebrae is only maintained in the cervical spine for morphological reasons.

The upper cervical cord segments are situated at approximately the same level as their corresponding vertebrae, so that their nerve roots pass transversely to exit from their intervertebral foramina above the pedicles of that same vertebral body. At lower cervical levels the spinal cord segments are one segment higher than the vertebral segment of the same number so that, for example, the C7 spinal nerve root arises at the C6 vertebral level. This causes the nerve roots of C7 to descend obliquely to reach their (C7) intervertebral foramen. Despite this, they still exit above the pedicle of their ipsisegmental vertebra (the C7 vertebral body), although below the level of the C7 intervertebral disk.

33. What is the anatomical origin of the spinal nerve, and why is encroachment within the intervertebral foramen more likely to cause sensory deficit?

The spinal nerves emerge as pairs from the cord at regular segmental intervals from between vertebrae consistent with chordates. At each segment of the neuraxis, a pair of nerves emerges from the right and left of vertical column that makes up the "H" of gray matter when viewed on cross section. On the right side, for example, pure motor fibers emerge from the right anterior horn while sensory fibers emerge from the left posterior horn. Before the joining of these fibers into a single mixed nerve, the sensory fibers merge into a bulbous ganglion* within the intervertebral foramen. Thus *because the preganglionic sensory fibers and ganglion take up relatively more space within the intervertebral foramen, encroachment of the foramen whether from osteophyte or disk protrusion is more likely to cause*

---

*In contrast to the brain that contains grey matter on the surface, and white matter in the interior, the spinal cord is organized into an H or butterfly shaped central region of gray matter surrounded by myelinated ascending and descending axon tracts of *white matter.* The central grey matter is composed of discrete collections of cell bodies of motor neurons located in the posterior (or dorsal) horns and are called *nuclei.* When viewed on cross section, the anterior (or ventral) horns of the butterfly shaped grey central portion are composed of central processes of sensory neurons. The cell bodies of sensory neurons are located outside the central nervous system in the dorsal roots of spinal nerves and hence termed *ganglions.*

sensory than motor signs and symptoms. Thus the post to ganglionic sensory fibers and the motor fibers join a short distance from the cord to form a single fixed nerve root within a canal between the adjacent vertebrae known as the intervertebral foramen.

34. What are the relevant nerve root innervations to the dermatomes and myotomes of the upper extremities?

Clinical confirmation of cervical spondylosis may be facilitated by electromyographic examination and a myelogram or other imaging techniques. Neurophysiologic testing, such as *electromyography* (EMG), accurately measures motor potentials. Two weeks after nerve injury or nerve root lesion, abnormal spontaneous electrical discharges known as *fibrillation potentials* and *positive sharp waves* appear in the resting muscle (such as the anterior spinal muscles or muscles of the lower extremity) and represent evidence of muscle denervation supplied by that root. Nerve conduction studies may show delayed or absent late waves (H or F waves) consistent with interruption of the sensory arc. These abnormal findings are evidence of muscle denervation that may result from herniated disks, nerve root avulsions, plexus or cord lesions, and peripheral nerve lesions. A myelogram will demonstrate a bulge in the spinal cord adjacent to that disk space.

Each of the gross motor movements of the upper extremity is almost exclusively mediated by a single root, so that it is not imperative to evaluate all muscles, which often exhibit redundant innervations. It is essential to learn to differentiate between a peripheral nerve lesion and a root lesion affecting upper limb function. Thus the clinician must distinguish whether sensory and motor signs lie in the territory supplied by a single nerve root or a single peripheral nerve or one of its branches.

C5 ROOT LESION

This will weaken the entire 180 degrees of shoulder abduction as the C5 root innervates both supraspinatus and the deltoid muscle (Fig. 63-9). Both muscles work in synergy to abduct the shoulder. The deltoid is supplied by the axillary nerve,* so that differentiating an axillary nerve lesion from a C5 root lesion depends on testing of the supraspinatus (which is difficult) and infraspinatus (which is also innervated by C5 and easier

---

*The axillary nerve also innervates teres minor.

to test) for external rotation, as these muscles are innervated by the suprascapular and not the axillary nerve.[25] Moreover, an axillary nerve lesion results in cutaneous loss of a circular portion over the middle deltoid region. In contrast, sensory changes secondary to spondylosis or disk lesion will demonstrate a C5 dermatomal pattern extending over the lateral arm from the summit of the shoulder to the elbow, as well as diminished biceps jerk (C5).

C6 ROOT LESION

This will weaken elbow flexion in both the supinated† and the half-pronated position of the forearm.‡ Both the musculocutaneous and radial nerves derive from C6. A C6 nerve root lesion will also manifest as weakness of the extensor carpi radialis longus and brevis, is also innervated by the radial nerve (Fig. 63-10), and will only weaken biceps and brachialis and spare brachioradialis. Moreover, a musculocutaneous nerve lesion will cause sensory loss in the distribution of the lateral cutaneous nerve to the forearm and not the C6 dermatome, which is characterized by paresthesias into the thumb, index finger, and radial half of the middle finger as well as the radial forearm. Finally, a C6 root lesion will result in a diminished supinator jerk (C6).

C7 ROOT LESION

This will weaken muscles affecting the shoulder, elbow, and wrist including: shoulder adduction (latissimus dorsi), elbow extension (triceps), wrist flexion (flexor carpi radialis) and wrist extension (extensor digitorum longus and extensor carpi ulnaris) (Fig. 63-11).[53] The C7 nerve root innervates an extensive portion of the upper extremity owing to its major contribution to both the radial and medial nerves. A radial nerve lesion cannot affect shoulder adduction or wrist flexion as these are innervated by the median nerve. Similarly, a median nerve lesion will not impact upon the strength of elbow extension. Moreover, the cutaneous innervation of these nerves maps a differing cutaneous distribution than the C7 dermatome, characterized by paresthesias in the forearm and dorsum of the hand, particularly to the middle finger.§ Finally, a C7 root lesion will result in a

---

†Achieved by biceps and brachialis via the musculocutaneous nerve.
‡Accomplished by brachioradialis via the radial nerve.
§However, as the middle finger is occasionally supplied by C6 and C8, there is no conclusive method of testing C7 sensation.

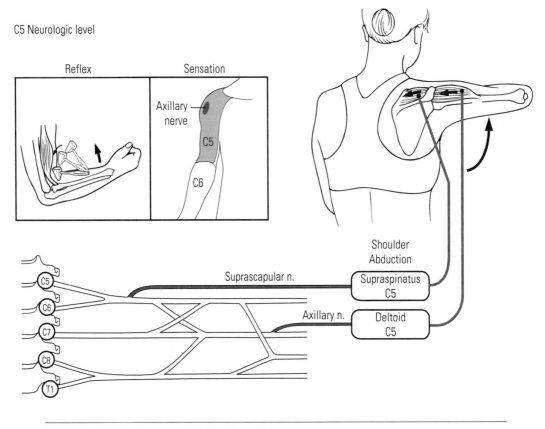

C5 Neurologic level

Reflex

Sensation

Axillary nerve

C5

C6

Shoulder Abduction

Suprascapular n.

Supraspinatus C5

Axillary n.

Deltoid C5

C5

C6

C7

C8

T1

FIG. 63-9 C5 nerve root lesion.

diminished triceps jerk (C7). Clinically differentiating between a C7 nerve root lesion and a radial nerve lesion is important as both lesions are common and occur from neck or shoulder trauma.

C8 ROOT LESION

This is uncommon, and causes muscles weakness of the long finger flexors as well as a diminished finger-jerk (C8). The extrinsics include flexor digitorum profundus and superficialis. Flexor digitorum profundus flexes the distal interphalangeal joints of the index, middle, ring, and little fingers, and assists in flexion of the proximal interphalangeal and metacarpophalangeal joints, as well as wrist flexion. As it is the only muscle that flexes the distal interphalangeal (IP) joints, weakness of this muscle manifests as diminished ability to flex the distal IP joints. While the ulnar half of profundus is conveyed through the ulnar nerve, the radial half is conveyed through the median nerve. The flexor digitorum super-

ficialis flexes the proximal interphalangeal joints of the second through the fifth digits, and assists in flexion of the metacarpophalangeal joints as well as the wrist. Weakness of the superficialis is noted as a diminished ability to flex the proximal interphalangeal (IP) joints with the distal IP joint extended. C8 innervation to the superficialis is conveyed through the median nerve. C8 involvement causes paresthesias to the little finger and distal half of the forearm (Fig. 63-12).[92]

T1 ROOT LESION

This will cause weakness of all the intrinsic hand muscles. Those muscles commonly identified with having the majority of innervation deriving from T1 are the dorsal interossei and the abductor digiti minimi (quinti), both of which are conveyed through the ulnar nerve.[50] The dorsal interossei abduct the index, middle, and ring fingers, while the abductor digiti minimi abducts the pinky finger.[92] T1 supplies sensation to the

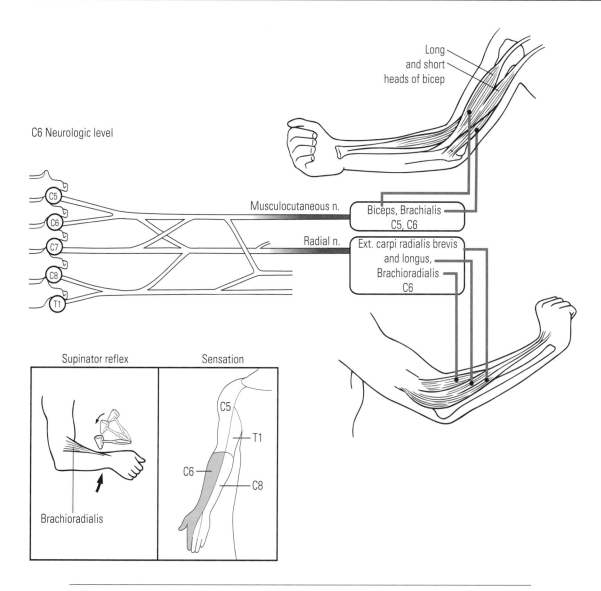

C6 Neurologic level

Long and short heads of bicep

Musculocutaneous n.

Biceps, Brachialis
C5, C6

Radial n.

Ext. carpi radialis brevis
and longus,
Brachioradialis
C6

Supinator reflex

Brachioradialis

Sensation

C5
T1
C6
C8

FIG. 63-10 C6 nerve root lesion. A musculocutaneous nerve lesion is uncommon and may occur from a humeral fracture.

upper half of the medial forearm and the medial portion of the arm. The T1 nerve root has no identifiable reflex associated with it (Fig. 63-13).

35. What are the reflexes of the upper extremity and what is their diagnostic value?

The term *reflex* means "bending back" in Latin because it refers to a sensory impulse that travels to the central nervous system only to "bend back" away from the central nervous along a motor nerve away to bring about a response. The specific nerve cell connection along which the nerve impulse travels from the initial sensation to the final response is the *reflex arc*. Most reflex arcs involve a three-neuron complex, in which a receptor neuron is connected to an effector neuron by means of an intermediate neuron called the connector neuron, which lies wholly within the central nervous system. Thus most spinal reflexes are polysynaptic in nature.

The reflex arc is automatic and involuntary and because of its simplicity, operates with no added input

C7 Neurologic level

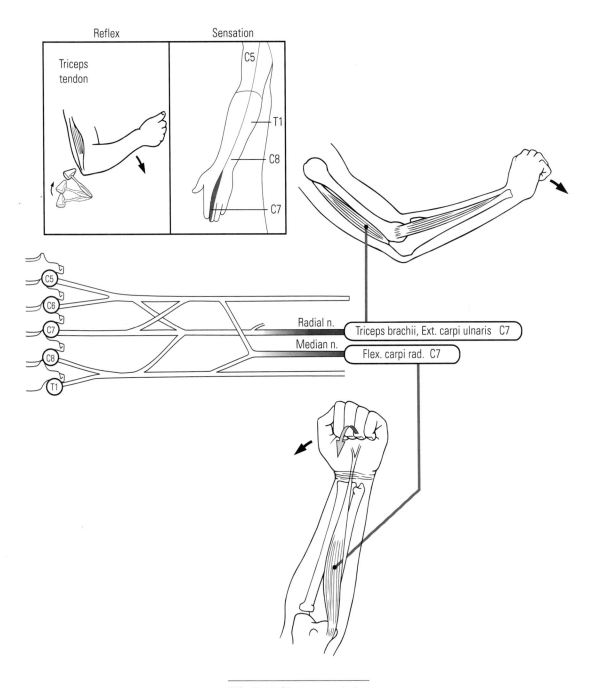

FIG. 63-11 C7 nerve root lesion.

C8 Neurologic level

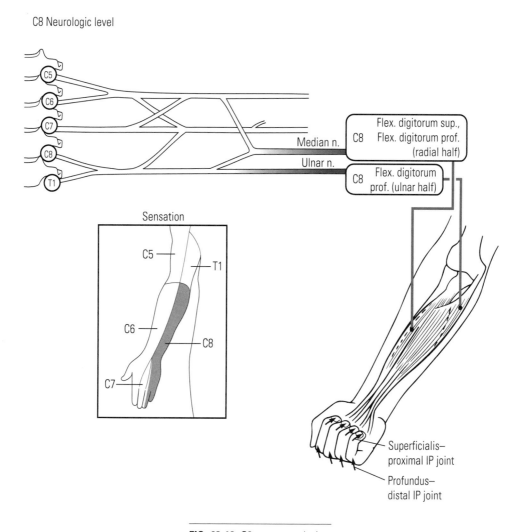

FIG. 63-12 C8 nerve root lesion.

from higher cortical levels.* The patellar reflex is un-usual in its simplicity as it only consists of two neurons (the sensory and the motor) without the benefit of the connector neuron. As such, the two-neuron reflex arc is primarily contained within the peripheral nervous system and may be said to be monosynaptic.

Reflexes are tested by holding the limb such that the tendon is placed on slight stretch. By tapping the tendon with a reflex hammer, the tendon stretches acutely to the point that the proprioceptive muscle spindles embedded within the muscle fire and cause ini-

tiation of the reflex arc. For example, in the biceps jerk the impulse is then carried across the motor axon of this same neuron through the emerging C5 nerve root and is conveyed through the musculocutaneous nerve that causes the biceps to contract and the elbow to flex.[92]

Diminishment (hyporeflexia) or loss of a reflex implies a disorder involving the portion of the nervous system through which the reflex arc travels. The disorders may be due to a disturbance in the muscle spindle, the muscle fibers, the peripheral nerve, or the spinal cord synapse. Bilateral comparison is essential because the degree of reflex activity varies from person to person. Reflexes may be documented as normal, elevated, or depressed. Diminished biceps (C5) and brachiora-dialis (C6) reflexes and an increased triceps (C7) jerk

---

*The independence of spinal reflexes from the brain is demonstrated by somewhat abnormal reflex preservation in quadriplegics.

T1 Neurologic level

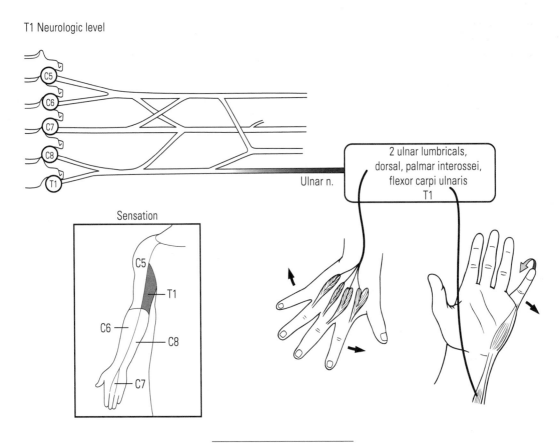

FIG. 63-13 T1 nerve root lesion.

is known as an *inverted radial reflex,* and is often a clue to cervical spondylosis and myelopathy at the C5/C6 interspace, causing segmental nerve root compression of C6 and pyramidal tract signs below that level.[19]

36. What are the deep tendon reflexes of the upper extremity and how are they elicited?

- *Biceps jerk.* The clinician should place their thumb on the biceps tendon in the cubital fossa of the elbow so as to place the tendon on slight stretch. With the elbow flexed to approximately 90°, tap the nail of the thumb with the narrow end of the reflex hammer to elicit contraction of the biceps and elbow flexion. This is an almost pure C5 reflex conveyed though the musculocutaneous nerve.
- *Supinator jerk.* This is also known as the brachioradialis reflex and performed with the patient's arm flexed at 90°. Using the flat end of the reflex hammer, the brachioradialis tendon is struck at the distal end of the radius, causing the forearm to jerk into elbow flexion. The supinator jerk is a C6 reflex conveyed through the radial nerve.
- *Triceps jerk.* This is performed with the patient's arm flexed at 90°. The triceps tendon is short and should be tapped with the point of the reflex hammer approximately one inch above the olecranon process. The triceps muscle will contract and the elbow will extend involuntarily. This is a pure C7 reflex that is, like the supinator jerk, also conveyed through the radial nerve.
- *Pectoralis jerk.* This reflex is elicited by placing one's fingers on the belly of the pectoralis major just medial to the deltoid and tapping one's fingers sharply with the reflex hammer. This is a C7/C8 reflex conveyed through both the lateral and medial anterior thoracic nerves.[12,35]
- *Finger jerk.* With the patient's palm upturned and the fingers in half-flexion, the tips of the fingers are held and then tapped. The patient's fingers are felt to flex, while the free thumb also flexes. The C8 reflex is conveyed through both the medial and ulnar nerve to the long finger flexors.[84]

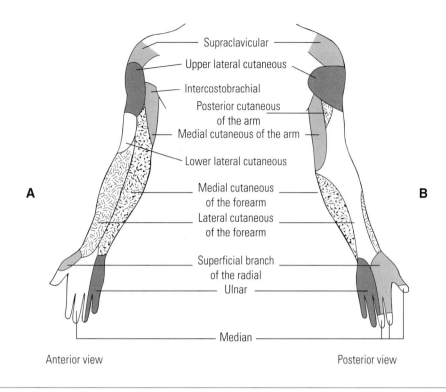

FIG. 63-14 Peripheral nerve cutaneous innervation of the upper limb. **A,** Anterior view. **B,** Posterior view.

37. What is the differential diagnosis of cervical disk disease?

A multitude of entities may masquerade as problems originating from the cervical spine, although careful attention to the history, physical examination, electromyographic abnormalities, and radiographic findings allows for differentiation and localization of the pathology. Nerve root pain may derive from spinal canal tumors, posterior fossa tumors, thoracic outlet syndrome, anterior interosseous syndrome, pronator teres syndrome, hemorrhage, apical lung carcinoma, cervical rib syndrome, or angina pectoris.[25] The more commonly encountered differential diagnoses involve compressive neuropathies of the upper extremity.[114] Finally, cervical nerve root compression may coexist with peripheral nerve root compression in a double-crush phenomenon.[28]

- *Peripheral entrapment neuropathy.* A number of entrapment neuropathies may occur along the length of the upper extremity and may be differentiated from cervical radiculopathy by several means. Peripheral neuropathies, such as carpal tunnel and similar syndromes rarely cause proximal pain, pain in the neck, scapular pain, or pain induced by neck movement.

Whereas patients with peripheral nerve disorders, such as carpal tunnel syndrome, often find pain relief by massaging, wringing their hands, immersion in water, or changing position, patients with cervical radiculopathy experience worsened pain with use of the hand and arm. Nerve conduction tests are almost always normal in cases of uncomplicated radiculopathy. Electromyographic tests performed on a number of arm muscles show changes in a myotomal pattern. Moreover, with cervical root disease, the paraspinous muscles may be denervated, confirming nerve root damage.[25] Finally, nondermatomal cutaneous innervation is manifest in patients with focal nerve damage (Fig. 63-14).

- *Shoulder disease.* This may be confused with cervical spine disease because radicular pain may refer to the shoulder region. However, the history and clinical presentation of shoulder disease differs from that of cervical disk disease and would demonstrate diminished glenohumeral joint range of motion, shoulder pain, a pain and weakness pattern that is not consistent with dermatomes and myotomes, and normal deep tendon reflexes.

- *Acute brachial neuritis.* Also known as *brachial plex-*

opathy, *Parsonage-Turner syndrome*,[102] *neuralgic amyotrophy,* or *serum neuritis* and is a relatively common cause of acute local shoulder pain followed by atrophy and weakness of the deltoid, and particularly of the serratus anterior muscles. This form of neuritis, characterized by dramatic symptoms and relatively good prognosis,[28] was prominent during the second world war when many soldiers were hospitalized due to an infectious disorder of the respiratory or alimentary tract, or recovering from a minor operation. Occurring most often in young men, this condition causes supraclavicular pain, weakness and diminished reflexes in myotomal and dermatomal patterns, and minor sensory abnormalities. This condition is believed to stem from an inflammatory condition involving the nerve roots, and often occurs as a sequel to immunization in which serum injection occurs directly into the deltoid muscles. The exact etiology is unknown, but this condition is believed to be related to a viral or immunological inflammatory process. Hence, this condition may follow inoculations, viral illness, and surgical procedures, but is not the result of a stretch injury or local trauma.[25] Pain, in the C5 through C7 dermatomes may be excruciating and is often worse at night when it disturbs sleep. After approximately a week to 10 days of pain, symptoms subside after which paralysis and atrophy of the affected muscles set in, and may be accompanied by profound weakness and rapid wasting. The primary muscles involved are the serratus anterior, deltoid, spinales, brachioradialis, biceps, and wrist extensors, although the majority of pain and weakness is localized to the shoulder girdle. The muscles that are usually spared include the pectorals, latissimus dorsi, biceps, triceps, and the muscles of the forearm and hand. Combinations of affected muscles may occur, the commonest being the deltoid and spinales on the same side. The most common sensory sign corresponds to a small ovoid zone of hypoesthesia over the middle deltoid muscles in the area of the cutaneous supply of the axillary nerve.[92] There is no accompanying neck stiffness. A hallmark of this condition is that electromyographic studies usually show changes indicating combined nerve root and peripheral nerve involvement.[25] The condition is bilateral in one third of patients.[6] The most consistent, and striking feature is singular involvement of the long thoracic nerve with paresis of the serratus anterior with scapular winging.[102] This condition does not cause focal slowing of nerve conduction,[20] and corticosteroids have no proven benefit.[95] The prognosis for recovery is good, although as much as a full year may be required before full muscle strength is restored in the paralyzed deltoid and serratus muscles. Recurrences in the same or opposite shoulder, while rare, may occur.[110]

- *Articular pillar fracture.* This refers to a chip fracture of the superior articular facet causing the patient to experience transient radicular pain often followed by mild to intense neck pain. Persistent radicular pain suggests displacement of the fragment into the dorsal root as it exits the intervertebral foramen.[119] This fracture is fairly common in the cervical spine and is frequently undetected.[113]

- *Apical lung tumor.* T1 level root damage may result from altered anatomy of the apical pleura due to apical lung tumor or cervical rib. Also known as pulmonary superior sulcus, or Pancoast tumor, this neoplasm is accompanied by rapid and severe weakness of all the small muscles of the hand, which, in advanced cases, results in radiographically visible cancerous erosion of the first and second ribs, as well as possible hoarseness owing to paralysis of one vocal cord.[67] A regular A-P radiograph may yield a false negative while apical views or CAT scan are more definitive.[109] Apical lung tumors ought to be especially suspect in patients who have a history of smoking.[111]

38. What is spinal cord neurapraxia?

Spinal cord neurapraxia refers to quadriplegia secondary to transient spinal cord injury due to forced hyperflexion, hyperextension or axial loading of the spine with rapid recovery of sensory and motor systems after five to ten minutes.[97] The mechanism of injury involves transient posterior overriding of the facets or transient posterior and inward buckling of the ligamentum flavum such that the cervical spinal cord is acutely pinched during extremes of neck movement or headbutting or spearing types of tackling. Athletes who already have preexisting cervical canal stenosis are predisposed toward developing this condition. Symptoms may be confined to the arms and legs, and may linger for as long as 48 hours after the injury as residual paresthesia or focal motor loss. Sensory symptoms include burning pain, numbness, tingling or complete anesthesia, whereas motor symptoms may range from weakness to complete paralysis. Neck pain should not be present at the initial clinical evaluation. Also known as spinal cord concussion, mild acute cervical spinal cord injury, transient quadriparesthesia, transient quadriparesis, and quadriburners,[112] this condition is most common in American football players, but has also been reported to occur in ice hockey, basketball, and boxing.[76,120] When encountered, the patient must not be treated any different than the patients with immediate complete quadriplegia until normal neurologic function is restored.[97] Athletes with a mid-sagittal cervical canal diameter of less than 14 mm are at risk for this transient condition and should be advised against participating in contact sports.[102] Radiographic findings include developmental stenosis, congenital fusion (Klippel-Feil syndrome), occult cervical instability, or intervertebral disk disease. Surgery is not indicated, while return to athletic participation is based upon severity and frequency of symptoms, duration of signs, and severity of radiographic stenosis.[122]

39. What is nerve-root neurapraxia?

Nerve root, or *brachial plexus neurapraxia,* also known as a "stinger" or "burner" injury[122] is the most common form of athletic cervical neurologic injury,[39] and represents a traction injury to the cervical nerve roots or brachial plexus. Frequently occurring in American football, or during wrestling, the usual mechanism of injury is identical to that of a brachial plexus injury, namely shoulder depression with lateral neck flexion to the contralateral side. Alternately, cervical spine extension, compression, and rotation toward the affected arm may produce this injury.[44] Occurring most commonly in the upper trunk of the plexus, patient with these injuries have a normal cervical range of motion, distinguishing this clinical entity from a classic neck-type injury. Symptoms include lancinating pain, burning sensation, numbness, and tingling extending from the shoulder to the hand that may travel as far as the base of the thumb.[25] Symptoms, including paralysis of the entire upper limb, typically last for several seconds to a few minutes. Athletic activity may resume once paresthesias have entirely abated. Patients with recurrent episodes, or unresolved episodes should undergo an electromyographic evaluation as well as stretching and strengthening of the neck musculature and shoulder girdle. Therapeutic exercises should initially focus on midline isometric strengthening exercises and active range of motion without resistance.

40. What is the clinical presentation of cervical spine disease and cervical sprain/strain?

The clinical symptoms of cervical sprain/strain deriving from cervical whiplash syndrome may not surface until 6 or more hours following the injury. Radiographs are typically normal, and the patient is often discharged home before the onset of symptoms. Symptoms include neck pain, shoulder and scapular pain, painful spinal motion, stiffness, exquisite neck muscle soreness, neck muscle spasm, headaches, back pain, dysphagia, as well as sleep and neurologic disturbances, including dizziness. Usually, there are no objective neurological findings in the upper extremity.[71] Other symptoms include vertigo, blurring of vision, nausea, tinnitus, unsteadiness of gait, and lack of concentration, if damage occurred to the vertebral artery or sympathetic ganglia. Shoulder, scapular, and occipital pain are usually referred pain from the spinal ligaments,[92] but may also be a result of C5 nerve root impingement, although the latter is ruled out by the assessment of relevant myotomes, dermatomes, and deep tendon reflexes. False root signs, especially C8, can be seen with spasm of the anterior scalenus muscles.[53] Muscular injuries most likely occur at the musculotendinous junction[73] rather than within the body of the cervical muscles. Hemorrhage from a tear at the musculotendinous junction results in an inflammatory response, muscle spasms, pain, and decreased range of motion. Dysphagia or swallowing problems may occur because the pharynx and esophagus are separated from the anterior aspect of the prevertebral fascia between which the retropharyngeal space is situated. Anteroposterior and lateral x-rays are indicated, as well as odontoid views when trauma to the upper cervical spine is suspected. The former offer valuable information regarding the magnitude of pre-existing degenerative changes.[103]

With cervical spondylosis, the patient may complain of a dull, aching-type of muscular pain that may extend to the scapular, interscapular, neck, posterior-auricular, and posterior-occipital pain (headache.) The posterior division of the cervical root may be responsible for painful radiation along the medial scapular borders, as well as anterior radiation in the prochordal region.[81] Alternately, the patient may feel pain in the affected root territory, that is provoked by neck movement or certain arm motions. Symptoms are generally worse on waking in the morning, and improve following a hot shower and mobility exercises. Symptoms often exacerbate after an unusual activity such as painting a ceiling. The C6, C7, and C5 nerve roots, in that order, are most often affected with cervical spondylosis. If an osteophyte extends laterally, encroaching on the vertebral artery foramen, vertebral artery occlusion symptoms may occur, including dizziness, tinnitus, intermittent blurring of vision and retro-ocular pain.[121] Roots

C3, C4, and T1 are so infrequently unaffected that their presentation merits suspicion of other possible causes.[41] The following provocative tests assess for radicular pain secondary to cervical spine disease:

CERVICAL COMPRESSION TEST

This is performed by pressing down on the patient's head and is considered positive if pain occurs or increases. Pain is caused by narrowing of the neural foramen, pressure on the facet joints, or provoking muscle spasm. The test may also refer pain down the upper extremity from the cervical spine, and may be followed by compression while tilting the head to that side. This has the effect of further diminishing the aperture of the intervertebral foramen and compressing the nerve root, thereby assisting in identifying the compressed root.

CERVICAL DISTRACTION TEST

This mimics spinal traction by placing one hand around the patient's chin and the other around the occiput and slowly lifting the head. A positive test is indicated if the pain is relieved or diminished, and indicates relieved pressure on the nerve roots secondary to widening of the cervical intervertebral foramina. This maneuver also helps relieves pressure on the joint capsules around the facet joints, and relieve muscle spasm by relaxing the contracted muscles involved.[41-44]

SHOULDER DEPRESSION TEST

This is performed by side-flexion of the patient's head while applying a downward pressure on the opposite shoulder. A positive test is indicated by increased pain secondary to irritation or compression of the nerve roots, foraminal encroachment on the nerve root from osteophytic overgrowth, or stretching of adhesions around the dural sleeves of the nerve and adjacent joint capsule.[48]

SPURLING MANEUVER

This reproduces arm pain by hyperextension and lateral cervical rotation[77] of the extended head toward the symptomatic arm (Fig. 63-15). This is followed by compression of the cervical spine. These combined movements decrease the diameter of the intervertebral foramen, and often exacerbate radicular symptoms.[42] When the maneuver produces neck pain only, the findings should be considered negative.[48]

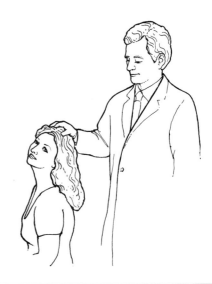

FIG. 63-15 *Spurling's maneuver.* (From Watkins RG: *The spine in sports,* St Louis, 1995, Mosby.)

41. What is the prognosis for cervical spine disease and cervical sprain/strain?

With early cervical spine disease, the patient usually complains of a dull, aching type of muscular pain that may extend to scapular, interscapular, neck, posterior-auricular, and posterior-occipital pain (headache.) This self-limiting phase improves in approximately 80% of patients presenting with axial neck pain, regardless of radiographic findings.[43] Management is conservative and focused upon the facets and muscles of the area. As the pathophysiologic changes associated with cervical disk disease evolve, the pain may become more severe, although encroachment of a nerve root and radiculopathic symptoms are usually self-limited and respond to conservative managment.[80] In patients with spondylosis with nerve root encroachment from multiple sources of hypertrophic bone changes, approximately one third of patients will not respond to conservative care.[66] With whiplash injuries, approximately 90% of patients are free of symptoms within 2 months.[98]

42. What imaging is indicated for patients with cervical spine disease?

Chondroosseous spurs along the vertebral end plates, uncovertebral and zygapophyseal joints are the radiographic hallmark of cervical spondylosis and are universally present to some degree in every asymptomatic patient over 55 years of age.[78] Oblique views allow for assessment of osseous foraminal patency. These osteo-arthritic changes tend to affect several adjacent spinal segmental levels. However, before the onset of spondylosis, suspected cervical disk disease in its early stages is confirmed by direct disk inspection via either magnetic resonance imaging and discography, whereas computerized tomography (CT), myelography, and CT enhanced myelography, at best, only visualize the canal and outer contours of the disk.[101] With cervical spine disease, effort must be made to match the clinical presentation to the appropriate radiographic or MRI studies. However, many individuals with entirely asymptomatic histories demonstrate abnormalities of the cervical spine with imaging studies.

43. What physical therapy is appropriate in the management of these patients?

Patients with nonmyelopathic neck pain should undergo an initial trial of conservative therapy as the results of nonoperative therapy are considered good.[17] The goals of therapy include pain reduction, improved range of motion, improved strength and flexibility, as well as improvement of daily activities of living. An eclectic treatment approach has been adopted here and may include:

REST

Following a sprain or strain of the soft tissues of the cervical region, 2 or 3 weeks of *rest* may be necessary in the event of severe injury. Generally, if significant pain is present after the first day, then the patient may find relief from several days to a week of *bed rest.*

CERVICAL COLLAR

Wear a soft *cervical collar* for 24 hours per day for 2 or 3 weeks, and then intermittently for 4 to 6 weeks. The collar should permit slight neck flexion and prevent extension. For cervical spine disease as well as whiplash injury. *Medications* may include muscle relaxants, nonsteroidal antiinflammatory medications, analgesics, or even sedatives.

EXERCISES

Cervical spine exercises restore normal muscle length to the scalene muscles. Exercises include cervical retraction, side flexions, cervical flexion and extension.

Patients should begin from either the position of minimal or absent pain, and proceed to the point of pain without pushing through their pain. If there is no pain felt, then the patient or therapist may apply gentle overpressure. Targeting tight structures is a major facet of the evaluation as well as treatment of this condition. Restoration of normal length of adaptively shortened tissue is paramount to successful treatment. Adaptively shortened tissue may either compress or prevent normal movement of the nerve roots and trunks. Lengthening of such tissue, provided inflammation has receded, is imperative to a successful treatment regimen. *Range of motion* in the nonpainful range exercises may be started as soon as they are tolerated and gradually increased. Once pain has subsided, the patient may perform *isometric exercises* and progress to progressive resisted neck motion[75] while utilizing rubber tubing.

STRETCHING

Correction of soft-tissue imbalance of trunk musculature and especially the lower extremity is imperative toward optimal maintenance of the cervical spine. Stretching of tightened soft-tissue structures such as levator scapulae,[38] pectoralis major and minor, as well as all neck musculature is an important part of management.[74] A self-stretching program of five to ten repetitions every 2 to 4 hours throughout the day is usually indicated. Each repetition ought to be performed from a position of rest or neutral to the point where pain is felt. The patient is warned not to push through the pain as this may exacerbate more inflammation and hinder progress. Between exercises, the patient may use the arm within tolerable limits or maintain the arm in the rest position.
- *Neck flexion.* This stretches the muscles and joint capsules in the back of the neck. Slowly bend the chin to the chest, hold for 5 seconds and relax, and return the head back to neutral.
- *Neck extension.* This stretches the muscles and joint capsules in the front of the neck. Slowly roll the head back so that the eyes are looking up. Hold for 5 seconds, relax, and move the head back to neutral.
- *Neck side bending.* This stretches the muscles and joint capsules on the opposite side of the neck and upper shoulder. Side-bend the neck gently, so that the ipsilateral ear drops toward the shoulder without lifting that shoulder. Hold for 5 seconds, relax, and move the head back to neutral.

- *Neck rotation.* This stretches the neck muscles and joint capsules. Turn the head to one side while keeping the eyes level by fixing them on one spot. Hold for 5 seconds and return to neutral. Repeat on the other side.
- *Middle back stretching.* This stretches the muscles in the mid-upper back. Gently pull one elbow toward the opposite shoulder. Hold for 5 seconds and relax, and repeat with the other arm.
- *Pectoral stretch.* This stretches the pectoralis musculature. Standing with the face toward a corner, place the palms against the wall, while keeping the hands and elbows at shoulder level. Lean toward the wall while keeping the heels firmly on the floor. Hold for 5 seconds and relax (see Fig. 18-8B).

MODALITIES

The utilization of physical modalities may help relieve the pain associated with the acute phase. In the subacute stage, *heat* and massage may be quite helpful. Cold therapy, appropriate for the acute stage, decreases spasm, inflammation, pain, and capillary blood flow, and is particularly helpful in cases of acute annular tears or ligament sprains. *Ice massage* may be applied for 8 to 10 minutes at regular intervals during the acute phase of inflammation. While the skin cools quickly, the rate of muscle cooling is directly proportionate to the thickness of overlying fat and may range from ten to thirty minutes.[16] The subacute or chronic states are preferably treated with thermotherapy such as deep heat (ultrasound, microwave, or shortwave) and, like heat, also minimize spasm and pain. Electrostimulation in the form of transcutaneous electrical nerve stimulation (TENS) or high volt galvanic stimulation (HVGS) may reduce acute muscle spasm, decrease edema, and relieve pain.[46] The mechanism for pain relief from TENS may involve raising the circulating levels of endogenous endorphins or by stimulating cutaneous afferents that block pain stimuli in the substantia gelatinosa.[57,96] Because the neck and shoulder muscles react to pain by undergoing involuntary spasm, these muscles may benefit from light *massage* that slowly progresses to a deeper soft-tissue massage.

MOBILIZATION

Articular mobilization is based on the concept that optimal joint mobility is necessary to achieve pain-free range of motion. The key concept to understanding

joint mobilizations and their benefit for regaining range of motion is that restricted motion is often due to soft-tissue contractures of the synovial and fibrous capsule surrounding the joint preventing osteokinematic motion. Joint mobilizations are small gliding or rotating movements within a joint should be performed before achieving gross ballistic movement. Joint mobilization techniques are used as an evaluative tool to assess joint play. Once limitations of the capsule have been identified, mobilization of the capsule commences. Grades I and II joint mobilizations are small amplitude oscillatory motions within resistance free range of motion that help improve movement as well as reduce pain. Grades III and IV mobilizations are larger amplitude forces that move the joint into its restricted range of motion and stretch the soft tissue surrounding the joint.

MANIPULATION

This is used by osteopaths, the occasional orthopedist,[58] physical therapists, and chiropractors and attempts to realign a subluxed facet joint and facilitate the release of entrapped synovial folds, relaxation of hypertonic muscle by sudden stretching, and disruption of entrapped synovial folds.[117] Manipulation may facilitate pain reduction and improved range of motion in patients with whiplash-related disorders.[1] The "cracking" noise associated with manipulation may correspond to joint cavitation in which the sudden thrust overcomes adhesive and cohesive forces within the synovial facet joints and releases subatmospheric gas within the joint from joint solution, and may be accompanied by a sudden "jump" due to joint separation. Within the scope of physical therapy, manipulation is a sharp movement of tiny amplitude representing overpressure and is carried out after the criterion position is reached. The joints involved are taken past their usual range of motion, but not beyond their anatomic range[30] in the direction opposite to the most painful movement. Manipulation should be preceded by stretching maneuvers to condition the tissue. The use of manipulative treatment in the presence of acute radiculopathy is controversial and has been associated with complications.[3] Moreover, manipulation of the upper cervical spine is particularly discouraged, particularly in the acute stage because of the risk of death or cerebrovascular accident from vertebrobasilar infarction[122] as well as damage to healing structures or neurologic elements. Other contraindications to manipulation include instability, fractures, high grade osteoporosis, senescence, and vascular problems. While a slightly bulging disk is not a contraindication to manipulative treatment, a herniated nucleus pulposus, with or without nerve root involvement is contraindicated.[62]

NERVE TRACT EXCURSION

Gentle gliding exercises of the brachial plexus, including the nerve roots, trunks, and terminal nerves to maintain free excursion of the nerve tracts within the upper extremity is an important part of management. The encroached nerve root in cervical spondylosis is tethered on either side of the intervertebral foramen. Its preforaminal length is a function of its emergence from the spinal cord. Beyond the intervertebral foramen, a peripheral nerve tenses it as it undulates along its course through the upper extremity. As a given nerve winds down its route to the distal extremity, it passes through various layers of muscle and other soft tissue. In the absence of adequate stretching to the upper extremity musculature, the major nerve tracts may be denied adequate mobility as they are tethered by a stiffened and nonpliant soft tissue that surrounds them. This increased nerve mobility relative to its surrounding soft tissue may help compensate for the encroachment of the nerve within the intervertebral foramen. Various movement combinations (see Fig. 18-5 on page 197) tense, and facilitate gliding of the median and radial nerve, in much the same way that straight leg raise tension-biases the sciatic nerve in the lower extremity. This maneuver involves superimposed movement sequences at the shoulder, elbow, and wrist joints that provoke pain by tensing the nerve. These same movements that have identified the tense nerve trunk are then used in treatment by gently stretching the nerve trunk in conjunction with stretching of the surrounding soft tissue. Inflammation of the nerve roots may cause adhesive binding of the plexus to surrounding tissue that may be become free with increased nerve root excursion.[56]

MYOFASCIAL RELEASING TECHNIQUES

These are based upon the idea that injury to the myofascial system, with resultant pain, swelling, and immobility may cause desiccation of the fascia with loss of elasticity. Similar to ligaments, myofascial tissue is composed of connective tissue that is itself comprised of layers of collagen and elastin in a ground substance matrix. All muscular and other soft tissues from the dermis to the periosteum are enveloped with fasciae. The deep fascia is thicker and stronger and designed for structure and support, whereas the superficial fascia is thinner and allows for more freedom of movement. The fascia functions to absorb shock, transmit mechanical force, exchange metabolites from fibrous elements to the circulatory and lymphatic systems, and join the various layers of muscle into a single functional unit. With loss of resiliency following injury, the fascial layers lose their normal ability to glide relative to each other resulting in increased cross-linking of fibers. Loss of mobility results in a diminished ability of the soft tissue surrounding the spine to function in a protective capacity. Myofascial release applies pressure and shear to the fascial layers, promoting improved elasticity, helps restores mobility between the fascial layers, and promotes flexibility.

POSTURAL EDUCATION

This is essential, particularly as a forward head posture abnormally affects muscle length-tension relationships and may cause further pain as a result of altered joint biomechanics about the head and neck. Moreover, the forward head posture may also lead to formation of traction spurs, which may exacerbate an already spondylitic cervical spine and may further encroach upon nerve roots or the supporting ligamentous structures.

ENDURANCE TRAINING

Cardiovascular and cardiopulmonary fitness are extremely important and may include brisk walking, jogging, swimming, tennis, and stationary bicycle activities. Many patient find that brisk walking eases their discomfort. Aerobic fitness activities should emphasize activities that avoid high-impact and ballistic-type spinal movements.

BIOFEEDBACK

This may be auditory or visual in which the magnitude of muscular contraction is conveyed to the patient through a speaker as high pitched sounds, or graphically represented on a display screen. With this sensory feedback, the patient learns how to decrease or increase muscular tension, and engenders heightened awareness at a threshold that might not otherwise be possible. Electromyographic biofeedback is helpful in teaching patients to inhibit excessive or unbalanced muscle activity by lowering muscular tension and thereby reducing pain intensity.

IMAGING

Utilizing imagery as a strategy for pain management is based on the premise that mental representations exert a profound influence on physical processes, emotions, and behavior. Because pain increases muscular tension, visualizing relaxing muscles may be helpful in relieving pain. Imaging may also be distracting as one visualizes a pleasant experience. Patient can be taught that seeing pain go away can help make it go away or at least make it less prominent in their lives. Success with imagery is thought to positively affect disease processes through a psychoimmunologic mechanism.

PATIENT EDUCATION

This includes teaching the patient to avoid neck extension (reaching above the head and looking up), to avoid riding in a car as much as possible, and the importance of sleeping on the side (never on the face) while in bed and having an adequate night's sleep. Anxiety, depression, fear, and anger act to exacerbate symptoms, while disputes with employers and workers compensation are negative factors in recuperation. These factors heighten emotional tension that may exacerbate headaches and increase symptoms in the neck.

CERVICAL TRACTION

Traction, with the head in slight flexion, may be helpful in relieving symptoms in patient with cervical spine sprain or strain. Traction is contraindicated for cervical sprain or strain in the acute state.

NECK SCHOOL

This is a formal educational setting, similar to back school, that aims to educate patients in a group setting. The group meets several times for 1 hour sessions over a period of 3 weeks to share information about relative anatomy, epidemiology, ergonomics, posture, stretching and strengthening exercises, pain medication and management, relaxation techniques, biofeedback, and coping mechanisms. Commonly given by a physical or occupational therapist, neck school attempts to empower the patient and foster a supportive environment.

Those patients with cervical radiculopathy unresponsive to physical therapy and who have intractable pain lasting for an intolerable period of time may be candidates for surgical intervention.

RECOMMENDED READING

Adams MA: Biomechanics of the cervical spine. In Gunzburg R, Szpalski M, editors: *Whiplash injuries: current concept in prevention, diagnosis, and treatment of cervical whiplash syndrome,* Philadelphia, 1988, Lippincott-Raven.

Bogduk N: The anatomy and pathophysiology of whiplash, *Clin Biomech* 1:92, 1986.

Oda J, Tanaba H, Tsyzuki N: Intervertebral disk changes with aging of human cervical vertebral from neonate to the eighties, *Spine* 13:1205, 1988.

REFERENCES

1. Achterberg J: *Imagery in healing,* Boston, 1985, New Science Library.
2. Adams MA: Biomechanics of the cervical spine. In Gunzburg R, Szpalski M, editors: *Whiplash injuries: current concept in prevention, diagnosis, and treatment of cervical whiplash syndrome,* Philadelphia, 1988, Lippincott-Raven.
3. Adler R editor: *Psychoneuroimmunology,* New York, 1981, Academic Press.
4. Babin E, Capesium P: Etude radiologique des dimensions du canal rachidien cervical et de leurs variations au cours des epreuves fonctionelles, *Annas Radiology* 19:457-462, 1976.
5. Bergmann TF, Peterson DH, Lawrence DJ: *Chiropractic technique,* New York, 1993, Churchill Livingstone.
6. Berkow R, Fletcher AJ editors: *The Merck manual of diagnosis and therapy,* ed 15, Rahway, N.J., 1987, Merck & Co.
7. Bland J: The cervical spine: from anatomy to clinical care, *Med Times* 117:15, 1989.
8. Bogduk N, Marsland A: The cervical Zygapophysial joints as a source of neck pain, *Spine* 13:610, 1988.
9. Bogduk N: The anatomy and pathophysiology of whiplash, *Clin Biomech* 1:92, 1986.
10. Bogduk N, Twomey LT: *Clinical anatomy of the lumbar spine,* ed 2, Melbourne, 1991, Churchill Livingstone.
11. Bolton PS, Stick PE, Lord RSA: Failure of clinical tests to predict cerebral ischemia before neck manipulation, *JMPT* 12:304, 1989.
12. Bora F, Osterman A: Compression neuropathy, *Clin Orthop* 163:23, 1982.
13. Breig A: *Adverse mechanical tension in the central nervous system,* Stockholm, 1978, Almqvist & Wiksell.
14. Breig A, Turnbull IM, Hassler O: Effects of mechanical stresses on the spinal cord in cervical spondylosis: a study of fresh cadaver material, *J Neurosurg* 25:45, 1966.
15. Brown MD, Tsaltos TT: Studies in permeability of the intervertebral disc during skeletal maturation, *Spine* 1:240, 1976.
16. Butler D: *Mobilisation of the nervous system,* Melbourne, 1991, Churchill Livingstone.

17. Cassidy JD, Lopes AS, Young-Hing K: The immediate effect of manipulation versus mobilization on pain and range of motion in the cervical spine: a randomized controlled trial, *J Manipulative Physiol Ther* 15:570, 1992.
18. Crowe H: Injuries to the cervical spine. Presentation to the annual meeting of Western Orhtopedic Association, San Francisco, 1928.
19. Cusick JF: *The cervical spine,* Philadelphia, 1989, JB Lippincott.
20. Czervionke L, Daniels DL, Ho PS et al: Cervical neural foramina: correlative anatomic and MR imaging study, *Radiology* 169:753, 1988.
21. Dai LY, Xu YK, Zhang WM et al: The effect of flexion-extension motion of the lumbar spine on the capacity of the spinal canal, *Spine* 14:523-525, 1989.
22. Dandy DJ: *Essential orthopaedics and trauma,* Edinburgh, 1989, Churchill Livingstone.
23. DataLink Inc.: *Car crash outcomes in rear impacts, appendix A to current issues of occupant protection in car rear impacts.* Washinton DC, 1989, DataLink.
24. DataLink Inc.: *Current issues of occupant protection in care rear impacts, prepared for the Office of Crashworthiness, Rulemaking, National Highway Traffic Safety Administration,* docket 89-20-No1-021, Washington DC, 1990, DataLink.
25. Dawson DM, Hallett M, Millender LH: *Entrapment neuropathies,* ed 2, Boston, 1990, Little, Brown and Company.
26. DeMyer WE: *Technique of the neurologic examination: a programmed text,* ed 4, New York, 1994, McGraw-Hill.
27. DePalma AF, Rothman RH: *The intervertebral disc,* Philadelphia, 1970, WB Saunders.
28. Dillin L, Hoaglund FT, Scheck M: Brachial neuritis, *J Bone Joint Surg* 67A:878, 1985.
29. Dopamine JL: The mechanism of ischemia in anteroposterior compression of the spinal cord, *Invest Radiol* 10:543, 1975.
30. Drukteinis AM: *The psychology of back pain: a clinical and legal handbook,* Springfield, IL, 1996, Charles C Thomas.
31. Dvorak J, Ablate L: Cervical spine injuries in Switzerland, *J Manual Med* 4:7, 1989.
32. Dvorak J, Panjabi MN, Gerber M et al: CT-functional diagnostics of the rotatory instability of upper cervical spine, *Spine* 12:197, 1987.
33. Dvorak J: Soft tissue injuries of the cervical spine. In Findlay G, Owen R, editors: *Surgery of the spine,* Oxford, 1992, Blackwellii Scientific.
34. Dwyer A, April C, Bogduk N: Cervical zygapophyseal joint pain patterns, I. A study in normal volunteers, *Spine* 15:453, 1990.
35. Dyck PJ, et al: *Peripheral neuropathy,* vols 1 and 2, Philadelphia, 1984, WB Saunders.
36. Farran H, Cosset J, Robertson G et al: The effects of torsion in the lumbar intervertebral joint: the role of torsion in production of disc degeneration, *J Bone Joint Surg* 52A: 468, 1970.
37. Farfan HG: *Mechanical disorders of the low back,* Philadelphia, 1973, Lea & Febiger.
38. Frumin LR, Balch RW: Wallenberg's syndrome following neck manipulation, *Neurology* 40:611, 1990.
39. Garrett WE, Tidball J: Myotedinous junction: structure, function, and failure, In *Injury and of the musculoskeletal soft tissues,* Park Ridge, IL, 1988, American Association of Orthopaedic Surgeons.
40. Gertzbein S, Seligman J, Holtby R et al: Centrode patterns and segmental instability in degenerative disc disease, *Spine* 10:257, 1985.
41. Gore DH, Sepic SB, Gardner GM et al: Neck pain: a long term follow-up of 205 patients, *Spine* 12:1, 1988.
42. Gore DR, Sepic S, Gardner G: Roentgenographic findings of the cervical spine in asymptomatic people, *Spine* 11(6):521, 1986.
43. Gore DR, Septic SB, Garner GM: Neck pain: a long-term follow-up study of 205 patients, *Spine* 12:1, 1987.
44. Gore DR, Sepic SB, Gardner GM et al: Roentgenographic findings of the cervical spine in asymptomatic people, *Spine* 11:521, 1986.
45. Gould JAIII: *Orthopaedic and sports physical therapy,* ed 2, St Louis, 1990, Mosby.
46. Greenman PE: *Principles of manual medicine,* Baltimore, 1989, Williams & Wilkins.
47. Greenstein GM: *Clinical assessment of neuromusculoskeletal disorders,* St Louis, 1997, Mosby.
48. Handal JA, Knapp J, Poletti S: The cervical spine. In White AH, Schofferman JA, editors: Spine care, vol 1, *Diagnosis and conservative treatment,* St Louis, 1995, Mosby.
49. Hasue M, Kikuchi S, Sakuyama Y et al: Anatomic study of the interrelation between lumbosacral nerve roots and their surrounding tissues, *Spine* 8:50, 1983.
50. Hauser SL, Levitt LP, Weiner HL: *Case studies in neurology for the house officer,* Baltimore, 1986, Williams & Wilkins.
51. Henderson C, Hennessy R: Posterolateral foraminotomy as an exclusive operative technique for cervical radiculopathy: a review of 846 consecutively operated cases, *Neurosurgery* 13:504, 1983
52. Hirsch SA, Hirsch PJ, Hiramoto H et al: Whiplash syndrome. Fact or fiction? *Orthop Clin North Am* 19:791, 1988.
53. Hoppenfeld S: *Orthopaedic neurology: a diagnostic guide to neurologic levels,* Philadelphia, 1977, JB Lippincott.
54. Ho PS, Yu SW, Sether LA et al: Ligamentum flavum: appearance on sagittal and coronal MR images, *Radiology* 168:469, 1988.
55. Hukins DWL, Kirby MC, Sikoryn TA et al: Comparison of structure, mechanical properties and functions of lumbar spinal ligaments, *Spine* 15:787, 1990.
56. Kamwendo K, Linton SJ: A controlled study of the effect of neck school in medical secretaries, *Scand J Rehab Med* 23(3):143-152, 1992.
57. Kapandji IA: *The physiology of the joints,* vol 3, ed 2, London, 1974, Churchill Livingstone.
58. Keefe FJ, Black AR, William RB Jr. et al: Behavioral treatment of chronic low back pain: clinical outcome and individual differences in pain relief, *Pain* 11:221, 1981.
59. Kelsey J, Githens PB, Walter SD et al: An epidemiological study of acute prolapsed cervical intervertebral disc, *J Bone Joint Surg* 66A:907, 1984.
60. Kirkaldy-Willis WH, Wedge JH, Hong-Ying K et al: Pathology and pathogenesis of lumbar spondylosis and stenosis, *Spine* 3: 319-328, 1978.

61. Kirkaldy-Willis WH: *Managing low back pain,* ed 2, New York, 1988, Churchill Livingstone.

62. Kisner C, Colby LA: *Therapeutic exercise: foundation and techniques,* ed 2, Philadelphia, 1990, FA Davis.

63. Korkala O, Gronblad M, Liesi P et al: Immunohistochemical demonstration of nociceptors in the ligament structures of the lumbar spine, *Spine* 10:156, 1985.

64. Langman J: *Medical embryology,* Baltimore, 1975, Williams & Wilkins.

65. LaRocca H: Cervical sprain syndrome. In Frymoyer JW, editor: *The adult spine: principles and practice,* New York, 1991, Raven Press.

66. Lehman J: Therapeutic heat and cold, *Clin Orthop* 99:207, 1974.

67. Lillegard WA, Rucker KS, editors: *Handbook of sports medicine: a symptoms-oriented approach,* Boston, 1993, Andover Medical Publishers.

68. Louis R: Spinal stability as defined by the three column spine concept, *Anat Clin* 7:33, 1985.

69. Louis R: *Surgery of the spine: surgical anatomy and operative approaches,* Berlin, 1983, Springer-Verlag.

70. Louis R: Vertebroradicular and vertebromedullar dynamics, *Anat Clin* 3:1-11.

71. McNab I: *The cervical spine,* Philidelphia, 1989, WB Saunders.

72. MacNab I: The whiplash syndrome, *Ortho Clin of N Am* 2:389, 1971.

73. Magee DJ: *Orthopedic physical assessment,* Philadelphia, 1987, WB Saunders.

74. Maigne Jean-Yves: Whiplash and spinal manipulation. In Gunzburg R, Szpalski M, editors: *Whiplash injuries: current concepts in prevention, diagnosis, and treatment of the cervical whiplash syndrome,* Philadelphia, 1998, Lippincott-Raven.

75. Maigne R: *Diagnosis and treatment of pain of vertebral origin. A manual medicine approach,* Baltimore, 1995, Williams & Wilkins.

76. Marks MR, Bell GR, Boumphrey FR: Cervical spine injuries and their neurologic implication, *Clin Sport Med* 9:263, 1990.

77. Meals RA: *One hundred orthopaedic conditions every doctor shoulder understand,* St Louis, 1992, Quality Medical Publishing.

78. Melzack R, Wall PD: Pain mechanisms: a new theory, *Science* 50:971, 1965.

79. Myklebust JB, Pintar F, Yoganandan N et al: Tensile strength of spinal ligaments, *Spine* 13(5):526, 1988.

80. Negri S, Holmes B, Leggett S et al: Treating cervical spondylosis, *Rehab Management,* February/March, 1992.

81. Netter FH: Nervous system, vol 1, part II, *Neurologic and neuromuscular disorders.* The Ciba Collection of Medical Illustrations, West Caldwell, NJ, 1986, CIBA-GEIGY.

82. Oda J, Tanaka H, Tsuzuki N: Intervertebral disc changes with aging of human cervical vertebra, *Spine* 11:1205, 1988.

83. Oliver J, Middleditch A: *Functional anatomy of the spine,* Oxford, 1991, Butterworth Heinemann.

84. Omer G, Spinner M: *Management of peripheral nerve problems,* Philadelphia, 1980, WB Saunders.

85. Ommaya AK, Faas F, Yarnell P: Whiplash injury and brain damage, *JAMA* 204:285, 1968.

86. Ommaya AR: The head: kinematics and brain injury mechanisms. In Aldman B, Chapon A, editors: *The biomechanics of impact trauma,* Amsterdam: 1984, Elsevier.

87. Pal GP, Cosio L, Routal RV et al: Trajectory architecture of the trabecular bone between the body and the neural arch in human vertebrae, *Anat Rec* 222:418, 1988.

88. Panjabi M, Dvorak J, Crisco J et al: Flexion, extension, and lateral bending of the upper cervical spine in response to alar ligament transections, *J Spine Disorders,* 4:157, 1991.

89. Panjabi M, Oxland T, Parks E: Quantitative anatomy of cervical spine ligaments. Part I. Upper cervical spine, *J Spine Disorders* 4:270, 1991.

90. Panjabi M, Oxland T, Parks E: Quantitative anatomy of cervical spine ligament. Part II. Middle and lower cervical spine, *J Spine Disorders* 4:277, 1991.

91. Parke W, Sherk H: *Normal adult in the cervical spine,* ed 2, Philadelphia, 1989, JB Lippincott.

92. Patten J: *Neurological differential diagnosis,* ed 2, London, 1996, Springer.

93. Porter RW: *Management of back pain,* ed 2, 1993, Churchill Livingstone.

94. Rauschning W: Anatomy and pathology of the cervical spine. In Frymoyer JW, editor: *The adults spine: principles and practice,* New York, 1991, Raven.

95. Renaudin J, Snyder M: Chip fracture through the superior articular facet with compressive cervical radiculopathy, *J Trauma* 18:66, 1978.

96. Rocabado M: Physical therapy and dentistry I and II. Course notes, 1979 and 1981.

97. Rockett FX: Observations on the "burner": traumatic cervical radiculopathy, *Clin Orthop* 164:18, 1992.

98. Roeser W, Meeks LW, Venis R et al: The use of transcutaneous nerve stimulation for pain control in athletic medicine: a preliminary report, *Am J Sports Med* 4:210, 1976.

99. Schonstrom NR, Hansson JH: Thickness of the human ligamentum flavum as a function of load: an in vitro experimental study, *Clin Biomech* 6.

100. Schneider RC, Cherry GR, Pantek H: Syndrome of acute central cervical cord injury with special reference to mechanisms involved in hyperextension injuries of the cervical spine, *J Neurosurg* 11:363, 1954.

101. Shekelle PG: Spinal manipulation, *Spine* 19:858, 1994.

102. Spillane JD, Spillane JA: *An atlas of clinical neurology,* ed 3, Oxford, 1982, Oxford University Press.

103. Spruling RG, Scoville WB: Lateral rupture of the cervical intervertebral discs, *Surg Gynecol Obstet* 78:350, 1944.

104. Stookey B: Compression of the spinal cord and nerve roots by herniation of nucleus pulposus in cervical region, *Arch Surg* 40:417, 1940.

105. Taylor JR: Growth and development of the human intervertebral disc, PhD Thesis, University of Edinburgh, 1973.

106. Taylor JR, Milne N: The cervical mobile segments. Proceeding of Whiplash Symposium. Adelaide: Orthopaedic Special Interest Group, Australian Physiotherapy Association, South Australian Branch, 1988.

107. Tesh KM, Shaw-Dunn J, Evans JH: The abdominal muscles and vertebral stability, *Spine* 12:501, 1987.

108. Tomita K, Kawahara N, Baba H et al: Circumspinal decompression for thoracic myelopathy due to combined ossification of the posterior longitudinal ligament and ligamentum flavum, *Spine* 15, 1990.

109. Torg JS, Sennett B, Vegso JJ et al: Axial loading injuries to the middle cervical spine segment: an analysis and classification of twenty-five cases, *Am J Sports Med* 19(1):6, 1991.

110. Torg JS, Fay CM: Cervical spinal stenosis with cord neurapraxia and transient quadriplegia. In Torg JS, editor: *Athletic injuries to the head, neck and face,* St Louis, 1991, Mosby.

111. Torg JS, Glasgow SG: Criteria for return to contact activity following cervical spine injury, *Clin J Sport Med* 1:12, 1991.

112. Torg JS: Management guidelines for athletic injuries to the cervical spine, *Clin Sports Med* 6:60, 1987.

113. Torg JS, Pavlov H, Genuario SE et al: Neuropraxia of the cervical spinal cord with transient quadriplegia, *J Bone Joint Surg* 68A:1354, 1986.

114. Tsairis P, Dyck PJ, Mulder DW: Natural history of brachial plexus neuropathy, *Arch. Neurol.* 27:109, 1972.

115. Twomey LT: *Clinical anatomy of the lumbar spine,* ed 2, Melbourne, 1881, Churchill Livingstone.

116. Wada E, Elsara S, Saito S et al: Experimental spondylosis in the rabbit spine: overuse could accelerate the spondylosis, *Spine* 17 (suppl): 1, 1992.

117. Warner L, McNeill ME: Mental imagery and its potential for physical therapy. *Physical therapy* 68(4), 1988.

118. Warwick R, Williams P editors: *Gray's anatomy,* British, ed 35, Philadelphia, 1973, WB Saunders.

119. Watkins RG, Dillin WH, Maxwell J: Cervical spine injuries in football players. In Hockhschuler SH, editor: *Spine: spinal injuries in sports,* Philadelphia, 1990, Hanley & Belfus.

120. Watkins RG: Neck injuries in foot ball players, *Clin Sports Med* 5:215, 1986.

121. Watkins RG: *The spine in sports,* St Louis, 1996, Mosby.

122. Weisberg LA, Garcia C, Strub R editors: *Essentials of clinical neurology,* ed 3, St Louis, 1996, Mosby.

123. Weisz GM: Lumbar spinal canal stenosis in Paget's disease, *Spine* 8, 1983.

124. White AA, Panjabi MM: *Clinical biomechanics of the spine,* Philadelphia, 1978, JB Lippincott.

125. Williams PL, Gray H: *Gray's anatomy,* ed 37, Edinburgh: 1989, Churchill Livingstone.

126. Yu S, Sether L, Haughton VM: Facet joint menisci of the cervical spine: correlative MR imaging and cryomicrotomy study, *Radiology* 164:79, 1987.

Index*

*Page numbers followed by: b indicates boxes, f in-
dicates illustration, and n indicates footnotes.